Neurotrauma and Critical Care of the Brain

Thieme

Neurotrauma and Critical Care of the Brain

Jack Jallo, MD, PhD, FACS
Associate Professor
Department of Neurosurgery
Temple University School of Medicine
Philadelphia, Pennsylvania

Christopher M. Loftus, MD, DHC (Hon.), FACS
Professor and Chairman
Department of Neurosurgery
Assistant Dean for International Affiliations
Temple University School of Medicine
Philadelphia, Pennsylvania

Thieme
New York • Stuttgart

Thieme Medical Publishers, Inc.
333 Seventh Ave.
New York, NY 10001

Executive Editor: Kay Conerly
Associate Editor: Ivy Ip
Vice President, Production and Electronic Publishing: Anne T. Vinnicombe
Production Editor: Print Matters, Inc.
Vice President, International Marketing and Sales: Cornelia Schulze
Chief Financial Officer: Peter van Woerden
President: Brian D. Scanlan
Compositor: Thomson Digital Services
Printer: Leo Paper Group

Library of Congress Cataloging-in-Publication Data

Neurotrauma and critical care of the brain / [edited by] Jack Jallo, Christopher M. Loftus.
p. ; cm.
Includes bibliographical references and index.
ISBN 978-1-60406-032-4 (alk. paper)
1. Brain damage. 2. Neurological intensive care. I. Jallo, Jack. II. Loftus, Christopher M.
[DNLM: 1. Brain Injuries—diagnosis. 2. Brain Injuries—therapy. 3. Critical Care—methods. WL 354 N494485 2009]
RC387.5.N493 2009
616.8'0428—dc22

2008043145

Important note: Medical knowledge is ever-changing. As new research and clinical experience broaden our knowledge, changes in treatment and drug therapy may be required. The authors and editors of the material herein have consulted sources believed to be reliable in their efforts to provide information that is complete and in accord with the standards accepted at the time of publication. However, in view of the possibility of human error by the authors, editors, or publisher of the work herein or changes in medical knowledge, neither the authors, editors, or publisher, nor any other party who has been involved in the preparation of this work, warrants that the information contained herein is in every respect accurate or complete, and they are not responsible for any errors or omissions or for the results obtained from use of such information. Readers are encouraged to confirm the information contained herein with other sources. For example, readers are advised to check the product information sheet included in the package of each drug they plan to administer to be certain that the information contained in this publication is accurate and that changes have not been made in the recommended dose or in the contraindications for administration. This recommendation is of particular importance in connection with new or infrequently used drugs.

Printed in China

5 4 3 2 1

ISBN 978-1-60406-032-4

Contents

Foreword

There is no greater pleasure for an academic than to see his student follow in his footsteps and ultimately to surpass him. I am therefore delighted to have the privilege of writing this brief foreword to a book that my former resident Jack Jallo, MD, has co-edited with my friend Chris Loftus, MD. These editors have brought together many of the current thought leaders in the field of traumatic brain injury (TBI) and by so doing have provided the reader with a succinct and valuable resource.

While it is true that we do not have a single agent that has been proven to improve the outcome from traumatic brain injury, there is little doubt that the outcomes from this common and often devastating condition have improved substantially over the past three decades. In the 1970s the mortality associated with severe TBI—even treated in some of the best centers—was approximately 50 percent. Several current series report mortalities of 30 percent or less. Furthermore, the quality of neurologic recovery also appears to be better. These dramatic improvements can be ascribed to a combination of factors including the introduction of seat belts and air bags, better rescue squads, more effective monitoring technologies, earlier CT scanning, prompt evacuation of intracranial hematomas, the growth of trauma centers, neurocritical care and neurorehabilitation, and the effect of evidence-based management guidelines, among others. It is highly unlikely that any single drug will exceed the cumulative effect of these diverse interventions. Nevertheless, it remains important to continue the search for agents that can modulate the many biochemical cascades that are set in motion by traumatic brain injury.

The diverse disciplines that impact on the care and outcome of the head-injured patient are concisely presented in this volume, which has been a labor of love for the authors and editors. It will no doubt serve as a very helpful starting point for the newcomer to the field, as well as a convenient source of up-to-date information for the seasoned neurotraumatologist.

Raj K. Narayan, MD
Mayfield Professor and Chairman
Department of Neurosurgery
University of Cincinnati School of Medicine
Cincinnati, Ohio

Preface

> Only as you do know yourself can your brain serve you as a sharp and efficient tool. Know your own failings, passions, and prejudices so you can separate them from what you see.
>
> *Bernard M. Baruch (1870–1965)*

We are confronted again and again with injury that renders the "efficient tool" into varying levels of uselessness. Our goal is to maintain the efficiency of this tool. Fortunately, our ability to treat brain and spinal cord injury continues to advance, allowing us to help our patients preserve the usefulness of this most precious tool. The ambition of this text is to provide a current and clear reference for the many physicians involved in the care of the patient with brain and spinal cord injury.

Despite significant advances in survival from severe head and spinal cord injury, there is no miracle drug for treating these patients. Care of these patients depends wholly on applying the best available treatment in the field, upon arrival to the emergency room, in the intensive care unit, the operating room, and finally, throughout their convalescence. While these elements have always been integral to the recovery of the patient, two major developments over the past decade are now affecting the care of the neurotrauma patient. Advances in critical care management and a push toward evidence-based medicine with the development of treatment guidelines are improving the care we provide to the brain injured patient.

Charting these new developments in a comprehensive guide to the care of individuals with brain injury suggested the structure for this text. In the early chapters, we focus on the science underlying daily practices and acute care and critical care management of the brain injured. We follow with chapters on nonacute care, outcomes, and socioeconomics. We place a particular stress on accepted guidelines and the evidence-based practice of medicine.

This book is not a quick read, and yet it is my hope that it will help my colleagues in the field as they confront the confounding problems associated with head and spinal cord injury.

Acknowledgments

In an undertaking such as this, there are many people to thank, because this is truly a collaborative effort. I wish to first thank all the contributors for their time and effort. Without them this text would not be possible. I understand that an undertaking such as this strains already busy schedules. I also want to acknowledge the staff at Thieme for their patience and support in making this text possible, especially Birgitta Brandenburg and Timothy Hiscock for getting us started and Ivy Ip and Dominik Pucek for seeing us through to the end. I wish to thank my research staff, Anuja Kulkarni, Julia Grayer, Rani Nasser, and Michael O'Malley. Additionally, this endeavor would not be possible without the training and education provided me by many mentors over the years. I am forever indebted to them. I also want to acknowledge my parents for their perseverance and for instilling in me a love of learning. Most importantly, none of this would be possible with out the support of my wife and children. Thank you.

Contributors

Opeolu M. Adeoye, MD
Assistant Professor
Departments of Emergency Medicine and Neurosurgery
University of Cincinnati School of Medicine
Cincinnati, Ohio

Mark A. Agostini, MD
Assistant Professor
Department of Neurology
University of Texas Southwestern Medical Center
Dallas, Texas

Rocco A. Armonda, MD
Director
Neurovascular Surgery and Interventional Neuroradiology Service
National Capital Neurosurgery Consortium
National Naval Medical Center
Walter Reed Army Medical Center
Bethesda, Maryland
Department of Radiology
Washington Hospital Center
Washington, D.C.

Julian E. Bailes, MD
Chair
Department of Neurosurgery
West Virginia University School of Medicine
Robert C. Byrd Health Sciences Center
Morgantown, West Virginia

Sylvia Bele, MD
Clinic of Neurosurgery
University of Regensburg
University Hospital Regensburg
Regensburg, Germany

Randy S. Bell, MD, MC, USN
Chief Resident
National Capital Neurosurgery Consortium
National Naval Medical Center
Bethesda, Maryland

Sharon M. Benedict PhD
Assistant Professor
Department of Physical Medicine and Rehabilitation
Clinical Assistant Professor
Department of Psychiatry
Virginia Commonwealth University School of Medicine
Polytrauma Rehabilitation Center
Hunter Holmes McGuire Richmond VA Medical Center
Richmond, Virginia

Alexander Brawanski, MD
Professor
Clinic of Neurosurgery
University of Regensburg
University Hospital Regensburg
Regensburg, Germany

M. Ross Bullock, MD, PhD
Professor
Neurological Surgery
Director
Clinical Neurotrauma
Miller School of Medicine University of Miami
Miami, Florida
Department of Neurosurgery
Virginia Commonwealth University School of Medicine
Richmond, Virginia

Heechin Chae, MD
Instructor
Department of Physical Medicine and Rehabilitation
Harvard Medical School
Medical Director
Spaulding Rehabilitation Hospital
Boston, Massachusetts

Randall M. Chesnut, MD, FCCM, FACS.
Professor
Department of Neurological Surgery
University of Washington School of Medicine
Harborview Medical Center
Seattle, Washington

David X. Cifu, MD
Professor and Chair
Department of Physical Medicine and Rehabilitation
Virginia Commonwealth University School of Medicine
Medical Director
Virginia Commonwealth University Rehabilitation and Research Center
Virginia Commonwealth University Medical Center
Richmond, Virginia

Victor G. Coronado, MD, MPH
Medical Officer
National Center for Injury Prevention and Control
Centers for Disease Control and Prevention
Atlanta, Georgia

Gerard J. Criner, MD
Chair, Professor, and Chief
Department of Medicine, Section of Pulmonary and Critical Care Medicine
Temple University School of Medicine
Philadelphia, Pennsylvania

Samuel Critides, MD, MC, USN
Attending Neurosurgeon
National Capital Neurosurgery Consortium
National Naval Medical Center
Walter Reed Army Medical Center
Bethesda, Maryland

Marek Czosnyka, PhD
Department of Clinical Neurosciences
University of Cambridge
Neurosurgical Unit
Addenbrooke's Hospital
Cambridge, United Kingdom

Abhishek Deshpande, MD
Department of Neurological Surgery
Cleveland Clinic
Cleveland, Ohio
School of Biomedical Sciences
Kent State University
Kent, Ohio

Ramon R. Diaz-Arrastia, MD, PhD
Professor
Department of Neurology
University of Texas Southwestern Medical Center
University of Texas Epilepsy Center
Parkland Memorial Hospital
Dallas, Texas

Mustapha A. Ezzeddine, MD
Director, Neurocritical Care
Director, Hennepin County Medical Center Stroke Center
Associate Professor of Neurology and Neurosurgery
Zeenat Qureshi Stroke Research Center
University of Minnesota
Minneapolis, Minnesota

Scott H. Faro, MD
Professor
Department of Radiology
Temple University School of Medicine
Temple University Health System
Philadelphia, Pennsylvania

Paul J. Ford, PhD
Assistant Professor
Department of Medicine
Cleveland Clinic Lerner College of Medicine of Case Western Reserve University
Department of Bioethics
Cleveland Clinic
Cleveland, Ohio

Thomas A. Gennarelli, MD
Professor and Chair
Department of Neurosurgery
Medical College of Wisconsin
Milwaukee, Wisconsin

Arlene I. Greenspan, DrPH, MPH
Senior Scientist
National Center for Injury Prevention and Control
Centers for Disease Control and Prevention
Atlanta, Georgia

Marinella Gugliotta, MD
Department of Neurosurgery
Virginia Commonwealth University School of Medicine
Richmond, Virginia

Joshua E. Heller, MD
Resident
Department of Neurosurgery
Temple University School of Medicine
Philadelphia, Pennsylvania

Delia Hendrie, MA
Senior Research Fellow
School of Public Health
Curtin University of Technology
Perth, Australia

Beverly L. Hershey, MD
Clinical Associate Professor
Department of Radiology
Temple University School of Medicine
Philadelphia, Pennsylvania

Jim Hitt, MD
Resident
Department of Anesthesiology
The State University of New York School of Medicine and Biomedical Sciences
Buffalo, New York

Peter Hutchinson, PhD
Senior Academy Fellow and Honorary Consultant Neurosurgeon
Department of Clinical Neurosciences
University of Cambridge
Neurosurgical Unit
Addenbrooke's Hospital
Cambridge, United Kingdom

Jack Jallo, MD, PhD, FACS
Associate Professor
Department of Neurosurgery
Temple University School of Medicine
Philadelphia, Pennsylvania

Peter J. Kirkpatrick, PhD, FMedSci
Lecturer and Honorary Consultant Neurosurgeon
Department of Clinical Neurosciences
University of Cambridge
Neurosurgical Unit
Addenbrooke's Hospital
Cambridge, United Kingdom

Jeffrey P. Kochan, MD
Professor
Departments of Radiology and Neurosurgery
Temple University School of Medicine
Chief
Diagnostic and Interventional Neuroradiology
Temple University Health System
Philadelphia, Pennsylvania

Frederick Levy, MD, JD
Assistant Professor
Department of Emergency Medicine
Johns Hopkins University School of Medicine
Johns Hopkins Hospital
Baltimore, Maryland

Christopher M. Loftus, MD, DHC (Hon.), FACS
Professor and Chair
Department of Neurosurgery
Assistant Dean for International Affiliations
Temple University School of Medicine
Philadelphia, Pennsylvania

Bennett Lorber, MD
Professor
Department of Medicine, Section of Infectious Diseases
Professor
Department of Microbiology and Immunology
Temple University School of Medicine
Philadelphia, Pennsylvania

Andrew I. R. Maas, MD, PhD
Professor and Chair
Department of Neurosurgery
University Hospital Antwerp
Edegem, Belgium

Christopher J. Madden, MD
Assistant Professor
Department of Neurological Surgery
University of Texas Southwestern Medical Center
Parkland Memorial Hospital
Dallas, Texas

Ubaldo Martin, MD
Assistant Professor
Department of Medicine, Section of Pulmonary and Critical Care Medicine
Temple University School of Medicine
Philadelphia, Pennsylvania

Gregory Mayro, MD
Department of Medicine
Jefferson Medical College
Thomas Jefferson University
Division of Infectious Disease
Albert Einstein Medical Center
Philadelphia, Pennsylvania

Shane D. McNamee, MD
Assistant Professor
Department of Physical Medicine and Rehabilitation
Virginia Commonwealth University School of Medicine
Medical Director
Polytrauma Rehabilitation Center
Hunter Holmes McGuire Richmond Veterans Administration Medical Center
Richmond, Virginia

Vincent J. Miele, MD
Department of Neurological Surgery
Center for Spine Health
Neurological Institute
Cleveland Clinic
Cleveland, Ohio

Ted R. Miller, PhD
Director
Public Services Research Institute
Pacific Institute for Research and Evaluation
Calverton, Maryland

Rani Nasser, MD
Medical Student
Department of Neurosurgery
Temple University School of Medicine
Philadelphia, Pennsylvania

Rosalyn Nguyen, MD
Spaulding Rehabilitation Hospital
Boston, Massachusetts

Erin O'Connor, MD
Assistant Professor
Department of Radiology
Temple University School of Medicine
Philadelphia, Pennsylvania

John D. Pickard, MCHIR, FMedSci
Professor
Department of Clinical Neurosciences
University of Cambridge
Neurosurgical Unit
Addenbrooke's Hospital
Cambridge, United Kingdom

Treven C. Pickett, PsyD, ABPP
Assistant Professor
Departments of Psychiatry and Physical Medicine and Rehabilitation
Virginia Commonwealth University School of Medicine
Assistant Professor
Department of Psychology
Virginia Commonwealth University
Mental Health Service
Hunter Holmes McGuire Richmond VA Medical Center
Richmond, Virginia

Adnan I. Qureshi, MD
Executive Director, Minnesota Stroke Initiative
Associate Head, Department of Neurology
Professor of Neurology, Neurosurgery, and Radiology
Zeenat Qureshi Stroke Research Center
University of Minnesota
Minneapolis, Minnesota

John Ragheb, MD
Director
Department of Neurosurgery
Miami Children's Hospital
Miami, Florida

Michael Rubin, MD
Clinical Instructor
Department of Neurology
Washington University in St. Louis School of Medicine
Division of Neurosciences
Barnes-Jewish Hospital
St. Louis, Missouri

Rafik Samuel, MD
Associate Professor
Department of Medicine, Section of Infectious Diseases
Temple University School of Medicine
Philadelphia, Pennsylvania

Pallav N. Shah, MD
Department of Radiology
Temple University School of Medicine
Temple University Health System
Philadelphia, Pennsylvania

Lori A. Shutter, MD
Associate Professor
Departments of Neurosurgery and Neurology
University of Cincinnati School of Medicine
Mayfield Clinic
Cincinnati, Ohio

David J. Thurman, MD, MPH
Neurologist and Medical Epidemiologist
Epilepsy Program
Division of Adult and Community Health
National Center for Chronic Disease Prevention and Health Promotion
Centers for Disease Control and Prevention
Atlanta, Georgia

Shelly D. Timmons, MD, PhD, FACS
Associate Professor, and Chief of Neurotrauma Division
Department of Neurosurgery
University of Tennessee Health Science Center
Semmes-Murphey Neurologic and Spine Institute
Memphis, Tennessee

Ryan S. Trombly, MD
Assistant Professor
Department of Neurological Surgery
Miller School of Medicine University of Miami
University of Miami Hospital
Miami, Florida

Alexander H. Vo, PhD
Senior Clinical Research Scientist
The University of Texas Medical Branch
Galveston, Texas

Nisha C. Wagle, JD, MA
Federal Appellate Attorney
U.S. Department of Veterans Affairs
Washington, D.C.

Marjorie C. Wang, MD, MPH
Assistant Professor
Department of Neurosurgery
Medical College of Wisconsin
Milwaukee, Wisconsin

Sheila Weaver, DO
Assistant Professor
Department of Medicine, Section of Pulmonary and Critical Care Medicine
Temple University School of Medicine
Philadelphia, Pennsylvania

Barbara M. Weissman
Associate Professor, Pediatrics
Emory University School of Medicine
Atlanta, Georgia

John S. Winestone, MD
Resident
Department of Neurosurgery
University of Tennessee Health Science Center
Memphis, Tennessee

Toshihiko Yanagawa, MD, PhD
Professor
School of Health and Nursing Science
Wakayama Medical University
Department of Pediatrics
Wakayama Medical University Hospital
Wakayama, Japan

Wengui Yu, MD, PhD
Assistant Professor
Departments of Neurological Surgery and Neurology
University of Texas Southwestern Medical Center
Dallas, Texas

Ross D. Zafonte, DO
Chair
Department of Physical Medicine and Rehabilitation
Harvard Medical School
Vice President of Medical Affairs
Spaulding Rehabilitation Hospital
Boston, Massachusetts

Eduard Zaloshnja, PhD
Research Scientist
Public Services Research Institute
Pacific Institute for Research and Evaluation
Calverton, Maryland

Introduction

1 Epidemiology

Victor G. Coronado, David J. Thurman, Arlene I. Greenspan, and Barbara M. Weissman

For the last 3 decades, researchers have used disparate methods, definitions, and case-inclusion criteria to study traumatic brain injury (TBI), especially its milder forms.[1–3] Epidemiologists at the Centers for Disease Control and Prevention (CDC) have developed standard definitions and methods for surveillance purposes to study TBI,[4,5] yielding data that lead to better understanding of this injury so that future prevention and research efforts can be focused on persons at greatest risk. CDC's analyses are based on the public health approach—define the problem, identify risk and protective factors, develop and test prevention strategies, and encourage widespread adoption of successful interventions.

TBI is defined as an injury to the head that results from blunt or penetrating trauma or acceleration or deceleration forces that temporarily or permanently disrupt the brain's function.[4,5] This chapter will describe what is known about the epidemiology of TBI worldwide—its magnitude (including prevalence and consequences), risk factors, impact on specified populations, trends in morbidity and mortality, and far-reaching economic impact. The chapter will also introduce how the data CDC collects, analyzes, and interprets can be used to increase understanding of TBI management, advance critical care, improve TBI outcomes, address socioeconomic concerns, and inform a broad range of disciplines whose interventions may help prevent TBI (e.g., engineering and design for the development of safer cars and homes, or behavioral change to reduce alcohol misuse).

Most of the epidemiological data presented in this chapter were estimated by researchers using data collected and maintained by CDC's National Center for Health Statistics (NCHS) and the National Center for Injury Prevention and Control (NCIPC). The NCHS systems include the Multiple Cause-of-Death Public-Use Data Files (MCD; for TBI-related deaths),[6–8] the National Hospital Discharge Survey (NHDS; for TBI-related hospitalizations),[8,9] the National Hospital Ambulatory Medical Care Survey (NHAMCS; for TBI-related emergency department [ED] and physician's office visits),[8,10–12] the National Ambulatory Medical Care Survey (NAMCS; for TBI-related physician's office and outpatient visits),[12] and the National Health Interview Survey (NHIS; for untreated TBI).[13] The NCIPC developed and maintains the CDC TBI Surveillance System (SS; for TBI-related deaths, hospitalizations, and ED visits).[4,5,14,15] Data presented include numbers and demographic characteristics of affected populations, risk factors, external causes or mechanisms of injury, injury severity, estimates of people living with the consequences of TBI, and economic impact.

The Burden of TBI

Injury, including TBI, is a leading cause of death and disability worldwide that affects people regardless of sex, age, income, race, or nationality.[16,17] CDC has estimated that each year in the United States, at least 1.4 million persons sustain a TBI[8]; of these, ~1.1 million are treated and released from EDs, 235,000 are hospitalized, and 50,000 die (**Tables 1.1** and **1.2**). The incidence of TBI in the U.S. is likely underestimated because ~25% of persons who sustain a TBI do not receive medical care.[13] The CDC figures also do not include TBIs treated in physicians' offices and outpatient facilities (~439,000 and 89,000 visits, respectively).[12] Worldwide, the burden of TBI is less documented and limited data are available.

TBI Definitions, Surveillance Methodology, Limitations, and Gaps

Since 1995, CDC/NCIPC has used standard definitions and surveillance guidelines to estimate the incidence of TBI in the United States.[4,5] CDC/NCIPC has both a code-based and a clinical case definition to collect TBI data for surveillance purposes. To identify TBI cases from coded hospital and ED discharge billing records and death certificates, CDC uses selected codes listed in the *International Classification of Diseases*, Ninth Revision, Clinical Modification (ICD-9-CM) and in the *International Statistical Classification of Diseases and Related Health Problems*, Tenth Revision (ICD-10).[5,18,19] TBI-related hospitalizations and ED visits are selected if the billing records have one or more

Table 1.1 Summary of TBI in the United States

Each year in the United States approximately:

- 1.9 million persons sustain a TBI (not counting those who do not seek medical care).
- 80,000 nonfatal TBI hospitalizations result in long-term disability.
- 50,000 die with a TBI-related diagnosis. TBI is the primary cause of death in 30 to 50% of all injury-related deaths.

Abbreviation: TBI, traumatic brain injury.

Table 1.2 Average Annual Numbers and Adjusted Rates of TBI per 100,000 Population by Sex, Age Group, Race/Ethnicity, and External Cause by Source. National Center for Health Statistics, U.S., 1995–2001

	Source			
Characteristics	**Death* Rates§ (Numbers)**	**Hospitalization† Rates§ (Numbers)**	**Emergency Department Visit‡ Rates§ (Numbers)**	**Aggregated Rates§ (Numbers)**
Overall	18.1 (49,900)	85.5 (235,000)	401.2 (1,111,000)	504.8 (1,396,000)
Sex				
Male	28.4 (36,922)	110.4 (146,000)	470.3 (652,000)	609.1 (835,000)
Female	8.9 (12,978)	60.7 (89,000)	329.3 (459,000)	398.9 (561,000)
Age group (years)				
0–4	5.7 (1,099)	79.9 (15,000)	1,035.0 (200,000)	1,120.7 (216,000)
5–9	3.1 (628)	53.0 (11,000)	603.3 (122,000)	659.3 (133,000)
10–14	4.8 (957)	56.9 (11,000)	567.0 (113,000)	628.6 (125,000)
15–19	24.3 (4,756)	129.1 (25,000)	661.1 (129,000)	814.4 (160,000)
20–24	27.5 (5,092)	98.7 (18,000)	429.3 (79,000)	555.5 (103,000)
25–34	18.9 (7,720)	73.6 (30,000)	357.6 (146,000)	450.2 (184,000)
35–44	17.2 (7,619)	66.5 (29,000)	291.0 (129,000)	374.7 (166,000)
45–54	16.4 (5,776)	57.6 (20,000)	211.3 (75,000)	285.2 (101,000)
55–64	17.0 (3,927)	61.6 (14,000)	150.9 (35,000)	229.5 (53,000)
65–74	22.5 (4,188)	86.8 (16,000)	158.1 (29,000)	267.4 (50,000)
≥75	50.6 (8,095)	272.1 (44,000)	336.4 (54,000)	659.1 (105,000)
Race/ethnicity				
Caucasians	18.1 (41,498)	63.8 (146,000)	404.9 (904,000)	486.8 (1,091,498)
African American	19.9 (6,878)	73.9 (26,000)	441.5 (173,000)	535.3 (205,878)
AI/AN A/PI	12.4 (1,524)	59.9 (7,000)	261.3 (35,000)	333.6 (43,524)
Other/unknown	—	24.1 (57,000)	—	24.1 (57,000)
External causes				
MVC-T‖	6.1 (16,800)	21.5 (59,000)	72.8 (204,000)	100.4 (280,000)
Falls	2.4 (6,426)	17.7 (48,000)	124.6 (343,000)	144.7 (398,000)
Assault	2.3 (6,499)	5.1 (14,000)	48.6 (135,000)	56.0 (156,000)
Struck by/against object	¶ (404)	¶ (6,000)	¶ (263,000)	¶ (269,000)
Other	¶ (19,413)	¶ (22,000)	¶ (127,000)	¶ (293,000)
Unknown	¶ (359)	¶ (85,000)	¶ (40,000)	¶ (293,000)

Abbreviations: AI/NA A/PI, American Indian or Native American, Asian or Pacific Islander; MVC-T, motor vehicle-traffic; TBI, traumatic brain injury.

*Death data were obtained from the Multiple Cause-of-Death public-use data files.

†Hospitalization data were obtained from the National Hospital Discharge Survey. In-hospital deaths were excluded.

‡Emergency department visit data were obtained from the National Hospital Ambulatory Medical Care Survey. Hospitalizations, deaths, transfers to another facility, or unknown dispositions were excluded.

§Rates per 100,000 population. Adjusted to the 2000 U.S. standard population.

‖Motor vehicle-traffic includes vehicle occupants, motorcyclists, pedal cyclists, pedestrians, other, and unspecified persons involved in motor vehicle-traffic incidents.

¶Rate not estimated.

Source: Adapted from Langlois JA, Rutland-Brown W, Thomas KE. Traumatic Brain Injury in the United States: Emergency Department Visits, Hospitalizations, and Deaths. Atlanta: Centers for Disease Control and Prevention, National Center for Injury Prevention and Control; 2006.

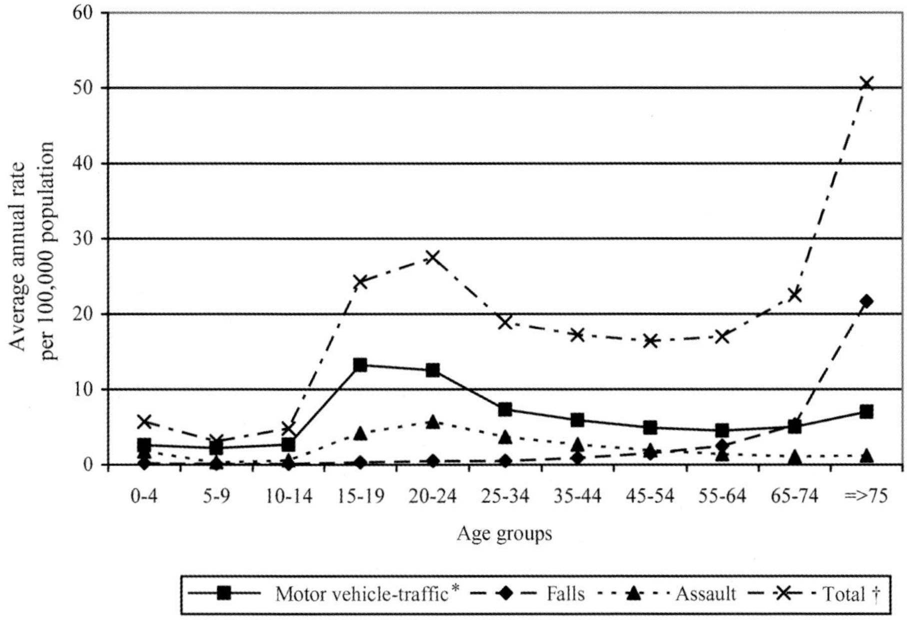

* Motor vehicle-traffic (MV-T) includes vehicle occupants, motorcyclists, pedal cyclists, pedestrians, other, and unspecified persons involved in MV-T incidents.
† Total includes 43 cases with missing age.
Note: Other/unknown external causes (not presented) include an annual average estimate of 404 struck by/against events (0.8% of total); 19,413 other events (38.9% of total); and 359 unknowns (0.7% of total).

Fig. 1.1 Average annual rates of TBI-related deaths by major external cause and age group. Multiple Cause-of-Death Public-Use Data Files. National Center for Health Statistics, U.S., 1995–2001. From: Langlois JA, Rutland-Brown W, Thomas KE. Traumatic brain injury in the United States: emergency department visits, hospitalizations, and deaths. Atlanta (GA): Centers for Disease Control and Prevention, National Center for Injury Prevention and Control; 2006.

of the following ICD-9-CM codes: 800.0–801.9, 803.0–804.9, 850.0–854.1, 950.1–950.3, 959.01, or 995.55. TBI-associated deaths are included if one or more of the following ICD-10 codes are listed as a contributing cause of death: S01.0–S01.9, S02.0, S02.1, S02.3, S02.7–S02.9, S04.0, S06.0–S06.9, S07.0, S07.1, S07.8, S07.9, S09.7–S09.9, T90.1, T90.2, T90.4, T90.5, T90.8, or T90.9. Although not considered valid in the United States, death codes T01.0, T02.0, T04.0, and T06.0 are included in the CDC TBI definition.[5,15] To determine the external causes (e.g., falls), injury locale (e.g., home), and whether the TBI resulted from violence or was unintentional, CDC uses the ICD-9-CM external causes of injury codes (E-codes) that are listed in hospital and ED discharge billing records classified by using CDC-recommended E-code groupings.[5,20,21] A case of TBI is recognized when a medical record documents one or more of the following conditions: observed or self-reported decreased level of consciousness, amnesia, skull fracture (a marker of TBI), objective neurological or neuropsychological abnormality, or intracranial lesion.[4,5] CDC has also developed surveillance definitions for mild TBI (MTBI).[3]

In the U.S., multiple data sources are used to estimate the national incidence (i.e., new cases) of TBI. MCD public-use data files are used to identify TBI-associated deaths if a TBI-related ICD-9 diagnosis code (1995–1998) or ICD-10 diagnosis code (1999–2001) is listed in Part I of the death certificate; external causes of death are obtained from the underlying cause-of-death field.[6–8,22] NHDS data are used to identify TBI-related hospitalizations if one of the seven diagnosis fields listed in each sampled record met the CDC criteria; in-hospital deaths were excluded from the analysis presented in **Table 1.2** and **Figs. 1.1** and **1.2**.[8] NHAMCS data are used to identify TBI-related ED visits and causes if one of three diagnosis fields and first E-code field listed in each sampled record met the CDC criteria; ED deaths and transfers to other facilities were excluded from the analysis presented in **Table 1.2** and **Figs. 1.1** and **1.3**.[8] Data from the NHIS, NHAMCS, and NAMCS are used to identify TBI untreated or treated in physician's offices or outpatient facilities.[12,13] The occurrence of untreated TBI was estimated using data from the 1991 NHIS[13]; a change in 1997 to the NHIS case inclusion criteria for medically attended conditions, however, precludes obtaining current estimates of untreated TBI. All of NCHS's surveys, except the MCD, allow estimating the occurrence of TBI at the national level only. NCIPC conducts the CDC TBI SS; currently, only 12 states conduct TBI surveillance.[4,5,15] The CDC TBI SS has two aspects: core and extended surveillance. Core surveillance data are obtained from unduplicated (i.e., account for multiple admissions) vital statistics and ICD-coded hospital billing records, which allows estimation of patient-level statistics.[5] For in-hospital deaths, reporting states provide ICD-9-CM or ICD-10 codes that are determined to be most complete.[5]

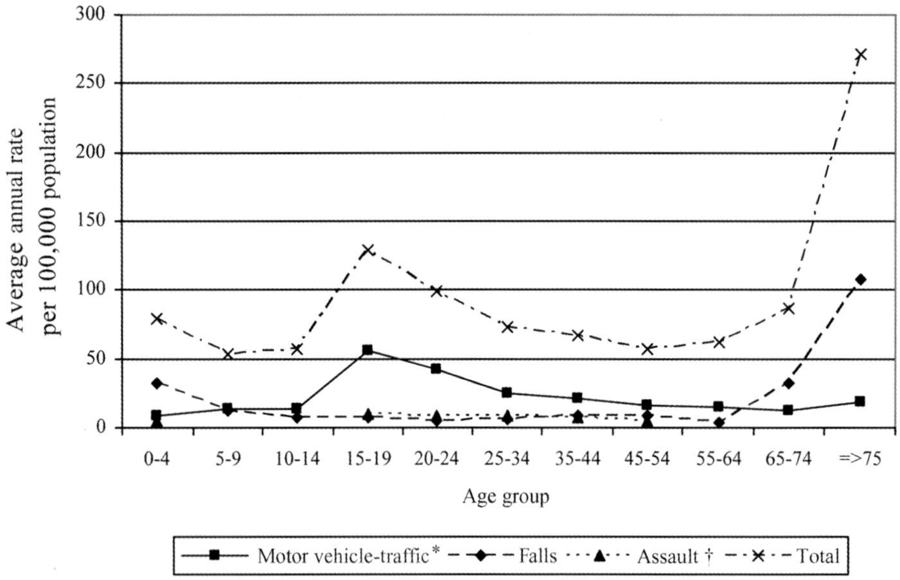

* Motor vehicle-traffic (MV-T) includes vehicle occupants, motorcyclists, pedal cyclists, pedestrians other, and unspecified persons involved in MV-T incidents.
† Assault rates for persons aged 5–9, 10–14, and 55 and older are not presented. The sample size for each excluded age group is less than 30, a value considered unstable.
Note: Other/unknown external causes (not presented) include an annual average estimate of 6,000 struck by/against events (2.4% of total); 22,000 other events (9.3% of total); and 85,000 unknowns (36.4% of total).

Fig. 1.2 Average annual rates of TBI-related hospitalizations by major external cause and age group. National Hospital Discharge Survey, National Center for Health Statistics, U.S., 1995–2001. From: Langlois JA, Rutland-Brown W, Thomas KE. Traumatic brain injury in the United States: emergency department visits, hospitalizations, and deaths. Atlanta (GA): Centers for Disease Control and Prevention, National Center for Injury Prevention and Control; 2006.

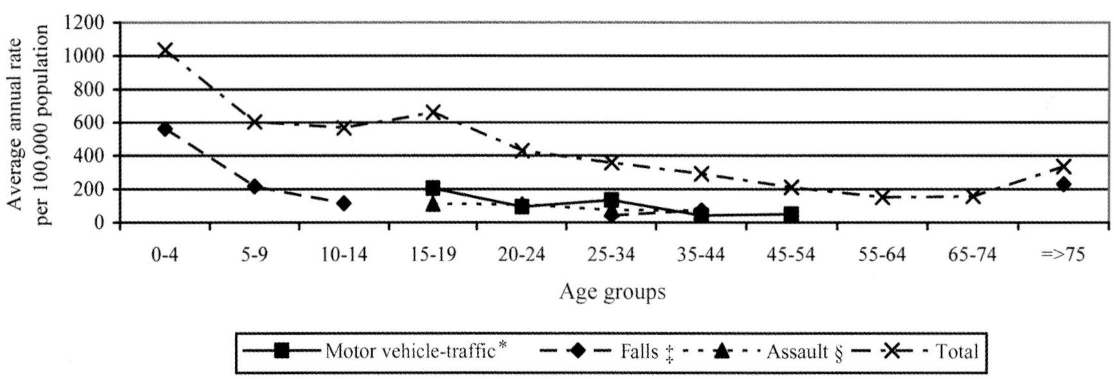

* Motor vehicle-traffic (MV-T) includes vehicle occupants, motorcyclists, pedal cyclists, pedestrians, other, and unspecified persons involved in MV-T incidents.
† MV-T rates for persons aged 0–14 and 55 and older are not presented. Because the sample size for each group is less than 30, the value is considered unstable.
‡ Fall rates for persons aged 15–24 and 45–74 are not presented. Because the sample size for each age group is less than 30, the value of the estimate is considered unstable.
§ Assault rates for persons aged 0–14 and 45 and older are not presented. Because the sample size for each age group is less than 30, the values of the estimate is considered unstable.
Note: Other/unknown external causes (not presented) include an annual average estimate of 263,000 struck by/against events (23.7% of total); 1,27,000 other events (11.4% of total); and 40, 000 unknowns (3.6% of total).

Fig. 1.3 Average annual rates of TBI-related emergency department visits by major external cause and age group. National Hospital Ambulatory Medical Care Survey, National Center for Health Statistics, U.S., 1995–2001. From: Langlois JA, Rutland-Brown W, Thomas KE. Traumatic brain injury in the United States: emergency department visits, hospitalizations, and deaths. Atlanta (GA): Centers for Disease Control and Prevention, National Center for Injury Prevention and Control; 2006.

Extended TBI surveillance data are obtained by a subset of participating states using sampling methodology and CDC's clinical criteria to obtain selected clinical information from a sample of medical records identified through core surveillance.[5]

In general, researchers who study TBI often use disparate methods and case inclusion criteria (e.g., patients who were hospitalized or seen in EDs).[1–3] Also, standard clinical and surveillance definitions are not universally employed, especially for MTBI. For example, ICD-9-CM–based CDC TBI surveillance definition includes fracture of the skull without neurological symptoms or head injury—not specified as proxies for TBI.[5] These criteria, however, are not fully accepted by researchers. To overcome these definition-related issues, CDC is conducting a sensitivity study to evaluate a proposed surveillance definition for MTBI[3] that can be applied to the general population. There is also lack of SSs that can ascertain, for example, untreated TBIs.[3] Data from the NHDS, NHAMCS, and NAMCS do not account for the multiple admissions that may occur for a single injury case; this limitation precludes estimating the incidence of TBI at the patient level. Also, in the United States, SSs rely mainly on ICD-coded data originally designed for reimbursement purposes; the coding validity and reliability of these data for TBI surveillance are being studied.[15,23] Despite that the incidence of TBI varies substantially by state, in 2002, only 12 states participated in the CDC TBI SS.[3,15] Estimates of incidence, external causes, and prevalence of TBI worldwide are not available. Approximations of the worldwide incidence and prevalence of TBI have been attempted by combining global estimates for fractures of the skull (including facial fractures) with short- and long-term intracranial injuries presented in *Global Health Statistics*.[24]

TBI Severity

Classification of TBI severity is crucial to understanding and describing the clinical management and burden of TBI. Several scoring systems can assess the initial neurological status of patients with TBI, including the Glasgow Coma Scale (GCS), the Trauma Score, the Trauma Score Revised, and the Abbreviated Injury Scale (AIS).[25–28] The GCS, despite its limitations,[29–32] is the most commonly used system. The GCS is a simple, practical scale used to determine an injured person's level of consciousness[25]; to predict outcomes for patients with TBI[33,34]; and to classify TBI as mild, moderate, or severe.[25] GCS scores of 3 to 8 are classified as severe; scores of 9 to 12 are classified as moderate; and scores of 13 to 15 are classified as mild. Modified versions of the GCS are used for infants and young children,[35–38] though none have adequately demonstrated reliability in predicting outcomes among children. Consequently, modified versions have not gained international acceptance. In general, most of the patients seen in EDs are treated and released, and as such are considered MTBI cases.[13] In hospital wards, the rate of MTBI was almost twice the rate of moderate or severe TBI (51; 21 and 19 per 100,000 population, respectively).[9] Data from the 1997 CDC TBI SS indicate that 74.9% of survivors suffered MTBIs; 9.6% were moderate, 9.8% were severe, and 5.7% were of unknown severity. Fatality statistics were not published for 1997.[14] Data from the 2002 CDC TBI SS indicate that 6% of patients hospitalized for a TBI died while hospitalized.[15]

Consequences of TBI

Persons who survive a TBI often experience neuropsychological and other problems, including disabilities, that affect their work or social activity; often these persons require extensive rehabilitation services and sometimes long-term care.[7] Each year, ~80,000 of the 230,000 nonfatal TBI-related hospitalizations result in long-term disability.[17] Quite likely, this figure underestimates the problem because most cases of TBI in the United States are mild[13,14] and do not result in hospital admission.[13] Still, an undetermined number of persons with MTBI may have adverse consequences, including long-term or permanent disability[2,3,39]; this is reflected, for example, in the high unemployment rate among previously employed MTBI survivors (34% at 3 months and 9% at 12 months post-TBI).[39,40]

The Incidence of Fatal and Nonfatal TBI

TBI-associated Deaths

TBI is the primary cause of death in ~30 to 50% of all injury-related deaths.[6] Data from the 1995–2001 MCD indicate that TBI is a major cause of death in the United States, especially among older adults (**Table 1.2**).[8] During this period, the average annual death rate was 18.1 per 100,000 population; the rate for males was approximately 3 times that for females (**Table 1.2**). The TBI-related death rate for persons aged 75 years or older was twice the rate of 65- to 74-year-olds and at least 60% higher than any other age group (**Table 1.2**).[8] The leading causes of TBI-related death were motor vehicle-traffic (MV-T) incidents, falls, and assaults; other causes (including firearm-related) accounted for ~40% of all deaths (**Table 1.2**). Also, between 1995 and 2001, 30% of MV-T-related TBI deaths occurred among persons aged 15 to 24 years, and 54% of fall-related TBI deaths occurred among adults 75 years or older (**Fig. 1.1**).[8] Interestingly, data from the 1989–1998 MCD indicate that the leading causes of TBI-related death were firearm-related injuries (40%), MV-T incidents (34%), and falls (10%).[7] These data also indicate that the overall

TBI-related death male/female ratio was 3:4; this ratio, however, was 6:1 for firearms and 2.5:1 each for MV-T incidents and falls.[7] Firearm-related injury was the leading cause of TBI-related deaths among 20- to 74-year-olds, especially among males.[7]

TBI-related Nonfatal Emergency Department Visits and Hospitalizations

From 1995 to 2001, the average annual rate of nonfatal TBI-related ED visits in the United States was more than 4 times higher than that of TBI-related hospitalization (**Table 1.2**)[8]; males had at least 1.4 times higher rates of nonfatal TBI-related hospitalizations and ED visits than females (**Table 1.2**).[8] Hospitalizations for TBI were highest for persons aged 75 or older; in contrast, TBI-related ED visits were highest among children ages 0 to 4 and 15 to 19 years (**Table 1.2**); these patterns were similar to those reported by CDC for 2003.[41]

TBI Untreated or Treated in Physicians' Offices or Outpatient Facilities

In the United States, most persons who sustain a TBI are not hospitalized.[13] NHIS data for 1991 indicate that ~1.5 million U.S. civilians sustained a TBI; of these, 25% received no medical care and 14% received care in outpatient facilities.[13] NAMCS and NHAMCS data for 1995–1997 indicate that almost 520,000 TBI-related visits were made to physician offices (439,000) and hospital outpatient departments (80,000).[12]

Findings of CDC's Hospital-Based TBI Surveillance System

Data from the 2002 CDC TBI SS indicate that 74,517 persons were hospitalized with a TBI-related diagnosis in the 12 participating states.[15] TBI hospitalization rates varied substantially by state; they were lowest in Nebraska and highest in Arizona (50.6 and 96.9 per 100,000, respectively).[15] Rates among males were almost twice that of females. Persons aged 75 or older, regardless of sex, had at least twice the rate of TBI hospitalizations as 15- to 24-year-olds, the group with the second highest rates; the high rates of both groups were associated with falls and MV-T incidents. Rates for falls were highest among persons aged 75 or older, 65 to 74, and 0 to 4 years (**Table 1.3**). Rates for MV-T incidents were highest among persons aged 15 to 34, and 75 years or older (**Table 1.3**). Most TBI survivors (66%) were discharged without needing follow-up health care; 17% were discharged to rehabilitation facilities or required in-home care; 3% were transferred to acute care hospitals; 1% left against medical advice; 6% died while hospitalized; and discharge disposition information was not available for 6%.[15] Despite including in-hospital deaths, the CDC TBI SS rates were generally lower than those reported using 1995–2001 NHDS data (79.0 vs. 85.5 per 100,000). Several factors may account for this difference: the CDC TBI SS may not reflect the occurrence of TBI nationally; participating states report TBI cases among state residents only.[5] NHDS may include multiple hospitalizations for the same TBI, whereas the CDC TBI SS usually does not; and advances in technology and treatment may have changed admission policies and practices for TBI over time.[9]

External Causes of TBI and Intentionality

Information about the external causes and injury intentionality are necessary to develop effective prevention strategies. Intentionality indicates if an injury was purposely inflicted by someone else with the aim of injuring (e.g., assault) or by oneself (e.g., suicide), or was unintentional (e.g., fall).[42,43] Between 1995 and 2002 falls, MV-T incidents, and assaults were the leading causes of TBI in the United States (**Tables 1.2** and **1.3**)[8,15]; most of the TBIs were unintentional (**Table 1.3**).[15]

Falls

Falls are a significant cause of TBI, especially in young children and older adults (**Table 1.4**). Between 1995 and 2001, falls were the leading cause of TBI-related ED visits and the second leading cause of TBI-related hospitalization and death in the United States (**Table 1.2**).[8] Overall, fall-related TBIs were higher in children younger than 15 years (with a peak in those aged 0–4 years) and among older adults, especially those aged 75 years or older (**Table 1.3**).[8] Interestingly, fall-related TBI hospitalizations increased with age in older adults; in fact, persons aged 85 years or older were 7 times more likely to be hospitalized than those aged 65 to 69 years (334.4 vs. 45.0 per 100,000 population; CDC TBI SS unpublished data). This age-group pattern prevailed among males and females; however, males always had a substantially higher rate than females. Falls were also the leading cause of TBI hospitalizations in children younger than 2 years of age, especially among those younger than 1 year.[44]

MV-T Incidents

During 1995 to 2001, MV-T incidents (including vehicle occupants, motorcyclists, pedal cyclists, pedestrians, and unspecified persons) were the leading cause of TBI-associated death and TBI hospitalization and the second cause of TBI-related ED visits in the United States (**Table 1.2**). Rates were higher among 15- to 44-year-olds, with a peak among 15- to 19-year-olds. Later in life, these rates increased in older adults (**Figs. 1.1, 1.2, 1.3, and 1.4**), especially for males (**Tables 1.3 and 1.4**).[8,15,45]

Table 1.3 Annual Incidence Rates of TBI-Related Hospitalization per 100,000 Population by Intent/Cause, Age Group, and Sex. Twelve States* Centers for Disease Control and Prevention TBI Surveillance System, 2002

Age Group (Years)	Unintentional			Assault	Other/ Unknown	Total
	Falls	Motor Vehicle-Traffic†	Struck by or against Object			
All						
0–4	33.7	10.1	4.0	5.8	7.6	61.2
5–14	11.2	16.0	4.3	1.1	9.5	42.0
15–24	10.5	60.4	3.9	14.5	13.9	103.3
25–34	8.6	32.9	1.9	10.8	8.7	62.9
35–64	17.9	24.3	1.7	7.3	9.8	60.9
65–74	58.6	21.7	2.1	2.8	12.7	97.9
≥75	203.9	30.3	3.5	1.9	24.8	264.4
Total	29.6‡	28.5‡	2.7‡	7.1‡	11.1‡	79.0‡
Males						
0–4	38.3	11.4	4.8	6.9	9.3	70.8
5–14	15.6	20.0	6.2	1.9	13.4	57.2
15–24	15.9	78.7	6.0	25.7	20.8	147.2
25–34	13.4	44.3	3.1	19.0	13.6	93.3
35–64	25.3	31.6	2.6	12.6	14.1	86.2
65–74	70.8	25.8	3.1	4.7	18.1	122.5
≥75	213.9	40.4	4.2	3.0	33.5	295.0
Total	36.3‡	36.9‡	4.0‡	12.2‡	16.0‡	105.3‡
Females						
0–4	28.9	8.6	3.1	4.8	5.8	51.2
5–14	6.5	11.8	2.2	0.3	5.3	26.1
15–24	4.8	40.9	1.5	2.7	6.5	56.5
25–34	3.7	21.2	0.7	2.2	3.7	31.4
35–64	10.7	17.2	0.8	2.1	5.6	36.4
65–74	48.5	18.3	1.3	1.2	8.2	77.5
≥75	197.9	24.2	3.1	1.3	19.6	246.1
Total	23.4‡	20.1‡	1.4‡	2.0‡	6.4‡	53.4‡

Abbreviations: MV-T, motor vehicle-traffic; TBI, traumatic brain injury.

*Alaska, Arizona, California, Colorado, Maryland, Minnesota, Nebraska, New Jersey, New York, Oklahoma, South Carolina, and Utah.

†Motor vehicle-Traffic (MV-T) includes drivers, passengers, pedestrians, motorcyclists, and bicyclists involved in MV-T incidents.

‡Age-adjusted to the 2000 U.S. standard population.

Source: Adapted from Coronado VG, Johnson RL, Faul M, Kegler SR. Incidence rates of hospitalization related to traumatic brain injury—12 states, 2002. MMWR 2006; 55(8):201–204.

Sports and Recreation

Limited comprehensive data are available to define the burden of sports- and recreation-related TBI in the United States; researchers have used multiple data sources, including NCHS's national surveys. Data from NHIS for 1991 indicate that ~300,000 of the 1.5 million TBIs reported in the United States resulted from sports- and recreation-related injuries (**Table 1.4**).[13] Of persons with sports-related TBIs, 12% were hospitalized; 55% were treated and released from EDs or outpatient facilities; and 34% did not receive medical attention.[13,46] MCD data for 1995 indicate that ~900 sports- and recreation-related deaths

Table 1.4 Summary of External Causes of TBI

• Falls, motor vehicle-traffic incidents (MV-T), and assaults are the leading causes of TBI.
• Fall TBIs are highest in children <15 years and in older adults. Rates are higher in males.
• MV-T TBIs are highest in 15–44-year-olds. Rates are higher in males and increase with age in older adults (65–74 year-olds to 75 and older).
• Assault TBIs are highest in 15–44-year-olds. Rates are higher in males. Peaks are also observed among 0–11-month-olds.
• Approximately 300,000 TBIs result from sports- and recreation-related injuries.

Abbreviations: MV-T, motor vehicle-traffic; TBI, traumatic brain injury.

occurred in the United States; these estimates, however, should be interpreted with caution because they depend on assumptions that cannot be verified; for example, the circumstances of the 500 bicycle-related deaths included in this figure cannot be verified.[46] Although these data suggest that most sports- and recreation-related TBIs are not severe, research suggests that concussions and repeated concussions may have potentially serious consequences—especially among persons participating in contact sports.[47] Although the number of TBIs that are repeat injuries is unknown, research shows that persons who have sustained a TBI are at greater risk for second (2.8–4.0 times) and third (7.8–9.3 times) TBIs.[48–50] These data are significant given the number of persons involved in sports and recreational activities. For example, a survey of 235 U.S. high schools found that boys' football and girls' basketball had the highest rates of concussion (3,660 and 1,040 per 100,000, respectively).[51] Head injury, especially among children and young adults, can occur during informal play; in 1991, ~58,000 such injuries were reported in U.S. EDs.[52] Special attention should be placed on the estimated 200,000 children treated in U.S. EDs for playground equipment–related injuries; 88% of these injuries were attributable to swings, climbers, and slides.[53]

Assaults

Assaults are the third leading cause of TBI-related deaths, hospitalizations, and ED visits in the United States (**Table 1.2; Figs. 1.1, 1.2, 1.3,** and **1.4**). Between 1995 and 2002, persons aged 15 to 44 years had the highest assault-related TBI rates, with a peak among those aged 15 to 19 years; these rates declined with increasing age (**Fig. 1.4, Tables 1.3** and **1.4**).[8,15] The rate of assault-related TBI hospitalizations

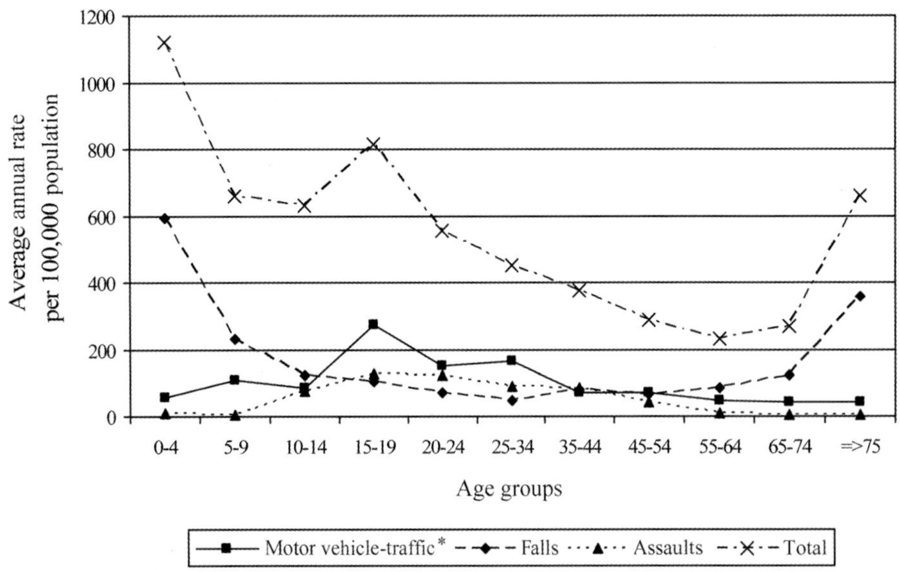

* Motor vehicle-traffic (MV-T) includes vehicle occupants, motorcyclists, pedal cyclists, pedestrians, other, and unspecified persons involved in MV-T incidents.
Note: External causes (not presented) include an annual average estimate of 269,000 struck by/against events (19.3% of total) and 293,000 other/unknown events (21.0% of total).

Fig. 1.4 Combined average annual rates of TBI by major external cause and age group. National Hospital Ambulatory Medical Care Survey, National Hospital Discharge Survey, and Multiple Cause-of-Death Public-Use Data Files. National Center for Health Statistics, U.S., 1995–2001. From: Langlois JA, Rutland-Brown W, Thomas KE. Traumatic brain injury in the United States: emergency department visits, hospitalizations, and deaths. Atlanta (GA): Centers for Disease Control and Prevention, National Center for Injury Prevention and Control; 2006.

for males was at least 6 times that for females (**Table 1.3**).[15] Interestingly, CDC TBI SS data for 2002 show that the rate of assault-related TBI hospitalizations for 0-to 4-year-olds was 4 times the rate for children aged 5 to 14 years (**Table 1.3**)[15]; and among children younger than age 2 years, 0-to 11-month-olds had significantly higher rates than 12- to 23-month-olds.[44]

Table 1.5 Summary of TBI Disability and Costs in the United States

- TBI disability: ~5 million Americans live with a TBI-associated disability.
- Cost of TBI in the United States: The lifetime cost of TBIs sustained in 2000 is almost $60.4 billion.

Abbreviation: TBI, traumatic brain injury.

Suicide and Homicide

In the United States, ~46,000 persons die each year from interpersonal (homicides) and self-inflicted (suicides) violence.[54] Homicide and suicide statistics, however, may not fully capture all violent deaths because many of these, particularly among women, children, and the elderly, may be attributed to other causes.[43] During 1989 to 1998, firearm-related TBIs were the leading cause associated to death; of these deaths, 68% were suicides, 27% were homicides, and 5% were of unintentional and of other or unknown intentionality.[7] Most of these deaths occurred among males (85%) aged 20 to 24 years. African Americans had the highest rate of firearm-related TBI death (11.1 per 100,000); of these, 70% were homicides. Males aged 20 to 24 years, regardless of race/ethnicity, had the highest rate of firearm-related TBI deaths.[7]

Impact of TBI

Although most fall-, MV-T–, and assault-related TBIs were nonfatal (**Table 1.1**), health effects ranging from temporary clinical problems to permanent disability occur in an unknown but substantial number of survivors. CDC has estimated that ~5 million Americans live with a TBI-associated disability (**Table 1.5**).[3]

Risk Factors

Persons who sustain a TBI are a heterogeneous group,[7–15] including substantial numbers of the very young and the elderly, as well as adolescents and young adults (**Tables 1.2** and **1.3; Figs. 1.1, 1.2, 1.3,** and **1.4**). Although some persons who sustained a TBI were healthy prior to their injury, others may have had one or more comorbid conditions that put them at risk.[45] The leading factors associated with risk for TBI (e.g., age, sex) are reviewed in **Table 1.6**.

Age

In general, persons aged 0 to 4 years, 15 to 19 years, and 75 years or older had the highest rates of TBI in the United States (**Table 1.6**).[8,15] These age-related rates likely reflect differences in exposure, particularly to falls and MV-T incidents (**Tables 1.2** and **1.3; Figs. 1.1, 1.2, 1.3,** and **1.4**).

Comorbid Conditions in Older Adults

Older adults tend to have more comorbid conditions[55] than younger patients.[56] CDC TBI SS data show that at least 70% of adults aged 65 years or older with fall- or MV-T–related TBI hospitalizations had one or more comorbid conditions.[45] Hypertension, diabetes mellitus, cardiac arrhythmias, and anemia were common in this age group, especially in persons with fall-related TBI (**Table 1.6**).[45] Alzheimer disease, other dementias, depression, and Parkinson disease were higher in older adults with fall-related TBI compared with those with MV-T–related TBI (**Table 1.6**).[45]

Table 1.6 Summary of TBI-Related Risk Factors

- Age: In the United States, persons aged 0–4, 15–19, and 75 years or older had the highest rates of TBI.
- Comorbid conditions in older adults: Hypertension, diabetes mellitus, cardiac arrhythmias, and anemia are common in older adults with TBI. Alzheimer disease, other dementias, depression, and Parkinson disease are higher in older adults with fall-related TBI.
- Sex: Males have substantially higher TBI rates than females.
- Race and ethnicity: African Americans and Hispanics in large metropolitan areas tend to have more violence and pedestrian-hit-by-car TBI. Nationally, TBI ED visits, hospitalizations, and deaths are higher in African Americans.
- Socioeconomic factors: Living alone was a risk factor for TBI among persons with annual income under $20,000.
- Alcohol/Drugs: Alcohol use is a factor for TBI-related MV-T incidents and falls.
- Lack of protective equipment (PE; e.g., seat belts, child seats, helmets, etc.): Use of PE may reduce injuries (including TBIs).

Abbreviations: ED, emergency department; MV-T, motor vehicle traffic; PE, protective equipment; TBI, traumatic brain injury.

Sex

Compared with women, men have approximately twice the rates of TBI-related hospitalizations and ED visits and 3 times the rate of TBI-related deaths in the United States (**Table 1.6**).[7,8,15] These patterns may reflect the higher overall rates of general injury among males, especially those related to falls, MV-T incidents, and firearm injuries,[7,57] and the male/female differences in risk-taking behavior and exposure to occupational hazards.[1,58]

Race and Ethnicity

Data on race and ethnicity are used to monitor trends, evaluate programs, understand the etiologic process and identify points of intervention, and monitor and enforce laws against discrimination.[59] Research indicates that TBI incidence is higher among certain racial/ethnic groups. Data from the National Model Systems Database (NMSD), a study of TBI-related disability in 20 U.S. medical centers located mainly in large urban areas, indicate that MV-T incidents were the leading cause of TBI in those urban areas; minority groups (i.e., African Americans and Hispanics), however, had more violence- and pedestrian-hit-by-car–related TBI than nonminority groups (i.e., Caucasians).[60] MCD data for 1989–1998 indicate that among all racial/ethnic groups, the greatest decline in TBI-associated mortality was observed among African Americans.[7] Data from NCHS for 1995–2001, however, indicate that African Americans have higher rates of TBI-related ED visits, hospitalizations, and deaths than other racial/ethnic groups (**Tables 1.2** and **1.6**).[8]

Socioeconomic Factors

There is an increased probability of injury[61] and injury mortality[62] associated with lower socioeconomic status. Research suggests that socioeconomic factors may influence the risk of TBI in the United States. Data from NHIS indicate that living alone was a risk factor for TBI among persons with annual income less than $20,000 (**Table 1.6**).[13] NMSD data indicate that minorities at risk for TBI are generally young, single, unemployed males with only high school education.[60]

Alcohol and Drugs

Alcohol is the leading risk factor for injury, contributing to unintentional and violent injury and mortality.[63,64] CDC TBI SS data for 1997 indicate that ~21% of MV occupants, 19% of motorcycle riders, and 10% of persons who fell and incurred a TBI had consumed alcohol or had blood alcohol concentration levels ≥0.01 g/dL[14]; these figures may be higher because data were missing for at least 24% of these reported cases (**Table 1.6**). Alcohol use is also a factor for TBI among older adults. CDC TBI SS data for 2002 showed clinical or laboratory evidence of alcohol use in 6% of MV-T– and 8% of fall-related TBI in adults aged 65 or older; these figures may be higher because alcohol use information was missing for nearly half of this population.[45]

Use of Personal Protective Equipment

The use of protective equipment (PE; e.g., car's seat belts and air bags; helmets and faceguards in transportation, sports, and recreation) substantially reduces the risk of head injury and TBI (**Table 1.6**).[65–68] CDC TBI SS data for 1997 indicate that ~46% of MV occupants, 53% of motorcyclists, and 41% of pedal cyclists injured in collisions were not using PE at the time of injury[14]; these figures may be higher because data were missing for 10 to 50% of the cases. These data can be used to support the need for legislation requiring use of PE or enforcement of existing legislation and reporting.

Other Comorbid Conditions

Persons with certain illnesses are at higher risk for a TBI; one of the most commonly associated disorders includes psychiatric illnesses and problems with attention. A case-control study of persons with and without psychiatric diagnoses preceding a TBI found that the adjusted relative risk (ARR) for TBI was 1.7 compared with those without psychiatric diagnosis.[69] The highest ARRs were for organic nonpsychotic and psychotic disorders (4.4 and 3.7, respectively) and somatoform disorders (2.8).[69] Likewise, attention deficit hyperactivity disorder (ADHD), a potential consequence of TBI, may also be a risk factor for TBI. An interview study of children with moderate and severe closed head injury found a premorbid prevalence of ADHD of 0.2, significantly higher than the reference population (0.045).[70] Socially dysfunctional behavior is also associated with TBI. A study of prisoners who reported a TBI in their lifetime showed that 36% had experienced TBI the previous year.[71] Thus, preventive measures for TBI should consider populations with potentially modifiable risk factors.

Incidence and External Causes of TBI Worldwide

The burden of TBI and its consequences can be reduced globally by a better understanding of its magnitude, external causes, risk factors, and the concerted efforts of those involved in TBI monitoring, prevention, and control. Data from the World Health Organization's (WHO) Global Health statistics suggest that 9.7 million TBIs (184.6 per

100,000) severe enough to require medical treatment or cause death occurred worldwide in 1990.[24] These estimates suggest that TBI rates ranged from 110.1 per 100,000 in China to 361.6 per 100,000 in countries in sub-Saharan Africa (SSA). Worldwide and in every region, MV-T incidents were the leading cause of TBI (60%; 111.7 per 100,000). Violence, the second leading cause of TBI (25%; 45.8 per 100,000), was highest in SSA (153.3 per 100,000). Falls were the third leading cause of TBI (16.1 per 100,000). Fall-related TBIs were highest in India (48.5 per 100,000). War-related TBI was relatively common in SSA (20.8 per 100,000) and in countries of the Eastern Mediterranean region such as Iraq, Iran, and Israel (13.3 per 100,000).[24] Rates of unintentional TBI were substantially greater worldwide than the rates of intentional injuries—except in SSA, where the two rates were almost the same. These data may underestimate the occurrence of TBI because persons who were injured but received no medical care were not included.[24]

Trends in TBI Morbidity and Mortality

Few studies have reported data describing the long-term trends in TBI occurrence. Two studies, using MCD data, have assessed U.S. mortality trends. The first indicated a 22% reduction in rates between 1979 and 1992 (from 24.6 to 19.3 per 100,000),[6] and the second indicated a further 4% reduction between 1992 and 1998.[7] The largest decline in TBI mortality occurred in the early 1980s and was attributed mostly to decreases in MV-related deaths.[6] During 1998 to 2003, these rates remained relatively unchanged.[41]

Trends in TBI morbidity are more difficult to interpret. TBI morbidity trends are assessed using rates of TBI-related hospitalization, which may be influenced not only by changes in actual incidence but also by changes in hospital admission criteria and the availability of hospital care. NHDS data indicate that TBI-related hospital discharge rates in the United States decreased 51% from 1980 to 1995 (from 199 to 98 per 100,000, respectively).[9] In Denmark, national hospital register data showed a 42% decline in rates from 1979 to 1993.[72] In New Zealand, national hospital discharge data indicated a similar decline of about ~53% from 1980 to 1998.[73] All three studies indicate decreases that were greatest among TBIs classified as less severe. Results also indicated greater reductions in rates of hospitalization than in deaths. Thus, the disproportionately larger decrease in rates of hospitalization in developed countries may be due in part to changes in hospital admission criteria requiring a higher threshold of severity. Notably, 1998 to 2003 NCHS data suggest that the number of TBI-related ED visits remained unchanged (~1.2 million per year); in contrast, TBI hospitalizations increased from 220,000 in 1998 to 290,000 in 2003.[41] The latter change, however, was not statistically significant and was attributed to small increases in the actual sample of cases reported.[41]

Prevalence of TBI-Related Disability and Methodological Issues

To help persons living with TBI-related disability, countries need better information to determine the magnitude and type of these disabilities. However, due to limitations in methodology, the prevalence of TBI-related disability in the United States and the world cannot be measured directly with confident results. Interview surveys that attempt to learn lifetime histories of TBI and link these to current disabilities are prone to underreporting because of poor recall of injuries in the remote past. Prospective cohort studies of representative populations of persons recently diagnosed with acute TBI offer more promise. One U.S. study examined the prevalence of disability in a population-based sample of persons one or more years after hospitalization for TBI.[74,75] Thirty-seven percent reported some disability (i.e., difficulties with one or more activities of daily living or instrumental activities of daily living severe enough to require assistance) at least 1 year postinjury. In principle, such information can be combined with TBI incidence data to yield estimates of the prevalence of TBI-related disability in a general population. In practice, such estimations are complicated by changes over time—changes in TBI incidence rates, severity distributions, general population age distributions, and life expectancies—and therefore may require several simplifying assumptions. By employing such methods, using earlier preliminary findings of this TBI follow-up study,[75] CDC has estimated that nearly 2% of the U.S. population has TBI-related disabilities (**Table 1.5**).[17] Approximating how many people worldwide live with TBI-related disabilities is more difficult.

Estimates of Cost (Incidence and Prevalence)

Data showing the economic costs of TBI are important so that policy makers can make informed decisions to allocate resources for injury prevention, acute care, and rehabilitation. However, knowledge of the current economic impact of TBI globally is limited. A U.S. study using 1985 incidence and cost data for TBIs that resulted in hospital admission or death[76] estimated that $37.8 billion would be incurred over the lifetimes of those injured. This estimate (in 1985 dollars) included $4.5 billion in direct medical cost and $33.3 billion in indirect cost, such as lost productivity and income. Using changes in the U.S. Consumer Price Index (160%; 1985–2000), the estimate may be adjusted for inflation, yielding $60.5 billion in 2000. This is comparable to a recent study of the lifetime cost of TBIs in the United States for 2000, estimating $9.2 billion in direct medical cost and $51.2 billion in indirect cost, totaling $60.4 billion.[77] Data on worldwide TBI cost are scarce. Extrapolating the U.S. cost of treatment to the world is unreliable due to differences in populations, health care systems, and access to health care and medical technology.

Other Methodological Issues and Gaps in TBI Epidemiology

Assessment of Risk and Contributing Factors: Data Sources, Quality, and Comparability

Although external cause of injury and injury locale information is a critical link in the public health approach to preventing injuries,[78] its completeness on hospital billing data varies in the United States by state (from 52.6 to 99.4%, averaging 87.2%).[79] Improving reporting, particularly in states with low completeness levels, can lead to the development of better prevention strategies that target specific causes of injury (e.g., helmet promotion and education programs in schools) and the evaluation of the effectiveness of intervention programs (e.g., the cost-effectiveness of helmet use programs in reducing bicycle-related injuries in children).[80]

Epidemiological Studies—Translating Data into Action

The Role of Public Health in the Prevention of TBI

Unintentional and violence-related TBI represents a significant burden in medical, economic, social, and personal terms. In the United States alone, for each person who dies with a TBI, approximately five are hospitalized, 22 are treated and released from EDs,[8] and two are permanently disabled.[17] These figures reflect the impact of general injury in the United States. For each person who dies of an injury, nine are hospitalized and 188 are treated and released from an ED (CDC unpublished data). Public health practitioners can lessen the burden of injury by developing, evaluating, and promoting effective surveillance systems and public health interventions. A matrix to systematically assess factors related to the occurrence and severity of injury by traditional epidemiological methods of host, agent, and environment—as well as a second dimension that examines each factor by preevent, event, and postevent periods—has been widely used in public health.[81] For example, factors in the preevent phase of an MV crash would decrease the likelihood of a crash occurring altogether (e.g., reduction in drivers' impairment by alcohol), whereas factors during the event phase would decrease the likelihood or severity of injury (e.g., seat belt use). The postevent phase would consist of factors that could influence the outcome after the injury occurs (e.g., comprehensive trauma care systems). Although the public perception that injuries are "accidents" that cannot be prevented hinders prevention efforts, public health and clinical practitioners and organizations, including CDC, conduct surveillance and research and strive to translate science into effective public health practice.[82,83]

TBI Prevention

Fall-Related Prevention

Falls are a leading cause of TBI among persons aged 65 years or older.[7,9,45] Consequently, as the size of this population continuous to grow, fall prevention becomes more important.[84–86] Guidelines for preventing falls among older adults focus on identifying modifiable risk factors such as impairments of balance or lower extremity function[86,87]; use of medications, especially psychotropic drugs[88,89]; concurrent medical conditions (e.g., arthritis, Parkinson disease, history of stroke,[45,90] cognitive impairment,[91] or visual impairment[92]); and hazards in the home (**Table 1.7**).[86]

Table 1.7 Summary of TBI Prevention

- Fall prevention: Identification and management of modifiable factors (e.g., use of multiple medications, especially psychotropic drugs, etc.) is important, especially in older adults.
- MV-T incident prevention: Mandated graduated driver's licensing reduces crashes among teenagers. Use of seat belts and cycle helmets, and adherence to speed limits, reduce injuries.
- Sports-related prevention: Improvements in protective equipment (e.g., helmets) may lead to lower rates of TBI, especially in contact sports. Adherence to rules for "return to play" after a mild TBI may reduce serious complications.
- Alcohol-related prevention: Patients with TBI may be screened for alcohol abuse and referred for counseling or treatment.
- Violence prevention: Initiatives are more effective when delivered in childhood and when the intervention is sustained over time.
- Prevention of comorbid conditions: Early treatment and management of comorbid conditions can reduce fall- and MV-T–related injuries.

Abbreviations: MV-T, motor vehicle-traffic; TBI, traumatic brain injury.

Because one-half to two-thirds of older adults fall in or around their homes,[93,94] CDC and other organizations have recommended ways to modify homes to help prevent falls (e.g., using nonslip mats in bathtubs and shower; installing handrails on both sides of stairways).[95–97]

Fall-related TBIs are also common among children,[11,15,44] though these rarely result in death.[98] Although successful fall-prevention strategies for older adults may be applicable worldwide, more research and prevention programs are needed to develop regionally appropriate prevention strategies for children. In India, for example, almost 40% of fatal TBI falls resulted from climbing trees,[99] a problem minimally encountered in the United States. Notably, data from the 1999 CDC TBI SS show that falls and assaults accounted for almost 75% of all nonfatal hospitalizations in children younger than 2 years of age.[44]

MV-T–Related Prevention

Worldwide, MV-T–related incidents are a leading cause of TBI.[16,100] In the United States, despite an increase in vehicles and hours driven, the rate of MV-T–related TBI fatalities decreased 42% from 11.4 per 100,000 in 1979 to 6.6 per 100,000 in 1992.[6] This decrease is likely due to safer cars (e.g., more vehicles equipped with air bags); changes in behavior (e.g., greater use of seat belts and child safety seats; decreased incidence of alcohol-impaired driving), and safer roads.[6,101–103] In North Carolina and Michigan, mandated graduated driver's licensing significantly reduced crashes among teenagers.[104,105] Although the rate of MV ownership in high-income countries exceeds that of low- and middle-income countries (527 vs. 26 per 1,000 people, respectively, in 1990),[106] developing countries accounted for more than 85% of MV-T–related deaths worldwide, especially among pedestrians, passengers in vehicles, and cyclists.[107–109] For example, between 1968 and 1983, road traffic mortality in Asian countries increased more than 150%, whereas in Europe, road traffic mortality decreased more than 20%.[108] Rates are higher in low- to middle-income countries for several reasons: locally designed vehicles lack features that prevent rollover or passenger ejection; roads lack pedestrian or vehicle lane separation or posted speed limits; and multi-use roads that carry vehicles, pedestrians, cyclists, animals, and trucks make road users, especially pedestrians and bicyclists, more vulnerable and prone to injuries.[109] To reduce MV-T incidents worldwide, low- and middle-income countries need to set and enforce effective laws and regulations (e.g., speed limits, use of seat belts, cycle helmets, alcohol and driving) and implement proven, cost-effective strategies to reduce injuries in populations at risk. Examples of beneficial strategies include improved design, construction, and maintenance of roads and vehicles; promotion of helmets for cyclists and reflective clothing for pedestrians; strict implementation of speed-control limits and measures; restriction of alcohol use; enforcement of laws; and separation of pedestrian and vehicle traffic on roadways (**Table 1.7**).[99,108,109]

Sports-Related Prevention

Sports-related TBI is an especially significant public health problem because of the large number of participants, high incidence of general injury each year, young age of injured patients (with possible long-term disability), and potential cumulative effect of repeated injuries.[46,110] Failure to recognize TBI, especially when it is mild, has implications in a rare but fatal event called second- impact syndrome. During this event, massive brain swelling may occur when the injured athlete receives a second blow to the head while still experiencing symptoms from the initial blow or concussion.[111] Therefore, the important factor is deciding when to return an athlete to play. Athletes are usually advised not to return to play until symptom free for at least 1 week[112–114]; with serious injuries, athletes are advised to end the season. These guidelines are supported by clinical studies including the National Collegiate Athletic Association (NCAA) study of recurrent concussions among collegiate football players.[47] CDC has developed an educational initiative called "Heads Up: Concussion in High School Sports" to educate high school coaches on how to prevent, recognize, and manage concussion.[115] CDC has also recommended several evidence-based strategies to prevent and control sports and recreation-related injuries.[116] Improvements in PE design may lead to lower rates of TBI in contact sports. For example, a new study has shown that newer-generation football helmets (e.g., the Riddell Revolution; Riddell Inc., Rosemont, IL) may reduce the risk of concussion in high school football players by 50% (**Table 1.7**).[117]

Alcohol-Related Prevention

Alcohol is an injury-related factor among patients admitted to trauma centers.[118] With 75,000 alcohol-attributable deaths,[119] excessive alcohol consumption is the third leading preventable cause of death in the United States; of these deaths, 18% occurred in MV-T incidents.[120] Alcohol consumption is associated with TBI[14,45]; alcohol abuse also decreases the likelihood of an affected person being able to live independently after a moderate to severe TBI.[121] Substance abusers are more likely to experience violence-related injuries,[122] to be repeat offenders, and to have poor outcomes.[123] Because substance and alcohol abuse greatly affect the incidence of TBI, efforts are under way to intervene when patients present to the trauma center or ED.[124–126] For example, patients with TBI might be screened for alcohol abuse and referred for counseling or treatment.[126] Other interventions include individually oriented interventions to change behavior (e.g., screening, brief intervention, and treatment); environmental interventions (e.g., reducing availability, zero tolerance laws); enforcement and education (e.g., sobriety checkpoints); and comprehensive community programs that combine several strategies (**Table 1.7**).[127]

Violence Prevention

Data indicate that interpersonal violence, including war-related and self-inflicted violence are important causes of TBI morbidity and mortality worldwide.[43] Violence is a multifaceted problem that needs to be addressed simultaneously at multiple levels and in multiple sectors of society. The most successful interventions tend to be those that are delivered in childhood and those that are sustained over time (**Table 1.7**). Preventive measures include those that target patients (e.g., incentives for students to complete secondary school or therapeutic programs for persons with psychiatric diseases), victims and perpetrators (e.g., training in parenting), the community (e.g., creating safe routes for children to and from school), and society (e.g., legislation against intimate violence).[43]

Prevention of Comorbid Conditions

Given the impact of TBI on morbidity, mortality, societal and health care costs, and the aging population, identifying comorbid conditions (e.g., psychiatric illness) as potentially modifiable risk factors for TBI is important to prevent TBI and its sequelae. Increased efforts should be made to educate medical practitioners, patients, and families about the increased risk of TBI associated with these comorbidities. Early treatment and management of these conditions can reduce fall- and MV-T–related injuries (**Table 1.7**).[90–92] Discussions can address ways to decrease behaviors that can raise the risk of TBI, and increase preventive measures, such as avoidance of psychoactive medications, in the elderly.[89]

The Role of Epidemiology in Future TBI Research and Prevention

Clearly, TBI is a public health problem of global proportions. Although epidemiological data from developing countries are limited, what is available demonstrates a significant problem. In general, estimated incidence and prevalence of TBI are higher in developing regions than in developed countries. To increase awareness of the public health importance of TBI and facilitate the implementation of cost-effective prevention programs, researchers need improved documentation and surveillance of TBI. Prevention efforts should focus on the leading causes of TBI: falls, MV-T incidents, and violence. For maximum effectiveness, public health practitioners should implement cost-effective prevention measures in an integrated and coordinated manner. They should also consider the social and cultural characteristics of the populations when trying to encourage acceptability and adoption of interventions. Findings from worldwide successful surveillance and injury prevention programs should be disseminated widely so that others can benefit from and emanate these proven programs to best suit regional needs.

Limited information is available on the long-term clinical history of TBI, especially its less-severe presentations; lack of information may compromise a patient's or health care provider's recognition of TBI's long-term consequences. Further understanding of the natural history of TBI, especially after the acute phase of an injury, is needed to determine its human and economic burden.[3]

Countries also need more information about the magnitude and consequences of TBI. Each year in the United States, an estimated 80,000 persons experience the onset of long-term disability after being hospitalized for a TBI. Available historic data for TBI-related disabilities are nearly a decade old[17]; a real need exists for more current information. Determining the needs of persons with TBI (e.g., effective rehabilitation methods and useful, readily available services) is essential to improving quality of life. Population-based longitudinal studies are needed to provide precise information on the sequelae of TBI. Evidence-based standardized measures for TBI outcomes are also needed to identify the adverse outcomes most amenable to prevention through rehabilitation and social support. Reducing TBI injury severity and improving outcomes require the availability of persons trained in emergency and prehospital care and rehabilitative services. The availability of these specialized services is even more pressing in developing countries. One study in India found that 40% of deaths occurred at the crash site or during transportation.[128] Rehabilitative services, especially in developing countries, need improvements that will allow TBI survivors to improve the quality of their recovery and to handle life more effectively.[99] To further reduce the impact of TBI, countries need to initiate strategies on multiple levels such as developing cost-effective TBI surveillance systems; adopting low-cost, integrated interventions; adhering to international safety standards; instituting a high level of political commitment; and fostering greater involvement of health professionals and the community in prevention, acute-injury care, and rehabilitation efforts.[99] Only through a better understanding of the magnitude of TBI, its root causes, and a concerted effort from those involved, can we hope to address and reduce the global burden of TBI.

Disclaimer The findings and conclusions in this chapter are those of the authors and do not necessarily represent the views the official views or policies of the U.S. Department of Health and Human Services (DHHS) and the Centers for Disease Control and Prevention (CDC). The inclusion of individuals, programs, or organizations in this chapter does not constitute endorsement by the U.S. federal government, DHHS, or CDC.

References

1. Kraus JF, McArthur DL, Silberman TA. Epidemiology of mild brain injury. Semin Neurol 1994;14:1–7
2. Dikmen SS, Levin HS. Methodological issues in the study of mild head injury. J Head Trauma Rehabil 1993;8:30–37
3. National Center for Injury Prevention and Control. Report to Congress on Mild Traumatic Brain Injury in the United States: Steps to Prevent a Serious Public Health Problem. Atlanta: Centers for Disease Control and Prevention; 2003
4. Thurman DJ, Sniezek JE, Johnson D, Greenspan A, Smith SM. Guidelines for Surveillance of Central Nervous System Injury. Atlanta: Centers for Disease Control and Prevention, National Center for Injury Prevention and Control; 1995
5. Marr AL, Coronado VG, eds. Central Nervous System Injury Surveillance. Data Submission Standards-2002. Atlanta: Centers for Disease Control and Prevention, National Center for Injury Prevention and Control; 2004
6. Sosin DM, Sniezek JE, Waxweiler RJ. Trends in death associated with traumatic brain injury, 1979 through 1992: success and failure. JAMA 1995;273:1778–1780
7. Adekoya N, Thurman DJ, White DD, Webb KW. Surveillance for traumatic brain injury deaths—United States, 1989–1998. MMWR Surveill Summ 2002;51(10):1–14
8. Langlois JA, Rutland-Brown W, Thomas KE. Traumatic Brain Injury in the United States: Emergency Department Visits, Hospitalizations, and Deaths. Atlanta: Centers for Disease Control and Prevention, National Center for Injury Prevention and Control; 2006
9. Thurman D, Guerrero J. Trends in hospitalization associated with traumatic brain injury. JAMA 1999;282:954–957
10. Guerrero JL, Thurman DJ, Sniezek JE. Emergency department visits associated with traumatic brain injury: United States, 1995–1996. Brain Inj 2000;14(2):181–186
11. Jager TE, Weiss HB, Coben JH, Pepe PE. Traumatic brain injuries evaluated in U.S. emergency departments, 1992–1994. Acad Emerg Med 2000;7:134–140
12. Schootman M, Fuortes LJ. Ambulatory care for traumatic brain injuries in the U.S., 1995–1997. Brain Inj 2000;14:373–381
13. Sosin DM, Sniezek JE, Thurman DJ. Incidence of mild and moderate brain injury in the United States, 1991. Brain Inj 1996;10:47–54
14. Langlois JA, Kegler SR, Butler JA, et al. Traumatic brain injury-related hospital discharges: results from a 14-state surveillance system, 1997. MMWR Surveill Summ 2003;52(4):1–20
15. Coronado VG, Johnson RL, Faul M, Kegler SR. Incidence rates of hospitalization related to traumatic brain injury–12 states, 2002. MMWR Morb Mortal Wkly Rep 2006;55(8):201–204
16. Krug EG, Sharma GK, Lozano R. The global burden of injuries. Am J Public Health 2000;90:523–526
17. Centers for Disease Control and Prevention. Traumatic Brain Injury in the United States: A Report to Congress. Atlanta: Centers for Disease Control and Prevention; 1999
18. U.S. Department of Health and Human Services. International Classification of Diseases, Ninth Revision, Clinical Modification (ICD-9-CM). Hyattsville, MD: National Center for Health Statistics; 2004. Available at: http:// www.cdc.gov/nchs/about/otheract/icd9/abticd9.htm
19. World Health Organization. International Statistical Classification of Diseases and Related Health Problems, 10th Revision (ICD-10). Geneva, Switzerland: World Health Organization; 1992
20. Centers for Disease Control and Prevention. Recommended Framework of E-code Groupings for Presenting Injury Mortality and Morbidity Data. Atlanta, GA: Centers for Disease Control and Prevention; 2003. Available at: http://www.cdc.gov/ncipc/whatsnew/matrix2.htm
21. Centers for Disease Control and Prevention. External Cause of Injury Mortality Matrix for ICD-10. Atlanta, GA: Centers for Disease Control and Prevention; 2002. Available at: http://www.cdc.gov/nchs/data/ice/icd10_transcode.pdf
22. U.S. Department of Health and Human Services. Mortality Data from the National Vital Statistics. Hyattsville, MD: National Center for Health Statistics; 2006. Available at: http://www.cdc.gov/nchs/deaths.htm
23. Shore AD, McCarthy ML, Serpi T, Gertner M. Validity of administrative data for characterizing traumatic brain injury-related hospitalization. Brain Inj 2005;19:613–621
24. Murray CJL, Lopez AD, eds. Global Health Statistics: A Compendium of Incidence, Prevalence, and Mortality Estimates for over 200 Conditions. Boston: Harvard School of Public Health; 1996
25. Teasdale G, Jennett B. Assessment of coma and impaired consciousness: a practical scale. Lancet 1974;2:81–84
26. Jennett B, Teasedale G. Aspects of coma after severe head injury. Lancet 1977;1:878–881
27. MacKenzie EJ, Shapiro S, Eastham JN. The Abbreviated Injury Scale and Injury Severity Score. Levels of inter- and intrarater reliability. Med Care 1985;23(6):823–835
28. Champion HR, Sacco WJ, Copes WS, Gann DS, Gennarelli TA, Flanagan ME. A revision of the trauma score. J Trauma 1989;29:623–629
29. Healey C, Osler TM, Rogers FB, et al. Improving the Glasgow Coma Scale score: motor score alone is a better predictor. J Trauma 2003; 54(4):671–678, discussion 678–680
30. Marion DW, Carlier PM. Problems with initial Glasgow Coma Scale assessment caused by prehospital treatment of patients with head injuries: results of a national survey. J Trauma 1994;36(1):89–95
31. Teasdale G, Kril-Jones R, van der Sande J. Observer variability in assessing impaired consciousness and coma. J Neurol Neurosurg Psychiatry 1978;41:603–610
32. Rowley G, Fielding K. Reliability and accuracy of the Glasgow Coma Scale with experienced and inexperienced users. Lancet 1991;337: 535–538
33. Gennarelli TA, Champion HR, Copes WS, Sacco WJ. Comparison of mortality, morbidity, and severity of 59,713 head injured patients with 114,447 patients with extracranial injuries. J Trauma 1994; 37(6):962–968
34. Marshall LF, Klauber GT, Eisenberg HM, et al. The outcome of severe closed head injury. J Neurosurg 1991;75:S28–S36
35. Duncan CC, Merit LR, Smith B, Ehrenkranz RA. A scale for the assessment of neonatal neurological status. Childs Brain 1981;8: 299–306
36. Raimondi AJ, Hirschauer J. Head injury in the infant and toddler: Coma scoring and outcome scale. Childs Brain 1984;11:12–35
37. Hahn YS, Chyung C, Barthel MJ, Bailes J, Flannery AM, McLone DG. Head injuries in children under 36 months of age. Childs Nerv Syst 1988;4:34–40
38. Simpson DA, Cockington RA, Hanieh A, Raftos J, Reilly PL. Head injuries in infants and young children: the value of the Paediatric Coma Scale. Review of the literature and report on a study. Childs Nerv Syst 1991;7:183–190

39. Rimel RW, Giordani B, Barth JT, Boll TJ, Jane JA. Disability caused by minor head injury. Neurosurgery 1981;9:221–228
40. Guthkelch AN. Posttraumatic amnesia, post-concussional symptoms and accident neurosis. Eur Neurol 1980;19:91–102
41. Rutland-Brown W, Langlois JA, Thomas KE, Xi YL. Incidence of traumatic brain injury in the United States, 2003. J Head Trauma Rehabil 2006;21:544–548
42. Annest LJ, Pogostin CL. A Training Module for Coding Mechanism and Intent of Injury for the NEISS All Injury Program. Atlanta: Centers for Disease Control and Prevention, National Center for Injury Prevention and Control; 2006
43. World Health Organization. World Report on Violence and Health: Summary. Geneva, Switzerland: World Health Organization; 2002
44. Eisele JA, Kegler SR, Trent RB, Coronado VG. Nonfatal traumatic brain injury-related hospitalization in very young children—15 states, 1999. J Head Trauma Rehabil 2006;21:537–543
45. Coronado VG, Thomas KE, Sattin RW, Johnson RL. The CDC traumatic brain injury surveillance system: characteristics of persons aged 65 years and older hospitalized with a TBI. J Head Trauma Rehabil 2005;20:215–228
46. Thurman DJ, Branche CM, Sniezek JE. The epidemiology of sports-related traumatic brain injuries in the United States: recent developments. J Head Trauma Rehabil 1998;13:1–8
47. Guskiewicz KM, McCrea M, Marshall SW, et al. Cumulative effects associated with recurrent concussion in collegiate football players: the NCAA Concussion Study. JAMA 2003;290:2549–2555
48. Annegers JF, Grabow JD, Kurland LT, Laws ER Jr. The incidence, causes, and secular trends of head trauma in Olmstead County, Minnesota, 1935–1974. Neurology 1980;30:912–919
49. Salcido R, Costich JF. Recurrent traumatic brain injury. Brain Inj 1992;6:293–298
50. Schulz MR, Marshall SW, Mueller FO, et al. Incidence and risk factors for concussion in high school athletes, North Carolina, 1996–1999. Am J Epidemiol 2004;160:937–944
51. Powell JW, Barber-Foss KD. Traumatic brain injury in high school athletes. JAMA 1999;282:958–963
52. Baker SP, Fowler C, Li G, Warner M, Dannenberg AL. Head injuries incurred by children and young adults during informal recreation. Am J Public Health 1994;84:649–652
53. Mack MG, Hudson S, Thompson D. A descriptive analysis of children's playground injuries in the United States 1990–4. Inj Prev 1997;3: 100–103
54. Minino AM, Smith BL. Deaths: preliminary data for 2000. Natl Vital Stat Rep 2001;49(12):1–40
55. Hannan EL, Mendeloff J, Farrell LS, Cayten CG, Murphy JG. Multivariate models for predicting survival of patients with trauma from low falls: the impact of gender and pre-existing conditions. J Trauma 1995;38: 697–704
56. Perdue PW, Watts DD, Kaufmann CR, Trask AL. Differences in mortality between elderly and younger adult trauma patients: geriatric status increases risk of delayed death. J Trauma 1998;45(4):805–810
57. Centers for Disease Control and Prevention. Web-Based Injury Statistics Query and Reporting System (WISQARS). Atlanta, GA: Centers for Disease Control and Prevention, National Center for Injury Prevention and Control; 2004. Available at: http://www.cdc.gov/ncipc/wisqars
58. Baker SP, O'Neill B, Ginsburg MJ, et al, eds. The Injury Fact Book. 2nd ed. New York: Oxford University Press; 1992:116
59. Physicians for Human Rights. The Right to Equal Treatment: An Action Plan to End Racial and Ethnic Disparities in Clinical Diagnosis and Treatment in the United States. Boston: Physicians for Human Rights; 2003. Available at: http://www.phrusa.org/research/domestic/race/race_report/report.html
60. Burnett DM, Kolakowsky-Hayner SA, Slater D, et al. Ethnographic analysis of traumatic brain injury patients in the national model systems database. Arch Phys Med Rehabil 2003;84:263–267
61. Ahmed N, Anderson R. Unintentional injury mortality and socioeconomic development among 15–44-year-olds: in a health transition perspective. Public Health 2000;114:416–422
62. Cubbin C, LeClere FB, Smith GS. Socioeconomic status and injury mortality: individual and neighbourhood determinants. J Epidemiol Community Health 2000;54:517–524
63. Maier RV. Controlling alcohol problems among hospitalized trauma patients. J Trauma 2005;59:S1–S2
64. Macdonald S, Cherpitel CJ, Borges G, DeSouza A, Giesbrecht N, Stockwell T. The criteria for causation of alcohol in violent injuries based on emergency room data from six countries. Addict Behav 2005;30: 103–113
65. McIntosh AS, McCrory P. Preventing head and neck injury. Br J Sports Med 2005;39:314–318
66. Siegel JH, Loo G, Dischinger PC, et al. Factors influencing the patterns of injuries and outcomes in car versus car crashes compared to sport utility, van, or pick-up truck versus car crashes: crash injury research engineering network study. J Trauma 2001;51:975–990
67. Hotz GA, Cohn SM, Popkin C, et al. The impact of a repealed motorcycle helmet law in Miami-Dade County. J Trauma 2002;52: 469–474
68. Sosin DM, Sacks JJ, Webb KW. Pediatric head injuries and deaths from bicycling in the United States. Pediatrics 1996;98:868–870
69. Fann JR, Leonetti A, Jaffe K, Katon WJ, Cummings P, Thompson RS. Psychiatric illness and subsequent traumatic brain injury: a case control study. J Neurol Neurosurg Psychiatry 2002;72:615–620
70. Gerring JP, Brady KD, Chen A, et al. Premorbid prevalence of ADHD and development of secondary ADHD after closed head injury. J Am Acad Child Adolesc Psychiatry 1998;37:647–654
71. Slaughter B, Fann JR, Ehde D. Traumatic brain injury in a county jail population: prevalence, neuropsychological functioning and psychiatric disorders. Brain Inj 2003;17:731–741
72. Engberg AW, Teasdale TW. Traumatic brain injury in Denmark 1979–1996: a national study of incidence and mortality. Eur J Epidemiol 2001;17:437–442
73. Stephenson S, Langley J, Cryer C. Effects of service delivery versus changes in incidence on trends in injury: a demonstration using hospitalized traumatic brain injury. Accid Anal Prev 2005;37:825–832
74. Brooks CA, Gabella B, Hoffman R, Sosin D, Whiteneck G. Traumatic brain injury: designing and implementing a population-based follow-up system. Arch Phys Med Rehabil 1997;78(8, Suppl 4):S26–S30
75. Whiteneck G, Brooks CA, Mellick D, Harrison-Felix C, Terrill MS, Noble K. Population-based estimates of outcomes after hospitalization for traumatic brain injury in Colorado. Arch Phys Med Rehabil 2004;85(Suppl 2):S73–S81
76. Max W, MacKenzie EJ, Rice DP. Head injuries: costs and consequences. J Head Trauma Rehabil 1991;6:76–91
77. Finkelstein EA, Corso PS, Miller TR. The Incidence and Economic Burden of Injury in the United States. New York: Oxford University Press; 2006
78. Sniezek JE, Finklea JF, Graitcer PL. Injury coding and hospital discharge data. JAMA 1989;262:2270–2272
79. Barrett M, Steiner C, Coben J. Healthcare Cost and Utilization Project (HCUP) E Code Evaluation Report, 2004. HCUP Methods Series Report # 2004–06. April 14, 2005. U.S. Agency for Healthcare Research and Quality. Available at: http://www.hcup-us.ahrq.gov/reports/methods.jsp
80. World Health Organization. Helmets: A Road Safety Manual for Decision Makers and Practitioners. Geneva, Switzerland: World Health Organization; 2006
81. Haddon W Jr. The changing approach to the epidemiology, prevention, and amelioration of trauma: the transition to approaches etiologically rather than descriptively based. Am J Public Health 1968;58:1431–1438
82. Sleet DA, Hopkins KN, Olson SJ. From discovery to delivery: injury prevention at CDC. Health Promot Pract 2003;4(2):98–102
83. Doll LS, Bonzo SE, Sleet DA, Mercy JA, Hass EN, eds. Handbook of Injury and Violence Prevention. New York: Springer; 2007
84. Randal J, German T, Ewing D, eds. The Ageing and Development Report: Poverty, Independence and the World's Older People. London: Earthscan Publications Ltd.; 1999
85. Taylor MD, Tracy JK, Meyer W, Pasquale M, Napolitano LM. Trauma in the elderly: intensive care unit resource use and outcome. J Trauma 2002;53:407–414

86. American Geriatrics Society, British Geriatrics Society, and American Academy of Orthopaedic Surgeons Panel on Falls Prevention. Guideline for the prevention of falls in older persons. J Am Geriatr Soc 2001;49:664–672
87. Lord SR, Tiedemann A, Chapman K, Munro B, Murray SM, Sherrington C. The effect of an individualized fall prevention program on fall risk and falls in older people: a randomized, controlled trial. J Am Geriatr Soc 2005;53:1296–1304
88. Ray WA, Griffin MR. Prescribed medications and the risk of falling. Top Geriatr Rehabil 1990;5:12–20
89. Cumming RG. Epidemiology of medication-related falls and fractures in the elderly. Drugs Aging 1998;12:43–53
90. Dolinis J, Harrison JE, Andrews GR. Factors associated with falling in older Adelaide residents. Aust N Z J Public Health 1997;21:462–468
91. Tromp AM, Pluijm SMF, Smit JH, Deeg DJH, Bouter LM, Lips P. Fall-risk screening test: a prospective study on predictors for falls in community-dwelling elderly. J Clin Epidemiol 2001;54:837–844
92. Lord SR, Dayhew J. Visual risk factors for falls in older people. J Am Geriatr Soc 2001;49:508–515
93. Wilkins K. Health care consequences of falls for seniors. Health Reports (Statistics Canada, Catalogue 82–003) 1999;10(4):47–55(ENG); 47–57(FRE)
94. Peek-Asa C, Zwerling C. Role of environmental interventions in injury control and prevention. Epidemiol Rev 2003;25:77–89
95. National Center for Injury Prevention and Control. Falls Among Older Adults: An Overview. Atlanta: Centers for Disease Control and Prevention; 2005. Available at: http://www.cdc.gov/ncipc/factsheets/adultfalls.htm
96. National Center for Injury Prevention and Control. Preventing Falls in Older Adults. Atlanta: Centers for Disease Control and Prevention; 2005. Available at: http://www.cdc.gov/ncipc/duip/preventadultfalls.htm
97. Rubenstein LZ, Stevens JA, Scott V. Interventions to prevent falls among older adults. In: Doll LS, Bonzo SE, Sleet DA, Mercy JA, Hass EN, eds. Handbook of Injury and Violence Prevention. New York: Springer; 2007:37–53
98. Kraus JF, Rock A, Hemyari P. Brain injuries among infants, children, adolescents, and young adults. Am J Dis Child 1990;144: 684–691
99. Gururaj G. Epidemiology of traumatic brain injuries: Indian scenario. Neurol Res 2002;24:24–28
100. Ahmed N, Anderson R. Differences in cause-specific patterns of unintentional injury mortality among 15–44-year-olds in income-based country groups. Accid Anal Prev 2002;34:541–551
101. Thurman DJ. The epidemiology and economics of head trauma. In: Miller LP, Hayes RL, eds. Head Trauma: Basic Preclinical and Clinical Aspects. New York: John Wiley and Sons; 2001:327–347
102. Loo GT, Siegel JH, Dischinger PC, et al. Airbag protection versus compartment intrusion effect determines the pattern of injuries in multiple trauma motor vehicle crashes. J Trauma 1996;41:935–951
103. McGwin G Jr, Metzger J, Rue LW III. The influence of side airbags on the risk of head and thoracic injury after motor vehicle collisions. J Trauma 2004;56:512–516, discussion 516–517
104. Foss RD, Feaganes JR, Rodgman EA. Initial effects of graduated driver licensing on 16-year-old driver crashes in North Carolina. JAMA 2001;286:1588–1592
105. Shope JT, Molnar LJ, Elliott MR, Waller PF. Graduated driver licensing in Michigan: early impact on motor vehicle crashes among 16-year-old drivers. JAMA 2001;286:1593–1598
106. World Bank. World Development Indicators. Washington, DC: World Bank; 2001
107. Nantulya VM, Reich MR. The neglected epidemic: road traffic injuries in developing countries. BMJ 2002;324:1139–1141
108. Soderlund N, Zwi AB. Traffic related mortality in industrialized and less developed countries. Bull World Health Organ 1995;73:175–182
109. Roberts I, Bliss A, Breen J, et al. Interventions. In: Peden M, Scurfield R, Sleet D, et al, eds. World Report on Road Traffic Injury Prevention. Geneva, Switzerland: World Health Organization; 2004:107–154
110. Centers for Disease Control and Prevention. Sports-related recurrent head injuries—United States. MMWR Morb Mortal Wkly Rep 1997; 46(10):224–227
111. Cantu RC. Head injuries in sport. Br J Sports Med 1996;30: 289–296
112. American Academy of Neurology. Practice parameter: the management of concussion in sports (summary statement). Report of the Quality Standards Subcommittee. Neurology 1997;48:581–585
113. Cantu RC. Cerebral concussion in sport: management and prevention. Sports Med 1992;14:64–74
114. Kissick J, Johnston KM. Return to play after concussion: principles and practice. Clin J Sport Med 2005;15:426–431
115. Centers for Disease Control and Prevention. Heads Up, Concussion in High School Sports: Guide for Coaches. Atlanta: Centers for Disease Control and Prevention; 2005
116. Gilchrist J, Saluja G, Marshall SW. Interventions to prevent sports and recreation-related injuries. In: Doll LS, Bonzo SE, Sleet DA, Mercy JA, Hass EN, eds. Handbook of Injury and Violence Prevention. New York: Springer; 2007:117–134
117. Collins M, Lovell MR, Iverson GL, Ide T, Maroon J. Examining concussion rates and return to play in high school football players wearing newer helmet technology: a three year prospective cohort study. Neurosurgery 2006;58:275–286
118. Moore EE. Alcohol and trauma: the perfect storm. J Trauma 2005; 59(Suppl 3):S53–S56
119. Centers for Disease Control and Prevention. Alcohol-attributable deaths and years of potential life lost—United States, 2001. MMWR Morb Mortal Wkly Rep 2004;53(37):866–870
120. Mokdad AH, Marks JS, Stroup DF, Gerberding JL. Actual causes of death in the United States, 2000. JAMA 2004;291:1238–1245
121. Macmillan PJ, Hart RP, Martelli MF, Zasler ND. Pre-injury status and adaptation following traumatic brain injury. Brain Inj 2002;16(1):41–49
122. Hingson RW, Swahn MH, Sleet DA. Interventions to prevent alcohol-related injuries. In Doll LS, Bonzo SE, Sleet DA, Mercy JA, Hass EN, eds. Handbook of Injury and Violence Prevention. New York: Springer: 2007:295–310
123. Silverman JG, Raj A, Mucci LA, Hathaway JE. Dating violence against adolescent girls and associated substance use, unhealthy weight control, sexual risk behavior, pregnancy, and suicidality. JAMA 2001; 286:572–579
124. Corrigan JD. Substance abuse as a mediating factor in outcome from traumatic brain injury. Arch Phys Med Rehabil 1995;76(4): 302–309
125. Schermer CR, Apodaca TR, Albrecht RM, Lu SW, Demarest GB. Intoxicated motor vehicle passengers warrant screening and treatment similar to intoxicated drivers. J Trauma 2001;51(6):1083–1086
126. Committee on Treatment of Alcohol Problems, Institute of Medicine. Broadening the Base of Treatment for Alcohol Problems. Washington, DC: National Academy Press; 1990
127. Hungerford DW, Pollock DA, eds. Alcohol Problems among Emergency Department Patients: Proceedings of a Research Conference on Identification and Intervention. Atlanta: Centers for Disease Control and Prevention, National Center for Injury Prevention and Control; 2002
128. Gururaj G, Sateesh VL. Assessment of facilities at casuality and emergency care services in Bangalore hospitals. J Acad Hosp Adm 1999; 11:9–11

II Science

2 Pathophysiology

M. Ross Bullock and Marinella Gugliotta

Traumatic brain injury (TBI) triggers a series of different events at the cellular and molecular level, thereby initiating reactive histochemical, molecular, and genetic responses that result in secondary insults, particularly ischemia, and exacerbate primary damage. On the other hand, some of these responses can also be neuroprotective. In this chapter we review the mechanisms, and complex biochemical, molecular, and genomic responses generated by primary impact acceleration forces when applied to the neuraxis.

Biomechanical Characteristics of Neurotrauma from Brain Movement during Impact

Subdural hematomas (SDHs) and diffuse axonal injuries (DAIs) are more lethal than most other brain lesions.[1] Gennarelli suggested that SDH was produced by the short duration and high amplitude of angular accelerations, whereas DAI was produced by a longer duration and low amplitude of coronal accelerations.[2] Using collision tests with cadavers, Löwenhielm hypothesized that bridging vein disruption due to an anterior-posterior rotational movement of the head is obtained when the angular acceleration exceeds 4.5 krad/s^2 and/or the change in angular velocity exceeds 50 krad/s^2.[3] More than 60 years ago, Holbourne examined the effects of acceleration/deceleration forces on a gelatin model of the human brain. Holbourne described how shear strains occurred in the brain, suggesting that rotational acceleration forces are the primary cause of injury and produce predictable damage to the brain.[4] Ommaya and Gennarelli suggested that acceleration/deceleration forces (also termed *impulsive loading*) cause mechanical strains that operate in a "centripetal sequence."[5] Injuries of this nature can occur when the head is propelled through space and is abruptly stopped by a solid object, such as the ground, or when the head is set into motion, for example, when a boxer is struck. With mild forces, the sequence begins at the surface of the brain and progressively affects deeper structures as forces become more severe (**Fig. 2.1**). Based on their original classification system, the authors made three predictions:

- When the degree of trauma is sufficient to produce loss of consciousness, the cortex and subcortical *systems* will be primarily affected, with damage being more severe than that found in the rostral brain stem.
- The damage to the rostral brain stem will not occur without more severe damage occurring in the cortex and subcortical *structures* because the mesencephalon is the last area to suffer trauma.
- Cognitive symptoms such as confusion and disturbance of memory can occur without loss of consciousness; however, the reverse cannot occur.

In addition to these critical predictions, the theory reinforced two important aspects of how TBI occurs and the potential effects different accelerlation/deceleration forces have on the brain:

- First, it reinforced the principle that the direction of force can determine the severity of the injury; specifically, rotational forces were believed to cause the most severe injuries.[4–6]
- Second, the direction of rotation was found to affect the severity of injury and recovery[1,6] with sagittal (front-to-back) injuries resulting in good recovery, lateral injuries (side-to-side) resulting in persistent coma

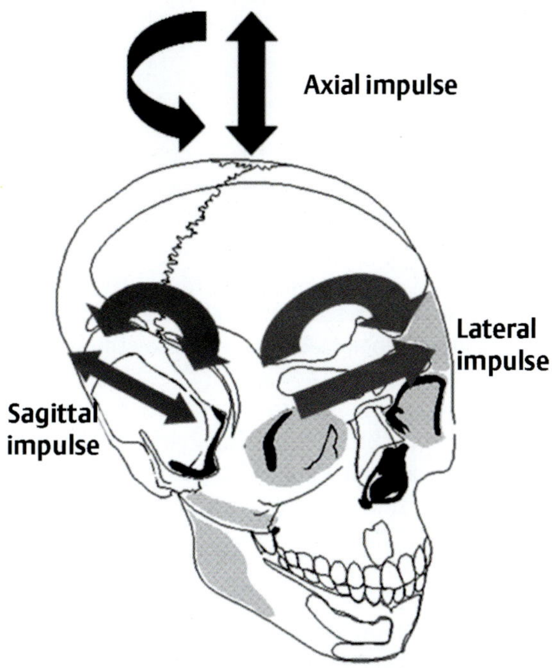

Fig. 2.1 Head motions as a result of impact forces. Sagittal impulses lead to posterior-anterior movement or posterior-anterior rotation, whereas axial and lateral impulses result in bending/stretching or axial rotation, respectively, in lateral movement and lateral rotation.

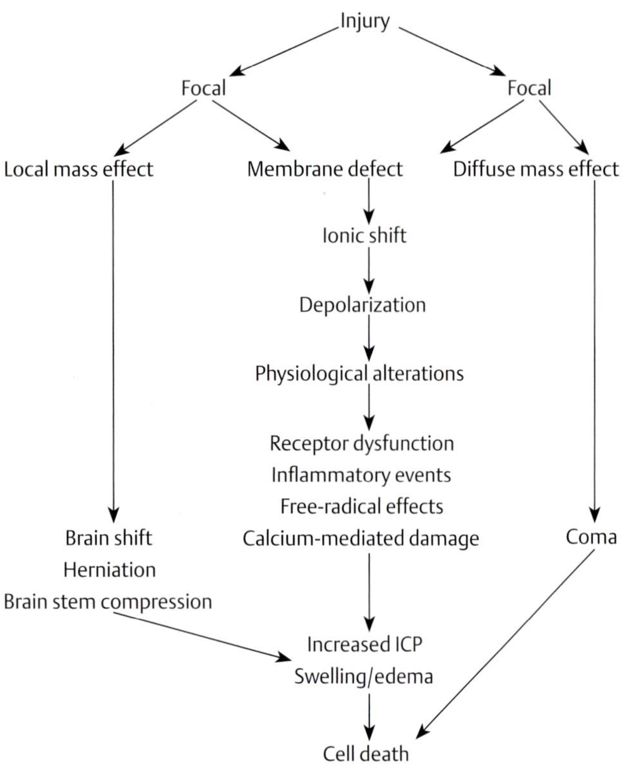

Fig. 2.2 Hypothetical cascade of events in TBI. (From Gennarelli T. Mechanisms of brain injury. J Emerg Med 1993;11(Suppl 1):5–11.)

or severe disability, and oblique injuries falling in between (**Fig. 2.2**).

Focal Injury

Focal brain injuries occur in the form of contusions or disruptions of brain tissue and also include hemorrhage and hematoma formation in the extradural, subarachnoid, subdural, and intracerebral areas.[6,7] According to Gennarelli and Graham, contusions are typically observed at the frontal poles, orbital frontal lobes, temporal poles, lateral and inferior surfaces of the temporal lobes, cortex above the sylvian fissure, and apex of the gyri. They appear as either multiple punctate hemorrhages or streaks of hemorrhage with an eventual progression of bleeding into adjacent white matter (see also **Table 2.1** and **Table 2.2** and **Fig. 2.3**).[8]

Following a contusion or hemorrhage, bleeding extends into adjacent cortical tissue where neurons undergo secondary necrosis due to ischemia.[8]

In most instances focal injuries are the result of the stationary cranium being struck by moving objects with relatively small mass such as sticks, baseball bats, or golf balls. Usually, impacts of this type do not cause prolonged unconsciousness; however, they may cause permanent focal neurological deficit due to the immediate effects of the penetrating/focal injury, or even death due to the

Table 2.1 Subdivisions of Contusions after TBI

- Contusions that occur directly beneath fractures
- Coup contusions that occur under the site of impact
- Contrecoup contusions that occur in regions distant to (but not always opposite of) the impact site
- Herniation contusions
- Gliding contusions, often associated with diffuse injuries

Abbreviation: TBI, traumatic brain injury.

delayed consequences of cerebral contusion or intracranial hematoma.

Effects of Shear Forces on Microvasculature

The work of Holbourne and Strich provided evidence that acceleration/deceleration injuries resulted in shear strains within the cranial vault, causing stretching and shearing of neurons and blood vessels.[4,9] The cerebral microvasculature is more resistant to shear damage than axons. In the majority of significant head injuries, however, focal concentrations of forces develop at the tips of the frontal and temporal poles that are of sufficient intensity to disrupt the pial vessels, causing a focal contusion. Thus, focal injury is superimposed on diffuse injury.[10]

Acute Subdural Hematoma

Acute SDHs complicate ~20% of severe head injuries and result in the worst outcome of any of the subgroups of severe head injury patients.

This complication is almost always caused by rupture of any of three types of surface vessel:

- Rupture of bridging veins
- SDH of arterial origin
- Rupture of parenchymal small vessels and bleeding from a contusion

Rupture of Bridging Veins

The most common type of SDH results from tearing of veins traversing the subdural space from the surface of the brain to the superior sagittal sinus when the cranium

Table 2.2 Categories of Hemorrhage after TBI

- Intracranial hematoma associated with a direct rupture of a blood vessel
- Extradural hematoma associated with skull fracture
- Acute subdural hematoma caused by a rupture of the bridging veins of the dura or possibly cortical arteries

Abbreviation: TBI, traumatic brain injury.

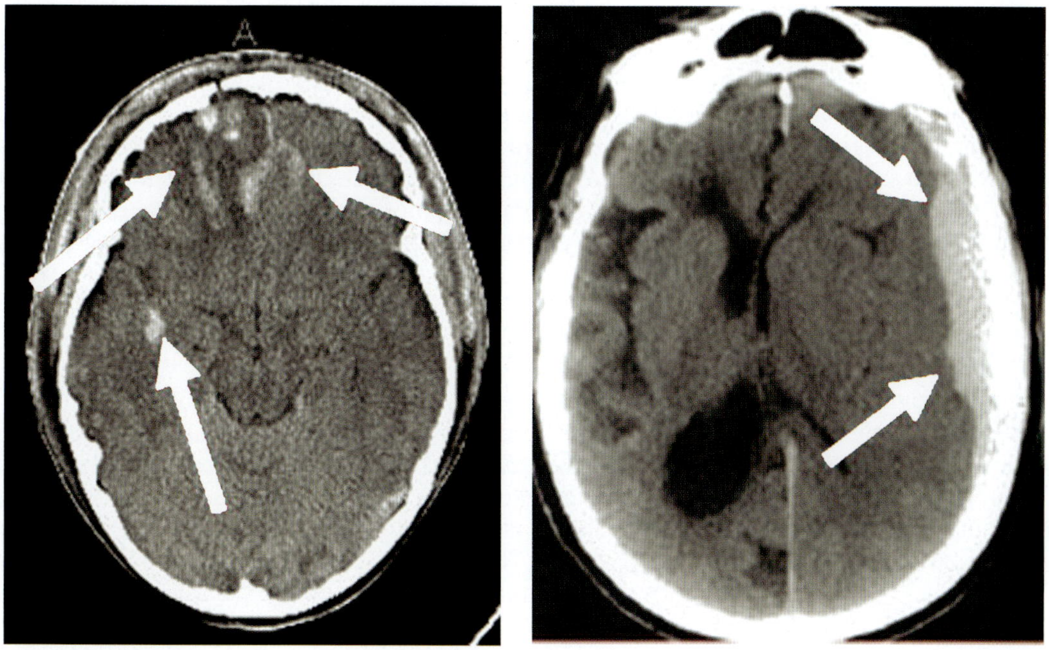

A B

Fig. 2.3 Computed tomography scan showing **(A)** intracerebral contusions frontal and temporal and **(B)** an acute subdural hematoma.

is rapidly decelerated with a relatively low magnitude of shear force applied.[1] These circumstances are given by a fall from standing height on to a solid surface such as a floor or in boxing injuries, that is, when rotational accelerations of the head occur.

Kleiven showed that the maximal strain occurred in the shortest bridging veins that are oriented in the plane of the motion and are angled in the direction of motion.[11] During a lateral impact, lower values of strain in the bridging veins are achieved compared with the occipital impacts. This could probably be explained by the supportive properties of the falx cerebri.[11] This is evident because the smaller relative motion between the brain and skull for a lateral impulse, compared with a corresponding sagittal one, suggests the influence of the falx cerebri, which may impinge upon adjacent structures such as the corpus callosum, potentially causing injury.[1] The supportive nature of the falx can also explain the smaller increase in the relative displacement between the skull and the brain when changing from a translational lateral motion to a corresponding rotational motion.[11] Furthermore, in clinical studies, Hirakawa et al reported that SDHs were rarely found in the occipital region, supporting the results that the largest strains were found for the parietally, centrally, or frontally located bridging veins for all impact directions.[12] However, avulsion of parasagittal and sylvian bridging veins is usually accompanied by a degree of diffuse axonal injury and polar contusion.[13]

Yet, the mechanism by which low-pressure venous bleeding can accumulate to form a hematoma of sufficient size to compress the brain is not completely understood. Episodes of coughing, straining, or vomiting may "pump out" sufficient blood to progressively tamponade the brain as clotting occurs. Another important fact is that these blood vessels are attached to the sagittal sinus, which is held open rather than compressed by the hematomas.

Subdural Hematomas of Arterial Origin

The classic "burst lobe" injury characterized by SDH, polar contusion, intracerebral hematoma, and hemispheric swelling is a result of extensive polar contusions that burst through the pia to accumulate in the subdural space.

Coalescence and Rupture of Parenchymal Small Vessels Bleeding from a Contusion

This kind of hematoma is frequently seen when a coagulation defect develops as a result of anticoagulant therapy or consumption of clotting factors (disseminated intravascular coagulation).[14] Such subdural events are usually associated with sizable intraparenchymal clots, and often recur after evacuation. Use of recombinant factor VII (NovoSeven; Novo Nordisk, Inc., Princeton, NJ) has revolutionized the care of these patients.

Penetrating Injury

Penetrating injuries may be caused by low-mass objects striking the cranium with high or very high velocity, for example, missiles or projectiles, or by sharp objects driven at low velocity into the cranial cavity. These stab wounds can damage vascular structures, cranial nerves, and white matter fiber tracts. As long as the wounding object remains imbedded within the skull and brain, the prognosis is very good with appropriate management. Angiography is usually needed to exclude vascular injury. However, if the object is levered free by the assailant, the resulting arc of blade movement within the brain may be devastating.[15]

Missile injuries and their effects on the brain are highly variable and unpredictable. The severity of the wound depends on the energy of the missile. Low-velocity missiles travel at <2000 m/s (civilian bullets) causing a damaging tract and cavity 4 times the size of the bullet. High-velocity military firearms (>2000 m/s) cause almost always fatal injuries because the kinetic energy of the bullet transmitted to the cranium is enormous. The effects of piercing projectiles traversing the intracranial contents are twofold:

- A pressure wave reverberates through the brain, transmitting extremely high pressure as the bullet enters, followed by low pressure of equal magnitude behind the missile's path. These pressure waves occur in proportion to the velocity of the projectile, and largely determine survival.
- Direct vascular and neural disruption results from the tearing effects of the bullet itself and in-driven skull fragments. These effects are similar to other forms of contusion, although the magnitude of vascular damage and consequent hematoma formation may be much greater.

Patients in persistent deep coma (Glasgow Coma Scale 3–5) after a bullet injury of high or low velocity have a 90 to 95% likelihood of a bad outcome (death or severe disability) unless an associated extraaxial hematoma can be removed.[16] Infratentorial missile injuries are very rare but are usually fatal if a midline trajectory is noted.[17] Many aspects of the pathophysiology and management of gun shots are common to blunt or closed cranial injury, mainly the transmission of kinetic energy through the brain, manifested as pressure waves of varying magnitude and duration, and the direct impact damage to small and large vascular structures and neurons close to the cortical surface.

Effect of Shear Forces on Synapses and Synaptic Function

We have shown in our laboratory that blockade of voltage-operated ion channels prior to TBI failed to ameliorate the negative neurological and behavioral effects of the trauma and produced only a modest effect on K^+-flux in the extracellular fluid (ECF), suggesting that agonist-operated ion channels are more important after TBI in mediating ionic events.[18] The behavioral changes that persist up to weeks or months after TBI, even in animals without any evidence of structural damage, have been taken as evidence to support functional changes at the synaptic level or in relation to second messenger systems.

Effect of Shear Forces on Axons

More than 40 years ago, neuropathological studies first demonstrated the accumulation of axoplasmic retraction "balls" at sites of axonal discontinuity,[9,19] chiefly found on large myelinated fibers in patients who were unconscious from the time of injury and subsequently died. These retraction balls were found in high density in white matter tracts in ~25% of severely head-injured patients.[13]

Diffuse brain injury may occur in the absence of impact forces but is dependent on inertial forces that are commonly produced by motor vehicle crashes and, in some cases, falls and assaults.[13,20–23] These inertial forces are a result of rapid head rotational motions, which deform the white matter and lead to DAI, commonly referred to as shearing brain injury.[23] These injuries are commonly called diffuse; however, the pattern of axonal damage in the white matter is more accurately described as multifocal, appearing throughout the deep and subcortical white matter, and is particularly common in midline structures including the splenium of the corpus callosum and brain stem.[23] In mild to low moderate DAI, there is often a remarkable absence of macroscopic pathology and the brains may appear normal upon radiological examination.[23–25] Nonetheless, microscopic examination of the brain tissue reveals the pathological signature of DAI: a multitude of swollen and disconnected axons.[23,26] In DAI at high severity, axonal pathology is accompanied by tissue tears in the white matter and intraparenchymal hemorrhage (**Fig. 2.4**).[5,23,27]

The principal mechanical force associated with the induction of DAI is rotational acceleration of the brain resulting from unrestricted head movement in the instant after injury.[1,23,27,28] This inertial loading to the brain induces dynamic shear, tensile, and compressive strains within the tissue, leading to dynamic tissue deformation. Under normal daily activities brain tissue is compliant and ductile to stretch and easily recovers its original geometry. In contrast, under severe circumstances, when the strain is rapidly applied, such as during an automobile crash, the brain tissue acts far stiffer.[23] Thus rapid uniaxial stretch or "tensile elongation" of axons is thought to result in damage of the axonal

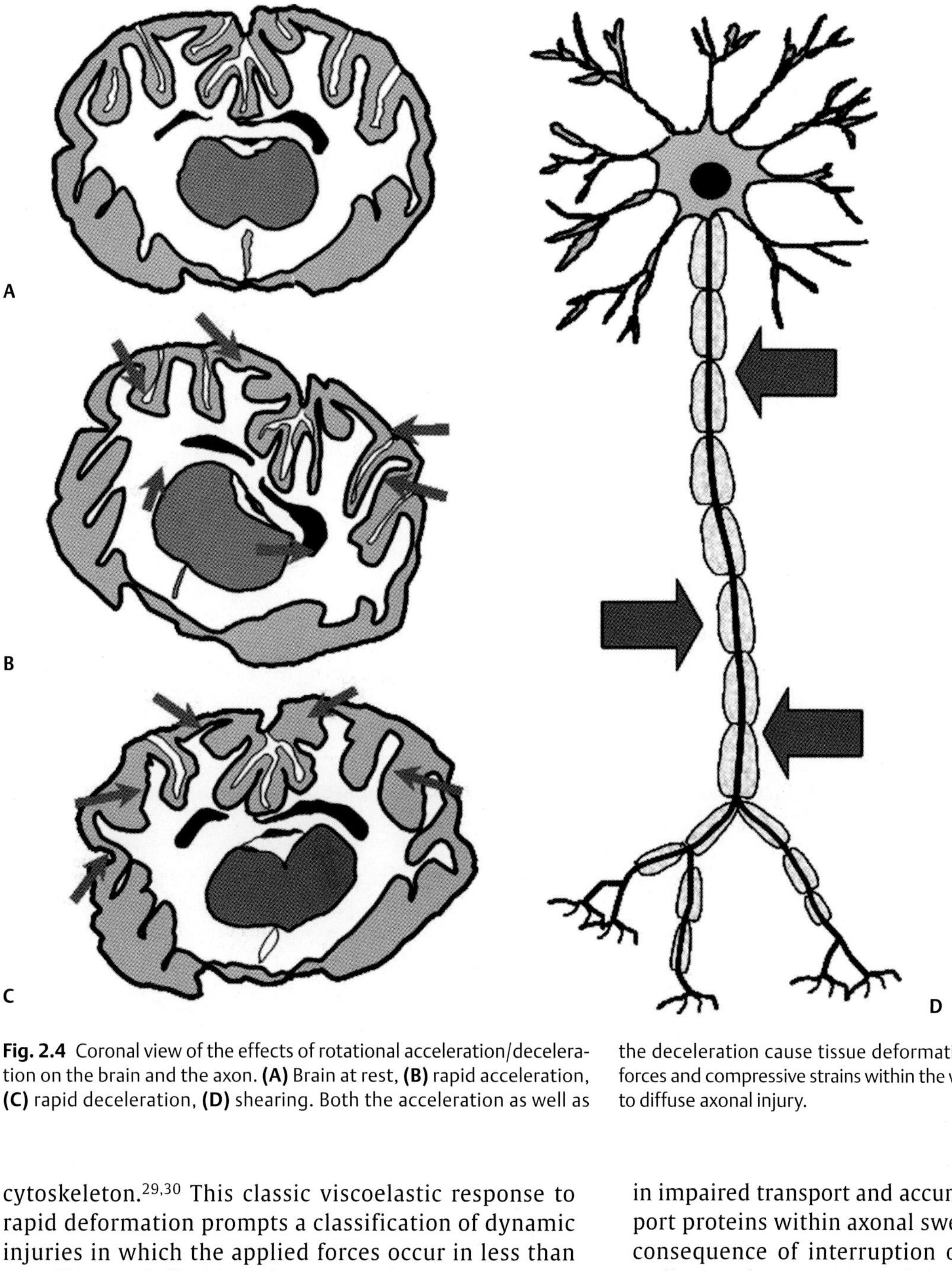

Fig. 2.4 Coronal view of the effects of rotational acceleration/deceleration on the brain and the axon. **(A)** Brain at rest, **(B)** rapid acceleration, **(C)** rapid deceleration, **(D)** shearing. Both the acceleration as well as the deceleration cause tissue deformation (*arrows*) induced by shear forces and compressive strains within the white matter leading ultimately to diffuse axonal injury.

cytoskeleton.[29,30] This classic viscoelastic response to rapid deformation prompts a classification of dynamic injuries in which the applied forces occur in less than 50 milliseconds.[31] Although axons may slowly recover to their prestretch orientation and shape, there is a characteristic evolution of physical and physiological changes. In particular, mechanical damage to sodium channels may result in massive influx of sodium with resultant swelling.[23,29] This sodium influx also triggers massive calcium entry through voltage-sensitive calcium channels. Adding to the immediate mechanical damage to the axonal cytoskeleton, further delayed damage may occur because of calcium-mediated proteolysis.[23] This acute and delayed cytoskeletal damage is thought to result in impaired transport and accumulation of axonal transport proteins within axonal swellings.[23,26,32,33] A further consequence of interruption of the axon is proximal wallerian degeneration of the affected neuron, while distally, the axon degenerates, fragments, and disappears, resulting in deafferentation of the affected neuronal fields. One of the functional consequences of this process may include seizures because of lack of inhibitory effects, spasticity, intellectual decline, and unmodulated behavior patterns. If the wallerian degeneration is widespread and many neurons are destroyed, the whole brain becomes atrophic, with ventriculomegaly and, in the worst case, a persistent vegetative state.[13]

Coma is the most common immediate impairment that has been associated with the severity of DAI. Indeed, an important difference between focal and diffuse brain injury is the source and character of posttraumatic coma resulting from these two general forms of injury: focal brain injury may include mass effects from hemorrhagic contusion or hematoma, which can induce herniation and brain stem compression.[34] Resultant coma may not be immediate but may develop in a secondary fashion. Much in contrast to these mechanisms of producing coma, in a landmark study, Gennarelli et al demonstrated that DAI can be a sole source for posttraumatic coma. Specifically, they observed that nonimpact rotational acceleration applied to the heads of nonhuman primates could induce an immediate and prolonged posttraumatic unconsciousness and DAI in the absence of mass lesions.[1] In particular, axonal injury in the brain stem appears to be a primary factor in the generation of coma with DAI.[23]

However, Blumbergs et al have recently shown that several patients who showed the features of DAI on examination of the brain at postmortem were actually lucid and conscious during part of their clinical course, suggesting that neurons and axons that subsequently show the changes of diffuse axonal injury may function after impact prior to degeneration, or that other, less affected, axon tracts do not progress to DAI.[35] These findings suggest that DAI may be amenable to therapeutic intervention, at least in the early phase.

Cytoskeletal Damage

The cytoskeleton consists of three main protein components:

- Microfilaments
- Neurofilaments
- Microtubules (MT)

Neurofilaments have been implicated in the maintenance of axonal caliber and many authors suggested that this is a simple function of their number.[36–38] But more recent work has questioned this general concept because neurofilament density, for example, has been documented to vary between central axons.[39] MTs, on the other hand, do not appear to play an important role in the regulation of axonal diameter but are dynamic components arranged along axons with side arms involved in fast axonal transport.[38]

Maxwell et al showed that axonal stretch injury is followed by a malalignment and distortion of the cytoskeletal components within minutes.[40] The consequences are a loss of MTs and an increased spacing of neurofilaments, especially at the node of Ranvier.

Biomechanical Effects of Vascular Damage in Response to Shear Forces and Age

Vulnerability, especially to vascular damage in response to shearing forces, is greatly increased at both extremes of the age spectrum. In the elderly, brain atrophy may result in reduced neuronal and astrocyte density with poorer support of vascular structures, with greater risk of progressive pericontusional hemorrhage and edema being greatly facilitated. In the premature neonate, for example, relative absence of myelination and reduced astrocyte maturity are probably responsible for the high incidence of periventricular white matter hemorrhage resulting from the shearing forces sustained during birth trauma.

Gender-Based Differences in TBI

Recent evidence from experimental models has shown a markedly reduced vulnerability of the female brain.[41,42] It has been postulated that the lesser vulnerability of female brain may be due to neuroprotective effects of estrogen[43–45] and progesterone.[41] It is not clear whether the proposed effects of estrogen are receptor or nongenomic based.

Mechanisms thought to mediate the neuroprotective effect of estrogens include:

- Preserved vascular autoregulatory capacity
- Antioxidant effect
- Attenuation of Aβ production
- Inhibitor of excitotoxicity
- Upregulation of proapoptotic *bcl-2*

Progesterone may mediate neuroprotective effects through a membrane-stabilizing antioxidant effect and suppression of neuronal excitability.[42]

Brain Swelling and Resolution of Edema

Edema is an important factor related to secondary brain injury, and in extreme cases, death is related to pressure and swelling within the cranial vault that produce herniation of structures in the brain stem. It occurs in most patients with severe brain injury, and in 5 to 10% of those with moderate injuries.[46,47] Unlike ischemia, edema can be caused by numerous factors and is the end point of several pathological processes that occur following injury.[6] According to Fishman, there are two primary types of edema: vasogenic and cytotoxic (**Fig. 2.5**).[48]

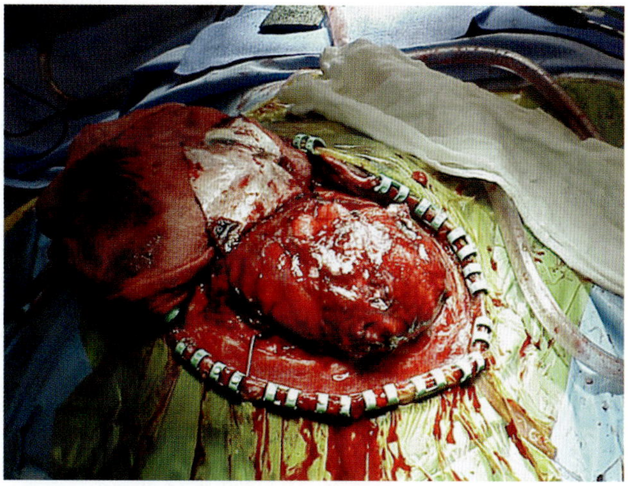

Fig. 2.5 Massive swelling and herniation of the brain during craniectomy.

One form of vasogenic edema occurs at the tight junctions of endothelial cells that limit the transfer of macromolecules across the blood–brain barrier (BBB). Moderate to severe injuries can result in hypertensive responses that can disrupt the BBB.[6] Factors related to the posttraumatic hypertensive response are the peak magnitude of blood pressure and the abruptness of the hypertensive onset.[49] Another form of vasogenic edema is related to the presence of arachidonic acid that causes minor vasomotor change, but more importantly causes increased endothelial cell permeability for small and large tracers and induces edema.[50]

Cytotoxic edema, on the other hand, does not strictly involve the BBB but involves all of the cellular elements of the brain. One form of cytotoxic edema occurs during hypoxic conditions where cells swell within a period of seconds after a hypoxic episode due to failure of the adenosine triphosphate (ATP) dependent Na^+/K^+ pump. As a result, Na^+ rapidly accumulates within cells, as does water due to osmotic pressure.[48,51] A second cause of cytotoxic edema is due to ion flux, due to increased amounts of extracellular excitatory amino acid neurotransmitters such as glutamate and glycine that can cause acute swelling in dendrites and cell bodies. The presence of high extracellular glutamate levels causes membrane channels to open, which in turn leads to Na^+ influx, membrane depolarization, and secondary influx of Cl^- and water resulting in excitotoxic swelling. This type of pathology, and the Ca^{2+} dependent late degeneration induced by glutamate, can act in isolation to produce irreversible neuronal injury.[6] Another cause of cytotoxic edema results directly from mechanical trauma and a deformation of the neuronal membrane. The latter causes massive K^+ efflux into the ECF with consequent astrocytic swelling as the astrocytes attempt to maintain cellular homeostasis.[52] At the worst end of the spectrum, brain tissue that is most severely injured is unable to restore ionic homeostasis because insufficient glucose can be delivered to the tissue via the microcirculation, and a vicious cycle may be set up whereby the microcirculation is squeezed by the astrocyte "end feet" that swell because of potassium uptake. Under these circumstances, intracranial pressure rises to further jeopardize global brain perfusion and cause death.

Disturbed ionic and neurotransmitter homeostasis seem to probably be the most important mechanisms contributing to secondary brain swelling following TBI. There is a net loss of potassium from injured tissue into the microvasculature that begins hours after onset. In mildly affected tissue, astrocyte swelling will begin to resolve after ~1 to 2 hours. In our own human ultrastructural studies, astrocytes around contusions appear to be shrinking by about the 5th day after injury.[51] Clearly, when the microcirculation is competent and cerebral blood flow (CBF) remains above ~20 mL/100 g/min, recovery of brain swelling will be much more rapid, and it is unlikely to occur at all when blood flow in the microcirculation is below these "threshold" levels.

Mechanisms of Secondary Brain Damage

As a consequence of the initial mechanical impact to the brain, cerebral metabolism, blood flow, and ion homeostasis are altered for a period of hours to days and even months (**Table 2.3**).[53]

Secondary Ischemic Neurological Damage

Inflammatory and cytotoxic mechanisms of injury are often the product of ischemia. Ischemia may be considered the most significant factor related to secondary damage that occurs following brain injury.[6,7] Focal injuries produce zones of profoundly reduced regional CBF that may be a factor in ischemic neuronal necrosis.[51] It is estimated that between 60 and 90% of patients who were severely head-injured and died show signs of ischemic brain damage postmortem.[54] The concept of delayed secondary neurological damage after head injury is also supported by the "lucid interval" statistics. Between 30 and 40% of severely head-injured patients who die will, at some time, have demonstrated a period of lucidity sufficient to obey commands or speak.[13] This implies that primary impact events were not sufficiently severe to damage the brain beyond the capacity for function, therefore emphasizing the importance of secondary damage.[55] The observation that ~70% of severely head-injured patients manifest high intracranial pressure during their

Table 2.3 Neuropathological Sequlae of TBI: Relationships between Neurochemical and Biomechanical Mechanisms

Immediate Onset Injury	Injury by Location	Cellular Pathophysiology
Primary injury	Focal	Cellular dysfunction
Skull fracture	Cortical contusion	Receptor dysfunction
Focal injury	Cortical laceration	Free-radical effect
Diffuse injury	Hematomas	Inflammatory events
Penetrating injury	Epidural	Calcium-mediated damage
	Subdural	
	Intracerebral	
Secondary injury	Diffuse	
Ischemia	Concussion	
Edema	Prolonged coma	
Neurochemical alterations	Diffuse axonal injury	

Abbreviation: TBI, traumatic brain injury.

Source: Adapted from McIntosh T. et al. Laboratory Investigations 1996;74:315–342 and Gennarelli T. Mechanism of brain injury. J Emerg Med 1993:11(Suppl 1)5–11.

clinical course in the intensive care unit is consistent with this concept.[56]

Mechanism by Which Reduced Cerebral Blood Flow Causes Tissue Damage

The landmark studies by Symon's group and Jones et al demonstrated a time-dependent hierarchy of neuronal events in response to progressive reduction of CBF.[57–59] In the healthy, normally autoregulating brain, cortical flow reduction down to levels around 20 mL/100 g/min may be tolerated without functional consequences, although the EEG may begin to slow and the subject may develop anxiety and drowsiness. Abruptly, at around 20 mL/100 g/min, consciousness is lost and the brain loses the capacity to make neurotransmitter substances, so that coma ensues.[58,60,61] When flow falls below 18 mL/100 g/min, ionic homeostasis becomes jeopardized because the energy-dependent Na/K-ATPase pump system, which maintains ionic gradient across the cell wall, cannot function. At this level, neurons move to anaerobic metabolism and lactate begins to be generated in large amounts. When flow falls further to levels around 10 mL/100 g/min, membrane integrity is lost, massive calcium influx begins, and the biochemical cascade of neuronal destruction becomes irreversible. The ultrastructural hallmarks of this process are mitochondrial swelling and perineuronal astrocytic process vacuolation, followed by swelling of the Golgi apparatus and intracellular cytoplasmic vesicles. Eventually, nuclear definition is lost (karyorrhexis).[54] In zones of focal cerebral contusion and beneath intracranial hematomas, flow may fall to levels close to the thresholds for ischemic brain damage.[59,62,63] The consequence of this together with an increase in glucose metabolism after TBI is an increased risk of damage to intracellular structures dependent upon continuous oxygen delivery, such as mitochondrial and various enzyme systems. These include, in particular, the enzyme systems that break down free radicals, thus leading to delayed damage in the hours that follow, especially during the reperfusion phase.[60,63,64] Therefore, it seems to be impossible for the most severely damaged tissue, which sustains the greatest magnitude of shearing injury, to be able to restore ionic homeostasis in spite of maximally increasing glycolytic activity. If tissue blood flow is reduced during this time of maximal metabolic need, the consequences are that tissue glucose and oxygen levels will fall to under threshold levels. This, again, will exacerbate tissue swelling, and ischemic necrosis will occur. Furthermore, cerebral blood flow may be further reduced at the tissue level by such processes as astrocytic swelling and generally by low blood pressure, high ICP, which itself is generated by cytotoxic swelling or intracranial hematomas causing distortion. Probably the effects of all these insults may be cumulative and occur to a varying extent in the majority of patients with severe head injury. Jenkins et al have shown that a mild global ischemic insult that is insufficient to cause neuronal death alone when combined with mild trauma causes massive hippocampal neuronal necrosis,[65] even when trauma and ischemia occur up to 24 hours apart. This sequence of events can be called ***double insult models and synergistic damage mechanisms after neurotrauma.***

This model may explain the relative success of therapies such as metabolic suppression using barbiturates or hypothermia, or raising cerebral perfusion and CBF by the use of vasopressors. Diuretics and rheological agents, such as mannitol, may help to improve tissue perfusion during these crucial early periods.[66] Ion channel blockade using agents directed at both voltage-dependent and agonist-operated channels may be important avenues for future therapy, as may be the use of hemoglobin substitutes (e.g., perfluorocarbons), which augment the oxygen carrying capacity of the microcirculation to damaged tissue.[18]

Infarction versus Selective Neuronal Loss

When flow is profoundly reduced (i.e., <5–10 mL/100 g/ min) within the distribution of one cerebral end artery for more than 60 to 90 minutes, infarction ensues. However, when the flow reduction is less marked (e.g., to levels around 15–18 mL/100 g/min) and when it persists for more than ~30 minutes, selective neuronal loss may occur.[67,68] The most vulnerable neuronal types are:

- Hippocampal neurons of the molecular layer, CA, and CA3 sectors
- Cerebellar granular cells
- Cortical neurons, particularly the larger cells, in areas such as the cuneate visual cortex

Within the context of head injury, this type of neuronal loss is especially important in patients with raised intracranial pressure, where cerebral perfusion pressure may be marginal (~30–40 mm Hg) for many hours, or even days. In such patients, recent studies have demonstrated an extremely high frequency of ischemic neuronal loss especially in the hippocampus.[54] Bilateral hippocampal loss and cerebellar damage may explain the high frequency of memory disorders and coordination difficulty seen in severely head-injured survivors.

Improving Cerebral Oxygenation

Enhancing oxygen availability in the (peri)ischemic region in the early phase may improve neuronal resistance against the ischemic attack. We were able to show that about one-third of severely head-injured patients demonstrated reduced brain oxygen tension (<25 mm Hg brain tissue partial pressure of oxygen [$P_{ti}O_2$]) for the first 6 to 24 hours following severe head injury.[69,70] For this group of patients with low brain $P_{ti}O_2$, outcome was significantly worse.[69,71] Such posttraumatic reduced cerebral oxygenation may arise from four mechanisms:

- Reduced oxygen delivery by reduced CBF
- Reduced oxygen uptake from the lungs (e.g., adult respiratory distress syndrome [ARDS] or severe lung disease)
- Reduced oxygen delivery by reduced hemoglobin content or hemoglobin function (e.g., carbon monoxide poisoning or anemia)
- Reduced oxygen unloading from the tissue (e.g., hypothermia)

Other important candidate mechanisms that may act focally include microvascular compromise due to astrocytic foot process swelling to cause reduced CBF (**Fig. 2.6**). Attempts have been made to raise CBF by use of vasopressors and by increasing cerebral perfusion pressure (CPP), but it remains unproven whether these treatments improve $P_{ti}O_2$, and in one study, increasing CPP to 70 mm Hg and above resulted in no increase in good outcome. An increase of tissue oxygen availability might be achieved by hyperbaric oxygenation, infusion of a modified oxygen carrier such as cross-linked hemoglobin, or administration of perfluorochemicals (PFCs) along with an increase of the inspired oxygen fraction.[72]

Perfluorocarbons have been studied as temporary blood substitutes for more than 3 decades[73,74] and have been used as contrast media.[75,76] They are insoluble in water, biologically inert, and a pharmacologically nonactive small molecule composed entirely of carbon and fluorine. They have the ability to dissolve in solution large quantities of gases, including oxygen and carbon dioxide. Therefore perfluorocarbons are especially attractive because they transport oxygen without the need for erythrocytes. The solubility of gases such as oxygen and carbon dioxide in PFC emulsions is much greater than that of plasma. Unlike hemoglobin, PFC emulsions do not bind oxygen. Oxygen is only physically dissolved in the emulsion and 90 to 100% is released by simple diffusion in response to low tissue partial pressure of oxygen (PO_2).[77,78] It is because of this simple physical transport system that PFC emulsions load and off-load oxygen twice as fast as does hemoglobin. Furthermore, the oxygen unloading occurring in nearby erythrocytes may be enhanced by an improved diffusion capacity of gases in the PFC emulsion. This enhanced diffusion capacity may be especially beneficial in low-flow states because the PFC emulsion releases oxygen to cerebral tissue on the basis of its diffusion gradient, such that the lower the oxygen tension, the more oxygen will be released.

Another important aspect of cerebral oxygenation that may be altered by TBI is capillary blood flow. Under normal conditions, most capillaries are perfused by a "single file" column of red blood cells (RBCs) known as rouleaux with limited O_2 transport by the plasma. With the addition of PFCs, however, the transport of O_2 can be expanded to the entire surface area of the capillary.[79] This mechanism may become important after TBI, when perivascular astrocyte foot process swelling occurs.[80,81]

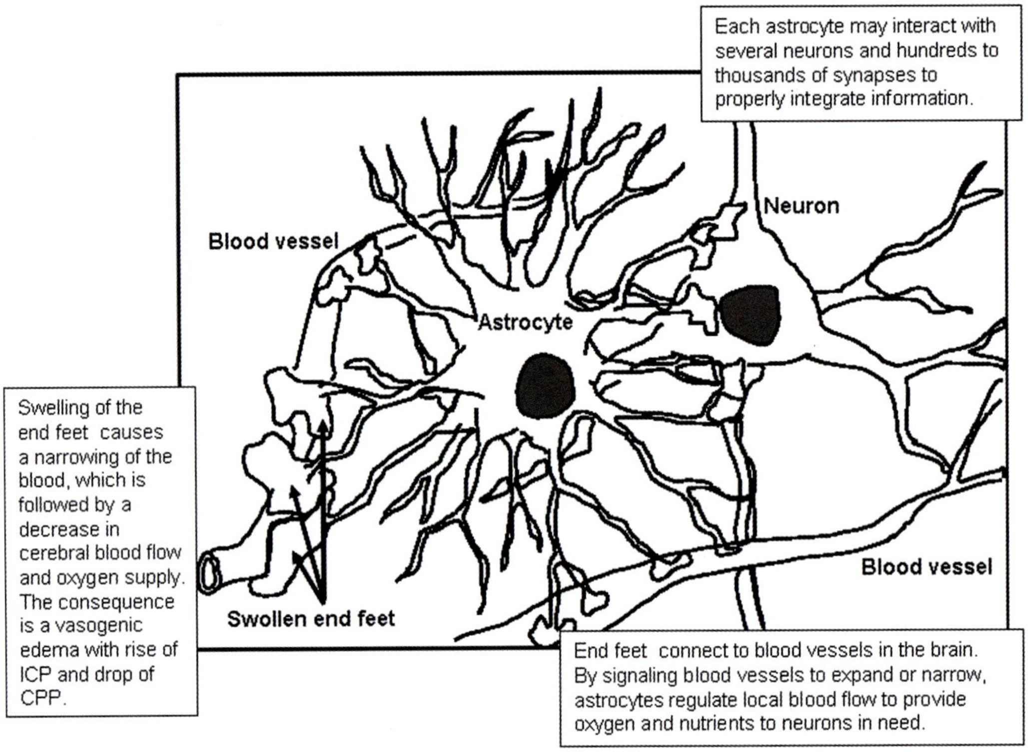

Fig. 2.6 Swelling of the end feet of the astrocytes around the capillaries leads to squeezing of the vessels with decrease in substrate supply to the brain. CPP, cerebral perfusion pressure; ICP, intracranial pressure.

Swelling of astrocyte end feet may in turn reduce the cross-sectional area of capillaries, thereby reducing normal RBC flow into the affected areas. In areas where RBC flow is thus excluded, PFCs may be able to continue delivery of O_2 because of their small particle size (1/35th the size of an RBC), thereby allowing perfusion of those tissues via cell-free plasma. They can thus possibly perfuse and oxygenate "pericontusional" brain tissue, in which it has been shown that capillaries are so narrowed as to impede RBC transport and, hence, introduce a new possibility for therapy.

Research led to the development of a first-generation PFC intravenous emulsion. The new third-generation perfluorocarbon emulsion can carry 5 times more oxygen than hemoglobin, unload oxygen, and take up carbon dioxide more efficiently than blood in a concentration-gradient–mediated manner according to Henry's Law. PFCs thus may be able to oxygenate tissues with narrowed capillaries, as occurs in brain contusions.

Recent studies also show that PFCs can reduce infarct volume and improve neurological function in experimental cerebral ischemic models with the PFC either administered intravenously or perfused through the ventriculosubarachnoid space.[82,83] Daugherty et al previously demonstrated that PFC combined with 100% O_2 treatment can significantly increase cerebral oxygenation.[84]

In a pilot study we were able to show that a few minutes after starting the PFC infusion an increase in brain $P_{ti}O_2$ could be observed, which continued for the next hours (**Fig. 2.7**).

Metabolic Consequences of TBI

The brain is dependent upon aerobic metabolism for substrate delivery (oxygen and glucose). Following severe head injury, impairment of oxygenation and perfusion occurs frequently, thus metabolic derangement is an extremely frequent and important consequence of TBI. Consequently, metabolic changes may be global, involving the whole brain, or focal, developing in the region of intracerebral and subdural hematomas and contusions. Immediately following impact, the shearing forces applied to neuronal tissues result in massive ion fluxes across neuronal membranes, widespread loss of resting membrane potential, and release of neurotransmitters into the extracellular space. A few minutes later, the brain attempts to restore ionic homeostasis by reuptake of neurotransmitters and ion pumping, which are intensely energy-dependent processes and result in an abrupt increase in glucose utilization.

Animal studies have shown that this increase in glucose metabolism, to facilitate ATP generation, is brief and

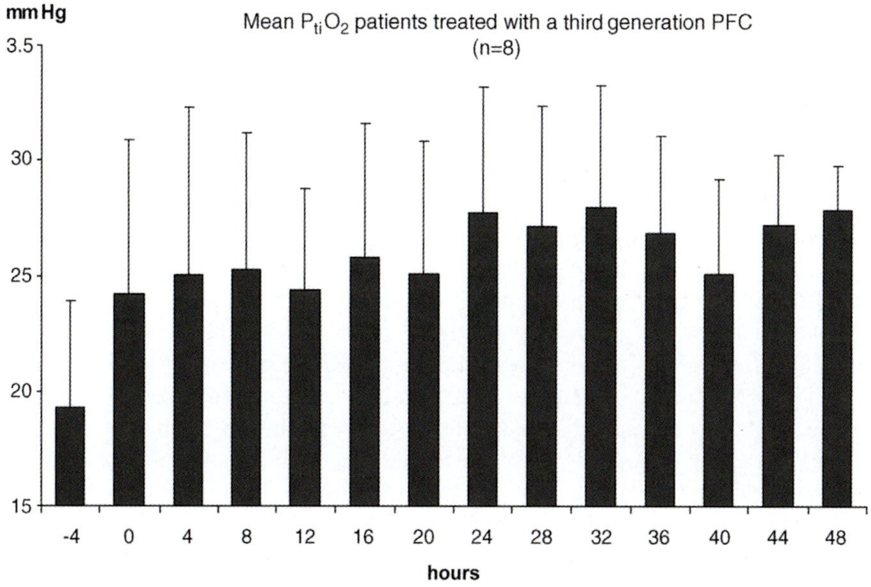

Fig. 2.7 Mean $P_{ti}O_2$ over 4-hour periods in patients (n = 8) treated with a third-generation perfluorocarbon. The infusion was given over ~30 minutes as a single shot.

maximally localized to those parts of the brain that are maximally deformed by the shearing forces.[85] Pellerin and Magistretti suggested that ionic pumping and glutamate surges in astrocytes both preferentially activate anaerobic glycolysis, thus producing lactate, especially in astrocytes, and this may be in the absence of severe ischemia.[86] This depletes ECF glucose. When focal lesions such as SDH, focal infarction, or cerebral contusion are present, then glucose use increases for a longer period in the "penumbral" border zone around the densely ischemic core of these lesions.[62,87]

Traditionally, aerobic glycolysis is the only form of metabolism considered in regard to cerebral metabolism. However, there is evidence now suggesting that astrocyts and glia may have the ability to use "coupled lactate metabolism" to meet their energy needs: Neurons and astrocytes are functionally coupled in their metabolic activity such that the astrocytic glucose is anaerobically metabolized to lactate, carried by the monocarboxilic transporter (MCT) to the neurons, where it is metabolized anaerobically to generate energy. As neuronal activity is increased, potassium and glutamate are released into the extracellular space and taken up by the astrocytes in an energy-dependent fashion, resulting in astrocytic glycolysis. Under extreme conditions, such as TBI, aerobic metabolism may be overwhelmed either by reduction in the oxygen delivery, mitochondrial impairment, or increased release of excitatory neurotransmitters resulting in increased lactate accumulation. Recently, we were able to show in an animal model that lactate uptake was significantly increased at the injury site where the metabolism is probably the greatest.[88] Lactate infusion initiated 30 minutes following a fluid percussion injury resulted in the animals demonstrating significantly reduced cognitive deficits when compared with saline-treated controls.[89]

Intracellular and Molecular Mechanism during Secondary Brain Injury

During the secondary injury high levels of glutamate, Ca^{2+}, and lactate are released, and cytokines are produced, leading to an inflammatory response, which all contributes to further tissue damage.[53,90] The disrupted homeostasis in energy and oxygen supply leads to activation of several systems. Transcription, growth, plasticity, differentiation, signaling, inflammation, and cell death genes are affected in different trauma models. The injury alters apoptotic and antiapoptotic factors such as caspases, *bax*, and *bcl-2*; immediate early genes such as c-*fos*, c-*jun*, and *jun* B; and inflammatory markers such as interleukins and heat shock proteins.

Cell Membranes and Ion Channels

The most common voltage-gated channels are closely linked functionally with the sodium/potassium ATPase pump.[91–93] Many types of ion channel are linked to the specific agonist-gated receptors, and others are linked within the cell with second messenger systems, such as adenylate cyclase and G proteins.[93] There is clear evidence that astrocytes are excitable, possess ion channels, and may be depolarized, though to a much lesser extent than neurons.[94–96] It seems that the majority of voltage-sensitive and agonist-gated ion channels are also sensitive to transient mechanical deformation by shearing forces. Some of these ion channels remain "leaky" for several hours after mechanical deformation.[97] Moreover, Tavalin et al showed that monolayer neuron and astrocyte cultures growing on a flexible plastic membrane, which are rapidly deformed by a brief air jet impulse, undergo rapid calcium entry and subsequent neuronal death, with efflux of lactate and potassium into the culture medium.[97]

We and other authors were able to show from in vivo trauma models such as fluid percussion injury and contusional impact models a massive rapid transient efflux of potassium into the ECF, associated with a fall in sodium content in ECF.[18,98–100] These changes may be explained by rapid alterations in the "pump leak" relationship that exists between voltage-dependent ion channels and the sodium-potassium–dependent ATPase pump, and the opening of agonist-gated channels. These data suggest that agonist-dependent ion channels and their receptors may be very sensitive to mechanical deformation with consequent increased leakiness due to their structural complexity. Astrocytes are known to function as potassium uptake buffers, having the capacity to rapidly take up potassium from the extracellular space.[95,101,102] However, this can result in rapid astrocyte swelling, which is the ultrastructural hallmark of both acute cerebral ischemia and focal cerebral contusion, and it is almost always seen in animal trauma.

Second Messenger Systems and Neurotrauma

Cyclic AMP is a recognized second messenger which are typically large molecules situated usually within the neuronal membrane or adjacent to its inner surface within the cytoplasm, and they mediate many cellular responses. Due to their large molecular size and complexity they are vulnerable to shear injury. Cyclic AMP was shown to inhibit apoptosis of cerebellar granule cells in a low K^+ medium.[103]

Intracellular Mechanisms

Calcium and Glutamate

In adjacent zones where ischemia may not reach critical levels, another process may occur that eventually leads to tissue damage and death.[6] Specifically, glutamate neurotoxicity may play a role in secondary ischemic damage. Hypoxia-related neuronal depolarization has been shown to increase extracellular levels of glutamate via increased release and decreased uptake.[104] Abnormally high levels of extracellular glutamate activate a wide variety of receptors that can cause depolarization of the cell membrane, allowing for the activation of voltage-dependent Ca^{2+} channels.[27] An influx of Ca^{2+} can propagate glutamate neurotoxicity in a positive feedback fashion by further stimulating the release of the transmitter glutamate.[104]

Calcium

Within minutes after trauma, there is a rapid and massive intracellular increase in free calcium ions.[85,100,105] One of the more recent perspectives regarding how Ca^{2+} enters the cell following stretch was a process labeled mechanoporation.[106] Mechanoporation was defined as the "development of transient defects in the cell membrane that are due to its mechanical deformation."[106] The mechanically induced pores were considered to be either transient or stable, the latter associated with long-term membrane leakage.[6] According to Gennarelli[106], ions were driven by diffusion through the pores and into cells with Ca^{2+} entering due to the large extracellular gradient. Calcium may enter cells also through many different channels that may be opened by several mechanisms, including voltage-dependent channel opening, induced by mechanical deformation of membrane and ion channels, and agonist-dependent channel opening, mediated by neurotransmitter substances released in excess into ECF.

Glutamate

Increases in cerebral ECF concentrations of the amino acid L-glutamate, a mostly excitatory neurotransmitter, as well as activation of glutamate receptors have been described after TBI, SAH and cerebral ischemic insults.[99,101,107–109] The massive glutamate release seen immediately after the trauma may be due to membrane depolarization caused by temporary deformation of transmembrane pore proteins. This event in turn could induce further glutamate release by other neurons, due to depolarization. An impaired reuptake of the neurotransmitter from the extracellular space might also be involved in this phenomenon, as the primary mechanism for glutamate removal from the synaptic cleft is an uptake into astrocytes via specific transporters. Massive release of glutamate after TBI, along with an associated efflux of potassium from the cells, seems to enhance astrocytic glycolysis, thus considerably affecting extracellular concentrations of glucose and lactate. The fundamental factor mediating the excitotoxic effects of glutamate overstimulation appears to be an intracellular calcium overload, primarily due to excessive calcium influx via N-methyl d-aspartate (NMDA)-receptor linked ion channels. The activation of intracellular calcium-dependent enzymes such as endonucleases, lipases, and proteases may trigger harmful cascades in cellular metabolism as well as the increased production of toxic products, such as free radicals.[110,111]

Free Radical Generation and Hydrogen Ions

Free radicals are highly reactive ionic molecules bearing an unpaired electron in their outer electron shell. These compounds are the normal by-product of oxidative metabolism within mitochondria, and they play important physiological roles within various tissues, such as polymorphonuclear-leukocyte–mediated destruction of bacteria.[61,112] On the other hand, free radicals can react with various structures within the cell membranes, proteins, and the genome. To prevent these damaging events, potent enzyme systems exist within all cells to break them down. Intracellular calcium inactivates some of these mechanisms, such as peroxidase and xanthine oxidase.[64] Most of these free radicals are derived from oxygen, thus these compounds seem to be generated especially in circumstances of postischemic reperfusion when the tissue is replete with oxygen, and after ischemic events when the protective enzymes may be inactivated. Free radical generation is also favored by the presence of free ferrous iron, which acts as a catalyst to the Haber–Weiss reaction depicted below[61]:

$$^{\bullet}O^{-}{}_{2} + Fe^{3+} \rightarrow O_2 + Fe^{2+}$$

$$H_2O_2 + Fe^{2+} \rightarrow OH^{-} + {}^{\bullet}OH^{+}Fe^{3+}$$

$$^{\bullet}O^{-}{}_{2} + H_2O_2 \rightarrow O_2 + OH^{-} + {}^{\bullet}OH$$

Free iron may be found in traumatized brain within a few hours of injury as repair mechanisms cleave iron from hemoglobin in breaking down red cells, which is an extremely frequent sequel of severe brain injury. High concentrations of hydrogen ions within cells appear to be harmful because they alter the function of intracellular enzymes. However, hydrogen ions in the extracellular space are also powerful cerebral vasodilators.[60]

However, there is no technique for demonstrating the existence of free radical species in the human brain after trauma, although studies using several indirect techniques have shown an increase in free radical activity following trauma and ischemia in various animal models.[60,113] It is likely that the large neuroprotective molecules directed against the free radical mechanism (tirilazad, an amino steroid) and polyethylene glycol–conjugated superoxide dismutase (PEG-SOD) do not penetrate extensively into brain tissue. This may in part explain their failure to benefit patients in clinical trials.

Stress Proteins

A most important group are the so-called heat shock proteins (Hsp). Hsp are highly conserved molecules that perform important functions in the folding and unfolding or translocation of proteins, as well as in the assembly and disassembly of protein complexes. Because of these helper functions, some Hsp have been termed *molecular chaperones*, protecting cells from environmental stress damage.[114–116] In nonstressed cells, Hsp are present in low concentrations, whereas in stressed cells they accumulate at high levels.[117] The heat shock response is elicited by a variety of stimuli, including thermal, chemical, and physical stress. Hsp are designated according to their approximate molecular weight.[115] The 70 kDa heat shock–related proteins compose a family of molecular chaperones that regulate cellular processes during normal and stress conditions.[114,115] Although typically regarded as intracellular proteins, it has been reported that Hsp can be released. Moreover, some investigators have suggested that circulating Hsp could be involved in the modulation of the immune system and in vivo responses to stress.[114,118] In the brain, Hsp70 is induced by a variety of pathological stimuli, including ischemia, excitotoxic insults, and inflammatory responses, major determinants of acute neural injury in TBI.[119–122] Increased expression of Hsp70 is suggested to play a role in cell survival and recovery after cerebral injuries.[122] Moreover, higher levels of Hsp70 within the first 20 hours after primary injury seem to be a sensitive biomarker of fatal outcome.[121] Upregulation of Hsp72 may be increased during neuronal injury and appears to be involved in cellular repair mechanisms and cytoprotection.[123] Hsp72 upregulation may also serve as a marker during neuronal injury.[124]

Inflammatory Response

Neuroinflammatory events are "delayed responses to TBI" and appear to display dual and opposing roles, promoting brain damage on one hand by the release of neurotoxic substances while on the other hand promoting repair of the injured tissue containing antigens and pathogens, such as viruses and bacteria. Accumulation of polymorphonuclear leucocytes begins in damaged brain tissue within 24 hours following acute injury, and they adhere to blood capillaries within minutes after trauma.[125,126] Thirty-six to 48 hours following injury, macrophages are seen[127] and secrete many factors, including cytokines.[128] Cytokines are vasoactive substances that have been shown to increase vascular permeability and induce edema formation,[129,130] and may have direct cytotoxic effects on glial and neuronal cells.[131] One cytokine, tumor necrosis factor α (TNFα), is upregulated in animal models of TBI from 1 to 4 hours following injury. This rapid response is thought to be due to the synthesis of TNFα by the primary cells of the central nervous system (CNS; glia and neurons) rather than by systemic inflammatory cells.[132] TNFα plays an important role in cell growth regulation, immunomodulation, inflammation, and autoimmune processes.[133] Furthermore,

TNFα and interleukin-1 β (IL-1β) may exert deleterious effects on the CNS through edema and delayed neuronal death.[134,135]

Apoptosis

Kerr et al described two types of cell death: one called cell necrosis, which results from injury and causes inflammation; the other, called apoptosis, is the normal developmental type with several distinct characteristics.[136,137] He described the morphological changes that occur during developmental cell death as cell shrinkage, membrane blebbing, chromatin condensation, and DNA fragmentation. These changes contrast with those found during cell death due to necorsis in which cells and their organelles tend to swell and rupture. From these findings, it was postulated that cells have the ability to self-destruct by activation of an intrinsic cellular suicide program when they are no longer needed or have become seriously damaged.[137] The recognition of apoptosis as a normal physiological process was the result of the genetic studies in the nematode *Caenorhabditis elegans*.

Neuronal and other brain cell death after TBI is thought to be composed of primary cell death, caused by mechanical destruction, and secondary or delayed cell death, caused by several pathological cascades initiated by trauma.[137] In humans, these cascades include ischemia, excitotoxicity, and inflammation, each of which can trigger apoptosis.[138,139] However, the complete biomechanical and molecular mechanisms are not completely understood.

Apoptosis can be followed by the TUNEL (terminal deoxynucleotidyl transferase-mediated dUTP nick end-labeling) method. The TUNEL labeling reflects only fragmented DNA, no matter how and why the DNA is fragmented, and thus lacks specificity for apoptosis. Another way to detect apoptosis is to monitor the degradation of poly(ADP-ribose) polymerase using appropriate antibodies[140] or through membrane phospholipids changes.[137] However, both in vitro and in vivo studies have suggested that the severity of injury can determine the type of neuronal death, that is, apoptosis or necrosis (**Table 2.4**).[141]

Genetic Regulation of Apoptosis

Genomic, that is, secondary molecular, responses to TBI include the regulation of genes that alter cellular architecture, upregulation of growth factors, induction of apoptosis, and regulation of transcriptional processes to generate proteins crucial to modulating the pathological responses to TBI.

The Oncosuppressor Gene p53

Apoptosis can be induced by the oncosuppressor protein p53.[142,143] This DNA binding protein, despite the short half-life of 5 to 20 minutes,[144] functions in genome surveillance, DNA repair, and as a transcription factor. The protein p53 commits to death cells that have sustained DNA damage. The mechanisms by which p53 induces apoptosis are largely unknown. However, p53 is a direct

Table 2.4 Comparative Features of Necrosis and Apoptosis

Necrosis	Apoptosis
Loss of cellular homeostasis	No initial major changes
Altered membrane permeability	Not seen, at least initially
Potassium loss; sodium entry; fall in membrane potential	No sodium influx; no change in potassium concentration in cell
Swelling of all cytoplasmic compartments	Cytosol condensation
Destruction of mitochondria and other organelles	Generally intact organelles
	Protruberances from cell surface separate to form apoptotic bodies
Depletion of cellular energy (ATP)	No depletion of cellular energy
Lowered macromolecular synthesis	Macromolecular synthesis activation is required
Affects tracts of contiguous cells	Affects scattered individual cells
Loose aggregates of chromatin	Highly condensed granular aggregates of chromatin
Passive atrophy	Active degeneration

Abbreviations: ATP, adenosine triphosphate.

Source: From Sastry PS, Rao KS. Apoptosis and the nervous system. J Neurochem 2000;74(1):1–20.

transcriptional activator of the *bax* gene[145] and a transcriptional repressor of the *bcl-2* gene.[146] In unstressed cells, the level of p53 protein is low. This protein exists in a latent, inactive form that requires modification to become active. Its levels can be increased because the rate of initiation of p53 mRNA translation is enhanced due to activation by DNA damage.[143] Increases in p53 levels are proportional to the extent of DNA damage, in which oncosuppressor protein functions as a DNA transcription factor.[142,143,145,146] *Bax*, a member of the *bcl-2* protooncogene family,[144] and redox-related genes are key transcriptional targets of p53 with regard to neuronal apoptosis.[145] *Bax* is thought to function by forming channels in mitochondrial membranes.[147] When active, these channels may allow the release of cytochrome c from mitochondria to the cytosol. In neuronal cell culture, *bax*-dependent, caspase-3 activation is a key determinant in p53-induced apoptosis.[148]

The Bcl-2 Gene Family

The *bcl-2* gene codes for a 25 kDa protein, a protooncogene. The *bcl-2* multigene superfamily includes antiapoptotic genes such as *bcl-2*, *bcl-xL*, and *bak*[149] and proapoptotic genes such as *bax*, *bad*, and *bcl-xs*.[141,150] *Bcl-2* is unique in that it has been shown to protect cells from a variety of insults such as treatment with calcium ionophores, glutamate, free radicals, and withdrawal of trophic factors.[141,151] It has been suggested that *bax* is an obligatory protein in programmed cell death. In a model of combined TBI and hypoxemia, Clark et al observed an upregulation of *bcl-2* in cortical neurons that survived the traumatic injury, whereas increased *bax* immunoreactivity was observed in apoptotic granule neurons in the dentate gyrus following controlled cortical impact injury.[138] An increase in *bax* mRNA and protein was observed in neurons in the peri-injured cortex. These observations suggest that neuronal survival may be compromised due to decreased expression of *bcl-2* and a concomitant increase in *bax* levels.

Bcl-2 has been observed to prevent both necrotic and apoptotic forms of cell death.[141] Increased *bcl-2* expression in vivo using viral transfection of the *bcl-2* gene reduced neuronal loss following focal ischemia.[20,152,153] Similarly, transgenic mice overexpressing human *bcl-2* are less susceptible to ischemic or traumatic brain injury.[154] Raghupathi et al observed acute decreases in *bcl-2* immunoreactivity in the absence of a concomitant alteration in *bax* immunoreactivity, supporting the hypothesis that altered cellular ratios of *bcl-2:bax* may be associated with cell death.[141] The same authors suggested that strategies to reverse the decrease in cellular *bcl-2* levels and/or to block the increase in *bax* mRNA may prevent, in part, TBI-induced neurodegeneration.

Cell death following TBI can occur due to the activation of multiple pathways that include the differential expression of the *bcl-2* family of genes. Control of the expression of these genes in neurons may confer resistance to trauma-induced death, thereby attenuating behavioral morbidity.[141]

Caspases

A set of genes called *ced*, the *ced*-3 genes have been shown to be essential for apoptosis to occur.[155] It was found that *ced*-3 encodes a cysteine protease that is homologous to interleukin-1b converting enzyme (ICE). These enzymes, called caspases, are cysteine proteases. Caspase-3 activation is thought to be a key committed step in the apoptotic cascade,[156] mediating apoptosis after

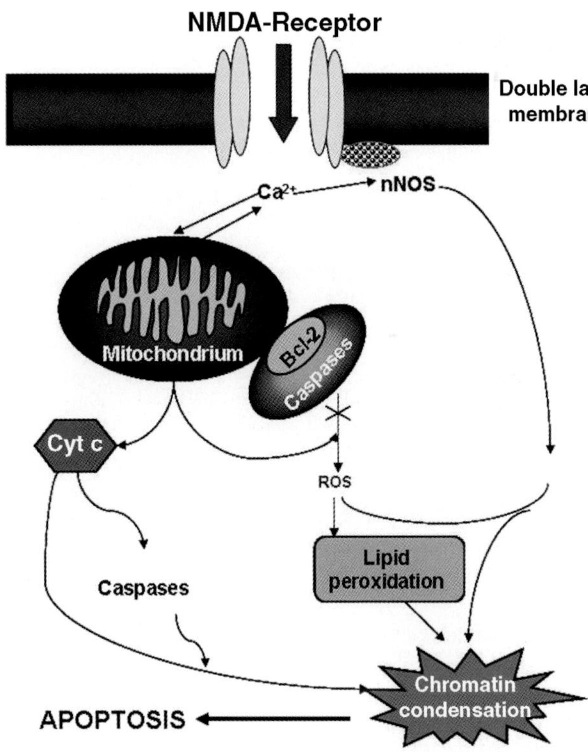

Fig. 2.8 Schematic representation of potential cascade of events leading to NMDA-induced apoptosis. NMDA receptor (NMDAA) overstimulation causes excessive Ca^{2+} influx. This leads to mitochondrial Ca^{2+} accumulation, energy loss, and subsequent mitochondrial membrane depolarization. In turn, ROS are formed with resulting lipid peroxidation. Tennetti et al showed that inhibition of caspases blocks the formation of ROS, lipid peroxidation, and chromatin condensation indicative of apoptosis, suggesting that caspases are upstream to these events. NO production leads to the production of peroxynitrite. (Abbreviations: cyt c, cytochrome c; NMDA, N-methyl d-aspartate; nNOS, neuronal NO synthase.) (From Tenneti L, D'Emilia DM, Troy CM, Lipton SA. Role of caspases in N-methyl-D-aspartate-induced apoptosis in cerebrocortical neurons. J Neurochem 1998;71(3):946–959.)

experimental TBI, for which pharmacological inhibition results in improved outcome.[139,156]

Cytochrome c

Cytochrome c is an integral component of the electron transport chain that, under conditions of cellular stress, can be released from mitochondria, whereupon it has the capacity to initiate apoptosis by activation of caspases.[137,156] Extracellular release of cytochrome c has been reported to be specific for apoptosis in humans and sufficient to induce apoptosis in cell culture.[156] However, its release does not appear to be sufficient to induce apoptosis in humans without the proapoptotic gene *bax*.[157] Thus, the presence of extramitochondrial cytochrome c can serve as a biomarker of apoptosis. Consequently, it seems possible that agents targeting the release cytochrome c serve as effective treatments for delayed neuronal death (**Fig. 2.8**).[156]

Conclusion

Mortality rates for severe brain injury have fallen ~10% per decade over the past 30 years. Yet, during this period, no single drug therapy has been shown to be clinically effective. Only by improving our understanding of the mechanisms of damage will we be able to devise effective therapies in TBI. Major advances have recently been made, and will begin to impact outcome over the next few years. Rational TBI management on a day-to-day basis also requires an understanding of the pathomechanistical events in TBI.

References

1. Gennarelli TA, Thibault LE, Adams JH, Graham DI, Thompson CJ, Marcincin RP. Diffuse axonal injury and traumatic coma in the primate. Ann Neurol 1982;12(6):564–574
2. Gennarelli TA. Head injury in man and experimental animals: clinical aspects. Acta Neurochir Suppl (Wien) 1983;32:1–13
3. Löwenhielm P. Strain tolerance of the vv. cerebri sup. (bridging veins) calculated from head-on collision tests with cadavers. Z Rechtsmed 1974;75(2):131–144
4. Holbourne AS. Mechanics of head injury. Lancet 1943;2:438–441
5. Ommaya AK, Gennarelli TA. Cerebral concussion and traumatic unconsciousness: correlation of experimental and clinical observations of blunt head injuries. Brain 1974;97(4):633–654
6. Gaetz M. The neurophysiology of brain injury. Clin Neurophysiol 2004;115(1):4–18
7. Gennarelli TA, Tipperman R, Maxwell WL, Graham DI, Adams JH, Irvine A. Traumatic damage to the nodal axolemma: an early, secondary injury. Acta Neurochir Suppl (Wien) 1993;57:49–52
8. Gennarelli TA, Graham DI. Neuropathology of the head injuries. Semin Clin Neuropsychiatry 1998;3(3):160–175
9. Strich SJ. Diffuse degeneration of the cerebral white matter in severe dementia following head injury. J Neurol Neurosurg Psychiatry 1956; 19(3):163–185
10. Kuijpers AH, Claessens MH, Sauren AA. The influence of different boundary conditions on the response of the head to impact: a two-dimensional finite element study. J Neurotrauma 1995;12(4): 715–724
11. Kleiven S. Influence of impact direction on the human head in prediction of subdural hematoma. J Neurotrauma 2003;20(4): 365–379
12. Hirakawa K, Hashizume K, Fuchinoue T, Takahashi H, Nomura K. Statistical analysis of chronic subdural hematoma in 309 adult cases. Neurol Med Chir (Tokyo) 1972;12(0):71–83
13. Adams JH, Doyle D, Ford I, Gennarelli TA, Graham DI, McLellan DR. Diffuse axonal injury in head injury: definition, diagnosis and grading. Histopathology 1989;15(1):49–59
14. Bullock R, Hanemann CO, Murray L, Teasdale GM. Recurrent hematomas following craniotomy for traumatic intracranial mass. J Neurosurg 1990; 72(1):9–14
15. du Trevou MD, van Dellen JR. Penetrating stab wounds to the brain: the timing of angiography in patients presenting with the weapon already removed. Neurosurgery 1992;31(5):905–911, discussion 911–912
16. Grahm TW, Williams FC Jr, Harrington T, Spetzler RF. Civilian gunshot wounds to the head: a prospective study. Neurosurgery 1990;27(5): 696–700, discussion 700
17. Nathoo N, Chite SH, Edwards PJ, van Dellen JR. Civilian infratentorial gunshot injuries: outcome analysis of 26 patients. Surg Neurol 2002; 58(3–4):225–232, discussion 232–233
18. Di X, Lyeth BG, Hamm RJ, Bullock MR. Voltage-dependent Na+/K+ ion channel blockade fails to ameliorate behavioral deficits after traumatic brain injury in the rat. J Neurotrauma 1996;13(9):497–504
19. Peerless SJ, Rewcastle NB. Shear injuries of the brain. Can Med Assoc J 1967;96(10):577–582
20. Adams JH, Doyle D, Graham DI, Lawrence AE, McLellan DR. Diffuse axonal injury in head injuries caused by a fall. Lancet 1984;2(8417–18): 1420–1422
21. Blumbergs PC, Jones NR, North JB. Diffuse axonal injury in head trauma. J Neurol Neurosurg Psychiatry 1989;52(7):838–841
22. Grady MS, McLaughlin MR, Christman CW, Valadka AB, Fligner CL, Povlishock JT. The use of antibodies targeted against the neurofilament subunits for the detection of diffuse axonal injury in humans. J Neuropathol Exp Neurol 1993;52(2):143–152
23. Smith DH, Meaney DF, Shull WH. Diffuse axonal injury in head trauma. J Head Trauma Rehabil 2003;18(4):307–316
24. Jane JA, Steward O, Gennarelli T. Axonal degeneration induced by experimental noninvasive minor head injury. J Neurosurg 1985;62(1): 96–100
25. Mittl RL, Grossman RI, Hiehle JF, et al. Prevalence of MR evidence of diffuse axonal injury in patients with mild head injury and normal head CT findings. AJNR Am J Neuroradiol 1994;15(8):1583–1589
26. Povlishock JT. Traumatically induced axonal injury: pathogenesis and pathobiological implications. Brain Pathol 1992;2(1):1–12
27. Gennarelli TA. Mechanisms of brain injury. J Emerg Med 1993; 11(Suppl 1):5–11
28. Ommaya AK, Hirsch AE. Tolerances for cerebral concussion from head impact and whiplash in primates. J Biomech 1971;4(1): 13–21
29. Wolf JA, Stys PK, Lusardi T, Meaney D, Smith DH. Traumatic axonal injury induces calcium influx modulated by tetrodotoxin-sensitive sodium channels. J Neurosci 2001;21(6):1923–1930
30. Smith DH, Wolf JA, Lusardi TA, Lee VM, Meaney DF. High tolerance and delayed elastic response of cultured axons to dynamic stretch injury. J Neurosci 1999;19(11):4263–4269
31. Metz H, McElhaney J, Ommaya AK. A comparison of the elasticity of live, dead, and fixed brain tissue. J Biomech 1970;3(4):453–458
32. Maxwell WL, Kosanlavit R, McCreath BJ, Reid O, Graham DI. Freeze-fracture and cytochemical evidence for structural and functional alteration in the axolemma and myelin sheath of adult guinea pig optic nerve fibers after stretch injury. J Neurotrauma 1999;16(4): 273–284

33. Hall GF, Lee VM. Neurofilament sidearm proteolysis is a prominent early effect of axotomy in lamprey giant central neurons. J Comp Neurol 1995;353(1):38–49
34. Adams JH, Graham DI, Gennarelli TA. Head injury in man and experimental animals: neuropathology. Acta Neurochir Suppl (Wien) 1983; 32:15–30
35. Blumbergs PC, Scott G, Manavis J, Wainwright H, Simpson DA, McLean AJ. Topography of axonal injury as defined by amyloid precursor protein and the sector scoring method in mild and severe closed head injury. J Neurotrauma 1995;12(4):565–572
36. Friede RL, Samorajski T. Axon caliber related to neurofilaments and microtubules in sciatic nerve fibers of rats and mice. Anat Rec 1970; 167(4):379–387
37. Reles A, Friede RL. Axonal cytoskeleton at the nodes of Ranvier. J Neurocytol 1991;20(6):450–458
38. Jafari SS, Maxwell WL, Neilson M, Graham DI. Axonal cytoskeletal changes after non-disruptive axonal injury. J Neurocytol 1997;26(4): 207–221
39. Szaro BG, Whitnall MH, Gainer H. Phosphorylation-dependent epitopes on neurofilament proteins and neurofilament densities differ in axons in the corticospinal and primary sensory dorsal column tracts in the rat spinal cord. J Comp Neurol 1990;302(2):220–235
40. Maxwell WL, Povlishock JT, Graham DL. A mechanistic analysis of nondisruptive axonal injury: a review. J Neurotrauma 1997;14(7): 419–440
41. Roof RL, Duvdevani R, Stein DG. Gender influences outcome of brain injury: progesterone plays a protective role. Brain Res 1993;607(1–2): 333–336
42. Roof RL, Hall ED. Estrogen-related gender difference in survival rate and cortical blood flow after impact-acceleration head injury in rats. J Neurotrauma 2000;17(12):1155–1169
43. Alkayed NJ, Murphy SJ, Traystman RJ, Hurn PD, Miller VM. Neuroprotective effects of female gonadal steroids in reproductively senescent female rats. Stroke 2000; 31(1):161–168
44. Wang Q, Santizo R, Baughman VL, Pelligrino DA, Iadecola C. Estrogen provides neuroprotection in transient forebrain ischemia through perfusion-independent mechanisms in rats. Stroke 1999;30(3):630–637
45. Pelligrino DA, Santizo R, Baughman VL, Wang Q. Cerebral vasodilating capacity during forebrain ischemia: effects of chronic estrogen depletion and repletion and the role of neuronal nitric oxide synthase. Neuroreport 1998;9(14):3285–3291
46. Miller JD, Butterworth JF, Gudeman SK, et al. Further experience in the management of severe head injury. J Neurosurg 1981;54(3):289–299
47. Marmarou A. Traumatic brain edema: an overview. Acta Neurochir Suppl (Wien) 1994;60:421–424
48. Fishman RA. Brain edema. N Engl J Med 1975;293(14):706–711
49. Hayes RL, Dixon CE. Neurochemical changes in mild head injury. Semin Neurol 1994;14(1):25–31
50. Wahl M, Schilling L. Regulation of cerebral blood flow—a brief review. Acta Neurochir Suppl (Wien) 1993;59:3–10
51. Bullock R, Maxwell WL, Graham DI, Teasdale GM, Adams JH. Glial swelling following human cerebral contusion: an ultrastructural study. J Neurol Neurosurg Psychiatry 1991;54(5):427–434
52. Schroder ML, Muizelaar JP, Bullock MR, Salvant JB, Povlishock JT. Focal ischemia due to traumatic contusions documented by stable xenon-CT and ultrastructural studies. J Neurosurg 1995;82(6):966–971
53. von Gertten C, Flores Morales A, Holmin S, Mathiesen T, Nordqvist AC. Genomic responses in rat cerebral cortex after traumatic brain injury. BMC Neurosci 2005;6:69
54. Graham DI. The pathology of brain ischaemia and possibilities for therapeutic intervention. Br J Anaesth 1985;57(1):3–17
55. Reilly PL, Graham DI, Adams JH, Jennett B. Patients with head injury who talk and die. Lancet 1975;2(7931):375–377
56. Becker DP, Miller JD, Ward JD, Greenberg RP, Young HF, Sakalas R. The outcome from severe head injury with early diagnosis and intensive management. J Neurosurg 1977;47(4):491–502
57. Astrup J, Siesjo BK, Symon L. Thresholds in cerebral ischemia—the ischemic penumbra. Stroke 1981;12(6):723–725
58. Branston NM, Symon L, Crockard HA, Pasztor E. Relationship between the cortical evoked potential and local cortical blood flow following acute middle cerebral artery occlusion in the baboon. Exp Neurol 1974;45(2):195–208
59. Jones TH, Morawetz RB, Crowell RM, et al. Thresholds of focal cerebral ischemia in awake monkeys. J Neurosurg 1981;54(6): 773–782
60. Siesjo BK. Pathophysiology and treatment of focal cerebral ischemia, I: Pathophysiology. J Neurosurg 1992;77(2):169–184
61. Siesjo BK. Pathophysiology and treatment of focal cerebral ischemia, II: Mechanisms of damage and treatment. J Neurosurg 1992; 77(3): 337–354
62. Kuroda Y, Bullock R. Failure of cerebral blood flow-metabolism coupling after acute subdural hematoma in the rat. Neurosurgery 1992; 31(6):1062–1071, discussion 1071
63. Schroder ML, Muizelaar JP, Kuta AJ. Documented reversal of global ischemia immediately after removal of an acute subdural hematoma: report of two cases. J Neurosurg 1994;80(2):324–327
64. Kontos HA, George E. Brown memorial lecture: oxygen radicals in cerebral vascular injury. Circ Res 1985;57(4):508–516
65. Jenkins LW, Moszynski K, Lyeth BG, et al. Increased vulnerability of the mildly traumatized rat brain to cerebral ischemia: the use of controlled secondary ischemia as a research tool to identify common or different mechanisms contributing to mechanical and ischemic brain injury. Brain Res 1989;477(1–2):211–224
66. Muizelaar JP, Wei EP, Kontos HA, Becker DP. Mannitol causes compensatory cerebral vasoconstriction and vasodilation in response to blood viscosity changes. J Neurosurg 1983;59(5):822–828
67. DeGirolami U, Crowell RM, Marcoux FW. Selective necrosis and total necrosis in focal cerebral ischemia: neuropathologic observations on experimental middle cerebral artery occlusion in the macaque monkey. J Neuropathol Exp Neurol 1984;43(1):57–71
68. Pulsinelli WA, Brierley JB, Plum F. Temporal profile of neuronal damage in a model of transient forebrain ischemia. Ann Neurol 1982; 11(5):491–498
69. Zauner A, Doppenberg E, Woodward JJ, et al. Multiparametric continuous monitoring of brain metabolism and substrate delivery in neurosurgical patients. Neurol Res 1997;19(3):265–273
70. Zauner A, Doppenberg EM, Woodward JJ, Choi SC, Young HF, Bullock R. Continuous monitoring of cerebral substrate delivery and clearance: initial experience in 24 patients with severe acute brain injuries. Neurosurgery 1997;41(5):1082–1091, discussion 1091–1093
71. Zauner A, Daugherty WP, Bullock MR, Warner DS. Brain oxygenation and energy metabolism, I: Biological function and pathophysiology. Neurosurgery 2002;51(2):289–301, discussion 302
72. Woitzik J, Weinzierl N, Schilling L. Early administration of a second-generation perfluorochemical decreases ischemic brain damage in a model of permanent middle cerebral artery occlusion in the rat. Neurol Res 2005;27(5):509–515
73. Sloviter HA, Kamimoto T. Erythrocyte substitute for perfusion of brain. Nature 1967;216(114):458–460
74. Geyer RP. Fluorocarbon-polyol artificial blood substitutes. N Engl J Med 1973;289(20):1077–1082
75. Franke RP, Reuter P, Rohlke W, et al. Interaction between a perfluorocarbon emulsion and radiographic contrast media. J Invasive Cardiol 2004;16(3):110–112
76. Satterfield R, Tarter VM, Schumacher DJ, Tran P, Mattrey RF. Comparison of different perfluorocarbons as ultrasound contrast agents. Invest Radiol 1993;28(4):325–331
77. Faithfull NS. Mechanisms and efficacy of fluorochemical oxygen transport and delivery. Artif Cells Blood Substit Immobil Biotechnol 1994;22(2):181–197
78. Faithfull NS. Oxygen delivery from fluorocarbon emulsions—aspects of convective and diffusive transport. Biomater Artif Cells Immobilization Biotechnol 1992;20(2–4):797–804
79. Padnick LB, Linsenmeier RA, Goldstick TK. Perfluorocarbon emulsion improves oxygenation of the cat primary visual cortex. J Appl Physiol 1999;86(5):1497–1504

80. Maxwell WL, Irvine A, Adams JH, Graham DI, Gennarelli TA. Response of cerebral microvasculature to brain injury. J Pathol 1988;155(4):327–335
81. Vaz R, Sarmento A, Borges N, Cruz C, Azevedo I. Ultrastructural study of brain microvessels in patients with traumatic cerebral contusions. Acta Neurochir (Wien) 1997;139(3):215–220
82. Osterholm JL, Alderman JB, Triolo AJ, D'Amore BR, Williams HD, Frazer G. Severe cerebral ischemia treatment by ventriculosubarachnoid perfusion with an oxygenated fluorocarbon emulsion. Neurosurgery 1983;13(4):381–387
83. Bell RD, Frazer GD, Brock DG, et al. Reduction of cerebral infarction using the third circulation. Crit Care Med 2002;30(12):2684–2688
84. Daugherty WP, Levasseur JE, Sun D, Spiess BD, Bullock MR. Perfluorocarbon emulsion improves cerebral oxygenation and mitochondrial function after fluid percussion brain injury in rats. Neurosurgery 2004;54(5):1223–1230, discussion 1230
85. Kawamata T, Katayama Y, Hovda DA, Yoshino A, Becker DP. Lactate accumulation following concussive brain injury: the role of ionic fluxes induced by excitatory amino acids. Brain Res 1995;674(2): 196–204
86. Pellerin L, Magistretti PJ. Glutamate uptake into astrocytes stimulates aerobic glycolysis: a mechanism coupling neuronal activity to glucose utilization. Proc Natl Acad Sci U S A 1994;91(22):10625–10629
87. Sutton RL, Hovda DA, Adelson PD, Benzel EC, Becker DP. Metabolic changes following cortical contusion: relationships to edema and morphological changes. Acta Neurochir Suppl (Wien) 1994;60:446–448
88. Chen T, Qian YZ, Rice A, Zhu JP, Di X, Bullock R. Brain lactate uptake increases at the site of impact after traumatic brain injury. Brain Res 2000;861(2):281–287
89. Rice AC, Zsoldos R, Chen T, et al. Lactate administration attenuates cognitive deficits following traumatic brain injury. Brain Res 2002; 928(1–2):156–159
90. Lenzlinger PM, Morganti-Kossmann MC, Laurer HL, McIntosh TK. The duality of the inflammatory response to traumatic brain injury. Mol Neurobiol 2001;24(1–3):169–181
91. Sachs F. Mechanical transduction by membrane ion channels: a mini review. Mol Cell Biochem 1991;104(1–2):57–60
92. Schwartz JHKE. Synaptic transmission mediated by second messengers. Principles of Neuroscience. New York: Elsevier Science; 1991;173–193
93. Siegelbaum SAKJ. Ion channels. Principles of Neuroscience. New York: Elsevier Science; 1991
94. Bowman CL, Ding JP, Sachs F, Sokabe M. Mechanotransducing ion channels in astrocytes. Brain Res 1992;584(1–2):272–286
95. Kimelberg HK, Norenberg MD. Astrocytes. Sci Am 1989; 260(4): 66–72,74,76
96. Orkand RK, Nicholls JG, Kuffler SW. Effect of nerve impulses on the membrane potential of glial cells in the central nervous system of amphibia. J Neurophysiol 1966;29(4):788–806
97. Tavalin SJ, Ellis EF, Satin LS. Mechanical perturbation of cultured cortical neurons reveals a stretch-induced delayed depolarization. J Neurophysiol 1995;74(6):2767–2773
98. Bullock R, Zauner A, Myseros JS, Marmarou A, Woodward JJ, Young HF. Evidence for prolonged release of excitatory amino acids in severe human head trauma: relationship to clinical events. Ann N Y Acad Sci 1995;765:290–297, discussion 298
99. Katayama Y, Becker DP, Tamura T, Hovda DA. Massive increases in extracellular potassium and the indiscriminate release of glutamate following concussive brain injury. J Neurosurg 1990;73(6):889–900
100. Nilsson P, Hillered L, Olsson Y, Sheardown MJ, Hansen AJ. Regional changes in interstitial K^+ and Ca^{2+} levels following cortical compression contusion trauma in rats. J Cereb Blood Flow Metab 1993;13(2): 183–192
101. Bullock R, Butcher SP, Chen MH, Kendall L, McCulloch J. Correlation of the extracellular glutamate concentration with extent of blood flow reduction after subdural hematoma in the rat. J Neurosurg 1991;74(5):794–802
102. Newman EA. High potassium conductance in astrocyte endfeet. Science 1986;233(4762):453–454
103. D'Mello SR, Galli C, Ciotti T, Calissano P. Induction of apoptosis in cerebellar granule neurons by low potassium: inhibition of death by insulin-like growth factor I and cAMP. Proc Natl Acad Sci U S A 1993;90(23):10989–10993
104. Choi DW. Glutamate neurotoxicity and diseases of the nervous system. Neuron 1988;1(8):623–634
105. Fineman I, Hovda DA, Smith M, Yoshino A, Becker DP. Concussive brain injury is associated with a prolonged accumulation of calcium: a 45Ca autoradiographic study. Brain Res 1993;624(1–2):94–102
106. Gennarelli TA. The spectrum of traumatic axonal injury. Neuropathol Appl Neurobiol 1996;22(6):509–513
107. Valadka AB, Goodman JC, Gopinath SP, Uzura M, Robertson CS. Comparison of brain tissue oxygen tension to microdialysis-based measures of cerebral ischemia in fatally head-injured humans. J Neurotrauma 1998;15(7):509–519
108. Persson L, Valtysson J, Enblad P, et al. Neurochemical monitoring using intracerebral microdialysis in patients with subarachnoid hemorrhage. J Neurosurg 1996;84(4):606–616
109. Bullock R, Zauner A, Woodward J, Young HF. Massive persistent release of excitatory amino acids following human occlusive stroke. Stroke 1995;26(11):2187–2189
110. Siesjo BK, Zhao Q, Pahlmark K, Siesjo P, Katsura K, Folbergrova J. Glutamate, calcium, and free radicals as mediators of ischemic brain damage. Ann Thorac Surg 1995;59(5):1316–1320
111. Lipton SA, Nicotera P. Calcium, free radicals and excitotoxins in neuronal apoptosis. Cell Calcium 1998;23(2–3):165–171
112. Kontos HA, Povlishock JT. Oxygen radicals in brain injury. Cent Nerv Syst Trauma 1986;3(4):257–263
113. Hall ED, Braughler JM. Central nervous system trauma and stroke, II: Physiological and pharmacological evidence for involvement of oxygen radicals and lipid peroxidation. Free Radic Biol Med 1989;6(3): 303–313
114. Rokutan K, Hirakawa T, Teshima S, et al. Implications of heat shock/stress proteins for medicine and disease. J Med Invest 1998; 44(3–4):137–147
115. Sarto C, Binz PA, Mocarelli P. Heat shock proteins in human cancer. Electrophoresis 2000;21(6):1218–1226
116. Takayama S, Reed JC, Homma S. Heat-shock proteins as regulators of apoptosis. Oncogene 2003;22(56):9041–9047
117. Zugel U, Kaufmann SH. Role of heat shock proteins in protection from and pathogenesis of infectious diseases. Clin Microbiol Rev 1999; 12(1):19–39
118. Pockley AG. Heat shock proteins as regulators of the immune response. Lancet 2003;362(9382):469–476
119. Dutcher SA, Underwood BD, Michael DB, Diaz FG, Walker PD. Heat-shock protein 72 expression in excitotoxic versus penetrating injuries of the rodent cerebral cortex. J Neurotrauma 1998;15(6):421–432
120. Reynolds LP, Allen GV. A review of heat shock protein induction following cerebellar injury. Cerebellum 2003;2(3):171–177
121. da Rocha AB, Zanoni C, de Freitas GR, et al. Serum Hsp70 as an early predictor of fatal outcome after severe traumatic brain injury in males. J Neurotrauma 2005;22(9):966–977
122. Guzhova I, Kislyakova K, Moskaliova O, et al. In vitro studies show that Hsp70 can be released by glia and that exogenous Hsp70 can enhance neuronal stress tolerance. Brain Res 2001;914(1–2):66–73
123. Amin V, Cumming DV, Latchman DS. Over-expression of heat shock protein 70 protects neuronal cells against both thermal and ischaemic stress but with different efficiencies. Neurosci Lett 1996; 206(1):45–48
124. Gonzalez MF, Shiraishi K, Hisanaga K, Sagar SM, Mandabach M, Sharp FR. Heat shock proteins as markers of neural injury. Brain Res Mol Brain Res 1989;6(1):93–100
125. Soares HD, Hicks RR, Smith D, McIntosh TK. Inflammatory leukocytic recruitment and diffuse neuronal degeneration are separate pathological processes resulting from traumatic brain injury. J Neurosci 1995;15(12):8223–8233
126. Biagas KV, Uhl MW, Schiding JK, Nemoto EM, Kochanek PM. Assessment of posttraumatic polymorphonuclear leukocyte accumulation

in rat brain using tissue myeloperoxidase assay and vinblastine treatment. J Neurotrauma 1992;9(4):363–371
127. Giulian D, Chen J, Ingeman JE, George JK, Noponen M. The role of mononuclear phagocytes in wound healing after traumatic injury to adult mammalian brain. J Neurosci 1989;9(12):4416–4429
128. Morganti-Kossmann MC, Rancan M, Otto VI, Stahel PF, Kossmann T. Role of cerebral inflammation after traumatic brain injury: a revisited concept. Shock 2001;16(3):165–177
129. Kim KS, Wass CA, Cross AS, Opal SM. Modulation of blood–brain barrier permeability by tumor necrosis factor and antibody to tumor necrosis factor in the rat. Lymphokine Cytokine Res 1992;11(6):293–298
130. Megyeri P, Abraham CS, Temesvari P, Kovacs J, Vas T, Speer CP. Recombinant human tumor necrosis factor alpha constricts pial arterioles and increases blood–brain barrier permeability in newborn piglets. Neurosci Lett 1992;148(1–2):137–140
131. Talley AK, Dewhurst S, Perry SW, et al. Tumor necrosis factor alpha-induced apoptosis in human neuronal cells: protection by the antioxidant N-acetylcysteine and the genes *bcl-2* and *crmA*. Mol Cell Biol 1995;15(5):2359–2366
132. Knoblach SM, Fan L, Faden AI. Early neuronal expression of tumor necrosis factor-alpha after experimental brain injury contributes to neurological impairment. J Neuroimmunol 1999;95(1–2):115–125
133. Merrill JE, Benveniste EN. Cytokines in inflammatory brain lesions: helpful and harmful. Trends Neurosci 1996;19(8):331–338
134. Gordon CR, Merchant RS, Marmarou A, Rice CD, Marsh JT, Young HF. Effect of murine recombinant interleukin-1 on brain oedema in the rat. Acta Neurochir Suppl (Wien) 1990;51:268–270
135. Selmaj K, Raine CS. Tumor necrosis factor mediates myelin damage in organotypic cultures of nervous tissue. Ann N Y Acad Sci 1988;540:568–570
136. Kerr JF, Wyllie AH, Currie AR. Apoptosis: a basic biological phenomenon with wide-ranging implications in tissue kinetics. Br J Cancer 1972;26(4):239–257
137. Sastry PS, Rao KS. Apoptosis and the nervous system. J Neurochem 2000;74(1):1–20
138. Clark RS, Chen J, Watkins SC, et al. Apoptosis-suppressor gene *bcl-2* expression after traumatic brain injury in rats. J Neurosci 1997;17(23):9172–9182
139. Clark RS, Kochanek PM, Chen M, et al. Increases in *Bcl-2* and cleavage of caspase-1 and caspase-3 in human brain after head injury. FASEB J 1999;13(8):813–821
140. Duriez PJ, Shah GM. Cleavage of poly(ADP-ribose) polymerase: a sensitive parameter to study cell death. Biochem Cell Biol 1997;75(4):337–349
141. Raghupathi R, Strauss KI, Zhang C, Krajewski S, Reed JC, McIntosh TK. Temporal alterations in cellular *Bax:Bcl-2* ratio following traumatic brain injury in the rat. J Neurotrauma 2003;20(5):421–435
142. Vogelstein B, Kinzler KW. p53 function and dysfunction. Cell 1992;70(4):523–526
143. Levine AJ. p53, the cellular gatekeeper for growth and division. Cell 1997;88(3):323–331
144. Martin LJ, Kaiser A, Yu JW, Natale JE, Al-Abdulla NA. Injury-induced apoptosis of neurons in adult brain is mediated by p53-dependent and p53-independent pathways and requires *Bax*. J Comp Neurol 2001;433(3):299–311
145. Miyashita T, Reed JC. Tumor suppressor p53 is a direct transcriptional activator of the human *bax* gene. Cell 1995;80(2):293–299
146. Miyashita T, Krajewski S, Krajewska M, et al. Tumor suppressor p53 is a regulator of *bcl-2* and *bax* gene expression in vitro and in vivo. Oncogene 1994;9(6):1799–1805
147. Antonsson B, Conti F, Ciavatta A, et al. Inhibition of *Bax* channel-forming activity by *Bcl-2*. Science 1997;277(5324):370–372
148. Cregan SP, MacLaurin JG, Craig CG, et al. *Bax*-dependent caspase-3 activation is a key determinant in p53-induced apoptosis in neurons. J Neurosci 1999;19(18):7860–7869
149. Boise LH, Gonzalez-Garcia M, Postema CE, et al. *bcl-x*, a *bcl-2*-related gene that functions as a dominant regulator of apoptotic cell death. Cell 1993;74(4):597–608
150. Oltvai ZN, Milliman CL, Korsmeyer SJ. *Bcl-2* heterodimerizes in vivo with a conserved homolog, *Bax*, that accelerates programmed cell death. Cell 1993;74(4):609–619
151. Reed JC. *Bcl-2* and the regulation of programmed cell death. J Cell Biol 1994;124(1–2):1–6
152. Linnik MD, Zahos P, Geschwind MD, Federoff HJ. Expression of *bcl-2* from a defective herpes simplex virus-1 vector limits neuronal death in focal cerebral ischemia. Stroke 1995;26(9):1670–1674, discussion 1675
153. Lawrence MS, Ho DY, Sun GH, Steinberg GK, Sapolsky RM. Overexpression of *Bcl-2* with herpes simplex virus vectors protects CNS neurons against neurological insults in vitro and in vivo. J Neurosci 1996;16(2):486–496
154. Martinou JC, Dubois-Dauphin M, Staple JK, et al. Overexpression of *BCL-2* in transgenic mice protects neurons from naturally occurring cell death and experimental ischemia. Neuron 1994;13(4):1017–1030
155. Ellis RE, Jacobson DM, Horvitz HR. Genes required for the engulfment of cell corpses during programmed cell death in *Caenorhabditis elegans*. Genetics 1991;129(1):79–94
156. Satchell MA, Lai Y, Kochanek PM, et al. Cytochrome c, a biomarker of apoptosis, is increased in cerebrospinal fluid from infants with inflicted brain injury from child abuse. J Cereb Blood Flow Metab 2005;25(7):919–927
157. Deshmukh M. Caspases in ischaemic brain injury and neurodegenerative disease. Apoptosis 1998;3(6):387–394

3 Biomarkers and Surrogate Markers

Sylvia Bele and Alexander Brawanski

Acute injuries to the brain, resulting from trauma, stroke, or cardiac arrest are the number one cause of death in people under the age of 40. Also, a large number of traumatic brain injury (TBI) survivors are permanently disabled, ~90,000 each year in the United States alone. This is a challenging situation, not only for the affected individuals but also for their families, and most importantly, for the society at large due to the rising health care costs. Thus, an accurate and reliable prediction of outcome following brain injury is important for head injury patients, clinicians, and society. So far, the outcome measurements most often used are the Glasgow Coma Scale (GCS) and the Glasgow Outcome Score (GOS) (see Chapter 6). Computed tomography (CT) or magnetic resonance imaging (MRI) is used to determine whether the TBI is localized or diffuse, without elucidating any of the biochemical cascades involved in brain injury following trauma. Furthermore, despite dramatically improved triage systems based on these outcome measures, most long-term survivors suffer lifelong impairment and are severely affected despite prediction of good outcome. Most limitations of current clinical assessment systems of brain injury are due to the fact that TBI is complex in pathology. It involves varying amounts of damaged tissue and/or different types of injury in each individual patient, and complex cellular and biochemical cascades are activated at the time of insult, leading to a variety of secondary injuries. Clinical assessments such as the GCS are often not helpful as anesthetics, sedatives, or other drugs applied at the trauma site might influence them. Neuroimaging methods such as CT or MRI have been proven to be valuable for detection and localization of acute brain damage. However, CT scans have limited sensitivity to mild injuries. MRI scanners, although they give higher resolution, are not widely available. All these aspects often limit the clinical evaluation of TBI patients.

Consequently, increasing effort is being devoted to the development of other tools to assess the severity of the initial brain injury, to identify patients at high risk for mortality and morbidity, and to predict outcome. The terms used for these tools are *biomarkers* or *surrogate markers*; surrogate markers are also termed *surrogate end points*.

By definition, a biomarker is a characteristic that is objectively measured and evaluated as an indicator of normal biological processes, pathological processes, or responses to a therapeutic intervention[1] (**Table 3.1**). It should appear in easily accessible material such as blood or cerebrospinal fluid (CSF) and should be highly sensitive and specific. It has its highest value in early efficacy and safety evaluations such as in vitro studies or in vivo studies in animal models.

A surrogate marker or end point is a marker that is intended to substitute for a clinical end point. It is expected to predict clinical benefit or harm (or lack of benefit or harm) based on epidemiological, therapeutic, pathophysiological, or other scientific evidence[1] (**Table 3.1**). Although all surrogate markers or end points can be considered biomarkers, it is likely that only a few biomarkers will achieve surrogate or end point status. The term *surrogate end point/marker* applies primarily to end points in therapeutic intervention trials; however, it is now applied in natural history of TBI to assess the initial severity of a trauma and possibly to predict outcome. In this application, surrogate markers need to be defined as highly sensitive for TBI and specifically connected with patient outcome.

Table 3.1 Definitions of Markers

Surrogate markers: Surrogate or end point markers are intended to substitute for a clinical end point. They are expected to predict clinical benefit or harm (or lack of benefit or harm) based on epidemiological, therapeutic, pathophysiological, or other scientific evidence.
Biomarkers: A biomarker is a characteristic that is objectively measured and evaluated as an indicator of normal biological processes, pathological processes, or responses to a therapeutic intervention. It should appear in easily accessible material such as blood or cerebrospinal fluid (CSF) and should be highly sensitive and specific.
Intention of using biomarkers or surrogate markers: The intention of using bio- or surrogate markers is to get new insights into the pathophysiology of brain trauma, that is, the effects of therapeutic interventions as well as the chance of a sufficient and efficient evaluation of patient outcome after traumatic brain injury at early time points.

To date, studies mostly focused on surrogate markers to predict outcome after TBI, using proteins that are expressed predominantly in the brain, released preferentially from damaged brain cells and transited into the CSF or into the blood stream via disrupted blood–brain barrier (BBB). Here, their quantity can be measured in correlation to the acute brain injury.

Evidence for efflux of brain proteins in humans was provided by reports showing that levels of certain neuronal and astroglial proteins are increased measurably in CSF or serum after TBI. The most extensively studied markers are the astroglial protein S-100β, myelin basic protein (MBP), neuron-specific enolase (NSE), and a proteolytic fragment of the microtubule associated protein tau, called cleaved-tau (C-tau). Unfortunately, high serum concentrations of those proteins have also been found with chronic disease unrelated to acute brain injury or even in its absence. Furthermore, not all kinds of brain injury occur with a measurable elevation in S-100β, MBP, NSE, or C-tau. Thus, none of those proteins has been established as a broadly accepted surrogate marker for acute brain injury.

Although brain-specific surrogate markers such as S-100β or C-tau may be useful clinical tools for predicting outcome, they provide no insight into neurobiochemical alterations mediating brain damage after TBI or ischemia. But biochemical signaling pathways underlying neurodegeneration could provide possible targets for developing mechanism-based markers for brain damage. It has been established that necrotic tissue injury of the brain is proportional to the primary insult, and outcome is related to the amount of tissue loss. But recent evidence suggests that besides necrotic cell death, programmed cell death (PCD) also occurs after TBI and may be involved in the complex mechanisms of secondary brain damage. Thus, there has been an increased interest in the development of biomarkers specific to different types of brain injury (focal or diffuse) to elucidate pathophysiological mechanisms operative in the traumatized brain. It is a widely accepted fact that treatment of brain injuries would benefit from understanding the pathobiochemical processes evoked by TBI, that is, the ability to monitor the beginning of secondary injuries and improvements concerning diagnosis at the time of onset of brain damage. This could possibly lead to more efficient interventions and the development of specially tailored therapies using surgical approaches or application of neuroprotective agents. These markers could also help to detect positive or negative treatment effects on patients. Because the development of neuroprotective agents is usually done in experimental TBI, biomarkers would also be a valuable tool for estimating the effects of neuroprotective agents used after TBI.

Surrogate Markers and Biomarkers of TBI

Due to the increasing numbers of bio- and surrogate markers, it is important to focus on those that are most promising for clinical application or those already used in clinical trials.

S-100β (Table 3.2)

S-100β is one of the most extensively studied potential markers for brain damage. It belongs to a family of Ca^{2+} binding protein of EF-hand type comprising 19 members so far, and is, together with S-100α, the most important subtype of this protein family. S-100 is a 21 kDa protein produced primarily by astrocytes and Schwann cells in the central nervous system and has been implicated in the Ca^{2+}-dependent regulation of a variety of intracellular functions such as protein phosphorylation, enzyme activities, cell proliferation and differentiation, dynamics of cytoskeleton constituents, structural organization of membranes, intracellular Ca^{2+} homeostasis, inflammation, and protection from oxidative cell damage. It has been documented that excessive S-100β levels promote the expression of inducible nitric oxide synthase or proinflammatory cytokines and exhibit detrimental effects on neurons (for review see Zimmer et al).[2] Studies using animal models of cerebral stroke or Alzheimer disease have suggested that the excessive S-100β produced by activated astrocytes precedes neurodegeneration.[3]

Table 3.2 S-100β

Advantages	• Ca^{2+} binding protein of the EF hand type
	• Most intensively studied surrogate marker
	• Easy to access in blood of CSF
	• Offers good clinical correlations and predictive value for unfavorable outcome after TBI in many studies, cut-off level $> 4\ \mu g/L$
Disadvantages	• Conflicting results
	• No better outcome prediction than CT scan
	• Extracranial sources
	• Available tests all cross-react with extracranial S-100.
	• No insight in trauma pathophysiology
Conclusion	Further studies with larger sample sizes are needed and the serum/CSF ratio of S-100 should be tested for higher predictive value

Abbreviations: CSF, cerebrospinal fluid; CT, computed tomographic; TBI, traumatic brain injury.

However, S-100β caught the eye of neuroscientists through cardiac surgery after miscellaneous interventions in cardiac surgery patients demonstrated elevated levels of S-100β.[4–6] Thirty to 50% of the patients showed neurological dysfunctions and up to 5% suffered from postoperative stroke. These patients also showed elevated levels of S-100β.[6,7] Hence, the study intensity concerning S-100β and its predictive value in the outcome of cardiac patients was extremely high, but the results were contradictory at times.[4–7] After bypass surgeries, S-100β showed a biphasic distribution pattern in which the early peak seemed to be connected to complications such as stroke. Studies in 2000 and 2001 show that most of the S-100β after cardiopulmonary bypass (CPB) with cardiotomy suction are due to extracranial sources[4,5] and vary according to whether the surgery was performed with or without the use of CPB.[8]

After these interesting initial findings, many groups have performed S-100β measurements in patients suffering from TBI (for examples, see references 9–20). TBI triggers a rapid increase in S-100β serum concentrations, which normalize 4 to 6 hour after a mild TBI but remain elevated 12 hours after severe TBI. The exact pathomechanisms of this time course still remain unclear, but it is believed that there is a continuous release of S-100β by injured glial cells and that the serum levels remain elevated due to a disrupted BBB. Studies from the last decade showed a relatively robust correlation between initial serum S-100β levels and outcome of patients after severe TBI.[9,11,20,21] Woertgen and Rothoerl showed an interesting correlation between elevated S-100β levels (> 2 µg/L) and the severity of damage shown in the CT or MRI as well as the outcome after TBI or polytrauma, revealing a serum level > 4 µg/L as an indicator for bad outcome.[9–11] Their data showed good clinical correlation and good specificity and sensitivity. These findings were backed by the data provided by Raabe et al.[20] In 2003 Raabe et al reviewed 18 clinical studies concerning S-100β levels and outcome.[21] Peak values of S-100β were demonstrated to have the highest correlation to any end point parameter. But despite these promising connections between outcome after TBI and serum S-100β levels, recent studies by Rothoerl et al[22] and Anderson et al[4,23] offered conflicting results, supported by the findings of Pelinka et al in 2003[24] and Routsi et al in 2006.[25] Patients from these studies showed significantly elevated S-100β serum levels without head injury,[22–25] thus suggesting that patient outcome and S-100β levels may not have any correlation at all.[26] Extracerebral sources of S-100β could be one reason for these inconsistent findings. Despite the fact that the brain contains the highest levels of S-100β, it is also found in fat tissue, skin, and muscle.[4,5,8,25] Thus, surgical procedures or bone and muscle injuries due to trauma could interfere with the measurement of S-100β. The most important finding of Anderson and colleagues was the detection that the S-100β monomer consists of two dimers, S-100α1β and S-100ßß.[4,23] Interestingly, almost all commercially available assays use the same antibody against the S-100 monomer, containing both dimers. Because isolated TBI is very rare, these findings cast doubt on the specificity and validity of increased S-100β concentrations as a selective marker for brain damage, especially in polytraumatized patients.

The most promising results were those found in children who underwent severe inflicted TBI[18,27,28] and in patients with isolated minor TBI.[29–31] However, even in these patient groups, some studies showed that S-100β was neither sensitive nor specific for inflicted TBI[32] or reflects only the findings of CT scans, GCS, and GOS, and that it is therefore not an independent surrogate marker for TBI.

Besides the lack of specificity, the other major shortcomings of S-100β are that it offers no direct insight in the pathomechanisms after TBI and that it did not correlate with trauma severity in experimental TBI.[33] These facts and the methodological problems surrounding the measurement of serum S-100β are a major concern among clinicians, averting the widespread clinical use of this marker. It would be helpful to develop an assay specifically detecting the S-100β form, which is concentrated much higher in brain tissue than in any other tissue of the body. In addition, further investigations with large patient numbers using CSF levels of S-100β and establishing a serum/CSF ratio of S-100β could be very helpful.[34] So far, S-100β provides useful additional information for outcome prediction, but only if used with care and not measured at a single time point because the time course of serum S-100β levels seems to give more reliable results.[16,35]

Neuron-Specific Enolase (NSE) (Table 3.3)

NSE is a glyceolytic enzyme localized primarily in the neuronal cytoplasm. In adults, NSE concentrations measured in CSF have served as markers of neuronal damage due to a variety of neurological disorders such as status epilepticus[36–38] or Creutzfeldt-Jacob disease.[39] Elevated NSE levels are also found in the CSF and serum[36,40–43] after TBI and were thus thought to be a possible surrogate marker for TBI. The findings of Yamazaki et al,[43] showing a good correlation between NSE serum levels > 50 ng/mL in blood samples from the jugular bulb vein and an unfavorable outcome after TBI, were weakened by the low number of patients and the fact that outcome scores were only performed at the time of hospital discharge. Later experiments clearly showed several shortcomings of NSE as a surrogate marker for TBI. Woertgen et al could clearly demonstrate that NSE serum levels reflect the severity of

Table 3.3 Neuron-Specific Enolase (NSE)

Advantages	• Glyceolytic enzyme located in the cytoplasm of neurons • Serum levels reflect severity of the initial trauma • CSF levels of NSE seem to reflect inflicted TBI in children and seem to reflect severity of the injury as well as outcome
Disadvantages	• All studies demonstrating a predictive value of NSE had low statistical significance • All studies had small sample sizes • No insight in trauma pathology • Extracranial sources of NSE (red blood cells, endocrine cells)
Conclusion	Further studies using larger sample sizes and using CSF as source of NSE levels are needed to establish NSE as an effective biomarker for TBI

Abbreviations: CSF, cerebrospinal fluid; NSE, neuron-specific enolase.

experimental TBI in rats,[44,45] but this has no clinical significance because NSE levels do not correlate with outcome in TBI patients.[46] NSE levels are not even an independent marker because they do not give better insights in trauma severity and outcome than the initial CT scan.

In 2004 Vos et al had promising results from a prospective study including 85 TBI patients measuring glial and neuronal proteins in serum and comparing their serum levels to clinical outcome.[40] They found a cut-off level of 21.7 µg/L for NSE predicting death or poor outcome better than clinical variables. The best results were obtained when NSE serum levels were used in combination with glial fibrillary acidic protein (GFAP) and GCS results, showing high sensitivity and specificity for prediction of unfavorable outcome. But a clinical trial by the same authors about surrogate markers after subarachnoid hemorrhage (SAH) proved that NSE serum levels from 67 patients did not reflect the severity of SAH or clinical outcome.[47] As regards the controversial results, almost all studies showing a connection between NSE levels and outcome after TBI[28,43,48] had several shortcomings such as small sample size, weak statistical significance, and outcome measurements only at the time of hospital discharge.

Another problem using NSE as a surrogate marker for brain injury arises from extracranial sources of NSE, mainly red blood cells, endocrine cells, or tumor cells, possibly falsifying the results. This could be avoided by using CSF levels of NSE for estimating trauma severity and outcome. A pilot study conducted by Berger et al[12] in 2002 revealed a specific NSE time course after severe inflicted TBI in children with robust elevation of NSE in CSF in two different peaks, the later time point possibly reflecting apoptotic neuronal death.[13] In their follow-up studies they found elevated NSE levels in serum or CSF in well-appearing infants after inflicted TBI.[28,32] They concluded that the correlation between CSF or serum levels of NSE and the severity of head trauma in children might be worth tracking because it offers the ability to identify inflicted TBI that might otherwise be missed. However, further investigations using larger sample sizes, different trauma types, and outcome measures after longer time periods are needed to find out if NSE holds true as a marker to screen for intracranial pathology after trauma and to identify occult TBI in children or in patients at risk after moderate or severe TBI.

Glial Fibrillary Acidic Protein (GFAP) (Table 3.4)

Early experiments focused on GFAP in CSF with promising results[49–52] but indicators of brain pathology measurable in blood are usually better because it is not always feasible or even possible to sample CSF. After van Geel and Missler published a method of GFAP measurement in blood,[53,54] GFAP became an interesting marker molecule. GFAP is a 50 kDa monomeric intermediate filament protein exclusively found in the astroglial skeleton that enters the circulation

Table 3.4 Glial Fibrillary Acidic Protein (GFAP) (50 kDa monomeric filament of astroglia skeleton)

Advantages	• Exclusively found in astroglia, therefore no extracranial sources • Marker of cell destruction • CSF levels showed very good correlation between severity of TBI • Even serum levels are a good predictor for mortality or disabilities or vegetative outcome after TBI, cut-off level 1.5 µg/L • Different expression patterns are found after different forms of brain injury • Good predictor for secondary brain damage after SAH
Disadvantages	• Studies had small sample sizes • Weak statistical significance in most studies • No correlation between initial GCS in most studies • Serum GFAP not easy to access (ELISA)
Conclusion	GFAP is an interesting and a promising marker for different kinds of brain injury, but, still, studies with higher patient numbers are needed, and maybe a combination between S-100 and GFAP is more predictive for patient outcome after TBI

Abbreviations: CSF, cerebrospinal fluid; ELISA, enzyme-linked immunosorbent assay; GCS, Glasgow Coma Scale; GFAP, glial fibrillary acidic protein; SAH, subarachnoid hemorrhage; TBI, traumatic brain injury.

upon loss of integrity of glial cells.[55] The existing data suggest that GFAP is in contrary to S-100β an indicator of cell destruction.[56–58] Because it is an exclusive central nervous system (CNS) expressed protein, no extracranial sources of GFAP could interfere with the results. This makes GFAP interesting for specifically estimating CNS damage. But can this protein hold up to the expectations?

Recent clinical studies revealed that GFAP is released to serum after TBI and the levels are related to trauma severity.[35,40,59,60] Pelinka's studies clearly showed that GFAP serum levels were related to the extent of brain damage, and that different patterns of TBI seemed to be associated with differences in GFAP release. They finally found that GFAP is a strong predictor in mortality and correlated well with severe disability and vegetative state.[35,59] These findings were supported by Vos et al who studied GFAP in comparison with S100-β and NSE after SAH.[47] They examined how closely the concentrations of those proteins in serum or CSF were associated with clinical severity. They concluded that the rise in serum levels of GFAP was congruent with the severity of the bleeding, rise in ICP, or higher CT-Fisher grade. Because it is known that SAH leads to loss of structural integrity of glial and neuronal cells and the release of cell-specific proteins into circulation, it is not very surprising that those proteins show higher levels in circulation. SAH patients have the potential for good recovery due to the limited degree of primary injury, but it is well known that secondary brain damage due to delayed cerebral ischemia (DCI) often impairs neurological outcome of those patients. Petzold et al reported that GFAP seems to be a very reliable marker for secondary brain damage after SAH because they found a typical second peak level of GFAP in CSF in patients undergoing vasospasm with unfavorable outcome and concluded from their results that GFAP may be a valuable marker for monitoring DCI in these patients.[61]

A recent study in TBI patients showed a 4.6-fold elevation of GFAP after severe trauma compared with controls, and GFAP levels were significantly higher in patients who died or had poor outcome 6 months later, with a cut-off level of 1.5 µg/L.[40] Interestingly, this study didn't show a significant correlation between serum GFAP and the hospital admission GCS. Thus, the authors suggested that brain-specific protein levels in serum might be good indicators for the initial severity of brain damage, if GCS scores cannot be obtained reliably in patients after TBI.

Nylen et al confirmed a clear correlation between levels of GFAP and unfavorable outcome after TBI even if samples were taken days after trauma.[60] This would be a useful clinical advantage because not all patients receive neurosurgical care in the first hours after TBI.

The problem with these studies is the low number of patients included, different results of GFAP time course (a range from 6 hours to days after TBI), as well as the problem that no clinician would really base his or her decision on a single potential biomarker. But especially in patients with unreliable GCS due to sedatives or intubation at the trauma scene, serum GFAP levels seem to be related to the severity of trauma and may be the most promising surrogate marker in this context for a first estimation of outcome.

Cleaved Tau (Table 3.5)

Surrogate or biomarkers reliably quantifying brain injury after experimental TBI are missing so far. Instead, histological assessment of lesion size and tissue loss is used to calculate trauma severity and the efficacy of neuroprotective drugs in experimental TBI. On the other hand, surrogate markers should also be potentially clinically applicable. Previous biomarkers NSE and S-100-β have failed to fulfill both requirements.

C-tau, a new and interesting marker, is a proteolytically cleaved form of the microtubule-associated protein tau (MAP-tau). MAP-tau is a neuronally localized cytoskeletal protein, targeted to the axonal compartment of

Table 3.5 Cleaved Tau (C-Tau)

Advantages	• Proteolytically cleaved form of the microtubule-associated protein tau (MAP-tau), a neuronally localized cytoskeletal protein, targeted to the axonal compartment of neurons
	• Exclusively found in the brain
	• Zemlan et al[68] and Shaw et al[70] demonstrated a direct connection between C-tau levels >0 in serum after TBI and unfavorable outcome
	• Elevated CSF levels >1000 ng/mL are related to poor outcome or death with almost 100% specificity and sensitivity
	• Offers insights in trauma pathology
	• Possible substrate for caspase-3
	• Serum levels may reflect integrity of blood–brain barrier after TBI
Disadvantages	• Studies (Chatfield et al,[73] Bazarian et al[74]) showed no correlation between c-TAU and outcome after TBI
	• All positive studies had small sample sizes, weak statistics
Conclusion	C-Tau seems to be a promising biomarker for evaluating the extent of neuronal damage in experimental TBI and may even be useful for testing the efficacy of neuroprotective agents, but so far the clinical implication is very limited

neurons.[62–66] Functionally MAP-tau binds to microtubules, resulting in the formation of axonal microtubule bundles, thus forming important parts of the cytoskeleton. These bundles are critical elements in the axoplasmic transport of proteins. Intact MAP-tau occurs in six isoforms in the CNS, resulting from alternative splicing of a single gene[67] with a molecular size of 48 to 68 kD. During neuronal injury in human TBI, MAP-tau is proteolytically cleaved on both the N- and C-terminals, resulting in a reduction of 18 kDa in all six isoforms[68,69] leading to a cleaved MAP-tau (C-tau) of 30 to 50 kD. Zemlan et al and Shaw et al showed that in human TBI C-tau levels were elevated 40,000-fold compared with neurological controls.[68,70] These studies indicated that MAP-tau undergoes proteolytic cleavage to produce C-tau after TBI in a reproducible manner. C-tau is released in the extracellular space gaining access to CSF and serum after axonal injury. In 2002, Shaw et al demonstrated in their pilot study that patients showing a C-tau serum level >0 after closed head injury, had significantly worse outcome compared with patients without C-tau in serum, independently from the CT findings.[70] The drawback of this study was the small sample size as well as the fact that the outcome was only measured at hospital discharge.

Also in 2002 Zemlan et al reported the correlation between elevated C-tau levels in CSF after human TBI and outcome at hospital discharge.[68] They were able to show an almost 100% sensitivity and specificity in patients after TBI with C-tau levels <1000 ng/mL and favorable clinical outcome as well as a significant correlation between unfavorable outcome and C-tau levels >1600 ng/mL. They also found out that a second peak in C-tau levels was often seen in patients developing elevated intracranial pressure (ICP) or secondary brain injury due to ischemia. However, even this study has limitations such as small sample size, and the fact that GOS was only taken at the time of hospital discharge despite the known fact that TBI patients often change in outcome over time, either showing improvement or worsening. In addition, only the relationship between initial C-tau levels and outcome was addressed, and the relationship of C-tau and other factors influencing the outcome after TBI such as patient age, injury severity, or presence of hematoma was not examined. After this primary assessment Zemlan et al performed another study in 2003 to examine the usability of C-tau as a marker for severity of induced neuronal injury in experimental TBI in rats.[71] They were able to demonstrate that C-tau levels in the rat brain as well as in the serum increased in a severity-dependent manner and therefore reflect the dynamic process of neuronal damage occurring after TBI. They compared histological data with C-tau levels to demonstrate neuronal injury after TBI. Brain C-tau levels increased in a time-dependent manner with peaks after 168 hours after injury. Similarly, histological measurements demonstrated a significant loss in cortical tissue at this time point. Interestingly the serum levels didn't show this time course. They were elevated 6 hours after TBI, but no significant increase was found after 24 hours or longer after injury. This might be due to the fact that the detection of biomarkers in serum is influenced by the integrity of the BBB. The BBB is maximally compromised within 6 hours of TBI in the rat suggesting that the normal serum C-tau levels after 24 hours may be associated with reestablishment of BBB integrity. The fact that in vitro evidence by Fasulo et al suggests that MAP-tau is a substrate of caspase-3 and that proteolytic tau fragments may be important effectors of apoptosis seems to support the connection between C-tau levels and neuronal damage.[72]

Chatfield et al[73] and Bazarian et al[74] reported C-tau being a very poor predictor of long-term outcome in patients with mild TBI, showing absolutely no correlation between initial serum or CSF levels and outcome.

According to these results, C-tau seems to be a very promising marker for neuronal damage and a possible test for the efficacy of neuroprotective agents in experimental TBI. But the clinical implication so far is very restricted because C-tau levels in CSF or serum seem to be unspecific in their predictive value for outcome after TBI. Further studies including larger sample sizes, short- and long-term survival or outcome, as well as different trauma severities are needed to rule out whether C-tau might be useful in clinical settings.

Spectrin Breakdown Products (SBDPs) (Table 3.6)

Despite the fact that focal and diffuse brain injuries can be evoked by different mechanisms, several studies to date have shown that similar biochemical cascades take part in the pathobiology of these different injury types. These studies have demonstrated increased activation of calpain and/or caspase-3 both after focal TBI[75–78] and diffuse brain injury.[79,80] Calpain and caspase-3 have also been shown to play an important role in the proteolytic cascades associated with several other CNS disorders such as stroke or ischemia.[81] Non-erythroid α II-spectrin, a major component of the cytoskeleton, is particularly abundant in axons and presynaptic terminals[82,83] and is a major substrate for both calpain and caspase-3 cysteine proteases.[84,85] Calpain-mediated cleavage of intact spectrin (280 kDa) occurs between Tyr1175 and Gly1177, resulting in 150 and 145 kDa fragments,[86] whereas the caspase-3–specific cleavage is linked to 150 and 120 kDa fragments,[84] called spectrin breakdown products (SBDPs). The use of selective α II-SBDPs antibodies has been used to demonstrate that brain regions with the highest accumulation of SBDPs also have the highest level of neuronal cell death.[75] Thus, the

Table 3.6 Apoptosis Markers

Advantages	• SBDP immunoblots offer concurrent information about calpain and caspase-3 activation after TBI • Offer good insights into the pathomachanisms after TBI • Farkas et al[87] showed significant correlation between high CSF levels of spectrin and unfavorable outcome • Possible monitoring of progression of damage after TBI
Disadvantages	• All studies used small sample sizes • Results not statistically significant • Difficult to assess • So far, only immunoblotting is able to detect SBDPs
Conclusion	For insights in trauma pathology, monitoring progression of damage, and even predicting outcome after TBI, SBDPs seem to be the most interesting molecules so far; however, for clinical use, there is a need for further advances in antibody-based specific and easy-to-use identification techniques so as to make identification of this marker easier for clinicians

Abbreviations: CSF, cerebrospinal fluid; SBDP, spectrin breakdown products; TBI, traumatic brain injury.

ubiquitous distribution of α II-spectrin in the brain coupled with the ability to utilize signature proteolytic fragments generated by either caspase-3 or calpain after TBI makes spectrin a potentially potent biomarker of brain damage. Using spectrins may also lead to an insight of biopathology after TBI. In 2001 Pike et al[85] demonstrated that after moderate TBI in rodents the calpain-specific SBDPs were elevated 244%, 530%, and 665% compared with sham operated control animals at 24, 48, and 72 hours, respectively, after TBI. In control animals no spectrin or SDBPs could be detected at any time point. This led to the conclusion that apoptotic changes or cell death after TBI is not only due to caspase activation but also to calpain activation after moderate TBI. They also found a correlation between the elevation in SBDPs and outcome of the animals after TBI.

In their 2005 article Farkas et al[87] provided promising insight into the possibilities that spectrin and its breakdown products may offer in clinical use. In their preliminary study conducted in patients with TBI, they could clearly demonstrate a connection between high levels of SBDPs in CSF and unfavorable outcomes. The samples taken from the control group showed no spectrin or SBDP at all. Interestingly, spectrin and SBDPs reached higher levels in TBI patients than in any other pathological condition associated with comparable ICP elevation, indicating that those changes are directly related to the trauma. Two patients showed a very interesting time course of spectrin and SBDP expression with a first peak level on day 2 and a second peak on day 7. Unfortunately, due to the small sample size no statistically significant conclusion could be drawn. Also, it has not yet been determined whether different kinds of brain traumas lead to different expression patterns or time courses of spectrin and its products.

SBDP immunoblots provide concurrent information about calpain[76] and caspase-3[88] activation, two of the most important regulators of cell death after TBI, thus offering interesting insight into the pathobiochemical mechanisms of trauma. Moreover, as the characteristic spectrin-derived products appear in easy accessible material, this may lead to a better monitoring of the progression of damage, response to medical intervention, and even prediction of patient outcome, thus making SSDPs a potential bio- and surrogate marker for TBI. Further advances in antibody-based specific identification technologies will facilitate development of fast, easy-to-use, and sensitive tests for research and clinical use.

Apoptosis Markers (Table 3.7)

The initial tissue injury of the brain is proportional to the primary impact; however, recent studies suggest that acute and chronic cell death after TBI may also be due to PCD or apoptosis (for details see Chapter 2). Apoptosis, a physiological cascade of strictly regulated cellular events, requires active initiation of transcription- and translation-dependent pathways and has been described in experimental models of TBI as well as in humans.[89–91] This kind of cell death is achieved through two caspase-dependent pathways, intrinsic and extrinsic, each of which is initiated by different mechanisms. The former by cytochrome c, the latter by binding of Fas ligand (FasL) to a death receptor such as Fas, leading to activation of caspases.[92] Because PCD is in most cases caspase-dependant, it seems logical to investigate activation of caspases, especially caspase-3, in TBI patients or after experimental TBI. Caspases are a family of cysteine proteases with at least 14 identified members, but few are fully characterized so far (for overview see Chowdhury et al[92]). Caspase-3 activation has been widely studied in experimental TBI using western blot analysis or immunocytochemistry.[88] Because

Table 3.7 Apoptosis Markers

- Offer interesting insights into pathomechanisms after traumatic brain injury
- May offer new targets for therapeutic interventions
- No significant correlations for, e.g., levels of sFAS and intracranial pressure or computed tomographic findings

there is a direct coherence between the amount of caspase activation and the number of apoptotic cell death, caspase-3 has become a valuable tool for recognizing secondary brain injury and for evaluation of possibly protective agents, capable of reduction of PCD.[93–96]

In 2006 Uzan et al[97] examined the CSF of 14 patients after TBI for caspase-3, sFas, and *bcl-2* and compared those results to the CSF of patients without trauma and to clinical findings such as GCS, GOS, and CT scans. They found that caspase-3 as well as another proapoptotic molecule, sFas, are significantly increased in the CSF of patients following severe TBI. Caspase-3 significantly correlated with ICP and cerebral perfusion pressure (CPP), which are good markers of severity of brain injury,[98] but not with initial CT findings. This was in accordance with the data reported by Harter et al[99] who also showed caspase-3 elevation with peak levels between days 2 and 5 after TBI.

The intrathecal release of proapoptotic molecules such as sFas, FasL, or *bcl-2* have been reported in a few research studies.[99–102] Fas, also called APO-1 or CD 95, is a membrane protein belonging to the tumor necrosis factor (TNF) receptor family, and whenever it interacts with FasL it will initiate the extrinsic cascade of apoptosis.[92] The results of Uzan et al[97] related to sFas were consistent to those of Ertel et al and Lenzlinger et al,[101,102] who demonstrated prolonged CSF release of sFAS for up to 2 weeks after trauma, but no detectable levels in control patients, suggesting that the presence of high sFAS levels reflects a pathological situation. Interestingly no correlations between sFAS levels and ICP, CPP, or CT findings were found, which is in contrast to Ertel et al who had demonstrated significant correlation between sFAS and ICP, CPP, and CT scans.[101] Those conflicting results may be attributed to insufficient sample size, which is a shortcoming of all these studies. The concordance between sFAS and caspase-3 level being highest on day 5 after TBI suggests that significant occurrence of PCD takes place at this time point. This allows interesting insights on the time frame of PCD after TBI and might show that there is a window for the application of potentially therapeutic substances that are able to inhibit apoptosis after trauma.

There is an increasing amount of PCD markers (for an overview, see Chapter 2),[92] but we focused on those molecules that give the most useful insights in brain pathology after TBI and that allow determination of biopathological pathways. Caspase-3 as effector, the pro-apoptotic Fas, or *bcl-2* as a potential antiapoptotic agent seem to be the most valuable candidates in this group of biomarkers. The parallel increase of these three molecules[97] may indicate that PCD plays a pivotal role in posttraumatic cell loss and edema and emphasize the significance of apoptosis markers as potential bio/surrogate markers for TBI. Further studies with larger sample sizes are needed to elucidate the role of posttraumatic apoptosis and may offer new targets for posttraumatic therapeutic intervention.

Conclusion

Despite several bio- or surrogate markers being available for several aspects of TBI, none of them so far meet the demands of an independent, highly specific, and sensitive marker for severity of TBI, which highlights the underlying pathomechanisms and estimates the outcome of patients. However, recent studies lead to the suggestion that it may be possible to develop a panel of clinically useful bio- and surrogate markers. These combinations of markers could provide better clinical information and help clinicians evaluate the prognosis of patients at early time points and may even help to identify patients at risk for clinical deterioration after mild TBI. Promising candidates such as SBDPs, apoptosis markers, and maybe a combination of two or more glial or neuronal markers (S-100-β, GFAP, NSE) need to be evaluated in future studies using larger sample sizes to be able to reach this goal.

References

1. Biomarkers Definitions Working Group. Biomarkers and surrogate endpoints: preferred definitions and conceptual framework. Clin Pharmacol Ther 2001;69(3):89–95
2. Zimmer DB, Cornwall EH, Landar A, Song W. The S100 protein family: history, function, and expression. Brain Res Bull 1995;37(4):417–429
3. Rothermundt M, Peters M, Prehn JH, Arolt V. S100B in brain damage and neurodegeneration. Microsc Res Tech 2003;60(6):614–632
4. Anderson RE, Hansson LO, Nilsson O, Liska J, Settergren G, Vaage J. Increase in serum S100A1-B and S100BB during cardiac surgery arises from extracerebral sources. Ann Thorac Surg 2001;71(5):1512–1517
5. Anderson RE, Hansson LO, Liska J, Settergren G, Vaage J. The effect of cardiotomy suction on the brain injury marker S100beta after cardiopulmonary bypass. Ann Thorac Surg 2000;69(3):847–850
6. Blomquist S, Johnsson P, Luhrs C, et al. The appearance of S-100 protein in serum during and immediately after cardiopulmonary bypass surgery: a possible marker for cerebral injury. J Cardiothorac Vasc Anesth 1997;11(6):699–703
7. Westaby S, Johnsson P, Parry AJ, et al. Serum S100 protein: a potential marker for cerebral events during cardiopulmonary bypass. Ann Thorac Surg 1996;61(1):88–92
8. Taggart DP, Bhattacharya K, Meston N, et al. Serum S-100 protein concentration after cardiac surgery: a randomized trial of arterial line filtration. Eur J Cardiothorac Surg 1997;11(4):645–649
9. Woertgen C, Rothoerl RD, Brawanski A. Early S-100B serum level correlates to quality of life in patients after severe head injury. Brain Inj 2002;16(9):807–816
10. Rothoerl RD, Woertgen C, Brawanski A. S-100 serum levels and outcome after severe head injury. Acta Neurochir Suppl (Wien) 2000;76:97–100
11. Woertgen C, Rothoerl RD. Serum S-100B protein in severe head injury. Neurosurgery 2000;46(4):1026–1027
12. Berger RP, Pierce MC, Wisniewski SR, et al. Neuron-specific enolase and S100B in cerebrospinal fluid after severe traumatic brain injury in infants and children. Pediatrics 2002;109(2):E31

13. Cotena S, Piazza O, Storti M. The S100B protein and traumatic brain injury. J Neurosurg 2006;104(6, Suppl)435–436, author reply 436
14. Townend W, Dibble C, Abid K, Vail A, Sherwood R, Lecky F. Rapid elimination of protein S-100B from serum after minor head trauma. J Neurotrauma 2006;23(2):149–155
15. Chen DQ, Zhu LL. Dynamic change of serum protein S100b and its clinical significance in patients with traumatic brain injury. Chin J Traumatol 2005;8(4):245–248
16. Pelinka LE, Toegel E, Mauritz W, Redl H. Serum S 100 B: a marker of brain damage in traumatic brain injury with and without multiple trauma. Shock 2003;19(3):195–200
17. Berger RP, Pierce MC, Wisniewski SR, Adelson PD, Kochanek PM. Serum S100B concentrations are increased after closed head injury in children: a preliminary study. J Neurotrauma 2002;19(11):1405–1409
18. Petzold A, Green AJ, Keir G, et al. Role of serum S100B as an early predictor of high intracranial pressure and mortality in brain injury: a pilot study. Crit Care Med 2002;30(12):2705–2710
19. Mussack T, Biberthaler P, Wiedemann E, et al. S-100b as a screening marker of the severity of minor head trauma (MHT)–a pilot study. Acta Neurochir Suppl (Wien) 2000;76:393–396
20. Raabe A, Grolms C, Seifert V. Serum markers of brain damage and outcome prediction in patients after severe head injury. Br J Neurosurg 1999;13(1):56–59
21. Raabe A, Kopetsch O, Woszczyk A, et al. Serum S-100B protein as a molecular marker in severe traumatic brain injury. Restor Neurol Neurosci 2003;21(3–4):159–169
22. Rothoerl RD, Woertgen C. High serum S100B levels for trauma patients without head injuries. Neurosurgery 2001;49(6):1490–1491, author reply 1492–149
23. Anderson RE, Hansson LO, Nilsson O, Dijlai-Merzoug R, Settergren G. High serum S100B levels for trauma patients without head injuries. Neurosurgery 2001;48(6):1255–1258, discussion 1258–1260
24. Pelinka LE, Szalay L, Jafarmadar M, Schmidhammer R, Redl H, Bahrami S. Circulating S100B is increased after bilateral femur fracture without brain injury in the rat. Br J Anaesth 2003;91(4):595–597
25. Routsi C, Stamataki E, Nanas S, et al. Increased levels of serum S100B protein in critically ill patients without brain injury. Shock 2006;26(1):20–24
26. Stapert S, de Kruijk J, Houx P, Menheere P, Twijnstra A, Jolles J. S-100B concentration is not related to neurocognitive performance in the first month after mild traumatic brain injury. Eur Neurol 2005;53(1):22–26
27. Meyer S, Gottschling S, Baghai A, Polcher T, Strittmatter M, Gortner L. The role of S100B-protein in neonatology, pediatric intensive care, and pediatrics. Klin Padiatr 2006;218(2):49–56
28. Berger RP, Adelson PD, Pierce MC, Dulani T, Cassidy LD, Kochanek PM. Serum neuron-specific enolase, S100B, and myelin basic protein concentrations after inflicted and noninflicted traumatic brain injury in children. J Neurosurg 2005;103(1, Suppl)61–68
29. De Kruijk JR, Twijnstra A, Leffers P. Diagnostic criteria and differential diagnosis of mild traumatic brain injury. Brain Inj 2001;15(2):99–106
30. Biberthaler P, Mussack T, Wiedemann E, et al. Evaluation of S-100b as a specific marker for neuronal damage due to minor head trauma. World J Surg 2001;25(1):93–97
31. Ingebrigtsen T, Romner B, Marup-Jensen S, et al. The clinical value of serum S-100 protein measurements in minor head injury: a Scandinavian multicentre study. Brain Inj 2000;14(12):1047–1055
32. Berger RP, Dulani T, Adelson PD, Leventhal JM, Richichi R, Kochanek PM. Identification of inflicted traumatic brain injury in well-appearing infants using serum and cerebrospinal markers: a possible screening tool. Pediatrics 2006;117(2):325–332
33. Rothoerl RD, Brawanski A, Woertgen C. S-100B protein serum levels after controlled cortical impact injury in the rat. Acta Neurochir (Wien) 2000;142(2):199–203
34. Hayakata T, Shiozaki T, Tasaki O, et al. Changes in CSF S100B and cytokine concentrations in early-phase severe traumatic brain injury. Shock 2004;22(2):102–107
35. Pelinka LE, Kroepfl A, Leixnering M, Buchinger W, Raabe A, Redl H. GFAP versus S100B in serum after traumatic brain injury: relationship to brain damage and outcome. J Neurotrauma 2004;21(11):1553–1561
36. DeGiorgio CM, Gott PS, Rabinowicz AL, Heck CN, Smith TD, Correale JD. Neuron-specific enolase, a marker of acute neuronal injury, is increased in complex partial status epilepticus. Epilepsia 1996;37(7):606–609
37. Schmitt B, Bandtlow C. Serum NSE in status epilepticus. Neurology 1996;46(6):1780–1781
38. Rabinowicz AL, Correale JD, Bracht KA, Smith TD, DeGiorgio CM. Neuron-specific enolase is increased after nonconvulsive status epilepticus. Epilepsia 1995;36(5):475–479
39. Kohira I, Tsuji T, Ishizu H, et al. Elevation of neuron-specific enolase in serum and cerebrospinal fluid of early stage Creutzfeldt-Jakob disease. Acta Neurol Scand 2000;102(6):385–387
40. Vos PE, Lamers KJ, Hendriks JC, et al. Glial and neuronal proteins in serum predict outcome after severe traumatic brain injury. Neurology 2004;62(8):1303–1310
41. Kleine TO, Benes L, Zofel P. Studies of the brain specificity of S100B and neuron-specific enolase (NSE) in blood serum of acute care patients. Brain Res Bull 2003;61(3):265–279
42. Ross SA, Cunningham RT, Johnston CF, Rowlands BJ. Neuron-specific enolase as an aid to outcome prediction in head injury. Br J Neurosurg 1996;10(5):471–476
43. Yamazaki Y, Yada K, Morii S, Kitahara T, Ohwada T. Diagnostic significance of serum neuron-specific enolase and myelin basic protein assay in patients with acute head injury. Surg Neurol 1995;43(3):267–270, discussion 270–261
44. Woertgen C, Rothoerl RD, Brawanski A. Neuron-specific enolase serum levels after controlled cortical impact injury in the rat. J Neurotrauma 2001;18(5):569–573
45. Woertgen C, Rothoerl RD, Wiesmann M, Missler U, Brawanski A. Glial and neuronal serum markers after controlled cortical impact injury in the rat. Acta Neurochir Suppl (Wien) 2002;81:205–207
46. Pelinka LE, Hertz H, Mauritz W, et al. Nonspecific increase of systemic neuron-specific enolase after trauma: clinical and experimental findings. Shock 2005;24(2):119–123
47. Vos PE, van Gils M, Beems T, Zimmerman C, Verbeek MM. Increased GFAP and S100beta but not NSE serum levels after subarachnoid haemorrhage are associated with clinical severity. Eur J Neurol 2006;13(6):632–638
48. Fridriksson T, Kini N, Walsh-Kelly C, Hennes H. Serum neuron-specific enolase as a predictor of intracranial lesions in children with head trauma: a pilot study. Acad Emerg Med 2000;7(7):816–820
49. Tullberg M, Rosengren L, Blomsterwall E, Karlsson JE, Wikkelso C. CSF neurofilament and glial fibrillary acidic protein in normal pressure hydrocephalus. Neurology 1998;50(4):1122–1127
50. Rosengren LE, Wikkelso C, Hagberg L. A sensitive ELISA for glial fibrillary acidic protein: application in CSF of adults. J Neurosci Methods 1994;51(2):197–204
51. Rosengren LE, Lycke J, Andersen O. Glial fibrillary acidic protein in CSF of multiple sclerosis patients: relation to neurological deficit. J Neurol Sci 1995;133(1–2):61–65
52. Noppe M, Crols R, Andries D, Lowenthal A. Determination in human cerebrospinal fluid of glial fibrillary acidic protein, S-100 and myelin basic protein as indices of non-specific or specific central nervous tissue pathology. Clin Chim Acta 1986;155(2):143–150
53. van Geel WJ, de Reus HP, Nijzing H, Verbeek MM, Vos PE, Lamers KJ. Measurement of glial fibrillary acidic protein in blood: an analytical method. Clin Chim Acta 2002;326(1–2):151–154
54. Missler U, Wiesmann M, Wittmann G, Magerkurth O, Hagenstrom H. Measurement of glial fibrillary acidic protein in human blood: analytical method and preliminary clinical results. Clin Chem 1999; 45(1):138–141
55. Eng LF, Ghirnikar RS, Lee YL. Glial fibrillary acidic protein: GFAP-thirty-one years (1969–2000). Neurochem Res 2000;25(9–10):1439–1451
56. Herrmann M, Vos P, Wunderlich MT, de Bruijn CH, Lamers KJ. Release of glial tissue-specific proteins after acute stroke: a comparative

analysis of serum concentrations of protein S-100B and glial fibrillary acidic protein. Stroke 2000;31(11):2670–2677
57. Valentim LM, Michalowski CB, Gottardo SP, et al. Effects of transient cerebral ischemia on glial fibrillary acidic protein phosphorylation and immunocontent in rat hippocampus. Neuroscience 1999;91(4): 1291–1297
58. Regner A, Alves LB, Chemale I, et al. Neurochemical characterization of traumatic brain injury in humans. J Neurotrauma 2001;18(8): 783–792
59. Pelinka LE, Kroepfl A, Schmidhammer R, et al. Glial fibrillary acidic protein in serum after traumatic brain injury and multiple trauma. J Trauma 2004;57(5):1006–1012
60. Nylen K, Ost M, Csajbok LZ, et al. Increased serum-GFAP in patients with severe traumatic brain injury is related to outcome. J Neurol Sci 2006;240(1–2):85–91
61. Petzold A, Keir G, Kerr M, et al. Early identification of secondary brain damage in subarachnoid hemorrhage: a role for glial fibrillary acidic protein. J Neurotrauma 2006;23(7):1179–1184
62. Brady RM, Zinkowski RP, Binder LI. Presence of tau in isolated nuclei from human brain. Neurobiol Aging 1995;16(3):479–486
63. Riederer BM, Binder LI. Differential distribution of tau proteins in developing cat cerebellum. Brain Res Bull 1994;33(2):155–161
64. Binder LI, Frankfurter A, Rebhun LI. The distribution of tau in the mammalian central nervous system. J Cell Biol 1985;101(4):1371–1378
65. Kosik KS. Traveling the tau pathway: a personal account. J Alzheimers Dis 2006;9(3, Suppl):251–256
66. Kosik KS. The molecular and cellular biology of tau. Brain Pathol 1993;3(1):39–43
67. Goedert M, Spillantini MG, Jakes R, Rutherford D, Crowther RA. Multiple isoforms of human microtubule-associated protein tau: sequences and localization in neurofibrillary tangles of Alzheimer's disease. Neuron 1989;3(4):519–526
68. Zemlan FP, Jauch EC, Mulchahey JJ, et al. C-tau biomarker of neuronal damage in severe brain injured patients: association with elevated intracranial pressure and clinical outcome. Brain Res 2002;947(1): 131–139
69. Zemlan FP, Rosenberg WS, Luebbe PA, et al. Quantification of axonal damage in traumatic brain injury: affinity purification and characterization of cerebrospinal fluid tau proteins. J Neurochem 1999;72(2): 741–750
70. Shaw GJ, Jauch EC, Zemlan FP. Serum cleaved tau protein levels and clinical outcome in adult patients with closed head injury. Ann Emerg Med 2002;39(3):254–257
71. Zemlan FP, Mulchahey JJ, Gudelsky GA. Quantification and localization of kainic acid-induced neurotoxicity employing a new biomarker of cell death: cleaved microtubule-associated protein-tau (C-tau). Neuroscience 2003;121(2):399–409
72. Fasulo L, Ugolini G, Visintin M, et al. The neuronal microtubule-associated protein tau is a substrate for caspase-3 and an effector of apoptosis. J Neurochem 2000;75(2):624–633
73. Chatfield DA, Zemlan FP, Day DJ, Menon DK. Discordant temporal patterns of S100beta and cleaved tau protein elevation after head injury: a pilot study. Br J Neurosurg 2002;16(5):471–476
74. Bazarian JJ, Zemlan FP, Mookerjee S, Stigbrand T. Serum S-100B and cleaved-tau are poor predictors of long-term outcome after mild traumatic brain injury. Brain Inj 2006;20(7):759–765
75. Newcomb JK, Kampfl A, Posmantur RM, et al. Immunohistochemical study of calpain-mediated breakdown products to alpha-spectrin following controlled cortical impact injury in the rat. J Neurotrauma 1997;14(6):369–383
76. Kampfl A, Posmantur RM, Zhao X, Schmutzhard E, Clifton GL, Hayes RL. Mechanisms of calpain proteolysis following traumatic brain injury: implications for pathology and therapy: implications for pathology and therapy: a review and update. J Neurotrauma 1997;14(3):121–134
77. Kampfl A, Posmantur R, Nixon R, et al. mu-calpain activation and calpain-mediated cytoskeletal proteolysis following traumatic brain injury. J Neurochem 1996;67(4):1575–1583
78. Pike BR, Zhao X, Newcomb JK, Posmantur RM, Wang KK, Hayes RL. Regional calpain and caspase-3 proteolysis of alpha-spectrin after traumatic brain injury. Neuroreport 1998;9(11):2437–2442
79. Buki A, Okonkwo DO, Wang KK, Povlishock JT. Cytochrome c release and caspase activation in traumatic axonal injury. J Neurosci 2000;20(8):2825–2834
80. Saatman KE, Bozyczko-Coyne D, Marcy V, Siman R, McIntosh TK. Prolonged calpain-mediated spectrin breakdown occurs regionally following experimental brain injury in the rat. J Neuropathol Exp Neurol 1996;55(7):850–860
81. Pike BR, Flint J, Dave JR, et al. Accumulation of calpain and caspase-3 proteolytic fragments of brain-derived alphaII-spectrin in cerebral spinal fluid after middle cerebral artery occlusion in rats. J Cereb Blood Flow Metab 2004;24(1):98–106
82. Goodman SR, Lopresti LL, Riederer BM, Sikorski A, Zagon IS. Brain spectrin(240/235A): a novel astrocyte specific spectrin isoform. Brain Res Bull 1989;23(4–5):311–316
83. Riederer BM, Lopresti LL, Krebs KE, Zagon IS, Goodman SR. Brain spectrin (240/235) and brain spectrin (240/235E): conservation of structure and location within mammalian neural tissue. Brain Res Bull 1988;21(4):607–616
84. Wang KK, Posmantur R, Nath R, et al. Simultaneous degradation of alpha II- and beta II-spectrin by caspase 3 (CPP32) in apoptotic cells. J Biol Chem 1998;273(35):22490–22497
85. Pike BR, Flint J, Dutta S, Johnson E, Wang KK, Hayes RL. Accumulation of non-erythroid alpha II-spectrin and calpain-cleaved alpha II-spectrin breakdown products in cerebrospinal fluid after traumatic brain injury in rats. J Neurochem 2001;78(6):1297–1306
86. Harris AS, Croall DE, Morrow JS. The calmodulin-binding site in alpha-fodrin is near the calcium-dependent protease-I cleavage site. J Biol Chem 1988;263(30):15754–15761
87. Farkas O, Polgar B, Szekeres-Bartho J, Doczi T, Povlishock JT, Buki A. Spectrin breakdown products in the cerebrospinal fluid in severe head injury: preliminary observations. Acta Neurochir (Wien) 2005;147(8):855–861
88. Beer R, Franz G, Srinivasan A, et al. Temporal profile and cell subtype distribution of activated caspase-3 following experimental traumatic brain injury. J Neurochem 2000;75(3):1264–1273
89. Liou AK, Clark RS, Henshall DC, Yin XM, Chen J. To die or not to die for neurons in ischemia, traumatic brain injury and epilepsy: a review on the stress-activated signaling pathways and apoptotic pathways. Prog Neurobiol 2003;69(2):103–142
90. Nathoo N, Narotam PK, Agrawal DK, et al. Influence of apoptosis on neurological outcome following traumatic cerebral contusion. J Neurosurg 2004;101(2):233–240
91. Ng I, Yeo TT, Tang WY, Soong R, Ng PY, Smith DR. Apoptosis occurs after cerebral contusions in humans. Neurosurgery 2000;46(4):949–956
92. Chowdhury I, Tharakan B, Bhat GK. Current concepts in apoptosis: the physiological suicide program revisited. Cell Mol Biol Lett 2006;11:506–525
93. Yrjanheikki J, Tikka T, Keinanen R, Goldsteins G, Chan PH, Koistinaho J. A tetracycline derivative, minocycline, reduces inflammation and protects against focal cerebral ischemia with a wide therapeutic window. Proc Natl Acad Sci U S A 1999;96(23): 13496–13500
94. Yrjanheikki J, Keinanen R, Pellikka M, Hokfelt T, Koistinaho J. Tetracyclines inhibit microglial activation and are neuroprotective in global brain ischemia. Proc Natl Acad Sci U S A 1998;95(26):15769–15774
95. Tikka TM, Koistinaho JE. Minocycline provides neuroprotection against N-methyl-D-aspartate neurotoxicity by inhibiting microglia. J Immunol 2001;166(12):7527–7533
96. Chen M, Ona VO, Li M, et al. Minocycline inhibits caspase-1 and caspase-3 expression and delays mortality in a transgenic mouse model of Huntington disease. Nat Med 2000;6(7):797–801
97. Uzan M, Erman H, Tanriverdi T, Sanus GZ, Kafadar A, Uzun H. Evaluation of apoptosis in cerebrospinal fluid of patients with severe head injury. Acta Neurochir (Wien) 2006;148(11):1157–1164

98. Saul TG, Ducker TB. Effect of intracranial pressure monitoring and aggressive treatment on mortality in severe head injury. J Neurosurg 1982;56(4):498–503
99. Harter L, Keel M, Hentze H, Leist M, Ertel W. Caspase-3 activity is present in cerebrospinal fluid from patients with traumatic brain injury. J Neuroimmunol 2001;121(1–2):76–78
100. Clark RS, Kochanek PM, Adelson PD, et al. Increases in *bcl-2* protein in cerebrospinal fluid and evidence for programmed cell death in infants and children after severe traumatic brain injury. J Pediatr 2000;137(2):197–204
101. Ertel W, Keel M, Stocker R, et al. Detectable concentrations of Fas ligand in cerebrospinal fluid after severe head injury. J Neuroimmunol 1997;80(1–2):93–96
102. Lenzlinger PM, Marx A, Trentz O, Kossmann T, Morganti-Kossmann MC. Prolonged intrathecal release of soluble Fas following severe traumatic brain injury in humans. J Neuroimmunol 2002;122(1–2):167–174

4 Noninvasive Monitoring

Michael Rubin, Wengui Yu, Mark A. Agostini, Christopher J. Madden, and Ramon R. Diaz-Arrastia

Acute management of patients with traumatic brain injury (TBI) remains a challenge. To minimize secondary injury and improve outcome, it is critical to detect neurological deterioration early, when it is potentially reversible. In awake and alert patients, monitoring evolution of brain injury can be effectively accomplished by astute clinicians and attentive nurses through the physical examination. In comatose, lethargic, or sedated patients, the examination is limited and additional studies are necessary to detect secondary deterioration, which is often subclinical. Secondary injury is a major cause of morbidity in brain trauma and may result from ischemic, inflammatory, or convulsive insults. The development of modern neuroscience intensive care units (neuro-ICUs),[1] allows intensive noninvasive bedside monitoring with the goal of obtaining real-time clinical data to optimize the management of trauma patients. The goal of noninvasive monitoring is to identify secondary insults early enough to allow the implementation of therapies designed to prevent further neurodegeneration. These methods attempt to gather vital information while minimizing invasiveness and complication risk. Additionally, they may help reduce the need to move the patient from the ICU to the computed tomography (CT) or magnetic resonance imaging (MRI) scanner and thus reduce the time away from the environment that is essential to his or her proper management.

A growing repertoire of noninvasive monitoring techniques have made their way into the management of TBI (see **Tables 4.1–4.7**). Although invasive probes serve essential functions in the ICU, the development of noninvasive technologies has been the major focus of much recent research. The oldest and most widely used noninvasive methods rely on recording of electroencephalographic potentials. This includes electroencephalography (EEG, **Table 4.2**), which has been available since the 1930s and continues to provide indispensable information to the neuroscience clinician. EEG has been updated by the use of digital recordings that allow long-term continuous monitoring, and computerized algorithms to assist in interpreting such data-intensive studies. EEG recordings are most valuable in the diagnosis of epileptic seizures, and recent findings indicate that seizures, both clinical and subclinical, are a common and significant comorbidity in comatose patients with TBI. Additionally, quantitative EEG (qEEG) analysis of particular frequency bands provides a measure of neuronal dysfunction and may be an early marker of cerebral ischemia. Continuous EEG monitoring, in tandem with qEEG analysis, may provide the neurointensivist information comparable to that available to a cardiologist following electrocardiogram (ECG) telemetry in the cardiac ICU.

Sensory evoked potentials (EPs, **Table 4.4**) have also been used in the ICU to monitor brain stem function and the integrity of thalamocortical connections. EPs differ from EEG in that instead of measuring scalp potentials of spontaneous cortical activity, they detect electrophysiological responses to an external stimulus that may or may not require a conscious response from the patient. For example, somatosensory EPs (SSEPs) measure EEG activity in a person stimulated at a distal extremity to analyze the entire pathway from nocioceptor to primary sensory cortex.

A major limitation of continuous EEG and EP monitoring is that application of electrodes and interpretation of the recordings requires highly trained EEG technologists

Table 4.1 Noninvasive Monitoring Technologies

Electrophysiological Measures	Abbreviation
Electroencephalography	EEG
Bispectral index	BIS
Evoked potentials (somatosensory, brain stem-auditory, visual)	EPS SSEP, BAEP, VEP
Vascular Monitoring Measures	
Transcranial doppler	TCD
Near-infrared spectroscopy	NIRS
Rhoencephalography	REG

Table 4.2 Electroencephalography and Quantitative Electroencephalography

Advantages	• Can provide continuous information with both temporal and spatial resolution
	• Alerts to many different types of physiological change: seizure, hypoxia, etc.
	• Well-established utility in treating seizures
Disadvantages	• Requires review by epileptologist of large amounts of data
	• Properly trained technician required to connect electrodes
	• Technical interference is common in the ICU
	• The significance of some waveform patterns is controversial

Table 4.3 Bispectral Index

Advantages	• Easy to set up • Single index value easy to interpret
Disadvantages	• Only provides an indication of level of awareness, does not provide data on specific events such as ischemia and seizure

Table 4.4 Evoked Potentials

Advantages	• Allows evaluation of an entire neurological pathway from stimuli transduction through cognitive processing • Can indicate subclinical deficits • Useful for prognostication
Disadvantages	• Evaluates a limited pathway at any one time

and clinical neurophysiologists, who are not practically available around the clock in the ICU. Another derivative EEG technology that has the potential to circumvent these limitations is bispectral index (BIS) monitoring (**Table 4.3**). BIS was originally created to measure depth of anesthesia, to assist anesthesiologists in the operating room. Recently BIS has being evaluated for its potential role in the ICU. BIS can be used to monitor changes in consciousness due to secondary injury, as well as help with the titration of sedative/hypnotic drugs by providing minimally sufficient sedation without overextending ICU recovery. Although it is unlikely that BIS will be useful in seizure detection, it may have a role in neurocritical care management because the electrodes can be readily applied by nursing staff, and its interpretation does not require an epileptologist.

In addition to the function of the brain parenchyma, prevention of secondary ischemic injury requires that the brain's blood supply be monitored. Subarachnoid hemorrhage, vasospasm, and reduced cerebral blood flow (CBF) are common complications of TBI. Three noninvasive technologies have been applied to these common complications. Transcranial Doppler (TCD; **Table 4.5**) is a form of ultrasound with a specific frequency range used to insonate the cerebral blood vessels. Like the other methods of noninvasive monitoring, TCD can be used at the bedside to prevent having to move the patient from the ICU for other means of investigation (in this case, for radiographic flow studies). Additionally, it can be used for the measurement of total CBF, and with new specialized mounting equipment can be adapted for serial or continuous monitoring. TCD has a well established place in the detection of vasospasm associated with aneurysmal subarachnoid hemorrhage. Near-infrared spectroscopy (NIRS; **Table 4.6**) uses light wavelengths that can penetrate several centimeters into scalp and bone to evaluate blood flow, similar to how TCD uses sound penetrance/absorbance to evaluate blood flow. Rhoencephalography (REG; **Table 4.7**) has been around for decades and has had a recent resurgence largely due to the efforts of the U.S. Department of Defense. REG uses EEG technology to evaluate vascular impedance, with the hope of providing a sturdy, battlefield-ready technique to measure intra-CBF.

Table 4.5 Transcranial Doppler

Advantages	• Can detect abnormalities of blood flow at the bedside • Useful for subarachnoid hemorrhage vasospasm and detection recanalization in stroke therapy • New equipment allows continuous monitoring
Disadvantages	• Accuracy is very operator dependent

Rationale for Noninvasive Neuro-ICU Monitoring

Secondary Neuronal Injury

The goal of neurocritical care is the prevention of secondary injury. Some series have shown rates of secondary injury in TBI to be as high as 91%.[2] Among the common causes of secondary injury detectable by noninvasive monitoring are seizures and ischemia. These insults are paroxysmal and transient, and techniques such as neuroimaging or brief electrophysiological studies that provide only snapshot assessments of cerebral function may miss clinically important but time-limited episodes. Thus, continuous monitoring is required to identify episodes that may produce secondary neuronal injury and require treatment.

Table 4.6 Near-Infrared Spectroscopy

Advantages	• Provides a single index value that can be easily interpreted • System is simple to set up
Disadvantages	• Does not provide specific information as to whether a hypoxic event is caused by a deficiency of flow or an excess of metabolic demand

Table 4.7 Rhoencephalography

Advantages	• Based on well-established electroencephalographic technology • Durable and less operator dependent then other vascular investigations
Disadvantages	• Insufficient data to establish validity

Seizures are a common mechanism of secondary neuronal injury. Seizures increase metabolic demand, and when they occur in the setting of marginal perfusion, an area of infarct much larger than the initial insult may result and lead to severe disability or death. Although convulsive seizures create complications by causing pyrexia and rhabdomyolysis, even nonconvulsive seizures (NCS) may result in secondary injury to cortical neurons due to extended neuronal firing and excessive release of excitatory amino acids and inflammatory mediators.[3] Seizures also increase glucose metabolism and raise intracranial pressure (ICP), which may lead to further secondary injury.

Ischemia is another common mechanism of secondary injury after TBI. Pathologically, most cases of lethal TBI demonstrate extensive laminar necrosis and ischemic neuronal death.[4] It is believed that ischemia is the most important cause of secondary injury, and incidence rates of up to 46% have been reported in TBI.[5] Thus, prevention of ischemic insults is a key goal of the neuro-ICU care of patients with TBI.

Another potential use of continuous noninvasive monitoring is their use as biomarkers in clinical trials. Studies on animal models provide convincing proof of the principle that therapies aimed at reducing secondary injury can significantly improve neurological outcome after TBI.[6] Despite this, clinical trials of neuroprotective agents such as polyethylene glycol–conjugated superoxide dismutase (PEG-SOD), tirilizad mesylate, calcium channel blockers, glutamate antagonists, and N-methyl d-aspartate (NMDA) antagonists have been successfully performed, but are so far negative.[7] It is likely that therapies may be effective only in some types of secondary injuries, and the ability to noninvasively monitor secondary ischemic or convulsive insults will be important in the early phases of clinical trials of therapies aimed at those injury mechanisms.

Advantages of Noninvasive Measurements

Noninvasive techniques have important advantages over other tools used in the management of the patient with TBI. Although they may never replace invasive techniques such as ICP monitoring, noninvasive tools may be superior under certain circumstances and should be included in the neuro-ICU repertoire. The most obvious advantages are that they are noninvasive and can be done at the bedside. The need for artificial ventilation, central venous and arterial access, and invasive parenchymal monitors provides many routes for infection and risk of organ system failure. Noninvasive monitoring devices do not penetrate skin nor provide added burden of systemic stress to patients in a fragile state. EEG monitoring is safe, the only risk being the less-than-pleasant smell of the adhesive glues used in the scalp probes of the EEG. TCD involves the application of high-frequency sound (albeit of low amplitude), which although incompletely studied, is unlikely to result in significant harm with long-term exposure.

The availability of noninvasive monitoring at the bedside also provides important advantages. The modern trauma ICU depends on highly skilled nurses and physicians and the proper equipment. Every minute the patient spends away from the unit results in increased vulnerability. Should a patient have a significant hemodynamic change or arrhythmia while in an elevator or in a CT scanner, the well-executed routine of critical care management might be disturbed to the detriment of the patient. If the patient is not in the critical care unit, it's difficult to administer critical care. Additionally, the need to transport patients to other parts of the hospital for imaging or other additional studies results in significant staffing demands in a busy trauma ICU and in some settings may negatively affect the quality of care.

The above considers the consequence of an event occurring coincidently during time spent away from the ICU; however, the transport itself might be deleterious. A patient may simply be so unstable that the idea of moving him or her is simply not acceptable and the intensivist has no choice but to use bedside examinations. Bekar et al took frequent measurements of patients with severe TBI on the way to CT scan and found an average 27% increase in ICP.[8] Others have compared secondary injury in ICU transport with ED transport of the same patient population and found that patients stabilized in the ICU had less secondary injury.[9] Put simply, a nurse and an assistant moving a bed, a ventilator, and IV poles posses a real risk to that patient. Research done to evaluate danger of transport is complex with numerous confounding variables of distance, equipment used, and personnel accompanying the patient, and it may not be definitive; however, it is clear that there are some patients who are simply too unstable to move, in which case there may be no choice but to rely on bedside testing.

Electrophysiological Monitoring

Electroencephalography (EEG)

EEG is unique in that it is the only investigative method that allows both spatial and temporal resolution simultaneously.[10] Spatial resolution refers to the anatomical localization of pathology; by comparing scalp electrode recordings to another electrode or ground, EEG creates a series of waveforms whose patterns differ due to where they originate and to which electrode they reach. This information can be used in conjunction with imaging to find if changes in waveform correspond to anatomical abnormalities. Unlike imaging, however, EEG can easily be recorded continuously and thereby provide temporal resolution, with measurements recorded as often as every 2 to 4 milliseconds.[10] Consequently, EEG can quantify pathology in all four dimensions versus a snapshot in time provided by CT.

The ability to measure neurological function on a continuous basis sets EEG apart. EEG is a summation of postsynaptic potentials modified by ascending diencephalic input. As the brain is altered by injury, so is the EEG; thus monitoring the EEG allows for continuous neurological surveillance. Although neurological examination is still the gold standard, it is of limited utility in a comatose or sedated patient. Complex partial seizures most commonly manifest as transient alterations in awareness, and they cannot be readily detected when a patient is obtunded or comatose at baseline. Although neurological examinations provide useful information, changes in neurological status might go undetected through physical examination until the next hourly neurological examination is performed.

EEG Monitoring of Early Posttraumatic Seizures

The primary and best-studied use of EEG in the neuro-ICU is for the detection of seizures. Seizures are hypersynchronus discharges of cortical neurons and represent both an immediate concern in the acute care and a long-term disabling sequelae of TBI. Although antiepileptic medications can be used to treat early posttraumatic seizure, they do not protect against the development of posttraumatic epilepsy. TBI results in potentially epileptogenic brain damage through several mechanisms, which may coexist within a single patient. Penetrating brain injury produces a cicatrix in the cortex and is associated with a risk of posttraumatic epilepsy of ~50%.[11] Nonpenetrating head injury may produce focal contusions and intracranial hemorrhages and is associated with a risk of posttraumatic epilepsy of up to 30%.[12] In this setting the mechanism of epileptogenesis may be partly related to the toxic effects of hemoglobin breakdown products on neuronal function.[13] Finally, closed head injury often produces diffuse concussive injury, with shearing of axons, diffuse edema and ischemia, and secondary cellular damage through the release of excitatory amino acids, cytokines, bioactive lipids, or other toxic mediators.[14] The incidence of posttraumatic epilepsy after diffuse head injury is less established but is likely to be in the order of 10% in patients who suffered loss of consciousness for >24 hours.[12] Epileptogenesis may arise from diffuse injury as a result of selective damage to vulnerable brain regions, such as the hippocampus.[15–17]

The best-studied indication for continuous EEG monitoring in the neuro-ICU is for the detection of subclinical NCS, which cannot reliably be identified through physical examination alone (**Fig. 4.1**). In animal models, seizures can lead to profound increases in ICP, CBF, cerebral

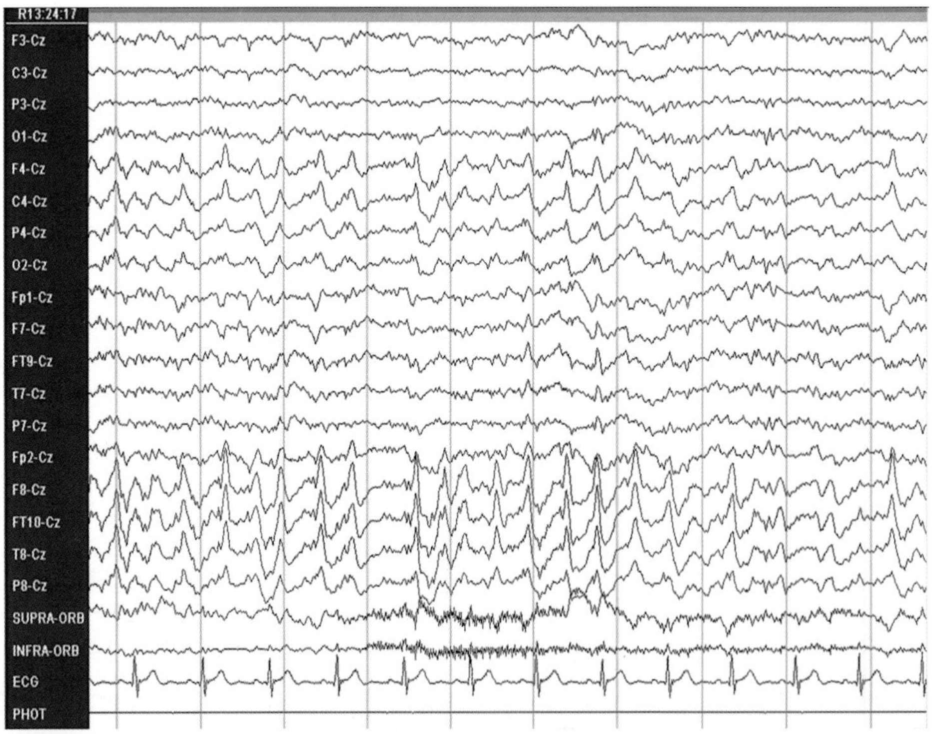

Fig. 4.1 Nonconvulsive seizure in 47-year-old man in coma after a motor-vehicle accident. Rhythmic sharp waves in the right temporal region lasted for 15 to 20 seconds and recurred every 3 to 4 minutes. There were no changes in behavior associated with these seizures noted by the intensive care unit staff.

metabolic demand, and may be associated with increased excitotoxic cell damage.[18–21] Thus, aggressive treatment of convulsive seizures during the acute postinjury period is the standard of care in all neurological and neurosurgical ICUs.[22] Further, prophylactic use of phenytoin, which decreases the incidence of early posttraumatic convulsive seizures,[23] is recommended by the Guidelines for the Management of Severe Head Injury[24], and is widely used in many centers. However, prophylactic antiepileptic drug therapy does not result in improved neurological outcome.[23,25,26] One criticism of these studies has been that because EEG monitoring was not performed during the acute hospitalization in these studies, subtle NCS could have persisted despite phenytoin therapy, and these subtle seizures may have resulted in a poor outcome. EEG studies are widely (if inconsistently) performed on patients with acute severe TBIs. These studies, which usually consist of 30-minute random samples of EEG, occasionally identify NCSs electrographically.[27,28] Litt et al[29] found that 11% of tracings contained NCS. A more recent study by Towne et al[30] identified NCS in 8% of 236 comatose patients who had EEGs as part of a prospective evaluation of coma. In most cases these were brief (30–60 minute) studies.

Improvements in EEG technology have made it possible to record and analyze EEG continuously for up to several days.[31] Such equipment is widely available and routinely used in epilepsy monitoring units for the characterization of seizures and the evaluation of patients with medically refractory epilepsy who are candidates for resective surgery. The use of such equipment in patients with TBI, or other forms of acute brain injury, has been less widespread. Several groups have used continuous EEG (cEEG) monitoring to determine the prevalence of NCS in patients with acute brain injuries. Young et al[32] found that 34% of 124 comatose neuro-ICU patients had NCS. Of these, 76% had nonconvulsive status epilepticus (NCSE). Patients with prolonged NCSE (>10 hours) had a dramatically increased risk of dying or being disabled (odds ratio [OR] 18, $p = 0.005$). Vespa et al[33] prospectively studied 94 patients consecutively admitted to their ICU with moderate-to-severe TBI. Seizures were identified electrographically in 21 patients (22%), and only six (6%) of these had clinically evident convulsive seizures. In this latter study, all six patients with NCSE died, compared with 19/88 (22%) of patients who did not have NCSE (relative risk [RR] 4.63, $p = 0.0002$). In the largest series to date, Claassen et al reviewed 570 cEEG recordings (including 51 patients with TBI) from the Columbia-Presbyterian Medical Center ICU over a 6.5-year period and found an overall prevalence of 19% for electrographic seizure; 92% of these were nonconvulsive, and 88% occurred within the first 24 hours.[34] For the 51 patients with TBI, nine (18%) had seizures, all of which were nonconvulsive. There is an emerging consensus from several leading neurocritical care centers that the prevalence of early seizures in TBI ranges from 19 to 44%, and the vast majority of these (52 to 92%) are nonconvulsive and would not be detected without cEEG monitoring (**Table 4.8**).[33–35]

Table 4.8 Prevalence of Seizures Detected by Continuous Electroencephalographic Monitoring

Study	Number of Patients	Percent of Patients with EEG Seizure	Percent of Seizures That were Nonconvulsive
Vespa et al, 1999[32]	94	22%	52%
Claassen et al, 2004[33]	570	19%	92%
Ronne-Engstrom and Winkler, 2006[34]	70	33%	Not reported
Jette 2006 (Critically ill children)	117	44%	75%

Although EEG has been used for decades to monitor seizures in patients with chronic epilepsy, the interpretation of cEEG recordings in the neuro-ICU continues to evolve. Whereas convulsive seizures with electrographic correlates are easily recognized even by a novice, some rhythmic waveform patterns seen in comatose patients in the neuro-ICU are controversial in their significance, terminology, and, most importantly, therapeutic implications. A committee of the American Clinical Neurophysiology Society met in 2004 to establish terminology of waveforms with less intrinsic implications.[36] For example, they advocated changing the term *PLED* (periodic lateralized epileptiform discharge) to *LPD* (lateral periodic discharge). That is, the term *epileptiform* was removed as it implies a particular significance of a PLED, which in the view of the committee remains controversial as to if and when they should be treated.[36] These guidelines have not yet won widespread acceptance.

It remains controversial when and for how long cEEG monitoring should be performed. It makes sense to start as soon as feasible after the brain injury. Claassen et al[34] found that most seizures were detected within 24 hours of starting the EEG record, and few additional seizures were found by recording >48 hours. However, the UCLA investigators[32] found that in 14% of patients seizures were found >2 days after injury, and advocate recording for up to 7 days.

The therapeutic implications of these NCS are unclear. NCS may contribute to secondary brain injury by resulting in excessive release of excitatory amino acids, oxygen free radicals, bioactive lipids, cytokines, or other potentially neurotoxic mediators.[18–21] Most investigators find that NCS, and particularly NCSE, is a poor prognostic sign.[33] However, it is also possible that these NCS are primarily a consequence of severe injury, and although they are associated with a poor outcome they may not contribute to neurodegeneration in a meaningful way. Thus, although most epileptologists favor treating NCS, the use of anesthetic doses of pentobarbital or propofol may not have a favorable risk-benefit ratio.[28] This is an important question for future research, which will have to overcome significant technical and methodological challenges.

EEG Monitoring of Cerebral Ischemia

cEEG recordings in comatose patients provide useful information beyond detection of NCS. EEG can alert to changes in blood flow, and δ slowing occurs when CBF falls below ~30 mL/100 g/min.[10,37] Such EEG findings have been correlated with decreased blood flow by use of positron emission tomography (PET) and xenon CT.[38] EEG can alert to the development of laminar necrosis in layers 3 and 6 after global ischemia[1] or to delayed cerebral ischemia in subarachnoid hemorrhage.[39] EEG changes are recognized to correlate well with significant infarcts, such as widespread polymorphic δ in hemiinfarction.[1] Subarachnoid hemorrhage results in diffuse δ/θ slowing with amplitude corresponding to level of consciousness.[39]

cEEG records can be analyzed quantitatively (qEEG) to provide information regarding cerebral ischemia while it is still reversible. The variability of the ratio of fast rhythm to slow rhythm (the relative α variability), may in fact precede such events as vasospasm.[40] The Columbia group has shown that the poststimulation α to δ ratio (PSADR; 8–13 hz:1–4 hz) corresponds with detection of delayed cerebral ischemia in subarachnoid hemorrhage by traditional means of TCD and angiography.[41]

Prognostic Information from EEG

EEG has also been extensively studied with the goal of providing prognostic information in TBI, which may have implications in decisions to continue aggressive care. For example, Vespa's group looked at a series of patients with Glasgow Coma Scale (GCS) ≤8 and found that a percentage of α variability of 0.1 or lower is predictive of poor outcome.[42] Similarly, EEG spectral analysis in post-TBI patients has been evaluated as an index of severity in a comparison with neuropsychiatry testing.[43] However, the evidence thus accumulated is not sufficient to reliably predict prognosis. Significant heterogeneity in the mechanism of TBI, complications, and hospital course make it impossible for one single investigative method to be dependable as a prognostic test. Whereas the clinical exam and individual patient-specific factors must be considered paramount in assessing prognosis, EEG may be useful in informing experienced clinicians attempting to counsel families and caregivers.

Technical Hurdles in Application of cEEG in the Neuro-ICU

Several technical hurdles limit the widespread use of cEEG in neuro-ICUs. cEEG remains a labor-intensive procedure that requires substantial technical and professional expertise to properly perform and interpret. Placement of electrodes requires highly skilled technicians, and the quality of the records must be continuously monitored and electrodes reapplied and regelled as required. Artifacts are common in the ICU environment because intravenous pumps, ventilators, and every device that uses electricity is a potential source of an interfering electromagnetic field. Further, nursing procedures such as repositioning and pulmonary toilet also produce artifacts that can be challenging to interpret. The use of video recordings in addition to cEEG is very helpful in assessing potential sources of artifact. Another major limitation is the lack of compatibility of many EEG electrodes with CT and MRI, which requires taking down an EEG set-up periodically. Whereas CT-compatible electrodes are available, MRI-compatible electrodes are not widely used. Attempts have been made to create compatible electrodes such as Ag-Ag/Cl wire electrodes that can be inserted subcutaneously.[44]

Probably of the greatest limitation to continuous EEG is the availability of qualified interpreters. Skilled interpretiion of EEG records requires a substantial amount of training, and it is impractical for a clinical neurophysiologist to monitor cEEG in real time. A solution to this problem may lie in the use of computer algorithms to analyze cEEG quantitatively using sophisticated software tools. Commercially available software programs create visual representations of EEG providing schemes that demonstrate seizure and cortical activity (see **Fig. 4.2**). Such programs could be used to signal an alarm when a waveform pattern is likely epileptogenic or could indicate early ischemia. At that point, a nurse or technologist can alert the neurophysiologist to confirm the finding and direct the ICU team to treat the event appropriately. Although similar technology has been used in epilepsy monitoring units for the seizure characterization of patients with chronic epilepsy as part of epilepsy surgery evaluations, the adaptation of such technologies to the ICU is still a work in progress even at leading institutions.

Bispectral Index Monitoring

As discussed above, a major limitation to the widespread use of cEEG recordings to assess neurological function in ICU patients with TBI is the technical and manpower requirements of this technology. An approach to this problem of EEG interpretation is to create a single index that represents the electrographic activity. Such is the

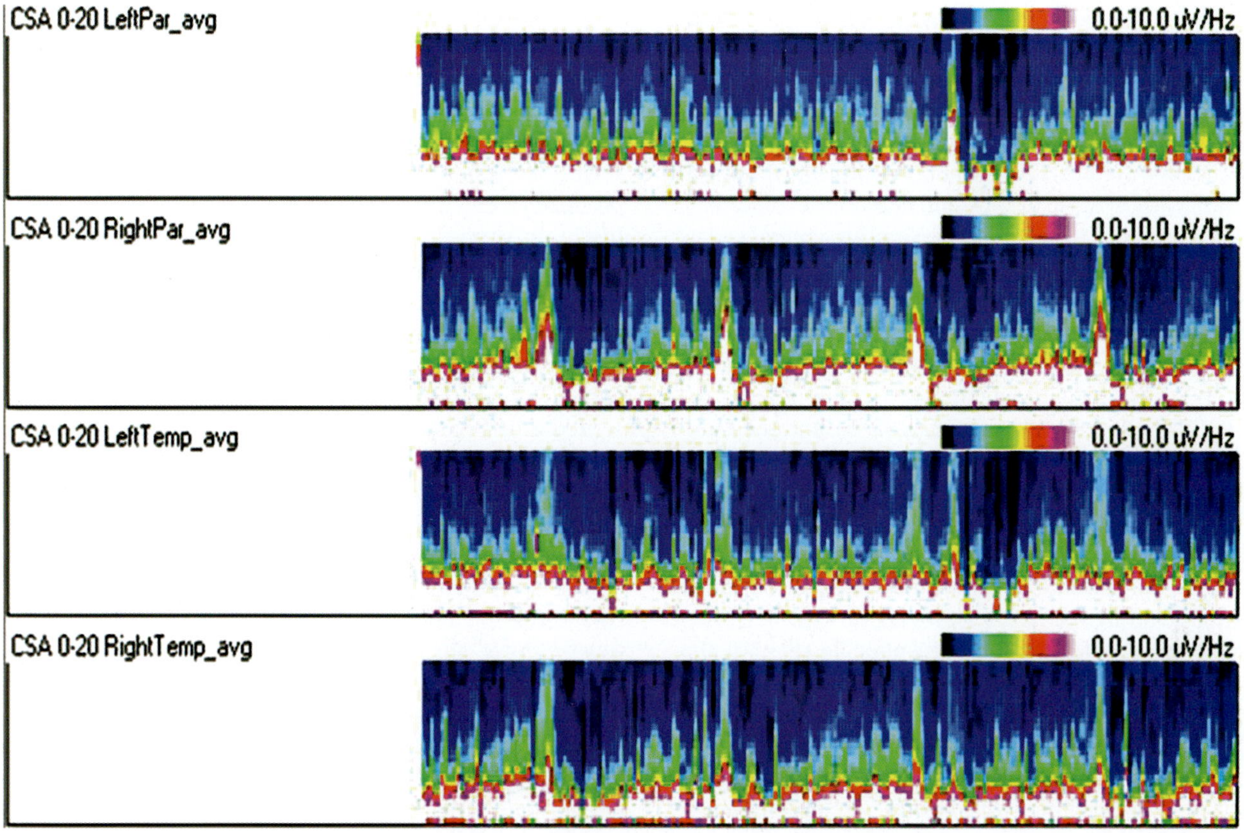

Fig. 4.2 Quantitative EEG (qEEG) analysis of a compressed spectral array, showing cyclic seizures manifesting as spikes in the power spectrum in the right parietal region. (Courtesy of Larry Hirsch, Department of Neurology, Columbia University).

rationale behind the use of BIS monitoring in the trauma ICU. Commercial devices initially developed to monitor depth of anesthesia in the operating room have been adapted to the neuro-ICU setting because they do not require expertise in placing the electrodes or interpreting the index. Although an index will never provide as much information as the full EEG, its ease of use makes it feasible for an ICU nurse to initiate a treatment protocol on the basis of a change in the BIS, if such a change can be demonstrated to indicate a real deterioration in the patient's status.

BIS was approved by the FDA in 1996 for monitoring depth of anesthesia and reducing the incidence of intraoperative awareness. The instrument has been widely adopted by anesthesiologists, and as of 2005 more than 25,000 units have been installed in U.S. hospitals.[44] The BIS system involves a four-electrode strip that is placed on the forehead and attached to a monitor that can be incorporated to a standard ICU monitor concurrently displaying a patient's vital signs and ICP. Bispectral analysis is a complex mathematical algorithm providing a weighted summation of multiple EEG parameters including time domain, frequency domain, and higher order spectral information. Interfrequency phase relationships are quantified providing a single 0 to 100 index value.[45,46] A value <70 represents a low likelihood of awareness and <60 an extremely low likelihood of awareness. Levels <40 are used for surgical hypnosis. BIS allows direct measurement of cerebral function to guide moment-to-moment titration of medication.

The ability of BIS to accurately report level of hypnosis has been extensively studied. Glass et al examined the ability of healthy patients to recall memory tasks after sedation with propofol, midazolam, isoflurane, and alfentanil with levels of sedation guided by BIS.[45] Multiple reviews have shown that BIS leads to a need for less anesthesia and improved recovery times postoperatively. Much of the information provided by BIS monitoring in the operating room applies to the ICU setting. Intensivists require the same balance between adequate anesthesia to reduce distress caused by awareness during ICU care and the need to allow for expeditious recovery from medication-induced anesthesia. Furthermore, BIS may provide a continuous value indicating level of consciousness that is useful in ICU patients, not only to guide sedation but also to gauge changes in neurological function. Recent publications have compared BIS with scales known to be valuable in assessing level of coma or near coma. Berkenbosch et al compared BIS values in a pediatric ICU population of 24 patients finding statistically significant correlation between BIS and PICU, Ramsay, and TSS scores.[47] Similarly, Gilbert et al studied 31 patients in a medical ICU with BIS monitoring, finding a correlation with APACHE III, GCS, and Reaction Level scale.[48] Consales et al chose to examine the Ramsay score of sedation in 40 patients and found a correlation to BIS.[49] As far as data specific to the TBI population, Deogaonkar et al studied 30 patients with TBI and measured every 6 hours their BIS and clinical neurological exam. These values were blinded to examiners of the patients; Richmond Agitation-Sedation Scale (RASS), Sedation-Agitation Scale (SAS), and the GCS, again finding statistically significant correlation.[50] A definitive review of these datasets has not been published, and there are some data to indicate that the correlation might not be valid.[51,52]

BIS has been examined in additional roles for patients with TBI, including its use as a prognostic indicator. For example, Haug et al looked at the use of BIS in TBI patients while they were still in the trauma bay of an emergency department. They found that of the 39 patients entered in the study, those with both a GCS <12 and a BIS <95 left the hospital with impairment.[53] Similarly, Fabregas showed that BIS could be used to predict which comatose patients were likely to recover consciousness.[54]

One of the limitations of BIS is that it requires frontal placement of the electrodes, which may interfere with other monitoring equipment, such as ICP monitors, or it may be in the field of a site of injury. If placed centrally or parietally, the BIS provides different values and changes the significance of the scale.[55] Thus, although there is promise that BIS monitoring may find a place in neuro-ICU care, particularly with regard to monitoring depth of sedation and potentially early detection of ischemia, much work remains to be done before its role in ICU monitoring is established.

Evoked Potentials in TBI

The effects of individual response to the external environment stimuli cannot be differentiated on conventional EEG. EPs allow detection of the cerebral response to an external stimulus, either auditory, visual, tactile, or motor action. In this manner, the electrophysiologist can determine the integrity of an entire function pathway from sensory transducer through afferent pathway, to CNS integration and response. Because the cerebral response to stimuli is of very low amplitude, they can be detected only by time-locking and averaging the signal from hundreds or thousands of stimulations, allowing the specific stimulus-evoked signal to summate while nonspecific EEG potentials that are randomly associated with the stimulus will cancel.[56]

EPs are designed to measure primary sensory pathways and the electrical response at the primary sensory cortex. Brain stem auditory EPs (BAEP or BAER) involve a series of clicks or tones heard through headphones that produce an electrophysiological measurement representing brain stem processing of those sounds. Amplitudes measure degree of response, and interpeak intervals represent processing time. BAEPs measure conduction time and relay potentials from the auditory signal to the eighth cranial nerve to the pons, midbrain, thalamus, and cortex.[55] Visual EPs involve a series of flashing lights presented to the patient with electrodes recording occipital lobe response. SSEPs involve the application of an external distal stimulus (typically to the median or peroneal nerves) and measurement of EPs along the spine and cerebral electrodes.

The components of the responses in EPs are indicated by a letter and a number. The letter, either a "P" for positive or an "N" for negative, represents the deflection on the EEG. The number indicates the milliseconds for the onset of that peak. For example, in BAEP, N1 represents the automatic CNS processing that occurs in 50 to 150 milliseconds. Waveforms are also delineated by Roman numerals. For example, in BAEP, a total of five waves are usually formed, with wave I representing the function of the cochlear nerve, wave II the cochlear cranial nerve nucleus and superior olivary complex, wave IV the lateral lemniscus, and wave V the inferior colliculus.[57]

EPs provide useful information in TBI for two main reasons. First, they can provide information as to subclinical deficits. That is, a person might not be aware of a posttraumatic hearing or visual deficit, but one may be detected in the EP. Furthermore, the specific location of the pathology on the pathway can be elucidated. The second use of EPs is for prognostic data in comatose patients. The comatose patient may provide little clinical data as to the likelihood of his or her chance of awakening because of a limited clinical exam, but electrophysiological testing might provide useful prognostic information.

Carter and Butt[58] published an extensive review in which SSEPs were compared with GCS, EEG, CT scanning, and pupil examination for predicting outcome of TBI. They found that in patients with good outcomes, SSEPs had superior sensitivity and specificity except for pupil exam (which had a superior sensitivity) and GCS (which had a superior specificity). In patients with bad outcomes, SSEPs had the best specificity. They concluded that with all cases of TBI overall, SSEPs were the best method for prognostication. SSEPs have been studied in the pediatric population for predicting outcome.[59] Amantini et al looked at awakening from coma in TBI over 7 days creating a grading system based on whether a hemisphere had normal, absent, or pathological SSEPs. The results were more reliable on either end of the spectrum, with a 93.1% positive predictive value (PPV) to awaken in those with normal studies or one hemisphere that was pathological and a 100% PPV for not awakening in those with both hemispheres having a pathological study or one with absent findings and the other either normal or pathological.[60] Fischer et al examined 346 coma patients (96 due to trauma) and found that 87% are likely to awaken if the N100 is present.[61]

For BAEPs, a prolongation of different waveforms in TBI has been reported (between I and III and between III and V.[46,50,51] Lew et al found in 11 TBI patients that not only did auditory but also visual event-related potentials had longer latency.[62] Plourde found that the 40 Hz auditory steady-state response provides a good measure of level of consciousness.[63]

Whereas EEG presents useful acute information, EPs delineate more specific pathways that have been shown to provide useful information as to level of impairment and prognosis. The implications of such studies are very significant: Although EPs initially are used to localize pathology, they provide information that can be used to help planning of future care of the TBI patient. Caution must be advised, however; treatment plans to discontinue care must not be made on just these studies alone. It would not be prudent, for example, to encourage the withdrawal of care of a comatose patient because an event-related potential predicts the likelihood of persistence of a vegetative state. The whole clinical picture must be considered.

Noninvasive Monitoring of Cerebral Blood Flow

Transcranial Doppler in TBI

TCD was first adopted from other ultrasound techniques to evaluate CBF. Before the onset of TCD, angiography was routinely required to evaluate flow in cerebral vessels. Although less invasive radiographic techniques have been developed, TCD has the advantage over angiography and nuclear testing in that it can be done at the bedside, allowing data to be gathered without having to remove the patient from the critical care unit. Likewise, TCD can be performed over extended periods with mounting equipment or simply frequently repeated without having to disturb the rest of a patient's critical care.

TCD was first used by Lee et al in 1997.[64] Using Doppler ultrasonography, a probe sends out a high-frequency pulse that undergoes a phase shift (the Doppler principle) as it contacts moving blood (primarily the cellular components). As it measures velocity only, the diameter of the vessel is needed to calculate flow. Use of TCD grew rapidly from its inception, and in 1990 the Academy of Neurology endorsed the value of TCD for diagnosis of intracranial stenosis, evaluation of collateral circulation, monitoring of vasospasm in subarachnoid hemorrhage, and determining brain death. Additionally, TCD can be used intraoperatively during vascular neurosurgery to help guide procedures. After the administration of tissue plasminogen activator (tPA), TCD can be used as a bedside measure to evaluate for recanalization. If an embolic source is determined to be likely during stroke, TCD can be used to find cerebral microembolic signals. In subarachnoid hemorrhage, TCD will help guide therapy in indicating the onset of vasospasm, so that therapy hemodilator hypervolume hypertension ("triple H") can be initiated to prevent infarction. Additionally, TCD can provide data on a patient in a barbiturate coma, whereas EEG would yield limited data as the patient's electrical activity is suppressed. TCD can be correlated to CBF, allowing approximation of ICP (assuming a constant mean arterial pressure [MAP]) without having to insert an ICP probe.

Conventional ultrasound uses a frequency of 3 to 10 MHz; however, these frequencies cannot penetrate bone.[64] In TCD, a 2 MHz frequency is used, with the probe applied over thinner areas of the skull, called insonation windows. The temporal window is commonly used, with the probe placed on the temporal bone above the zygomatic arch to insonate the middle cerebral artery (MCA) and anterior cerebral artery (ACA). Other windows used include through the eyes, below the jaw, and at the back of the head to insonate through the foramen magnum to evaluate the posterior cerebral artery (PCA), vertebral artery (VA), basilar artery (BA), and internal carotid artery (ICA).[65] The Doppler ultrasound is represented visually with different colors corresponding to changes in blood velocity (see **Fig. 4.3**).

Vasospasm is a serious complication of both aneurysmal and traumatic subarachnoid hemorrhage which occurs in 45 to 62% of patients.[66,67] Extravascular blood acts as an irritant to vessels and as they spasm exposes the brain to altering levels of flow that may induce ischemia. The so-called triple H therapy can reverse this complication by increasing the flow through vessels to stabilize them. Alternatively, interventional angioplasty may be performed to stabilize the vessels. TCD performs a vital function by indicating when such therapy should be initiated. Vasospasm is defined by an flow velocity (maximal) [FVm] above 200 cm/s and suspected if between 140 and 200 cm.[68] Lee et al found a significantly worse outcome in 152 TBI patients with vasospasm by TCD, which was confirmed by 133Xe cerebral blood flow imaging.[67] In patients with craniocerebral gunshot wounds, Kordestani et al found by TCD and 133Xe that 42% of the patients had vasospasm.[68] Through many studies comparing its findings to 133Xe cerebral flow, TCD has been shown to be a valuable bedside examination for the identification of vasospasm, of both the aneurysmal and the traumatic type.

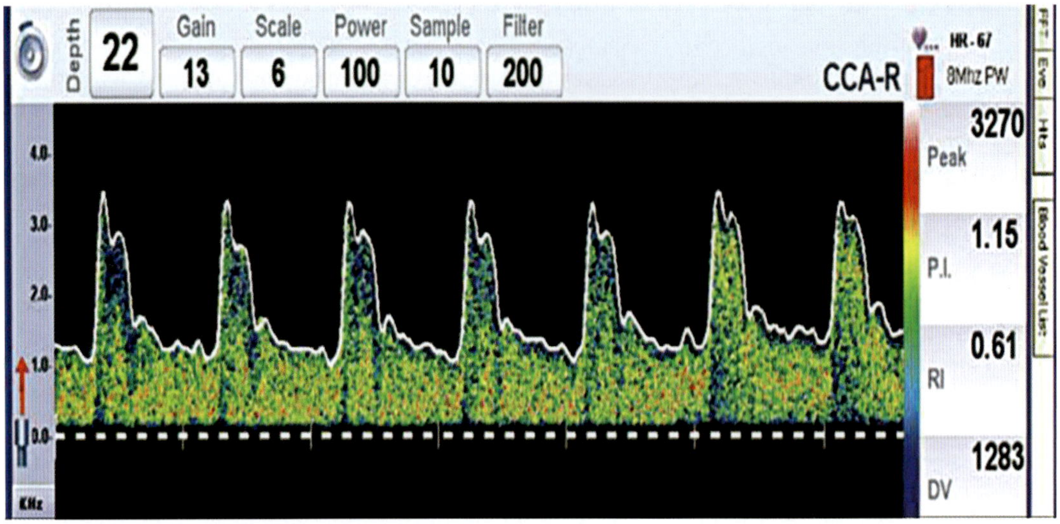

Fig. 4.3 Transcranial Doppler (TCD) waveforms.

Another application of TCD to TBI is the detection of cerebral ischemia before infarction occurs, giving time for interventions such as the use of pressors. Although radiographic evaluations will clearly delineate the presence of a cerebral infarction, and flow studies are useful for quantifying blood flow, they require removing the patient from the ICU. The validity of TCD for ischemia evaluation has been confirmed by comparison with such devices as the Licox probe (Integra Lifesciences Corp., Plainsboro, NJ). Licox is an invasive probe that measures parenchymal $P_{ti}O_2$. Van Santbrink et al compared Licox measurements in 57 patients with TBI and a GCS less then 8 with TCD measurements in the first 72 hours after insult and found that 63% had low flow by TCD, which corresponded to hypoxia by Licox.[69]

Another use of TCD is to indirectly monitor ICP by measuring CBF. As ICP rises in TBI, the concern is that the brain will be inadequately perfused and suffer from ischemia, eventually causing parenchymal infarction. Traditionally, an ICP monitor is placed in either the parenchyma or a ventricle to indicate when medical or surgical management must be changed during the edema and hydrocephalus that commonly occur in TBI. If TCD values can be correlated accurately with cerebral perfusion pressure (CPP) or ICP, the need for an invasive device might be avoided. Voulgaris et al used a concept called the pulsatility index (PI) to investigate such a correlation.[71] The PI is the difference between the systolic and the diastolic flow velocities divided by the mean velocity, and it provides a single value to compare with ICP. The researchers took 37 patients with a GCS <8 and measured the PI and compared it with ICP measured by an invasive device. They found a significant correlation between PI, CPP, and ICP.[70]

TCD has found use in brain death determination in TBI and other catastrophic neurological insults. The clinical exam and apnea test are often conclusive in determination of brain death; however, an occasion might arise where either an exam is inconclusive or concern for lingering medication levels leads the determination unproven. With TCD, lack of flow can be shown to corroborate the determination. Kuo et al studied 101 comatose patients determined to be clinically brain dead and found the basilar artery to be a valuable predictor of brain death with a sensitivity of 77.2% and a specificity of 100%.[71]

Despite the utility of TCD in detecting spasm and flow, it does have the limitations of being dependent on skilled technicians. Furthermore, although its use for flow is certain, using it to determine oxygenation of tissue in the evaluation of ischemia is limited in that it requires a significant inference: that perfusion equates to sufficient oxygenation. If hemoglobin concentration and alveolar oxygenation are not normal (which is often the case in critically ill patients) the flow delivered might be insufficient for metabolic need. A more recently developed technology, near-infrared spectroscopy (NIRS), might address this need.

Near-Infrared Spectroscopy

NIRS involves a light-emitting diode with one or two detectors a few centimeters away that measures the ratio of oxyhemoglobin (HbO_2) to total hemoglobin (THb) and creates an absolute regional oxygen saturation index (rSO_2).[72] Whereas visible light (450–700 nm) is almost completely absorbed by soft tissue and bone, near-infrared uses wavelengths of 700 to 1100 nm, which is able to penetrate ~10 cm of scalp and bone to reach the cerebral blood vessels.[73] Depending on the amount of light absorbed and returned, oxygenation can be determined intracranially.[72]

McLeod et al helped validate this technology by comparing jugular oxygen saturation, invasive tissue brain oxygenation, and NIRS in eight severe TBI patients.[73] Values of the three measures were compared at a fraction of inspired oxygen (FIO_2) of 1.0, 0.6, and 0.02 to 0.05 less than their baseline requirements. All three measures correlated in this small population sample.[74] Other studies have shown contrary results.[75] Clearly, more extensive studies are required.

An obvious comparison could be made to pulse oximetry. The difference is that multiple transducers are used because a straight line cannot be obtained with NIRS, which requires the geometric extrapolation of returning energy to determine the ratio of oxygenation. Furthermore, pulse oximetry depends on pulsatile flow, whereas NIR does not.[73] NIRS does require more ancillary equipment than a pulse oximeter including fiber optic cabling and its own computer; however, this could eventually be integrated to an ICU multimonitoring apparatus.

Although NIRS is in its infancy, its applications might be very beneficial. It can be used continuously, does not require much daily maintenance, and can produce a single index. If multiple transducers are used, oxygenation specific to a hemisphere or lobe might be determined, potentially warning the ICU team of an impending ischemic episode. It has advantages over invasive probes in that it doesn't risk infection and tissue damage. Whereas pulse oximetry is a well established technology, it does not indicate central oxygen delivery; in a patient on pressors, peripheral oxygenation might be compromised but CNS oxygenation may be adequate. The major limitation in NIRS is that it provides a ratio of oxygenation without indicating whether it is because of inadequate perfusion or excessive metabolic use.[72]

Rhoencephalography

The last method of monitoring vascular neurology is a new adaptation of an older technology. REG was initially developed in the 1950s as a bedside measure of CBF. The principle is measuring with an EEG scalp electrode the electrical impedance of brain and blood as they change with heart rhythm.[76] Two different methods are used: REG I (one pair of recording electrodes) and REG II (two pairs of recording electrodes).[76] As an arterial pulse passes between the electrodes, the recorded EEG waveforms are compared with calculate impedance and from that blood flow. Much debate exists as to which algorithm to use for signal calculation, and there is much concern that the method might inadvertently measure scalp blood vessels. Although this technology has been available for 5 decades, it was largely abandoned until a recent resurgence, mostly by the U.S. military to discover a battlefield-ready method to measure cerebral flow.[77]

Conclusion

Cerebral tissue is extremely unforgiving and fragile. Numerous threats loom over the TBI patient. A constant concern for seizure and ischemia must be attended. In an already damaged brain the ideal method of prevention would require keeping a patient in the critical care environment, provide useful and reliable information, and not expose the patient to any further risk. We are on the horizon of a paradigm shift in neurocritical care where tools of electrophysiology will not be used just piecemeal but as a continuous means of interrogating the CNS. With improvements in detection of secondary injury we can apply the improvements in TBI management, and ultimately reach our goal of improving the outcome of TBI patients.

Acknowledgments Work in Dr. Diaz-Arrastia's laboratory was supported by NIH-NICDH grants (R01 HD48179, U01 HD42652), and a U.S. Dept. of Education grant (H133 A020526) (to RD-A).

References

1. Jordan KG. Continuous EEG monitoring in the neuroscience intensive care unit and emergency department. J Clin Neurophysiol 1999;16: 14–39
2. Jones PA, Andrews PJ, Midgley S, et al. Measuring the burden of secondary insults in head-injured patients during intensive care. J Neurosurg Anesthesiol 1994;6:4–14
3. Vespa P, Prins M, Ronne-Engstrom E, et al. Increase in extracellular glutamate caused by reduced cerebral perfusion pressure and seizures after human traumatic brain injury: a microdialysis study. J Neurosurg 1998;89:971–982
4. Graham DI, Ford I, Adams JH, et al. Ischaemic brain damage is still common in fatal non-missile head injury. J Neurol Neurosurg Psychiatry 1989;52:346–350
5. Sahuquillo J, Poca MA, Garnacho A, et al. Early ischaemia after severe head injury: preliminary results in patients with diffuse brain injuries. Acta Neurochir (Wien) 1993;122:204–214
6. McIntosh TK, Juhler M, Wieloch T. Novel pharmacologic strategies in the treatment of experimental brain injury. J Neurotrauma 1998;15:731–769
7. Narayan RK, Michel ME, The Clinical Trials in Head Injury Study Group. Clinical trials in head injury. J Neurotrauma 2002;19:503–557
8. Bekar A, Ipekoglu Z, Tureyen K, Bilgin H, Korfali G, Korfali E. Secondary insults during intrahospital transport of neurosurgical intensive care patients. Neurosurg Rev 1998;21:98–101
9. Andrews PJ, Piper IR, Dearden NM, Miller JD. Secondary insults during intrahospital transport of head-injured patients. Lancet 1990;335: 327–330
10. Scheuer ML. Continuous EEG monitoring in the intensive care unit. Epilepsia 2002;43(Suppl 3):114–127
11. Salazar AM, Jabbari B, Vance SC, Grafman J, Amin D, Dillon JD. Epilepsy after penetrating head injury, I: Clinical correlates: a report of the Vietnam Head Injury Study. Neurology 1985;35: 1406–1414
12. Jennett WB, Lewin W. Traumatic epilepsy after closed head injury. J Neurol Neurosurg Psychiatry 1960;23:295–301
13. Willmore LJ. Post-traumatic epilepsy: cellular mechanisms and implications for treatment. Epilepsia 1990;31(Suppl. 3):S67–S73

14. Graham DI, McIntosh TK. Neuropathology of brain injury. In: Evans RW, ed. Neurology and Trauma. Philadelphia: W.B. Saunders; 1996:53–90
15. Coulter DA, Rafiq A, Shumate M, Gong QZ, DeLorenzo RJ, Lyeth BG. Brain injury-induced enhanced limbic epileptogenesis: anatomical and physiological parallels to an animal model of temporal lobe epilepsy. Epilepsy Res 1996;26:81–91
16. Diaz-Arrastia R, Agostini MA, Frol AB, et al. Neurophysiologic and neuroradiologic features of intractable epilepsy after traumatic brain injury in adults. Arch Neurol 2000;57:1611–1616
17. Hudak AM, Caesar RR, Frol AB, et al. Functional outcome scales in traumatic brain injury: a comparison of the Glasgow Outcome Scale (Extended) and the Functional Status Examination. J Neurotrauma 2005;22:1319–1326
18. Meldrum BS, Horton RW, Brierley JB. Epileptic brain damage in adolescent baboons following seizures induced by allylglycine. Brain 1974;97:407–418
19. Meldrum BS. Excitotoxicity and selective neuronal loss in epilepsy. Brain Pathol 1993;3:405–412
20. Wasterlain CG, Fujikawa DG, Penix L, Sankar R. Pathophysiological mechanisms of brain damage from status epilepticus. Epilepsia 1993;34(Suppl 1):S37–S53
21. Sloviter RS. Permanently altered hippocampal structure, excitability, and inhibition after experimental status epilepticus in the rat: the "dormant basket cell" hypothesis and its possible relevance to temporal lobe epilepsy. Hippocampus 1991;1:41–66
22. Jallo JI, Narayan RK. Craniocerebral trauma. In: Bradley WG, Daroff RB, Fenichel GM, Marsden CD, eds. Neurology in Clinical Practice. 3rd ed. Boston: Butterworth Heinemann; 2000:1055–1087
23. Temkin NR, Dikmen SS, Wilensky AJ, Keihm J, Chabal S, Winn HR. A randomized, double-blind study of phenytoin for the prevention of post-traumatic seizures. N Engl J Med 1990;323:497–502
24. Brain Trauma Foundation. Guidelines for the management of Severe Traumatic Brain Injury, Third Edition. 2007. Neurotrauma 24(Suppl 1) S1–S106
25. Temkin NR, Dikmen SS, Anderson GD, et al. Valproate therapy for prevention of posttraumatic seizures: a randomized trial. J Neurosurg 1999;91:593–600
26. Dikmen SS, Machamer JE, Winn HR, Anderson GD, Temkin NR. Neuropsychological effects of valproate in traumatic brain injury. Neurology 2000;54:895–902
27. Jordan KG. Nonconvulsive status epilepticusin acute brain injury. J Clin Neurophysiol 1999;16:332–340
28. Drislane FW. Presentation, evaluation, and treatment of nonconvulsive status epilepticus. Epilepsy Behav 2000;1:301–314
29. Litt B, Dizon L, Ryan D. Fatal non-convulsive status epilepticus in the elderly. Epilepsia 1994;35(Suppl 8):10
30. Towne AR, Waterhouse EJ, Boggs JG, et al. Prevalence of nonconvulsive status epilepticus in comatose patients. Neurology 2000;54:340–345
31. Nuwer M. Assessment of digital EEG, quantitative EEG, and EEG brain mapping. Neurology 1997;49:277–292
32. Young GB, Jordan KG, Doig GS. An assessment of nonconvulsive seizures in the intensive care unit using continuous EEG monitoring: an investigation of variables associated with mortality. Neurology 1996;47:83–89
33. Vespa PM, Nuwer MR, Nenov V, et al. Increased incidence and impact of nonconvulsive and convulsive seizures after traumatic brain injury as detected by continuous electroencephalographic monitoring. J Neurosurg 1999;91:750–760
34. Claassen J, Mayer SA, Kowalski RG, Emerson RG, Hirsch LJ. Detection of electrographic seizures with continuous EEG monitoring in critically ill patients. Neurology 2004;62:1743–1748
35. Ronne-Engstrom E, Winkler T. Continuous EEG monitoring in patients with traumatic brain injury reveals a high incidence of epileptiform activity. Acta Neurol Scand 2006;114:47–53
36. Hirsch LJ, Brenner RP, Drislane FW, et al. The ACNS subcommittee on research terminology for continuous EEG monitoring: proposed standardized terminology for rhythmic and periodic EEG patterns encountered in critically ill patients. J Clin Neurophysiol 2005;22:128–135
37. Astrup J, Siesjo BK, Symon L. Thresholds in cerebral ischemia—the ischemic penumbra. Stroke 1981;12:723–725
38. Tolonen U, Sulg IA. Comparison of quantitative EEG parameters from four different analysis techniques in evaluation of relationships between EEG and CBF in brain infarction. Electroencephalogr Clin Neurophysiol 1981;51:177–185
39. Claassen J, Mayer SA, Hirsch LJ. Continuous EEG monitoring in patients with subarachnoid hemorrhage. J Clin Neurophysiol 2005; 22:92–98
40. Vespa PM, Nuwer MR, Juhasz C, et al. Early detection of vasospasm after acute subarachnoid hemorrhage using continuous EEG ICU monitoring. Electroencephalogr Clin Neurophysiol 1997;103:607–615
41. Claassen J, Hirsch LJ, Kreiter KT, et al. Quantitative continuous EEG for detecting delayed cerebral ischemia in patients with poor-grade subarachnoid hemorrhage. Clin Neurophysiol 2004;115:2699–2710
42. Vespa PM, Boscardin WJ, Hovda DA, et al. Early and persistent impaired percent alpha variability on continuous electroencephalography monitoring as predictive of poor outcome after traumatic brain injury. J Neurosurg 2002;97:84–92
43. Thatcher RW, North DM, Curtin RT, et al. An EEG severity index of traumatic brain injury. J Neuropsychiatry Clin Neurosci 2001;13:77–87
44. Ives JR. New chronic EEG electrode for critical/intensive care unit monitoring. J Clin Neurophysiol 2005;22:119–123
45. Johansen JW. Update on bispectral index monitoring. Best Pract Res Clin Anaesthesiol 2006;20:81–99
46. Glass PS, Bloom M, Kearse L, Rosow C, Sebel P, Manberg P. Bispectral analysis measures sedation and memory effects of propofol, midazolam, isoflurane, and alfentanil in healthy volunteers. Anesthesiology 1997;86:836–847
47. Berkenbosch JW, Fichter CR, Tobias JD. The correlation of the bispectral index monitor with clinical sedation scores during mechanical ventilation in the pediatric intensive care unit. Anesth Analg 2002;94: 506–511
48. Gilbert TT, Wagner MR, Halukurike V, Paz HL, Garland A. Use of bispectral electroencephalogram monitoring to assess neurologic status in unsedated, critically ill patients. Crit Care Med 2001;29:1996–2000
49. Consales G, Chelazzi C, Rinaldi S, De Gaudio AR. Bispectral Index compared to Ramsay score for sedation monitoring in intensive care units. Minerva Anestesiol 2006;72:329–336
50. Deogaonkar A, Gupta R, DeGeorgia M, et al. Bispectral Index monitoring correlates with sedation scales in brain-injured patients. Crit Care Med 2004;32:2403–2406
51. Simmons LE, Riker RR, Prato BS, Fraser GL. Assessing sedation during intensive care unit mechanical ventilation with the Bispectral Index and the Sedation-Agitation Scale. Crit Care Med 1999;27: 1499–1504
52. De Deyne C, Struys M, Decruyenaere J, Creupelandt J, Hoste E, Colardyn F. Use of continuous bispectral EEG monitoring to assess depth of sedation in ICU patients. Intensive Care Med 1998;24:1294–1298
53. Haug E, Miner J, Dannehy M, Seigel T, Biros M. Bispectral electroencephalographic analysis of head-injured patients in the emergency department. Acad Emerg Med 2004;11:349–352
54. Fabregas N, Gambus PL, Valero R, et al. Can bispectral index monitoring predict recovery of consciousness in patients with severe brain injury? Anesthesiology 2004;101:43–51
55. Pandin P, Van Cutsem N, Tuna T, D'hollander A. Bispectral index is a topographically dependent variable in patients receiving propofol anaesthesia. Br J Anaesth 2006;97:676–680
56. Gaetz M, Bernstein DM. The current status of electrophysiologic procedures for the assessment of mild traumatic brain injury. J Head Trauma Rehabil 2001;16:386–405
57. Lew HL, Lee EH, Miyoshi Y, Chang DG, Date ES, Jerger JF. Brainstem auditory-evoked potentials as an objective tool for evaluating hearing dysfunction in traumatic brain injury. Am J Phys Med Rehabil 2004;83: 210–215

58. Carter BG, Butt W. Are somatosensory evoked potentials the best predictor of outcome after severe brain injury? A systematic review. Intensive Care Med 2005;31:765–775
59. Schalamon J, Singer G, Kurschel S, Hollwarth ME. Somatosensory evoked potentials in children with severe head trauma. Eur J Pediatr 2005;164:417–420
60. Amantini A, Grippo A, Fossi S, et al. Prediction of "awakening" and outcome in prolonged acute coma from severe traumatic brain injury: evidence for validity of short latency SEPs. Clin Neurophysiol 2005;116: 229–235
61. Fischer C, Luaute J, Adeleine P, Morlet D. Predictive value of sensory and cognitive evoked potentials for awakening from coma. Neurology 2004;63:669–673
62. Lew HL, Lee EH, Pan SS, Date ES. Electrophysiologic abnormalities of auditory and visual information processing in patients with traumatic brain injury. Am J Phys Med Rehabil 2004;83:428–433
63. Plourde G. Auditory evoked potentials. Best Pract Res Clin Anaesthesiol 2006;20:129–139
64. Lee JH, Martin NA, Alsina G, et al. Hemodynamically significant cerebral vasospasm and outcome after head injury: a prospective study. J Neurosurg 1997;87:221–233
65. DeWitt LD, Wechsler LR. Transcranial Doppler. Stroke 1988;19: 915–921
66. Martin NA, Doberstein C, Zane C, Caron MJ, Thomas K, Becker DP. Posttraumatic cerebral arterial spasm: transcranial Doppler ultrasound, cerebral blood flow, and angiographic findings. J Neurosurg 1992;77:575–583
67. Oertel M, Boscardin WJ, Obrist WD, et al. Posttraumatic vasospasm: the epidemiology, severity, and time course of an underestimated phenomenon: a prospective study performed in 299 patients. J Neurosurg 2005;103:812–824
68. Kordestani RK, Counelis GJ, McBride DQ, Martin NA. Cerebral arterial spasm after penetrating craniocerebral gunshot wounds: transcranial Doppler and cerebral blood flow findings. Neurosurgery 1997;41: 351–359
69. van Santbrink H, Schouten JW, Steyerberg EW, Avezaat CJ, Maas AI. Serial transcranial Doppler measurements in traumatic brain injury with special focus on the early posttraumatic period. Acta Neurochir (Wien) 2002;144:1141–1149
70. Voulgaris SG, Partheni M, Kaliora H, Haftouras N, Pessach IS, Polyzoidis KS. Early cerebral monitoring using the transcranial Doppler pulsatility index in patients with severe brain trauma. Med Sci Monit 2005;11:CR49–CR52
71. Kuo JR, Chen CF, Chio CC, et al. Time dependent validity in the diagnosis of brain death using transcranial Doppler sonography. J Neurol Neurosurg Psychiatry 2006;77:646–649
72. Adelson PD, Nemoto E, Scheuer M, Painter M, Morgan J, Yonas H. Noninvasive continuous monitoring of cerebral oxygenation periictally using near-infrared spectroscopy: a preliminary report. Epilepsia 1999;40:1484–1489
73. Ward KR, Ivatury RR, Barbee RW, et al. Near infrared spectroscopy for evaluation of the trauma patient: a technology review. Resuscitation 2006;68:27–44
74. McLeod AD, Igielman F, Elwell C, Cope M, Smith M. Measuring cerebral oxygenation during normobaric hyperoxia: a comparison of tissue microprobes, near-infrared spectroscopy, and jugular venous oximetry in head injury. Anesth Analg 2003;97:851–856
75. Lewis SB, Myburgh JA, Thornton EL, Reilly PL. Cerebral oxygenation monitoring by near-infrared spectroscopy is not clinically useful in patients with severe closed-head injury: a comparison with jugular venous bulb oximetry. Crit Care Med 1996;24:1334–1338
76. Perez JJ, Guijarro E, Sancho J. Spatiotemporal pattern of the extracranial component of the rheoencephalographic signal. Physiol Meas 2005;26:925–938
77. Bodo M, Pearce FJ, Baranyi L, Armonda RA. Changes in the intracranial rheoencephalogram at lower limit of cerebral blood flow autoregulation. Physiol Meas 2005;26:S1–S17

5 Monitoring of the Brain: Pressures, Flows, and Brain Tissue Probes

Marek Czosnyka, Peter Hutchinson, Peter J. Kirkpatrick, and John D. Pickard

In contrast to experimental studies of head injury and cerebral ischemia, the scientific basis of clinical management of head trauma patients is still poorly documented. After traumatic brain injury clinical manifestations vary, hence large numbers of observations are required before significant convergence of data is achieved, providing a consistent picture. The injury usually triggers a variety of pathophysiological mechanisms that in turn create a highly heterogeneous pattern of changes within the brain. Ischemic brain damage may arise from primary or secondary insults.[1,2] Episodes of intracranial hypertension, arterial hypotension, vasospasm, hypoxemia, spreading depression, and many other phenomena are commonly listed.[3–5]

From the point of view of control theory, all self-sustaining complex systems require stabilizing negative feedback loops. Following brain trauma, the system of cerebrovascular circulation usually works without feedback information. Moreover, physiological negative feedback loops are converted to positive vicious circles.[6] For example, cerebral pressure autoregulation, a major brain self-protective mechanism,[7] may fail, with endothelial dysfunction, vasospasm, and free radical generation playing potential roles. With impaired autoregulation, the brain is more vulnerable to the effects of secondary insults and less capable of delivering an optimal cerebral blood flow (CBF), stabilizing blood volume, and maintaining the correct metabolic balance, resulting in worse outcome.[8,9] Initial failure of autoregulation may result in an increase in cerebral blood volume, intracranial hypertension, ischemia, more endothelial stress, deeper dysautoregulation, deeper intracranial hypertension, etc.

The aim of intensive care monitoring[10] is to provide missing data, closing the disrupted control loop by an appropriate therapy controlled by doctors' decisions.

The continuous monitoring of comatose head-injured patients in neurological intensive care provides information regarding spontaneous fluctuations in cerebral hemodynamic and metabolic function. The capture and understanding of this information demands at the front end a simple, reliable monitoring system, internally incorporating sophisticated signal analysis.[11] Because secondary insults may be frequent and of short duration (a few minutes[7,12]), continuous observation is an essential component with 1 minute epochs being generally accepted as the basic period for averaging. User-dependent selection of the modalities for monitoring, and their subsequent integrated on-line interpretation, requires considerable computer support.

An ideal monitoring system (**Table 5.1**) should not only detect the secondary insults but also identify states of cerebral dysfunction that render the brain more susceptible to such insults. Therefore, testing of cerebral pressure autoregulation and cerebrovascular reactivity has a very special place among the techniques used in brain monitoring. Most of the tests are based on the observation of the specific response of CBF to increase or decrease in arterial blood pressure, therefore they can be repeated with limited frequency. In the previous decade, the methods suitable for continuous assessment of autoregulatory reserve, utilizing endogenous variations in cerebral perfusion or arterial pressure, have been described.[13]

The value of continuous monitoring of different variables such as intracranial pressure (ICP), arterial blood pressure (ABP), jugular venous bulb oxygen saturation ($S_{jv}O_2$), have been studied for many years. More recently, the continuous monitoring of relative changes in CBF using indirect methods such as transcranial Doppler (TCD)[14,15] and laser Doppler flowmeter (LDF)[16] have been included. Finally, real time monitoring of the cerebral oxygenation and metabolic state using near-infrared spectroscopy (NIRS),[17] direct cerebral tissue oxygenation,[4,18,19] and microdialysis[5,20] have been introduced to neurological intensive care (**Table 5.2**).

A user of multimodality monitoring systems is frequently confronted with huge volumes of data, much of which may not be of clinical relevance. Identifying the most important parameters in subgroups of head-injured patients is therefore a future priority. Various data formats

Table 5.1 Ideal Monitoring System

1. Displays changes (time trends) of vital brain modalities
2. Identifies states of cerebral dysfunction that render brain more susceptible to insults
3. Involves testing cerebral pressure autoregulation and/or cerebrovascular reactivity
4. Supports optimization of cerebral perfusion pressure
5. Stores raw data for optional postprocessing
6. Detects secondary insults according to flexible criteria

Table 5.2 Methods for Brain Monitoring

Method	Continuous	Resolution	Invasive	Quantitative	Remarks
Intracranial pressure	Yes	Global	Yes	Yes	Intraparenchymal probes; intraventricular catheter, subdural drain, and epidural sensors are available
Cerebral perfusion pressure	Yes	Global	Yes	Yes	Requires simultaneous ICP and direct arterial pressure monitoring
CBF velocity: Transcranial Doppler ultrasonography	Yes	MCA (ACA/PCA)	No	No	Problems with probe holders; it may provide information on autoregulation and asymmetry of CBF
Brain temperature	Yes	Regional	No	Yes	
CBF jugular thermodilution	Yes	Global	Yes	Yes	
CBF laser Doppler flowmetry	Yes	Local (1–2 mm^3)	Yes	No	Unknown physiological zero
CBF thermal diffusion	Yes	Local	Yes	Yes	Cortical probe; with parenchymal probe a bigger region can be monitored (5cm^2)
NIRS	Yes	Regional	No	No	Technology yet to be refined; some machines prone to extracranial contamination; % tissue oxygen saturation is debatable
$S_{jv}O_2S_{jv}O_2$	Yes	Global	Yes	No	Requires frequent (every 2 hours?) co-oximetry
Brain tissue PO_2	Yes	Local	Yes	No	
Microdialysis	No	Regional	Yes	No	Various compounds can be monitored

Abbreviations: ACA, anterior cerebral artery; CBF, cerebral blood flow; MCA, middle cerebral artery; NIRS, near-infrared spectroscopy; PCA, posterior cerebral artery; $S_{jv}O_2$, jugular venous bulb oxygen saturation.

Source: Adapted from Steiner LA, Czosnyk M. Should we measure cerebral blood flow in head-injured patients? Br J Neurosurg 2002;16:429–439.

have been used.[12,13] All the brain monitoring techniques generate artifacts that are frequently difficult to identify with certainty. However, because each modality measures independent variables, their artifacts are unlikely to coincide in time. Therefore multimodal systems can help in discriminating relevant events from contaminated readings.

In contrast to brain imaging techniques (which provide high spatial resolution at a selected time point, usually with a ±1 hour random deviation), bedside monitoring provides dynamic readings with poor spatial, but high temporal, resolution. Therefore they allow detection of short-lasting cerebral events that generally affect large areas within the supratentorial compartment.

In terms of directing treatment, the monitoring of only one component may be misleading. The inability to reliably distinguish hyperemia from vasospasm using TCD ultrasonography is an example of where an inappropriate and potentially dangerous response could occur. In both cases blood flow velocity is elevated, hence a second modality (such as SjO_2 monitoring) is necessary for differentiating these two terminally different states. The potential for hyperventilation to reduce ICP and to improve cerebral perfusion pressure (CPP), with its concomitant risk of generating cerebral lactate acidosis, is another example where multimodality monitoring has identified a well-rehearsed therapy, which has been subsequently shown to be potentially harmful.[21]

Subsequent parts of this chapter contain short descriptions of the clinical aspects of montoring brain pressures, CBF, metabolism, and biochemical makeup. Methods of testing of cerebral autoregulation are discussed toward the end. The subject is large, therefore the chapter includes references for further reading.

Brain Pressures (Table 5.3)

Although most neuroscientists, both clinical and basic, are familiar with the concepts of ICP and CPP, there are other pressures that can be measured within the brain. How many are there? Are they all clinically relevant?

In addition to ICP, cerebral intraparenchymal pressure can be monitored nowadays using microsensors with the intention to approximate the gold standard ICP- ventricular cerebrospinal fluid (CSF) pressure.[22]

Cerebral venous pressure is the pressure of venous blood in cortical or bridging veins. This pressure follows ICP as long as CBF is preserved.[23] Under certain conditions,

Table 5.3 Other Pressures Measured (in Addition to ICP and CPP)

Pressure	Uses
Cerebral intraparenchymal pressure	Approximate gold standard for ICP-ventricular CSF pressure
Cerebral venous pressure	Measures pressure of venous blood in cortical and bridging veins; follows ICP as long as cerebral blood flow is preserved; not measured directly in clinical practice
Dural sinus pressure	Recorded in patients with idiopathic intracranial hypertension
Critical closing pressure	Purely conceptual pressure; assessed using transcranial Doppler ultrasonography
Other pressures of clinical relevance	Transparenchymal pressure gradients, pressure gradients between cisterna magna and lumbar CSF space in Arnold-Chiari malformation, and pressure within spinal cord syrinxes in syringomyelia

Abbreviations: CSF, cerebrospinal fluid; ICP, intracranial pressure.

coupling between cerebral venous pressure and ICP can be disrupted, for example, when ICP falls below sagittal sinus pressure due to excessive drainage of CSF.[24]

The pressure in the dural sinuses is rarely measured. Increase in this pressure can be recorded in patients with idiopathic intracranial hypertension, sometimes in association with stenosis of part of the transverse or posterior part of the sagittal sinuses.[25]

In other intracranial pathologies, where further compartmentalization of intracranial space may occur, different pressures may have clinical relevance, for example, transparenchymal pressure gradients in noncommunicating hydrocephalus, pressure gradients between the cisterna magna and the lumbar CSF space in Arnold-Chiari malformation, or pressure within spinal cord syrinxes in syringomyelia.

All the pressures listed above can be measured with adequately placed pressure transducers, regardless of whether such a measurement is clinically feasible or not. There are also pressures that are purely conceptual. They emerge from various models describing the brain circulation or from methods of their estimation. The best example here is critical closing pressure (CCP), which can be assessed using TCD ultrasonography. It cannot be measured directly under physiological circumstances; it can only be estimated from the waveform of blood flow velocity and arterial pressure.

This chapter summarizes the most important points related to various brain pressures after head trauma and is based on both the literature and the author's own experience.

Intracranial Pressure (Table 5.4)

ICP is derived from both CBF and CSF circulation. It can be symbolically represented as a sum of hypothetical vascular component (ICP_{vasc}) and CSF circulatory component (ICP_{CSF}).

$$ICP = ICP_{vasc} + ICP_{CSF} \qquad \text{(Eq. 5.1)}$$

However, it is not clear whether a "sum" in a strict mathematical sense is adequate. The CSF circulatory component describes part of ICP, which conforms to the Davson's equation[26]:

$$ICP_{CSF} = (\text{CSF formation rate} \times R_{CSF}) + \text{sagittal sinus pressure} \qquad \text{(Eq. 5.2)}$$

where R_{CSF} is the resistance to CSF outflow.

The vascular component[27] is derived from the pulsatile fraction of CBF.[28] Its sudden disappearance can be observed after cardiac arrest or during longer periods of

Table 5.4 Intracranial Pressure: $ICP = ICP_{vasc} + ICP_{CSF}$ (Normal Range = 7.5–13 mm Hg)

Component	Characteristics
CSF component (ICP_{CSF})	• Conforms to Davson's equation: ICP_{CSF} = (CSF formation rate × R_{CSF}) + sagittal sinus pressure
	• Average CSF formation rate = 0.3–0.4 mL/min
	• Normal resistance to CSF outflow = 6–10 mm Hg/(mL/min)
	• Normal sagittal sinus pressure = 5–8 mm Hg
	• Contributes to interpretation of clinical problems associated with hydrocephalus, whereas in head trauma, ICP requires both CSF and vascular components
Vascular component (ICP_{vasc})	• Derived from pulsatile fraction of cerebral blood flow
	• Magnitude depends on vascular tone, heart rate, autoregulatory reserve, etc.

Abbreviations: CSF, cerebrospinal fluid; ICP, intracranial pressure.

asystole. The magnitude of this component depends, in a difficult to express manner, on vascular tone, heart rate, autoregulatory reserve, etc. Mathematical models of CSF and CBF dynamics seem to be helpful in better understanding this concept.[29]

The normal ICP ranges from 7.5 to 13 mm Hg (this is the 95% confidence range in patients without obvious intracranial pathology[30]). An average normal CSF formation rate is 0.3 to 0.4 mL/min, normal resistance to CSF outflow is from 6 to 10 mm Hg/(mL/min),[31] and a value of normal sagittal sinus pressure varies from 5 to 8 mm Hg.[30]

Cerebral venous sinus pressure may, however, not always stay constant. The measurements performed during an infusion study in patients with idiopathic intracranial hypertension may demonstrate a parallel increase in sinus pressure when CSF pressure increases (**Fig. 5.1**). If such a coupling is possible in idiopathic intracranial hypertension, it may potentially happen in other pathologies where ICP is elevated.

ICP depends on body position. Normal values given above were measured in horizontal body position. ICP in the upright body position may fall to −5 mm Hg[32] and probably even lower (−10 mm Hg; Czosnyka et al, 2006, unpublished data).

The CSF circulatory component contributes to interpretation of clinical problems related to hydrocephalus, whereas in head injury a combination of both circulatory and vascular components determines ICP.[33]

The gold standard definition of ICP is a CSF pressure in brain ventricles.[22,34] However, in clinical practice intraparenchymal microsensors are commonly used.[2,34,35] Intraparenchymal pressure may differ from CSF pressure in the ventricles as it does not conform to Pascal's law. It is not propagated equally in all directions; it is no longer a scalar but is rather a vector of forces (tensor). Direction of this vector relative to the surface of pressure transducer may influence pressure readings. Regional gradients of the intraparenchymal pressure can be demonstrated experimentally but less common clinically.[36,37]

The outcome following head injury depends on averaged ICP.[38–41] The distribution of mean ICP in different outcome groups shows significantly greater value of ICP

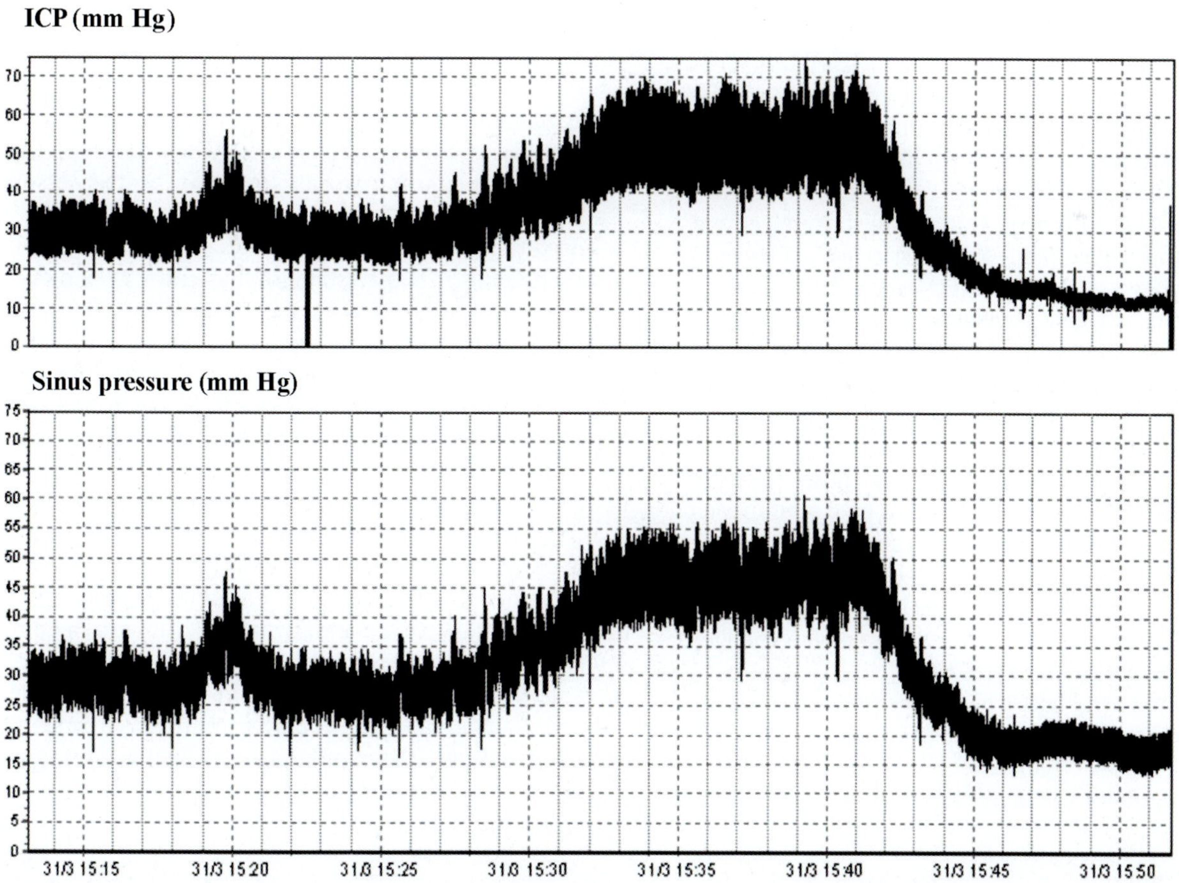

Fig. 5.1 Simultaneous recording of lumbar cerebrospinal fluid pressure [intracranial pressure (ICP)] and sagittal sinus pressure during infusion into the lumbar space of a patient with idiopathic intracranial hypertension. There is obvious coupling between the two pressures, probably caused by collapsing transverse sinuses when ICP was forced to rise. X-axis: time in hours and minutes. (From Higgins N, Pickard JD, Czosnyka Z&M, unpublished data, 2005.)

in patients who died in comparison with those who survived. The critical range of increased ICP in TBI is between 20 and 25 mm Hg. Mean ICP does not differentiate patients who achieved good, moderate outcome or persisted in a severely disabled state. Therefore it is likely that ICP-oriented therapies improve first of all the mortality rate.[42]

Important diagnostic information is included in ICP waveforms[2,43,44]: pulse, respiratory, and slow waves (slow variations of ICP having periods from 20 seconds to 3 minutes) (**Fig. 5.2**).

The ICP-volume curve may explain the relationship between pulse amplitude and mean ICP (**Fig. 5.3**),[2,38,43] but it is not the only possible explanation.[45] Augmentation of transmission of arterial pulse to CSF compartment (when CPP falls and vasodilatation increases the compliance of the arterial bed) is another potential mechanism explaining this relationship.

The correlation coefficient between slow changes in pulse amplitude of ICP and slow waves of mean ICP (so-called RAP coefficient; do not mix with so-called Resistance Area Product assessed using TCD) may indicate where on the pressure-volume curve the current working point of cerebrospinal space is positioned.[45]

The pressure-reactivity index (PRx; the correlation coefficient between slow waves in ICP and mean arterial pressure) describes the level of disturbance in physiological vascular responses to change in arterial pressure (**Fig. 5.4**).[45,46] The mortality rate is higher in patients with positive PRx (absent reactivity) than in those in whom reactivity is preserved (i.e., PRx is negative).[39] Disturbed PRx is associated with low $CMRO_2$ and greater oxygen extraction fraction.[47] PRx correlates well with cerebral autoregulation assessed with positron emission tomography (PET)-CBF[48] and with TCD ultrasonography[45] (**Table 5.5**).

Slow waves in ICP (20 second to 3 minute period) correlate with outcome: Low content of these waves is associated with increased mortality after head injury.[39] Plateau waves of ICP are provoked by spontaneous increases in cerebral blood volume. Various models have been proposed in the past.[7] During the wave both CBF and cerebrovascular resistance decrease (**Fig. 5.5**). However, the majority of ICP variations are associated with changes in arterial pressure or CBF (**Fig. 5.6**).

ICP following head injury has a tendency to decreases with age. Severe intracranial hypertension occurs more frequently in females than males. This probably explains the greater mortality rate in females than in males.[49]

Cerebral Perfusion Pressure (Table 5.6)

CPP is defined as the difference between cerebral arterial pressure and pressure in the cerebral venous bed just before outlet to the sagittal sinus, that is, in cortical or bridging veins.

CPP is the pressure driving blood through the cerebrovascular bed.[50] As the pressure in bridging veins is difficult to measure and can be approximated by ICP,[24] the clinical definition of CPP is:

$$CPP = MAP - meanICP \qquad \text{(Eq. 5.3)}$$

Too low CPP causes ischemia, too high causes hyperemia. Autoregulation of CBF works within certain CPP limits (lower and upper) (**Fig. 5.7**).[8]

Therefore, decreasing CPP is particularly dangerous after head injury: It both decreases the driving force for cerebral blood to flow and destroys autoregulation.

CPP-oriented therapy has been introduced to decrease risk of ischemia in postinjury care.[51] An alternative concept, the so-called Lund protocol,[42] is aimed at lowering ICP, even sacrificing the principle of maintaining CPP above 60 mm Hg.

The distribution of mean CPP for different outcome groups post–head injury is equivalent to the distribution of mean ICP.[39] In patients who died, mean CPP was significantly lower. Other outcome groups have similar CPP levels.

Optimal CPP

Autoregulation of CBF is one of the most important intrinsic mechanisms of brain protection following head injury. As long as autoregulation works, the brain protects itself against ischemia.[8,10,52]

The relationship between the PRx (or autoregulation assessed using TCD ultrasonography[9] and CPP shows a U-shaped curve (**Fig. 5.8**).

The curve indicates that too low or too high CPPs are associated with failure of autoregulation. Therefore the optimal CPP, in which cerebral autoregulation is strongest,[46] may be identified by plotting PRx against CPP in individual cases (from the moving time window of the past few hours). Patients with the greater distance between their averaged CPP and post hoc assessed optimal CPP had a worse outcome after head trauma.[46]

An algorithm has been proposed to modify CPP-oriented therapy to trace optimal CPP in 4- to 6-hour intervals and maintain current CPP close to optimal level (see Steiner et al[46]). It remains to be demonstrated whether such a strategy is able to improve outcome. If clinical benefit was documented, individualized optimal CPP would form a consensus between CPP therapy[51] and the Lund concept.[42]

Critical Closing Pressure (Table 5.7)

CCP is the blood pressure below which cerebral arteries close and blood flow ceases.[53] CCP is supposed to be equal

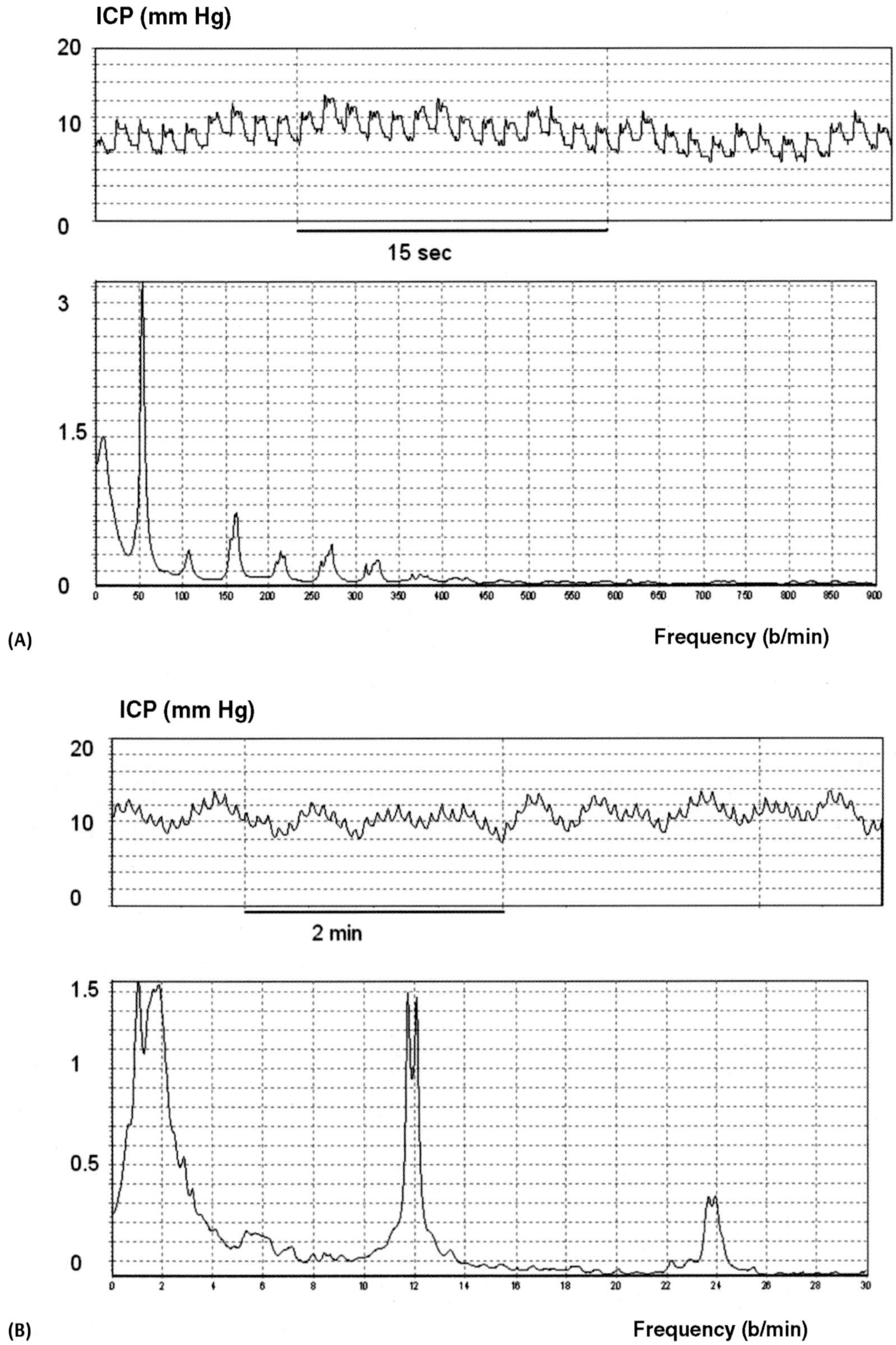

Fig. 5.2 Waveforms of intracranial pressure (ICP) and their spectral representations. **(A)** Pulse wave in time domain and results of spectral analysis (*y*-axis shows the equivalent amplitude of the component in mm Hg; *x*-axis shows frequency in cycles per minute). Low-frequency hump represents respiratory and slow waves (combined). First sharp peak: fundamental harmonic of pulse amplitude with at least seven higher harmonic components equally spaced along frequency axis. **(B)** In different time domain, respiratory wave and regular slow waves (B waves). Pulse component was filtered out. Frequency spectrum shows hump at 2 cycles per minute representing slow waves. Respiratory component forms a maximum at 12 cycles per minute (with the second harmonic).

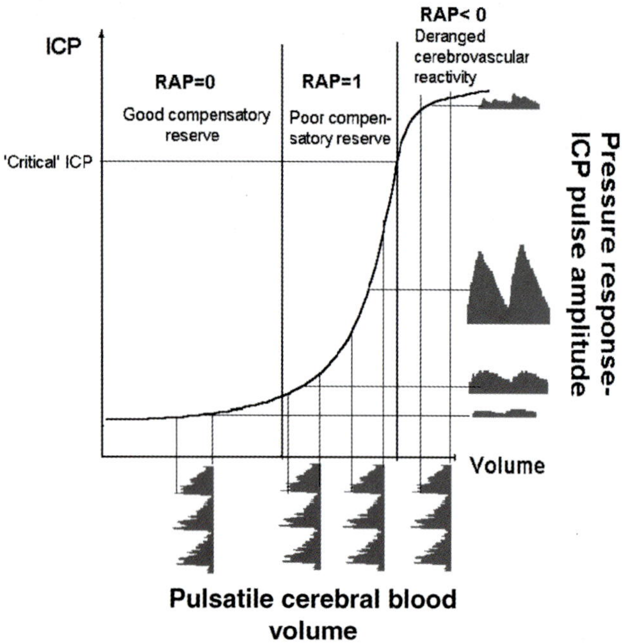

Fig. 5.3 In a simple model, pulse amplitude of intracranial pressure (ICP) (expressed along the *y*-axis on the right side of the figure) results from pulsatile changes in cerebral blood volume (expressed along the *x*-axis) transformed by the pressure-volume curve. This curve has three zones: a flat zone, expressing good compensatory reserve, an exponential zone, depicting poor compensatory reserve, and a flat zone again, seen at very high ICP (above the "critical" ICP) depicting derangement of normal cerebrovascular responses. The pulse amplitude of ICP is low and does not depend on mean ICP in the first zone, resulting in values of RAP close to zero. The pulse amplitude increases linearly with mean ICP in the zone of poor compensatory reserve, resulting in RAP close to +1. In the third zone, the pulse amplitude starts to decrease with rising ICP; RAP theoretically becomes negative. (Adapted from Avezaat CJ, van Eijndhoven JH, Wyper DJ. Cerebrospinal fluid pulse pressure and intracranial volume-pressure relationships. J Neurol Neurosurg Psychiatry. 1979;42(8):687–700).[43]

to ICP plus a factor resulting from the tension of arterial walls[54]:

$$CCP = ICP + \textit{tension of arterial walls} \quad \text{(Eq. 5.4)}$$

The measurement of CCP relies on linear interpolation between systolic and diastolic values of blood flow velocity (FV) and arterial pressure waveforms. The intercept point between this line and the *x*-axis (arterial pressure) signifies CCP. As exact detection of systolic and diastolic maximal flow velocity may be prone to contamination, alternative methods relying on the analysis of the first harmonic of ABP and FV[55] or linear regression between flow velocity and ABP pulse waveform are also used.

The methods based on pulse wave analysis of ABP and FV provide the same results as using the definition of CCP, which can be measured during cardiac arrest.[55]

Correlation between CCP and ICP is significant but weak in head-injured patients.[56] During cerebrovascular spasm CCP decreases and often reaches negative values.[57] CCP correlates much better with cerebrovascular resistance (calculated as FV divided by CPP) than with ICP.[58] Changes in CCP correlate well with changes in tension of arterial blood CO_2.[59]

However, in individual cases after head injury, changes in ICP in time may correlate spectacularly well with changes in CCP (**Fig. 5.9**). With bilateral TCD, CCP can be monitored simultaneously on both sides. Asymmetry in left-right CCP correlates with asymmetry seen in computed tomography (CT) scan (unilateral contusion, midline shift, etc.).[60]

Assessment of CCP is only theoretically independent of the angle of insonation of the vessel. In fact, the quality of TCD waveform and how the peripheral arterial pulse has approximates the intracerebral pulse has important influence on the accuracy of CCP estimation. In clinical practice, negative values of CCP or values well below measured ICP (although negative arterial walls tension is difficult to imagine) are not uncommon.

Noninvasive CPP and ICP

The middle cerebral artery is a big vessel with elastic walls. It can be imagined as a membrane transducer able to detect changes in transmural pressure. Unfortunately, the tension of the membrane is unknown and may be variable in time. Therefore the value of its calibration coefficients, linearity, and geometry of the membrane are also unknown.

The CPP affects the shape of the blood flow velocity waveform.[14] However, the arterial pulse waveform, heart rate, the tension of arterial CO_2, distal vascular resistance, and even age affect the FV waveform as well.

Some simple formulas to assess CPP noninvasively from ABP and FV waveforms have been proposed in the past.[61,62]

Of these formulas, one in particular has reached possible satisfactory accuracy (error <10 mm Hg in >80% measurements in a large group of head-injured patients)[63]:

$$nCCP = MAP \times FVd / FVmean + 14 \quad \text{(Eq. 5.5)}$$

(*FVd*: diastolic FV; *FVmean*: mean FV).

Noninvasive CPP (nCPP) is useful both to estimate absolute CPP and to monitor changes in CPP in time (**Fig. 5.10**). The 95% confidence limit for estimation of CPP is 12 mm Hg.[63] Although this seems to be acceptable for CPP, such a precision would not be good enough to estimate ICP (**Table 5.8**).

ICP can be measured noninvasively using various methods: tympanic membrane displacement,[64] time of flight of

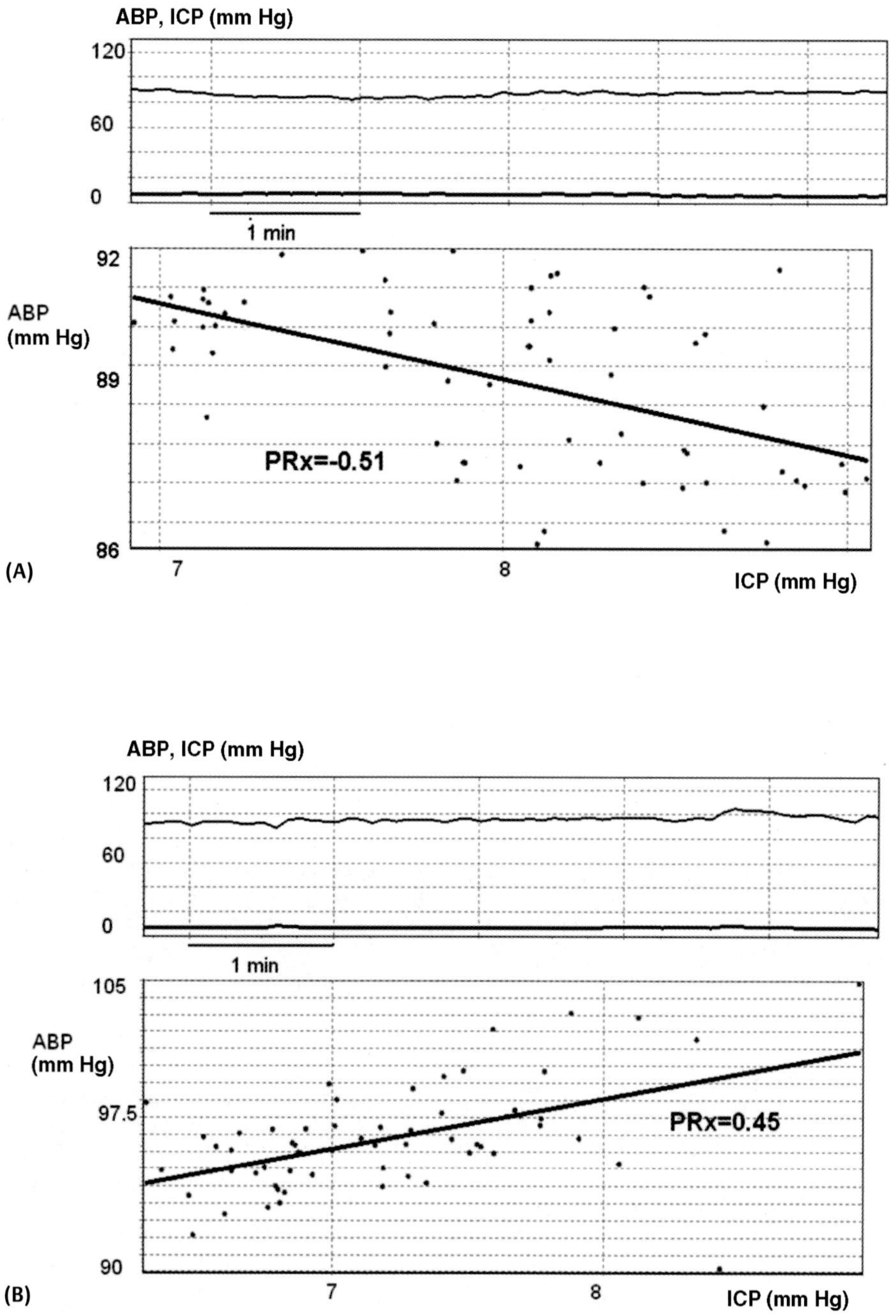

Fig. 5.4 Relationship between slow waves in intracranial pressure (ICP) and arterial blood pressure (ABP). **(A)** Negative relationship signifies active cerebrovascular volume control. Correlation coefficient PRx is negative **(B)** Passive relationship between spontaneous changes in ABP and ICP signifies disturbed vascular reactivity [pressure reactivity index (PRx) positive]).

Table 5.5 Pressure Reactivity Index (PRx)

Defined	Correlation coefficient between slow waves in intracranial pressure (ICP) and MAP. Slow waves: periods from 20 seconds to 3 minutes
Function	Describes level of disturbance in physiological vascular responses to changes in arterial pressure
Outcome	Worse outcome in patients with a positive PRx (absent reactivity) compared with those with a negative PRx (preserved reactivity)
Disturbed PRx	Associated with a low $CMRO_2$ and greater O_2 extraction fraction. Also during plateau waves of ICP, during refractory intracranial hypertension, hyperemia, too low or too high cerebral perfusion pressure
Correlation	Correlates well with cerebral autoregulation assessed with positron emission tomography–cerebral blood flow and with transcranial Doppler ultrasonography

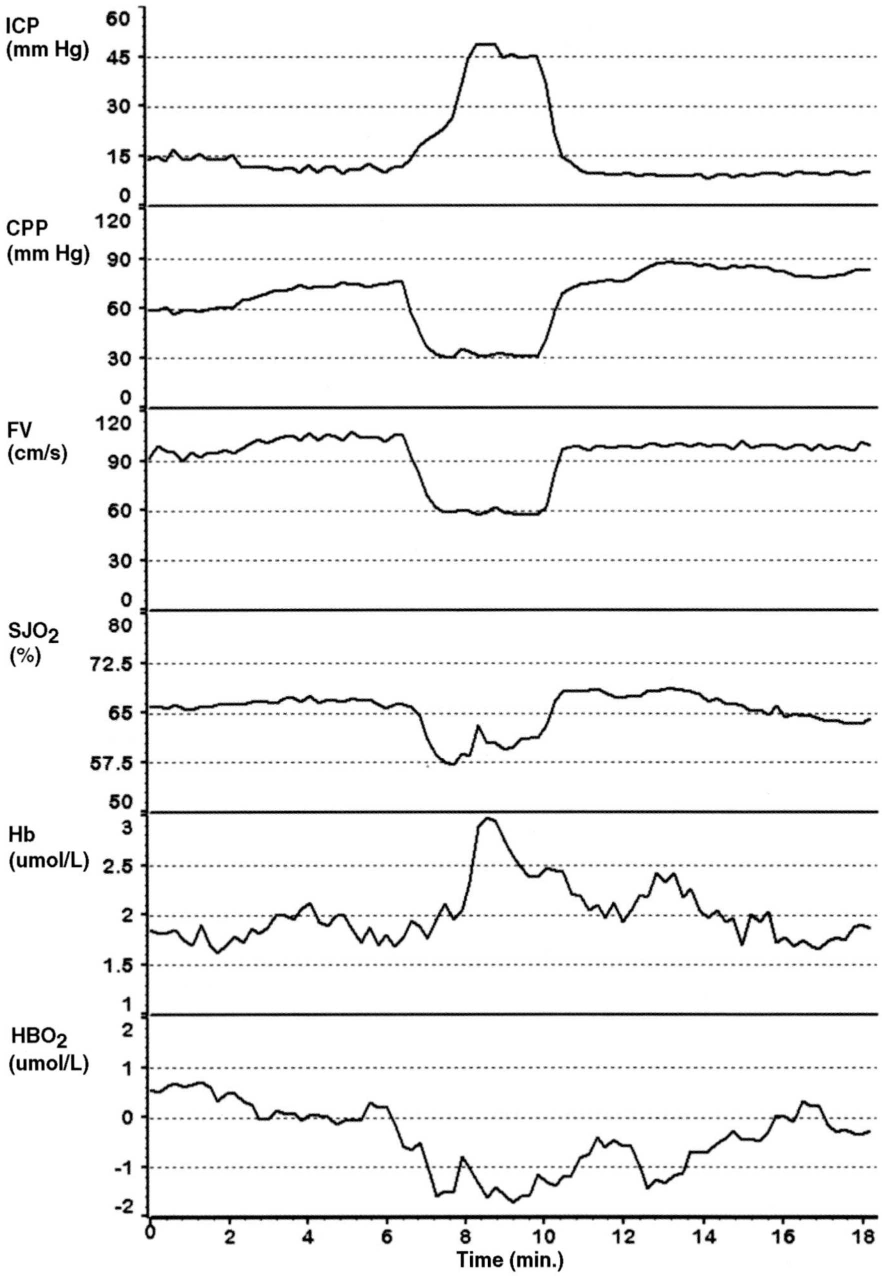

Fig. 5.5 Decrease in transcranial Doppler blood flow velocity (FV), jugular bulb oxygenation (S_jO_2), deoxygenated (Hb), and oxygenated hemoglobin (HbO_2) using near-infrared spectroscopy during short-term intracranial pressure (ICP) plateau wave (duration of 4 minutes).

ultrasound through the skull,[65] change in skull diameter[66]), change in blood flow velocity in the straight sinus,[67] or by analysis of pulse waveform of TCD[61,68,69] (**Table 5.9**).

The pulsatility index (PI) increases with rising ICP.[44] Prediction of absolute ICP using PI is not accurate enough as many other factors may influence PI [arterial pulse, heart rate, partial pressure of carbon dioxide, arterial ($PaCO_2$), vascular tone, proximal stenosis, spasm, etc]. However, the value of the PI above 1.5 in normocapnic patients may always raise doubts regarding adequate CPP or meaningful intracranial hypertension.

Estimation of ICP using the equation[61]:

$$ICP = MAP - A1 / F1 \times FVmean \qquad \text{(Eq. 5.6)}$$

(where F1 and A1 are first harmonic components of FV and arterial pressure pulse waveforms) gives 95% confidence limit of approximately ±25 mm Hg.

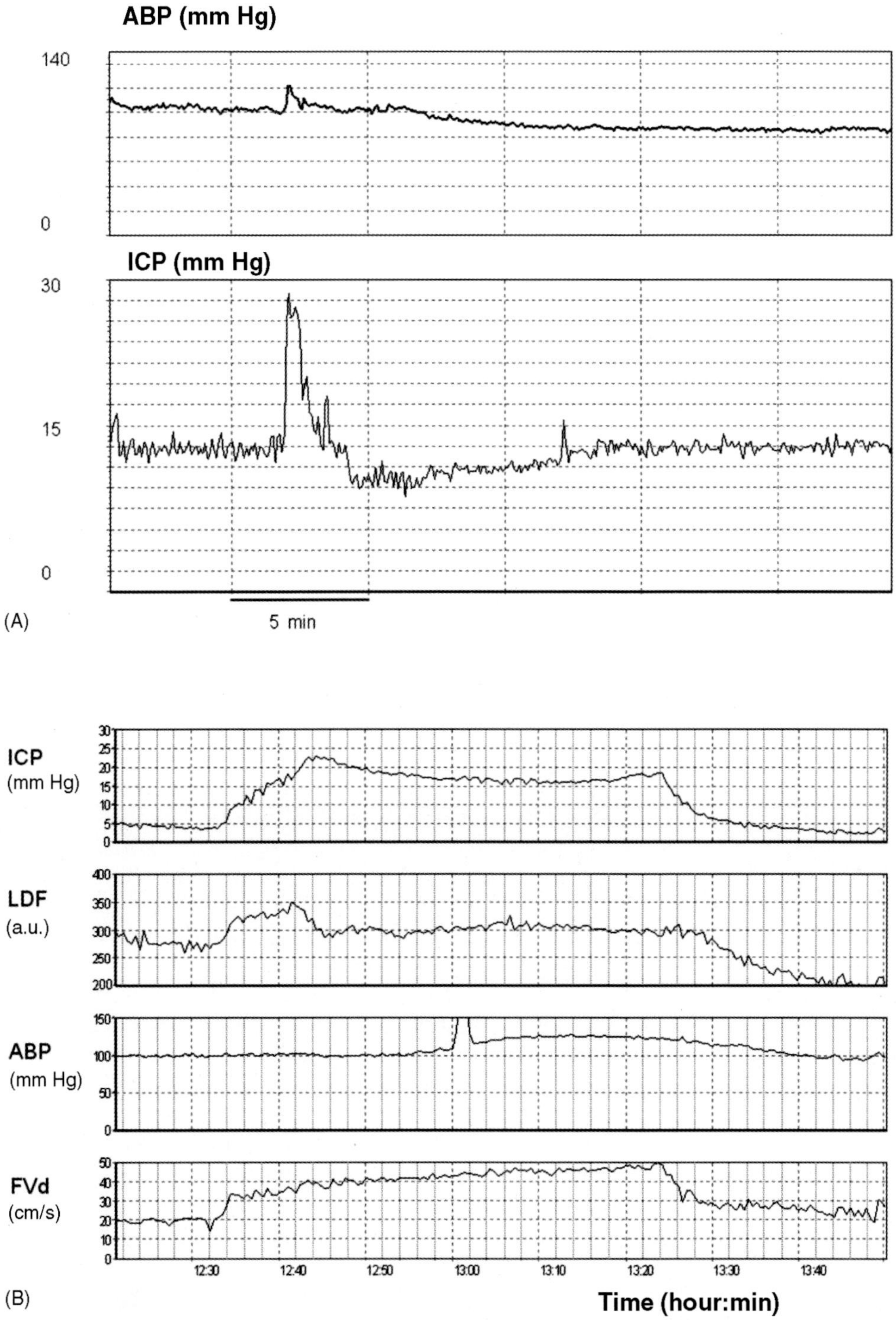

Fig. 5.6 Example of waves of intracranial pressure (ICP) **(A)** associated to variable arterial pressure; **(B)** caused by increase in cerebral blood flow. ABP, arterial blood pressure; FVd, diastolic FV; LDF, laser Doppler flowmeter

The moving-average model of transmission between ABP and ICP, modified by the relationship between ABP and FV, gives lower mean absolute error (~8 mm Hg[69]). The method is based on analysis of a large database of patients with homogeneous pathology who underwent full ICP, ABP, and FV direct monitoring and is most probably pathology dependent. Changes in $PaCO_2$, spasm, and proximal stenosis are confounding factors.

Table 5.6 Cerebral Perfusion Pressure (CPP) (*CPP = MAP – Mean ICP*)

Defined	Difference between cerebral arterial pressure and mean ICP
Function	Pressure driving blood through the cerebrovascular bed
Implications	• Too low CPP = ischemia • Too high CPP = hyperemia • Autoregulation works within upper and lower CPP limits • Thus, a decrease in CPP is dangerous following head trauma as it decreases the driving force for cerebral blood flow and destroys autoregulation. • Excessively high CPP causes intracranial hypertension secondary to transcapillary water leak aggravating brain edema.
Therapy	• CPP-oriented = decreased risk of ischemia postinjury • Lund protocol = alternative concept aimed at decreasing ICP
Optimal CPP	• Where cerebrovascular reactivity is the strongest • Identified by plotting PRx against CPP in individual cases

ICP, intracranial pressure; PRx, pressure reactivity index.

Intracerebral Pressure Gradients

As long as CSF communicates freely among different fluid cavities within the brain there should not be any substantial differences in regionally measured ICP.[70]

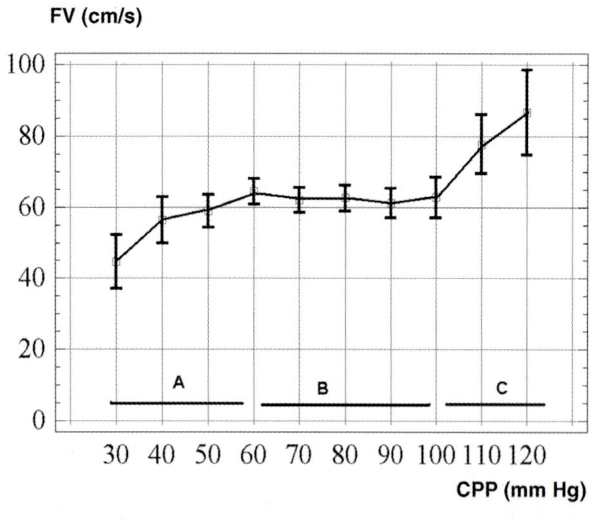

Fig. 5.7 Autoregulatory curve. Flow velocity (FV) measurement points were averaged from almost 300 head-injured patients monitored over periods from 10 minutes to 2 hours day by day. CPP, cerebral perfusion pressure.

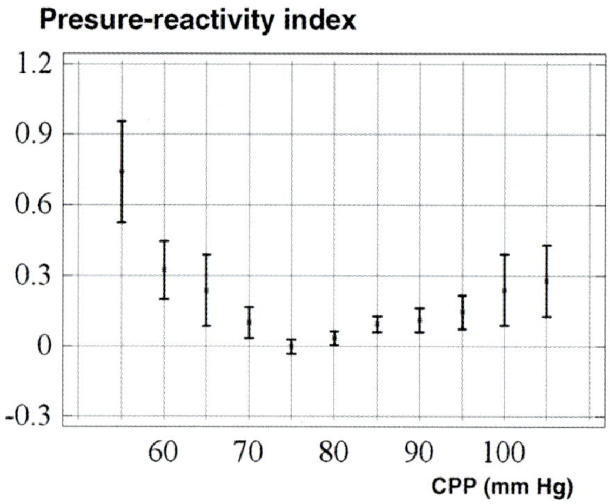

Fig. 5.8 Pressure-reactivity index plotted against cerebral perfusion pressure (CPP) (*N* = 220 patients after head trauma) shows that for low CPP (<65 mm Hg) autoregulation gets worse. But for CPPs >80 mm Hg it also gradually deteriorates. Is there any "optimal CPP" for individual patients?

Direct measurements of pressures in two CSF compartments are performed rarely; however, in head injury intrahemispherical pressure gradients have been reported.[36]

There are intrahemispherical pressure gradients in CCP and nCPP associated with midline shift, side of contusion (assessed using CT), or side of craniectomy.[60,63]

Both nCPP and CCP measurements indicate that cerebral perfusion (nCPP) or level of cerebral dilatation (CCP) is greater on the side of contusion or expanding brain in the case of midline shift or on the side of craniectomy. This may support the hypothesis that it is not a volume expansion of brain tissue but a rather vascular expansion that is associated with side-to-side differences seen on CT scan.[69] This hypothesis is further supported by the fact that cerebral autoregulation is worse on the side of contusion or brain expansion.[71]

Asymmetry in nCPP correlates with worse outcome following head injury.[69]

There are other brain pressures that have not been discussed here. Following head injury, the most useful clinically are ICP and CPP. Although there is no class I evidence that monitoring of these pressures improves outcome, both ICP- or CPP-oriented therapies indicate that strict adherence to protocols improves outcome following head injury.

Cerebral Blood Flow and Autoregulation (Table 5.10)

Direct Methods

Continuous Jugular Thermodilution

Contemporary techniques for the quantitative determination of global CBF include continuous jugular thermodilution,[72] or a double-indicator method based on injections

Table 5.7 Critical Closing Pressure (*CCP = ICP + Active Tension of Arterial Walls*)

Defined	MBP below which cerebral arteries close and blood flow ceases
Measured	Can be measured in three different ways: • Linear interpolation between systolic and diastolic values of blood flow velocity and arterial pressure waveforms • Analysis of first harmonic ABP and FV • Linear regression between flow velocity and ABP pulse waveforms
Correlation with ICP	Weak but significant in head trauma patients (may vary among individual patients)
Correlation with cerebrovascular resistance	Much stronger correlation than with ICP
Correlation with arterial blood CO_2	Correlates well with changes in tension of arterial blood CO_2

Abbreviations: ABP, arterial blood pressure; CO_2, carbon dioxide; FV, flow velocity; ICP, intracranial pressure.

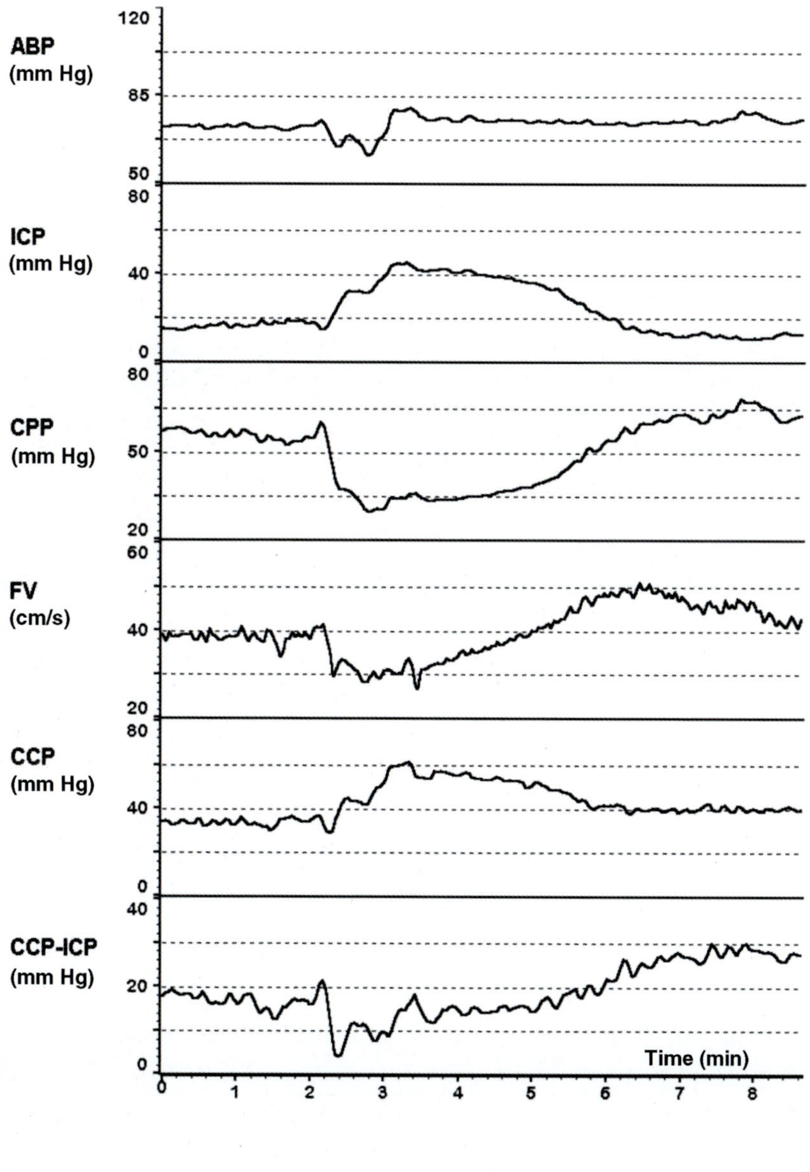

Fig. 5.9 Although absolute value of critical closing pressure (CCP) inaccurately approximates intracranial pressure (ICP), time-related changes in CCP and the difference between CCP and ICP (theoretical value describing tension of arterial walls) during plateau wave of ICP well reflect underlying physiological phenomena. Tension of arterial walls (CCP–ICP) decreases during the wave signifying vasodilation, which in turn increases ICP. ABP, arterial blood pressure; CPP, cerebral perfusion pressure; FV, flow volume.

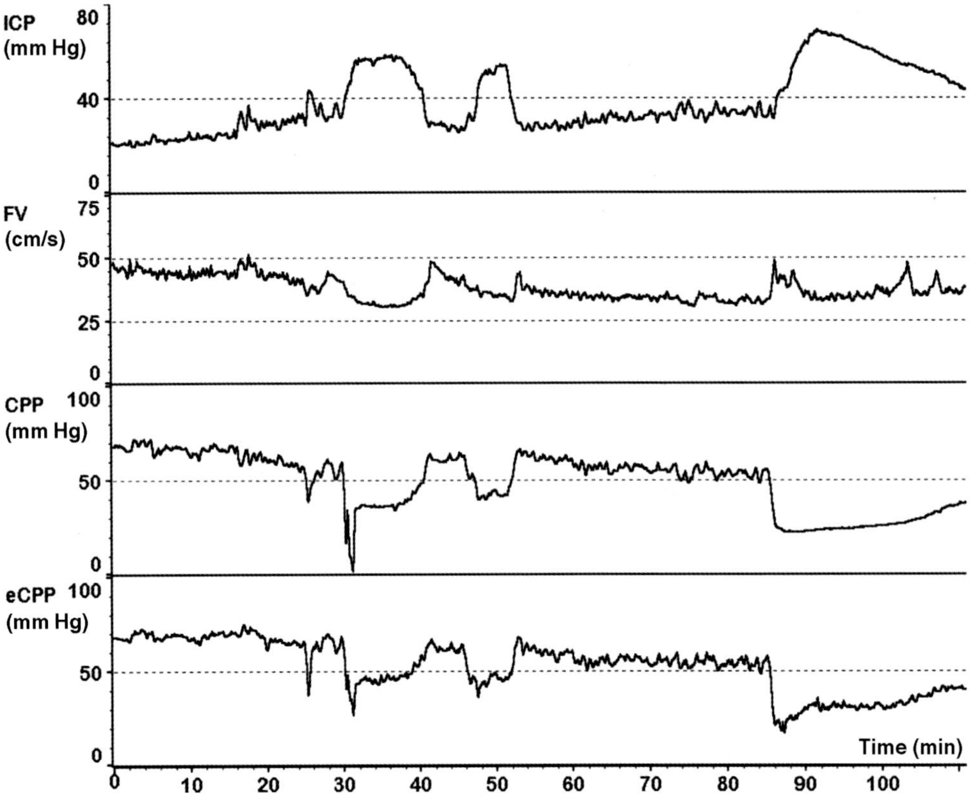

Fig. 5.10 Well-correlated changes in noninvasive cerebral perfusion pressure (nCPP) and real CPP during 2-hour monitoring, including several plateau waves of intracranial pressure (ICP). FV, flow volume.

of dye or iced water providing noncontinuous measurements.[73] Both methods are novel and require wider validation in clinical practice.

Thermal Diffusion (TD)

Thermal diffusion (TD) monitors focal cortical blood flow. A probe is inserted through a bur hole and placed in a cortical region of interest. Recently, an improved version of this technique using an intraparenchymal probe with thermistors has been evaluated in brain-injured patients.[74]

Doppler Flow

More recently, a method based on two angled probes to measure both Doppler flow velocity and the diameter of the internal carotid artery has been introduced for direct blood flow measurement.[75]

Table 5.8 Noninvasive CPP

Formula	*nCPP* = *MAP* × *FVd*/*FVmean* + 14
	• *FVd* = diastolic FV
	• *FVmean* = mean FV
Uses	• Estimate absolute CPP
	• Monitor changes in CPP over time

Abbreviations: CPP, cerebral perfusion pressure; FV, flow volume; nCPP, noninvasive CPP.

Brain Imaging Methods

Brain imaging methods such as xenon-CT, single photon emission computed tomography (SPECT), PET, CT-perfusion, and perfusion magnetic resonance imaging

Table 5.9 Noninvasive ICP

Simple formula	*ICP* = *MAP* − *A*1/*F*1 × *FVmean*
	• *F*1 and *A*1 are first harmonic components of flow velocity and arterial pressure pulse waveforms. This estimator can be interpreted as critical closing pressure (see **Table 5.7**) calculated using first harmonics of FV and ABP.
	• 95% confidence limit large (>20 mm Hg)
Other noninvasive methods	1. Tympanic membrane displacement
	2. Time-of-flight ultrasound through skull
	3. Change in skull diameter
	4. Change in flow velocity in straight sinus
	5. Analysis of pulse waveform of TCD

Abbreviations: ABP, arterial blood pressure; ICP, intracranial pressure; FV, flow volume; MAP, mean arterial blood pressure; TCD, transcranial doppler.

Table 5.10 Direct and Indirect Methods of Measuring Cerebral Blood Flow and Autoregulation

Direct	
1. Continuous jugular thermodilution and double indicator method	Novel, requiring wider validation
2. Thermal diffusion	Monitors focal cortical blood flow, does not work if brain temperature >39°C
3. Doppler carotid artery flow	Direct blood flow measurement
4. Brain imaging methods	Cannot be used for continuous monitoring; provides "snapshot pictures" of distribution of cerebral blood flow (CBF), brain metabolism, or cerebral blood volume
Indirect Methods	
1. Jugular bulb oximetry	Provides information about adequacy of global CBF in relation to metabolic demands
2. Transcranial Doppler ultrasonography	Easy to use, noninvasive, no ionizing radiation; measures blood flow velocity instead of CBF
3. Near-infrared spectroscopy (NIRS)	Measures cerebral hemoglobin saturation via photon scattering in not precisely defined target volume
4. Laser Doppler flowmetry (LDF)	Invasive, continuous, real-time measurements of local perfusion; two major disadvantages: uses small sample volume and only relative changes can be assessed
5. Brain tissue PO_2	Estimates local adequacy of perfusion in a small, focal volume of brain
6. Microdialysis	Measures consequence of raised intracranial pressure and hypoxia on tissue metabolism
7. Brain temperature probes	Controlling brain hypothermia and avoiding pyrexia

(MRI) cannot be used for continuous monitoring. Rather than dynamic information, they provide precision "snapshot pictures" of the distribution of CBF, brain metabolism, or cerebral blood volume.

Indirect Methods

Jugular Bulb Oximetry

Jugular bulb oximetry provides information about the adequacy of global CBF in relation to metabolic demands. The clinical usefulness of $S_{jv}O_2$ monitoring is debatable; although a publication earlier this decade found that $S_{jv}O_2$ monitoring does not substantially influence the management of head-injured patients,[76] other studies indicate a clear and practical benefit.[77]

Transcranial Doppler (TCD)

TCD ultrasonography is easy to use, noninvasive, does not involve ionizing radiation, and can therefore be used repeatedly and also over a longer time period.[15] However, it measures blood flow velocity (BFV) instead of CBF, and the linear relationship between CBF and BFV (CBF = BFV × area of the insonated vessel × cosine of angle of insonation) is only valid if neither the diameter of the insonated vessel nor the angle of insonation change during the examination. This assumption is probably fulfilled in most situations where examinations of the basal cerebral arteries are performed, with the exception of cases of subarachnoid hemorrhage with vasospasm. Monitoring of BFV is possible over even longer periods (several hours); however, problems with reliable fixation of ultrasound probes have not been technically solved. The technique is very useful in continuous monitoring of cerebral autoregulation (see the last section), noninvasive estimation of CPP or ICP and assessment of interhemispherical asymmetry of cerebral hemodynamics.[60,71]

Near-Infrared Spectroscopy (NIRS)

NIRS measures the chromophore level of oxygenated and deoxygenated hemoglobin (i.e., cerebral hemoglobin saturation) via photon scattering, albeit in a target volume that cannot be clearly defined.[17] Changes in these parameters have been used to estimate relative changes in CBF or brain tissue oxygen saturation, with variably enthusiastic reports. There is continuous ongoing technical development in this area, stimulated by excellent cooperation between scientists and industry. New models of NIRS monitors can estimate percent oxygen saturation of mixed cortical blood and provide information with faster resolution, probably allowing continuous monitoring of autoregulation of CBF. However, more clinical studies need to be conducted to unequivocally prove the utility of this interesting technology.

Laser Doppler Flowmetry (LDF)

LDF allows invasive, continuous, real-time measurements of local perfusion (red cell flux) with excellent dynamic resolution.[16,78] It has two major disadvantages: the sample volume is small (1–2 mm^3) and only relative changes can be assessed. However, technique seems to be suitable in continuous assessment of autoregulation of CBF.[78]

Brain Tissue PO_2 ($P_{ti}O_2$)

Brain tissue PO_2 ($P_{ti}O_2$) has been used as an estimator of local adequacy of perfusion.[9] The method is promising because of its good temporal resolution. In some centers, clear clinical benefit has been reported.[19] Brain tissue PO_2 differs from jugular venous oxygen saturation in that it monitors oxygen metabolism in a small, focal volume of brain. Careful consideration therefore needs to be given to sensor location (location in "normal" appearing brain on CT vs. pericontusional location). Increasing experience with this technique enabled thresholds for brain tissue oxygen to be established of 1 to 1.5 kPa.[18] Also, first reports on "optimal CPP"—the perfusion pressure at which $P_{ti}O_2$ achieves maximal level, apparently well correlated with the optimum in PRx—are available (Jaeger 2006, unpublished report). Attempts have been made to integrate tissue oxygen sensor with CO_2, pH,[79] and temperature, but experience has demonstrated that although efficient in research studies,[80] routine clinical monitoring has been hampered by several factors, including sensor fragility. New sensors integrating brain tissue oxygen with temperature and ICP are currently being developed.

Microdialysis

The consequence of raised ICP and hypoxia on tissue metabolism can be monitored using the technique of microdialysis. Pioneered in the laboratory, this technique has now been introduced into the clinical arena.[5,81–84] Bedside monitors enable the extracellular concentrations of glucose, lactate, pyruvate, glutamate and glycerol to be determined. Increasing experience from a number of centers has identified the lactate:pyruvate ratio as a marker of ischemia and glycerol as an indicator of cell membrane integrity. Derangement in biochemistry has been studied in relation to outcome following head injury. The next stage in evaluation of microdialysis is to investigate which therapeutic maneuvers influences the chemistry favorably. Examples include hyperoxia and augmentation of CPP. Recommendation for an application of microdialysis to patients with traumatic brain injury and subarachnoid hemorrhage have been produced in a consensus statement.[85] The temporal resolution of microdialysis is limited, and the position of the probe will influence results.

Brain Temperature

Brain temperature probes may be used alone or in combination with other intraparenchymal sensors (such as the Camino ICP monitor or Neurotrend). They are important in controlling brain hypothermia (although use of hypothermia protocols is still controversial) and avoiding pyrexia.[86]

Cerebral Autoregulation

Two essential brain-protecting reserves may be described (**Table 5.11**).

1. Compensatory reserve can be understood as the hypothetical maximal cerebral volume load below which we do not notice any substantial (exponential) increase in ICP.
2. Autoregulatory reserve represents how far the CPP can be reduced without substantial decrease in CBF.

Although compensatory reserve may be assessed using continuous monitoring of brain compliance[87] and perhaps ICP pulse waveform analysis,[45] TCD ultrasonography can be used to assess the brain autoregulatory reserve. Although cerebral autoregulation is frequently disturbed following head injury, the extent of this disturbance may fluctuate with time.[88,89] Regular assessment is therefore an essential component of this type of evaluation. Several methods are available (**Table 5.12**).

Static Test of Autoregulation

Static test of autoregulation relies on recording MCA flow velocity during changes in MAP (mean arterial blood pressure) induced by an infusion of vasopressors. The static rate of autoregulation (SRoR) is calculated as the percentage increase in vascular resistance (CPP/BFV) divided by the percentage rise in CPP. The common error here is considering only changes in MAP instead of CPP—this may

Table 5.11 Two Essential Brain-Protecting Reserves

	Description	How Measured
Compensatory reserve	Hypothetical maximum cerebral volume load in which no substantial increase in ICP is seen	Measured via continuous monitoring of brain compliance or ICP pulse waveform analysis
Autoregulatory reserve	How far the CPP can be decreased without a significant change in CBF	Measured via transcranial Doppler ultrasonography or monitored using pressure reactivity

Abbreviations: CBF, cerebral blood flow; CPP, cerebral perfusion pressure; ICP, intracranial pressure.

Table 5.12 Methods for Assessing Extent of Autoregulation in the Event of a Head Injury

Test	Function
Static test of autoregulation (SRoR)	Calculated as a percentage change in vascular resistance (CPP/BFV) divided by the percentage change in CPP (100% SroR = fully intact autoregulation; 0% = no autoregulation)
CO_2 cerebrovascular reactivity	Correlates significantly with worse outcome following head injury
Dynamic rate of autoregulation	Measures quickness of cerebral vessels reacting to sudden change in MBP. Can be measured using leg-cuff test or spontaneous fluctuations in ABP. Can be graded using autoregulation index (ARI: 9 = good autoregulation, 0 = absent autoregulation)
Transient hyperemic response test (THRT)	Presence of response correlates with better outcomes
Phase shift between superimposed respiratory and arterial BP waves	Noninvasive method of deriving autoregulation status from natural fluctuations in MCA flow velocity • 0° phase shift = absent autoregulation • Positive phase shift = intact autoregulation
Continuous monitoring	Allows calculation of mean index (Mx) = correlation coefficient between mean CPP and mean BFV • Positive coefficient signifies a positive association between BFV and CPP = disturbed autoregulation • Zero or negative correlation = intact autoregulation

Abbreviations: ABP, arterial blood pressure; BFV, blood flow velocity; CPP, cerebral perfusion pressure; MAP, mean arterial blood pressure; SRoR, static rate of autoregulation.

lead to "false autoregulation" when ICP changes proportionally to the testing step-increase in MAP. An SRoR of 100% indicates fully intact autoregulation, whereas an SoR of 0% indicates that autoregulation is fully exhausted.[90]

CO_2 Cerebrovascular Reactivity

Testing for CO_2 cerebrovascular reactivity has been shown to have an important application in the assessment of severely head-injured patients as well as other cerebrovascular diseases. Although cerebral vessels are reactive to changes in $PaCO_2$ even when cerebral pressure autoregulation is impaired, disturbed CO_2 reactivity correlates significantly with worse outcome following head injury.[91]

Dynamic Rate of Autoregulation (RoR)

A method in which a step decrease in arterial blood pressure is achieved by the deflation of compressed leg cuffs while simultaneously measuring TCD flow velocity in the MCA allows calculation of the so-called dynamic rate of autoregulation (RoR).[90] It describes how quickly cerebral vessels react to the sudden fall in blood pressure.

Transient Hyperemic Response Test (THRT)

Short-term compression of the common carotid artery produces a marked decrease in the ipsilateral MCA flow velocity. If autoregulation is intact, the distal cerebrovascular bed dilates during compression. Upon release of compression, a transient hyperemia lasting for a few seconds occurs until the distal cerebrovascular bed constricts to its former diameter. This sequence of events, which underlies the transient hyperemic response test (THRT), indicates a positive autoregulatory response (see **Fig. 5.11**). A positive correlation between the presence of a hyperemic response and better outcome following head injury has been demonstrated.[92]

Phase Shift between the Superimposed Respiratory and Arterial Blood Pressure Waves

An interesting noninvasive method of deriving autoregulatory status from natural fluctuations in MCA flow velocity involves the assessment of phase shift between the superimposed respiratory and arterial blood pressure waves during slow and deep breathing. A zero degree phase shift indicates absent autoregulation, whereas a phase shift of 90 degrees indicates intact autoregulation.[93]

Continuous Monitoring

By continuous monitoring over 60 consecutive 5- to 10-second periods, a correlation coefficient between mean CPP and mean BFV can be calculated. This coefficient has been termed the *mean index* (Mx). A positive coefficient signifies a positive association between BFV and CPP, that is, disturbed autoregulation. A zero or negative correlation coefficient signifies an absent or negative association, implying intact autoregulation. Mathematical interpretation is exactly the same as for the PRx. Suitable illustration would be exactly the same as in **Fig. 5.4**, with the exception of variables plotted against the y- and x-axis. This time it should be BFV (y) and CPP (x). This index seems to

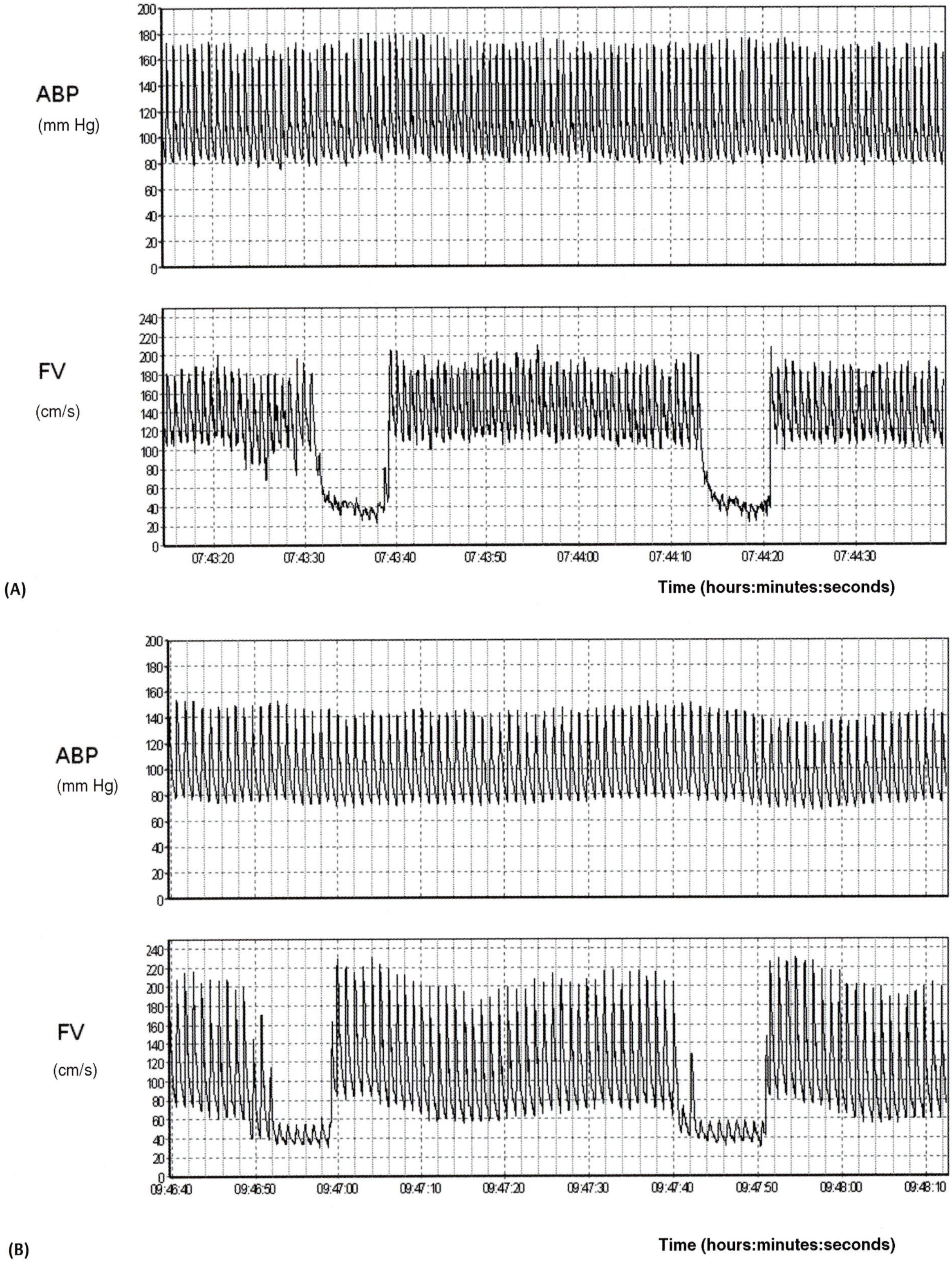

Fig. 5.11 Transient hyperemic response test. There is no hyperemia after release of common carotid artery compression in **(A)** indicating failure of cerebral autoregulation. In contrast, in **(B)** a short period of elevated blood flow velocity following release of compression signifies intact autoregulation. ABP, arterial blood pressure; FV, flow volume.

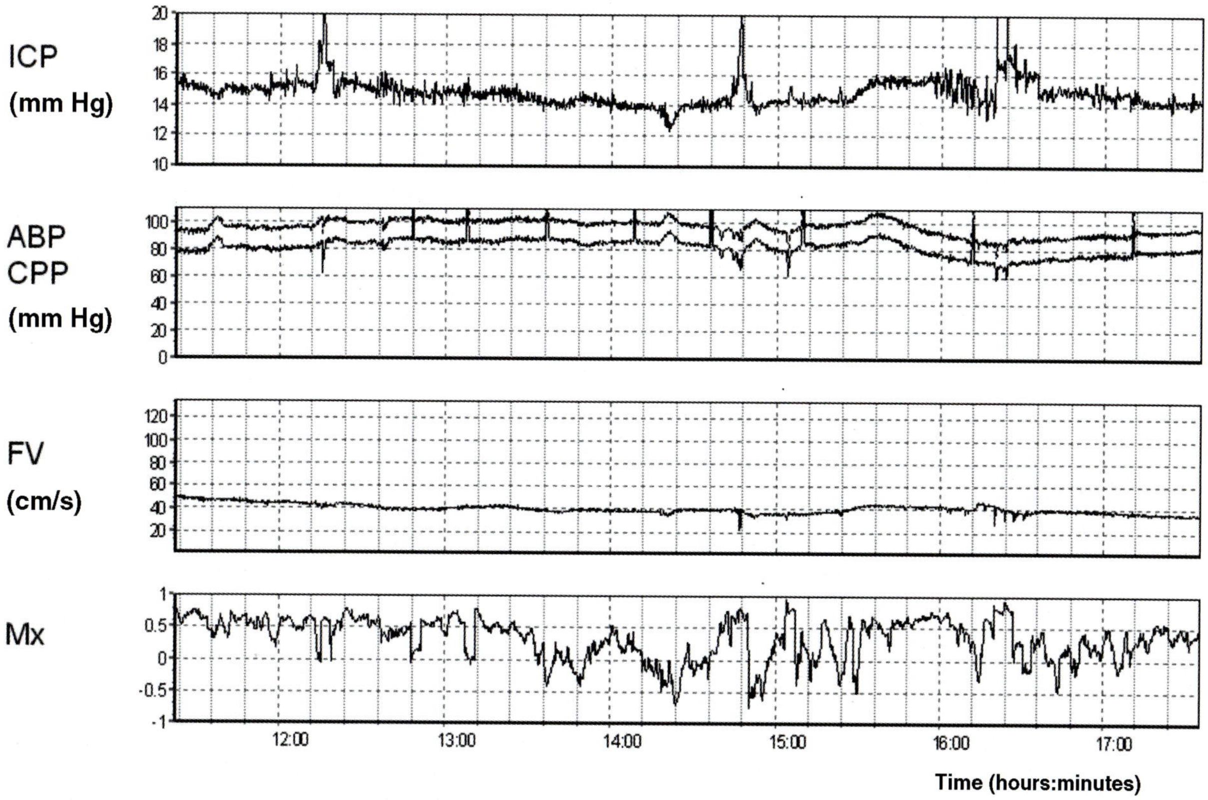

Fig. 5.12 Example of 6 hours of monitoring of Mx (mean index) in patient after head injury. Autoregulation is first disturbed (12:00 to 13:30), then improves, then gets worse and again gets slightly better at the end of recording. Mx is (like PRx) quite noisy and requires time-averaging. At the same time it seems to respond to temporary elevations of intracranial pressure (ICP) (approximately 14:40 and 16:30). ABP, arterial blood pressure; CPP, cerebral perfusion pressure; FV, flow volume.

be ideal for monitoring transient changes in autoregulation in response to a cerebral intrinsic phenomena (see **Fig. 5.12**). Group analysis has demonstrated that the autoregulation index averaged daily was related to clinical outcome following head injury; a positive Mx (disturbed autoregulation) was associated with worse outcome.[9] Similar methods, based on transfer function, coherence function, or phase shift analysis are becoming popular in multiple clinical applications.[11,93–95]

Other ultrasound Doppler modalities have been recently used for estimation of autoregulatory index: LDF, brain tissue oxygenation, or NIRS. Although these new techniques look promising, more clinical data are needed to validate them fully.

Conclusion

Brain monitoring techniques are able to facilitate clinical decision making in posttraumatic clinical care. A mixture of invasive and noninvasive methods, monitoring of cerebral autoregulation, and a multimodal approach are emerging themes, requiring further clinical validations. There are trends toward the individualization of fixed management protocols in posttraumatic intensive care, according to available monitoring results.

Acknowledgments Many thanks to our colleagues who participated in the head injury monitoring program in Cambridge, UK in 1991–2006, whose experience, knowledge, and clinical material helped us to write this review:

Mrs. P. Al-Rawi, Mrs. D. Chattfield, Mrs. C. Turner, Dr. Balestreri, Miss. M. Hiler, Dr. P. Smielewski, Dr. S. K. Piechnik, Dr. L. A. Steiner, Mr. E. Guazzo, Mr. P. C. Whetfield, P. Minhas, Dr. M. Soehle, Mr. R. Kett-White, Dr. E. Schmidt, Dr. B. Schmidt, Mr. A. Kumar, Mr. A. Raabe, Mr. M. Schuhmann, Dr. F. K. Matta, Professor A. Gupta, Professor D. K. Menon, the nursing and research staff from the Neuro Critical Care Unit and the Wolfson Brain Imaging Centre.

Grant support: Medical Research Council No G9439390 ID 65883.

Dr. M. Czosnyka is on leave from Warsaw University of Technology, Poland.

Dr. P. J. Hutchinson is supported by Academy of Medical Sciences Health Foundation Senior Surgical Fellowship.

References

1. Miller JD, Becker DP. Secondary insults to the injured brain. J R Coll Surg Edinb 1982;27:292–298
2. Pickard JD, Czosnyka M. Management of raised intracranial pressure. J Neurol Neurosurg Psychiatry 1993;56:845–858
3. Robertson CS, Contant CF, Narayan RK, Grossman RG. Cerebral blood flow, AVDO2, and neurologic outcome in head-injured patients. J Neurotrauma 1992;9(Suppl 1):S349–S358
4. Unterberg AW, Kiening KL, Hartl R, Bardt T, Sarrafzadeh AS, Lanksch WR. Multimodal monitoring in patients with head injury: evaluation of the effects of treatment on cerebral oxygenation. J Trauma 1997; 42(5, Suppl):S32–S37
5. Ungerstedt U. Microdialysis: principles and applications for studies in animals and man. J Intern Med 1991;230:365–373
6. Rosner MJ, Necker DP. Origin and evolution of plateau waves. J Neurosurg 1984;60:312–324
7. Lassen NA. Cerebral blood flow and oxygen consumption in man. Physiol Rev 1959;39:183–238
8. Czosnyka M, Smielewski P, Piechnik S, Steiner LA, Pickard JD. Cerebral autoregulation following head injury. J Neurosurg 2001;95: 756–763
9. Overgaard J, Tweed WA. Cerebral circulation after head injury, I: Cerebral blood flow and its regulation after closed head injury with emphasis on clinical correlation. J Neurosurg 1974;41:531–541
10. Czosnyka M, Whitehouse H, Smielewski P, Kirkpatrick P, Pickard JD. Computer supported multimodal monitoring bed-side in neuro intensive care. Int J Clin Monit Comput 1994;11:223–232
11. Smielewski P, Czosnyka M, Steiner L, et al. ICM+: software for on-line analysis of bedside monitoring data after severe head trauma. Acta Neurochir Suppl (Wien) 2005;95:43–49
12. Howells TP, Piper IR, Jones PA, Souter M, Miller JD. Design of a research database for the study of secondary insults following head injury. J Neurotrauma 1995;12:471
13. Panerai RB, White RP, Markus HS, Evans DH. Grading of cerebral dynamic autoregulation from spontaneous fluctuations in arterial blood pressure. Stroke 1998;29:2341–2346
14. Chan KH, Dearden NM, Miller JD, Midgley S, Piper IR. Transcranial Doppler waveform differences in hyperemic and nonhyperemic patients after severe head injury. Surg Neurol 1992;38:433–436
15. Manno EM. Transcranial Doppler ultrasonography in the neurocritical care unit. Crit Care Clin 1997;13:79–104
16. Kirkpatrick PJ, Smielewski P, Czosnyka M, Pickard JD. Continuous monitoring of cortical perfusion by laser Doppler flowmetry in ventilated patients with head injury. J Neurol Neurosurg Psychiatry 1994;57(11): 1382–1388
17. Kirkpatrick PJ, Smielewski P, Czosnyka M, Menon DK, Pickard JD. Near-infrared spectroscopy use in patients with head injury. J Neurosurg 1995;83:963–970
18. Gupta AK, Hutchinson PJ, Fryer T, et al. Measurement of brain tissue oxygenation performed using positron emission tomography scanning to validate a novel monitoring method. J Neurosurg 2002;96(2):263–268
19. van den Brink WA, van Santbrink H, Steyerberg EW, et al. Brain oxygen tension in severe head injury. Neurosurgery 2000;46:868–876
20. Hutchinson PJ, O'Connell MT, Al-Rawi PG, et al. Clinical cerebral microdialysis: a methodological study. J Neurosurg 2000;93(1):37–43
21. Steiner LA, Czosnyka M. Should we measure cerebral blood flow in head-injured patients? Br J Neurosurg 2002;16:429–439
22. Zhong J, Dujovny M, Park HK, Perez E, Perlin AR, Diaz FG. Advances in ICP monitoring techniques. Neurol Res 2003;25(4):339–350
23. Pedley TJ, Luo XY. Modelling flow and oscillations in collapsible tubes. Theor Comput Fluid Dyn 1998;10:277–294
24. Piechnik SK, Czosnyka M, Richards HK, Whitfield PC, Pickard JD. Cerebral venous blood outflow: a theoretical model based on laboratory simulation. Neurosurgery 2001;49:1214–1222
25. Higgins JN, Cousins C, Owler BK, Sarkies N, Pickard JD. Idiopathic intracranial hypertension: 12 cases treated by venous sinus stenting. J Neurol Neurosurg Psychiatry 2003;74(12):1662–1666
26. Davson H, Hollingsworth G, Segal MB. The mechanism of drainage of cerebrospinal fluid. Brain 1970;93:665–678
27. Marmarou A, Maset AL, Ward JD, et al. Contribution of CSF and vascular factors to elevation of ICP in severely head injured patients. J Neurosurg 1987;66:883–890
28. Czosnyka M, Richards HK, Czosnyka Z, Piechnik S, Pickard JD. Vascular components of cerebrospinal fluid compensation. J Neurosurg 1999;90:752–759
29. Piechnik SK, Czosnyka M, Harris NG, Minhas PS, Pickard JD. A model of the cerebral and cerebrospinal fluid circulations to examine asymmetry in cerebrovascular reactivity. J Cereb Blood Flow Metab 2001;21(2):182–192
30. Ekstedt J. CSF hydrodynamic studies in man: normal hydrodynamic variables related to CSF pressure and flow. J Neurol Neurosurg Psychiatry 1978;41:345–353
31. Albeck MJ, Borgesen SE, Gjerris F, Schmidt JF, Sorensen PS. Intracranial pressure and cerebrospinal fluid outflow conductance in healthy subjects. J Neurosurg 1991;74(4):597–600
32. Chapman PH, Cosman ER, Arnold MA. The relationship between ventricular fluid pressure and body position in normal subjects and subjects with shunts: a telemetric study. Neurosurgery 1990;26:181–189
33. Marmarou A. Increased intracranial pressure in head injury and influence of blood volume. J Neurotrauma 1992;9(Suppl 1):S327–S332
34. Narayan RK, Kishore PR, Becker DP, et al. Intracranial pressure: to monitor or not to monitor? A review of our experience with severe head injury. J Neurosurg 1982;56(5):650–659
35. Piper I, Barnes A, Smith D, Dunn L. The Camino intracranial pressure sensor: is it optimal technology? An internal audit with a review of current intracranial pressure monitoring technologies. Neurosurgery 2001;49:1158–1164
36. Chambers IR, Kane PJ, Signorini DF, Jenkins A, Mendelow AD. Bilateral ICP monitoring: its importance in detecting the severity of secondary insults. Acta Neurochir Suppl (Wien) 1998;71:42–43
37. Wolfla CE, Luerssen TG, Bowman RM. Regional brain tissue pressure gradients created by expanding extradural temporal mass lesion. J Neurosurg 1997;86(3):505–510
38. Balestreri M, Czosnyka M, Steiner LA, et al. Intracranial hypertension: what additional information can be derived from ICP waveform after head injury? Acta Neurochir (Wien) 2004;146(2):131–141
39. Balestreri M, Czosnyka M, Hutchinson P, et al. Impact of intracranial pressure and cerebral perfusion pressure on severe disability and mortality after head injury. Neurocrit Care 2006;4(1):8–13
40. Saul TG, Ducker TB. Effect of intracranial pressure monitoring and aggressive treatment on mortality in severe head injury. J Neurosurg 1982;56(4):498–503
41. Uzzell BP, Obrist WD, Dolinskas CA, Langfitt TW. Relationship of acute CBF and ICP findings to neuropsychological outcome in severe head injury. J Neurosurg 1986;65(5):630–635
42. Eker C, Schalen W, Asgeirsson B, Grande PO, Ranstam J, Nordstrom CH. Reduced mortality after severe head injury will increase the demands for rehabilitation services. Brain Inj 2000;14:605–619
43. Avezaat CJ, van Eijndhoven JH, Wyper DJ. Cerebrospinal fluid pulse pressure and intracranial volume-pressure relationships. J Neurol Neurosurg Psychiatry 1979;42(8):687–700
44. Piper IR, Miller JD, Dearden M, Leggate JRS, Robertson I. System analysis of cerebrovascular pressure transmission: an observational study in head injured patients. J Neurosurg 1990;73:871–880
45. Czosnyka M, Guazzo E, Whitehouse H, et al. Significance of intracranial pressure waveform analysis after head injury. Acta Neurochir (Wien) 1996;138:531–542
46. Steiner LA, Czosnyka M, Piechnik SK, et al. Continuous monitoring of cerebrovascular pressure reactivity allows determination of optimal cerebral perfusion pressure in patients with traumatic brain injury. Crit Care Med 2002;30(4):733–738
47. Steiner LA, Coles JP, Czosnyka M, et al. Cerebrovascular pressure reactivity is related to global cerebral oxygen metabolism after head injury. J Neurol Neurosurg Psychiatry 2003;74(6):765–770

48. Steiner LA, Coles JP, Johnston AJ, et al. Assessment of cerebrovascular autoregulation in head-injured patients: a validation study. Stroke 2003;34:2404–2409
49. Balestreri M, Steiner LA, Czosnyka M. Sex-related differences and traumatic brain injury. J Neurosurg 2003;99(3):616–617
50. Miller JD, Stanek A, Langfitt TW. Concepts of cerebral perfusion pressure and vascular compression during intracranial hypertension. Prog Brain Res 1972;35:411–432
51. Rosner MJ, Rosner SD, Johnson AH. Cerebral perfusion pressure: management protocol and clinical results. J Neurosurg 1995;83:949–962
52. Obrist WD, Langfitt TW, Jaggi JL, Cruz J, Gennarelli TA. Cerebral blood flow and metabolism in comatose patients with acute head injury: relationship to intracranial hypertension. J Neurosurg 1984;61:241–255
53. Burton AC. On the physical equilibrium of the small blood vessels. Am J Physiol 1951;164:319–329
54. Dewey RC, Pieper HP, Hunt WE. Experimental cerebral hemodynamics: vasomotor tone, critical closing pressure, and vascular bed resistance. J Neurosurg 1974;41:597–606
55. Aaslid R, Lash SR, Bardy GH, Gild WH, Newell DW. Dynamic pressure–flow velocity relationships in the human cerebral circulation. Stroke 2003;34(7):1645–1649
56. Czosnyka M, Smielewski P, Piechnik S, et al. Critical closing pressure in cerebrovascular circulation. J Neurol Neurosurg Psychiatry 1999;66: 606–611
57. Soehle M, Czosnyka M, Pickard JD, Kirkpatrick PJ. Critical closing pressure in subarachnoid hemorrhage: effect of cerebral vasospasm and limitations of a transcranial Doppler–derived estimation. Stroke 2004;35(6):1393–1398
58. Richards HK, Czosnyka M, Pickard JD. Assessment of critical closing pressure in the cerebral circulation as a measure of cerebrovascular tone. Acta Neurochir (Wien) 1999;141:1221–1227
59. Gooskens I, Schmidt EA, Czosnyka M, et al. Pressure-autoregulation, CO_2 reactivity and asymmetry of haemodynamic parameters in patients with carotid artery stenotic disease: a clinical appraisal. Acta Neurochir (Wien) 2003;145(7):527–532
60. Kumar A, Schmidt EA, Hiler M, Smielewski P, Pickard JD, Czosnyka M. Asymmetry of critical closing pressure following head injury. J Neurol Neurosurg Psychiatry 2005;76(11):1570–1573
61. Aaslid R, Lundar T, Lindegaard K-F. Estimation of erebral perfusion pressure from arterial blood pressure and transcranial Doppler recordings. In: Miller JD, Teasdale GM, Rowan JO, Galbraith SL, Mendelow AD eds. Intracranial Pressure VI. Berlin, Heildelberg: Springer Verlag; 1986:229–231
62. Czosnyka M, Matta BF, Smielewski P, Kirkpatrick P, Pickard JD. Cerebral perfusion pressure in head-injured patients: a non-invasive assessment using transcranial Doppler ultrasonography. J Neurosurg 1998;88:802–808
63. Schmidt EA, Czosnyka M, Gooskens I, et al. Preliminary experience of the estimation of cerebral perfusion pressure using trascranial Doppler ultrasonography. J Neurol Neurosurg Psychiatry 2001;70:198–204
64. Reid A, Marchbanks RJ, Martin R, Pickard JD, Bateman N, Brightwell R. Mean intracranial pressure monitoring by an audiological technique—a pilot study. J Neurol Neurosurg Psychiatry 1989;52:610–612
65. Petkus V, Ragauskas A, Jurkonis R. Investigation of intracranial media ultrasonic monitoring model. Ultrasonics 2002;40:829–833
66. Torikoshi S, Wilson MH, Ballard RE, et al. Ultrasound measurement of transcranial distance during head-down tilt. J Gravit Physiol 1995; 2(1):P145–P146
67. Schoser BG, Riemenschneider N, Hansen HC. The impact of raised intracranial pressure on cerebral venous hemodynamics: a prospective venous transcranial Doppler ultrasonography study. J Neurosurg 1999; 91(5):744–749
68. Klingelhofer J, Conrad B, Benecke R. Evaluation of intracranial pressure from transcranial Doppler studies in cerebral disease. J Neurol 1988;235:159–162
69. Schmidt B, Klingelhofer J, Schwarze JJ, Sander D, Wittich I. Noninvasive prediction of intracranial pressure curves using transcranial Doppler ultrasonography and blood pressure curves. Stroke 1997;28(12): 2465–2472
70. Stephensen H, Tisell M, Wikkelso C. There is no transmantle pressure gradient in communicating or noncommunicating hydrocephalus. Neurosurgery 2002;50(4):763–771
71. Schmidt EA, Czosnyka M, Steiner LA, et al. Asymmetry of pressure autoregulation after traumatic brain injury. J Neurosurg 2003;99(6): 991–998
72. Melot C, Berre J, Moraine JJ, Kahn RJ. Estimation of cerebral blood flow at bedside by continuous jugular thermodilution. J Cereb Blood Flow Metab 1996;16:1263–1270
73. Wietasch GJ, Mielck F, Scholz M, von Spiegel T, Stephan H, Hoeft A. Bedside assessment of cerebral blood flow by double-indicator dilution technique. Anesthesiology 2000;92:367–375
74. Sioutos PJ, Orozco JA, Carter LP, Weinand ME, Hamilton AJ, Williams FC. Continuous regional cerebral cortical blood flow monitoring in head-injured patients. Neurosurgery 1995;36:943–949
75. Soustiel JF, Glenn TC, Vespa P, Rinsky B, Hanuscin C, Martin NA. Assessment of cerebral blood flow by means of blood-flow-volume measurement in the internal carotid artery: comparative study with a 133 xenon clearance technique. Stroke 2003;34:1876–1880
76. Latronico N, Beindorf AE, Rasulo FA, et al. Limits of intermittent jugular bulb oxygen saturation monitoring in the management of severe head trauma patients. Neurosurgery 2000;46:1131–1138
77. Gopinath SP, Robertson CS, Contant CF, et al. Jugular venous desaturation and outcome after head injury. J Neurol Neurosurg Psychiatry 1994;57:717–723
78. Lam JM, Hsiang JN, Poon WS. Monitoring of autoregulation using laser Doppler flowmetry in patients with head injury. J Neurosurg 1997;86: 438–445
79. Gupta AK, Zygun DA, Johnston AJ, et al. Extracellular brain pH and outcome following severe traumatic brain injury. J Neurotrauma 2004; 21(6):678–684
80. Charbel FT, Du X, Hoffman WE, Ausman JI. Brain tissue PO_2, PCO_2, and pH during cerebral vasospasm. Surg Neurol 2000;54:432–437
81. Hutchinson PJ, Gupta AK, Fryer TF, et al. Correlation between cerebral blood flow, substrate delivery, and metabolism in head injury: a combined microdialysis and triple oxygen positron emission tomography study. J Cereb Blood Flow Metab 2002;22(6):735–745
82. Hutchinson PJ, O'Connell MT, Kirkpatrick PJ, Pickard JD. How can we measure substrate, metabolite and neurotransmitter concentrations in the human brain? Physiol Meas 2002;23(2):R75–R109
83. Kett-White R, Hutchinson PJ, Al-Rawi PG, et al. Cerebral oxygen and microdialysis monitoring during aneurysm surgery: effects of blood pressure, cerebrospinal fluid drainage, and temporary clipping on infarction. J Neurosurg 2002;96(6):1013–1019
84. Nordstrom CH, Reinstrup P, Xu W, Gardenfors A, Ungerstedt U. Assessment of the lower limit for cerebral perfusion pressure in severe head injuries by bedside monitoring of regional energy metabolism. Anesthesiology 2003;98:809–814
85. Bellander BM, Cantais E, Enblad P, et al. Consensus meeting on microdialysis in neurointensive care. Intensive Care Med 2004;30: 2166–2169
86. Dietrich WD. The importance of brain temperature in cerebral injury. J Neurotrauma 1992;9(Suppl 2):S475–S485
87. Kiening KL, Schoening W, Stover J, Unterberg AW. Continuous monitoring of intracranial compliance after severe head injury: relation to data quality, intracranial pressure and brain tissue PO_2. Br J Neurosurg 2003;17:311–318
88. Kirkpatrick PJ, Smielewski P, Piechnik S, Pickard JD, Czosnyka M. Early effects of mannitol in patients with head injuries assessed using bedside multimodality monitoring. Neurosurgery 1996;39(4): 714–720
89. Muizelaar JP, Ward JD, Marmarou A, Newlon PG, Wachi A. Cerebral blood flow and metabolism in severely head-injured children, II: Autoregulation. J Neurosurg 1989;71:72–76
90. Strebel S, Lam AM, Matta B, Mayberg TS, Aaslid R, Newell DW. Dynamic and static cerebral autoregulation during isoflurane, desflurane, and propofol anesthesia. Anesthesiology 1995;83:66–76

91. Lee JH, Kelly DF, Oertel M, et al. Carbon dioxide reactivity, pressure autoregulation, and metabolic suppression reactivity after head injury: a transcranial Doppler study. J Neurosurg 2001;95:222–232
92. Smielewski P, Czosnyka M, Kirkpatrick P, Pickard JD. Evaluation of transient hyperaemic response test in head injured patients. J Neurosurg 1997;86:773–778
93. Diehl RR, Linden D, Lucke D, Berlit P. Spontaneous blood pressure oscillations and cerebral autoregulation. Clin Auton Res 1998;8:7–12
94. Hu HH, Kuo TB, Wong WJ, et al. Transfer function analysis of cerebral hemodynamics in patients with carotid artery stenosis. J Cereb Blood Flow Metab 1999;19:460–465
95. Steinmeier R, Bauhuf C, Hubner U, et al. Slow rhythmic oscillations of blood pressure, intracranial pressure, microcirculation, and cerebral oxygenation: dynamic interrelation and time course in humans. Stroke 1996;27:2236–2243

6 Classification Systems

Marjorie C. Wang and Thomas A. Gennarelli

There is no classification system for brain injury that meets every need. The corollary of this principle is that different classification systems meet differing needs (**Table 6.1**). To determine which type of classification system is best for individual circumstances demands consideration of several facts.

Why Classify

Patients could need to be categorized for different purposes such as for triage, for treatment, or for outcomes research. Triage may itself require different systems depending on whether classification is necessary at a sporting venue (football or soccer fields, for instance), on a battlefield (with multiple possible scenarios, depending on the battle), or in single, multiple, or mass civilian casualties. These systems will have as their principal purpose a rough determination of injury severity so that patients can be brought to the most appropriate medical facility. Undertriage is not sensitive enough and allows too few to be delivered to a higher care facility, whereas overtriage will deliver too many patients with minor injuries to a high-level facility. In general, the complexity of the physiological derangement is the most important property for triage, the type of injury being of less importance. However, when classifying patients regarding treatment, the type of injury may be of predominant importance. Thus, immediate classification regarding the need for urgent surgery is dependent on whether a mass lesion or open wound is present and not on whether diffuse axonal injury exists. Finally, different variables are important when classifying the outcome of patients with brain injury than are used when classifying injury severity. Thus, outcomes definitions and outcomes research must use systems that are less dependent on acute physiological changes and more dependent on functional capacity, impairments, or brain function and disability.

Table 6.1 Traumatic Brain Injury Classification Systems

Different classification systems are useful for different purposes.

Advantages

- Facilitates triage, treatment, and research
- Provides a tool for communication between providers
- Allows for measurement of change over time with repeat administration of classification tools

Disadvantages

- No system meets every need.
- Personnel administering classification instruments need to be trained to classify consistently and correctly.
- The optimal time to classify patients is unknown and depends on the purpose of classification.

Who Classifies

Given that there must be different classification systems for different purposes, it follows that many different types of personnel must be involved in determining a patient's classification. Each must be trained in the nuances of the systems he or she uses. Thus, an athletic trainer must understand mild traumatic brain injury (MTBI) classification used in the sports arena whereas an emergency medical services provider, emergency department nurse or physician, or trauma surgeon must understand the Glasgow Coma Score (GCS) instead. To this, the neurosurgeon must also understand the anatomic and physiological derangements and scale them appropriately for treatment.

What to Classify

For most purposes classification systems target the immediate postinjury problems (these are the injury severity scales) or the long-term consequences of the injuries (these are the outcome scales).

Types of Classification Systems

Classification systems can be constructed in many ways. There is a general hierarchy of scaling systems from *categorical* (or nominal, where names are assigned to subcategories; injury classified by gender is an example), to *ordinal* (where classes are rank ordered, often with a numeric descriptor, and where the "distance" between the numbers is not necessarily equal; the Abbreviated Injury Scale [AIS] and GCS are examples), to *continuous* scales (sometimes subdivided into interval and ratio systems, where the distance between the numbers is the same, such as age). Other than for age, there are few clinical brain injury classification systems that use continuous descriptors. Most systems in use are either ordinal or categorical. Although widely violated, to be correct, these latter systems should use non-parametric statistical methods for analysis (median, mode, etc.) than continuous systems, where mean values, standard deviations, etc., are appropriate.

This chapter will review some of the classification systems currently in use with an emphasis on the severity classification systems.

Severity Classification Systems

Glasgow Coma Scale (Table 6.2)

The GCS was originally designed by Teasdale and Jennett to describe unconsciousness after brain injury.[1] The GCS includes an assessment of eye opening, best motor response, and verbal response. The total GCS score is a sum of the three components. TBI patients are typically divided into subgroups based on total score: severe (GCS 3–8), moderate (GCS 9–12), and mild (GCS 13–15). However, more recently, some have argued that moderate should include GCS 9–13 and mild, GCS 14–15. GCS is widely used in the field as well as in the hospital, and it has also been incorporated into other trauma classification systems such as the Revised Trauma Score because of its general relationship to death.

Table 6.2 Glasgow Coma Scale (GCS)

Advantages	• Most widely used classification system for traumatic brain injury • Assesses eye opening, best motor response, and verbal response • Motor component strongly associated with outcome • Incorporated into other trauma classification systems
Disadvantages	• Summation of score results in loss of information • Pupillary reaction and lateralization of exam not included in score • Reliability of score questionable in the setting of sedative and paralytic use • Optimal timing of measurement unclear
Conclusion	GCS is the most commonly used classification system for traumatic brain injury. Use of the GCS is enhanced by including other information such as pupillary reaction and lateralization of motor responses. A change in GCS score may be more relevant than a single measurement in time.

Limitations of the Glasgow Coma Scale

Criticism of the GCS has included the loss of information with summation of the score, lack of inclusion of pupillary reaction, lateralization of motor responses and brain stem reflexes, numerical weighting of the scale toward motor responses, and lack of interrater reliability in scoring.[2] Summation of the score results in loss of information because multiple combinations of eye, motor, and verbal scores can equal the same total score. As prehospital intubation and use of sedatives and paralytics have become more prevalent, use of the GCS has come into question because components such as the verbal score cannot be reliably measured. To circumvent this issue, regression modeling has been used to calculate the Glasgow verbal score from the eye and motor scores.[3,4] Other authors have used multiple imputation to calculate GCS from other variables in a trauma registry database.[5] The motor component of the GCS has also been reported to be the strongest predictor of outcome,[6,7] and a simplified motor score based on the Glasgow motor score has been proposed and found to perform similar to the full GCS.[8–11] Finally, timing of measurement is also controversial, but this applies to many classification schemes. A change in score may be more relevant than a single measurement in time.[12]

Other Severity Classification Systems Based on GCS (Table 6.3)

Other classification systems have revised or added to the three components in GCS to address some of its limitations. These are briefly reviewed. The Reaction Level Scale (RLS85) combines the eye, motor, and verbal components into a single 8 point scale.[13] The Glasgow-Liege Scale adds an assessment of five brain stem reflexes to the GCS.[14,15]

The Clinical Neurologic Assessment Tool includes response to verbal or tactile stimulation, ability to follow commands, posture, muscle tone, and reflex responses such as chewing.[16] The Comprehensive Level of Consciousness Scale includes the components of GCS plus pupillary reaction, eye position and movements, posture, and general responsiveness.[17] The Head Injury Watch Sheet supplements the GCS with pupillary reaction and stimulus to awaken.[18] The Innsbruck Coma Scale includes a pupillary exam as well as eye movements, motor responses, responses to sound, and oral automatisms.[19] The Leeds Coma Scale includes the GCS components plus age, pupillary exam, intracranial pressure, systolic blood pressure, extracranial injuries, and computed tomography (CT) findings.[20] The Maryland Coma Scale includes the GCS components, brain stem reflexes, pupillary response, lateralization of the motor exam, and intensity of stimulation needed for response.[21] The Neurosurgical Watch Sheet is a 100 point scale that includes GCS components,

Table 6.3 Classification Systems for Traumatic Brain Injury (brief overview)

Classification System	Eye Opening	Verbal Response	Motor Response	Brain Stem Reflexes	Pupillary Exam	Clinical Variables
Glasgow Coma Scale	Y	Y	Y			
Glasgow Liege Scale	Y	Y	Y	Y		
Clinical Neurologic Assessment Tool	Y	Y	Y			Response to stimulation, ability to follow commands, cooperativity, muscle tone, body position and movement, chewing and yawning, lateralization
Comprehensive Level of Consciousness Scale	Y	Y	Y		Y	Posture, eye position, general motor functioning including yawning, chewing, etc., abnormal ocular movements, general responsiveness
Head Injury Watch Sheet		Y	Y		Y	Stimulus to awaken, quality of consciousness, ability to move
Innsbruck Coma Scale	Y		Y		Y	Reaction to acoustic stimuli and pain, posture, eye position and movement, oral automatisms
Leeds Coma Scale	Y	Y	Y		Y	Age, intracranial pressure, systolic blood pressure, other extracranial injuries, CT findings
Maryland Coma Scale	Y	Y	Y	Y	Y	Lateralization of motor exam, intensity of stimulus needed for response
Neurosurgical Watch Sheet	Y	Y	Y		Y	Vital signs including temperature, stimulus needed to awaken, strength of extremities
Reaction Level Scale (RLS85)*	Y	Y	Y			

*8-point scale

vital signs, and a pupillary exam.[22] The reliability and validity of many of these systems have been reviewed.[23]

GCS still remains the most widely used classification system for TBI.

Computed Tomography Classification of Traumatic Brain Injury (Table 6.4)

As CT technology improved and became more widespread, utilization also increased, providing a wealth of information not incorporated into physiological classification systems such as the GCS.[24] To enhance classification of severity of injury, information from neuroimaging studies began to be added to the use of GCS. Gennarelli et al evaluated outcome after severe TBI, incorporating both GCS and CT findings. This classification system divided patients on the basis of their lesion on CT (focal or diffuse), their GCS, and the length of coma. Subdural hematomas and diffuse injuries with >24 hour coma were associated with the highest mortality.[25] Lobato et al also found that subdural hematomas and multiple brain contusions were associated with the highest mortality after severe TBI.[26]

In 1991, Marshall et al described another CT classification system based on information gathered from severe TBI patients in the Traumatic Coma Data Bank.[27] The Marshall classification divided focal lesions on the basis of surgical evacuation and volume, and divided diffuse

Table 6.4 Image-Based Classification Systems

• Computed tomography • Magnetic resonance imaging • Positron emission tomography • Single-photon emission computed tomography	
Advantages	• Includes information not incorporated into physiologic classification systems like GCS • Individual CT characteristics are correlated with mortality • Repeat imaging can be used to assess change
Disadvantages	• Optimal timing of imaging unknown • Resource intensive and time consuming • Misclassification may be common • Relationship to outcome not well-defined
Conclusion	Imaging provides useful information for classification of injury. However, the relationship between imaging findings and outcome, and questions about reliability and validity are issues for ongoing research.

lesions on the basis of midline shift, cistern compression, and the volume of the high- or mixed-density lesion. Diffuse Injury IV, >5 mm of midline shift with no high- or mixed-density lesion >25 cc, was associated with the highest mortality.[27] In a later study, Vos et al evaluated the reliability of the Marshall classification system in the Traumatic Coma Data Bank. Interrater and intrarater reliability was high (0.80 and 0.85, respectively), although they were higher for mass lesions than diffuse lesions (0.94 and 0.91 vs. 0.71 and 0.67).[28]

Individual CT characteristics have also been found to correlate with outcome. Appearance of the cisterns and brain stem were used as a 5 point grading scale by Liu et al and found to correlate with Glasgow Outcome Score (GOS) and mortality.[29] Fearnside et al found cerebral edema, cistern compression, intraventricular blood, and degree of midline shift on CT to be significantly associated with mortality in patients with severe TBI. After taking clinical variables into account using logistic regression, brain swelling, amount of midline shift, and intraventricular blood were significantly correlated with mortality.[30] Wardlaw et al also found clinical variables, the presence of subarachnoid hemorrhage, and a grading of the overall appearance of the CT to be predictive of outcome in TBI patients of all severity.[31]

Maas et al evaluated the Marshall classification system in comparison with the use of individual CT findings for prognosis after TBI.[32] They used data gathered from the International and North American Tirilazad Trials, which included both moderate (GCS 9–12) and severe (GCS- 8) TBI patients. CT classification was based on the admission CT performed within 4 hours of injury. Midline shift >5 mm, compressed or absent basal cisterns, intraventricular blood, and traumatic subarachnoid hemorrhage were significantly associated with mortality. Midline shift >5 mm and absent or compressed basal cisterns were associated with the highest mortality. Of note, the authors also found inconsistencies in categorization using the Marshall system. For example, midline shift >5 mm was reported as absent in 30% of patients classified as Diffuse Injury IV, which is defined as midline shift >5 mm and no high- or mixed-density lesion >25 cc. Although the authors found these discrepancies to be less pronounced in studies with a central review process, they still noted that after central review, 7% of patients with absent midline shift were still classified as Diffuse Injury IV. This may allow misclassification.[32]

Other Neuroimaging Techniques and Traumatic Brain Injury (Table 6.4)

Magnetic resonance imaging (MRI), although more sensitive for detection and localization of cerebral injury, is not widely utilized for imaging after acute TBI at this time.[33,34] MRI scanning is more resource intensive, requires a longer imaging time, and is often technically difficult for an unstable trauma patient. Likewise, positron emission tomography (PET) and single-photon emission computed tomography (SPECT) scanning are not typically used in the acute phase of TBI.[33] More research is needed to correlate these neuroimaging findings with outcome.[33]

Mild Traumatic Brain Injury (Table 6.5)

Classification of MTBI is a controversial topic. Patients with a total GCS of 13 to 15 have been categorized as MTBI. However, many researchers have modified the GCS criteria to include other factors such as loss of consciousness, posttraumatic amnesia, seizures, CT criteria, and length of hospital stay. Others have documented heterogeneity within the GCS definition of MTBI and recommended that GCS 15 patients be classified differently from GCS 13 and 14 patients.[35] No standard definition of MTBI exists, complicating standardization of clinical care as well as attempts to study the pathophysiology, epidemiology, and outcomes of MTBI.[36–39] In addition, MTBI has many other labels, including concussion[36] and minor head injury.[40]

One of the earliest definitions of MTBI was made by Ommaya and Gennarelli in 1974: "a graded set of clinical syndromes following head injury wherein increasing severity of disturbance in level and content of consciousness is caused by mechanically induced strains affecting the brain in a centripetal sequence of disruptive effect on function and structure."[41] MTBI was divided into six categories based on confusion, amnesia, and coma. This system related clinical symptoms to pathology. Grades I through III included less severe injuries with confusion, and were hypothesized to not affect the reticular activating system. The more severe grades were associated with diffuse cerebral damage not necessarily localized to the mesencephalon. This grading system enabled prediction of the extent and location of injury to the cortex and was supported by experimental observations.

Another classification system was described in 1981 by Rimel et al to include a history of unconsciousness ≤20 minutes, GCS 13 to 15, and length of hospital stay of ≤48 hours. At 3 month follow-up, headaches and persistent deficits in memory and cognition were noted, as well as higher unemployment among those who worked prior to injury.[40,42] Litigation did not appear to have a strong relationship with this outcome.[40] This was one of the earliest studies to document significant postinjury deficits.

Several definitions of MTBI have since been published. The American Congress of Rehabilitation Medicine published their criteria in 1993 (**Table 6.5**). These criteria did not make loss of consciousness a necessary component for defining MTBI. The American Congress of Rehabilitation Medicine (ACRM) criteria were also accepted by the World

Table 6.5 Mild Traumatic Brain Injury Classification Systems

Classification System	Glasgow Coma Scale	Loss of Consciousness	Loss of Memory	Alteration of Mental State	Other
American Congress of Rehabilitation Medicine and World Health Organization	≥13 sustained	≤30 minutes	≤24 hours	Time of accident (dazed, disoriented, confused)	Focal neurological deficit: not necessarily transient
Centers for Disease Control, MTBI Work Group, conceptual definition	≥13, Abbreviated Injury Severity Scale score = 2	≤30 minutes	≤24 hours	Transient confusion, disorientation or impaired consciousness	Seizures and/or symptoms such as irritability, fatigue, headache, dizziness
Diagnostic and Statistical Manual for Mental Disorders (DSM-IV) post–concussive disorder		>5 minutes	>12 hours	Difficulty in memory and attention	New seizures or worsening of preexisting seizure disorder within 6 months of injury; at least 3 months of symptoms such as headache, dizziness, disordered sleep
European Federation of Neurological Societies	≥13	Graded by category 0 to 3; <30 minutes	Graded by category 0 to 3; <1 hour		Risk factors for intracranial complications visualized on CT (e.g., severe headache, vomiting, seizure, coagulation disorder, age, etc. included in categories)

Health Organization Collaborating Centre for Neurotrauma Task Force on MTBI, with the caveat that the GCS be measured at the first available opportunity by a qualified health care provider[39] rather than at 30 minutes postinjury.

In contrast, in 1994, the fourth edition of the *Diagnostic and Statistical Manual for Mental Disorders* (DSM IV) defined a concussion to include a 5 minute loss of consciousness. Because of this contradiction, the DSM IV criteria were divided into three levels to better match the ACRM criteria.[43,44]

The Centers for Disease Control Mild Traumatic Brain Injury Work Group also published a definition of MTBI similar to the ACRM criteria[37] but without GCS criteria. The CDC conceptual definition also included symptoms that are found under Post-Concussive Disorder criteria such as irritability, fatigue, headache, and dizziness.[45]

The European Federation of Neurological Societies (EFNS) criteria include GCS, loss of consciousness, posttraumatic amnesia, and risk factors for intracranial findings on CT, including age, severe headache, vomiting, seizure, coagulation disorder, etc.[46]

Neuroimaging and MTBI Classification

Other authors have expanded the MTBI criteria to include CT or MRI findings. Patients are classified as "complicated MTBI" if they have findings on MR or CT.[34,47,48] CT criteria were noted to correlate with GOS at 6 months.[48] Borgaro et al defined complicated MTBI patients as those with a GCS of 13 to 15 and a space-occupying lesion on CT or MRI.[47] In a pilot study of 28 patients, they assessed neuropsychological testing (speech and language, orientation, attention and concentration, visuospatial and visual problem solving, learning and memory, affect, and awareness vs. performance testing) and found that complicated MTBI patients performed worse than uncomplicated MTBI patients on speech and language testing, but both groups performed worse than control patients on affect and awareness testing. Levin et al also studied 20 patients and found that lesions localized on MRI corresponded to deficits on neuropsychological testing. For example, patients with left frontal lesions had less verbal fluency than patients with right frontal lesions. Improved performance was also noted to correlate with improved MRI appearance on 1 to 3 month follow-up.[34]

Anatomically Based Severity Classification

Abbreviated Injury Scale (AIS) (Table 6.6)

The AIS is an anatomically based, consensus-derived, global severity scoring system that classifies each injury by body region according to its relative importance on a 6 point ordinal scale.[49,50] It was conceived more than 30 years ago as a system to describe the severity of injuries throughout the body and has subsequently become

Table 6.6 Anatomically Based Severity Classification: Abbreviated Injury Scale (AIS)

- Anatomically based, global severity scoring system
- Classifies injuries by body region using a 6 point ordinal scale
- Subcategories describe location and etiology of injury.
- Measured once, time invariant
- AIS deals only with the "usual" injury severity in a healthy young adult.
- AIS may be scored using *International Classification of Disease-Clinical Modification* codes in administrative databases.
- Secondary AIS-based classification systems include the maximum AIS (MAIS), the injury severity score (ISS), the New Injury Severity Score (NISS), the anatomical profile, and the Trauma Score–Injury Severity Score (TRISS)

the most prevalent of injury scoring systems throughout the world. It is now used in every trauma-receiving hospital in the developed world and by most transportation departments in many countries. The initial intention was to map a series of anatomically defined injury descriptions by several parameters (energy dissipation, threat to life, permanent impairment, treatment period, incidence). In 1971 the original AIS was thus created (all references can be found in reference[49]). By 1975–76, the first injury coding dictionary was developed and published, consisting of a list of ~500 injuries and severity levels ranging from 1 (least severe) to 6 (most severe). By the mid-1970s, the AIS had been adopted as the standard for crash investigation teams funded by the U.S. Department of Transportation as well as many university and industry research teams in the United States, Europe, and Australia. In 1980 the injury dictionary was expanded by threefold and the descriptions of many injuries were improved. The brain injury section was updated to parallel contemporary research in head injury. The 1985 version also introduced a numeric system that assigned a unique code number to each injury description to facilitate computerized use of the AIS.

The current AIS (2005) defines 2018 injuries, with 286 injuries to the head subdivided into the cranial nerves, blood vessels, brain stem, cerebellum, cerebrum, skull, and concussive injuries. Subcategories for injury type (such as contusion subdural hematoma, etc.) and for injury size determine the 1 through 6 severity score. The example in **Table 6.7** is for cerebral contusion. The six digit number before the decimal (or "dot") is a code number for computer use that is distinct to each injury and defines the body region, structure (vessel, brain, skull, etc.), and specific injury. The "post dot" number that follows the decimal defines the injury severity level from 1 to 6 (or with 9 if no severity is assigned). Additional postdot numbers are available to further specify location and etiology of injury (**Table 6.7**).

Thus, not only does the AIS serve as a severity scoring system, but it also serves as the most precise international dictionary of injuries for the head and all other body regions. Over the years, variants of the AIS have been used to define the severity of more than one injury

Table 6.7 Examples of Postdot Scale Severity in AIS System

140602.3	Contusion not further specified (NFS)
140604.3	Single NFS
140605.2	Tiny; each <1 cm diameter
140606.3	Small; superficial; <30 cc or <15 cc if age <10; 1–4 cm diameter, 1–2 cm if age <10; midline shift <5 mm
140608.4	Large; deep; 30–50 cc or 15–30 cc if age <10; >4 cm diameter or 2–4 cm if age <10; midline shift >5 mm
140610.5	Extensive; massive; >50 cc if age >10; >30 cc or >4 cm diameter if age <10
140611.3	Multiple NFS
140612.3	Multiple, on same side but NFS
140613.2	Tiny; each <1 cm diameter
140614.3	Small; superficial; total volume <30 cc or <15 cc if age <10; midline shift <5 mm
140616.4	Large; total volume 30–50 cc or 15–30 cc if age <10; midline shift >5 mm
140618.5	Extensive; massive; total volume >50 cc or >30 cc if age <10
140620.3	Multiple, at least one on each side but NFS
140621.2	Tiny; each <1 cm diameter
140622.3	Small; superficial; total volume <30 cc or <15 cc if age <10
140624.4	Large; total volume 30–50 cc or 15–30 cc if age <10
140626.5	Extensive; massive; total volume >50 cc or >30 cc if age <10

to the body. These secondary classifications include the maximum AIS (MAIS), the Injury Severity Score (ISS), the New Injury Severity Score (NISS), the anatomical profile, and the Trauma Score–Injury Severity Score (TRISS).[49,51]

The AIS and its derivatives have certain limitations and differences from physiologically bases systems such as the GCS. First, the AIS is determinable only once; it is time invariant. This, in fact, is its purpose: to provide an assessment of injury severity soon after the event occurs without the effect or consequences of injury or complicating features. Second, there can be wide variations in physiological response, especially in the brain, in an anatomical injury of a certain size in a certain location. The AIS only deals with the "usual" severity in a healthy young adult. Third, there are many similar AIS-defined injuries with the same severity score. This was done purposefully, in case outcomes were different for injuries of the same severity.

International Classification of Diseases (ICD)

The *International Classification of Diseases* (ICD) and its clinical modification (ICD-CM) are used by hospitals throughout the world to code the diagnoses of patients on discharge. Currently, the ICD version 10 is in use, but its clinical modification has not yet been released, so for injury purposes ICD9-CM is still in use. Because discharge data are readily available from large administrative and hospital discharge databases, it was felt that the coding from ICD9-CM could be used as a surrogate for injury severity assessment. To some degree and with considerable limitations this system ICD can be applied for mortality classification.[51,52] The system is highly dependent on the specific database used and is subject to the coding peculiarities of the ICD9-CM system, which were not designed to define injuries, especially for the head.

Classification by Outcome after TBI (Table 6.8)

Glasgow Outcome Scale

Classification of traumatic brain injury patients by outcome is an active area of research. Traditionally, the GOS has been used to categorize patients, and the score has been dichotomized into GOS 3 to 5 versus GOS 1 to 2.[53] Although the 5 point GOS score has been criticized for lacking sensitivity and for having a ceiling effect,[54,55] it is still the most widely used instrument for classifying outcome after TBI. Most TBI patients fall into the extremes of the scale, good recovery or death.[56] The GOS has undergone several revisions and was extended to an 8 point scale to address some of these limitations.[57–59] Both the GOS and the extended form (GOSe) have been extensively used and shown to have validity and reliability in measurement of outcome by trained staff and structured interview.[59–62] GOS and GOSe also correlate with other measures of disability, mental status, and neurobehavioral functioning, such as the Controlled Oral Word Association and Grooved Pegboard tests.[63,64] GOS and the SF-36 are also recommended for assessment of quality of life after multiple trauma.[65]

Outcome after TBI is multifactorial and best assessed with a multidisciplinary approach. Outcome relates to the severity of injury, comorbid conditions, preinjury status, social factors, and patient age.[66,67] Although definitions of quality of life and outcome vary, overall recommendations include using a battery of instruments to measure different domains. Each instrument should have validity and reliability, and results should be compared with normative values, taking into account the specific characteristics of the TBI population.[67,68]

Although no accepted guidelines exist at this time, the American Brain Injury Consortium recommended that outcome measurement include the GOSe and neuropsychological testing as well as the Neurobehavioral Functional Inventory to assess quality of life.[56,69]

General Measures of Outcome

The SF-36, Sickness Impact Profile, Nottingham Health Profile, EuroQoL and WHO-QoL are measures of outcome that are also used in other illnesses, including multiple trauma.[66,70–74] In addition, measurements of pain are recommended and are included in the SF-36 or with the addition of a Visual Analog Scale.[71] MacKenzie et al studied the SF-36 with a supplementary assessment of cognitive function. In a multiple trauma population with TBI, the cognitive supplement was found to measure a domain of health not included in the SF-36.[72]

Table 6.8 Outcome Classification Systems for Traumatic Brain Injury

- Classification can be made using disease-specific instruments (e.g., GOS) or general health instruments (e.g., SF-36).
- Outcome is multifactorial and is best assessed using a multidisciplinary approach.
- Outcome assessment should be performed using a battery of instruments, including neuropsychological tools to assess various skills.
- Timing of measurement, reliability and validity of instruments, length of the test battery, impaired self-reflection among TBI patients, and inclusion of input from caregivers or significant others remain areas of ongoing research.

Other outcome measures have been developed to relate to the AIS. These include the Injury Impairment Scale (IIS)[50] and the more recent Functional Capacity Index (FCI).[50] In both, each AIS injury is assigned a score that defines the average impairment of functional capacity that would occur in 80% of survivors at 1 year from injury. The FCI is another instrument that was designed to measure physical and cognitive limitations after multiple trauma.[75] After blunt multiple trauma, the Functional Capacity Index was found to correlate well with the Sickness Impact Profile and SF-36, and to also correlate well with AIS grades of TBI severity.[76]

Quality of life has proven a difficult measure to define and quantify. In general, it is recommended that quality-of-life instruments measure physical, psychological, social and cognitive domains, especially with TBI patients.[77] Measurement of quality of life is typically performed using instruments such as the SF-36.[78] This has been validated and found to correlate well with GOS.[56]

Traumatic Brain Injury Measures of Outcome

The Disability Rating Score (DRS) has also been commonly used to assess outcome although it was originally created to measure recovery after severe TBI. It is a 30 point scale that includes assessment of factors such as self-care, employability, and GCS.[55,79] Although some studies have shown increased sensitivity in comparison with the GOS, others have not confirmed this.[55,80] Choi et al also found that the DRS did not act as an ordinal scale, so that there was overlap in DRS score for patients classified as severely disabled and vegetative patients by GOS.[80] Other instruments include the Rancho Los Amigos Levels of Cognitive Function Scale (LCFS),[81] although this has been criticized for lack of sensitivity and concerns about reliability and validity[82,83]; the Functional Independence Measure, an instrument designed to measure changes in function during rehabilitation but also criticized for significant ceiling effects[84–86]; and the Functional Status Examination, which was developed to evaluate a change in everyday life activities after TBI, and which correlated well with the GOSe. This instrument is designed to assess limitations in the physical, social, and psychological domains.[54,87] Numerous other instruments exist.

Neuropsychological Outcome Measures

Many neuropsychological instruments have been used in the TBI population. Typically, a battery of tests is administered to address various skills, samples of which are listed. Cognitive function (Wechsler Adult Intelligence Scale III (WAIS III), composite score includes a verbal and performance IQ; language function (Verbal Fluency Test, Benton Controlled Oral Word Association Test [COWAT]); nonverbal function (Digit Symbol Subtest of WAIS III); attention and concentration; learning and memory (Rey Auditory Verbal Learning Test, Buschke Selective Reminding Test, California Verbal Learning Test); executive functioning (Wisconsin Card Sorting Test, Controlled Oral Word Association Test, Ruff Figural Fluency Test, Porteus Maze, Stroop Color Word Naming Test, Trail Making Test Parts A and B); visual and auditory deficits; motor and dexterity function (Finger Tapping Test, Grooved Pegboard Test); and emotional functioning and impact on caregivers (Katz Adjustment Scale, Revised; Neurobehavioral Rating Scale (NBRS), Portland Adaptability Inventory (PAI).[67]

Issues with Outcome Measurement

Measurement of outcome after TBI is a growing area of research. It is generally agreed that studies should take into account the reliability and validity of the instruments, the timing of measurement, the length of the test battery, effects of impaired self-reflection among TBI patients, impairment preventing participation in testing, and inclusion of input from caregivers or significant others.[67,68] The optimal timing of measurement of outcome is not known. Some studies have shown that recovery improves over the first 6 months, then plateaus.[88] The TBI Consensus Group divided postinjury timing into three groups: T1 acute phase, 3 months postinjury; T2 rehabilitation phase; and T3 long-term outcome phase, reintegration. Measurement of quality of life during T2 and T3 was recommended.[66]

Conclusion

Although multiple generic and disease-specific instruments exist to measure outcome and quality of life after TBI, the GOS is the most widely used. It is recommended that assessment of outcome include a battery of other instruments; however, their role in categorizing TBI patients by outcome is not yet clear.

References

1. Teasdale G, Jennett B. Assessment of coma and impaired consciousness: a practical scale. Lancet 1974;2(7872):81–84
2. Gill MR, Reiley DG, Green SM. Interrater reliability of Glasgow Coma Scale scores in the emergency department. Ann Emerg Med 2004; 43(2):215–223
3. Rutledge R, Lentz CW, Fakhry S, Hunt J. Appropriate use of the Glasgow Coma Scale in intubated patients: a linear regression prediction of the Glasgow verbal score from the Glasgow eye and motor scores. J Trauma 1996;41(3):514–522
4. Meredith W, Rutledge R, Fakhry SM, et al. The conundrum of the Glasgow Coma Scale in intubated patients: a linear regression prediction

of the Glasgow verbal score from the Glasgow eye and motor scores. J Trauma 1998;44(5):839–844, discussion 844–845
5. Moore L, Lavoie A, LeSage N, et al. Multiple imputation of the Glasgow Coma Score. J Trauma 2005;59(3):698–704
6. Choi SC, Narayan RK, Anderson RL, Ward JD. Enhanced specificity of prognosis in severe head injury. J Neurosurg 1988;69(3):381–385
7. Healey C, Osler TM, Rogers FB, et al. Improving the Glasgow Coma Scale score: motor score alone is a better predictor. J Trauma 2003;54(4):671–678, discussion 678–680
8. Eftekhar B, Zarei MR, Ghodsi M, et al. Comparing logistic models based on modified GCS motor component with other prognostic tools in prediction of mortality: results of study in 7226 trauma patients. Injury 2005;36(8):900–904
9. Gill M, Steele R, Windemuth R, Green SM. A comparison of five simplified scales to the out-of-hospital Glasgow Coma Scale for the prediction of traumatic brain injury outcomes. Acad Emerg Med 2006;13(9): 968–973
10. Gill M, Windemuth R, Steele R, Green SM. A comparison of the Glasgow Coma Scale score to simplified alternative scores for the prediction of traumatic brain injury outcomes. Ann Emerg Med 2005; 45(1):37–42
11. Haukoos JS, Gill MR, Rabon RE, et al. Validation of the Simplified Motor Score for the Prediction of Brain Injury Outcomes after Trauma. Ann Emerg Med 2007;50:18–24
12. Davis DP, Serrano JA, Vilke GM, et al. Predictive value of field versus arrival Glasgow Coma Scale score and TRISS calculations in moderate-to-severe traumatic brain injury. J Trauma 2006;60(5):985–990
13. Starmark JE, Stalhammar D, Holmgren E. The Reaction Level Scale (RLS85): manual and guidelines. Acta Neurochir (Wien) 1988;91(1–2): 12–20
14. Born JD. The Glasgow-Liege Scale: prognostic value and evolution of motor response and brain stem reflexes after severe head injury. Acta Neurochir (Wien) 1988;91(1–2):1–11
15. Born J, Hans P, Dexters G, et al. Evaluation pratique du dysfonctionnement encephalique chez le traumatise cranien. Neurochirurgie 1982;28:1–7
16. Crosby L, Parsons LC. Clinical neurologic assessment tool: development and testing of an instrument to index neurologic status. Heart Lung 1989;18(2):121–129
17. Stanczak DE, White JG III, Gouview WD, et al. Assessment of level of consciousness following severe neurological insult: a comparison of the psychometric qualities of the Glasgow Coma Scale and the Comprehensive Level of Consciousness Scale. J Neurosurg 1984;60(5): 955–960
18. Yen JK, Bourke RS, Nelson LR, Popp AJ. Numerical grading of clinical neurological status after serious head injury. J Neurol Neurosurg Psychiatry 1978;41(12):1125–1130
19. Benzer A, Mitterschiffthaler G, Marosi M, et al. Prediction of non-survival after trauma: Innsbruck Coma Scale. Lancet 1991;338(8773):977–978
20. Gibson RM, Stephenson GC. Aggressive management of severe closed head trauma: time for reappraisal. Lancet 1989;2(8659):369–371
21. Salcman M, Schepp RS, Ducker TB. Calculated recovery rates in severe head trauma. Neurosurgery 1981;8(3):301–308
22. Bouzarth WF. Neurosurgical watch sheet for craniocerebral trauma. J Trauma 1968;8(1):29–31
23. Segatore M, Way C. The Glasgow Coma Scale: time for change. Heart Lung 1992;21(6):548–557
24. Wiest PW, Locken JA, Heintz PH, Mettler JA. CT scanning: a major source of radiation exposure. Semin Ultrasound CT MR 2002;23(5): 402–410
25. Gennarelli TA, Spielman GM, Langfitt TW, et al. Influence of the type of intracranial lesion on outcome from severe head injury. J Neurosurg 1982;56(1):26–32
26. Lobato RD, Cordobes F, Rivas JJ, et al. Outcome from severe head injury related to the type of intracranial lesion: a computerized tomography study. J Neurosurg 1983;59(5):762–774
27. Marshall L, Marshall S, Klauber M, et al. New classification of head injury based on computerized tomography. J Neurosurg 1991;75:S14–S20
28. Vos PE, van Voskuilen AC, Beems T, et al. Evaluation of the traumatic coma data bank computed tomography classification for severe head injury. J Neurotrauma 2001;18(7):649–655
29. Liu HM, Tu YK, Su CT. Changes of brainstem and perimesencephalic cistern: dynamic predictor of outcome in severe head injury. J Trauma 1995;38(3):330–333
30. Fearnside MR, Cook RJ, McDougall P, McNeil RJ. Westmead Head Injury Project outcome in severe head injury: a comparative analysis of pre-hospital, clinical and CT variables. Br J Neurosurg 1993;7(3):267–279
31. Wardlaw JM, Easton VJ, Statham P. Which CT features help predict outcome after head injury? J Neurol Neurosurg Psychiatry 2002;72(2): 188–192, discussion 151
32. Maas AI, Steyerberg EW, Butcher I, et al. Prognostic value of computerized tomography scan characteristics in traumatic brain injury: results from the IMPACT study. J Neurotrauma 2007;24(2):303–314
33. Lee B, Newberg A. Neuroimaging in traumatic brain imaging. NeuroRx 2005;2(2):372–383
34. Levin HS, Amparo E, Eisenberg HM, et al. Magnetic resonance imaging and computerized tomography in relation to the neurobehavioral sequelae of mild and moderate head injuries. J Neurosurg 1987;66(5):706–713
35. Culotta VP, Sementilli ME, Gerold K, Watts CC. Clinicopathological heterogeneity in the classification of mild head injury. Neurosurgery 1996;38(2):245–250
36. von Wild K, Terwey S. Diagnostic confusion in mild traumatic brain injury (MTBI): lessons from clinical practice and EFNS-Inquiry. Brain Inj 2001;15(3):273–277
37. Gerberding J, Binder S. Report to Congress on Mild Traumatic Brain Injury in the United States: Steps to Prevent a Serious Public Health Problem. Atlanta, GA: Centers for Disease Control and Prevention; 2003
38. Dikmen S. Methodological issues in the study of mild head injury. J Head Trauma Rehabil 1993;8(3):30–37
39. Carroll LJ, Cassidy JD, Holm L, et al. Methodological issues and research recommendations for mild traumatic brain injury: the WHO Collaborating Centre Task Force on Mild Traumatic Brain Injury. J Rehabil Med 2004;43(Suppl):113–125
40. Rimel RW, Giordani B, Barth J, et al. Disability caused by minor head injury. Neurosurgery 1981;9(3):221–228
41. Ommaya AK, Gennarelli TA. Cerebral concussion and traumatic unconsciousness: correlation of experimental and clinical observations of blunt head injuries. Brain 1974;97(4):633–654
42. Barth JT, Macciocchi SN, Giordani B, et al. Neuropsychological sequelae of minor head injury. Neurosurgery 1983;13(5):529–533
43. Ruff R. Two decades of advances in understanding of mild traumatic brain injury. J Head Trauma Rehabil 2005;20(1):5–18
44. Ruff RM, Jurica P. In search of a unified definition for mild traumatic brain injury. Brain Inj 1999;13(12):943–952
45. Moore EL, Terryberry-Spohr L, Hope DA. Mild traumatic brain injury and anxiety sequelae: a review of the literature. Brain Inj 2006;20(2): 117–132
46. Vos PE, Battistin L, Birbamer G, et al. EFNS guideline on mild traumatic brain injury: report of an EFNS task force. Eur J Neurol 2002;9(3): 207–219
47. Borgaro SR, Prigatano GP, Kwasnica C, Rexer JL. Cognitive and affective sequelae in complicated and uncomplicated mild traumatic brain injury. Brain Inj 2003;17(3):189–198
48. Williams DH, Levin HS, Eisenberg HM. Mild head injury classification. Neurosurgery 1990;27(3):422–428
49. Gennarelli TA, Wodzin E. The Abbreviated Injury Scale 2005. Barrington, IL: Association for the Advancement of Automotive Medicine; 2005
50. Gennarelli TA, Wodzin E. AIS 2005: a contemporary injury scale. Injury 2006;37:1083–1091
51. Meredith JW, Evans G, Kilgo P, et al. A comparison of the abilities of the nine scoring algorithms in predicting mortality. J Trauma 2002; 53(4):621–629
52. Osler T, Rutledge R, Deis J, Bedrick E. ICISS: an international classification of disease-9 based injury severity score. J Trauma 1996;41:380–386
53. Jennett B, Bond M. Assessment of outcome after severe brain damage. Lancet 1975;1(7905):480–484

54. Dikmen S, Machamer J, Miller B, et al. Functional status examination: a new instrument for assessing outcome in traumatic brain injury. J Neurotrauma 2001;18(2):127–140
55. Hall K, Cope DN, Rappaport M. Glasgow Outcome Scale and Disability Rating Scale: comparative usefulness in following recovery in traumatic head injury. Arch Phys Med Rehabil 1985;66(1):35–37
56. Bullock MR, Merchant RE, Choi SC, et al. Outcome measures for clinical trials in neurotrauma. Neurosurg Focus 2002;13(1):ECP1
57. Jennett B, Snoek J, Bond MR, Brooks N. Disability after severe head injury: observations on the use of the Glasgow Outcome Scale. J Neurol Neurosurg Psychiatry 1981;44(4):285–293
58. Levin HS, Boake C, Song J, et al. Validity and sensitivity to change of the extended Glasgow Outcome Scale in mild to moderate traumatic brain injury. J Neurotrauma 2001;18(6):575–584
59. Wilson JT, Pettigrew LE, Teasdale GM. Structured interviews for the Glasgow Outcome Scale and the extended Glasgow Outcome Scale: guidelines for their use. J Neurotrauma 1998;15(8):573–585
60. Anderson SI, Housley AM, Jones PA, et al. Glasgow Outcome Scale: an inter-rater reliability study. Brain Inj 1993;7(4):309–317
61. Pettigrew LE, Wilson JT, Teasdale GM. Reliability of ratings on the Glasgow Outcome Scales from in-person and telephone structured interviews. J Head Trauma Rehabil 2003;18(3):252–258
62. Teasdale GM, Pettigrew LE, Wilson JT, et al. Analyzing outcome of treatment of severe head injury: a review and update on advancing the use of the Glasgow Outcome Scale. J Neurotrauma 1998;15(8):587–597
63. Clifton GL, Kreutzer JS, Choi SC, et al. Relationship between Glasgow Outcome Scale and neuropsychological measures after brain injury. Neurosurgery 1993;33(1):34–38, discussion 38–39
64. Wilson JT, Pettigrew LE, Teasdale GM. Emotional and cognitive consequences of head injury in relation to the Glasgow outcome scale. J Neurol Neurosurg Psychiatry 2000;69(2):204–209
65. Neugebauer E, Bouillon B, Bullinger M, Wood-Dauphinee S. Quality of life after multiple trauma–summary and recommendations of the consensus conference. Restor Neurol Neurosci 2002;20(3–4):161–167
66. Bullinger M, Azouvi P, Brooks N, et al. Quality of life in patients with traumatic brain injury-basic issues, assessment and recommendations. Restor Neurol Neurosci 2002;20(3–4):111–124
67. Ruff R. Sequelae of traumatic brain injury. In: Winn, HR, ed. Youmans Neurological Surgery. Vol. 4. Philadelphia: Saunders; 2003:5181–5201
68. Dijkers MP. Quality of life after traumatic brain injury: review of research approaches and findings. Arch Phys Med Rehabil 2004;85(4, Suppl 2):S21–S35
69. Marmarou A. Conduct of head injury trails in the United States: the American Brain Injury Consortium. Acta Neurochir Suppl (Wien) 1996;66:118–121
70. von Steinbuechel N, Richter S, Morawetz C, Riemsma R. Assessment of subjective health and health-related quality of life in persons with acquired or degenerative brain injury. Curr Opin Neurol 2005;18(6): 681–691
71. Bouillon B, Kreder HJ, Eypasch E, et al. Quality of life in patients with multiple injuries—basic issues, assessment, and recommendations. Restor Neurol Neurosci 2002;20(3–4):125–134
72. MacKenzie EJ, McCarthy ML, Ditunno JF, et al. Using the SF-36 for characterizing outcome after multiple trauma involving head injury. J Trauma 2002;52(3):527–534
73. Temkin N, McLean A Jr, Dikmen S, et al. Development and evaluation of modifications to the Sickness Impact Profile for head injury. J Clin Epidemiol 1988;41(1):47–57
74. Dimopoulou I, Anthi A, Mastora Z, et al. Health-related quality of life and disability in survivors of multiple trauma one year after intensive care unit discharge. Am J Phys Med Rehabil 2004;83(3):171–176
75. MacKenzie EJ, Damiano A, Miller T, Luchter S. Development of the Functional Capacity Index. J Trauma 1996;41(5):799–807
76. MacKenzie EJ, Sacco WJ, Luchter S, et al. Validating the Functional Capacity Index as a measure of outcome following blunt multiple trauma. Qual Life Res 2002;11(8):797–808
77. Berger E, Leven F, Pirente N, et al. Quality of Life after traumatic brain injury: systematic review of the literature. Restor Neurol Neurosci 1999;14(2–3):93–102
78. Johnston MV, Miklos CS. Activity-related quality of life in rehabilitation and traumatic brain injury. Arch Phys Med Rehabil 2002;83(12, Suppl 2):S26–S38
79. Rappaport M, Hall KM, Hopkins K, et al. Disability rating scale for severe head trauma: coma to community. Arch Phys Med Rehabil 1982;63(3):118–123
80. Choi SC, Marmarou A, Bullock R, et al. Primary end points in phase III clinical trials of severe head trauma: DRS versus GOS. The American Brain Injury Consortium Study Group. J Neurotrauma 1998;15(10): 771–776
81. Hagen C, Malkmus D, Durham P, Stenderup K. Communication Disorders Service. Rancho Los Amigos Hospital; 1974
82. Duff D. Review article: altered states of consciousness, theories of recovery, and assessment following a severe traumatic brain injury. Axone 2001;23(1):18–23
83. Gouvier WD, Blanton PD, LaPorte KK, Nepomuceno C. Reliability and validity of the Disability Rating Scale and the Levels of Cognitive Functioning Scale in monitoring recovery from severe head injury. Arch Phys Med Rehabil 1987;68(2):94–97
84. Hall K. Functional measures after traumatic brain injury: ceiling effects of FIM, FIM+FAM, DRS, and CIQ. J Head Trauma Rehabil 1996; 11:27–39
85. Hamilton B, Granger C, Sherwin F, et al. A uniform national data system for medical rehabilitation. In: Fuhrer M, ed. Rehabilitation Outcomes: Analysis and Measurement. Baltimore: Paul H. Brookes; 1987
86. van Baalen B, Odding E, van Woensel MP, Roebroeck ME. Reliability and sensitivity to change of measurement instruments used in a traumatic brain injury population. Clin Rehabil 2006;20(8):686–700
87. Hudak AM, Caesar RR, Frol AB, et al. Functional outcome scales in traumatic brain injury: a comparison of the Glasgow Outcome Scale (Extended) and the Functional Status Examination. J Neurotrauma 2005;22(11):1319–1326
88. Choi SC, Barnes TY, Bullock R, et al. Temporal profile of outcomes in severe head injury. J Neurosurg 1994;81(2):169–173

7 Introduction to Brain Injury Imaging

Beverly L. Hershey, Scott H. Faro, Pallav N. Shah, and Erin O'Connor

One of the greatest advances in the diagnosis of brain trauma has been the in the field of neuroimaging. Imaging of acute head trauma is important not only in diagnosing the extent of injury but also in expediently determining the appropriate therapy, particularly to determine if a surgically treatable lesion is present. Imaging modalities in use for the evaluation of the acute head trauma patient include computed tomography (CT), magnetic resonance imaging (MRI), and digital subtraction angiography (DSA) (**Table 7.1**). Skull x-rays are not indicated, as low-risk patients rarely have x-ray findings, and negative x-rays in high-risk patients do not exclude significant intracranial pathology, therefore requiring CT.[1] Each of the modalities has advantages and drawbacks in the diagnosis of trauma-induced pathology. The strengths and weaknesses of these modalities will be addressed. Appearances of posttraumatic lesions will be discussed. Imaging assessment of herniation syndromes, pediatric head trauma, and imaging of the sequelae of head trauma with attention to advanced imaging techniques will be discussed.

Imaging Modalities for Acute Head Trauma

Computed Tomography (CT)

CT utilizes ionizing radiation with detectors to produce images. In the 1970s, CT became the preeminent imaging modality for head trauma victims, at that time with a single detector and relatively lengthy scanning times. However, for the first time, relatively fast noninvasive imaging to detect intracranial hemorrhage and posttraumatic mass lesions was possible. In the late 1980s, helical or spiral CT scanning was introduced, allowing more rapid acquisition of data, with the beam and detectors tracing a spiral path around the patient. In the head trauma patient, this advance allowed for shorter imaging times necessary in uncooperative patients and for the assessment of intra- and extracranial vascular structures by CT angiography (CTA). Multidetector CT (MDCT) was introduced in 1998, at that time collecting two slices of data in a single revolution using subsecond scanning times. Today, various multidetector row scanners are available for clinical use up to 64 slices. Although MDCT is not essential in routine imaging of the head trauma patient, certain injuries are better assessed with the additional applications available with MDCT, including high-quality two-dimensional (2-D) and three-dimensional (3-D) reconstructions and CTA.

The basic principle behind CT is similar to that of plain film radiography. An x-ray tube is used to generate a beam of photons, which is passed through the patient. This beam is highly collimated to allow detailed spatial resolution of the body part being imaged. The beam is rotated through many angles with a row of detectors placed at 180 degrees opposite the tube to detect the number of photons passing through the patient. The higher the x-ray attenuation of the tissue the beam passes through, the greater the absorption and therefore the fewer photons transmitted. An absorption value is calculated for every point along the beam path, from every angle scanned. Using a projection reconstruction mathematical algorithm, an image is reconstructed. Matrix refers to the number of imaging partitions in the x–y plane of a single axial slice. Field of view is the centimeters of tissue imaged. For a head CT a common field of view is 20 cm with a matrix of 512×512. The pixel size, or 2-D unit, for which x-ray beam attenuation is being measured is the field of view in millimeters divided by the matrix. Therefore a typical pixel size is 0.39 mm. This number is indicative of the spatial resolution of the image. A voxel is a 3-D imaging unit, the third dimension being the slice thickness. Multidetector CT can collect up to 64 slice locations in one gantry rotation.

Table 7.1 Imaging Modalities Used in Brain Trauma Evaluation

Computed Tomography (CT)

- Utilizes ionizing radiation with detectors to produce images
- Basic principle similar to that of plain film radiography. Images obtained according to tissue attenuation of X-rays (Hounsfield units)

Magnetic Resonance Imaging (MRI)

- Utilizes a high (or sometimes mid to low) field strength magnet and radiofrequency pulses to generate images
- Images obtained according to relaxation factors of protons

Digital Subtraction Angiography (DSA)

- Intravascular injection of iodinated contrast
- Digital equipment capable of rapid image acquisition to follow a bolus of contrast material through the arterial, capillary, and venous phases
- Resultant image shows vessels without any other structures

Advantages of MDCT include greater areas of patient coverage, reduction of motion artifacts, enhanced image quality due to thinner slices with improved spatial resolution, decreased scan time, and advanced image postprocessing including multiplanar reformatting, maximum intensity projection, volume rendering techniques, and quantitative analysis for tissue perfusion. MDCT imaging provides the capability to image the neural axis in seconds and allows reformatting in multiple planes within a few additional minutes. This reduction in imaging time reduces motion artifact, which can compromise assessment of subtle intracranial injury.[2] In the event the patient moves during the study, individual slices could be repeated within seconds. Data obtained in the axial plane can be viewed in multiple other planes, including coronal, sagittal and oblique projections using 2-D multiplanar reformatting. Maximum intensity projection (MIP) technique allows for 3-D visualization of vascular structures, or CTA, by combining axial slices and displaying the pixels with the highest density following rapid administration of a bolus of iodinated contrast material. Thin slab MIP displays can be used to eliminate surrounding structures such as bone, which can be of attenuation similar to contrast material. Viewing angles can be changed in small increments to create a rotating display of images, which can be viewed in a cine loop. Volume rendering techniques reconstruct a 3-D image from a stack of axial images. A wider variety of tissue structures of varying gray scales are displayed allowing for greater image detail. With both MIP and volume rendering techniques, images can be viewed from multiple angles. CTA and perfusion imaging are particularly useful to identify arterial injuries and to determine if there are associated ischemic sequelae. Multiplanar reformats are more useful in evaluating the spine in trauma patients, and in combination with volume rendering techniques are particularly helpful in displaying fractures of the calvaria and facial bones.

Indications for head CT in the traumatized patient include moderate to severe traumatic brain injury (TBI) with Glasgow Coma Scale (GCS) score of 12 or below, headache, vomiting, age greater than 60 or less than 2, drug or alcohol intoxication, deficits in short-term memory, physical evidence of trauma above the clavicles, coagulopathy, and seizure (**Table 7.2**). Approximately two-thirds of patients with head trauma in the United States are classified as mild TBI with a GCS of 13 or better, and less than 10% of these cases have positive CT findings, with less than 1% requiring surgical intervention. Mild head injuries are more commonly seen in patients greater than 60 years of age or young males who are intoxicated. CT is useful in mild TBI to identify the rare circumstance of clinically occult major intracranial pathology, allowing for safe early discharge.[3]

Typical head CT technique includes 4 to 5 mm thick axial slices from slightly below the foramen magnum to the vertex, angled parallel to the orbitomeatal line.

Table 7.2 Indications for Various Imaging Modalities

Computed Tomography (CT)

- Moderate to severe traumatic brain injury (TBI) with Glasgow Coma Scale (GCS) score of 12 or below
- Headache
- Vomiting
- Age greater than 60 or less than 2 years
- Drug or alcohol intoxication
- Short-term memory deficits
- Physical evidence of trauma above the clavicles
- Coagulopathy
- Seizure

Magnetic Resonance Imaging (MRI)

- Evaluation of patients with mild TBI
- Evaluation of chronic neurological and neuropsychological deficits
- Particularly useful when the neurological status of the patient does not match the computed tomographic (CT) scan and diffuse axonal injury is suspected
- MRI as an adjunct to CT is useful in the identification of small extradural hematomas, low-grade subarachnoid hemorrhage (SAH) and traumatic parenchymal lesions, particularly in the brain stem.
- In pediatric patients for assessment of nonaccidental head injury (NAHI).

Digital Subtraction Angiography (DSA)

- Used to be the gold standard for vascular injury related to head trauma
- Primary modality when patients present with evidence of vascular injury creating unstable hemodynamics
- Can be used when computed tomographic angiography (CTA) is negative but clinical suspicion of an arterial injury remains high
- For endovascular therapy if vascular occlusion/thrombosis, arterial dissection/transection, pseudoaneurysm, or carotid fistula are diagnosed by CTA

Images are reconstructed using a soft tissue algorithm and a bone algorithm. These algorithms include postprocessing features that allow "smoothing" of the structures of interest. The images are viewed at various window widths and levels, the window width (WW) referring to the range of the gray scale, whereas the window level (WL) is chosen by the Hounsfield units of the structure being visualized (i.e., brain, hematoma or contrast material, bone or calcium). The soft tissue algorithm is viewed at "brain" windows optimized for displaying the attenuation differences between white and gray matter (WW 80, WL 40) and at "subdural" windows (WW 150, WL 50) optimized for accentuating thin, acute subdural

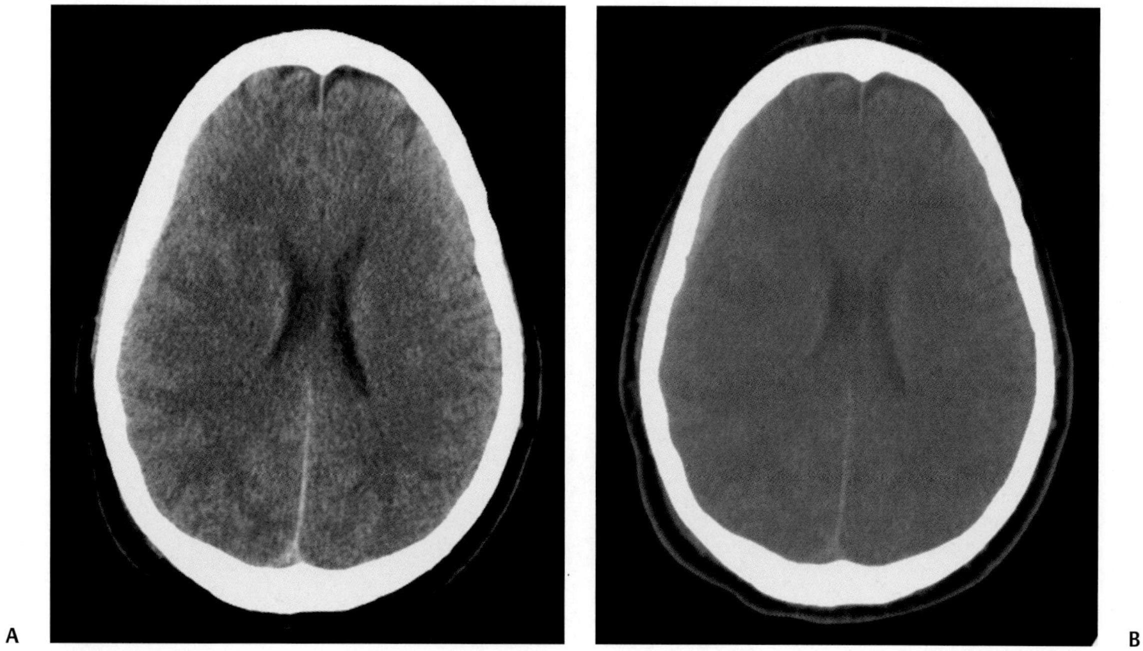

Fig. 7.1 Acute right frontal convexity subdural hematoma. **(A)** The lesion is invisible on the brain windows. **(B)** Subdural windows are necessary for identification.

hematomas (SDHs) adjacent to the calvarian that may be overlooked at the narrower brain window (**Fig. 7.1**). The subdural windows should not be used to evaluate more subtle parenchymal lesions. Bone algorithm images are optimal for identifying fractures of and soft tissue abnormalities within the sinuses and temporal bones, and are viewed at WWs of 1000 to 2000 and WL of 500 (**Fig. 7.2**). Intravenous iodinated contrast material should not be given prior to head scanning, as acute intracranial hemorrhage may be obscured by contrast enhancement of normal arteries and veins, as well as dural structures (**Fig. 7.3**). Therefore, if CT scanning of

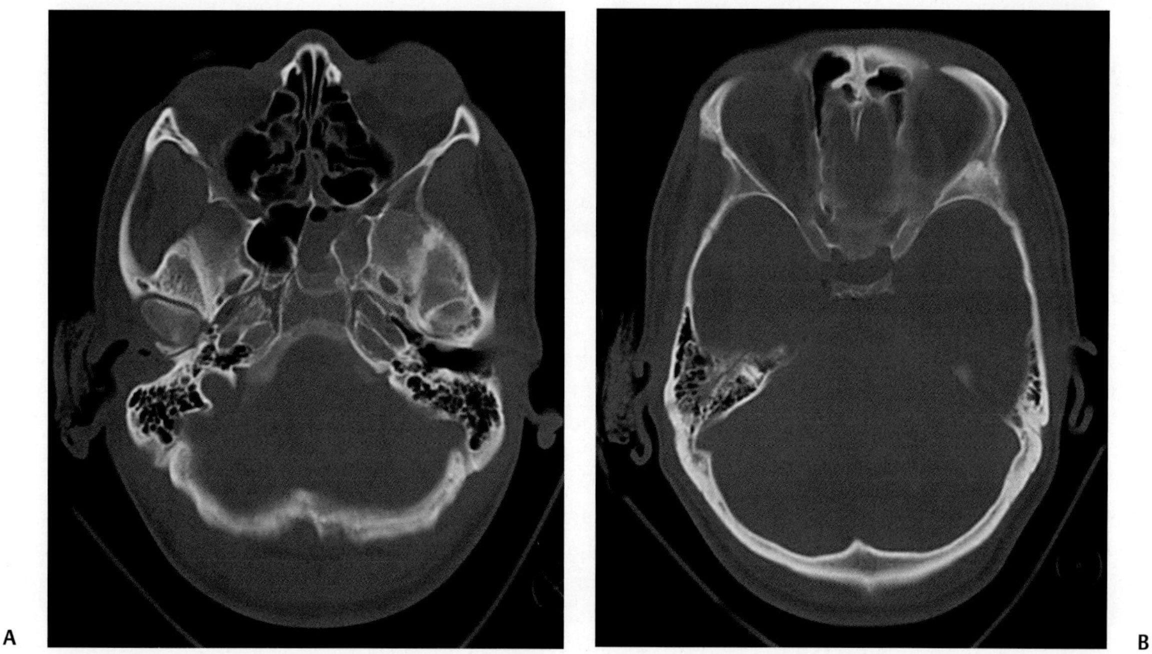

Fig. 7.2 Unhelmeted motorcyclist status post–motor vehicle accident. **(A)** Basilar skull fracture traverses foramen lacerum on the right with extension into the sphenoid sinus. An air-fluid level is seen in the sphenoid sinus indicating hemorrhage. **(B)** Longitudinal right temporal bone fracture with pneumocephalus.

(Continued on page 100)

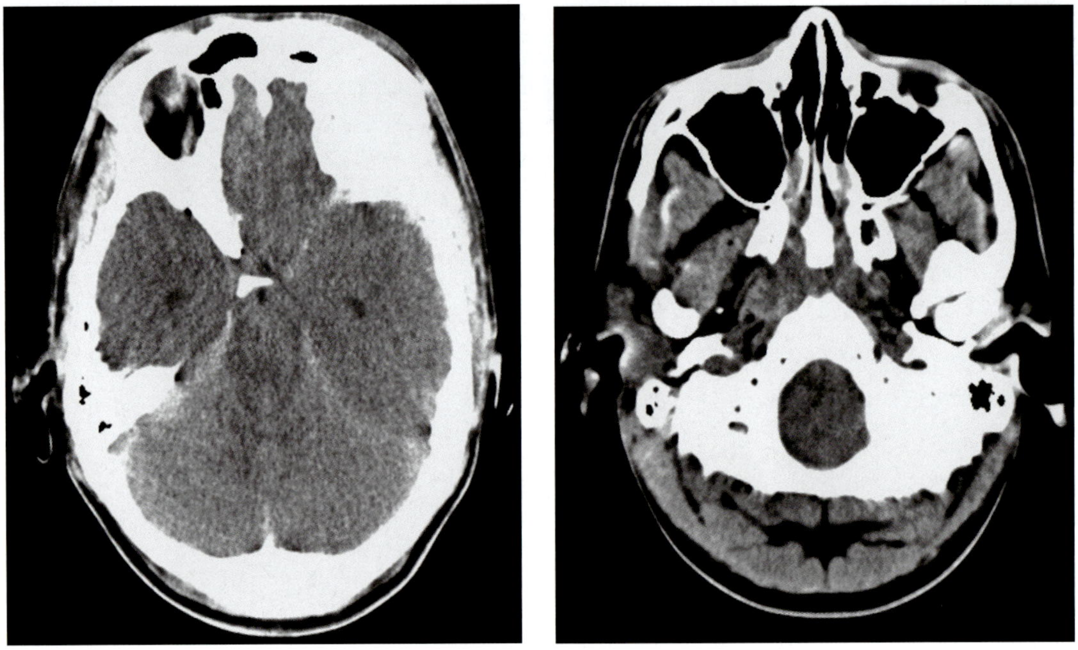

C D

Fig. 7.2 *(Continued)* **(C)** Cerebral edema. The reversal sign is seen with hyperattenuation of the cerebellum in relation to the cerebral hemispheres. Basal cisterns are effaced from central transtentorial herniation. A thin, acute left subdural hematoma is present. **(D)** Cerebellar tonsillar herniation is seen with complete effacement of cisterns in the foramen magnum.

the chest, abdomen, and pelvis is to be performed, the head must be the first body part examined.

Serial CT scanning of the head is indicated in several different clinical settings. Patients with severe head injury should be reexamined within 24 hours postinjury, as 25% of those patients with a normal head CT initially will demonstrate abnormalities on the follow-up scan.[1] Those with clinical deterioration should be scanned as soon as possible after the deterioration is observed. Two-thirds of patients deteriorating after 48 hours will have new hemorrhagic lesions, either intra- or extraaxial. These delayed lesions are associated with a poorer outcome; however, prognosis is improved by earlier recognition and treatment. Patients taken to the operating room receive baseline scans immediately after surgery. More than 50% of patients will develop new hemorrhages following decompression due to release of the tamponade effect created by the initial lesion (**Fig. 7.4**).

Magnetic Resonance Imaging (MRI)

MRI typically utilizes a high (or sometimes mid to low) field strength magnet and radiofrequency pulses to generate images. MRI images are obtained according to relaxation factors of protons. Currently fast spin echo techniques with multiple echo train lengths are employed to reduce imaging time. Imaging sequences required for complete assessment of the head trauma patient include T1, T2, fluid attenuated inversion recovery (FLAIR), gradient recalled echo (GRE) or T2*, diffusion weighted imaging (DWI) and apparent diffusion coefficient (ADC) mapping. Multiple planes of imaging are obtained for best identification of lesions at the base of the anterior, middle, or posterior cranial fossae, at the vertex or along the tentorium. FLAIR images, T2-weighted images with cerebrospinal fliud (CSF) nulling, are used to detect nonhemorrhagic cortical contusions, subdural hemorrhages particularly adjacent to the base of the brain, subarachnoid hemorrhage (SAH), and diffuse axonal injuries (DAIs).[4,5] GRE, also known as fast field echo, a pulse sequence utilizing a rephasing gradient pulse after the initial flip-angle magnetization used in spin echo imaging, is the most sensitive for detection of small parenchymal hemorrhages due to the paramagnetic effects of hemoglobin in its various stages.[6] DWI and ADC mapping are newer techniques sensitive to restriction of water diffusion across cell membranes. These images are obtained in seconds, rather than the minutes for other imaging sequences; however, they require echo-planar hardware, now standard on high field strength MRIs. Gradient echo pulses are added before and after the 180 degree refocusing pulse of the standard spin echo sequence. Random water motion causes a greater signal drop; conversely, restriction of random motion lessens the signal drop. In the setting of acute trauma, DAI, ischemia from vascular injury, and hypoxic-ischemic injury all show restricted diffusion, seen as a high signal intensity on DWI. Due to a reduced

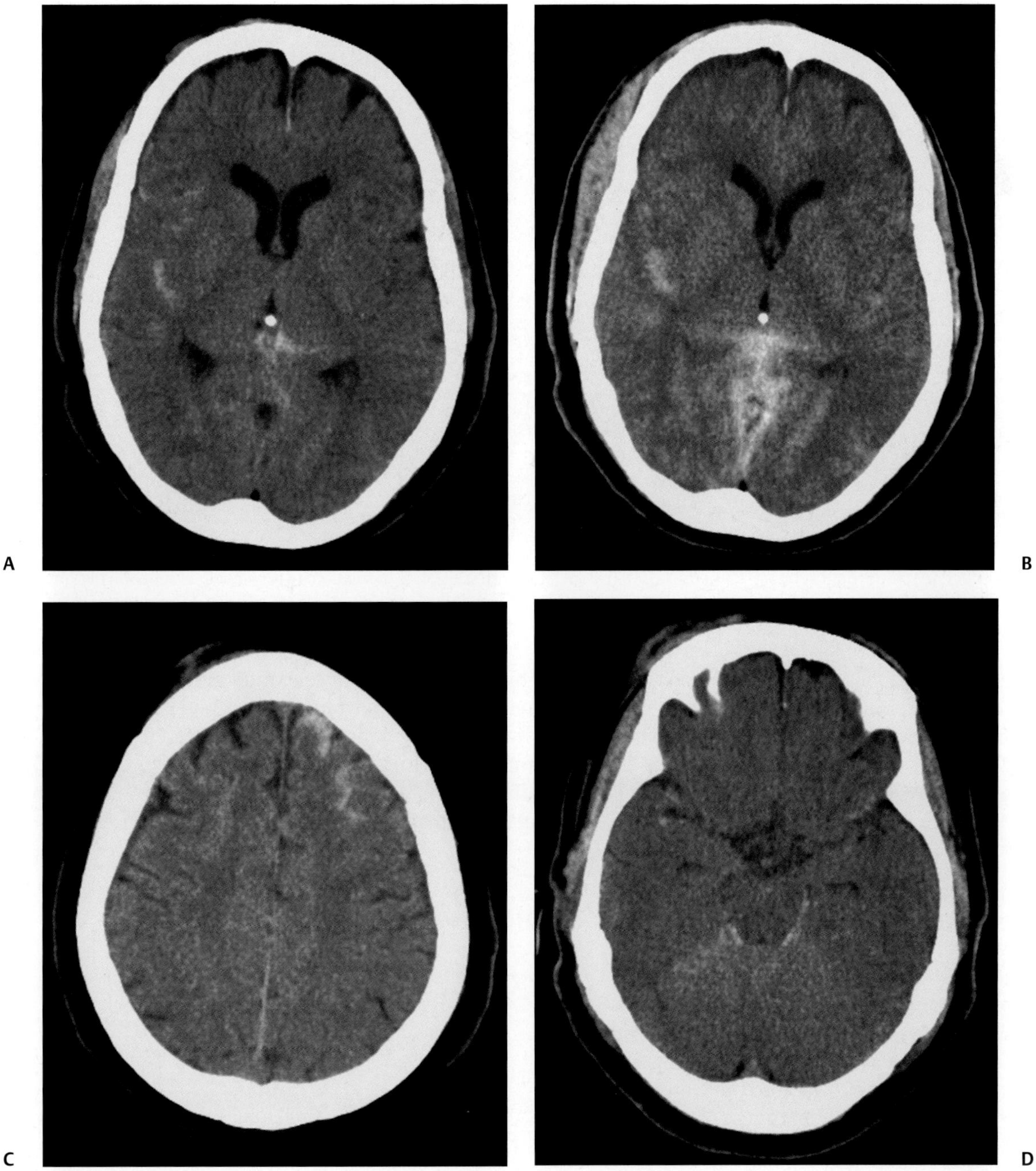

Fig. 7.3 Acute traumatic subarachnoid hemorrhage (SAH). **(A)** Initial scan demonstrates hemorrhage in the quadrigeminal plate cistern posterior to the pineal gland and in the right sylvian fissure. **(B)** Follow-up scan performed 7 hours later reveals increasing hyperattenuation along the tentorium. Intravenous contrast had been administered at the time of the first study for body computed tomography (CT) and computed tomographic angiography (CTA). The presence of contrast in vascular and meningeal structures limits assessment for progression of subarachnoid hemorrhage. Note also development of bilateral frontal subdural hygromas. **(C)** Hyperattenuating SAH is seen in the superior frontal sulci. **(D)** Minimal SAH is seen in the sylvian fissures and perimesencephalic cistern with relative sparing of the suprasellar cistern. Most supratentorial aneurysmal hemorrhages have a significant component in the suprasellar cistern.

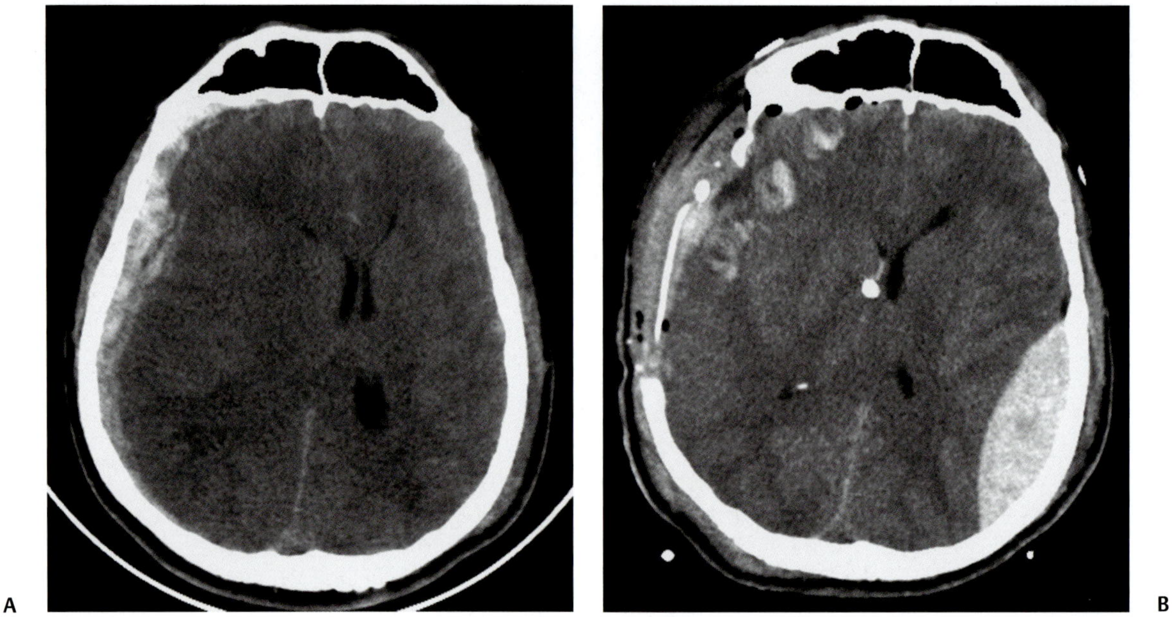

Fig. 7.4 Tamponade effect. **(A)** Large, right subdural hematoma (SDH) associated with subfalcine herniation. **(B)** Following evacuation of right SDH, a left epidural hematoma and right frontal parenchymal hemorrhages are evident.

ADC, these same areas will appear dark on ADC maps. MRI is particularly useful in the evaluation of patients with mild TBI or those with chronic neurological or neuropsychological deficits (see **Table 7.2**).

CT versus MRI (Table 7.3)

Although it is commonly acknowledged that MRI is superior to CT in the detection of posttraumatic brain lesions in the acute setting, CT remains the mainstay of imaging of the acute head trauma patient. MRI is more commonly used to assess brain trauma patients a few days to years postinjury for several reasons. MRI is less available and more costly, imaging times are longer, and severely injured patients are more difficult to get into the scanner as MRI compatible life support equipment must be utilized. MRI does not offer advantages in the identification of potentially surgical mass lesions. Patients must be carefully screened for MRI. However, MRI as an adjunct to CT in the acute setting has greater sensitivity in the identification of small extraaxial hematomas, low-grade SAH,[7] and traumatic parenchymal lesions, particularly in the brain stem. MRI is particularly useful when the neurological status of the patient does not match the CT scan and DAI is suspected. In the pediatric patient, MRI adds additional information in assessment of the victim of nonaccidental head injury (NAHI). MRI is not limited in evaluation of areas of the brain near the skull base by the beam hardening artifacts seen on CT. These artifacts are generated by transmission of the x-ray beam through structures of significantly different attenuation or between bony structures such as the petrous apices. However, CT is superior in imaging the cranium and associated maxillofacial trauma. CT also does not exclude patients with contraindications such as pacemakers, certain vascular clips, metallic implants, and ocular foreign bodies.

Imaging Vascular Injuries

Digital Subtraction Angiography versus Computed Tomographic Angiography versus Magnetic Resonance Angiography (Table 7.4)

DSA relies on the intravascular injection of iodinated contrast and digital equipment capable of rapid image acquisition to follow a bolus of contrast material through the arterial, capillary, and venous phases. Mask images are acquired prior to the injection of the contrast to be used to subtract bone and any other preexisting radiodensities such as bullets from the images obtained following the contrast injection. The resultant image is that of the vessels without any other structures. DSA is expensive, invasive, and not immediately available, as it requires the mobilization of a team of professionals including the neuroradiologist, angiographic technologist, and a nurse to administer and monitor sedation. Once the gold standard for evaluation of vascular injury related to head trauma, DSA is being supplanted by CTA for diagnosis of

Table 7.3 CT versus MRI in the Evaluation of Head Trauma

	CT	MRI
Use in acute head trauma	Method of choice. Not the most sensitive for all post-traumatic brain injury (TBI) lesions; serial computed tomographic (CT) scanning of the head increases detection of lesions	Usually not the first choice. However, magnetic resonance imaging (MRI) is superior to CT in detection of post-TBI lesions. More commonly used to assess brain trauma patients a few days to years postinjury
Use in mild TBI	Useful in mild TBI to identify the rare circumstance of clinically occult major intracranial pathology and allow for early patient discharge when negative	Useful in the evaluation of patients with mild TBI or those with chronic neurological or neuropsychological deficits
Use in moderate to severe TBI	Head CT indicated in moderate to severe TBI with Glasgow Coma Scale (GCS) score of 12 or below	Severely injured patients are more difficult to get into the scanner as MRI-compatible life support equipment must be utilized
Availability	Readily available in most facilities	Not as readily available as CT
Cost	Relatively less expensive	More expensive
Imaging time	Shorter imaging times	Longer imaging times
Patient selection	• Usually well tolerated by most patients • Can be used in patients with pacemakers, certain vascular clips, metallic implants, and ocular foreign bodies	• Careful patient screening required • Cannot be used in patients with pacemakers, vascular clips, metallic implants, and ocular foreign bodies

Table 7.4 Evaluation of Vascular Injuries

Digital Subtraction Angiography (DSA)

- Used to be the gold standard for vascular injury related to head trauma
- Primary modality when patients present with evidence of vascular injury creating unstable hemodynamics
- Can be used when computed tomographic angiography (CTA) is negative but clinical suspicion of an arterial injury remains high
- For endovascular therapy if vascular occlusion/thrombosis, arterial dissection/transection, pseudoaneurysm, or carotid cavernous fistula are diagnosed by CTA
- Disadvantage: expensive, invasive, and not immediately available

Computed Tomographic Angiography (CTA)

- Has replaced DSA for diagnosis of vascular pathologies including occlusion/thrombosis, arterial dissection, complete transection, pseudoaneurysm, or carotid cavernous fistula
- CTA can be performed to assess vascular injuries while the patient is still in the CT scanner in any of the following situations:
  - Routine noncontrast head CT demonstrates a basilar skull fracture, or
  - Fracture involving the middle meningial arterial groove, or
  - Clinical symptoms indicate territorial infarction suggesting more proximal arterial injury with thrombosis/embolization

Magnetic Resonance Angiography (MRA)

- Least invasive and most simply performed of the vascular imaging techniques
- Contrast material is generally not administered for intracranial MRA
- MRA in the presence of ICH must be performed as soon as possible
- MRA supplemented by T1-weighted axial images is the most accurate test in demonstrating carotid dissection.[8]
- Disadvantage: MRA takes longer to perform
- Limited role in the evaluation of the acutely injured patient for the same reasons that MRI is uncommonly used in the acute setting

vascular pathologies including occlusion/thrombosis, arterial dissection, complete transection, pseudoaneurysm, or carotid cavernous fistula. If routine noncontrast head CT demonstrates a basilar skull fracture or one involving the middle meningeal arterial groove, or clinical symptoms indicate territorial infarction suggesting more proximal arterial injury with thrombosis/embolization, CTA can be performed to assess for vascular injuries while the patient is still in the CT scanner. As previously discussed, the advent of MDCT has revolutionized CTA allowing for detection of more subtle lesions.

CTA is generally performed with the intravenous injection of 100 mL nonionic iodinated contrast material through an 18 gauge needle in adults. A 22 gauge needle may be used in children, with a contrast dose not to exceed 2 mL/kg. The contrast injection is generally followed by a saline flush to maximize the delivery of contrast material. Axial images are reconstructed at thin increments (at our institution 0.6 mm) with 3-D images performed on a separate workstation. These 3-D images can be viewed at various angles or in a cine loop. Depending on the level of injury, CTA of the cervical as well as the intracranial arteries can be obtained. CT perfusion can be performed at the same sitting by splitting the contrast dose between the two studies. CT perfusion must be performed prior to CTA to avoid having a background of contrast material in the brain.

Magnetic resonance angiography (MRA) is the least invasive and most simply performed of the vascular imaging techniques. However, MRA takes longer to perform. An intracranial MRA generally takes at least 5 minutes to obtain. Techniques employed in MRA include 2-D time of flight (TOF) or 3-D TOF. Time of flight imaging exploits the signal void that flowing blood creates on routine MRI images. By suppressing the signal of background tissues, images of only the vascular structures are created. Imaging of arteries excluding the venous structures is obtained by adding a saturation pulse that eliminates signal from blood flowing from superior to inferior. Two-dimensional TOF acquires images in the axial plane one slice at a time, as compared with the 3-D technique, acquiring a volume of information in all directions. Three-dimensional reconstructions are performed using the MIP algorithm, which includes only signals above a predefined threshold. MRA of the cervical arteries is initially obtained with a 2-D technique, as this technique is most useful in vessels with flow perpendicular to the axial plane. Three-dimensional TOF is more sensitive to multiplanar flow and is used for imaging of intracranial vessels. This technique is also used for the common carotid artery bifurcations and is helpful in evaluating flow in arteries running parallel to the axial plane, sometimes encountered in the proximal segment of the internal carotid artery. The length of anatomy that can be covered using the 3-D TOF technique is limited in comparison with the 2-D technique, such that the two sequences are complementary to each other. Caution should be exercised in evaluating the distal vertebral arteries at the C1 to C2 level where flow in the axial plane is seen, as inplane dephasing of arterial spins leads to artifactual loss of signal. Administration of intravenous contrast using a gadolinium chelate optimizes imaging of the aortic arch and cervical arteries with acquisition of images in the coronal plane. The addition of intravascular contrast allows for visualization of flow in all planes, as physiological flow artifacts are diminished. Contrast material is generally not administered for intracranial MRA, as intracranial venous structures will overlap and obscure the arterial structures. As MRA sequences are T1 weighted, any substance with short T1 relaxation properties such as fat or methemoglobin will be visualized on the images. Fat in the marrow of the skull base must be subtracted during postprocessing of the images. Fat in the clivus, petrous apices, underaerated sphenoid sinus, and clinoid processes may obscure the proximal intracranial arteries. MRA in the presence of intracranial hemorrhage must performed as soon as possible, as after the first few days methemoglobin will appear making identification of arteries in or around the hemorrhage difficult. Likewise, the T1 shortening associated with intracranial hemorrhage will overlap distant arteries as the MIP images are rotated.

DSA is utilized as the primary modality when patients present with evidence of vascular injury creating unstable hemodynamics. DSA can also be used for cases where CTA is negative but clinical suspicion of an arterial injury remains high, and for endovascular therapy if one of the above conditions is diagnosed by CTA. MRA plays a limited role in the evaluation of the acutely injured patient for the same reasons that MRI is uncommonly used in the acute setting. MRA supplemented by T1-weighted axial images, however, is the most accurate test in demonstrating carotid dissection with a sensitivity of 95% and a specificity of 99% in a study by Levy et al.[8]

Imaging Intraaxial Injury (Table 7.5)

Diffuse Axonal Injury

DAI occurs with acceleration/deceleration injury that results in mechanical forces that damage the integrity of axons. The distribution of lesions tends to be at points of maximum shearing stress along white matter tracts. Nearly two-thirds of lesions occur in lobar white matter at the corticomedullary junction.[9] The corpus callosum is another common site of involvement, particulary the splenium.

This is explained by the rigid attachment of the corpus callosum to the falx rendering the corpus callosum significantly less mobile than the cerebral hemispheres. When

Table 7.5 Imaging of Intraaxial Injuries

	CT	MRI
Diffuse axonal injury (DAI)	Limited value when diffuse axonal injury is suspected (sensitivity 20%)[12]	Particularly useful (sensitivity 97%)[12] when the neurological status of the patient does not match the CT scan and DAI is suspected
Contusion	Image findings determined by age of blood products. Initial findings may be subtle or absent. Serial computed tomographic (CT) scans may be used.	Image findings determined by age of blood products. Magnetic resonance imaging (MRI) obtained in the hyperacute stage (<3 hours after trauma) may be less sensitive than CT.
Intraparenchymal hematoma (penetrating trauma)	Intraparenchymal hematoma will appear as a well-defined hyperdense mass in the acute stages.	Missile trauma with metallic objects may preclude imaging with MRI. Lysis of clot will follow signal characteristics on MRI as for contusions, except somewhat slower.
Cerebral edema	Early signs are lack of visualization of the sulci and basilar cisterns. These are followed by homogeneous decreased attenuation and increased T2-weighted signal intensity on CT and MRI, respectively, with loss of gray–white differentiation.	

mechanical forces are applied to the head, the rigid falx prevents the cerebral hemispheres from moving across the midline, and shear strains develop at the corpus callosum. Less strain develops anteriorly where the falx is shorter and can allow transient displacement of portions of the brain across the midline. Posteriorly the falx is broader and effectively prevents this displacement, allowing greater shear and tensile strains to develop within the fibers of the corpus callosum.[10] Brain stem shearing injury is also commonly seen, predominantly in the dorsolateral aspect of the brain stem, sparing the ventral aspect. With more severe head trauma, involvement of the cerebellar hemispheres, basal ganglia, and thalami can also be seen.

CT scan is often initially normal. When CT findings are evident in axonal shear injury, they include multiple discrete foci of low density, typically measuring less than 1 cm in size. When hemorrhagic shear injury lesions are present, they may be easily identified on CT due to their hyperdense appearance (**Fig. 7.5A**). However, hemorrhagic foci are often more easily detected on delayed than on initial CT scans.

The value of CT is limited when there is clinical suspicion of DAI as studies have shown discrepancies between the findings on CT and the neurological status of patients after head trauma. Mittl et al[11] report that 30% of patients with a negative head CT scan result will have radiographic evidence of DAI on MRI. Study by Orrison et al[12] showed the sensitivity of MRI (97%) was significantly higher than that of CT (20%) for detection of DAI. Thus, it is now recommended that all patients with moderate to severe head injury get an MRI within the first 2 weeks of injury for better evaluation of the full extent of brain involvement.[13]

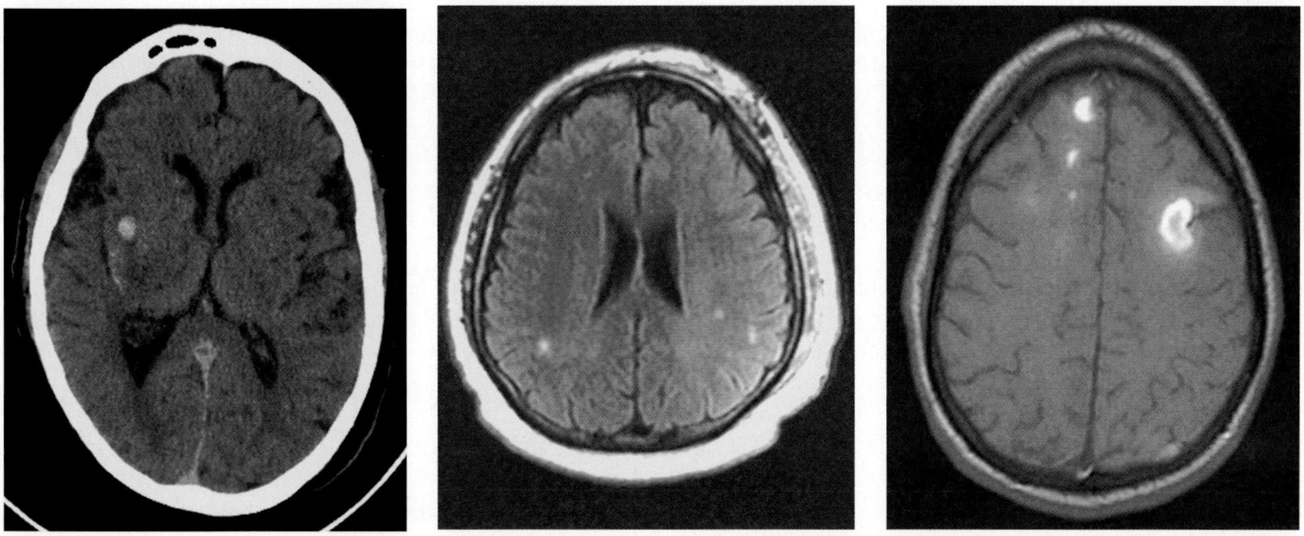

Fig. 7.5 Diffuse axonal injury (DAI). **(A)** Axial computed tomography. A hemorrhage is identified at the junction of the right lentiform nucleus and external capsule. A small amount of subarachnoid hemorrhage is seen in the right sylvian fissure. **(B)** Axial fluid attenuated inversion recovery reveals punctuate hyperintensities at the corticomedullary junctions. **(C)** In a second patient, T1-weighted image through the centrum semiovale demonstrates multiple T1 hyperintense lesions at the corticomedullary junction.

(Continued on page 106)

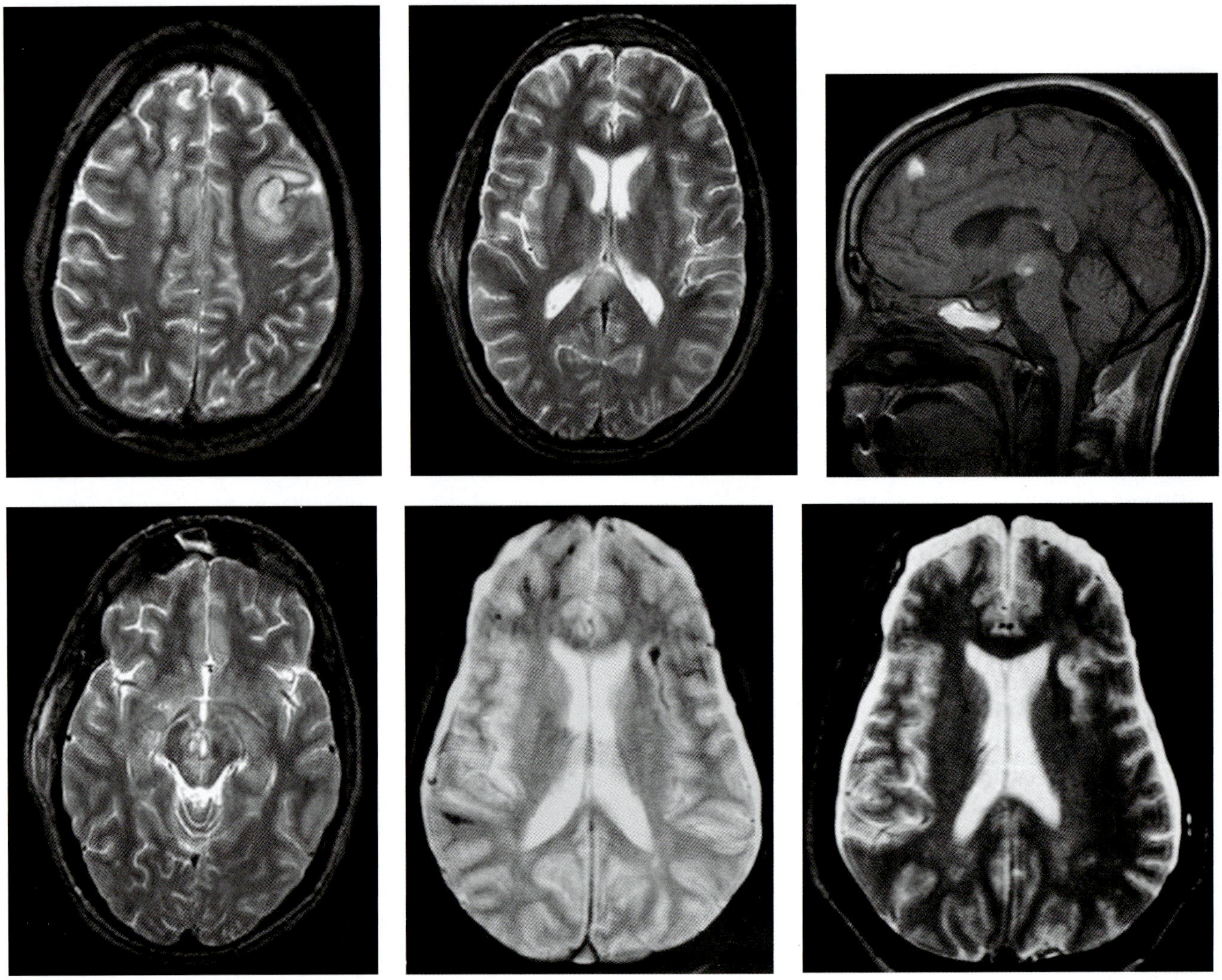

D–F

G–I

Fig. 7.5 *(Continued)* **(D)** Axial T2-weighted image at the same level shows T2 hyperintensity in the lesions. The combination of TI hyperintensity and T2 hyperintensity indicates extracellular methemoglobin (metHgb) of subacute hemorrhage. Surrounding T2 hyperintensity is consistent with edema. **(E)** T2-weighted axial magnetic resonance imaging (MRI) reveals T2 hyperintensity in the splenium of the corpus callosum. **(F)** Sagittal T1-weighted image reveals T1 hyperintensity consistent with hemorrhage at the posterior callosal–septal junction. The lesion in the splenium is isointense. Additional hemorrhagic lesions are seen in the frontal lobe and midbrain. **(G)** Axial T2-weighted image demonstrates T2 hyperintensity in the tegmentum of the right midbrain, another common site for DAI. **(H)** In a third patient, gradient recalled echo axial image reveals multiple T2 hypointensities at the gray–white junction representing hemorrhages secondary to shearing injury. **(I)** T2-weighted axial image at the same level fails to demonstrate these hemorrhages.

Although, the neuropathological literature suggests that DAI is typically accompanied by small hemorrhages,[14,15] most MRI studies of TBI state that most DAI lesions are nonhemorrhagic.[6,11] Conspicuity of a lesion on MRI depends on many factors, including its location, size, presence of hemorrhage, and the pulse sequence used. The most sensitive sequence for detection of nonhemorrhagic lesions of DAI is FLAIR. On these sequences, the lesions will typically be small areas of increased signal with the most common locations including the gray–white matter interface, the corpus callosum, and the dorsolateral brain stem (**Figs. 7.5B–7.5G**). T2-weighted gradient echo sequences are useful for detecting microbleeding associated with DAI, which causes marked signal loss due to magnetic susceptibility (**Figs. 7.5H** and **7.5I**). Although hyperacute hematomas are composed primarily of oxyhemoglobin, which has little magnetic susceptibility effects, this stage of hemoglobin only lasts for the first several hours after injury. Deoxyhemoglobin, methemoglobin (when intracellular), and hemosiderin in the subsequent stages of traumatic hemorrhage do have magnetic susceptibility and thus will have corresponding signal loss on T2-weighted gradient echo sequences.

Contusion

Contusions are bruises of the brain that occur when the brain contacts a dural ridge or bony protuberance. Thus, they have very characteristic locations, most commonly seen in the frontal lobes and anterior temporal lobes. When acceleration/deceleration forces are applied to the head, brain parenchyma strikes an osseous ridge or dural fold, and hemorrhagic contusion results.[13] Contusions are often categorized into coup and contrecoup injuries, the former occurring at the site of impact and the latter distant or opposite to the site of impact (**Fig. 7.6**).

Nearly 50% of all cases involve the temporal lobes, the temporal tip most frequently, inferior surface, and cortex around the sylvian fissure. One-third of contusions occur in the frontal lobes, particularly along the inferior surface and around the frontal poles. In these cases injury results from brain moving over the floor of the anterior cranial fossa and striking the sphenoid wings and petrous ridges. Twenty-five percent are parasagittal in location, caused by brain striking paramedian bony irregularities. The inferior surfaces of the cerebellar hemispheres are less common sites of cortical contusion. Focal contusions are also seen in association with depressed skull fractures (**Fig. 7.7**).

Contusions occur in up to 43% of patients with blunt or nonpenetrating head injuries.[13] With this high percentage of affected patients compared with DAI, combined with the fact that contusions are less frequently associated with loss of consciousness, noncontrast CT is the most reasonable exam to obtain on initial evaluation of these patients. Initially findings on CT may be subtle or absent. Early findings include ill-defined areas of low attenuation if hemorrhage is absent, which represents edematous brain, and small patchy areas of high attenuation surrounded by low attenuation representing petechial hemorrhage with surrounding edema. Petechial cortical contusions tend to coalesce into larger hemorrhagic foci, thus frequently becoming more evident on follow-up CT obtained 24 to 48 hours after the initial trauma.[16,17] These follow-up studies often show more lesions than initially seen as well. In 20% of cases, delayed hemorrhages develop in what previously appeared as areas of low attenuation without hemorrhage.[13] Edema and mass effect generally increase during the first few days after trauma and then gradually subside.

Imaging findings on MRI will vary greatly depending on the time elapsed after trauma and the presence or absence of hemorrhage. Nonhemorrhagic contusions will manifest as areas of increased signal intensity on T2-weighted and FLAIR sequences; there may be corresponding areas of low T1 signal intensity but these are much less conspicuous. These foci of abnormal signal intensity represent areas of edematous brain. Again the edema tends to increase within the first few days following the trauma and then subsides.

In the presence of hemorrhage, the imaging findings will be determined by the age of the blood products. MRI obtained in the hyperacute stage (<3 hours after trauma) is less sensitive than CT because diamagnetic intracellular oxyhemoglobin will have signal characteristics similar to

A

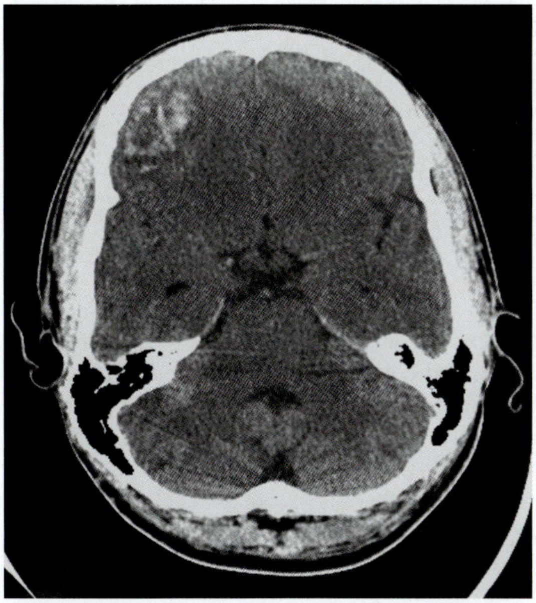

B

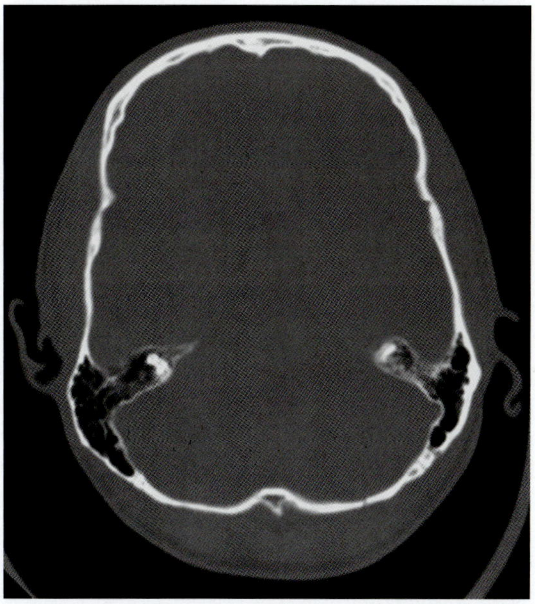

Fig. 7.6 Right frontal hemorrhagic contusion 1 day status postassault. **(A)** Brain window reveals hyperdense hemorrhage mixed with hypodense edema consistent with hemorrhagic contusion. **(B)** Bone window shows linear left occipital fracture at the site of impact. The contusion represents a contrecoup injury.

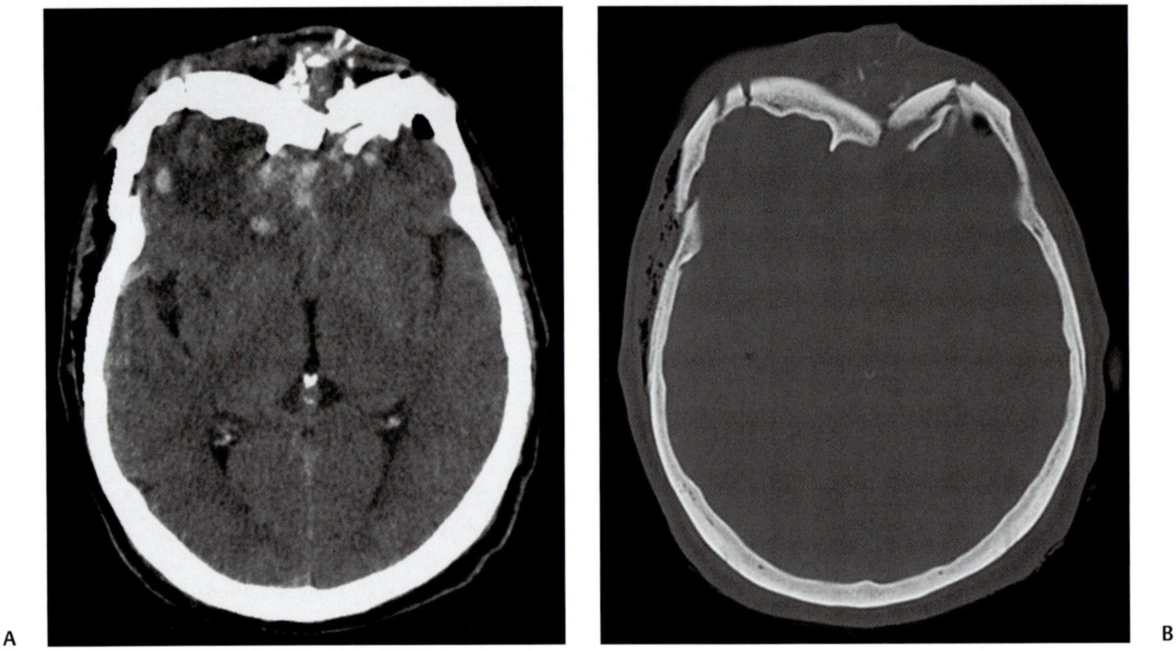

Fig. 7.7 Contusions associated with depressed fracture. (A) Brain window demonstrates hemorrhagic contusion in the frontal lobes. (B) Bone window shows depressed, comminuted frontal bone fracture fragments. A small amount of left frontal pneumocephalus is seen.

that of brain, specifically normal to slightly lower signal on T1-weighted images and slightly higher signal on T2-weighted images, thus injury may be masked.[9]

Clot resorption begins at the peripheral margins and moves inward and thus the change in signal characteristics that accompanies the degradation of blood products will be seen first in the periphery, then progressing centrally.

Acute hemorrhagic contusions (1 to 3 days old) are composed predominantly of paramagnetic intracellular deoxyhemoglobin, which will demonstrate signal characteristics of isointense signal to brain on T1-weighted images and hypointense signal to brain on T2-weighted images; the areas of abnormal signal intensity will be more conspicuous on T2* gradient echo images due to magnetic susceptibility artifact.

With the continued evolution of blood products, hemorrhagic contusions in the early subacute stage will have predominantly intracellular methemoglobin, manifesting as hyperintense T1 signal and hypointense T2 signal. Methemoglobin may appear in the periphery of the hematoma as early as 2 to 3 days after injury, and then it gradually fills in over the next several days.[18] This is followed by erythrocyte membrane breakdown and extracellular migration of methemoglobin. Extracellular methemoglobin will be hyperintense on both T1- and T2-weighted images, and these signal characteristics may persist for several weeks to even months. During this stage, intense enhancement may be seen on both contrast-enhanced CT and MRI along the margins of lesions. This can be explained by the process of neovascularization, where the new blood vessels at the periphery of the lesion lack the tight endothelial junctions of an intact blood–brain barrier.[19]

In the final phase of the breakdown of blood products, hemosiderin will have slightly low signal intensity on T1-weighted images and marked low signal intensity on T2-weighted images. With clot resorption, necrotic tissue is sloughed and cystic cavities are formed over the next 6 to 12 months. Focal atrophy is characterized by volume loss of the cortical gyri, enlargement of the local subarachnoid spaces, and ex vacuo dilatation of the adjacent ventricle.[9]

Intraparenchymal Hematoma

Intraparenchymal hematomas unrelated to contusions are generally the result of penetrating trauma. Although many bullets now are nonferromagnetic, it is important to consider that missile trauma with metallic objects may preclude imaging with MRI.[9] On CT, intraparenchymal hematoma will appear as a well-defined hyperdense mass in the acute stages (**Fig. 7.8A**). Surrounding vasogenic edema will be hypodense and generally peaks between 3 and 5 days. Subacute hematomas 3 to 7 days of age may demonstrate fluid-blood levels within the hematoma.[9] Because clot resorption begins in the periphery and progresses inward, there is corresponding decreased attenuation

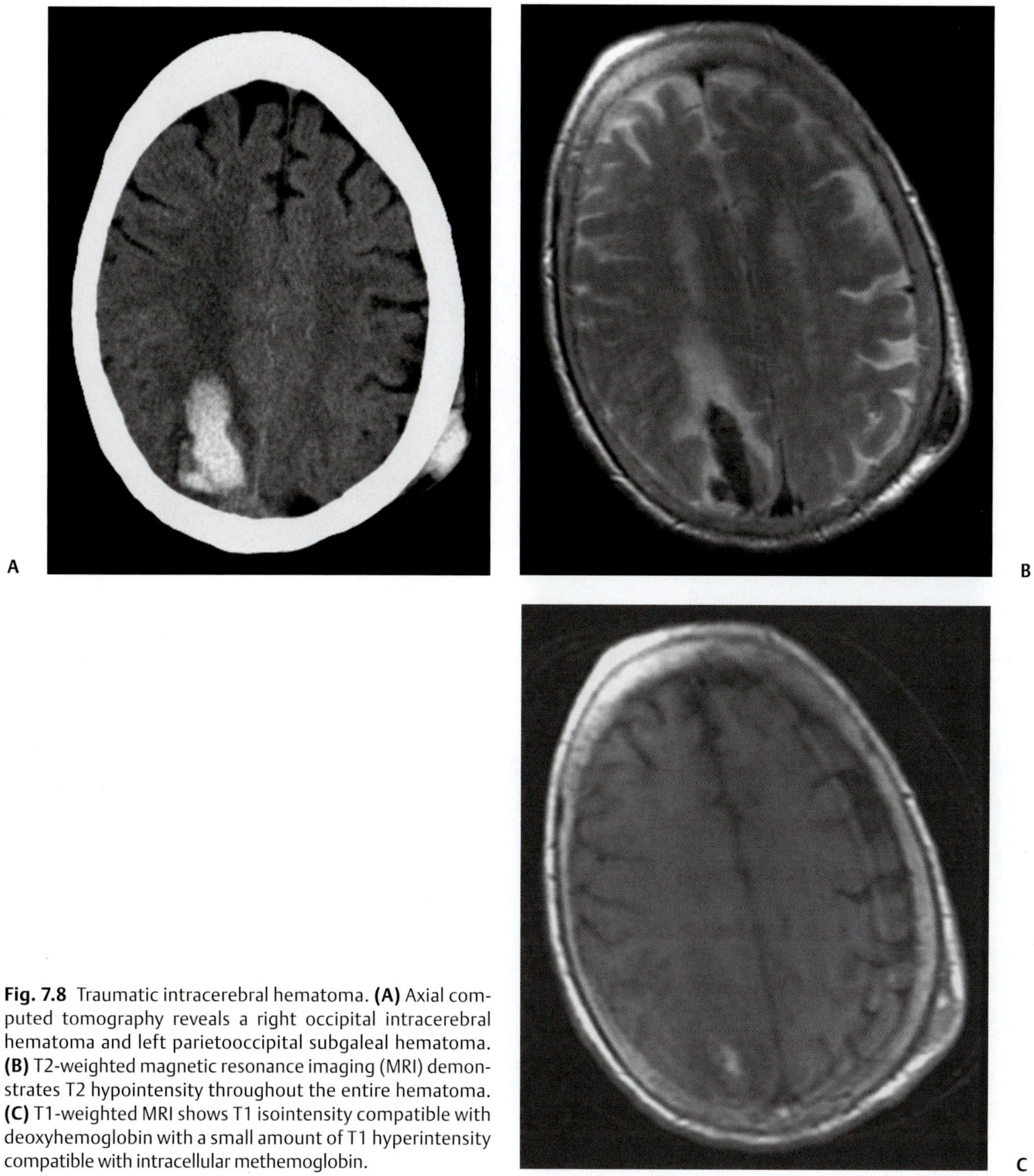

Fig. 7.8 Traumatic intracerebral hematoma. **(A)** Axial computed tomography reveals a right occipital intracerebral hematoma and left parietooccipital subgaleal hematoma. **(B)** T2-weighted magnetic resonance imaging (MRI) demonstrates T2 hypointensity throughout the entire hematoma. **(C)** T1-weighted MRI shows T1 isointensity compatible with deoxyhemoglobin with a small amount of T1 hyperintensity compatible with intracellular methemoglobin.

on CT, first in the periphery and then moving inward as degradation of blood products continues. This decreased attenuation in the periphery is usually seen around 7 to 10 days, and by 3 to 10 weeks, hematoma in its chronic phase is near completely isodense to normal brain parenchyma. With continued proteolysis and phagocytosis, the hematoma is eventually replaced by an area of encephalomalacia.[9]

Lysis of clot with breakdown of blood products will generally follow the signal characteristics on MRI as described earlier for contusions but may have a somewhat slower time course because the intraparenchyal hematomas tend to be larger in size relative to contusions (**Figs. 7.8B** and **7.8C**).

When intraparenchymal hematomas are extensive, they may burst through the pia to accumulate in the subdural space. The term *burst lobe* is sometimes used to describe the appearance of intracerebral hematoma mixed with necrotic brain tissue, rupturing out into the subdural space with associated hemispheric swelling (**Fig. 7.9**).

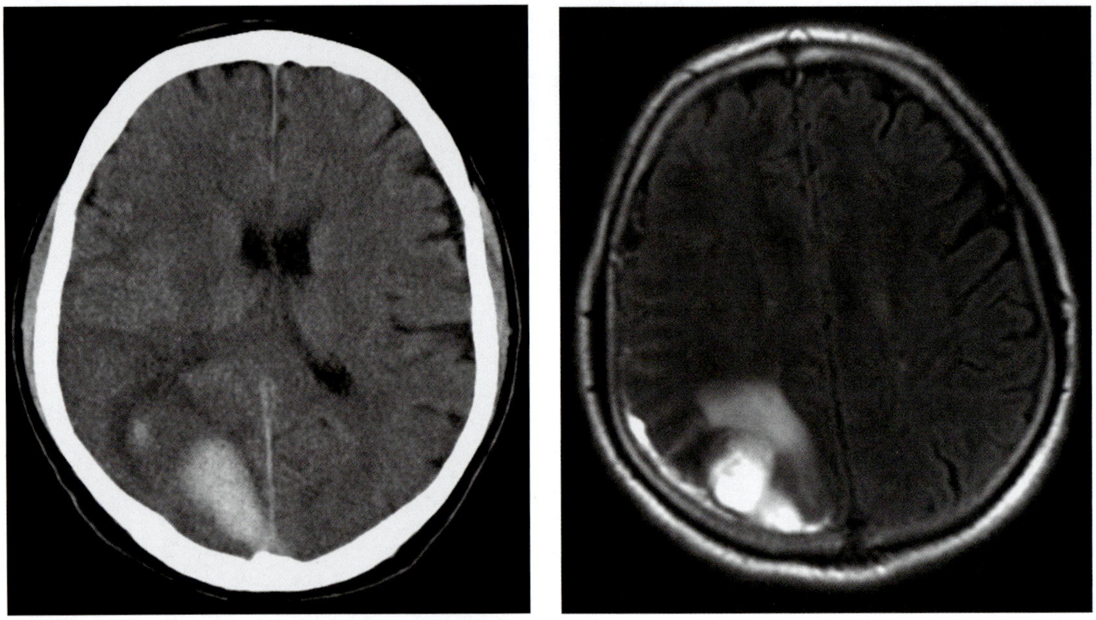

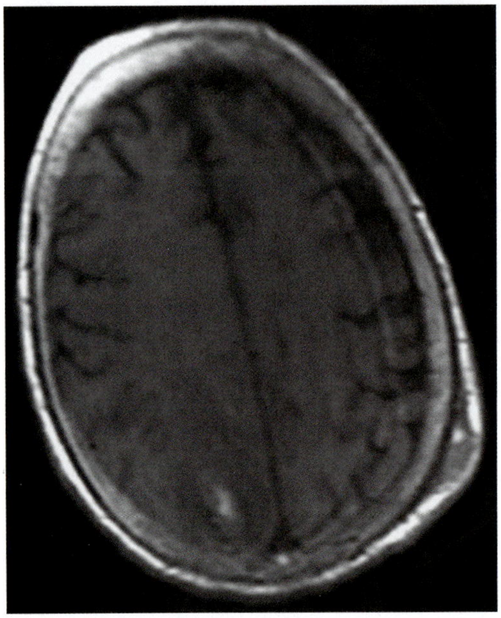

Fig. 7.9 Burst lobe. **(A)** Axial computed tomography demonstrates hyperdense acute intracerebral hematoma in the right parietooccipital lobe. **(B)** Axial fluid attenuated inversion recovery image demonstrates T2 hyperintensity within the hematoma with extension into the adjacent subdural space. Edema is seen in the adjacent parenchyma. **(C)** Axial T1 image reveals T1 hyperintensity in the anterior aspect of the hematoma and around its margins with T1 isointensity posteriorly compatible with a mixture of intra- and extracellular methemoglobin (metHgb) in this evolving hemorrhage.

Cerebral Edema

Diffuse cerebral edema is seen in 10 to 20% of severe brain injuries and occurs nearly twice as often in children compared with adults.[20] It usually takes 24 to 48 hours after the traumatic insult for severe cerebral edema to develop.

Diffuse cerebral edema in the setting of trauma is similar to cerebral edema seen in other clinical scenarios. The earliest manifestations will be lack of visualization of the sulci and basilar cisterns. The ventricles may appear smaller than usual. These early signs are followed by homogeneous decreased attenuation and increased T2-weighted signal intensity on CT and MRI, respectively, with loss of gray–white differentiation.

On occasion, the cerebellum may appear hyperdense on CT relative to the edematous cerebral hemispheres (**Fig. 7.2C**). This finding is caused by relative sparing of the cerebellum and brain stem from cerebral ischemia and is often associated with extracranial trauma such as drowning or strangulation.[21]

Of course with increased intracranial pressure, herniation of brain from one compartment to another may occur. Imaging characteristics of the various types of herniations are discussed in this chapter in the section, "Imaging Cerebral Herniation Syndromes."

Imaging Extraaxial Hemorrhage (Table 7.6)

Subdural Hematoma

Subdural hemorrhage is the most common type of intracranial hemorrhage. SDHs are seen in 10 to 20% of patients with head trauma as opposed to the 11% of TBI patients who develop SAH. The mortality rate, however, is significantly higher (50–85%) in patients with complicated subdural hemorrhage than in patients with SAH.[9] The most commonly encountered operable intracranial hematoma is an acute SDH, with or without associated cerebral contusion.[22]

A subdural collection is found between the pia–arachnoid membrane and the overlying dura of the inner table. Hemorrhage into this potential space is secondary to tearing of fixed bridging veins being stretched by the moveable brain, which is experiencing rotational forces. The subdural portion of the vein is not ensheathed with arachnoid trabeculae and therefore is the weaker segment of the vein. SDHs are classified as simple (without associated brain parenchymal injury) or complicated (with parenchymal injury). Imaging characteristic of SDHs are dependent on the age of the blood products that have been clinically classified into acute, subacute, and chronic stages that range from time of injury to 3 days, 3 days to 3 weeks, and greater than 3 weeks.

Imaging features of an acute SDH include hyperattenuation on CT and a medially concave margin. This is often referred to as crescentic extraaxial density (**Figs. 7.1** and **7.4A**). The thickness of the hematoma can be quite variable, ranging from pencil thin to large. Rarely, an acute subdural hemorrhage can present as an isodense or hypodense extracerebral mass on CT. This has been seen in patients who are profoundly anemic (hemoglobin level of 8–10 g/dL). Also, this imaging feature of an acute subdural hemorrhage has also been reported in patients who are suffering from disseminated intravascular coagulopathy or in patients who have concomitant tears of the arachnoid membrane, which as a result, dilute the concentration of red blood cells with CSF.

Table 7.6 Imaging of Extraaxial Injuries

Subdural hematoma	• Hemorrhage in the potential space between the pia–arachnoid membrane and the overlying dura of the inner table
	• Imaging characteristic of subdural hematomas are dependent on the age of the blood products that have been clinically classified into acute, subacute, and chronic stages
	• *Acute* (injury to 3 days): hyperattenuation on computed tomography (CT) and medially concave margin (crescentric extraaxial density)
	• *Subacute* (3 days to 3 weeks) and chronic (>3 weeks): layering with differential attenuation and convex margin with inward displacement of the convexity veins
	• Magnetic resonance imaging (MRI) allows further classification of subacute into early versus late
Subdural hygroma	• Fluid collections that are isoattenuation on CT or nearly isosignal on all MRI pulse sequences to cerebrospinal fluid within the subdural space
	• *Common causes*: trauma with tear in the arachnoid membrane or degradation of subdural hematomas
	• Differentiated from arachnoid cyst by lack of scalloping of calvarial inner table
	• May be impossible to distinguish from chronic subdural hematoma
Epidural hematoma	• Hemorrhage in the potential space between the inner table of the calvaria and the dura
	• *Common causes*: temporal bone fracture with a tear of the middle meningeal artery
	• CT imaging demonstrates high density biconvex extraaxial mass
	• Acute epidural hematomas are hyperdense on CT, whereas chronic are generally hypodense
	• On MRI, extraaxial hemorrhage demonstrates different signal characteristics based on the age of the blood products
Subarachnoid hemorrhage	• Most common cause is trauma
	• More commonly seen in the elderly or in infants (enlarged subarachnoid spaces)
	• Chronic subarahnoid hemorrhage cannot be identified on CT; MRI with gradient echo is more sensitive
	• Well-known complication of chronic subarachnoid hemorrhage is pial siderosis, which can be identified on MRI with T2W1

Subacute and chronic hematomas may display layering with differential attenuation. The supernatant portion of the collection is usually of lower attenuation due to the settling of cells and cellular debris. Whereas the acute hematomas often demonstrate a concave inner margin, the subacute and chronic hematomas may develop a convex margin with inward displacement of the convexity veins, which are found along the inner surface of the arachnoid. SDHs are not confined by sutures as are epidural hematomas (EDHs). Although they usually are found over the convexities, they can also be seen within the posterior fossa, middle cranial fossa, and/or along the tentorium. At times, thin isodense subdurals are difficult to separate from the inner table of the calvaria. However CT postprocessing features of intermediate WLs on the Picture Archiving and Communication System (PACS) can be utilized to increase conspicuity. This, however, is not an issue with MRI. MRI can also further separate and date blood products based on their ionic properties (ferrous vs. ferric iron states of the hemoglobin). This allows further characterization of the subacute hematomas into early versus late. Subacute SDHs may be isodense to low density, but mass effect remains a prominent feature. Following contrast administration, the wall of the hematoma will demonstrate enhancement. The enhancement is caused by the vascularization of the subdural membranes. The enhancement is frequently thicker on the outer margin than on the inner margin. This usually occurs between the first and third week after the initial trauma. These vascularized membranes contain vessels that do not have endothelial tight junctions and can leak contrast. These leaky vessels may also tear easily, resulting in various blood products and growth patterns to a subdural collection. Repeat episodic bleeding into the subdural collection leads to the formation of fibrous septa, which can result in loculated compartments. Delayed scans may reveal layering within extracerebral collections. Hematomas may also occur between the leaves of the tentorium and often have a characteristic pattern of fading laterally while maintaining an abrupt medial margin.

Chronic subdurals are usually of low attenuation but recurrent or repeat rebleeding may result in fluid of variable attenuation (**Fig. 7.10**). Chronic SDHs are commonly seen in the very young or very old, with more than 75% occurring in patients over the age of 50. Causes of chronic subdurals include birth injury, vitamin K deficiency, child abuse, or coagulopathy. Rarely, chronic subdurals have been reported to contain fat or reported to ossify.

Patients who have bilateral isodense SDHs can be particularly challenging for the radiologist (**Fig. 7.11A**). In these instances it is important to evaluate the equivocal finding in the context of the patient's age and additional findings such as ventricular position. Elderly patients will generally demonstrate enlarged sulci due to atrophy; therefore, loss

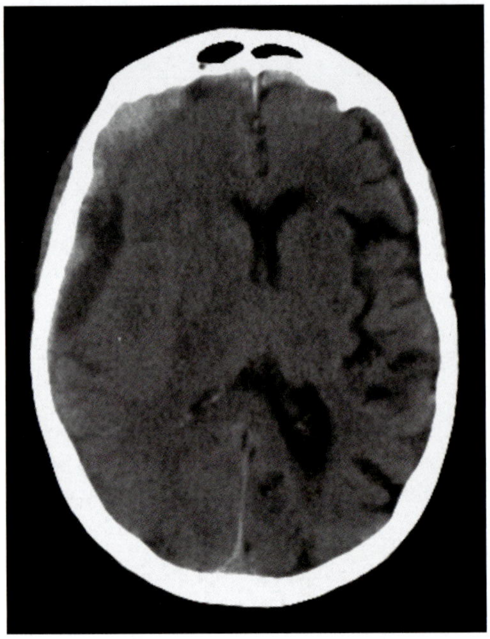

Fig. 7.10 Acute on chronic subdural hematoma. Hypoattenuating subdural collection is seen along the right convexity. Areas of high attenuation represent acute hemorrhage. Compression of underlying sulci and the right lateral ventricle is seen with subfalcine herniation. The collection is partially biconvex due to the underlying chronic component.

of sulcation is a key finding in making the appropriate diagnosis. When bilateral, the subdurals may exert equal mass effect on the ventricular system, resulting in symmetrically small and possibly medially deviated lateral ventricles. In addition, the gray–white matter interfaces remain intact and the cortex appears buckled, implying an extraaxial mass lesion. With an intraaxial space-occupying lesion, the gray–white interface should be obscured and the overlying cortex is generally expanded. Contrast administration will also be helpful in demonstrating the inwardly displaced cortical veins.

On MRI, SDHs have characteristic signal intensities to easily differentiate acute, subacute, and chronic stages. With MRI, SDHs follow the intensity of blood. Acute SDHs are isointense on T1-weighted images and hypointense on T2-weighted images. Subacute subdurals will generally be of higher intensity on T1- and T2-weighted images. Imaging of the subacute subdural hemorrhage on T2 sequences, however, can be variable depending on whether the methemoglobin molecule is intra- or extracellular. If it is intracellular, the blood products will be hypointense on T2WI, but if it is extracellular, implying a slightly older stage of hemorrhage, it will remain hyperintense on T2-weighted images. However, over time, the higher intensity on T1-weighted images will gradually diminish to an isointenisty similar to the underlying brain parenchyma (**Fig. 7.11B** and **7.11C**). Such collections can be confused with subdural empyemas, and because either

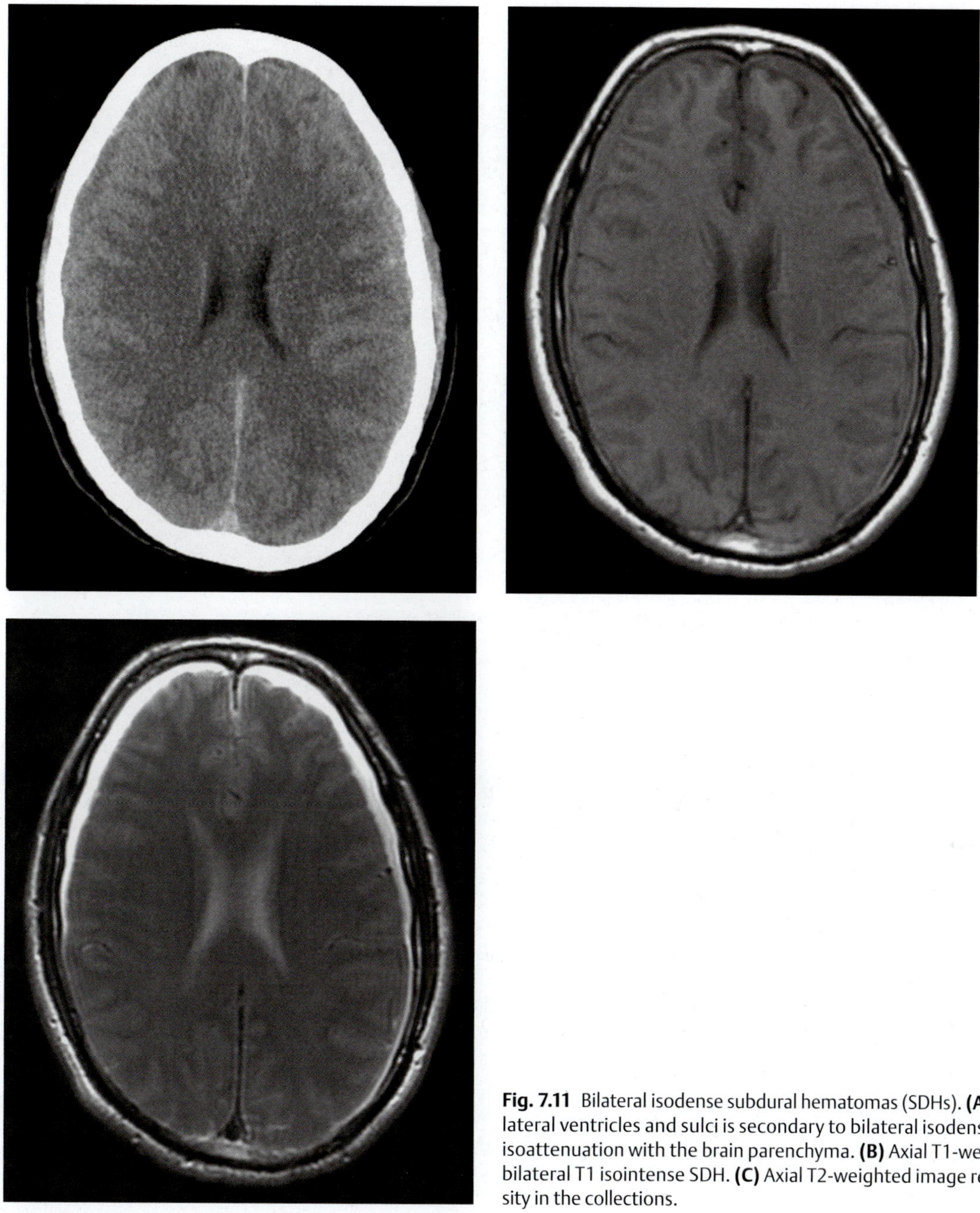

A B C

Fig. 7.11 Bilateral isodense subdural hematomas (SDHs). **(A)** Compression of the lateral ventricles and sulci is secondary to bilateral isodense SDHs that are near isoattenuation with the brain parenchyma. **(B)** Axial T1-weighted image reveals bilateral T1 isointense SDH. **(C)** Axial T2-weighted image reveals T2 hyperintensity in the collections.

could demonstrate contrast enhancement, they can be hard to distinguish. However, diffusion imaging would demonstrate restriction with an empyema and the clinical presentation should be quite different. Chronic SDHs will generally be hypointense on T1- and T2-weighted images.

Subdural Hygroma

Fluid collections that are isoattenuation on CT or nearly isosignal on all MRI pulse sequences to CSF within the subdural space are termed *hygromas* (**Fig. 7.12**). They may demonstrate slightly higher signal intensity on FLAIR and proton-weighted sequences, depending on their protein content. These fluid collections are the result of trauma and can occur acutely from tears in the arachnoid membrane, or can result from the degradation of SDHs. One, however, may find it difficult to distinguish a chronic SDH or CSF subdural hygroma from atrophy. The differentiating finding will be the position of the cortical veins. If the superficial cortical veins are displaced inward, the fluid collection is more likely to represent a CSF hygroma or chronic subdural, whereas if the cortical veins traverse the fluid collection, it is more likely to represent enlarged subarachnoid spaces from atrophy. In addition, the

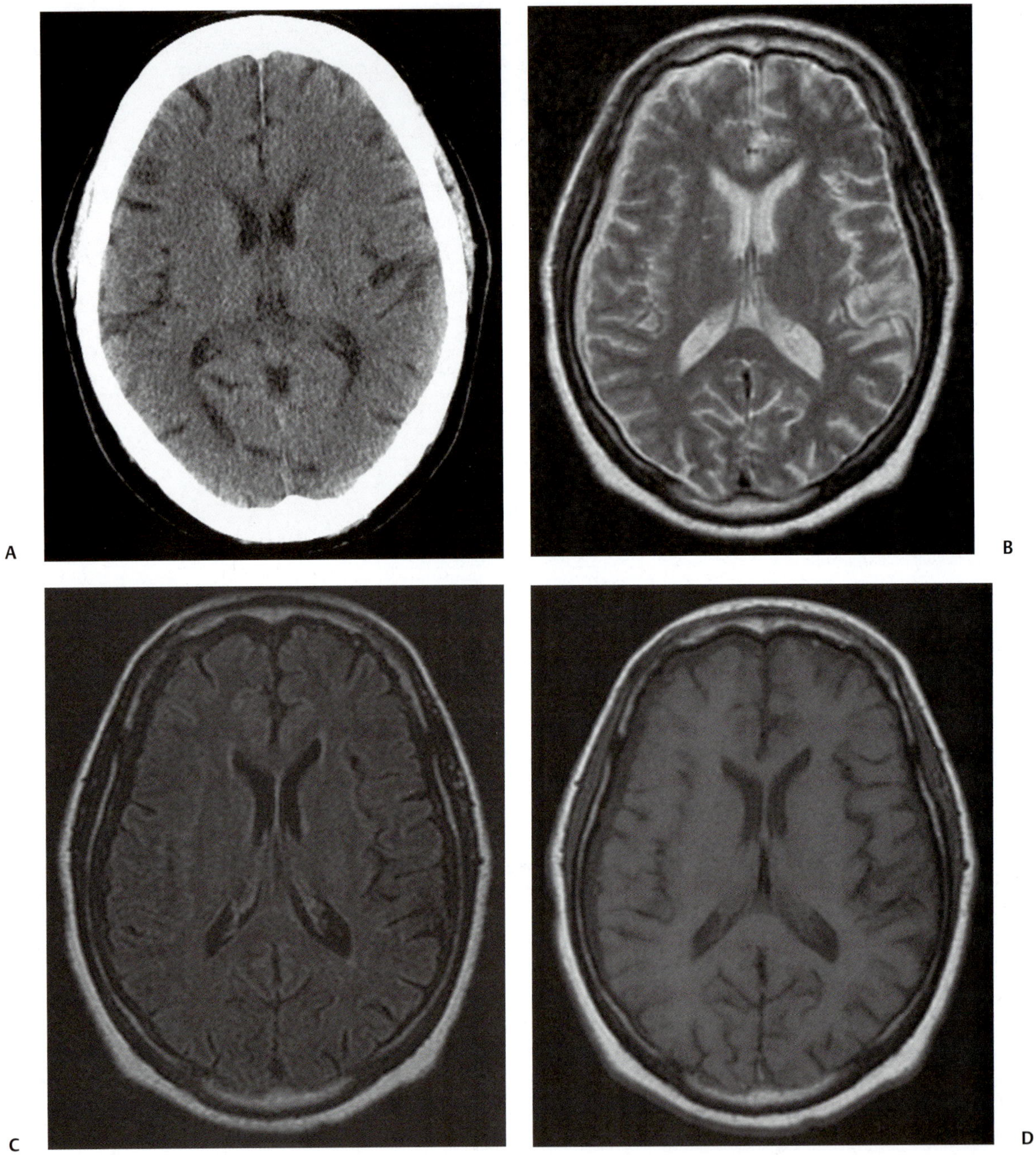

Fig. 7.12 Delayed subdural hygromas. (A) Initial computed tomographic scan reveals no evidence of extraaxial collections. (B–D) Axial T2, fluid attenuated inversion recovery, and T1-weighted images 9 days later reveal bilateral right larger than left isointense to cerebrospinal fluid subdural collections.

chronic subdural will demonstrate decreased signal intensity (or blooming) on gradient echo imaging due to the presence of hemosiderin from prior hemorrhage. One additional consideration for a CSF attenuating extraaxial fluid collection, which may or may not be secondary to trauma, is an arachnoid cyst. However, a key differentiating feature will be the presence or absence of bony scalloping. Whereas the arachnoid cyst may cause bony remodeling, the chronic hygroma or hematoma will never demonstrate scalloping of the inner calvarial table. Differentiating chronic SDHs from chronic subdural hygroma, however, may be almost impossible at times because the former may evolve into the latter.[23]

Epidural Hematoma

The potential space between the inner table of the calvaria and the dura is termed the *epidural space*. The most common cause of hemorrhage in this space is a temporal (squamosal) bone fracture with a tear of the middle meningeal artery. Ninety percent of EDHs in this location are associated with calvarial fractures. The exception, however, can be seen in children who may still retain elasticity to their calvaria, permitting tears of the meningeal vessels without the presence of a fracture. Although a majority of EDHs are secondary to artery disruption (60–90%), some are the result of tears in the middle meningeal vein, venous sinus, or diploic vein (10–40%). In this situation the epidural would be of venous, rather than arterial, origin and may present with slow or rapid accumulation of hemorrhage. Children are reported to have a higher incidence of venous epidurals, particularly in the posterior fossa. Epidurals are either biconvex or demonstrate a medial convex margin, secondary to the firm adherence of the dura to the inner table. They do not cross calvarial sutures but are not confined by the interhemispheric falx, and therefore they can cross the midline. In the case of a venous posterior fossa epidural, there is often a tear of the transverse dural venous sinus with a collection extending on both sides of the tentorium. Therefore, the hemorrhage can be in the supratentorial or infratentorial compartment (**Figs. 7.13A** and **7.13B**). In addition, the epidural is of arterial origin and found in the temporal parietal region. Delayed complications of fistula or pseudoaneurysm formation have been reported when both the middle meningeal artery and vein or simply the artery has been torn.

CT imaging of acute EDH will demonstrate a high-density biconvex extraaxial mass. At times, one may find some low-density regions in the acute hemorrhagic mass, which is thought to represent serum extruded from the clot (**Fig. 7.13C**). In these cases, it is important to perform CT imaging with a specific bone kernel setting to optimize the detection of an associated skull fracture (**Fig. 7.13D**). In addition, one should evaluate the scout image for oblique calvarial fractures and upper cervical spine subluxation, which may not be visible on the axial images.

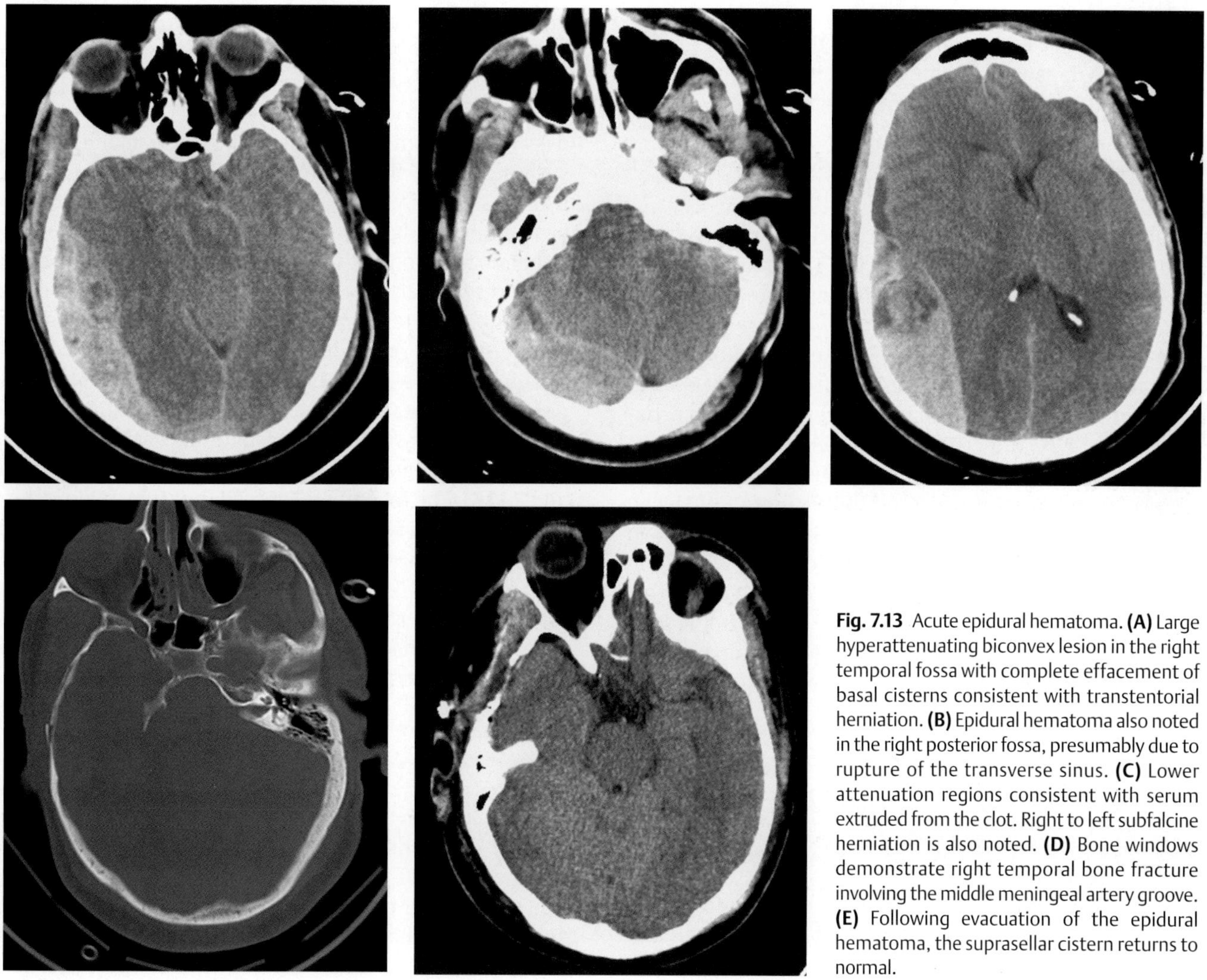

Fig. 7.13 Acute epidural hematoma. **(A)** Large hyperattenuating biconvex lesion in the right temporal fossa with complete effacement of basal cisterns consistent with transtentorial herniation. **(B)** Epidural hematoma also noted in the right posterior fossa, presumably due to rupture of the transverse sinus. **(C)** Lower attenuation regions consistent with serum extruded from the clot. Right to left subfalcine herniation is also noted. **(D)** Bone windows demonstrate right temporal bone fracture involving the middle meningeal artery groove. **(E)** Following evacuation of the epidural hematoma, the suprasellar cistern returns to normal.

Whereas acute EDHs are hyperdense on CT, chronic epidurals are generally hypodense and may even demonstrate a concave medial margin, similar to a chronic subdural hematoma. On MRI, the extraaxial hemorrhage will demonstrate different signal characteristics based on the age of the blood products. Acute EDHs, similar to subdurals, will demonstrate isointensity to the gray matter on T1-weighted images and hypointensity on T2-weighted images. A few days after the injury, the subacute EDH will demonstrate increased signal on T1-weighted images. It is not the signal intensity on the MRI that helps one diagnose the epidural, but rather its configuration, which has frequently been described as biconvex or "lenticular" in the acute stage. The classic clinical presentation, seen in ~30% of cases, is a brief initial period of loss of consciousness, followed by a lucid interval, and subsequent rapid neurological decline, which may lead to coma or death. Loss of consciousness is seen in 50% of patients, and ~66% of patients with EDHs will have associated diffuse axonal injury.[24] Because shallow EDHs spontaneously resolve in 1 to 3 weeks, surgeons have often used the measurement of 1.5 cm width as a threshold to apply conservative management. A craniotomy is generally indicated for an acute EDH that is either greater than 2.0 cm, is acutely bleeding, or is impending herniation with or without corresponding neurological deficit.

Subarachnoid Hemorrhage

Trauma is the most common overall cause of SAH. It can be associated with skull fracture but is not always found at the site of direct impact. SAH is more commonly seen in the elderly or in infants, both of whom demonstrate enlarged subarachnoid spaces. Frequent locations of intracranial hemorrhage include the frontal or temporal cerebral sulci, interpeduncular cistern, or sylvian fissures (**Figs. 7.3C** and **7.3D**). Chronic SAH cannot be identified on CT imaging and its only remnant may be a dystrophic focus of calcification. MRI with gradient echo imaging is more sensitive to chronic SAH. A well-known complication of chronic SAH is pial siderosis, which can be identified on MRI with T2-weighted images. In this condition, patients present with either hearing loss or ataxia, and a thin rim of hypointensity can be seen "coating" the brain stem or the cisternal segments of the cranial nerves.

Imaging Cerebral Herniation Syndromes (Table 7.7)

Cerebral herniation is the displacement of brain tissue from one intracranial compartment to another seen as a complication of focal traumatic intracranial mass lesions such as hematomas, or more diffuse mass-producing lesions such as cerebral edema. Variables that affect the degree of herniation include the size of the mass, the location of the mass, rate at which the mass develops, intracranial pressure, and degree of preexisting atrophy. Herniation accounts for significant morbidity and mortality in head injury patients. Displacement of brain by mass lesions leads to compression of vascular structures resulting in infarction, compression of cranial nerves leading to palsy, or compression of the brain stem, a potentially fatal complication.[25]

Lateral Descending Transtentorial Herniation (LDTH)

Lateral transtentorial herniation refers to displacement of the medial temporal lobe, anteriorly the uncus, or posteriorly the parahippocampus, over the tentorial edge, or petroclinoid ligament. Smaller temporal lobe lesions or somewhat larger lesions of the frontal or parietal lobes or adjacent extraaxial spaces can lead to LDTH (**Fig. 7.14A**). The third cranial nerve lies in close proximity to the uncus and may be entrapped by uncal herniation, giving rise to pupillary dilatation. Compression of the cerebral peduncle leads to contralateral hemiparesis. Loss of consciousness results from compression of the reticular activating system. Due to displacement of the midbrain the contralateral cerebral peduncle and corticospinal tract may be compressed against the other tentorial margin, leading to hemiparesis on the same side as the lesion. As the posterior cerebral artery runs in the perimesenphalic cistern adjacent to the tentorial margin, it can be compressed by the herniating uncus leading to infarction (**Fig. 7.14B**). Imaging studies reveal encroachment on the lateral aspect of the suprasellar cistern by the medially deviated uncus. Compression of the ipsilateral cerebral peduncle leads to contralateral brain stem displacement (**Fig. 7.13A** and **7.13E**). The ipsilateral cerebellopontine angle cistern is widened as a result. Masses in the posterior temporal or occipital lobes cause posterior LDTH of the parahippocampus with compression of the midbrain tectum rather than the cerebral peduncle. In this herniation the ambient and quadrigenial plate cisterns will be effaced without compression of the lateral suprasellar cistern.[26]

Central Descending Transtentorial Herniation

Central descending transtentorial herniation refers to displacement of the brain stem inferiorly through the tentorial incisura and occurs in the presence of bilateral supratentorial masses, hydrocephalus, or midline masses. In addition to third nerve palsy, posterior cerebral artery

Table 7.7 Imaging of Various Cerebral Herniation Syndromes*

Lateral descending transtentorial herniation (LDTH)

- Displacement of medial temporal lobe (uncus or parahippocampus) over the tentorial edge
- Imaging studies reveal encroachment on the lateral aspect of the suprasellar cistern; compression of the ipsilateral cerebral peduncle leads to contralateral brain stem displacement

Central descending transtentorial herniation

- Displacement of the brain stem inferiorly through the tentorial incisura occurs in the presence of bilateral supratentorial masses, hydrocephalus, or midline masses
- May lead to hemorrhage in the pontine tegmentum: Duret hemorrhage
- Recognized by effacement of basal cisterns, downward displacement of the pineal gland, and deformity of the midbrain

Subfalcine herniation

- Produced by unilateral frontal, parietal, or temporal mass lesions
- Greater degrees may compress the foramina of Monro leading to dilatation of the contralateral ventricle with the ipsilateral ventricle compressed by the mass
- On imaging, evaluated by measuring the amount of shift of the septum pelludicum to the contralateral side

Tonsillar herniation

- Displacement of cerebellar tonsils through the foramen magnum due to posterior fossa mass lesions
- Most dangerous form of herniation because death results from compression of the medulla
- MRI is the best test, but thin-section CT of the skull base may also identify this herniation

Ascending transtentorial herniation

- Displacement of the vermis upward through the tentorial incisura due to posterior fossa mass lesions or trapping and massive enlargement of the fourth ventricle
- Cerebral aqueduct becomes obstructed, leading to hydrocephalus of lateral and third ventricles

Transphenoidal herniation

- Less common form of herniation
- Descending type is caused by far anterior frontal lesions
- Ascending type is seen with middle cranial fossa masses

External herniation

- Herniation of brain and meninges through craniectomy defects or skull fractures
- Both CT and MRI can identify; however, MRI more accurately identifies contents of herniation

*Cerebral herniation is the displacement of brain tissue from one intracranial compartment to another seen as a complication of focal traumatic intracranial mass lesions such as hematomas, or more diffuse mass-producing lesions such as cerebral edema.

entrapment and midbrain compression, stretching and tearing of the pontine perforating arteries of the brain stem may lead to hemorrhage in the pontine tegmentum known as Duret hemorrhage. This type of herniation is recognized by effacement of the basal cisterns, downward displacement of the pineal gland, and deformity of the midbrain (**Fig. 7.2A**).

Subfalcine Herniation

Unilateral frontal, parietal, or temporal mass lesions produce subfalcine herniation (**Figs. 7.4A, 7.13,** and **7.14A**). The falx is attached anteriorly to the crista galla and fans out to a broad insertion into the region of the straight sinus within the tentorium. The falx does not extend deeply in the anterior aspect of the interhemispheric fissure, allowing for displacement of the cingulate gyrus under the falx with compression of the corpus callosum. The pericallosal branch of the anterior cerebral artery can be compressed by shifting of the frontal lobe, leading to infarction in the parasagittal posterior frontal lobe. Greater degrees of subfalcine herniation compress the foramina of Monro leading to hydrocephalus. Commonly, the ipsilateral ventricle is compressed by the mass and the contralateral lateral ventricle, particularly the temporal horn, is dilated. On

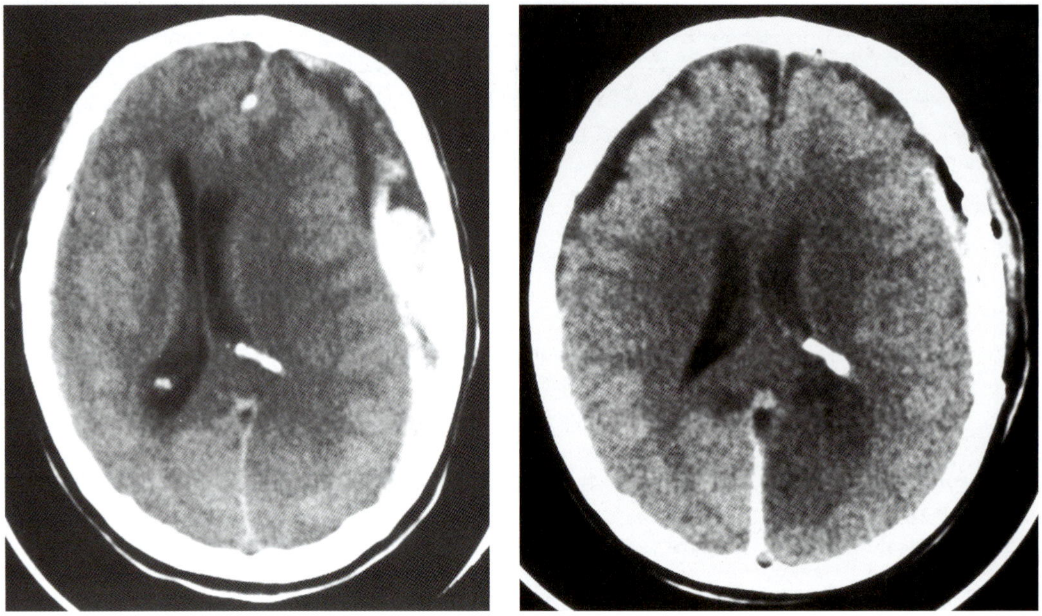

Fig. 7.14 Posterior cerebral artery infarct secondary to lateral descending transtentorial herniation. **(A)** Large acute on chronic subdural hematoma along the left convexity is seen causing left to right subfalcine herniation with compression of the left lateral ventricle and trapping of cerebrospinal fluid in the right lateral ventricle. Lateral descending transtentorial herniation was also present in this patient. **(B)** Postoperative scan shows hypoattenuation in the left occipital lobe posterior cerebral artery territory compatible with acute infarction.

imaging studies, subfalcine herniation is evaluated by measuring the amount of shift of the septum pellucidum to the contralateral side. This measurement should be performed on the image obtained at the level of the foramen of Monro. With worsening degrees of subfalcine herniation, descending transtentorial herniation may develop.

Tonsillar Herniation

Posterior fossa mass lesions can cause displacement of the cerebellar tonsils through the foramen magnum. A large degree of supratentorial mass effect may also cause tonsillar herniation. As the posterior fossa is a small and tightly enclosed space, smaller masses can cause significant herniation. Tonsillar herniation is the most dangerous form of herniation, as death results from compression of the medulla. Although MRI is the best test to identify the position of the tonsils, thin section CT of the skull base can also identify tonsillar herniation as effacement of the cisterna magna and medullary cistern with extension of the tonsils below the level of the posterior lip of the foramen magnum (**Fig. 7.2D**). Compression of the posterior inferior cerebellar artery may lead to infarction.

Ascending Transtentorial Herniation

Posterior fossa mass lesions or trapping and massive enlargement of the fourth ventricle may also cause displacement of the vermis upward through the tentorial incisura, referred to as ascending transtentorial herniation. The superior vermian and quadrigeminal plate cisterns are effaced by upward displacement of the cerebellar vermis (**Fig. 7.15**). With greater degrees of herniation, the tectum of the midbrain is compressed. The cerebral aqueduct becomes obstructed, leading to hydrocephalus of the lateral and third ventricles. Compression of the posterior cerebral or superior cerebellar arteries against the tentorium can be seen in ascending as well as descending transtentorial herniation.

Transphenoidal Herniation

This less common form of herniation may be descending or ascending. Descending transpehnoidal herniation is caused by far anterior frontal lesions. The frontal lobe is displaced over the sphenoid wing from the anterior cranial fossa into the middle cranial fossa. Imaging demonstrates effacement of the cistern of the middle cerebral artery, which lies behind the sphenoid wing. Ascending transphenoidal herniation is seen with middle cranial fossa masses elevating the temporal lobe and displacing it over the sphenoid wing into the anterior cranial fossa. Arterial compression may result in infarction in the ipsilateral middle cerebral artery territory.

External Herniation

Craniectomy defects or skull fractures may allow the herniation of brain and meninges through a defect, known as

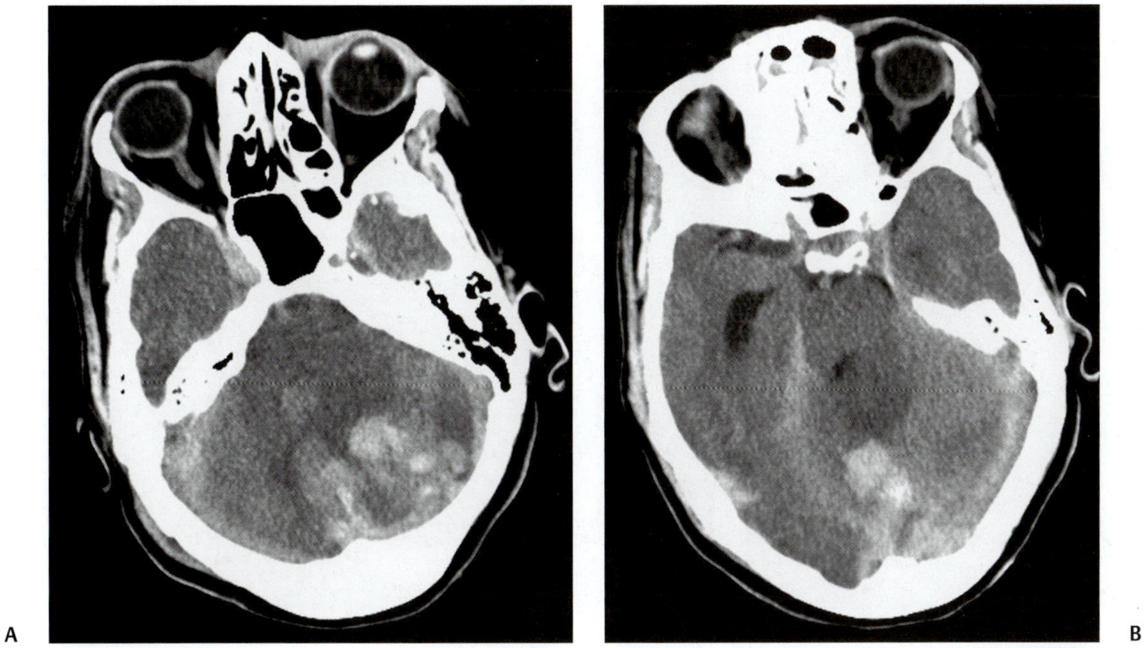

Fig. 7.15 Cerebellar parenchymal hematoma with upward herniation. **(A)** Large hyperattenuating hemorrhage is seen in the left posterior fossa. The fourth ventricle is nearly completely effaced and displaced anteriorly and to the right. **(B)** A slightly more superior image demonstrates compression of the pontine–midbrain junction, partial compression of the superior fourth ventricle, and dilatation of the right temporal horn indicating obstructive hydrocephalus.

external herniation. Craniectomies may be performed to allow for external herniation as a mechanism to relieve severe intracranial herniations as a life saving maneuver. Both CT and MRI can identify these herniations; however, MRI is more accurate to determine if actual brain tissue is extending through the defect. Infection or infarction may accompany external herniation (**Fig. 7.16**).

Imaging Cranial Gunshot Wounds and Other Penetrating Injuries (Table 7.8)

Gunshot wounds represent the most common form of penetrating injury; however, a variety of other objects including knives, metal objects such as rods, wooden objects such as chopsticks or pencils, and nails from nail guns (usually self inflicted) have been reported to enter the cranial vault.[27–29] Missiles can penetrate the calvaria anywhere owing to their high velocity, whereas other objects gain entry through the orbits; paranasal sinuses, particularly through the transoral route; and temporal bone via the mastoids or external auditory canal. Bullet wounds may be superficial, confined to the scalp and/or skull; tangential, or grazing injuries; penetrating with the bullet entering and stopping within the cranial vault; and perforating where both entrance and exit wounds can be identified.

Imaging assessment is performed with CT whether or not there is clinical evidence of penetration or perforation, as superficial or tangential injuries may be associated with intracranial hemorrhage or displacement of bone fragments related to calvarial fracture. The major limitation of CT in these kinds of injuries relates to the metallic streak artifact generated by the objects due to their much higher x-ray attenuating characteristics in relation to brain (**Fig. 7.17A**). Entire multiple contiguous axial images may be uninterpretable if the object is large, or only portions of one image may be degraded if the object is small. Inspection of the scout image generated by the CT scanner may be helpful to identify fractures and position of metal fragments that may be obscured by streak artifact on the axial CT images. Repeating the scan with a different gantry angulation to avoid the metallic objects is another way to reduce artifacts. MRI may be useful in the subacute to chronic phases of penetrating injury and should be performed only if the foreign bodies from the penetrating injury are known to be nonferromagnetic. Whereas most commercial bullets are nonferromagnetic, bullets used in assault weapons, increasingly popular on the streets, do contain ferromagnetic materials and therefore may move when placed in the magnetic field. Cases are considered for MRI on an individual basis, and only if the bullet type is known to be nonferromagnetic. Nonferromagnetic bullets do not generate significant artifact, and in this regard location of fragments is more precise

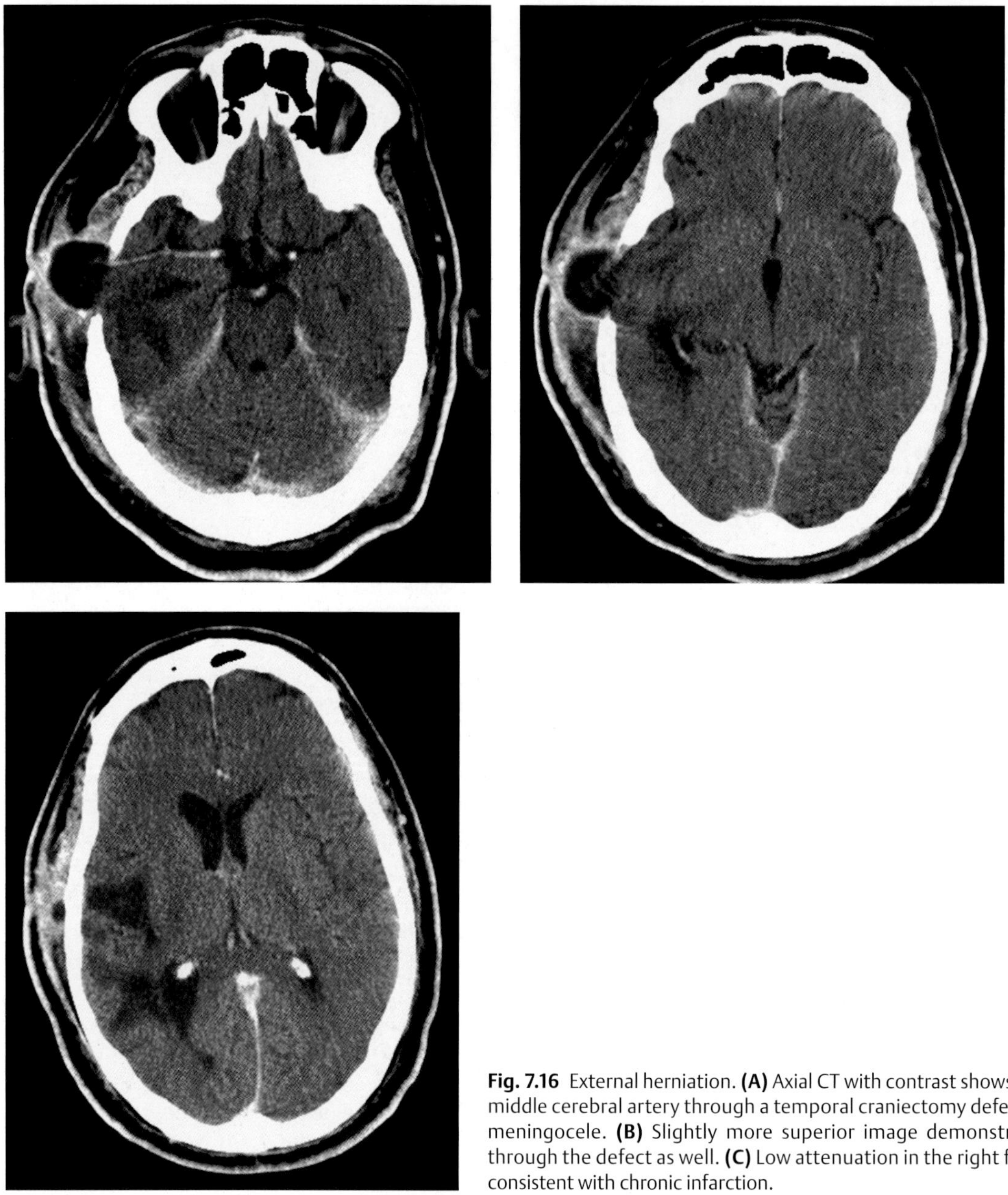

Fig. 7.16 External herniation. **(A)** Axial CT with contrast shows extension of the right middle cerebral artery through a temporal craniectomy defect with an extracranial meningocele. **(B)** Slightly more superior image demonstrates brain extending through the defect as well. **(C)** Low attenuation in the right frontotemporal lobe is consistent with chronic infarction.

due to lack of streak artifact encountered on CT. MRI has been shown to better document the extent of intracranial injury by a penetrating object entering through the orbit after removal of the object, and can more accurately define the cause of lesions seen on CT.[27]

Scalp injuries may consist of subcutaneous, subgaleal, or subperiosteal hematomas. Subperiosteal hematomas are confined by attachment of the periosteum at suture lines and therefore are lenticular in shape. Subcutaneous and subgaleal hematomas are more diffuse; subgaleal hematomas are more common. On CT, these hematomas are hyperattenuating, similar to intracranial hematomas. Subgaleal hygromas, or collections of CSF, may form through a fracture and associated meningeal laceration with connection of the subarachnoid space to the scalp.

A variety of skull fracture patterns may be seen with missile injuries, including linear, stellate, depressed, and comminuted. Fractures are seen at entrance and exit sites; however, they may be remote to the site of direct injury. Entrance wounds associated with penetrating or perforating injuries demonstrate comminution of the inner table with beveled edges (**Fig. 7.17B**). Stellate fractures may be seen at the entrance site. Fracture fragments from the inner table, metal fragments, and blood will be scattered along the path of the bullet (**Figs. 7.17C** and **7.17D**). Exit wounds of perforating injuries demonstrate

Table 7.8 Cranial Gunshot Wounds and Other Penetrating Injuries

- *Causes*: gunshot wounds (most common), knives, metal objects such as rods, wooden objects such as chopsticks or pencils, and nails from nail guns (usually self-inflicted)
- Imaging assessment for bullet wounds is performed with computed tomography; cases are considered for magnetic resonance imaging (MRI) on individual basis only if bullet is known to be nonferromagnetic
- MRI may be useful in subacute to chronic phases of penetrating injury
- Scalp injuries may consist of subcutaneous, subgaleal, or subperiosteal hematomas
- Variety of skull fracture patterns: linear, stellate, depressed, and comminuted
- *Other complications*: intracerebral, epidural, subdural, subarachnoid, and intraventricular hemorrhage, nonhemorrhagic contusion, cerebral edema/swelling, infarction, and pneumocephalus
- Infection is a common complication of missile injuries (11%)[32]
- Hemorrhage along the bullet path is widest at the point of entry and tapers along path
- Cerebrospinal fluid leaks are seen in 9% of cases[30]
- Hydrocephalus is seen in acute, subacute, or chronic phases of penetrating injury secondary to intracranial hemorrhage, infection, intraventricular missile, or bone fragments
- Aneurysms as a result of gunshot injury seen in 3–4% of cases[30]
- *Poorer prognosis*: intracerebral hematoma or intraventricular hemorrhage; transventricular injury; transtentorial herniation or subfalcine herniation > 10 mm; gas, bone, or bullet fragments remote from missile track, infection

beveling and comminution of the outer table. The size of the exit wound is typically larger than the size of the entrance wound. Penetrating missiles commonly richocet, therefore fracturing the inner table at multiple sites (**Fig. 7.17D**). Superficial or tangential injuries may also cause comminuted and depressed skull fractures. *Spallation* is a term used to describe inbending and fracture of the inner table of the skull without fracture of the outer table. Guttering, or grooving of the calvaria, may also occur with tangential bullet paths.

Skull-base fractures if not well seen are suspected when fluid is seen in the paranasal sinuses, mastoids, or tympanic cavity. MDCT with axial reconstructions of 0.6 to 0.75 mm allows for detailed coronal reformats aiding in detection of more subtle fractures, which should be suspected if there is CSF otorrhea or rhinorrhea, facial nerve palsy, hearing loss, or vertigo. Fractures of the sphenoid sinus wall may be associated with cranial nerve palsies of the nerves in the cavernous sinus or carotid artery injury, including dissection, transaction, or carotid-cavernous fistula.

In addition to intracranial bone and bullet fragments, other complications include intracerebral, epidural, subdural, subarachnoid, and intraventricular hemorrhage, nonhemorrhagic contusion, cerebral edema/swelling, infarction, and pneumocephalus. In penetrating or perforating injuries, hemorrhage along the bullet path is widest at the point of entry and tapers along the path. Bullet tracks can be nonhemorrhagic as well. Intracerebral hematomas develop as a result of direct or transmitted vascular injury, or from contusions. Intracerebral hematomas have been reported with an incidence of ~25%. These are associated with a lower survival rate as compared with patients with extraaxial hemorrhages. EDHs are unusual, reported with an incidence of less than 3%. SDHs are more common, seen in ~20% of cases. SAH is the most common intracranial hemorrhage seen, between 31 and 59% of cases.[30] Traumatic pseudoaneurysm may present with either delayed SAH or SDH. Delayed intracranial hemorrhage may also be seen with disseminated intravascular coagulation, a complication seen in 25% of head trauma patients.[31]

Cerebral contusion may develop from direct energy transmission from the missile or by direct contact of the brain adjacent to focal inbending of the calvaria. Contusions are bruises and are composed of cytotoxic edema, which is low attenuation on CT, or high attenuation if hemorrhage is present. Nonhemorrhagic contusions are better identified by MRI than by CT, particularly with the use of diffusion imaging. DAI is seen in more extensive injury; it is seen only if hemorrhagic on CT.

Intraventricular hemorrhage results from direct involvement by the missile, transmitted force with shearing of vessels in the ventricular wall, or extension from parenchymal hemorrhage. Intraventricular hemorrhage can be identified as a hyperdensity forming a layer with low attenuation CSF, or as high attenuation clots in the choroid or forming casts of the ventricle (**Fig. 7.17E**). Patients with intraventricular hemorrhage have a poorer prognosis, due to the extensive brain injury suffered.

Global anoxic/ischemic encephalopathy is a common complication of missile injury due to apnea induced by pressure waves transmitted to the brain stem. Direct vascular injury by the missile or bone fragments, vasospasm, and thrombosis are mechanisms leading to cerebral ischemia. CT is typically normal for the first 12 to 24 hours in cerebral ischemia with hypoattenuation seen in affected areas after that time due to increasing cytotoxic edema accompanied by developing vasogenic edema. MRI with DWI is abnormal much earlier, even within 1 hour of the insult.

Intracranial hypertension develops within minutes, related to hyperemia, edema, intra- and/or extraaxial hemorrhage, and ventricular obstruction. Hyperemia is seen as hyperattenuation in the cortex, as compared with edema, which is identified by hypoattenuation. Intracranial

Birth Trauma

Intracranial injury is seen in infants delivered by forceps or vacuum extraction or by cesarean section more commonly than with spontaneous vaginal delivery. Breech delivery and cephalopelvic disproportion are additional risk factors. SDH is the most common intracranial complication of birth trauma. Posterior fossa SDHs arise from tentorial tears with rupture of the vein of Galen or straight or transverse sinus, or from occipital diastasis. CT demonstrates hyperdense extraaxial collections along the tentorium, which can become large enough to cause brain stem compression. Laceration of the falx at its junction with the tentorium can also cause SDH, but it is not as common as laceration of the tentorium. Bleeding arises from the inferior sagittal sinus with hematoma in the posterior inferior interhemispheric fissure.(**Fig. 7.18**). SDH along the convexity is seen from tearing of superficial cortical veins and may be associated with SAH and cerebral contusion.

Skull injuries occur in newborns and children up to the age of 2 with relatively minor trauma due to the soft, thin nature of the calvarial bones. Overriding of calvarial bones at the sutures can be seen following delivery and usually resolves with growth over time. Instrumentation can cause depressed fractures, most commonly the parietal and frontal bones. The amount of depression can be measured on CT, and evaluation for underlying injuries can be made. Scalp hemorrhage is common in traumatic deliveries, *caput succedaneum* referring to hemorrhage in the skin and seen as hyperdensity in the scalp crossing suture lines. Subgaleal hemorrhage occurs between the aponeurosis of the scalp and the periosteum, seen as scalp hyperdensity, which may be quite large and diffuse, leading to significant blood loss. Cephalohematomas are subperiosteal in location and are bound by sutures due to the firm attachment of the periosteum. Follow-up x-ray or CT will show ossification at the margins of a cephalohematoma.

Nonaccidental (NA) versus Accidental Trauma (Table 7.10)

The radiologist may play a vital role in the diagnosis of nonaccidental head trauma. Many infants present with nonspecific findings such as seizures or encephalopathy, and histories are intentionally misleading. Imaging findings vary depending on the mechanism of injury, including blunt impact, shaking with or without impact, strangling, smothering, stabbing, drowning, or poisoning.[33] SDHs, particularly multifocal, chronic, of mixed age, interhemispheric, or tentorial; and/or cerebral edema; and a combination of old and new skull fractures or fractures that are multiple, complex, bilateral, or that cross sutures are highly suspicious for NAHI.

Skull Fracture

Skull fractures are unusually the result of accidental trauma in children. Accidents in young children usually involve falls from distances less than 3 feet, and if fracture does occur it is typically linear. Linear fractures are also

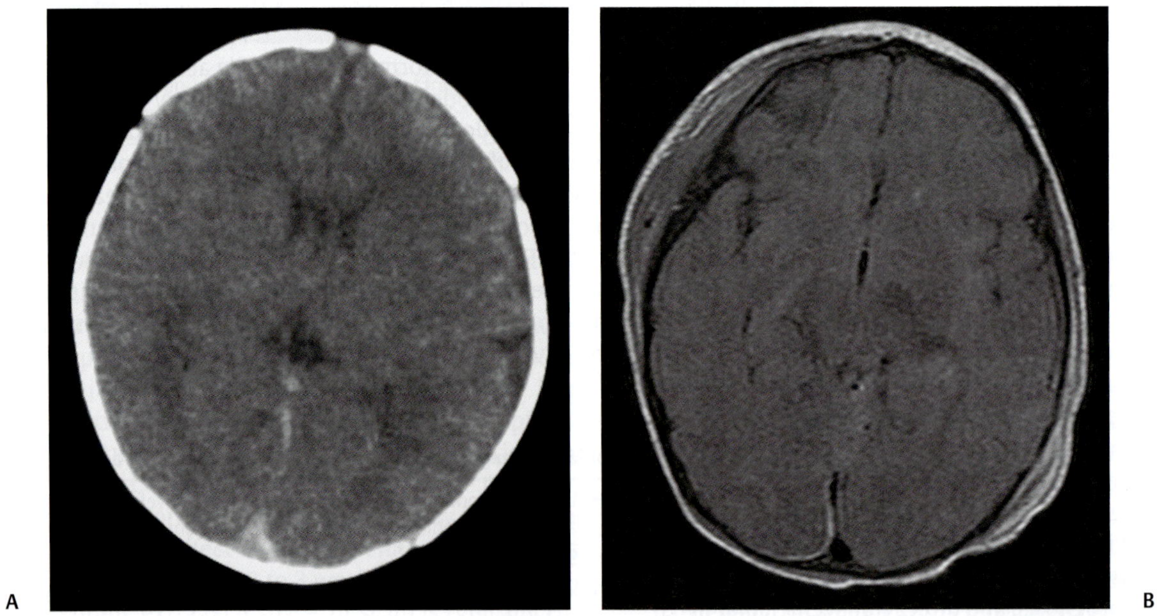

Fig. 7.18 Birth trauma. **(A)** Axial computed tomographic image demonstrates a posterior interhemispheric fissure (IHF) subdural hematoma. **(B)** Axial fluid attenuated inversion recovery magnetic resonance imaging reveals a thin subdural hemorrhage in the posterior interhemispheric fissure.

Table 7.10 Nonaccidental versus Accidental Trauma in Children

Skull fracture	• Skull fractures unusual in accidental trauma
	• A combination of old and new skull fractures, or fractures that are multiple, complex, bilateral, or that cross sutures: suspicious of nonaccidental head injury (NAHI)
	• If fractures occur, they are typically linear (both in trauma and NAHI)
	• Stellate, depressed, diastatic (>1 mm width) and/or comminuted fractures more common in NAHI
	• Direct impact can cause ping-pong fracture with indenting of the membranous calvarial bone
	• X-rays are the gold standard for identification of skull fractures; computed tomography (CT) may miss linear fracture but is the study of choice for underlying intracranial lesions
Intracranial hemorrhage	• Acute subdural hemorrhage, particularly at multiple locations, should raise suspicion for NAHI
	• Magnetic resonance imaging recommended in all patients with suspected NAHI (combination of CT and MRI increases accuracy)
	• Subarachnoid hemorrhage (SAH) seen in nearly all serious head trauma; SAH seen in interpeduncular cisterns and sylvian fissures
	• SAH in the setting of NAHI seen in the sulci along the falx or as focal hyperdense clots within the cerebral hemispheric sulci
	• Acute subdural hemorrhage due to accidental trauma is rare
	• Epidural hematomas rare and usually venous in origin
	• Cortical contusions may be seen in both accidental and NAHI.
Cerebral edema/infarct	• Cerebral edema in NAHI usually diffuse. Infarction in NAHI tends to be multifocal or involving multiple lobes.
	• Infants with edema may also develop watershed infarct, usually between the anterior and middle cerebral artery territories
	• Multifocal SDH in combination with diffuse ischemic change is highly suspicious for NAHI
	• Strangulation is associated with cerebral infarcts from compression of common carotid artery in the neck
	• Retinal hemorrhages seen funduscopically are classic of NAHI but are rarely seen on imaging

seen in NAHI, most common in the parietal and occipital bones. Direct impact can cause the so-called ping-pong fracture with indenting of the membranous calvarial bone. Depressed, comminuted fractures or skull-base fractures occur with increasing severity of impact, such as with falls from greater heights or NAHI. Stellate, depressed, diastatic, and/or comminuted fractures are seen more commonly in NAHI as compared with accidental injuries. Diastatic fractures or fractures greater than 1 mm wide are seen in the NAHI patient population.[34] In a young child, healing takes several months; in older children healing may take up to 3 years. Fractures are seen in 45% of NAHI victims[35]; however, 50% of patients will have intracranial injury without fracture.

X-rays are the gold standard for identification of skull fractures, although x-rays may miss fractures in young infants due to poor ossification of the calvaria. As fractures of the long bones are more common than skull fractures in NAHI patients, skull x-ray is performed as part of the skeletal survey in suspicious cases. CT may miss linear fractures that are in the axial plane parallel to the angle of imaging; however, is the study of choice in suspected NAHI patients as underlying lesions including convexity SDH and/or hemorrhagic contusion can be seen (**Fig. 7.19**). Fractures more than 5 mm wide at time of diagnosis may expand, the so-called growing fracture or leptomeningeal cyst. X-rays demonstrate a wide lucency in the skull. CT shows extension of a CSF attenuation mass through the wide calvarial defect compatible with herniation of meninges and subarachnoid CSF (**Fig. 7.20A**). Due to CSF pulsations the size of the calvarial lucency and degree of meningeal herniation increase over time. The parietal bone is the most commonly involved. Three-dimensional CT using a bone algorithm is useful in defining the relationship of the leptomeningeal cyst to the sutures[33] (**Fig. 7.20B**).

Intracranial Hemorrhage

Acute subdural hemorrhage in the setting of accidental trauma is rare in children, particularly at multiple locations. If this pattern is seen, NAHI should be highly suspected.[21] Whiplash shaking injury was initially described by Guthkelch[36] and named shaken baby syndrome by Caffey in 1946[37] to include the findings of retinal hemorrhages in association with subarachnoid and/or subdural hemorrhage. The acceleration-deceleration forces that arise in whiplash shaking are transmitted to the draining

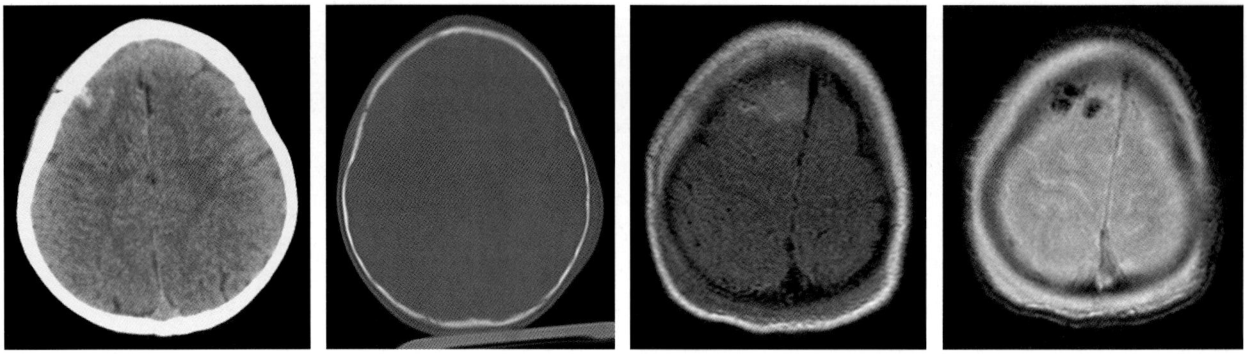

A–D

Fig. 7.19 "Accidental" trauma in a 4-month-old. **(A)** Axial computed tomography demonstrates small acute right frontal hemorrhagic contusion. **(B)** Bone window demonstrates diastatic fracture of the right coronal suture. **(C)** Axial fluid attenuated inversion recovery image reveals T2 hyperintensity in the contusion. **(D)** Gradient recalled echo image shows magnetic susceptibility related to acute blood products.

veins bridging the infant's generous subarachnoid space and dura resulting in tearing and intracranial hemorrhage, specifically in these two spaces. Interhemispheric SDHs secondary to shaking with whiplash are seen more commonly in the posterior aspect than anteriorly. Acute SDH in the interhemispheric fissure can be identified by an asymmetric linear hyperdensity seen on one side of the falx with a flat edge along the falx and a slightly convex margin laterally (**Fig. 7.21A**). Acute SDH also occurs in the parietooccipital regions and may extend over or under the cerebral hemispheres. CT images must be inspected at subdural windows to avoid missing thin subdural hemorrhages adjacent to the inner table of the calvaria. Thin SDH under or over the hemispheres may be entirely missed by axial CT due to plane of imaging and beam hardening artifacts that tend to occur in these regions. Low attenuation areas seen within acute SDH may represent unclotted blood or CSF entering through a rent in the arachnoid. SDHs containing hemorrhage of varying ages and therefore varying densities from hypo- (chronic) to iso- (subacute) to hyper- (acute) dense are nearly pathognomonic for NAHI. MRI is recommended in all patients with suspected NAHI to identify small subdural hemorrhages, as well as to estimate the age of the subdural hemorrhage. Factors affecting rate of change of the CT attenuation or MRI signal of subdural hemorrhage include volume of blood present, patient's hemoglobin at the time of the hemorrhage, or intervention such as subdural

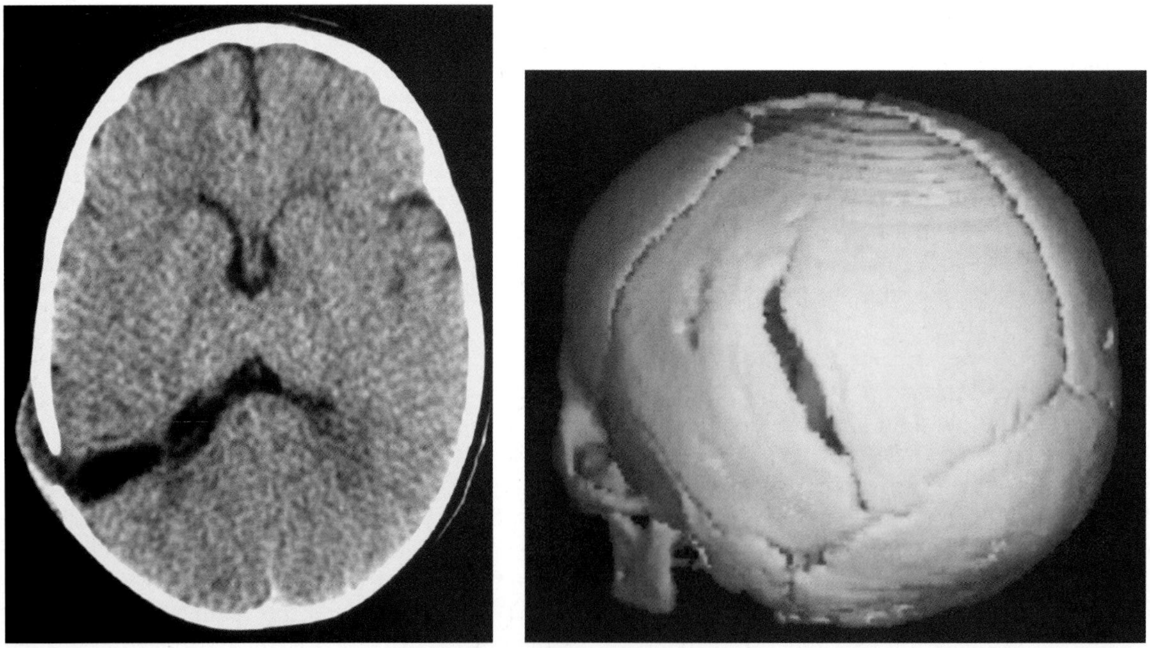

A B

Fig. 7.20 Leptomeningeal cyst (growing fracture). **(A)** Axial computed tomography demonstrates a cerebrospinal fluid–filled cleft in the right parietal lobe with extension through a fracture. **(B)** Posterior oblique 3-D reconstruction reveals the relationship of the fracture to the sutures.

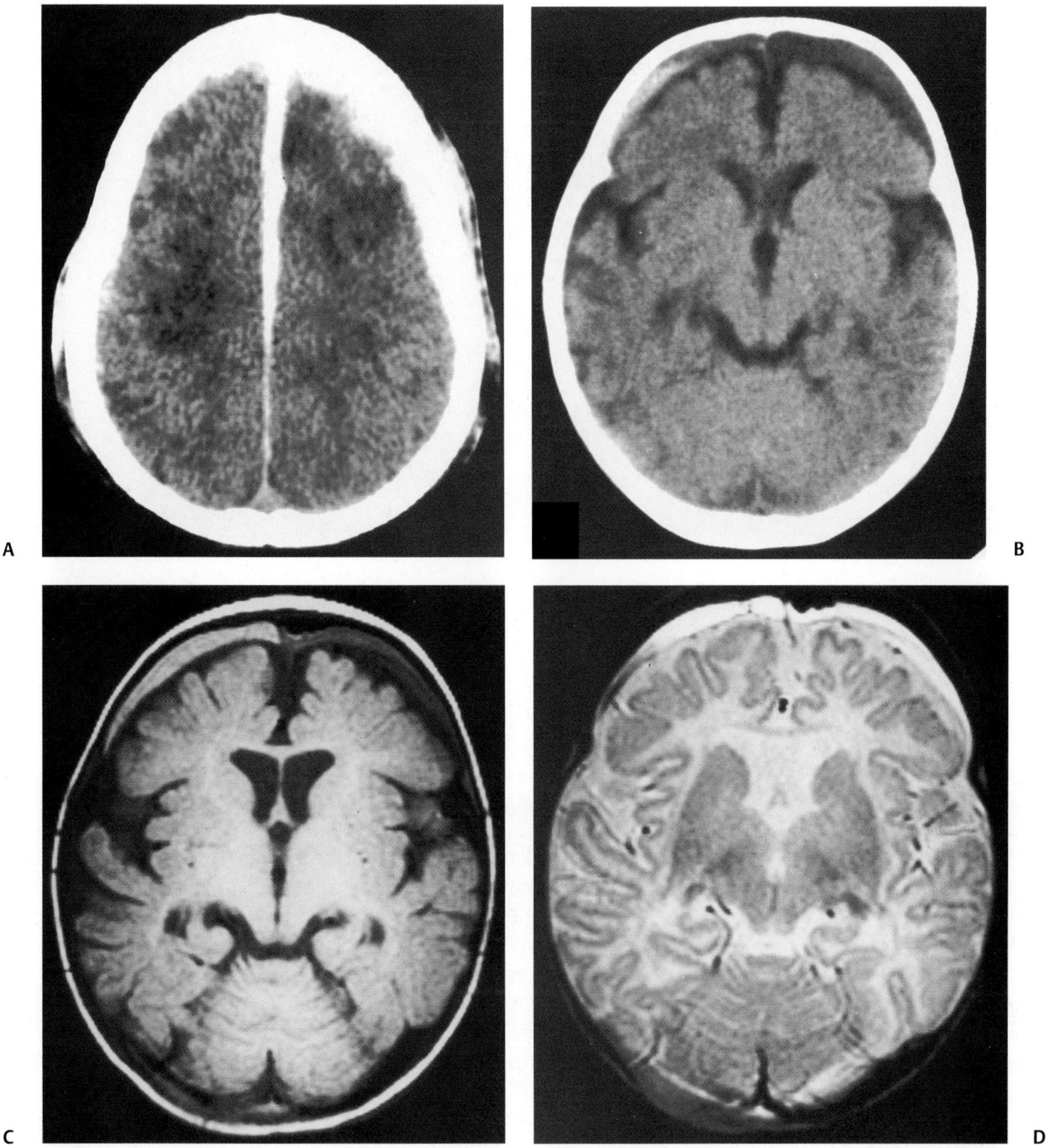

Fig. 7.21 Subdural hematomas of varying ages in nonaccidental head injury. **(A)** Acute interhemispheric subdural hematoma. Blood is seen along the falx and left frontal convexity. **(B)** Computed tomography demonstrates a right frontal acute on chronic subdural hematoma. Left frontal hematoma is mainly hypoattenuating consistent with chronicity; however, haziness within the collection indicates a subacute component. **(C)** T1-weighted axial image demonstrates T1 shortening (bright signal) in the right frontal subdural hematoma with mixed T1 prolongation in the left subdural hematoma. These collections are superimposed on dilated subarachnoid spaces indicating atrophy. **(D)** T2-weighted axial image demonstrates T2 prolongation brighter than cerebrospinal fluid in both frontal subdural hematomas.

tap.[38] The combination of CT and MRI increases the accuracy in determining the age of SDHs[39] (**Figs. 7.21B–7.21D**).

SAH is seen in nearly all serious head trauma. SAH is seen in the setting of NAHI in the sulci along the falx or as focal hyperdense clots within the cerebral hemispheric sulci. In accidental trauma, SAH is seen in the interpeduncular cisterns and sylvian fissures. Vascular injuries will cause greater degrees of SAH. SAH is best identified by CT. MRI FLAIR images can also identify acute SAH in these locations.

In children, EDHs are more often venous in origin than arterial and less common than they are in adults. Sources of venous bleeding include the dura and its sinuses, and the diploic space. Therefore, childhood EDH is more

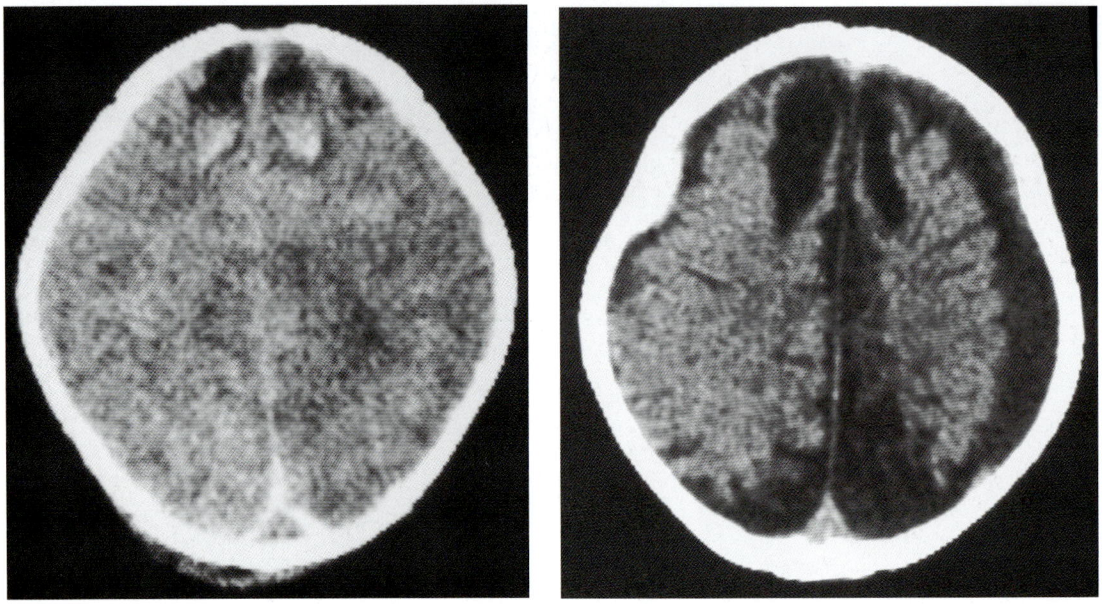

A B

Fig. 7.22 Nonaccidental head injury. **(A)** Acute hemorrhage in bilateral frontal contusions and in the posterior interhemispheric fissure is seen. **(B)** Follow-up computed tomography 4 months later demonstrates an acute right frontal epidural hematoma superimposed on bilateral chronic subdural hematomas and parafalcine encephalomalacia related to prior contusion.

commonly seen in the posterior fossa or adjacent to the tentorium, as opposed to adult EDH seen in the middle cranial fossa. Venous EDHs accumulate more slowly, and their onset is more insidious. Rapid deterioration may occur after a period of lucidity. Arterial EDHs are less common in children as the middle meningeal artery is not yet fixed in its groove, which is not as deep as it is in adults, and there is greater plasticity of the skull. EDH is less commonly the result of nonaccidental trauma. EDH is recognized on CT as a hyperattenuating biconvex extraaxial mass that does not cross suture lines.

Cortical contusions are seen in the inferior frontal and anterior temporal lobes due to direct impact with the bone in both accidental injury and NAHI. Gliding contusions occur in the subcortical white matter of the frontal lobes, particularly in infants less than 5 months old, as the floor of the anterior cranial fossa is relatively smooth. Contusions may also occur in brain adjacent to dural structures (**Fig. 7.22**). Intraparenchymal hematoma and DAI involving the white–gray matter junction of the centrum semiovale, corpus callosum, and brain stem is seen more commonly in the accidental head trauma patient. Intraparenchymal hematomas are seen most commonly in the frontal and temporal lobes. Rupture of the lenticulostriate or thalamoperforating arteries may cause petechial hemorrhages in the basal ganglia and thalami. Infants are particularly susceptible to DAI due to their relatively larger heads and weak neck musculature. As in adults, this injury is most commonly seen with high-speed motor vehicle accidents and is less commonly seen in NAHI. The accidental injury group more commonly has focal or unilateral injuries.

Cerebral Edema/Infarct

Cerebral edema in the setting of NAHI is usually diffuse, although it may be focal as well. Mechanisms for the development of edema are poorly understood. Acute cerebral edema may be visualized on CT within the first 12 hours as loss of gray–white matter differentiation and decreased size of the ventricles and subarachnoid spaces. Over time, decreasing attenuation of the cerebral hemispheres and basal ganglia is more apparent. Due to autoregulation with relative sparing of the posterior circulation in the early stages of ischemia, the "reversal sign" is seen with a hyperdense appearance of the cerebellum and thalami.[40] MRI may demonstrate bright signal on DWI due to intracellular water accumulation, with concomitant low signal on the ADC maps. T2-weighted images may be insensitive to edema, as the unmyelinated infant white matter has high water content. These findings are indicative of hypoxic-ischemic encephalopathy and are seen in cases of accidental or nonaccidental strangulation, suffocation, and drowning. Infants with cerebral edema may also develop watershed infarct, usually between the anterior and middle cerebral artery territories.[41] This is seen on CT as focal hypoattenuation in a wedge shape extending from the frontal horn to the cortex and in the centrum semiovale overlying the body of the lateral ventricle, and on MRI as diffusion positive T2 prolongation in

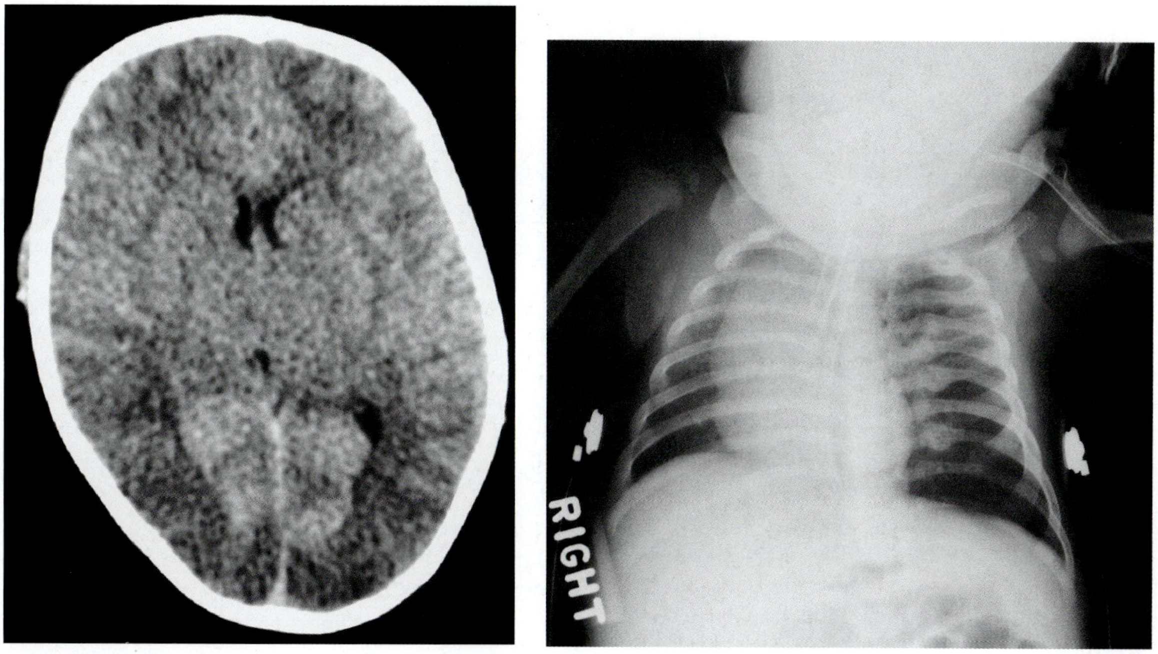

A B

Fig. 7.23 Nonaccidental head injury. **(A)** Axial computed tomography demonstrates acute bilateral posterior cerebral artery distribution infarcts. **(B)** Chest x-ray in the same patient demonstrates multiple healed left posterior rib fractures.

the same area. Cortical necrosis may develop in one hemisphere underlying an acute SDH.[42] Serial imaging of NAHI survivors reveals edema resolving after 1 week, with development of cerebral infarction in up to 50% and atrophy in 100%.[43] The presence of multifocal subdural hemorrhage in combination with diffuse hypoxic-ischemic parenchymal changes is highly suspicious for NAHI victims and helps distinguish them from patients with perinatal asphyxia.

Strangulation is associated with cerebral infarcts arising from direct compression of the common carotid artery in the neck. Bilateral carotid compression results in diffuse bilateral cerebral hemispheric infarct. Due to the coexisting mechanism of shaking, subdural and/or SAH may be present and may aid in identification of the true cause of infarction. Whereas retinal hemorrhages visible at funduscopy are present in the classic case of NAHI, hyperdensity in the orbital globe signifying acute hemorrhage is uncommonly seen. Infarction in NAHI victims tends to be multifocal or involve multiple lobes. The posterior aspects of the cerebral hemispheres tend to be involved (**Fig. 7.23**).

Vascular Injury

Arterial injury caused by nonpenetrating injury in the pediatric population is rare. The same spectrum of injuries that occur in adults may occur in children as well, including carotid or vertebral dissection, carotid-cavernous fistulas, venous occlusion, or rupture. Dissections are most commonly associated with penetrating injury, skull-base fractures involving the carotid canal, or cervical spine fractures involving the foramen transversarium. Seemingly minor traumatic flexion or extension forces may cause dissection of the extracranial arteries, involving the internal carotid artery just above the common carotid artery bifurcation, or the vertebral artery at the C1–2 level. Arterial occlusion or embolization from dissection causes cerebral infarction, visualized on diffusion-weighted MRI within hours of the event.

Carotid-cavernous fistula may initially be recognized by dilatation of the cavernous sinus and superior ophthalmic vein on the affected side. DSA demonstrates the fistula and allows for closure by neurointerventional methods.

Advanced Imaging Techniques and Outcomes (Table 7.11)

Conventional imaging techniques have been studied for their ability to predict clinical outcomes of TBI patients. Neurobehavioral outcome of patients with mild TBI (GCS 13–15) and CT abnormalities has been reported to be similar to that of patients with GCS in the moderate range, and significantly worse than mild TBI patients with no CT abnormalities.[44] One study using FLAIR and GRE images in severe TBI patients 60 to 90 days later found total lesion volume on FLAIR images correlated significantly with

Table 7.11 Advanced Imaging Techniques and Outcomes

1. Perfusion CT or MRI
2. Diffusion weighted imaging, diffusion tensor imaging, and fractional anisotropy
3. MR spectroscopy (MRS)
4. Functional MRI
5. Magnetization transfer
6. Quantitative imaging (volumetry): CT or MRI
7. Nuclear medicine: SPECT, PET
8. Susceptibility weighted imaging (SWI)
9. Magnetic source imaging (MSI)

clinical outcome, whereas that on GRE did not.[45] Hughes et al[46] found that standard MRI techniques are not helpful in identifying patients with mild TBI who are likely to have delayed recovery, and that nonspecific MRI abnormalities are frequently seen. Enlarged high-convexity Virchow-Robin spaces (VRSs) are one nonspecific finding, seen in mild TBI patients in both early and late stages.[47] A study of patients with primary brain stem injuries revealed good outcomes as measured by the Glasgow Outcome Scale (GOS) in patients with ventral or dorsal superficial brain stem lesions, whereas poor outcomes were seen in deep dorsal brain stem lesions.[48] A prospective study by Scheid et al[49] at 3T found that the total amount of microbleeds from DAI identified by GRE T2* images as well as involvement of the corpus callosum correlated with GCS but not GOS.

The observation of poor clinical outcomes without notable neuroimaging findings in some patients on conventional MRI and CT particularly after mild TBI has spurred investigations utilizing advanced imaging techniques to aid in predicting clinical outcomes, and to determine which of these techniques is most useful in prognosis. Findings of these investigations may be helpful in guiding therapy in the acute phase of TBI to improve outcomes, as well as to determine predictability of outcomes following TBI of any severity, with or without acute imaging findings.

Perfusion CT or MRI

CT or MRI perfusion is performed utilizing a bolus of contrast administered rapidly, with continuous rapid scanning of a few slices selected at the level of the basal ganglia and lateral ventricular bodies to include portions of the anterior, middle, and posterior cerebral artery territories. Wash-in and wash-out of the contrast bolus is analyzed by computer to generate color-coded quantitative images of brain perfusion. rCBF, rCBV, and MTT are calculated to demonstrate areas of ischemia, cerebral blood flow being the most sensitive parameter. In a perfusion CT study of patients with GCS of 8 or less, Wintermark demonstrated a higher sensitivity for cerebral contusions compared with noncontrast CT.[50] Perfusion alterations are also seen in patients with extraaxial hemorrhages and cerebral edema (**Fig. 7.24**). Furthermore, patients with intracranial hypertension (ICP of >18 mm Hg or CT evidence of herniation) tended to show more arterial territories with low rCBV or increased MTT.

Perfusion CT results compared with GOS scores 3 months post–head trauma revealed the patients with the best functional outcome were those with normal perfusion or hyperemia (high rCBV and rCBF values). Those with low rCBV and rCBF values (oligemia) had unfavorable clinical outcomes.[50] A study using perfusion MRI demonstrated poorer clinical outcomes in two groups of patients, those with reduced rCBV in regions of focal pathology seen on conventional MRI and increased rCBV in surrounding normal-appearing brain, as well as those with reduced rCBV in normal-appearing areas of brain remote from visible abnormality.[51]

Diffusion-Weighted Imaging, Diffusion Tensor Imaging, and Fractional Anisotropy

DWI is a physiological measure of differences in diffusion rate of water molecules. DWI utilizes a gradient echo technique to assess ease of water diffusion and is therefore sensitive to cytotoxic edema. Restriction of water diffusion (and therefore low apparent diffusion coefficient) corresponds to high signal intensity on DWI and low signal intensity on ADC maps. Vasogenic edema possesses a high apparent diffusion coefficient and is bright on ADC maps, whereas typically a decreased signal on DWI is seen. Any lesion with prolonged T2 values may mimic an area of restricted diffusion on DWI, a phenomenon known as T2 shine-through. Comparison of DWI images with the ADC map is essential in identifying areas of true restricted diffusion.

DWI can detect ischemia before other imaging modalities. TBI patients develop lesions demonstrating restricted diffusion due to ischemia as well as DAI. Inspection of the lesion location and distribution is helpful in distinguishing between ischemic lesions secondary to vascular injury and DAI.[50] In trauma patients DWI can distinguish between vasogenic edema typically associated with hematomas and cytotoxic edema seen with DAI or acute infarction.[52–56] This has implications for treatment with cerebral perfusion pressure therapy.[57] Whole brain ADC values may be abnormal even when conventional MRI is normal, and correlate significantly with GCS in patients with TBI.[57]

Diffusion tensor imaging (DTI) exploits the fact that diffusion of water is anisotropic or nonrandom along axonal white matter pathways. DTI is unique in its ability

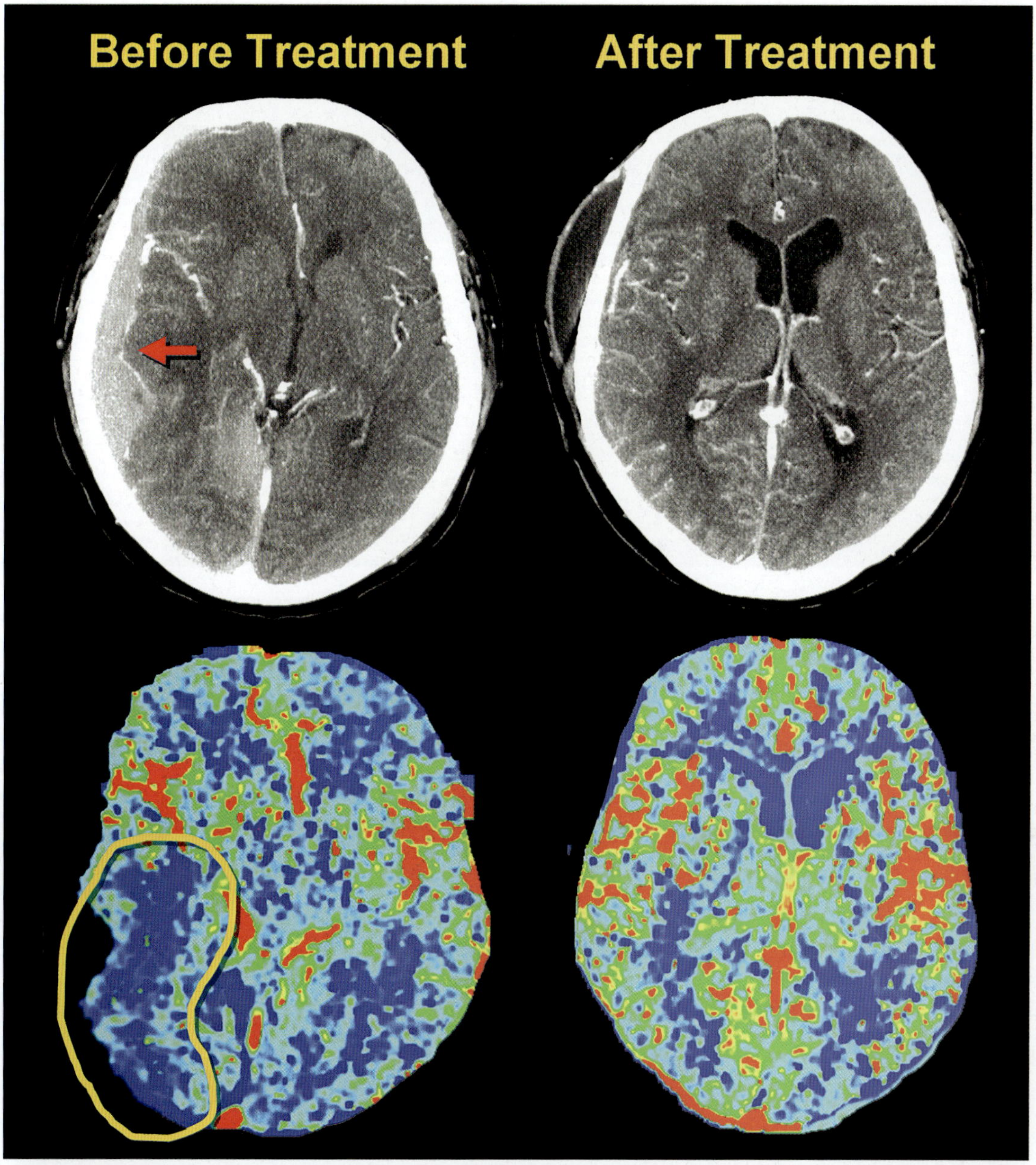

Fig. 7.24 Brain ischemia underlying acute subdural hematoma. Axial computed tomography (CT) images demonstrate acute right convexity subdural hematoma before and after evacuation. Corresponding perfusion CT color images demonstrate decreased perfusion in the right posterior temporal lobe (*outlined*) that reverts to normal perfusion following evacuation. (Courtesy of Max Wintermark, M.D., and Alisa D. Gean, M.D.)

to provide visualization of white matter pathways and measure their functional integrity. Diffusion gradients are placed in at least six directions, and calculations of the diffusion tensor in 3-D space are performed. Directionally encoded color maps of the diffusion tensors are made (**Fig. 7.25**). Fractional anisotropy (FA) is calculated using the multidirectional apparent diffusion coefficients, a value of 1 signifying total anisotropy, and 0, total isotropy.

DTI and FA may be able to detect abnormalities early or later in the course of TBI in areas of normal-appearing brain.[58–61] Multiple studies of TBI patients with GCS scores ranging from 15 to 3 using DTI and FA have shown a correlation between abnormalities and outcome.[62–64] Fiber tracking performed on one patient with DAI in the corpus callosum showed disappearance of upward frontal and parietal white matter fibers that worsened while GCS improved. At 4 months, the patient's level of consciousness did not improve, suggesting that fiber tracking was more useful in predicting outcome.[65] The combination of DTI and fiber tracking can differentiate between edema and fiber disruption. Fiber tracking has identified intact fibers in the splenium, which correlated with better clinical outcome.[66]

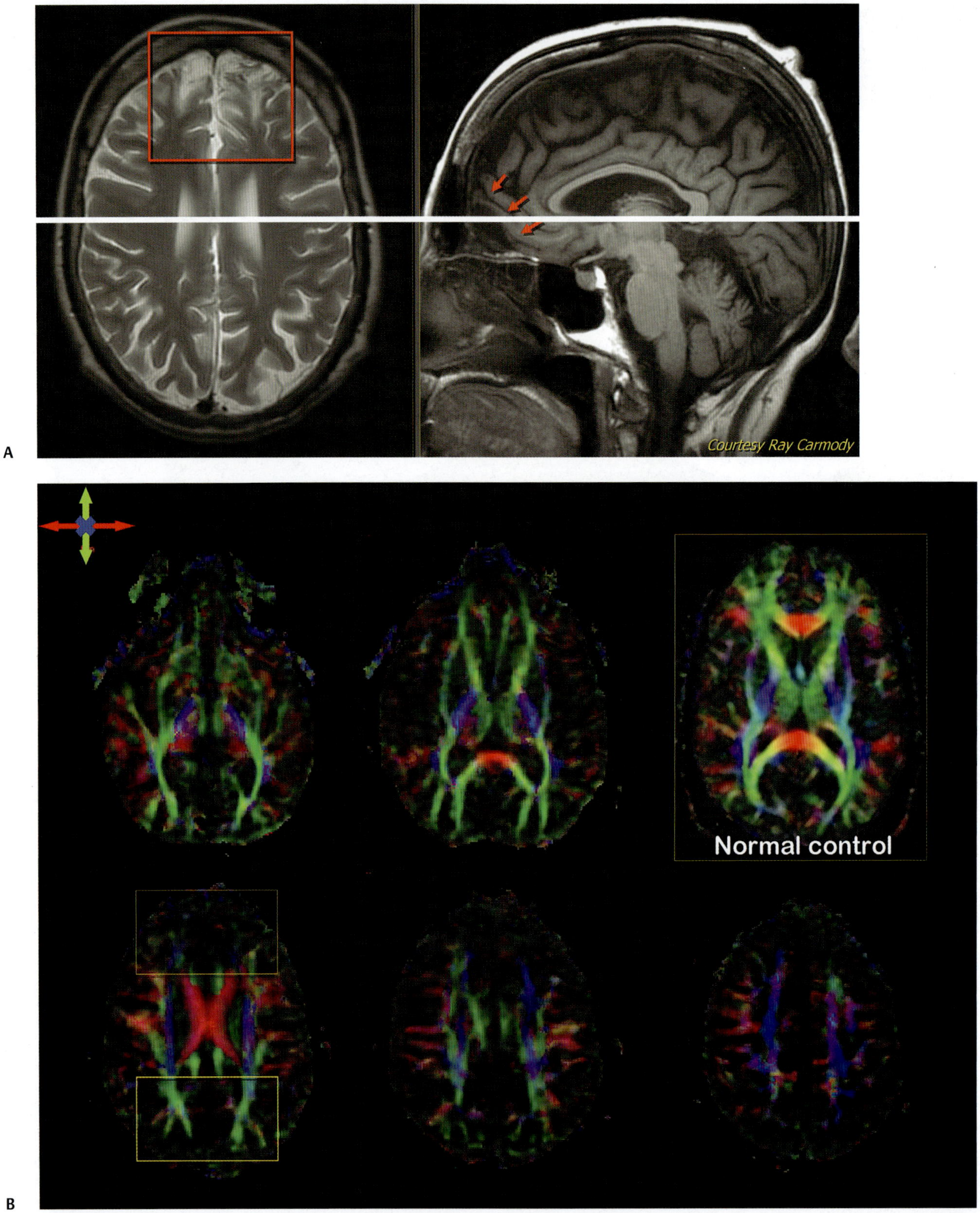

Fig. 7.25 Diffusion tensor imaging (DTI) in chronic traumatic brain injury. **(A)** Axial T2- and sagittal T1-weighted images demonstrate bilateral frontal lobe encephalomalacia. **(B)** Color encoded DTI maps demonstrate reduced fractional anisotropy in the genu of the corpus callosum, adjacent frontal white matter, and splenium of the corpus callosum in comparison to a normal control. (Courtesy of Ray Carmody, M.D. and Alisa D. Gean, M.D.)

Okumura et al[67] studied patients with memory and cognitive impairment with DTI and positron emission tomography (PET). Reduction in glucose metabolism in the anterior cingulated association cortex revealed by PET was felt to indicate deprived neuronal activation caused by impaired neuronal connectivity as demonstrated by DTI (**Fig. 7.26**).

MR Spectroscopy (MRS)

MRS is used to investigate the chemical environment of the brain. MRS is acquired using the same head coil as for routine MRI with software designed for spectral analysis. Hydrogen (proton) spectroscopy is the most widely used element due to its abundance. Signal from water protons is suppressed allowing detection of signals from protons in other metabolites. Each of these metabolites' protons resonates at a particularly frequency allowing for plotting on the horizontal axis of a graph, the vertical peak representing relative metabolite concentrations and measured in parts per million. Spectra are obtained using short and long echo times. Seven key metabolites are measured in order of decreasing abundance, N-acetyl aspartate (NAA) at 2.0, creatine (Cr) at 3.03, choline (Cho) at 3.22, myoinositol (mI) at 3.56, glutamate/glutamine at 2.05 to 2.5, lactate at 1.33, and lipids at 0.9 to 1.2. Lactate and lipids are not observed in normal brain but are important in detection of pathology. Spectra can be acquired in one large voxel (single voxel spectroscopy or SVS), or by multiple smaller voxels (multivoxel spectroscopy). Hunter's angle refers to the 45 degree angle formed by the peaks mI, Cr, Cho, and NAA when present in normal proportions.

It has been shown that the balance of the brain chemicals is perturbed in DAI.[68] Typical findings are reduced NAA resulting from axonal injury or metabolic depression, as well as elevated choline due to breakdown products appearing after the shearing of myelin and cellular membranes. This results in loss of Hunter's angle (**Fig. 7.27**). This is seen in patients with DAI in normal-appearing and hemorrhagic corpus callosum.[69] In some patients normal levels of NAA have returned 6 months after injury, suggesting a partially reversible process. Sustained reduction of gray matter NAA is a marker of irreversible or continued secondary neuronal loss. Several studies have found that lower NAA:choline ratios in TBI patients correlated with cognitive function.[69–71] NAA:Cr ratio was decreased in normal-appearing brain to a greater

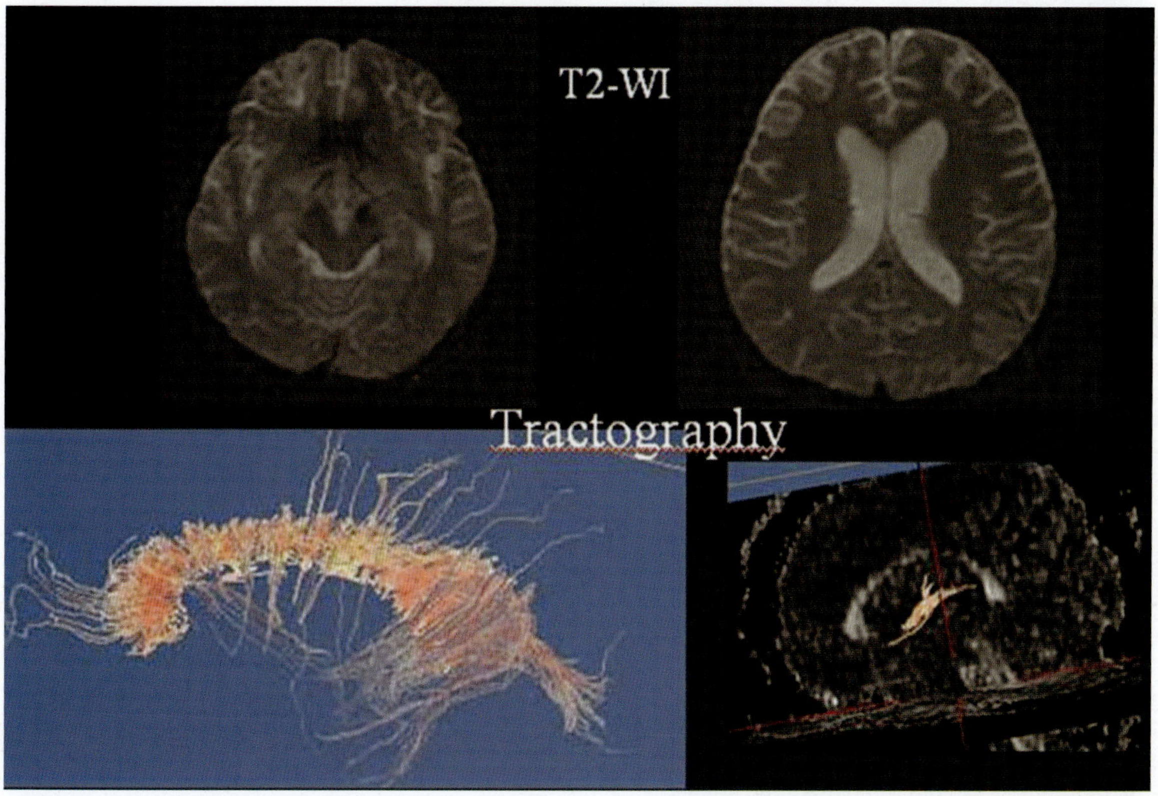

A

Fig. 7.26 Anatomical and functional images of a patient with moderate to severe traumatic brain injury. **(A)** Axial magnetic resonance T2-weighted images show mild diffuse cortical brain atrophy. Tractology of corpus callosum and fornix from diffusion tensor images show coarsening and thinning of the axonal nerve tracts in comparison with those of a normal subject.

(Continued on page 134)

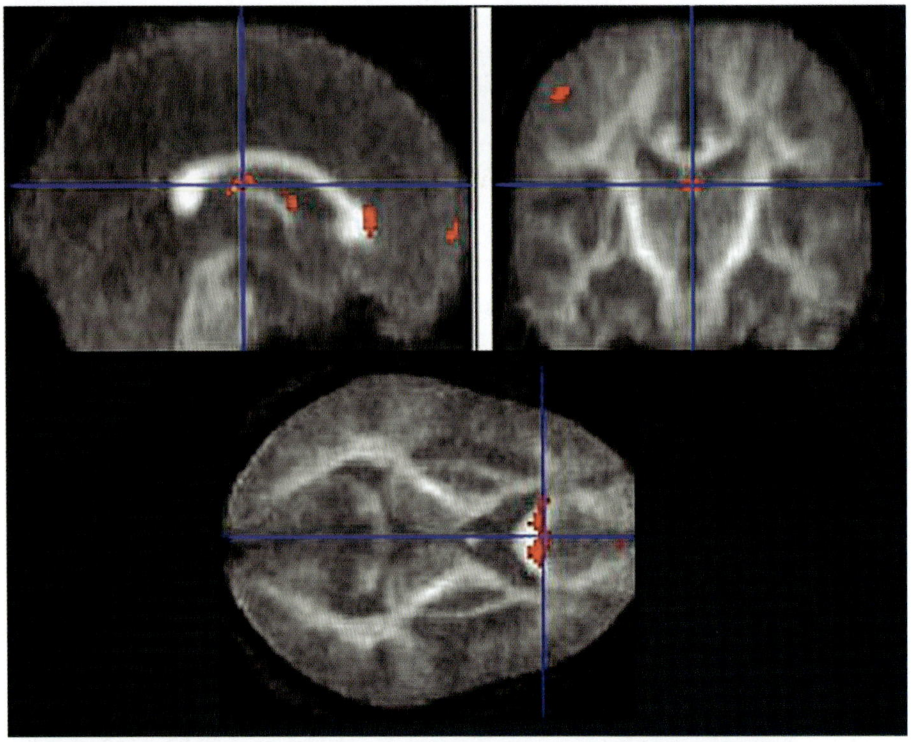

B

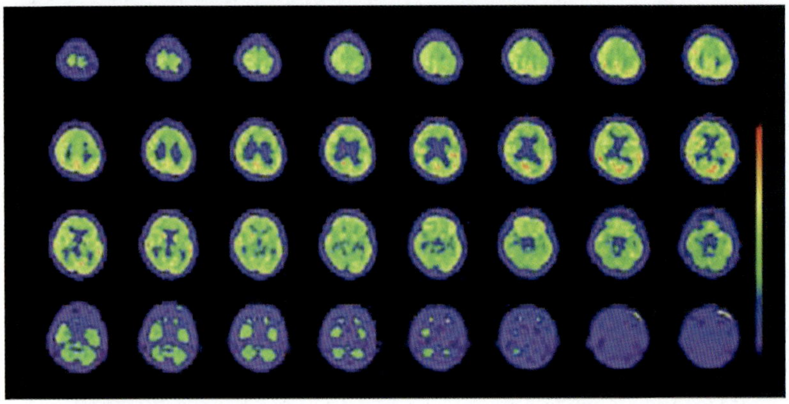

C

Fig. 7.26 *(Continued)* **(B)** Fractional anisotropy (FA), SPM analysis of this case shows reduced FA in the column of fornix (Sagittal) in the genu of corpus callosum (Coronal, axial). **(C)** Fluorodeoxyglucose–positron emission tomography shows views of cerebral metabolism that are superimposed on brain surface images of each hemisphere. Color scale indicates degree of significance (red>green>blue). This map shows decreased metabolism in mesiofrontal cortex, including anterior cingulated cortex. (Courtesy of Okumura, M.D., Ph.D.)

degree in patients with poor outcomes; however, ratios were similarly altered in visibly injured brain for all outcomes. Persistent elevated choline levels at 3 and 6 months suggesting continued inflammation are seen in patients with less favorable outcomes.[72] In patients with more favorable outcomes, choline levels tend to normalize at 6 months.[73]

Gray matter glutamate/glutamine elevation has been reported to be the single strongest predictor of poor outcomes when measured 2 to 3 days postinjury[74] with normalization at 6 to 12 months. Diffusely elevated lactate levels in normal-appearing tissues on MRI have been correlated with poor clinical outcome in adults and children[75,76]; however, increased lactate confined to areas of injury did not correlate with a poor outcome.[75] Another metabolite, myo-inositol has been found to be elevated in TBI patients, likely representing astrogliosis or a disturbance in osmotic function, and has been found to be associated with poor outcomes.[77,78]

However, at least one study[79] did not find a correlation between MRS abnormalities and outcome. Reduced NAA:Cr, increased Cho:Cr, and reduced NAA:Cho ratios were found; however, metabolite ratios did not significantly correlate with GCS score at admission or GOS at 6 months after injury and weakly correlated with GOS at discharge.

Functional MRI

The blood oxygen level–dependent (BOLD) technique is the most commonly employed for functional MRI (fMRI), based on the greater magnetic susceptibility of

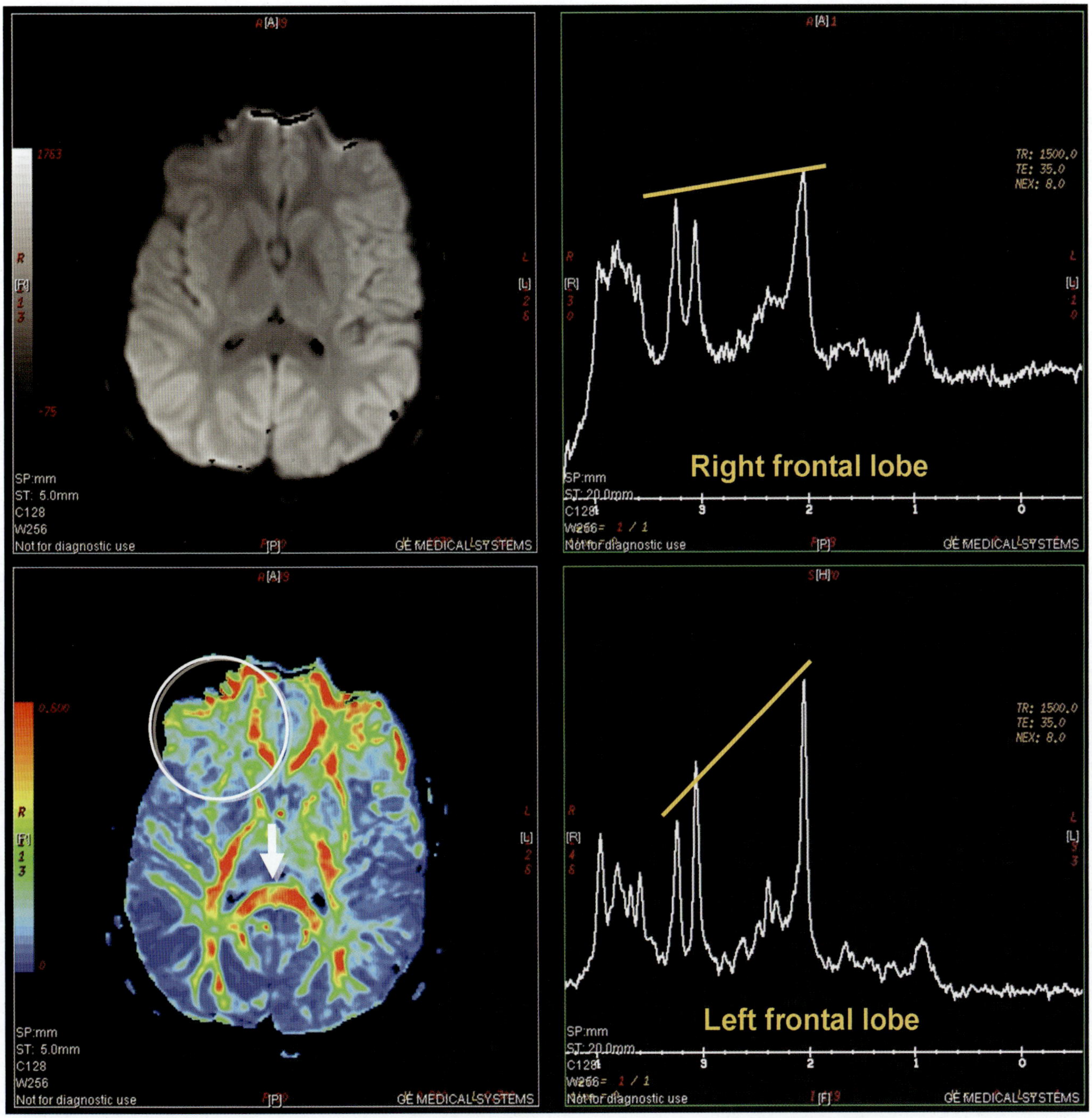

Fig. 7.27 Spectroscopy and diffusion tensor imaging (DTI) in chronic traumatic brain injury. DTI reveals decreased fractional anisotropy in the right frontal lobe and splenium of the corpus callosum. Spectroscopy of the right frontal lobe show loss of Hunter's angle with reduced N-acetyl aspartate and increased choline. MVA: motor vehicle accident. (Courtesy of Alisa D. Gean, M.D.)

deoxyhemoglobin than oxyhemoglobin. Increased regional neuronal activity related to the performance of a task results in increased perfusion, and surplus oxyhemoglobin. An alteration in the ratio of oxyhemoglobin to deoxyhemoglobin is the basis for BOLD contrast. T2* echoplanar images with BOLD contrast are acquired and compared with T1-weighted 3-D scans for anatomical localization. Compared with PET and single photon emission computed tomography (SPECT), fMRI has superior spatial and temporal resolution and absence of exposure to radiation. This allows for noninvasive, repeatable mapping of brain activation. Drawbacks include sensitivity to patient motion, need for complex postprocessing, and susceptibility artifact in areas of air–brain interface such as the inferior frontal lobe, which is a significant limitation in the evaluation of the TBI patient.

Research on TBI patients with fMRI has been performed to assess attention, memory, and sensorimotor tasks. fMRI is of particular interest for prediction of neurological outcomes in TBI patients. In 2001, Moritz et al[80] reported the initial use of fMRI to predict brain function in a comatose TBI patient who demonstrated intact task-correlated response to stimuli, and at 3 months recovered many cognitive and sensorimotor functions.

Activation fMRI has revealed areas of both hypo- and hyperactivation in TBI patients.[81–83] fMRI may increase sensitivity to concussion and memory deficits when compared with neuropsychological evaluation, previously felt to be the gold standard in evaluating deficits in patients with mild TBI. Brain activation differs in patients with mild and moderate TBI even though task performance does not[84–86] (**Fig. 7.28**).

Multiple researchers have found that subjects recruit other brain areas to perform tasks, a finding not seen in control groups.[83,87] TBI patients in response to sensory or motor tasks showed activation of areas adjacent to the damaged brain as well as areas in the contralateral hemisphere when compared with control subjects.[88,89] These findings suggest reorganization and neuromodulation of the brain accounting for behavioral recovery in some patients.

Magnetization Transfer Imaging

Magnetization transfer imaging has been used to assess the biochemical macromolecular composition of lesions. Protons bound in macromolecules exhibit T1 relaxation coupling with protons in free water. A suppressor pulse is given to saturate the magnetization of the macromolecular protons, which then exchange their longitudinal magnetization with free water protons. Signal intensity detected from these free protons is reduced. The magnetization transfer effect may be quantified by calculating the magnetization transfer ratio (MTR). MT imaging is sensitive to the presence of edema, demyelization, and wallerian degeneration. This technique is sensitive to dysfunctional neuronal tissue in the absence of visible structural change. Gadolinium administration enhances detection of white matter lesions and local areas of breakdown of the blood–brain barrier. A series of 28 patients

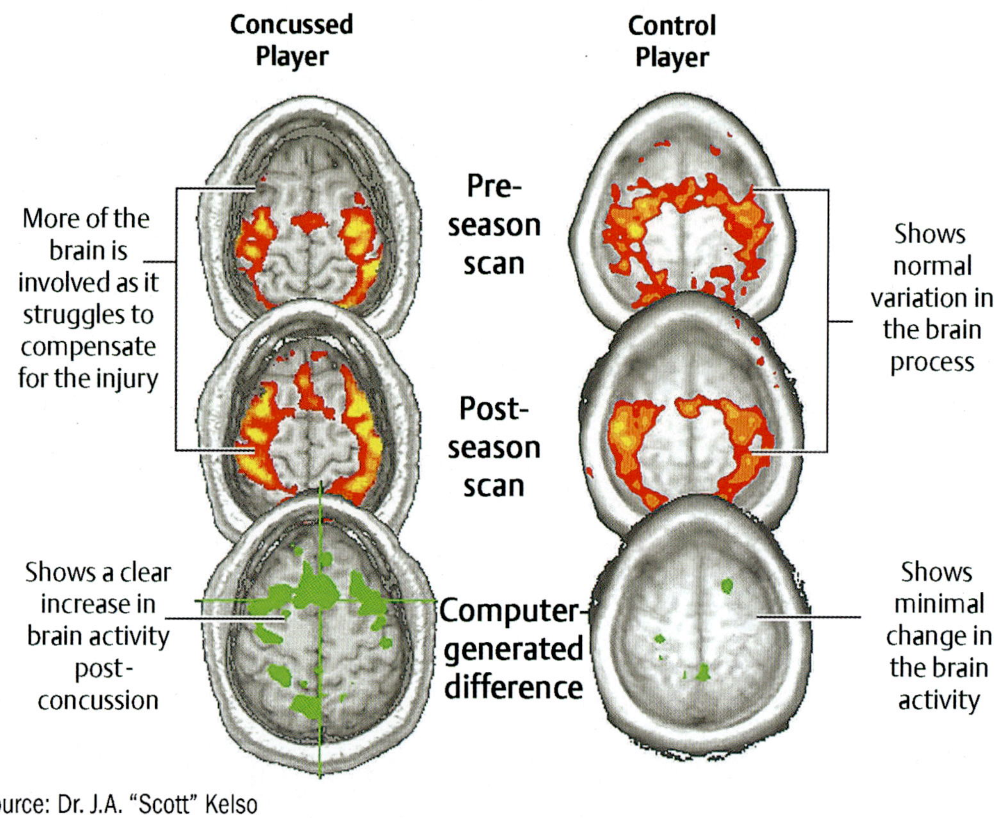

Fig. 7.28 Functional magnetic resonance imaging in traumatic brain injury demonstrates increased brain activity in concussed football player versus control. (Courtesy of Kelly J. Jantzen, Ph.D., and Scott Kelso, Ph.D.)

with TBI and loss of consciousness (LOC) demonstrated reduced MTR values in all locations (normal and T2 abnormal white matter (WM)) in patients with persistent neurological deficits as compared with those without. Regions of reduced MTR in NAWM were only detected in patients with persistent neurological deficits. Patients with good outcomes, even those with abnormalities detected on T2-weighted and gradient echo images all demonstrated normal MTR values in normal appearing white matter (NAWM). This study concluded low MTR in the characteristic locations suggest a poorer prognosis and appears more specific for prognosis than the abnormalities seen on T2.[90] Patients with an MT abnormality beyond a T2 abnormality have been shown to have significantly higher intractability of seizures compared with an MT abnormality within a T2 abnormality.[91] Patients with mild TBI and without abnormality on routine MRI have shown lower MTR in the splenium with impairment on neuropsychological tests.[92]

Quantitative Imaging (Volumetry)

Quantitative imaging of the brain can be performed either by CT or by MRI. MRI with its multiplanar capability and high spatial resolution allows volumetric quantification of structures commonly injured in brain trauma such as the corpus callosum or hippocampus. Ventricular size can be assessed by either imaging technique, although more accurately with MRI. Volume analysis is performed with a software program possessing an region of interest (ROI) feature that yields a count of gray matter, white matter, and CSF pixels. Regions of interest include the hippocampus, parahippocampal gyrus, fusiform gyrus, temporal gyri and sulci, temporal horn, and sylvian fissure.

Multiple authors have documented diffuse and focal atrophy in TBI patients. Whole brain atrophy occurs after mild or moderate TBI and is evident at an average of 11 months, before injury producing loss of consciousness leads to more atrophy.[93] Atrophy is found in both closed and penetrating head injury groups.[94,95] Significant hippocampal, fornix, and corpus callosal atrophy has been demonstrated.[96,97] Length of coma correlates with volume reduction in the corpus callosum.[97]

A correlation between atrophy and cognitive outcome as well as severity of injury has been demonstrated. Severe TBI patients without obvious neuroradiological lesions demonstrate volume reductions in the hippocampus, fornix, and corpus callosum, which significantly correlate with memory test scores. Verbal memory deficits correlate with hippocampal and fornix volume loss, and may be associated with an increased risk for development of dementia.[98,99] Postinjury IQ testing correlates to third ventricular and temporal horn size.[100] Neuropsychological test performance has demonstrated a strong correlation with gray and white matter volume loss in patients with moderate to severe brain injury with or without large focal lesions.[101] Pediatric patients may demonstrate reduced growth of brain structures typically affected by TBI including the corpus callosum.[102] A poorer outcome measured by GOS has been correlated with decreased frontotemporal volume in pediatric patients with moderate to severe TBI.[103]

Nuclear Medicine (SPECT and PET)

SPECT using a photon emitting radioisotope (most commonly technetium-99m-HMPAO) detected by a gamma camera allows for in vivo detection and mapping of regional cerebral blood flow. Regional counts must be normalized to an area that is free of injury. Resolution is less than that of PET imaging. Regional cerebral metabolism is measured by PET either at rest using the tracer [18F]-fluorodeoxyglucose (FDG) or during the performance of various cognitive tasks using 15O (oxygen-15-water). PET has been considered the gold standard for functional neuroimaging but requires access to a cyclotron and is expensive. One drawback in assessing TBI patients is that patients with persistent postconcussive complaints have psychiatric comorbidity, which has been demonstrated to be associated with SPECT/PET abnormalities.

SPECT has been shown to be superior to CT and MRI in detecting number of lesions and lesion size after TBI.[104] SPECT by detecting cortical perfusion abnormalities may more accurately reflect the size and extent of damaged tissue than CT. In a recent study using SPECT performed within 72 hours of TBI, researchers found a higher number of perfusion abnormalities in patients with posttraumatic amnesia, loss of consciousness, or postconcussion syndrome.[105] SPECT also demonstrates superior correlation with neuropsychological testing when compared with structural imaging after severe TBI; however, there is no particular SPECT profile that is pathognomonic or reliable for brain injury.[106]

Studies in patients in vegetative states have demonstrated deep reduction in global glucose metabolism.[106,107] Hypometabolism is most pronounced in patients in a vegetative state as compared with a minimally conscious state, and least in those with higher levels of function although still cognitively impaired.[106]

PET has provided insight into the areas of brain with reduced metabolism in TBI patients demonstrating deficiencies on neuropsychological testing but with no abnormality on MRI.[108,109]

Functional PET may be more sensitive to deficits than resting PET in patients with mild TBI with persistent postconcussion symptoms and normal CT and MRI.[110]

Functional PET studies show findings similar to those of fMRI in terms of neuronal reorganization in TBI patients.[111]

Susceptibility Weighted Imaging

Susceptibility weighted imaging (SWI) is a technique of postprocessing 3-D high-resolution GRE images to increase visualization of magnetic susceptibility effects, particularly to identify lesions containing hemorrhage.[112] SWI detects smaller areas of hemorrhagic DAI than conventional GRE imaging[113] (**Fig. 7.29**).

A larger number and volume of DAI lesions detected by this technique, as well as lesions in deeper areas of brain, have been demonstrated in patients with poorer performance on neuropsychological tests.[114]

Magnetic Source Imaging (MSI)

Magnetoencephalography (MEG) measures electrical currents from dendritic activity. These data can be combined with anatomical data from conventional MRI, which allows for better spatial localization of abnormal signals. Lewine et al[115]

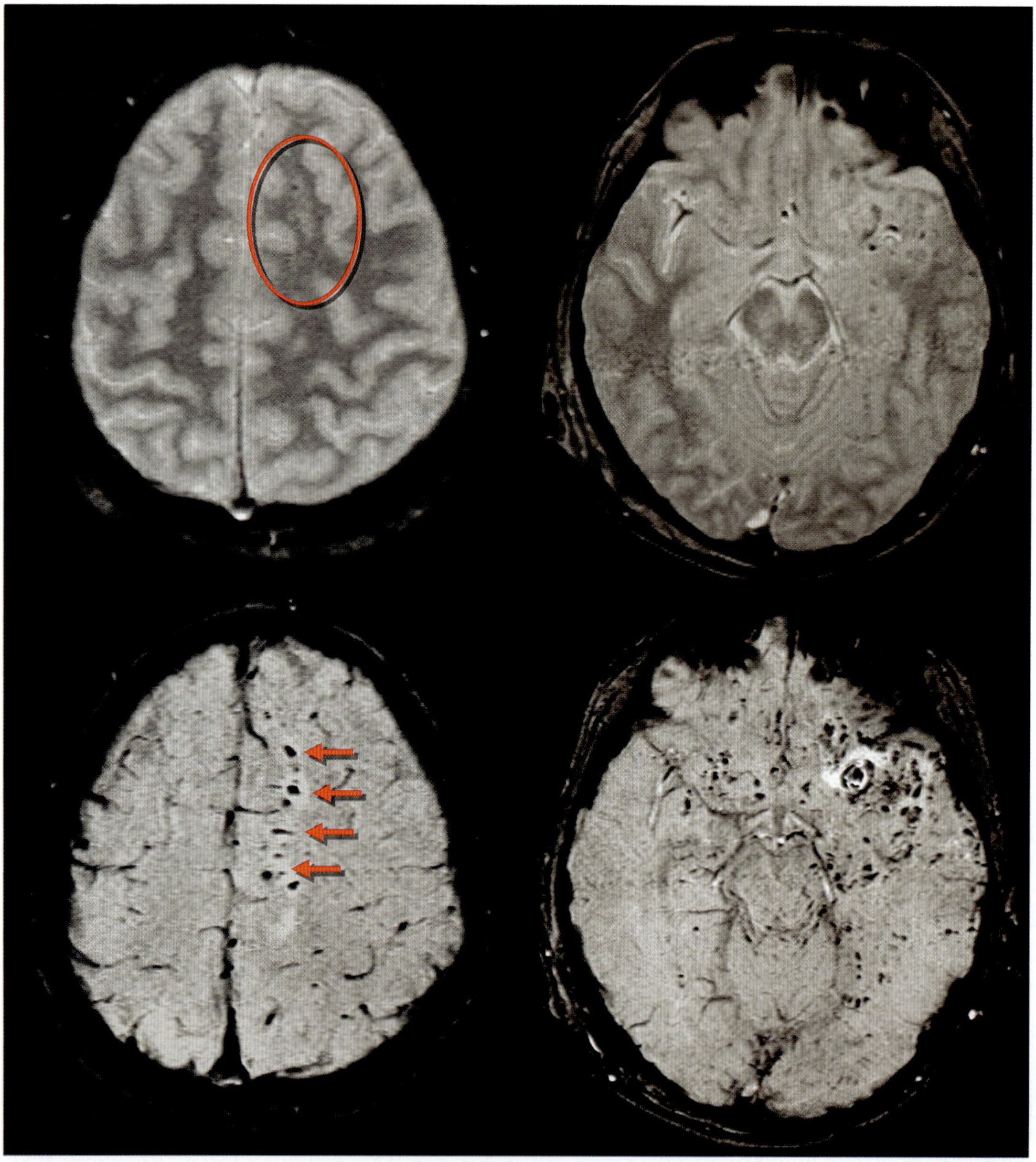

Fig. 7.29 Susceptibility weighted imaging (SWI) versus gradient recalled echo. SWI images (*bottom*) demonstrate many more microhemorrhages related to chronic diffuse axonal injury. (Courtesy of Karen Tong, M.D., and Alisa D. Gean, M.D.)

used MEG, MRI, and electroencephalogram (EEG) data to assess mild TBI patients 2 to 38 months postinjury without and with postconcussive symptoms. They found MSI abnormalities in 13 of the 20 symptomatic, mild TBI patients.

Conclusion

Recent studies using a variety of newer imaging techniques offer promise in the evaluation of TBI patients. Several of these techniques have found abnormalities in areas of normal appearing brain by conventional studies of TBI patients, and these patients tend to have poorer outcomes. Functional studies may be able to identify changes in mild TBI patients that until recently have commonly not demonstrated neuroimaging findings.

Moderate to severe TBI patients may benefit from imaging that can identify the physiological changes associated with head trauma to guide therapy with the goal of improving outcomes.

References

1. Le TH, Gean AD. Imaging of head trauma. Semin Roentgenol 2006;41:177–189
2. Jones TR, Kaplan RT, Lane B, Arlas SW, Rubin GD. Single versus multidetector row CT of the brain: quality assessment. Radiology 2001;219:750–755
3. Stiell IG, Wells GA, Vendemheen K, et al. The Canadian CT Head Rule for patients with minor head injury [see comment]. Lancet 2001;357:1391–1396
4. Kelly AB, Zimmerman RD, Snow RB, Gandy SE, Heier LA, Deck MD. Head trauma:comparison of MR and CT—experience in 100 patients. AJNR Am J Neuroradiol 1988;9(4):699–708
5. Ashikaga R, Araki Y, Ishida O. MRI of head injury using FLAIR. Neuroradiology 1997;39:239–242
6. Yanagawa Y, Tsushima Y, Tokumaru A, et al. A quantitative analysis of head injury using T2*-weighted gradient-echo imaging. J Trauma 2000;49:272–277
7. da Rocha AJ, da Silva CJ, Gama HP, et al. Comparison of magnetic resonance imaging sequences with computed tomography to detect low-grade subarachnoid hemorrhage: role of fluid-attenuated inversion recovery sequence. J Comput Assist Tomogr 2006;30:295–303
8. Levy C, Laissy JP, Raveau V, et al. Carotid and vertebral artery dissections: three-dimensional time-of-flight MR angiography and MR imaging versus conventional angiography. Radiology 1994;190:97–103
9. Young RJ, Destian S. Imaging of traumatic intracranial hemorrhage. Neuroimaging Clin N Am 2002;12:189–204
10. Gentry LR, Thompson B, Godersky JC. Trauma to the corpus callosum: MR features. AJNR Am J Neuroradiol 1988;9:1129–1138
11. Mittl RL, Grossman RI, Hiehle JF, et al. Prevalence of MR evidence of diffuse axonal injury in patients with mild head injury and normal heat CT findings [see comment]. AJNR Am J Neuroradiol 1994;15: 1583–1589
12. Orrison WW, Gentry LR, Stimac GK, Tarrel RM, Espinosa MC, Cobb LC. Blinded comparison of cranial CT and MR in closed head injury evaluation. AJNR Am J Neuroradiol 1994;15:351–356
13. Gentry LR, Godersky JC, Thompson B. MR imaging of head trauma: review of the distribution and radiopathologic features of traumatic lesions. AJR Am J Roentgenol 1988;150:663–672
14. Graham KI, Gennarelli T. Trauma. In: Graham DI, Lantos PL eds. Greenfield's Neuropathology. 6th ed. London: Arnold; 1997:197–262
15. Graham DI, Gennarelli T. Pathology of brain damage after head injury. In: Cooper PR, Golfinos JG, eds. Head Injury, 4th ed. New York: McGraw-Hill; 2000:133–153
16. Pierallini A, Pantano P, Fantozzi LM, et al. Correlation between MRI findings and long-term outcome in patients with severe brain trauma. Neuroradiology 2000;42:860–867
17. Huneidi AH, Afshar F. Delayed intracerebral haematomas in moderate to severe head injuries in young adults. Ann R Coll Surg Engl 1992;74:345–349
18. Gomori JM, Grossma RI, Goldberg HI, Zimmerman RA, Bilaniuk LT. Intracranial hematomas: imaging by high-field MR. Radiology 1985;157:87–93
19. Gentry LR. Imaging of closed head injury. Radiology 1994;191:1–17
20. Aldrich EF, Eisenberg HM, Saydjari C, et al. Diffuse brain swelling in severely head-injured children: a report from the NIH Traumatic Coma Data Bank. J Neurosurg 1992;76:450–454
21. Harwood-Nash, DC. Abuse to the pediatric central nervous system. AJNR Am J Neuroradiol 1992;13:569–575
22. Gutman MB, Moulton RJ, Sullivan I, Hotz G, Tucker WS, Muller Pj. Risk factors predicting operable intracranial hematomas in head injury. J Neurosurg 1992;77:9–14
23. Grossman RI, Yousem DM. Head trauma. In: Grossman RI, Yousem DM. Neuroradiology: Requisites 2003. 2d ed. New York: Mosby; 2003:243–245
24. Koeller KK, Levy AD, Woodward PJ, Lonergan GJ, Galvin JR, Murphey MD. Imaging of head trauma. In: Koeller KK, Levy AD, Woodward PJ, Lonergan GJ, Galvin JR, Murphey MD, eds. Radiologic Pathology. 1st ed. Washington, DC: Armed Forces Institute of Pathology; 2002:724–726
25. Johnson PL, Eckard DA, Chason DP, Breicheisen MA, Batnitzky S. Imaging of acquired cerebral herniations. Neuroimaging Clin N Am 2002;12:217–228
26. Grossman RI, Yousem DM. Head trauma. In: Grossman RI, Yousem DM. Neuroradiology: Requisites 2003. 2d ed. New York: Mosby; 2003:261–263
27. Uemura A, O'uchi T, Yashiro N. Usefullness of gradient-echo T2*-weighted MR imaging in evaluation of transorbital penetrating cerebral injury. Clin Imaging 2001;25:163–166
28. Taniura S, Tatebayashi K, Akatsuka K, et al. Transoral penetration of a half-split chopstick between the basion and the dens. AJNR Am J Neuroradiol 2004;25:871–872
29. Litvack ZN, Hunt MA, Weinstein JS, West GA. Self-inflicted nail-gun injury with 12 cranial penetrations and associated cerebral trauma: case report and review of the literature. J Neurosurg 2006;104:828–834
30. Kim PE, Go JL, Zee CS. Radiographic assessment of cranial gunshot wounds. Neuroimaging Clin N Am 2002;12:229–248
31. Stein SC, Smith DH. Coagulopathy in traumatic brain injury. Neurocrit Care 2004;1:479–488
32. Aarabi B, Taghipour M, Alicaii E, Kamgarpour A. Central nervous system infections after military missile head wounds. Neurosurgery 1998;42:500–507
33. Woodcock RJ, Davis PC, Hopkins KL. Imaging of head trauma in infancy and childhood. Semin Ultrasound CT MR 2001;22:162–182
34. Chen CY, Zimmerman RA, Rorke LB. Neuroimaging in child abuse: a mechanism-based approach. Neuroradiology 1999;41:711–722
35. Hobbs CJ. Skull fracture and the diagnosis of abuse. Arch Dis Child 1984;59:246–252
36. Guthkelch AN. Infantile subdural hematoma and its relationship to whiplash injuries. BMJ 1971;2:430–431
37. Caffey J. On the theory and practice of shaking infants: its potential residual effects of permanent brain damage and mental retardation. Am J Dis Child 1972;124:161–169
38. Stoodley N. Neuroimaging in nonaccidental head injury: if, when, why and how [see comment]. Clin Radiol 2005;60:22–30

39. Barnes PD. Ethical issues in imaging nonaccidental injury: child abuse. Top Magn Reson Imaging 2002;13:85–93
40. Han BK, Towbin RB, De Courten-Myers G, McLaurin RL, Ball WS Jr. Reversal sign on CT: effect of anoxic/ischemic cerebral injury in children. AJNR Am J Neuroradiol 1989;10:1191–1198
41. Gilles EE, Nelson MD Jr. Cerebral complications of nonaccidental head injury in childhood. Pediatr Neurol 1998;19:119–128
42. Poussaint TY, Moeller KK. Imaging of pediatric head trauma. Neuroimaging Clin N Am 2002;12:271–294
43. Zimmerman RA, Bilaniuk LT, Bruce D, Schut L, Uzzell B, Goldberg HI. Computed tomography of craniocerebral injury in the abused child. Radiology 1979;130:687–690
44. Temkin NR, Machamer JE, Dikmen SS. Correlates of functional status 3–5 years after traumatic brain injury with CT abnormalities. J Neurotrauma 2003;20:229–241
45. Pierallini A, Pantano P, Fantozzi LM, et al. Correlation between MRI findings and long-term outcome in patients with severe brain trauma. Neuroradiology 2000;42:860–867
46. Hughes DG, Jackson A, Mason DL, Berry E, Hollis S, Yates DW. Abnormalities on magnetic resonance imaging seen acutely following mild traumatic brain injury: correlation with neuropsychological tests and delayed recovery. Neuroradiology 2004;46:550–558
47. Inglese M, Bomsztyk E, Gonen O, Mannon LJ, Grossman RI, Rusinek H. Dilated perivascular spaces: hallmarks of mild traumatic brain injury. AJNR Am J Neuroradiol 2005;26:719–724
48. Shibata Y, Matsumura A, Meguro K, Narushima K. Differentiation of mechanism and prognosis of traumatic brain stem lesions detected by magnetic resonance imaging in the acute stage. Clin Neurol Neurosurg 2000;102:124–128
49. Scheid R, Preul C, Gruber O, Wiggins C, von Cramon DY. Diffuse axonal injury associated with chronic traumatic brain injury: evidence from T2*-weighted gradient-echo imaging at 3T. AJNR Am J Neuroradiol 2003;24:1049–1056
50. Wintermark M, Chiolero R, Van Melle G, et al. Cerebral vascular autoregulation assessed by perfusion CT in severe head trauma patients. J Neuroradiol 2006;33:27–37
51. Garnett MR, Blamire AM, Corkill RG, et al. Abnormal cerebral blood volume in regions of contused and normal-appearing brain following traumatic brain injury using perfusion magnetic resonance imaging. J Neurotrauma 2001;18:585–593
52. Huisman TA. Diffusion-weighted imaging: basic concepts and application in cerebral stroke and head trauma. Eur Radiol 2003;13:2283–2297
53. Hanstock CC, Faden AI, Bendall MR, Vink R. Diffusion-weighted imaging differentiates ischemic tissue from traumatized tissue. Stroke 1994;25:843–848
54. Alsop DC, Murai H, Detre JA, McIntosh TK, Smith DH. Detection of acute pathologic changes following experimental traumatic brain injury using diffusion-weighted magnetic resonance imaging. J Neurotrauma 1996;13:515–521
55. Barzo P, Marmarou A, Fatouros P, Hayasaki K, Corwin F. Contribution of vasogenic and cellular edema to traumatic brain swelling measured by diffusion-weighted imaging. J Neurosurg 1997;87:900–907
56. Liu AY, Maldjian JA, Bagley LJ, Sinson GP, Grossman RI. Traumatic brain injury: diffusion-weighted MR imaging findings [see comments]. AJNR Am J Neuroradiol 1999;20:1636–1641
57. Pasco A, Ter Minassian A, Chapon C, et al. Dynamics of cerebral edema and the apparent diffusion coefficient of water changes in patients with severe traumatic brain injury: a prospective MRI study. Eur Radiol 2006;16:1501–1508
58. Shanmuganathan K, Gullapalli RP, Mirvis SE, Roys S, Murthy P. Whole-brain apparent diffusion coefficient in traumatic brain injury: correlation with Glasgow Coma Scale score. AJNR Am J Neuroradiol 2004;25: 539–544
59. Field AS, Hasan K, Jellison BJ, Arfanakis K, Alexander AL. Diffusion tensor imaging in an infant with traumatic brain swelling. AJNR Am J Neuroradiol 2003;24:1461–1464
60. Chan JH, Tsui EY, Peh WC, et al. Diffuse axonal injury: detection of changes in anisotropy of water diffusion by diffusion-weighted imaging. Neuroradiology 2003;45:34–38
61. Arfanakis K, Haughton VM, Carew JD, Rogers BP, Dempsey RJ, Meyerand ME. Diffusion tensor MR imaging in diffuse axonal injury. AJNR Am J Neuroradiol 2002;23:794–802
62. Inglese M, Makani S, Johnson G, et al. Diffuse axonal injury in mild traumatic brain injury: a diffusion tensor imaging study. J Neurosurg 2005;103:298–303
63. Salmond CH, Menon DK, Chatfield DA, et al. Diffusion tensor imaging in chronic head injury survivors: correlations with learning and memory indices. Neuroimage 2006;29:117–124
64. Huisman TA, Schwamm LH, Schaefer PW, et al. Diffusion tensor imaging as a potential biomarker of white matter injury in diffuse axonal injury. AJNR Am J Neuroradiol 2004;25:370–376
65. Lee JW, Choi CG, Chun MH. Usefulness of diffusion tensor imaging for evaluation of motor function in patients with traumatic brain injury: three case studies. J Head Trauma Rehabil 2006;21:272–278
66. Ducreux D, Huynh I, Fillard P, et al. Brain MR diffusion tensor imaging and fibre tracking to differentiate between two diffuse axonal injuries. Neuroradiology 2005;47:604–608
67. Okumura A, Yasokawa Y, Nakayama N, Miwa K, Shinoda J, Iwama T. The clinical utility of MR diffusion tensor imaging and spatially normalized PET to evaluate traumatic brain injury patients with memory and cognitive impairments. No To Shinkei 2005;57:115–122
68. Ross BD, Ernst T, Kreis R, et al. 1H MRS in acute traumatic brain injury. J Magn Reson Imaging 1998;8:829–840
69. Holshouser BA, Tong KA, Ashwal S. Proton MR spectroscopic imaging depicts diffuse axonal injury in children with traumatic brain injury. AJNR Am J Neuroradiol 2005;26(5):1276–1285
70. Hunter JV, Thornton RJ, Wang ZJ, et al. Late proton MR spectroscopy in children after traumatic brain injury: correlation with cognitive outcomes. AJNR Am J Neuroradiol 2005;26:482–488
71. Friedman SD, Brooks WM, Jung RE, Hart BL, Yeo RA. Proton MR spectroscopic findings correspond to neuropsychological function in traumatic brain injury. AJNR Am J Neuroradiol 1998;19:1879–1885
72. Brooks WM, Stidley CA, Petropoulos H, et al. Metabolic and cognitive response to human traumatic brain injury: a quantitative proton magnetic resonance study. J Neurotrauma 2000;17:629–640
73. Brooks WM, Friedman SD, Gasparovic C. Magnetic resonance spectroscopy in traumatic brain injury. J Head Trauma Rehabil 2001;16:149–164
74. Shutter L, Tong KA, Lee A, Holshouser BA. Prognostic role of proton magnetic resonance spectroscopy in acute traumatic brain injury. J Head Trauma Rehabil 2006;21:334–349
75. Condon B, Oluoch-Olunya D, Hadley D, Teasdale G, Wagstaff A. Early 1H magnetic resonance spectroscopy of acute head injury: four cases. J Neurotrauma 1998;15:563–571
76. Yoon SJ, Lee JH, Kim ST, Chum MH. Evaluation of traumatic brain injured patients in correlation with functional status by localized 1H-MR spectroscopy. Clin Rehabil 2005;19:209–215
77. Ashwal S, Holshouser BA, Shu SK, et al. Predictive value of proton magnetic resonance spectroscopy in pediatric closed head injury. Pediatr Neurol 2000;23:114–125
78. Ashwal S, Holshouser B, Tong K, et al. Proton spectroscopy detected myoinositol in children with traumatic brain injury. Pediatr Res 2004;56:630–638
79. Govindaraju V, Gauger GE, Manley GT, Ebel A, Meeker M, Maudsley AA. Volumetric proton spectroscopic imaging of mild traumatic brain injury. AJNR Am J Neuroradiol 2004;25:730–737
80. Moritz CH, Rowley HA, Haughton VM, Swartz KR, Jones J, Badie B. Functional MR imaging assessment of a non-responsive brain injured patient. Magn Reson Imaging 2001;19:1129–1132
81. Levine B, Fujiwara E, O'Connor C, et al. In vivo characterization of traumatic brain injury neuropathology with structural and functional neuroimaging. J Neurotrauma 2006;23:1396–1411
82. Soeda A, Nakashima T, Okumura A, Kuwata K, Shinoda J, Iwama R. Cognitive impairment after traumatic brain injury: a functional magnetic resonance imaging study using the Stroop task. Neuroradiology 2005;47:501–506
83. Chen JK, Johnston KM, Frey S, Petrides M, Worsley K, Ptito A. functional abnormalities in symptomatic concussed athletes: an fMRI study. Neuroimage 2004;22:68–82

84. Jantzen KJ, Anderson B, Steinberg FL, Kelso JA. A prospective functional MR imaging study of mild traumatic brain injury in college football players. AJNR Am J Neuroradiol 2004;25:738–745
85. McAllister TW, Sparling MB, Flashman LA, Guerin SJ, Mamourian AC, Saykin AJ. Differential working memory load effects after mild traumatic brain injury. Neuroimage 2001;14:1004–1012
86. Hammoud DA, Wasserman BA. Diffuse axonal injuries: pathophysiology and imaging. Neuroimaging Clin N Am 2002;12:205–216
87. Ricker JH, Hillary FG, DeLuca J. Functionally activated brain imaging (O-15 PET and fMRI) in the study of learning and memory after traumatic brain injury. J Head Trauma Rehabil 2001;16:191–205
88. Cioni G, Montanaro D, Tosetti M, Canapicchi R, Ghelarducci B. Reorganisation of the sensorimotor cortex after early focal brain lesion: a functional MRI study in monozygotic twins. Neuroreport 2001;12: 1335–1340
89. Wiese H, Tonnes C, deGrieff A, Nebel K, Diener HC, Stude P. Self-initiated movements in chronic prefrontal traumatic brain injury; an event-related functional MRI study. Neuroimage 2006;30:1292–1301
90. Bagley LJ, McGowan JC, Grossman RI, et al. Magnetization transfer imaging of traumatic brain injury. J Magn Reson Imaging 2000;11:1–8
91. Kumar R, Gupta RK, Husain M, et al. Magnetization transfer MR imaging in patients with posttraumatic epilepsy. AJNR Am J Neuroradiol 2003;24:218–224
92. McGowan JC, Yang JH, Plotkin RC, et al. Magnetization transfer imaging in the detection of injury associated with mild head trauma [see comment]. AJNR Am J Neuroradiol 2000;21:875–880
93. MacKenzie JD, Siddiqi F, Babb JS, et al. Brain atrophy in mild or moderate traumatic brain injury: a longitudinal quantitative analysis. AJNR Am J Neuroradiol 2002;23(9):1509–1515
94. Himanen L, Portin R, Isoniemi H, Helenius H, Kurki T, Tenovuo O. Cognitive functions in relation to MRI findings 30 years after traumatic brain injury. Brain Inj 2005;19:93–100
95. Hammoud DA, Wasserman BA. Diffuse axonal injuries: pathophysiology and imaging. Neuroimaging Clin N Am 2002;12:205–216
96. Gale SD, Johnson SC, Bigler ED, Blatter DD. Nonspecific white matter degeneration following traumatic brain injury. J Int Neuropsychol Soc 1995;1:17–28
97. Tomaiuolo F, Carlesimo GA, DiPaola M, et al. Gross morphology and morphometric sequelae in the hippocampus, fornix, and corpus callosum of patients with severenon-missile traumatic brain injury without macroscopically detectable lesions: a T1 weighted MRI study. J Neurol Neurosurg Psychiatry 2004;75:1314–1322
98. Blatter DD, Bigler ED, Gale SD, et al. MR-based brain and cerebrospinal fluid measurement after traumatic brain injury: correlation with neuropsychological outcome. AJNR Am J Neuroradiol 1997;18:1–10
99. Bigler ED, Blatter DD, Anderson CV, et al. Hippocampal volume in normal aging and traumatic brain injury. [see comment] AJNR Am J Neuroradiol 1997;18:11–23
100. Bigler ED, Johnson SC, Blatter DD. Head trauma and intellectual status: relation to quantitative magnetic resonance imaging findings. Appl Neuropsychol 1999;6:217–225
101. Levine B, Fujiwara E, O'Connor C, et al. In vivo characterization of traumatic brain injury neuropathology with structural and functional neuroimaging. J Neurotrauma 2006;23:1396–1411
102. Levin HS, Benavidez DA, Verger-Maestre K, et al. Reduction of corpus callosum growth after severe traumatic brain injury in children. Neurology 2000;54:647–653
103. Wilde EA, Hunter JV, Newsome MR, et al. Frontal and temporal morphometric findings in mild traumatic brain injury. J Neurotrauma 2005;22:333–344
104. McAllister TW, Sparling MB, Flashman LA, Saykin AJ. Neuroimaging findings in mild traumatic brain injury. J Clin Exp Neuropsychol 2001;23:775–791
105. Gowda NK, Agrawal D, Bal C, et al. Technetium Tc-99m ethyl cysteinate dimer brain single-photon emission CT in mild traumatic brain injury: a prospective study. AJNR Am J Neuroradiol 2006;27: 447–451
106. Nakayama N, Okumura A, Shinoda J, Nakashima T, Iwama T. Relationship between regional cerebral metabolism and consciousness disturbance in traumatic diffuse brain injury without large focal lesions: an FDG-PET study with statistical parametric mapping analysis. J Neurol Neurosurg Psychiatry 2006;77:856–862
107. Plum F, Schiff N, Ribary U, Linas R. Coordinated expression in chronically unconscious persons. Philos Trans R Soc Lond B Biol Sci 1998; 353:1929–1933
108. Azouvi P. Neuroimaging correlates of cognitive and functional outcome after traumatic brain injury. Curr Opin Neurol 2000;13: 665–669
109. Fontaine A, Azouvi P, Remy P, Bussel B, Samson Y. Functional anatomy of neuropsychological deficits after severe traumatic brain injury. Neurology 1999;53:1963–1968
110. Chen SH, Kareken DA, Fastenau PS, Trexler LE, Hutchins GD. A study of persistent post-concussion symptoms in mild head trauma using positron emission tomography. J Neurol Neurosurg Psychiatry 2003; 74:326–332
111. Ricker JH, Hillary FG, DeLuca J. Functionally activated brain imaging (O-15 PET and MRI) in the study of learning and memory after traumatic brain injury. J Head Trauma Rehabil 2001;16:191–205
112. Sehgal V, Delproposto Z, Haacke EM, et al. Clinical applications of neuroimaging with susceptibility-weighted imaging. J Magn Reson Imaging 2005;22:439–450
113. Tong KA, Ashwal S, Holshouser BA, et al. Hemorrhagic shearing lesions in children and adolescents with posttraumatic diffuse axonal injury: improved detection and initial results. Radiology 2003;227: 332–339
114. Babikian T, Freier MC, Tong KA, et al. Susceptibility weighted imaging: neuropsychological outcome and pediatric head injury. Pediatr Neurol 2005;33:184–194
115. Lewine JD, Davis JT, Sloan JH, Kodituwakku PW, Orrison WW Jr. Neuromagnetic assessment of pathophysiologic brain activity induced by minor head trauma. AJNR Am J Neuroradiol 1999;20: 857–866

8 Endovascular Therapy

Jeffrey P. Kochan

Newer imaging modalities now enable improved visualization of traumatic neurovascular pathology. Notably, the development of noninvasive vascular imaging techniques, for example, computed tomographic angiography (CTA) and magnetic resonance angiography (MRA) provide greater insight as to the status of major arterial and venous vascular anatomy that until now often required more invasive diagnostic angiography. Both these newer modalities are capable of demonstrating the entire cervical-cerebral vasculature and are not limited to the midcervical region as is the more traditional sonographic examination. CTA in particular is now commonly utilized in both blunt and penetrating head and neck trauma, and as a result, more vascular pathology is being identified. As a consequence, invasive conventional angiography is now performed more frequently on patients with vascular injuries diagnosed by CTA and MRA. Invasive angiography is therefore more commonly positive and is used as part of a planned intervention rather than as the screening tool it has been in the past. CT perfusion (CTP) provides even more information as to the cerebral ischemic consequences of vascular injuries, information useful in determining the efficacy of management of underlying vascular injuries (**Fig. 8.1**). For example, a CTP examination demonstrating no perfusion in an area of the brain due to a more proximal occlusion of greater than 6 hours' duration might suggest the futility and added risk of attempting to reopen an occluded vessel. Conversely, with reduced perfusion in an event of 3 hours' duration, one might anticipate a significant benefit to the patient with revascularization procedures. In the following paragraphs, we will stress the value of the various imaging modalities and their impact on endovascular treatment planning.

Modern trauma suites in most level 1 trauma centers are fully equipped to sustain life in the severely traumatized patient. Any decision to move a critical patient from that controlled environment should take into account

A–D

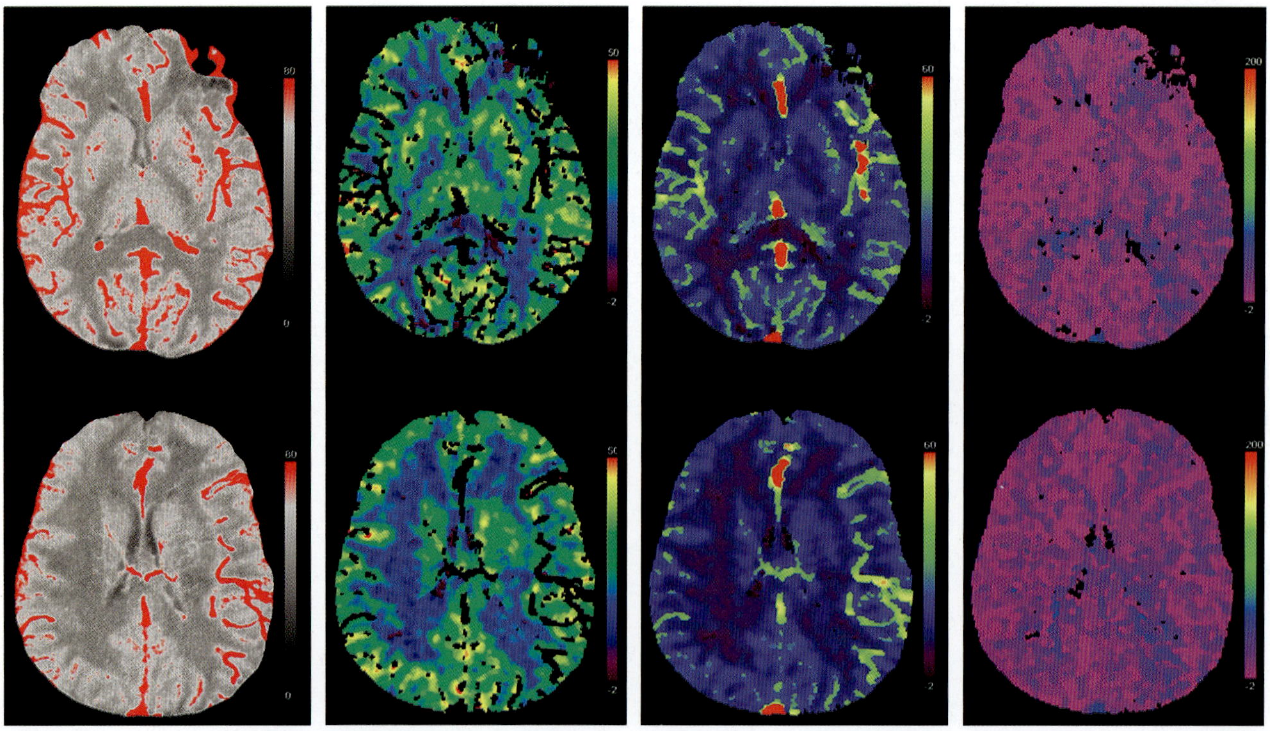

Fig. 8.1 Computed tomographic Perfusion (CTP) imaging can provide rapid information about the cerebral ischemic consequences of head and neck trauma. Selected datasets include **(A)** MIP, **(B)** flow, **(C)** peak enhancement, and **(D)** time to start images. Two separate levels are assigned a color-coded index and are assessed for blood perfusion and blood volume. This study can be obtained during the initial CT workup of the trauma patient with only a minimal investment in additional time.

the risks to the patient by losing that control, even if temporarily. Attention is directed toward which patients should leave the emergency room setting for radiographic examinations and when. Particular imaging modalities requested in any given situation should provide answers to specific questions regarding the patient's medical problem and lead to the determination of an optimal approach to treatment. Studies should be tailored to answer such questions as presence or absence of bleeding and which vessel is the likely source, presence of fractures or foreign bodies, location of the abnormality, what have been the consequences of the injury on the underlying neural, osseous, and vascular structures, what procedures might be helpful in stabilizing the patient, and what would be the best approach to effect a surgical repair. Although these are all important questions to be answered, imaging should not as a rule be the first course of management of the traumatized patient. A thorough clinical evaluation will narrow the area of interest, limiting unnecessary imaging of unaffected parts of the body and incorrect selection of an imaging modality. A more focused area of interest usually results in more detailed information about that given area. Conversely, a very wide area of interest usually results in less detail in any one particular area. Imaging is most effective when used to confirm a clinical diagnosis rather than as the primary means of making a diagnosis. In the acute trauma setting, a trip to the radiology department may represent a temporary reduction in control of the patient. Not uncommonly, a trauma patient will experience a sudden decline while in the radiology department where the appropriate equipment for dealing with a crisis may not be readily available. The patient must be therefore either stable, or unable to be stabilized before being transported out of the emergency room environment.

Imaging Modalities and Endovascular Treatment Planning

The easiest imaging studies to obtain are those that can be provided in the trauma suite without moving the patient. Plain film radiography has traditionally been the study of first election. This modality is quite effective at identifying radiopaque foreign bodies, fracture deformities, masses, and free air, but it is inherently weak at identifying soft tissue injuries, hemorrhage, and nonradiopaque foreign bodies such as glass, wood, and plastic, and it may be relatively insensitive at identifying nondisplaced linear fractures, especially in obese and osteoporotic patients. Generally, plain film radiography is of little or no value in the determination of soft tissue injury to the nervous system or in the identification of the hemorrhagic sequelae of head and neck trauma.

Ultrasound, although portable and readily available in the trauma suite, may be useful in the evaluation of abdominal and pelvic injuries but has no role in the workup of a neurological injury. Doppler sonography is certainly of value in identifying vascular lesions of the midcervical region, but in the trauma setting, vascular assessment must include imaging of not only the entire course of the carotid and vertebral arteries from the aortic arch to the skull base, but should also include the major intracranial arterial and venous anatomy, specifically the presence or absence of the communicating arteries in determining the integrity of the circle of Willis. If a vascular intervention is contemplated the presence or absence of these key collateral vessels is crucial in risk assessment. While useful in the evaluation of the carotid bifurcation, proximal and distal arterial injuries and an assessment of the end organ (e.g., brain or spinal cord) for the consequences of a vascular injury cannot be assessed by ultrasound and would therefore require an additional study to answer those questions. A Doppler study would therefore be redundant and an ineffective use of critical time and resources. Ultrasound therefore has no role in the workup of acute head and neck trauma.

The remaining imaging alternatives are not routinely available in the trauma suite and would require an out of emergency room experience. At this point the risk versus benefit of pursuing additional studies should be considered.

CT is unquestionably the most useful imaging tool in acute trauma. With respect to head trauma, CT is the fastest, most convenient means of identifying intracranial hemorrhage and linear skull fractures. The newer 16 and 64 multislice scanners and pending 128 and 320 slice scanners can provide this information in less time than would be possible with the older single slice systems. The advent of multislice CT scanning has also provided us with two additional modalities, CTA and CTP imaging, both of which can be offered to patients at the same time as their initial CT evaluation with only a minimal additional investment of time. These two modalities provide useful prognostic information in subsequent treatment planning and should therefore be considered in all cases of head and neck trauma.

Noncontrast cranial CT scans should always be performed first. Once contrast has been administered, it may be difficult to distinguish between hemorrhage and contrast enhancement. Depending on the manufacturer and model, CTA source images are then acquired in contiguous 0.75 mm sections on the 16 slice scanners or 0.5 to 0.6 mm thick slices on the 64 slice scanners in the axial projection. The source images are obtained 10 seconds following bolus infusion of 100 mL of iodinated contrast followed by a bolus of 12 mL of saline. The initial submillimeter axial images are reformatted to more conventional 3 mm thick contrast enhanced slices that can then be reconstructed in the axial, coronal, and sagittal planes. The submillimeter source images are then transmitted to workstations where they are then manually post processed into two- (2-) and three-dimensional (3-D) reconstructed images that are then filmed in varying degrees of magnification and projection. With these remarkably thin source images, reconstructions can be provided in any plane with a greater degree of resolution than was possible on the third- and fourth-generation single slice scanners and, as such, this technology has all but eliminated the need for direct coronal scanning. This in turn means less time on the scanner for critically ill patients and a reduction in total radiation dose.

CTP (**Fig. 8.1**) can also be obtained as part of the acute trauma workup. An initial noncontrast CT examination of the brain is first performed. Currently, two axial images, usually at and above the level of the basal ganglia, are then scanned dynamically over 40 seconds following the bolus administration of 40 mL of Omnipaque 300 (Iohexol, GE Healthcare) at 8 mL/s. Parametric color maps of cerebral blood flow, cerebral blood volume, and mean transit times are then obtained. Perfusion imaging of the entire brain as a single volume is anticipated shortly. Like CTA, little investment of additional time is required. In patients who present with neurological deficits or in whom vascular injuries of the head or neck have been identified, CTP can offer valuable information as to the cerebral consequence of those injuries. For example, abnormal perfusion to a hemisphere on the same side as a cervical arterial lesion would imply an ischemia either as a result of absence of collateral flow such as is associated with an incomplete circle of Willis, or as a thromboembolic consequence of cervical vascular injury. If identified within the first few hours of the event, an intervention, either surgical or endovascular, would then become a more pressing priority. The severity and distribution of a perfusion defect in conjunction with the neurological presentation and duration of the deficits may also provide some indication as to whether the ischemic injury is reversible with probable neurological recovery or more profound and less likely to be reversible or neurologically recoverable. Conversely, a normal CTP study in the face of a known cervical arterial injury suggests that the brain has tolerated the vascular injury well. If no clinically detectable neurological alteration is identified, the lesion may be best treated with conservative medical management. In this instance, conventional angiographic confirmation may not be indicated.

Interventional Neuroradiology

Interventional neuroradiology is a relatively new subspecialty that offers minimally invasive therapies for lesions of the head, neck, spine, brain, and spinal cord.[1–4] A significant percentage of endovascular therapies deal with the hemorrhagic and thromboembolic consequences of penetrating and blunt trauma. Endovascular therapies generally include (1) embolotherapy, with which the goal is the occlusion of abnormal blood vessels, such as traumatic vascular rupture with active extravasation, vascular malformations, and aneurysms; and (2) cervical-cerebral revascularization, where occluded or narrowed normal vessels are reopened.[5–8] Although the practice of embolotherapy has existed for ~30 years, active consideration of this therapy continues to evolve for the emergent management of vascular injury and aneurysms as well as adjunctive preoperative management of vascular malformations and tumors. The progressive increase in demand is principally the result of the development and refinement of newer microcatheter delivery systems and of safer and more varied embolic agents and implants. The newer microcatheters provide increased superselectivity, which in turn improves target-specific embolization with greater preservation of adjacent normal vascular anatomy. These microcatheters can be used to deliver all currently available embolic agents, including particulate emboli, coils, balloons, tissue adhesives, nonadhesive liquid embolic agents, sclerosing agents, and chemotherapeutic agents. Microcatheters also provide the conduit for devices designed to recanalize occluded vessels, such as mechanical thrombectomy devices, foreign body retrieval devices, angioplasty, and stent delivery.

Ideally, patients suffering from acute and severe neurovascular injuries are best managed with the joint participation of the trauma and neurosurgical services while in the interventional angiography suite. Any intervention contemplated is not performed in a vacuum. Once the diagnostic portion of the exam has been completed, the findings are discussed among the referring services prior to commencement of any treatment. The decision to treat should be based on an evaluation of the risk of the procedure versus the potential benefit. The same question should be asked with respect to the risk versus benefit of a surgical repair versus endovascular repair versus medical management. The course of therapy then will be determined by a consensus of opinions as to the best way to proceed based on the expertise of each of the involved specialists. The product of this discussion, patient status permitting, is then presented to patient family members.

Patient Preparation and Triage

It is of course preferable that the patient be stabilized prior to transfer out of the more controlled environment of the trauma suite or intensive care unit, but often the patient will be referred because he or she cannot be stabilized. In these cases, advanced preparation will facilitate a more rapid intervention at lower risk to the patient and with the least amount of time out of the intensive care unit (ICU) or trauma suite. For patients with hemorrhagic emergencies, a recent hemoglobin, hematocrit, and platelet count should be available. Depending on the severity of the injury, patients should also be typed and cross matched for possible transfusion with packed red blood cells (pRBCs) and platelets during the endovascular procedure. Patients should also be maintained as normotensive as possible until the extent of vascular injury has been determined and endovascular repair is initiated.

Rapid control of hemorrhage is essential, especially in the hemodynamically unstable patient. Manual extrinsic compression or mechanical control of any persistent superficial bleeding with compression devices, temporary gauze packing, electrocautery, and/or hemostat clamping of bleeding vessels in injuries of the face and scalp should be achieved prior to departing the emergency room setting.

Upon arrival in the angiography suite, vascular access should be achieved as quickly as permissible. In unstable patients, a no. 5 or 6 French (6F) arterial sheath should be placed at the start of the procedure. This will provide vascular access in the event resuscitation is required without the need to abandon distal catheterization required to treat the source of bleeding. Every effort should be made to achieve hemodynamic stability while vascular access to the bleeding site is achieved. Both processes should be addressed simultaneously. Either distal vascular access without stabilizing the patient or stabilizing the patient without addressing distal control of hemorrhage could both lead to disastrous outcomes in the angiography suite. Once the vascular injury is identified, temporary hemostasis can occasionally be achieved by wedging the diagnostic catheter into a small parent vessel proximal to the site of a more distal arterial injury. This may provide a short-term stasis of bleeding while the microcatheter is being prepared and delivered more distally to the site of injury. Alternatively, similar control, although not as quickly accomplished, can be achieved with the use of nondetachable balloon occlusive guide catheters or with the tandem placement of a microballoon catheter. These latter techniques are more suitable when treating high-flow arterial-venous fistula in a state of flow arrest when a greater degree of precision and control is required.

Embolic Agents

Once the abnormal vessel has been identified and selectively catheterized, there are several therapeutic options available for the treatment of that vessel. A wide variety of agents and devices may then be employed to provide the desired result in the treatment of a specific vascular abnormality.

Particulate agents are the embolic materials of choice for occluding the microvascular supply of many craniofacial hemorrhagic conditions, notably, epistaxis and penetrating injuries to the face (**Fig. 8.2**).[2] These agents are divided into two general categories: absorbable and nonabsorbable agents. Absorbable agents, as their name implies, do not permanently occlude vessels and therefore are of value in the achievement of hemostasis in the emergent setting while not significantly impeding the wound healing process. Materials in this category include gelatin sponge (Gelfoam; Pfizer, Inc., New York, NY), which is available in pledgets or as a powder of 40 to 60 microns in particulate diameter. Microfibrillar collagen (Avitene; CR Bard, Inc., Murray Hill, NJ) is supplied as a powder with a particle size of ~50 microns. Avitene is widely used as a topical thrombotic agent in conventional surgery; however, when prepared as a colloidal suspension with contrast, collagen can produce a rapid thrombosis of a selected vessel. An admixture of Avitene and a more permanent agent such as polyvinyl alcohol (PVA) offers an effective compromise between speed of occlusion and permanence of the occlusion.

On occasion, absorbable embolic agents can be used to protect normal vessels (**Fig. 8.3**). In this technique, the normal branching vessels are temporarily occluded, allowing the operator to direct the flow of permanent embolic agents into the abnormal vessels. An autologous blood clot may be used for temporary, protective occlusion as it rapidly recanalizes. Likewise, a pledget of gelatin sponge (Gelfoam) can be placed in the origin of a normal arterial branch to ensure that the more permanent embolic agents infused proximally do not enter that vessel; rather they are flow-directed to the abnormal vessels. The vessel occluded with autologous clot and/or pledget recanalizes in a short time, reestablishing flow to its normal territory. Abnormal vessels embolized with nonabsorbable agents will remain occluded for a longer period of time.

The nonabsorbable particulate agents most commonly used are PVA particles (Ivalon, Nycomed Laboratories, Paris, France; PVA, Biodyne, Inc., El Cajon, CA; PVA, Cook Medical, Bloomington IN; Contour Emboli, Target Therapeutics, Inc./Boston Scientific Corp., Naticle, MA) Particle sizes are typically 150 to 1000 microns in diameter. The smaller particle sizes are most frequently used to embolize bleeding from hyperemic soft tissue injury, whereas the large sizes are most useful in occluding larger, higher flow vascular lesions. Microcoils can be used to build a framework or mesh against which microparticulate agents may accumulate.

Vessels embolized with PVA alone tend to recanalize after a few weeks. Although the particle itself is nonabsorbable, the extremely irregular surface of each particle creates a high coefficient of surface friction, which often results in a more proximal adhesion of the particles to the wall of the vessel. Blood flow is usually eliminated

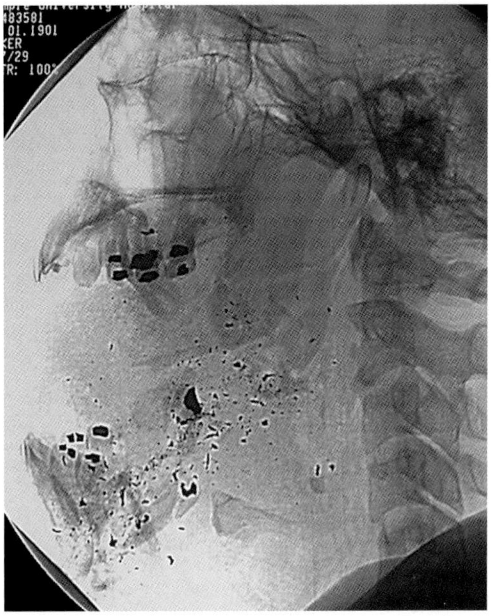

A

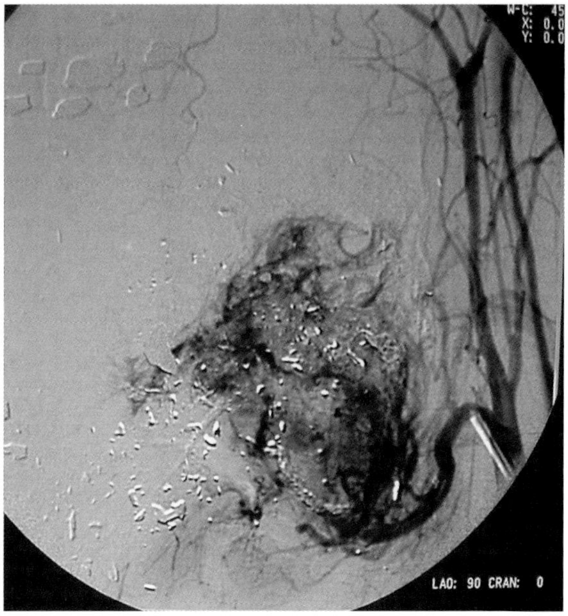

B

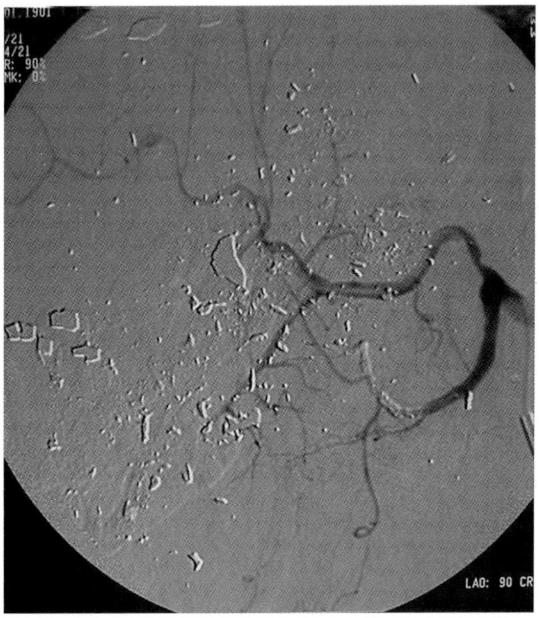

C

Fig. 8.2 **(A)** A 32-year-old male patient with extensive injury secondary to a transfacial gunshot wound to the mandible. **(B)** Diffuse soft tissue injury was evident bilaterally on selective lingual and facial angiography. **(C)** Following embolization with PVA particles and coils angiography shows occlusion of the abnormal branches. As embolizations were performed on the same branches bilaterally, the patient suffered from impaired wound healing of the tongue during his recovery.

initially; however, the thrombus that forms between the particles may eventually recanalize. A more permanent occlusion may be achieved by packing the vessel with high concentrations of smaller PVA particles followed by proximal occlusion with platinum microcoils to reduce arterial pulsations against the occlusive particles that would promote recanalization. In the face of acute trauma, however, a temporary occlusion may be preferable, providing hemostasis in the acute setting, while allowing for revascularization necessary for the healing process over the next few days to weeks.

Another alternative combination to extend the duration of the embolization is a mixture of PVA particles and microfibrillar collagen (Avitene, Microfibrillar collagen. Davol, Inc., Cranston, RI). As previously mentioned, this combination offers several advantages. When mixed in contrast material, microfibrillar collagen forms a colloidal suspension in which the PVA particles remain suspended and somewhat evenly dispersed. This suspension, in turn, facilitates delivery of the particles through the small lumen of the microcatheter, decreasing the likelihood of impacting particles in the catheter and occluding it. This

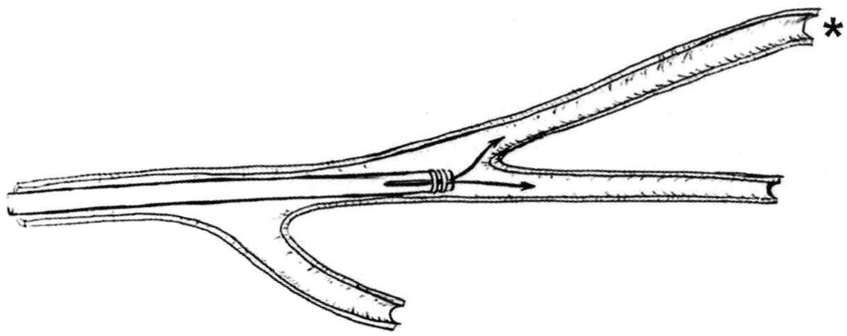

A

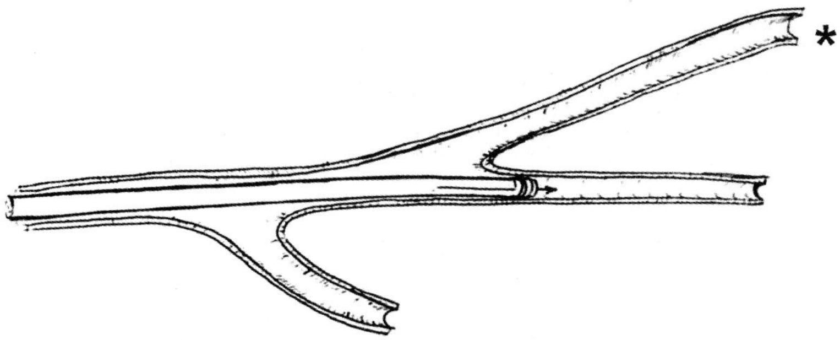

B

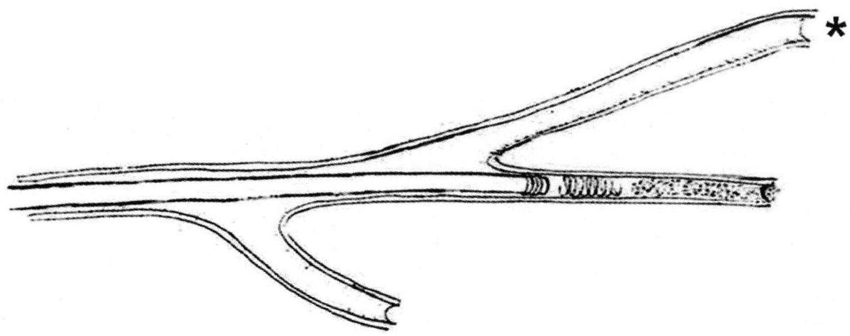

C

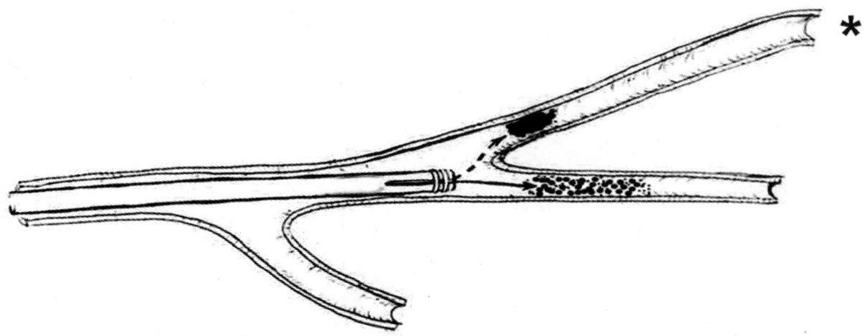

D

Fig. 8.3 (A–C) Selective versus protective embolotherapy. The microcatheter is advanced as selectively as possible into the vessel to be embolized. **(D)** Occasionally, the target vessel cannot be selectively catheterized. The normal branch (*) may be selectively embolized with an absorbable agent such as Gelfoam or autologous blood clot. The abnormal branch can then be embolized from a proximal catheter position with more permanent agents while the temporarily occluded vessel will recannulize within hours.

advantage helps to avoid a time-consuming exchange of catheters. In addition, a more rapid vessel occlusion is achieved. With an average particle size of 50 microns, microfibrillar collagen fills the gaps between the PVA particles to provide a more complete occlusion. Histological studies have shown that microfibrillar collagen in occluded vessels forms a collagen matrix that adheres to both the endothelium and the PVA particles. This combination offers an advantage in that it produces little patient discomfort and it is less likely to pass through

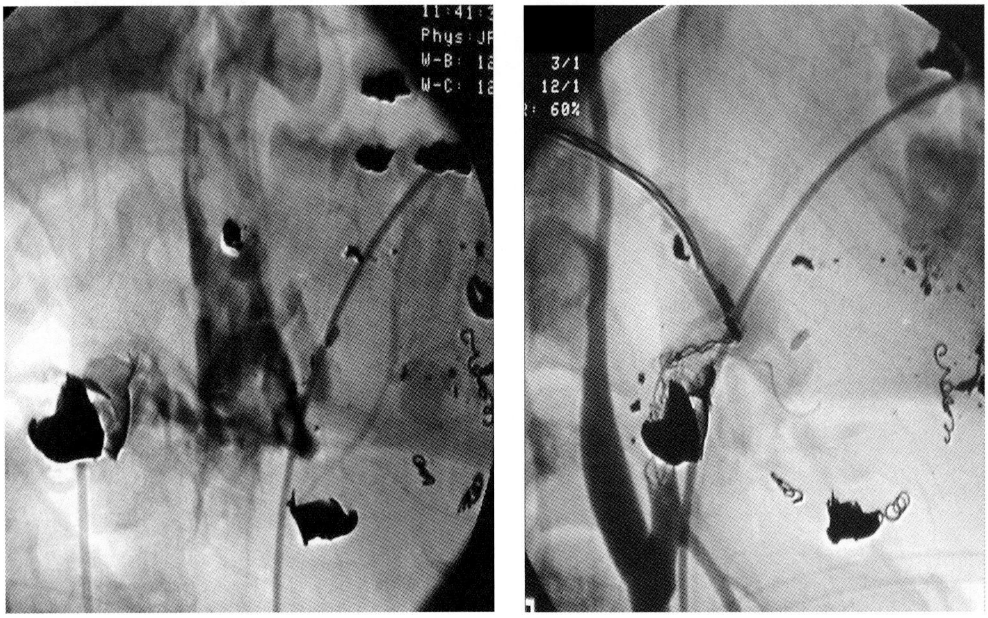

A B

Fig. 8.4 Transcervical gunshot wound resulting with perioral hemorrhage as a result of a carotid-pharyngeal fistula. Control of the patient's airway was provided with intubation. Multiple external carotid artery branches were then embolized with fibered platinum microcoils until hemostasis was achieved.

small anastomoses and injure adjacent normal tissue, yet is significantly faster in occluding vessel than PVA alone.

A new class of particulate microembolic agent has recently become available. Soft, smooth, deformable particles (Embosphere microspheres; BioSphere Medical, Rockland, MA) and liquid PVA compressible microspheres (Bead Block; Terumo, Tokyo, Japan) tend to ovalize when confined, a trait that makes these agents effective in distal embolotherapy. Unlike crystalline PVA particles, they do not adhere to vascular walls. With a lower coefficient of friction, they are more likely to pass more distally in the vascular bed. In the trauma setting, this trait may make these agents less effective at achieving stasis than crystalline PVA.

Coils

Gianturco coils (Cook Inc., Bloomington, IN) were used in the past to reduce flow in large arteriovenous malformations (AVMs) of the extracranial circulation. Fibered, stainless steel Gianturco coils are considerably larger than the microcatheter delivery systems currently used. Vortex (Target Therapeutics/Boston Scientific, Natick, MA) and Nestor coils are the fibered platinum equivalent. Catheters 4F or larger are required with these 0.035 and 0.038 in. coils. Catheters of this size severely limit the distance into which a vessel can be cannulized. The coil itself often does not produce complete thrombosis of the vessel, and may secondarily inhibit further embolization with other agents. Therefore, use of the large coils is limited to occlusion of large vessels in the neck and skull base, usually occurring after penetrating trauma. Larger coils also serve to provide a backup proximal occlusion to impede recanalization of a more distal particulate embolization. MR-compatible platinum coils have largely replaced MR-incompatible stainless steel coils.

A variety of microcoils have been developed for use with the microcatheter systems to facilitate distal deployment in small vessels of the head, neck, and spine. Hilal coils (Cook Inc., Bloomington, IN), the earliest of the fibered microcoils, were effective, but they were relatively stiff and made of stainless steel. These were later replaced by a soft, platinum version that was MR compatible. Platinum microcoils 0.010 in. and 0.016 in. in diameter, with and without polyester fibers, are available for use with microcatheter systems and are supplied in a variety of shapes and lengths (Cook Inc., Bloomington, IN; Cordis Endovascular, Inc., Miami, FL; Boston Scientific, Natick, MA) (**Figs. 8.4–8.12**). Most of these are woven with small polyester fibers to increase their thrombogenicity. These small coils can be deployed just proximal to the nidus of a malformation if it is accessible with a microcatheter. Smaller coils can also be flow directed or floated peripherally if direct access to the nidus cannot be achieved.

The soft, Berenstein Liquid coils (Target Therapeutics/Boston Scientific, Natick, MA) are the most compliant of

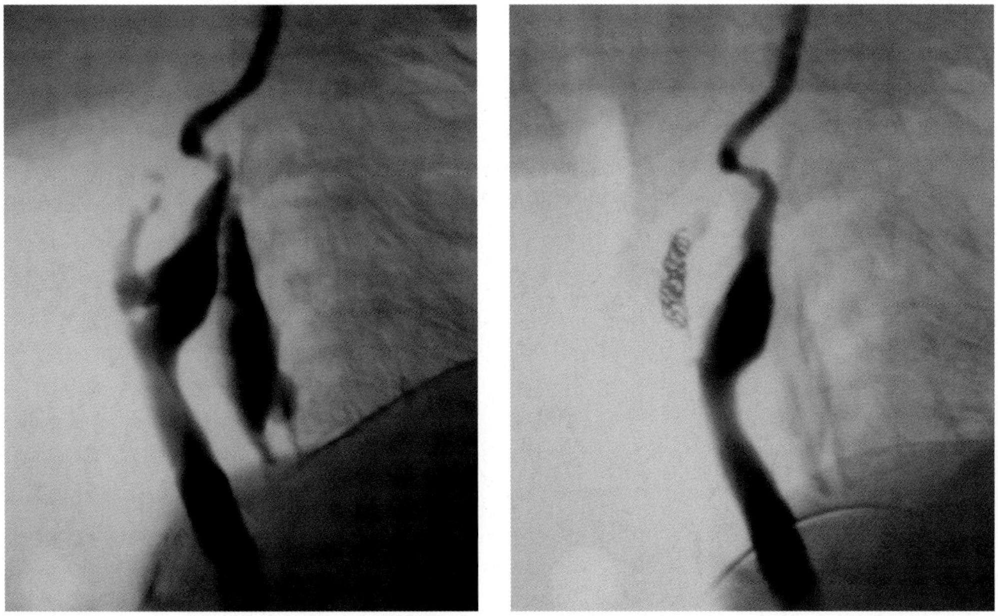

A B

Fig. 8.5 (A) A 26-year-old male with a stab wound to the neck resulting in a carotid-pharyngeal fistula. **(B)** The lesion was successfully treated by external carotid artery sacrifice with fibered platinum microcoils. The injury to the postbulbar internal carotid artery was not felt to require treatment in the acute setting.

all coils and lack fibers (**Fig. 8.13**). These are intended to flow further into an abnormal vessel than the more rigid fibered coils. Because of the small size and extremely soft nature of these coils, distal occlusion is more effectively achieved. In the rare instance where complete stasis cannot be achieved, flow velocity may otherwise be reduced to a point where subsequent particulate or liquid embolization will provide a thorough occlusion of the abnormal vessels. As previously mentioned, coils are frequently deposited proximally in a vessel after particulate embolization to reduce the likelihood of recanalization.

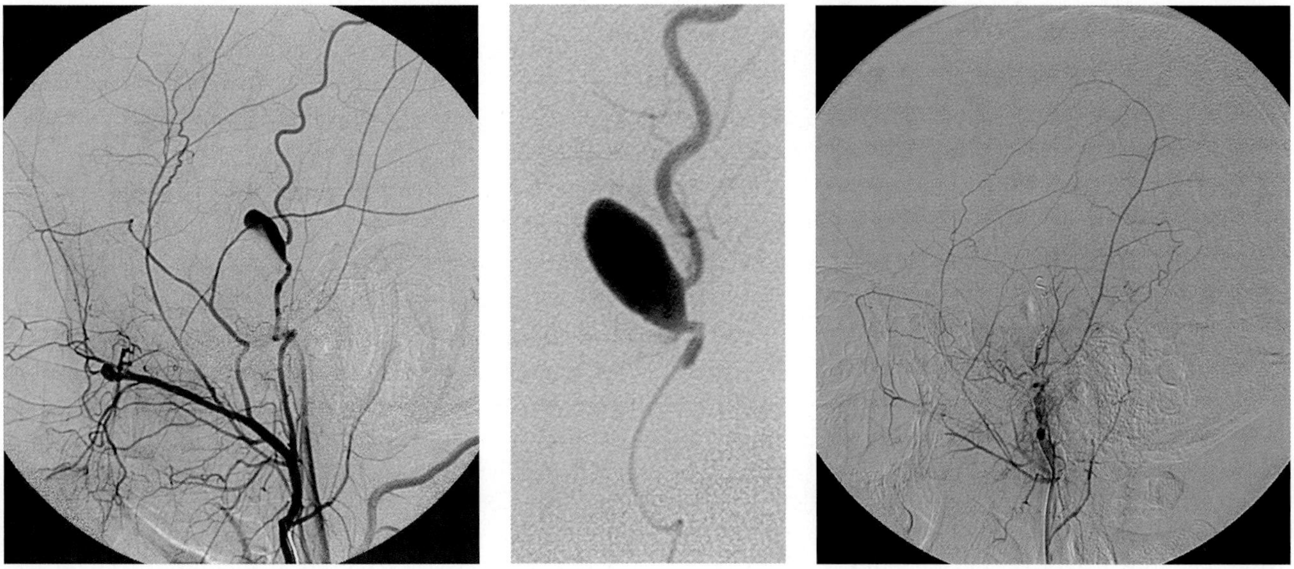

Fig. 8.6 (A) Blunt trauma to the head in a teenage male resulting in formation of a pseudoaneurysm of the superficial temporal artery (STA). **(B)** Selective catheterization of the STA and **(C)** external carotid arteriogram following coil embolization.

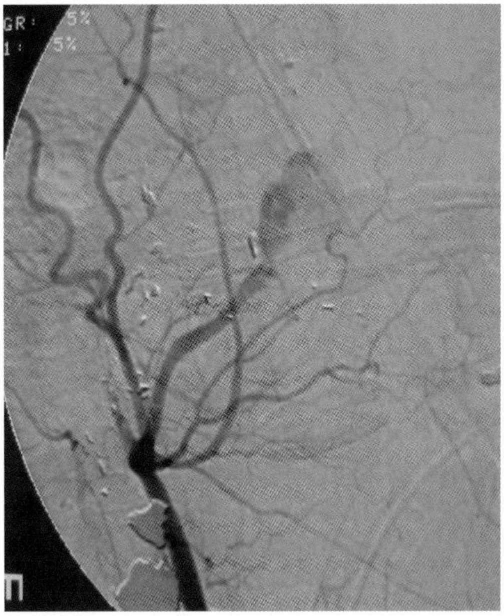

A

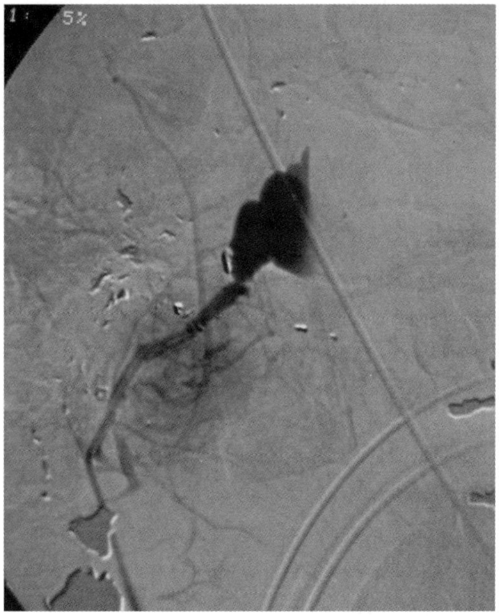

B

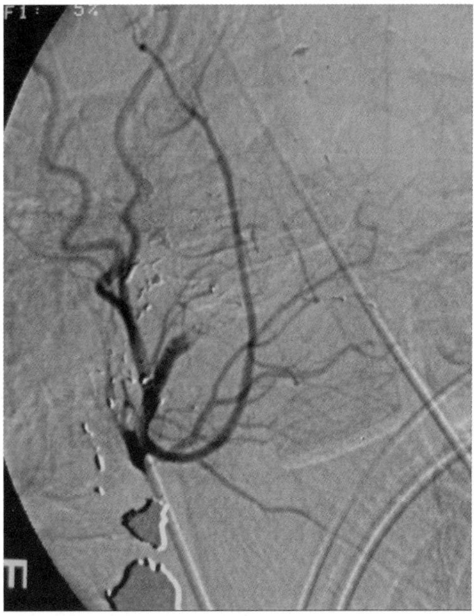

C

Fig. 8.7 A teen-aged male presented to the emergency room with an oronasal hemorrhage following a gunshot wound to the face. **(A)** External carotid artery angiography showed what appeared to be minor bleeding from the internal maxillary artery. **(B)** Selective injection of that vessel, however, demonstrated pseudoaneurysm formation and brisk extravasation of contrast. **(C)** Hemostasis was achieved following the deposition of several fibered platinum microcoils.

The choice of micro- or macrocoils is dependent on the size of the vessel being treated. In the larger cervical arteries in situations where the artery cannot be reconstructed, the larger macrocoils are most effective in achieving hemostasis. The addition of microcoils will provide a more densely packed coil mass. Macrocoils can be used to provide a framework in which to hold the smaller coils in place. Smaller fibered microcoils and "liquid" coils work best in the more distal branches. When occluding larger vessels such as the cervical carotid arteries in which there is still antegrade flow, the operator should anticipate the possibility of distal emboli. When deploying these thrombogenic foreign bodies within the lumen of a still flowing artery, the occlusion is not immediate and may not occur until after several coils have been deployed. During this short period of time, this progressive occlusion predisposes to the formation of thrombus on the surface of the coil mass that can be liberated and embolize the distal vasculature. This risk persists until the target artery has been completely occluded. This risk can be minimized with the use of anticoagulants or flow arrest techniques; however, advanced preparation having several coils available on the

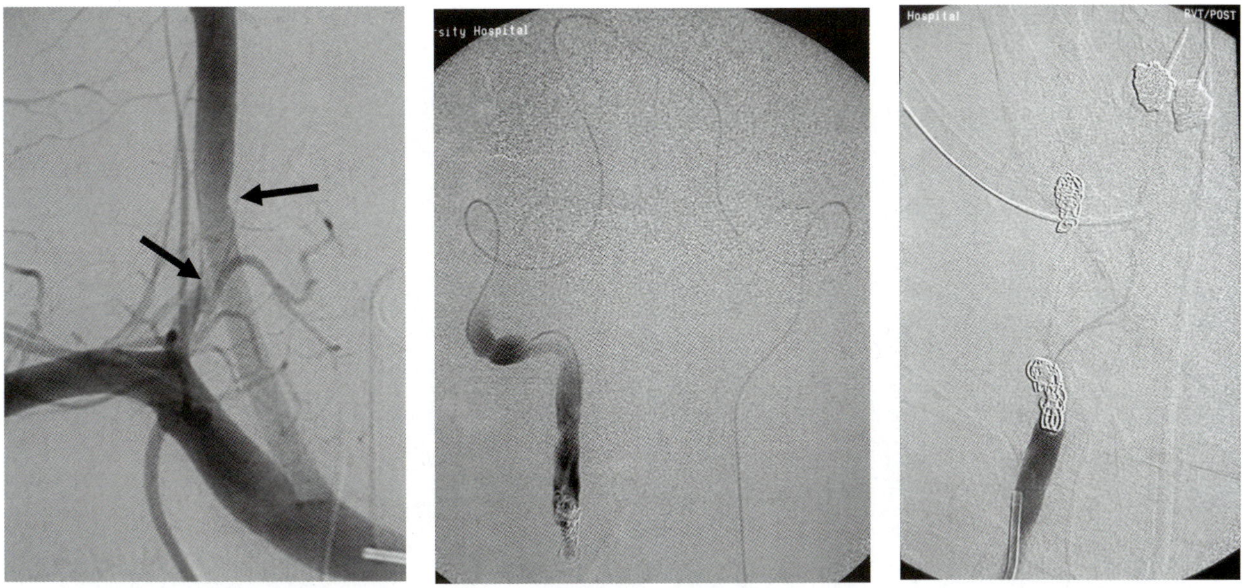

A-C

Fig. 8.8 **(A)** A 23-year-old male patient with gunshot wound to zone 2 of the neck with transection of the right vertebral artery and arterial hemorrhage out both the entrance and exit wounds. Hemostasis of both ends of the transected segment is essential to prevent either antegrade and/or retrograde extravasation. **(B)** Distal control was accomplished by retrograde catheterization via the contralateral left vertebral artery. **(C)** Both proximal and **(B)** distal occlusion was accomplished with multiple fibered platinum microcoils.

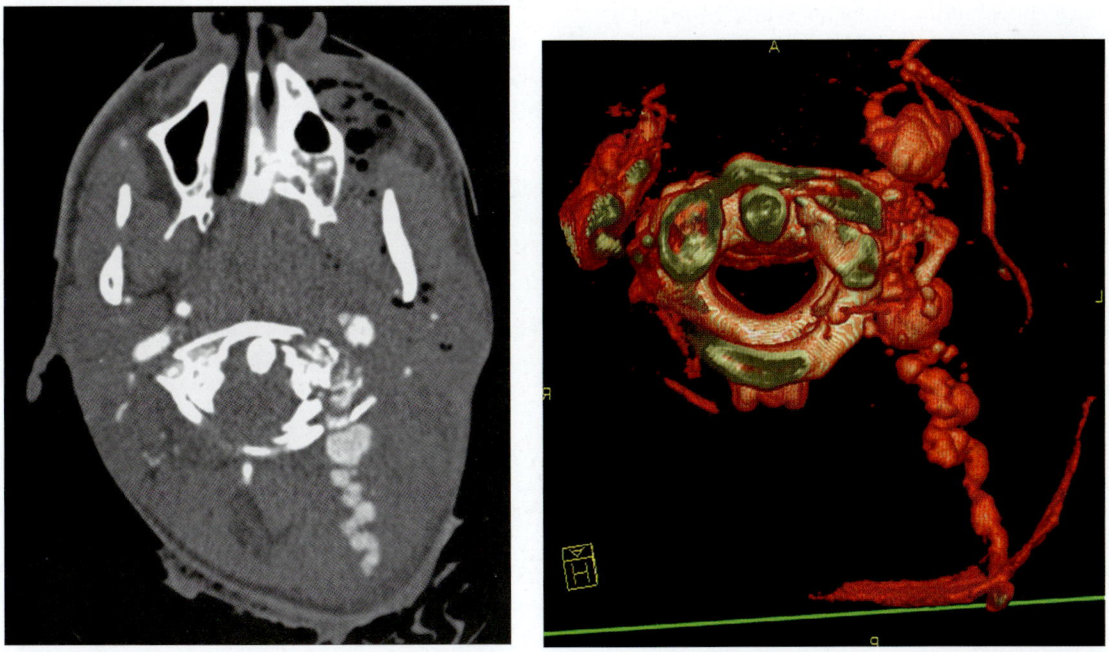

A B

Fig. 8.9 **(A)** Transcervical gunshot wound entering the left maxillary sinus and exiting the ipsilateral side of the upper neck posteriorly. Although no active bleeding was noted on transport to computed tomography (CT), initial source images of the CT angiography (CTA) examination showed the patient had begun to hemorrhage out her exit wound. **(B–D)** Axial and 3-D reconstructed images suggested the hemorrhage was from the carotid and/or vertebral arteries. An incidental finding of a contralateral PCOM aneurysm was also identified (not shown). Temporary hemostasis was achieved by placing a finger in the exit wound as the patient was transported from CT to special procedures.

(Continued on page 152)

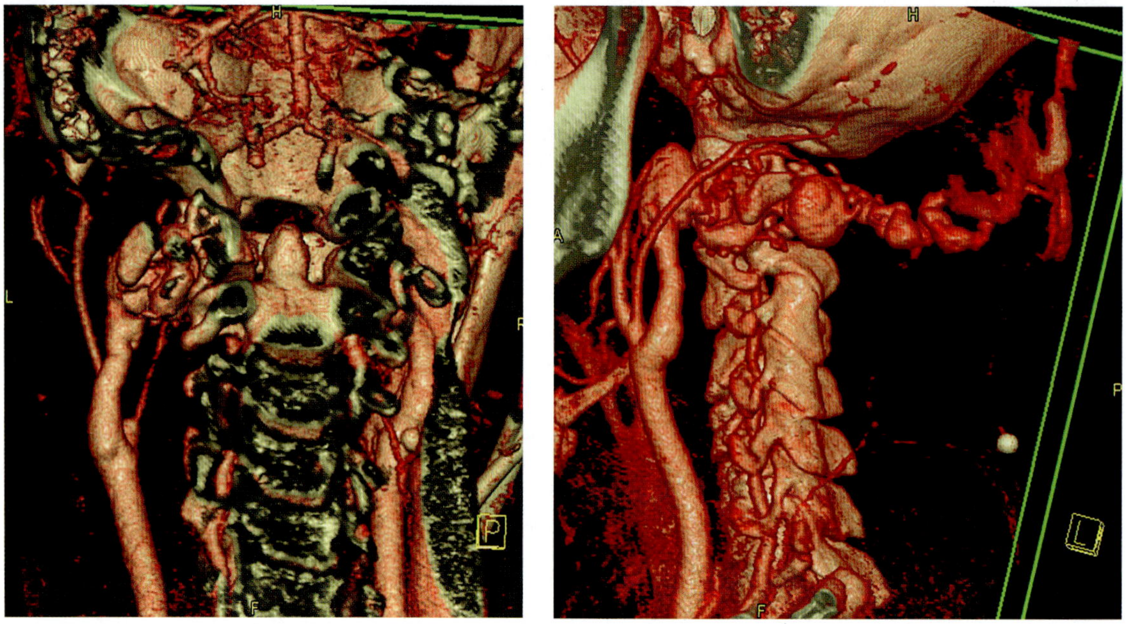

C D

Fig. 8.9 *(Continued)*

bench for deployment in rapid succession is often the most effective measure. Examples of this situation include the embolization of partially transected arteries that are not amenable to stent repair and in the management of the larger carotid-cavernous sinus fistula in which carotid artery sacrifice might be deemed the best therapeutic alternative. The interventional management of aneurysms with platinum detachable coils is distinctly different from management with nondetachable coils. This will be discussed in greater detail in the section, "Aneurysms."

Balloons

The advantages of balloon embolization include (1) the ability to occlude a vessel at a precise location; (2) the ability to flow navigate attached, partially inflated

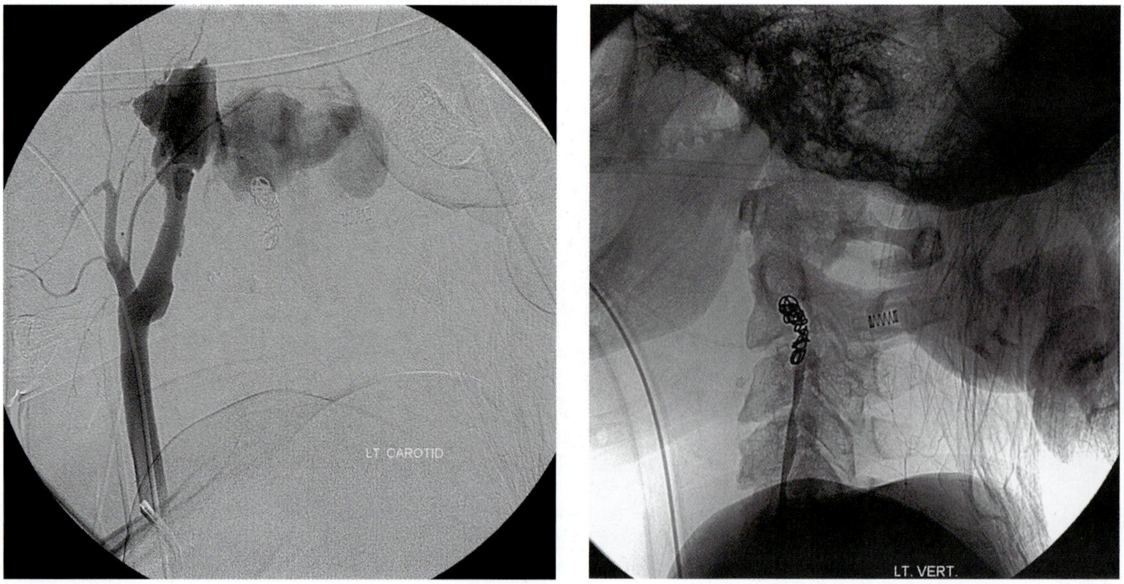

A B

Fig. 8.10 **(A)** With the finger of the physician volunteer still in the exit wound, angiography demonstrated transections of both the left internal carotid and **(B)** left vertebral arteries as well as the left jugular vein. A large fistulous tract to the exit wound was evident **(A)**. **(C)** The carotid and vertebral arteries were successfully embolized with fibered platinum coils

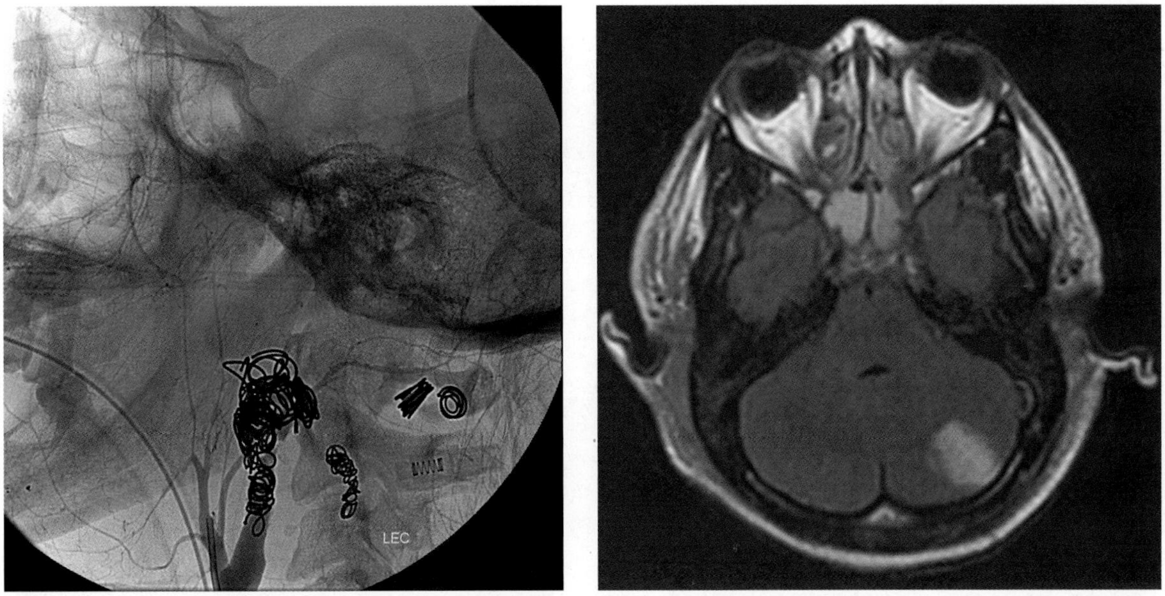

C D

Fig. 8.10 *(Continued)* Cerebral perfusion was maintained by the right internal carotid and vertebral arteries via patent anterior and both posterior communicating arteries. **(D)** The patient survived the event with only a minor cerebellar infarct.

balloons to distal locations along a tortuous course; (3) the ability to rapidly occlude large vessels; and (4) the ability to repeatedly inflate, deflate, and reposition the balloon until the desired position is achieved (**Figs. 8.14, 8.15, 8.16, 8.17, 8.18, 8.19,** and **8.20**).

The original latex balloons were manually bound to microcatheter assemblies with latex ligatures. Although effective, this technique was tedious and time consuming. Latex (Gold Valve; Nycomed Ingenor, Paris, France) and silicone elastomer (detachable silicone balloon [DSB]; Target Therapeutics) balloons with mitered valves were subsequently developed to facilitate preparation, attachment, and detachment. Although silicone detachable balloons are no longer in production, a rerelease of the device is anticipated in the near future.

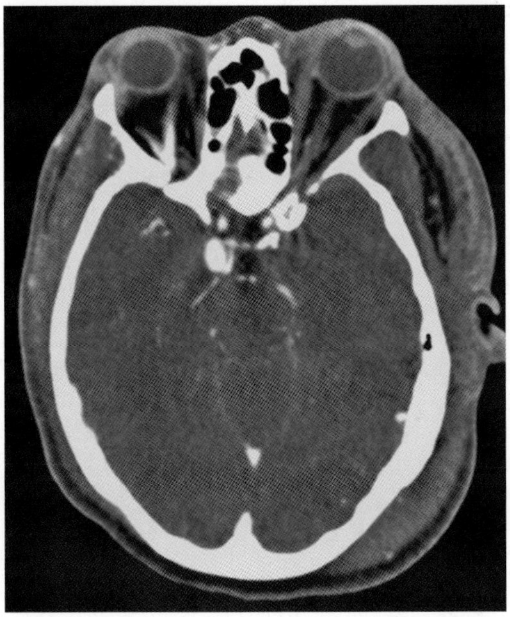

A

Fig. 8.11 Twenty-four hours following embolization of the carotid-vertebral-cutaneous fistula, repeat computed tomographic angiography confirmed occlusion of the fistula and better defined the contralateral right posterior communicating artery aneurysm on **(A)** 2-D and

(Continued on page 154)

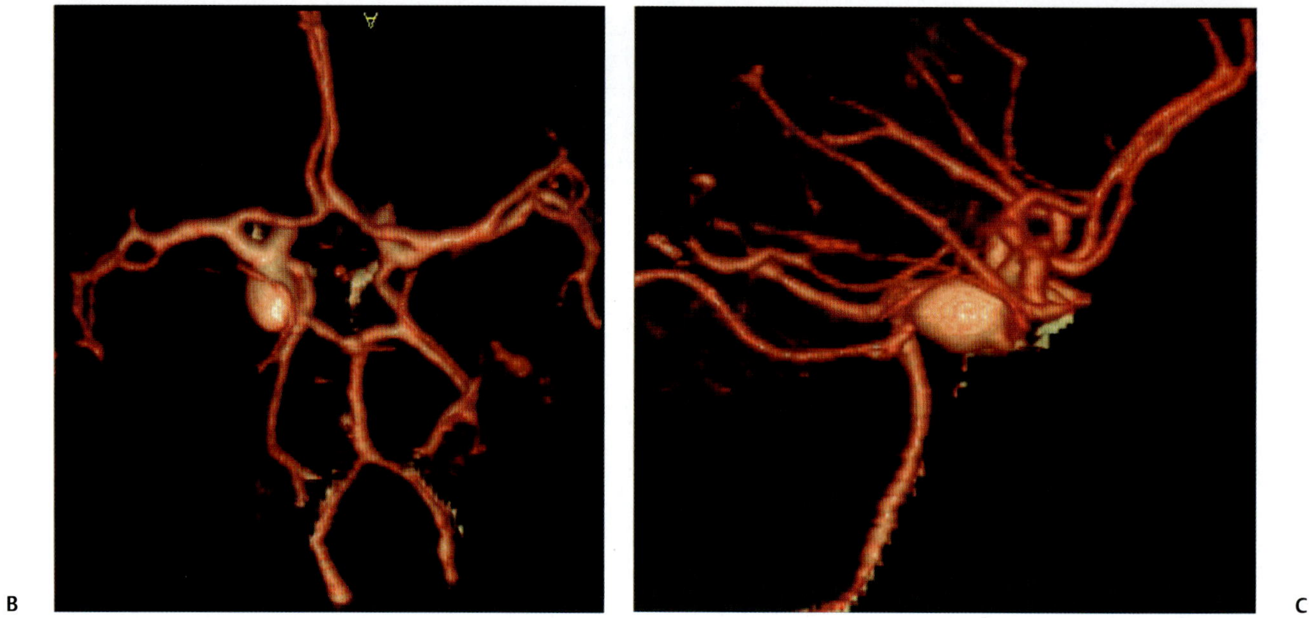

Fig. 8.11 *(Continued)* **(B, C)** 3-D CT angiography.

Latex and silicone balloons have different properties with respect to distensibility, time to deflation, and surface-friction characteristics, features to be considered when selecting a balloon for a specific pathology. Latex balloons are more distensible and compliant than silicone balloons and therefore will more readily conform to the shape of a vessel while reducing the risk of vascular rupture. Latex also has a far greater coefficient of surface friction than that of silicone balloons, a feature that reduces the likelihood of balloon migration. These properties make latex balloons the preferred device for occluding large, high-flow vessels, as in trapping procedures, and for treating carotid-cavernous sinus fistula.[7]

Silicone balloons, on the contrary, are relatively noncompliant and inflate to a preformed shape. Therefore, they are less likely than latex balloons to mold to the vascular contour. Because of their lower coefficient of friction, they are more likely than latex balloons to migrate after detachment. Because the Silastic (Dow Corning Corp., Midland, MI) material in silicone balloons is less porous than latex, silicone balloons tend to remain inflated longer, averaging greater than 24 weeks versus 2 to 4 weeks to deflation time of latex balloons.

Liquid Embolic Agents

Among the most notable liquid embolic agents are *N*-butyl cyanoacrylate (NBCA), (Histocryl; B. Braun, Melsungen, Germany) and an FDA-approved acrylic tissue adhesive (Trufill; Cordis Endovascular, Inc., Johnson & Johnson, Miami, FL). The acrylic tissue adhesive rapidly polymerizes on contact with any ionic substance, such as blood, saline, ionic contrast medium, and vascular epithelium. To extend working time, polymerization time may be prolonged with the mixture of glacial acetic acid and/or oil-based contrast agents such as ethiodized oil (Ethiodol; Savage Laboratories, Malville, NY).

The flow velocity of an arteriovenous shunt may be reduced with other agents such as coils before NBCA is infused to minimize the risk of errant passage of glue into the venous system. The main advantage of this tissue adhesive is its ability to rapidly occlude high-flow AVMs with a result more permanent than that possible with particulate agents. NBCA is more likely than particulate agents to reach and occlude the nidus of an AVM.

NBCA has several disadvantages. First, the catheter must be rapidly withdrawn after each injection of NBCA, resulting in frequent, time-consuming catheter exchanges. Second, if the lesion was difficult to access initially, considerable time may be required to reposition a microcatheter into the vessel a second or third time if additional infusions are required. Third, failure to withdraw the catheter rapidly augments the risk of gluing the catheter in place. Fourth, complications secondary to incorrect polymerization time are associated with risks. Too short a polymerization time may result in adhesion of the catheter to the vessel wall or an occlusion too proximal to the nidus allowing for collateralization. A too prolonged polymerization time may result in passage of glue beyond

A
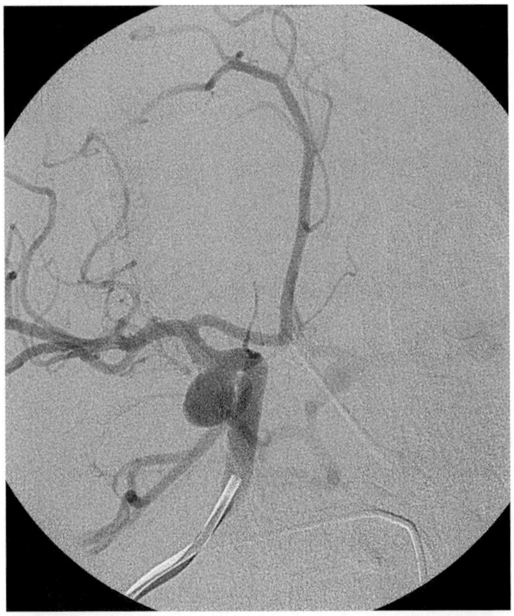
B
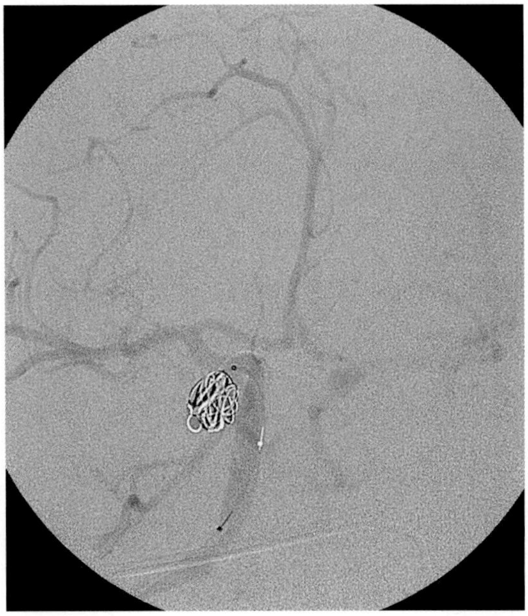
C
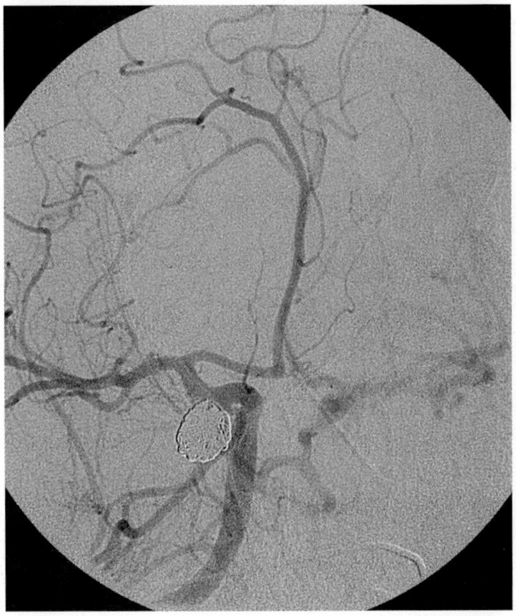

Fig. 8.12 (A) The following day, having stabilized from her gunshot wound, the patient's right posterior communication artery aneurysm was **(B,C)** successfully coil embolized with detachable platinum coils.

the target lesion and may result in a pulmonary embolus or solidification in the venous outflow tract of a malformation prior to arterial control, which increases the risk of periprocedural hemorrhage. Fifth, because the resultant glue cast is rigid, patient discomfort and a foreign-body sensation could occur after embolization of lesions of the face, mouth, tongue, or neck. These characteristics make the endovascular use of acrylic adhesives in the acute trauma setting far less practical.

The increased demand for interventional procedures has spurred extensive research to develop embolic agents and devices that are safer and more permanent than the current options. One newly released nonadhesive liquid embolic system (Onyx; MicroTherapeutics, Inc., Irvine, CA) appears to be safer and more effective than NBCA in the treatment of high-flow arterial venous shunts. As a nonadhesive, flexible polymer, Onyx offers all the advantages of NBCA without the risk of gluing a catheter in place or the need to exchange catheters after each infusion. The risk of a distal embolic event is still of concern. For these reasons, the use of NBCA or Onyx is limited to the occlusion of high-flow AVMs of the brain

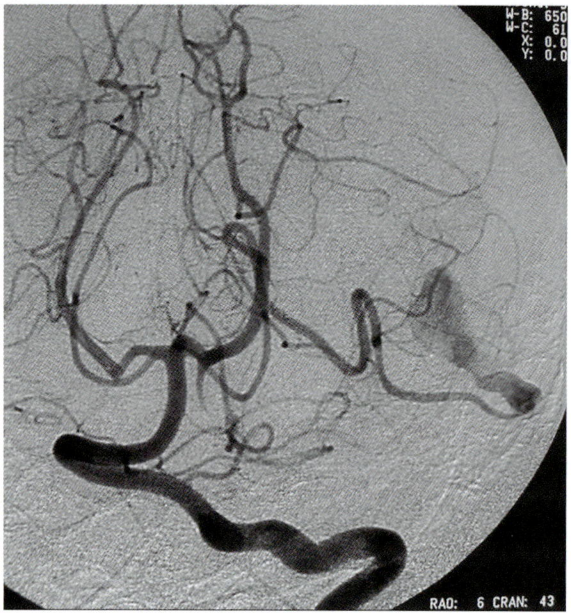

A

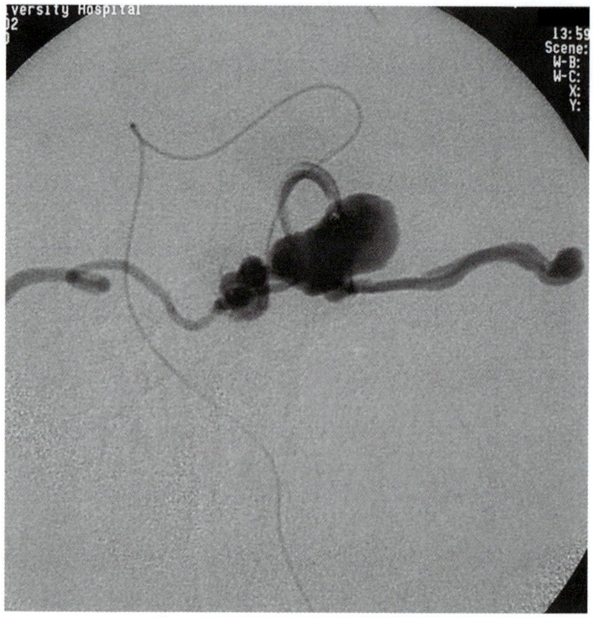

B

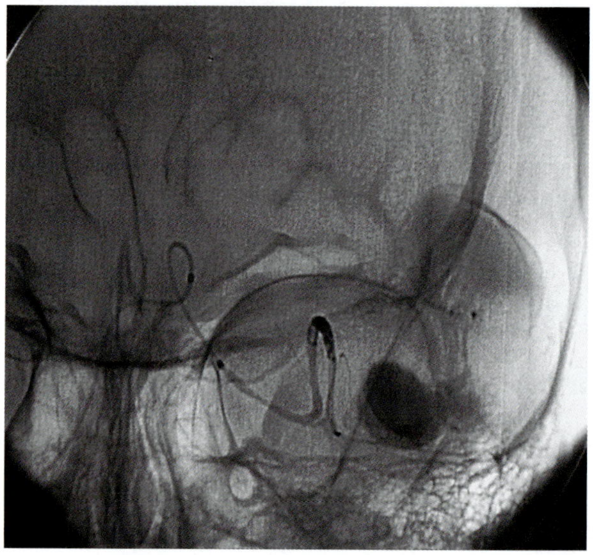

C

Fig. 8.13 A female college athlete suffered an intracranial hemorrhage following a relatively trivial head injury during a sports event. **(A,B)** Diagnostic angiography revealed a small arterial venous fistula of the posterior temporal artery in the base of the left temporal lobe. **(C)** Although the artery was successfully embolized with multiple injectable platinum microcoils, the patient suffered an unfortunate intraprocedural rehemorrhage that required urgent surgical evacuation.

and spinal canal. Although subject to personal preference, liquid embolic agents have no role in the acute trauma setting.

Sclerosing Agents

Absolute ethanol is the prototypic sclerosing agent. Solutions opacified with metrizamide powder have produced excellent results in the obliteration of large vascular malformations. Sodium tetradecyl sulfate (Sotradecol; Bioniche Pharma, Lake Forest, IL) behaves similarly to alcohol but with less associated pain. Alcohol has been included in particulate admixtures, most notably with microfibrillar collagen (Avitene; Davol Inc.) and PVA particles, as previously discussed. Aggressive clinical monitoring during embolotherapy by an anesthesiologist is essential to reduce pain, and to preserve an airway when lesions of the oropharynx and neck are treated.

The result of embolotherapy with ethanol compared with the particulate agents and with NBCA has been a more permanent occlusion of abnormal vessels without the inherent risks associated with tissue adhesives. The use of ethanol in acute trauma is discouraged as particulate agents and coils are simply faster to use and at lower risk to the patient when a rapid stasis of bleeding is the principle goal.

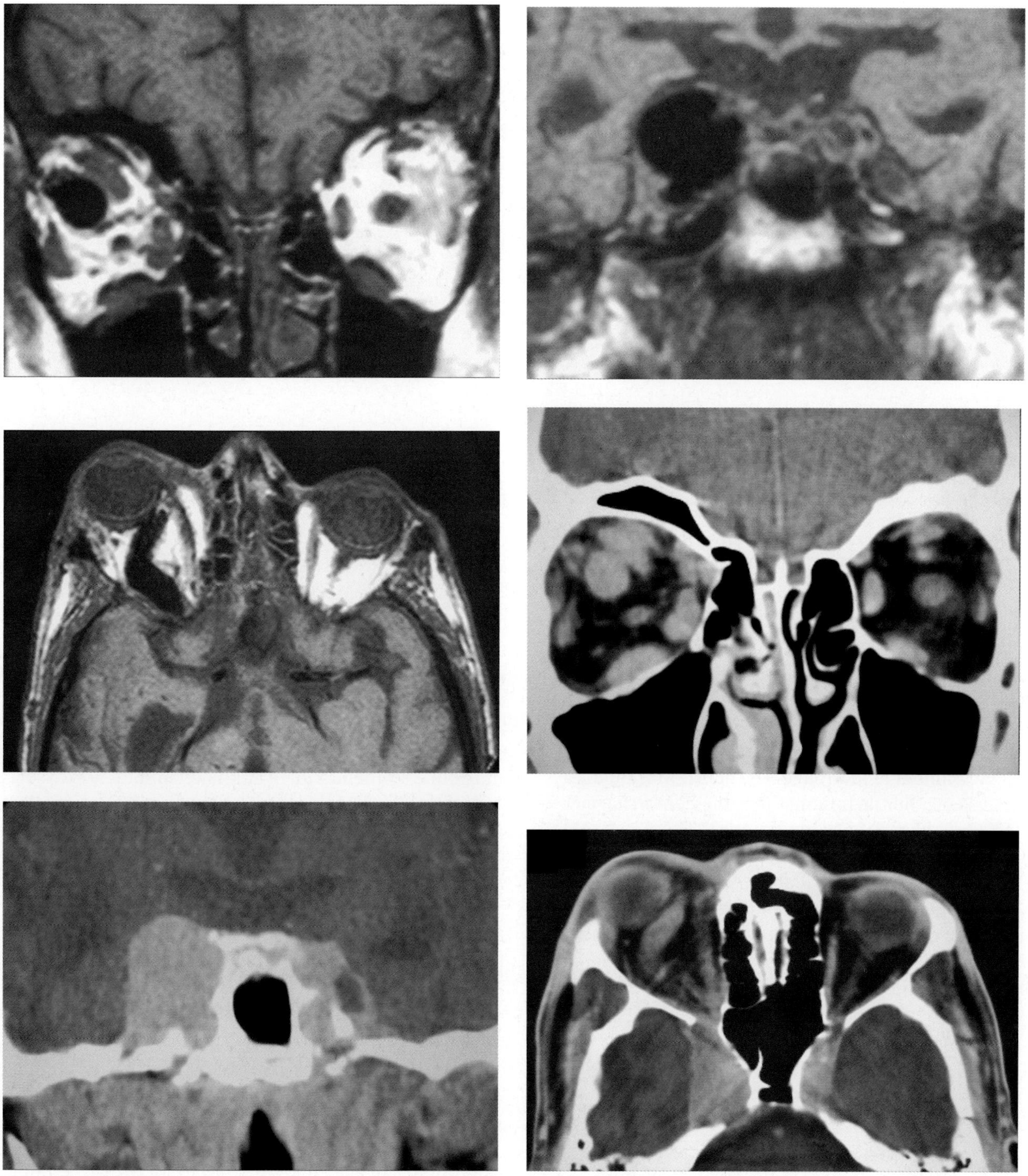

B

D

F

Fig. 8.14 Carotid–cavernous sinus fistula is usually diagnosed on the basis of history and physical examination. The diagnosis can be confirmed by both computed tomography (CT) and magnetic resonance imaging (MRI). **(A,B)** Coronal MRI and **(D,E)** CT images demonstrate enlargement of the superior ophthalmic vein with engorgement of the cavernous sinus. **(C)** Axial MRI and **(F)** CT images demonstrate how the enlarged veins produce the exophthalmia. The marked signal void noted on MRI denotes high velocity flow.

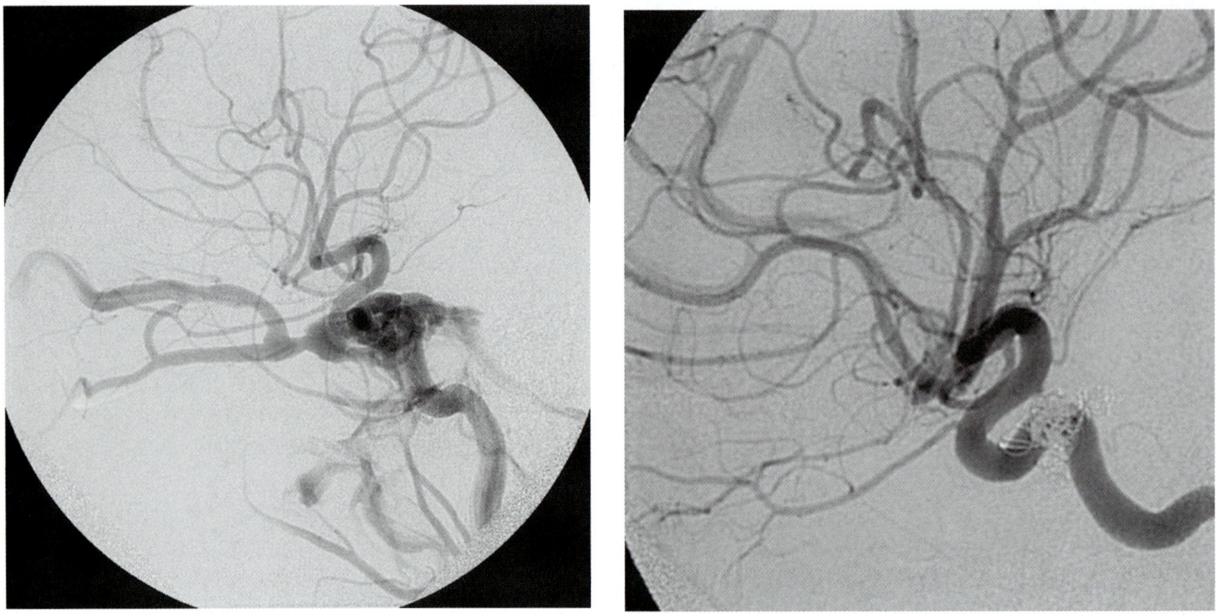

A B

Fig. 8.15 A middle-aged male presented to the emergency room with a painful, pulsatile exophthalmia following a head injury sustained in an automobile accident. **(A)** Angiography confirmed the presence of a direct carotid-cavernous sinus fistula that was subsequently treated with **(B)** multiple detachable platinum coils.

Aneurysms

Not infrequently, a patient will present with a head injury and a subarachnoid hemorrhage. The question should always be asked, "Did the trauma cause the hemorrhage or did the hemorrhage lead to the trauma?" These patients usually present with a poor neurological status, and a reliable history is often not available. All trauma patients who present with a subarachnoid hemorrhage would benefit from a CTA examination at the time of their initial CT assessment. If an aneurysm is identified, conventional angiography should become a priority with the intent of treating either endovascularly or with conventional surgery. The urgency to treat an aneurysm is based on two clinical concerns: (1) the physician cannot determine with certainty whether the aneurysm or the trauma was the cause of the hemorrhage. If the aneurysm was the cause, the risk of rerupture over the next 2 months is nearly 50%; and (2) regardless of the etiology, all patients with subarachnoid hemorrhage are at risk of vasospasm over the ensuing 2 weeks. As the principle treatment for vasospasm is volume expansion and hypertension, patients with untreated aneurysms are at increased risk of rupture whether the aneurysm was the cause of the bleed or not. In the face of an acute subarachnoid hemorrhage, it should be assumed that the aneurysm identified is the cause of the hemorrhage and it should be treated as early as possible before vasospasm occurs.

Historically, endovascular management of aneurysms was based on the endosaccular deployment of appropriately sized latex balloons. Developed in Russia by Dr. Fedor Serbinenko in 1974, the technique was associated with a high incidence of aneurysmal rupture. This complication was believed to be as a result of the rigid balloons exerting an asymmetric pressure on the wall of the aneurysm. The resulting deformity of the aneurysm frequently led to rupture. Although the use of balloons to treat aneurysms quickly fell out of favor, Dr. Serbinenko's work provided the momentum that eventually led to the fields of interventional neuroradiology and endovascular neurosurgery. The detachable-balloon technique was eventually replaced with a detachable-coil technique developed by Dr. Guido Guglielmi in 1991. Numerous modifications of the Guglielmi detachable coil (GDC; Target Therapeutics/Boston Scientific) have been made over the years, but the basic design remains the most widely used device for embolotherapy of intracranial aneurysms to date.

The endovascular management of aneurysms requires a coil with unique properties, including control and recoverability, softness, conformability, and maximum packability. GDC coils are long, nonfibered platinum microcoils fused to a guidewire. These coils, the first to gain FDA approval, can be positioned, withdrawn, and repositioned repeatedly until the desired position is obtained. Detachment is then achieved by passing

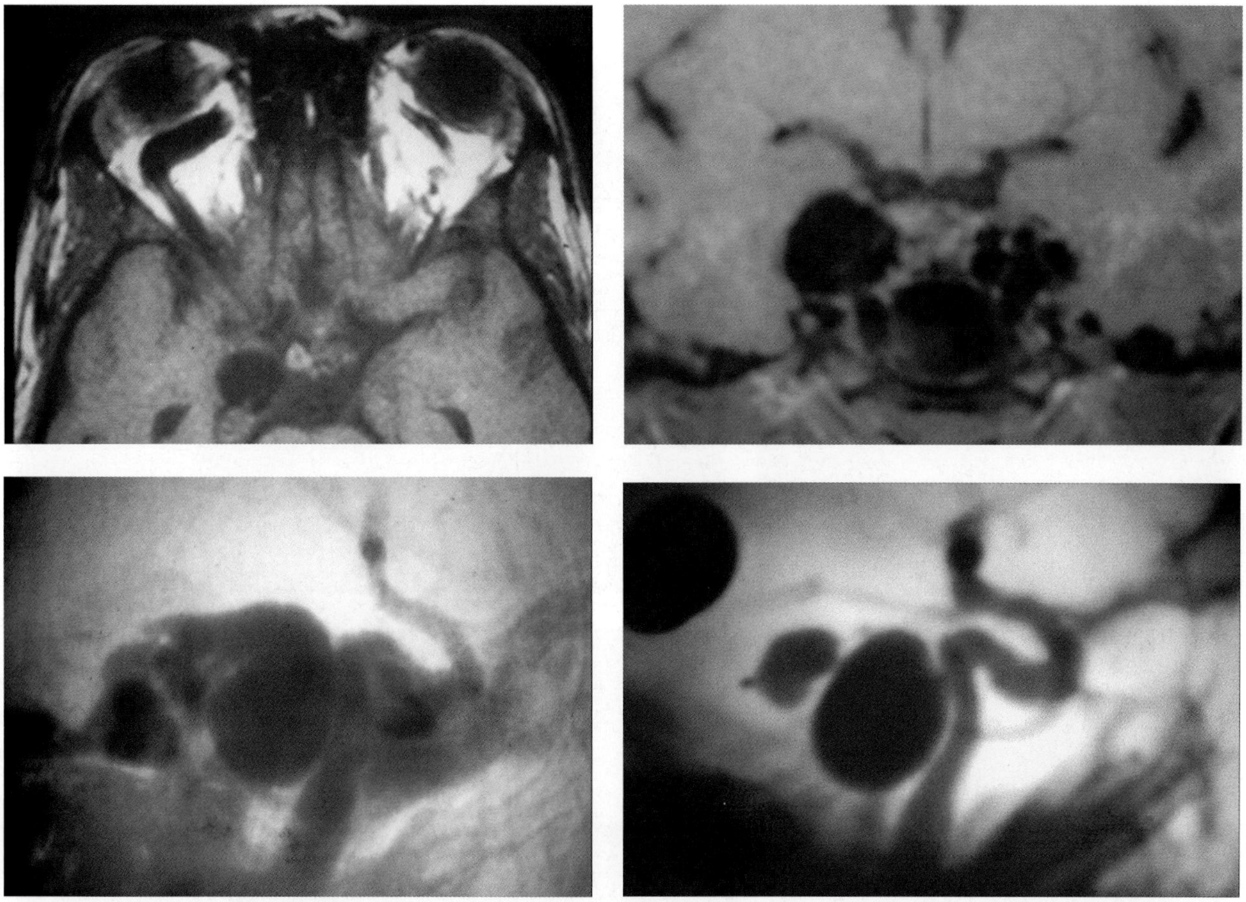

B

D

Fig. 8.16 A 39-year-old female with bilateral, painful pulsatile exophthalmia following an automobile accident. **(A,B)** Magnetic resonance imaging and **(C)** conventional angiography, confirmed the presence of a carotid–cavernous sinus fistula that was then treated with **(D)** detachable latex balloons .

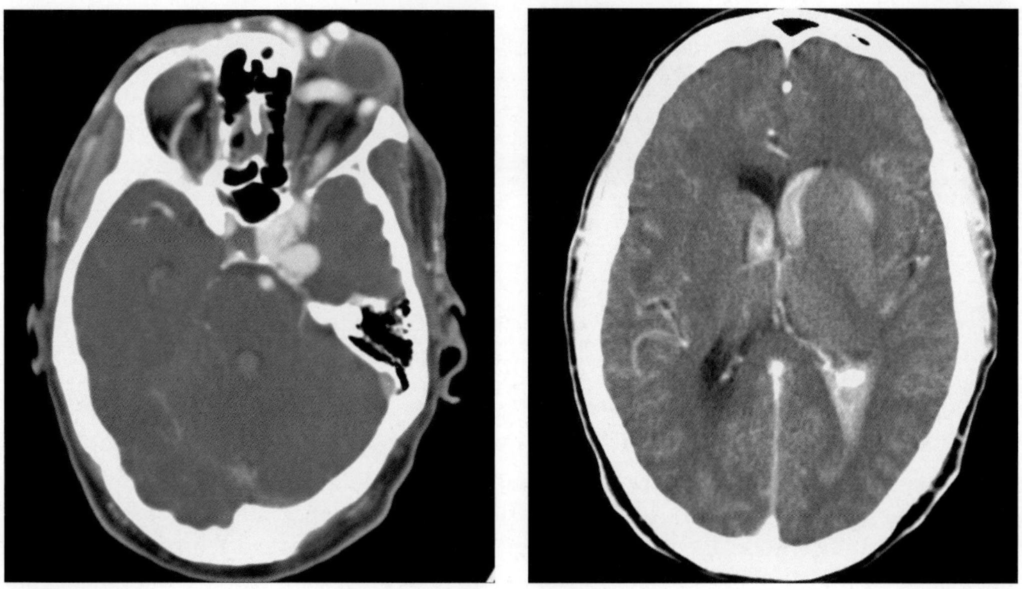

A

B

Fig. 8.17 This 44-year-old male presented with a severe headache. **(B,E)** His radiographic workup showed subarachnoid and intraventricular hemorrhage. **(A)** Two-dimensional and **(D)** 3-D computed tomographic (CT) angiography revealed not only a left anterior cerebral artery aneurysm but also a C-C fistula of the ipsilateral internal carotid artery. **(C,F)** CT perfusion imaging was normal.

(Continued on page 160)

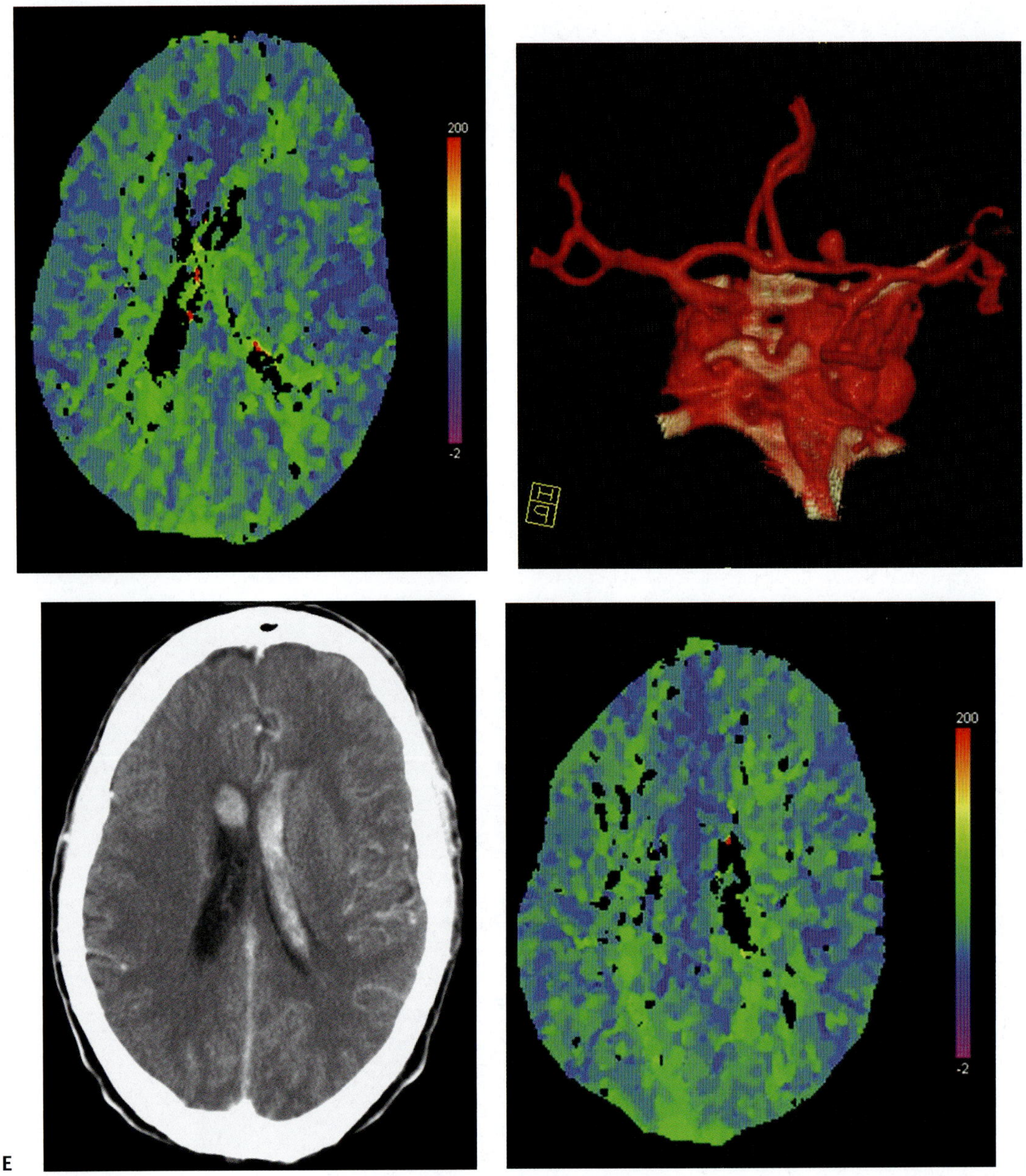

C D E F

Fig. 8.17 *(Continued)*

a low-voltage, low-amperage current through the guidewire to hydrolyze the connection between the guidewire and the coil. The current also initiates platelet and RBC aggregation, theoretically promoting thrombosis. This coil has been used principally in the endovascular treatment of aneurysms because the conformable platinum coil exerts a minimal and symmetrical pressure on the wall of the aneurysm. This feature reduces the risk of rupture, a problem inherent with the use of rigid coils and balloons.

A newer GDC coil called the Matrix coil is coated with a bioactive copolymer that is intended to promote fibrosis of the occluded lumen and improve the permanence of the occlusion. Micrus Corporation (San, Jose, CA) produces a line of coils including a platinum coil and a bioactive coil containing a copolymer core (Cerecyte). Functionally similar to the GDC coil, they differ in that they are detached thermally rather than hydrolytically, and the copolymer is in the core of the coil rather than on the surface, a feature that appears to reduce the risk of recanalization. Another device, the Hydrocoil (MicroVention, Aliso Viejo, CA) is unique in that it is coated with a hydrogel that expands after deployment.

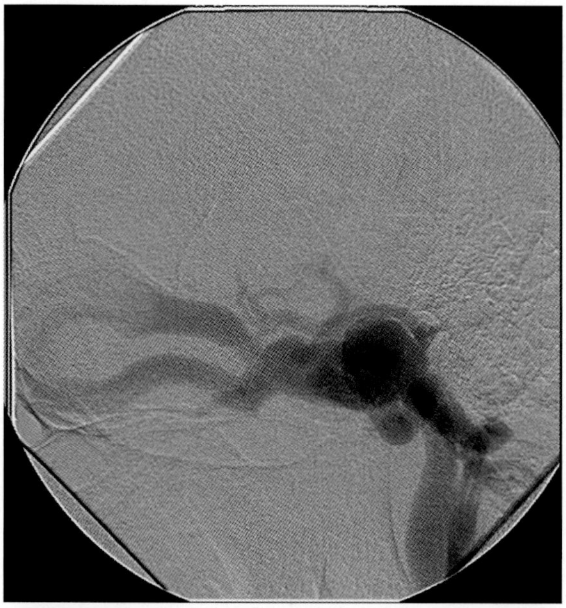

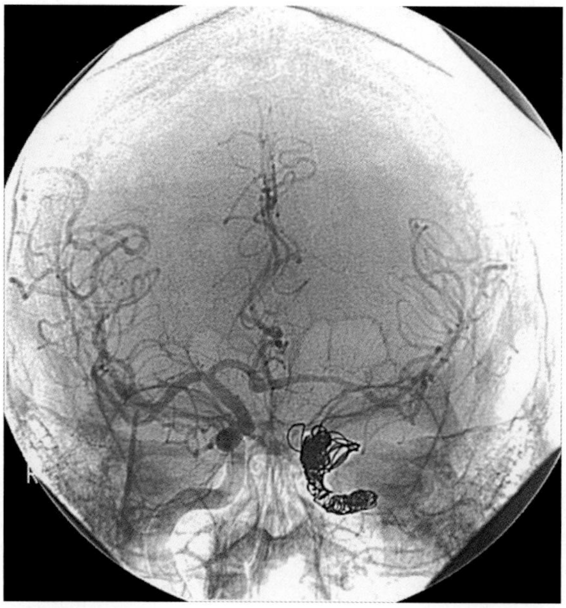

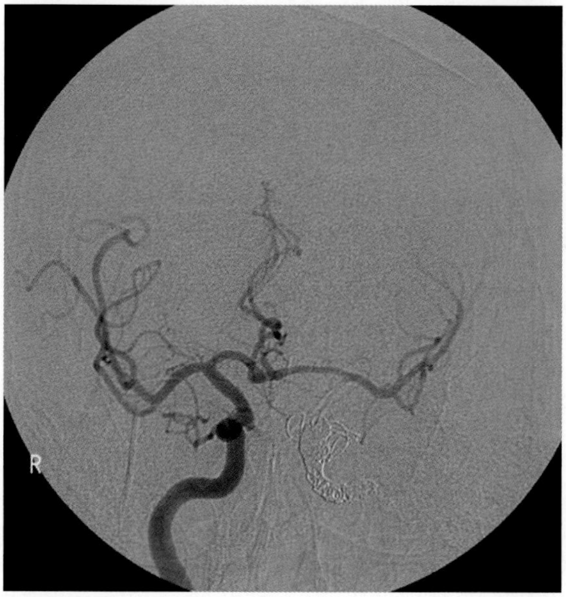

Fig. 8.18 **(A)** Angiography confirmed the carotid–cavernous sinus fistula, but did not demonstrate antegrade flow to the left anterior cerebral artery aneurysm from the left internal carotid artery. In the face of an acutely ruptured aneurysm, occlusion of the fistula and reestablishment of flow to the distal left internal carotid artery was deemed to pose a high risk of rerupture of the aneurysm. A carotid sacrifice was therefore performed with placement of coils across the point of fistulization. **(B,C)** Postembolization angiography of the right internal carotid artery showed collateral flow to the left anterior and middle cerebral arteries but nonvisualization of the aneurysm. This was felt to be as a result of reversal of flow. On follow-up, the aneurysm did not recanalize.

Until recently, endovascular therapy could be offered only to patients with aneurysms of a configuration that were amenable to coiling. The aneurysm had to have a relatively small neck that could hold the detached coils in place in the lumen of the aneurysm and out of the parent artery. The balloon-assist technique uses extremely soft, compliant, nondetachable balloon catheters made of a silicone-based Silastic elastomer (Hyperform; Micro Therapeutics, Inc., Irvine, CA). When inflated across the neck of an aneurysm, this balloon catheter facilitates coil packing in aneurysms with wide necks that were previously considered untreatable from an endovascular approach. The development of the Neuroform stent (Target Therapeutics/Boston Scientific, Fremont, CA) further increased the number of wide-necked aneurysms that would be amenable to embolotherapy. The soft, self-expanding nitinol stent is deployed across the neck of the aneurysm. If the aneurysm is unruptured, the stent is left in place for several weeks to allow for assimilation of the ends of the stent into the arterial walls distal and proximal to the aneurysm neck. This assimilation stabilizes the stent so that subsequent coil embolization through the interstices of the stent can be performed more safely. Covered stents have yet to be

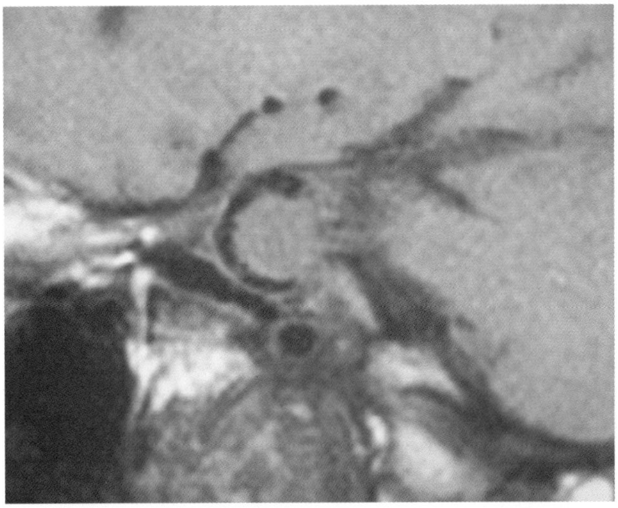
A

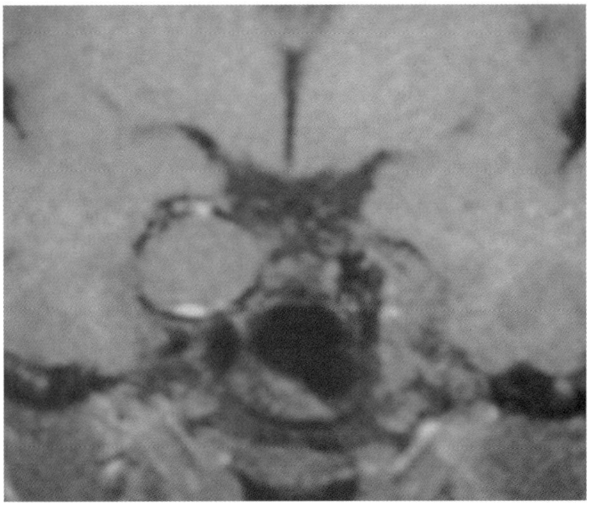
B

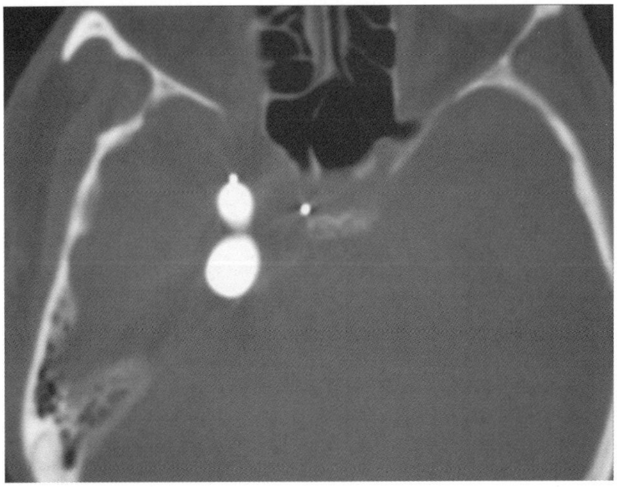
C

Fig. 8.19 Cross-sectional imaging can also be useful in following patients treated who have undergone endovascular therapy. **(A,B)** Two patients treated for C-C fistula, magnetic resonance imaging and magnetic resonance angiography can identify reestablishment of flow, whereas **(C)** computed tomography can monitor the position of the implants. Computed tomographic angiography may be helpful in following patients with nonmetallic implants; however, the metallic artifact inherent with platinum coils limits the utility of this modality in postprocedural assessment following coil embolization.

developed for use intracranially, although the Jostent covered coronary graft stent (Abbott Laboratories, Abbott Park, IL) and the Wallgraft covered stent (Boston Scientific) have been used to successfully treat pseudoaneurysms in the cervical segments of the carotid and vertebral arteries.

Technically, coil embolization of aneurysms is accomplished with the coaxial catheterization of the aneurysm lumen with microcatheters of 2.7F outer diameter or less (**Figs. 8.11** and **8.12**). Once catheter position is confirmed with an endolumenal aneurysmogram, the coils are then slowly advanced into the aneurysm lumen. Although extremely soft, coils are constructed with either a spiral shape or a more complex configuration designed to promote deployment within the aneurysm and to promote a higher packing density. Unlike coil embolization of large arteries, aneurysms may thrombose with only a solitary coil even if very little platinum is present. In this situation, the aneurysm will likely recanalize and leave the patient at risk of rerupture. Further coil embolization once the aneurysm has thrombosed may lead to a displacement of the thrombus back into the parent artery, possibly resulting in a distal thromboembolic complication, which in the acute traumatic setting may not be amenable to thrombolytic therapy. It is therefore recommended that patients be anticoagulated during the embolization procedure. To minimize the risk of intraprocedural hemorrhage, it is our practice to heparinize the patient with an intravenous bolus of 2000 to 3000 units after the first coil has been deployed. If the aneurysm is wide necked and there is a large surface of coil mass abutting the parent artery lumen, the patient may also be placed on a 500 unit/hour infusion of heparin over the next 12 hours to reduce the risk of periprocedural thrombus formation. The extent of the patient's concurrent traumatic injuries will factor in to this decision. Beyond 12 hours, anticoagulant therapy appears to be of little added benefit. It would seem counterintuitive to anticoagulate a patient

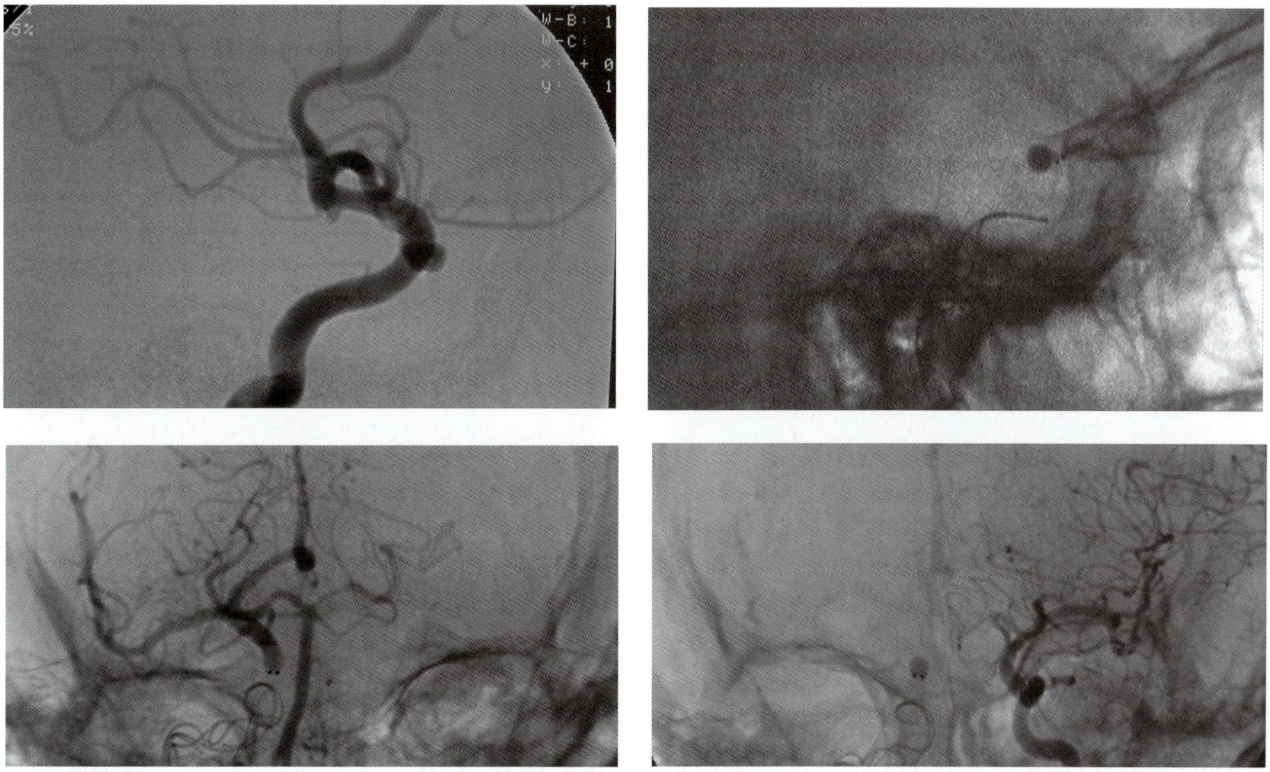

B

D

Fig. 8.20 **(A)** Pseudoaneurysm as a complication of a transsphenoidal resection of a macroadenoma. **(B)** Trapping procedure with deployment of a solitary latex balloon distal to the lesion followed by coil embolization proximal to the lesion. **(C)** Collateral supply to the right internal carotid artery is via the right PCOM and **(D)** to a lesser extent by the ACOM. With the subsequent development of small covered stents, this lesion would have been amenable to stent placement with preservation of the internal carotid artery.

with a ruptured aneurysm, but the incidence of intraprocedural hemorrhage appears to be no greater, whereas the incidence of thromboembolic complication has been considerably lower in patients who have been anticoagulated.

Detachable coils have also proven quite useful in the treatment of carotid–cavernous sinus fistula when preservation of the carotid artery is considered possible (**Fig. 8.18**). The feature of controlled detachment is of great advantage over nondetachable coils in avoiding the possibility of distal migration of the coil mass. The coil can be positioned, withdrawn, and repositioned repeatedly until a satisfactory configuration of the coil is achieved. Deployment by electrolytic, thermal, or hydraulic means can often be accomplished more safely. With each additional coil deployed, the risk of migration declines. Similarly, closure of fistula with preservation of the parent artery can also be achieved with detachable balloons (**Figs. 8.14, 8.15, 8.16, 8.17, 8.18,** and **8.19**). Although a much older technique, it has been a reliable method for treating carotid–cavernous sinus fistula. The risks are somewhat different and include valve failure with premature deflation and migration of the balloon and the need for a larger-caliber delivery system.

Although all traumatized patients with aneurysms should be evaluated for endovascular management, not all are best served with this therapy. Conventional surgical clipping is still a consideration. In selecting appropriate therapy, the physician should consider the configuration of the aneurysm and its neck, the location and accessibility of the aneurysm, the number of aneurysms, and the patient's preference and overall physical condition (e.g., ability to tolerate anesthesia and surgery). The decision as to the course of treatment is as a result of the consensus of opinions of both the neurointerventionalist and the neurosurgeon.

Cerebral Revascularization

Thromboembolic stroke, like intracerebral hemorrhage, may present either as the result of a trauma or as a cause of a trauma. Thromboemboli may result from severe chest trauma or more commonly from a traumatic neck injury that results in an arterial dissection or fragmentation of an atherosclerotic plaque. Intravenous thrombolysis with tissue plasminogen activator (tPA), the only thrombolytic therapy approved by the Food and Drug Administration, can be offered within 3 hours of onset of a neurological deficit but is generally not an option in the acute trauma setting. Alternative therapies include the more traditional volume expansion and anticoagulation therapies or the newer endovascular therapies.

Statistically, the American Stroke Association defines stroke as the third most common cause of death in North America. Approximately 730,000 strokes occur each year in the United States. Of these, 500,000 patients will present with a first stroke and 230,000 with a recurrent stroke. There are more than 160,000 stroke-related deaths per year. This equates to approximately one stroke every 45 seconds and one stroke death every 3 minutes. Stroke carries a 17% 30 day mortality and a 40% 5 year mortality. These rates translate to an enormous expense in terms of human and financial costs. Medical care for patients with stroke had historically focused on limiting the extent of the stroke with volume expansion and anticoagulation followed by rehabilitation. Until recently, no therapy directed at stroke reversal has been available to this large segment of the population. Given the tremendous strides made in the areas of cardiac and limb salvage over the past 2 decades, several modalities are now directed at reestablishing cerebral blood flow. If accomplished quickly enough, neurological function may be restored.

Intraarterial cerebral revascularization incorporates several new technologies and new applications of techniques that have been well established in peripheral revascularization.[5,7–9] Historically, the most commonly used agents are those classified as plasminogen activators and include streptokinase (Streptase; Behring, Marburg, Germany), urokinase (Abbokinase; Abbott Laboratories), and recombinant tissue-type tPA (r-tPA) (Alteplase; Genentech, South San Francisco, CA). Streptokinase is no longer widely used because of its tendency to cause hypersensitivity reactions. Although quite effective, urokinase is also no longer available (**Figs. 8.21, 8.22,** and **8.23**). Prourokinase, (Abbott Laboratories), a genetically engineered fibrin-specific variant of urokinase, has been shown to be quite effective in the endovascular treatment of acute stroke, but it has yet to be made available for clinical use.

Several protocols are in effect for the intravenous (IV) administration of thrombolytic agents, most notably r-tPA. These methods establish a systemic lytic state with large doses of thrombolytic agents. Risks include lysis of thrombi anywhere in the body, including the musculature, lungs, and abdominal viscera, as well as in peptic ulcers and recent wounds and puncture sites. Evidence suggests an increased incidence of hemorrhagic conversion of strokes older than 6 hours when they are treated with IV r-tPA. However, the U.S. Food and Drug Administration (FDA) approved the use of r-tPA in strokes of less than 3 hours in duration. To date, this protocol is the only thrombolytic protocol to receive FDA approval. Although trauma is not included in the FDA approved, American Heart Association (AHA) recommended list of exclusionary criteria, most physicians are reluctant to offer this therapy in the acutely traumatized patient out of concern for the increased risk of hemorrhage in any traumatized portion of the body.

The intraarterial delivery of thrombolytic agents allows for the administration of decreased volumes of a higher concentration of thrombolytic agent over a shorter period of time. Concurrent anticoagulant therapy and platelet inhibition appear to augment the effects of locally infused lytic agents; however, the FDA has only approved the use of intravenous tPA within the first three hours of clinical onset of stroke. The FDA has not approved either the concurrent use of heparin with IV-tPA of the intra-arterial delivery of tPA. The arterial route offers the distinct advantage of infusing the drug directly into the clot, accelerating the restoration of flow. A systemic lytic state is not produced; therefore, the risk of hemorrhage at other sites, although not eliminated, is markedly reduced. Extensive research is under way to develop agents that are clot specific and that can lyse thrombi quickly with fewer adverse effects. The author recently completed a study to evaluate an in vitro technique to preactivate the inactive precursor plasminogen to the active form, plasmin. Utilizing this technique with combinations of lytic agents resulted in an acceleration of the rate of thrombolysis and reestablishment of arterial flow with smaller volumes of lytic drug(s) over a shorter period of time. The technique appears to improve neurological recovery with a lowered risk of hemorrhagic complication.

Selective intraarterial dissolution of thrombus has also been achieved with the newer antiplatelet agents. Abciximab (ReoPro; Eli Lilly, Indianapolis, IL) is an antiplatelet agent that also has thrombolytic properties similar to those of the plasminogen activators. The incidence of hemorrhagic complication appears to be less than that associated with the use of plasminogen activators. In the face of an acute thromboembolic stroke associated with a serious trauma, the benefits of selective intraarterial thrombolytic therapy may outweigh the risks, but each case should be evaluated individually.

In the acute trauma setting, the risk of hemorrhagic complication of chemothrombolysis is greater than in the nontraumatized stroke patient. Therefore, alternative mechanical thrombolytic techniques may be preferable in the recanalization of larger-caliber occluded vessels of the neck and skull base. Nonthrombolytic techniques include low-pressure angioplasty of the thrombus and mechanical thrombectomy. A variety of compliant and noncompliant balloon catheters are

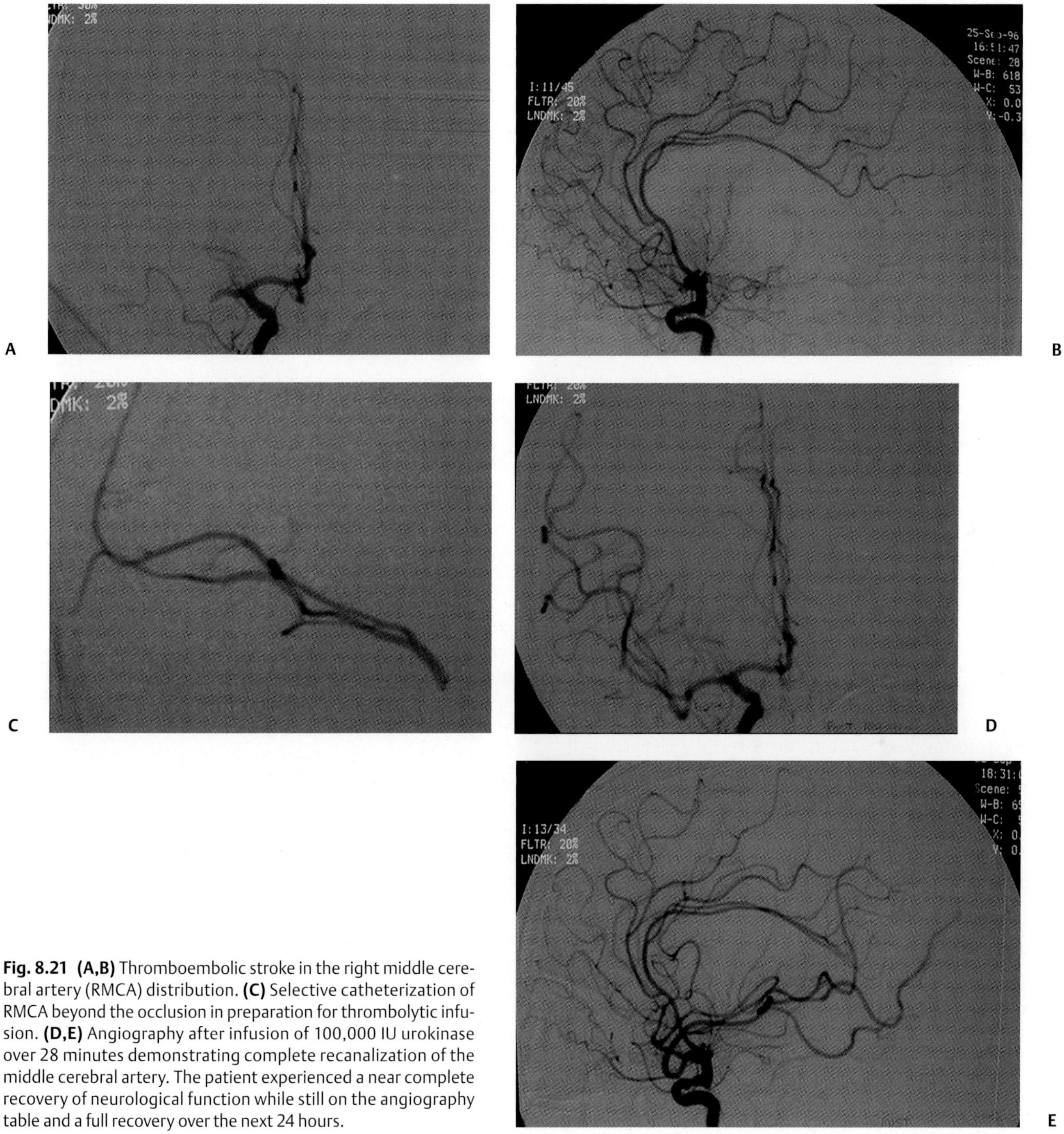

Fig. 8.21 (A,B) Thromboembolic stroke in the right middle cerebral artery (RMCA) distribution. **(C)** Selective catheterization of RMCA beyond the occlusion in preparation for thrombolytic infusion. **(D,E)** Angiography after infusion of 100,000 IU urokinase over 28 minutes demonstrating complete recanalization of the middle cerebral artery. The patient experienced a near complete recovery of neurological function while still on the angiography table and a full recovery over the next 24 hours.

available in sizes of 2 to 10 mm to allow access to both the cervical carotid and vertebral arteries and primary branches of the major intracranial arterial anatomy. Risks include distal embolization of fragmented thrombus and occlusion of small perforator branches of the circle of Willis. Mechanical thrombectomy devices (**Fig. 8.24**) most notably include the Angiojet and Neurojet devices (Possis Medical, Minneapolis, MN) and the Merci device (Concentric Medical; Mountain View, CA). These tend to be most effective in treating the larger vessels of the neck and proximal intracranial vasculature and have led to a significant reduction in the volume of thrombolytic drugs necessary to treat more distal cerebral arterial thromboembolic complications.

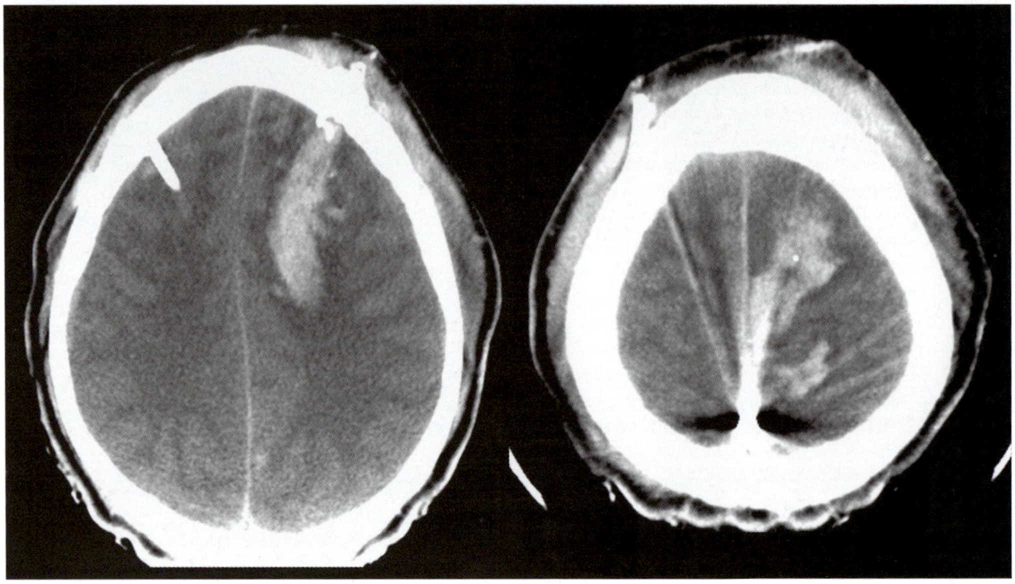

A B

Fig. 8.22 Young male patient status post–gunshot wound to head, presented with a sudden decline in his neurological exam on the second day of admission. Repeat computed tomography demonstrated no change from the prior study other than minor progression of edema surrounding the hematoma.

Angioplasty and Stent Placement

An integral part of cerebral revascularization is treating the source of the embolus or hypoperfusion. In the acutely traumatized patient, an arterial dissection or thrombosis is most likely[10,11]; however, other nontrauma-related etiologies such as a cardiogenic thromboemboli and carotid or vertebral atherocclusive disease should also be considered. Recent technological advances have made angioplasty and stenting of proximal arterial stenoses in carotid or vertebral vessels possible. Dilation of the thromboembolic foci increases cerebral perfusion pressure and reduces the risk of reembolization and reocclusion.

Carotid stenting has been practiced for more than 15 years as an off-label application of an FDA-approved device. In 2004, the FDA approved the use of the Acculink stent (Abbott Laboratories) and Accunet distal filtration guidewire (Guidant Corp., St Paul, MN/Boston Scientific, Natick, MA). In 2005, the Xact stent (Abbott Laboratories) was also approved. This approval, however, is limited to the treatment of symptomatic atherosclerotic lesions of the carotid artery bifurcation. In the repair of traumatic vascular injuries, the use of stents remains as an off-label application of an FDA-approved device (**Figs. 8.25, 8.26,** and **8.27**).

Stenting has also been proven to be an effective means of treating the vascular sequela of blunt and penetrating injuries of the neck. Stents can be rapidly deployed in the management of large vessel dissections (**Figs. 8.26** and **8.27**). Stenting appears to be the most efficient means of reapplying a detached intimal lining of an artery to the wall of the vessel. Covered stents have also proven quite useful in the repair of penetrating injuries to the cervical arterial anatomy (**Fig. 8.25**). Partial transactions can result in carotid-pharyngeal or carotid/vertebral-cutaneous fistula. In the acute setting, manual external compression or flow arrest with a balloon catheter can help buy the time needed to deploy a covered stent over the lacerated arterial segment.

If compatible with the patient's overall condition, patients without active hemorrhage are usually pretreated with aspirin 325 mg and clopidogrel 300 mg before the procedure to reduce the risk of thromboembolic complication of stent placement. In the face of active bleeding, this step is logically deferred. During the procedure, an activated clotting time (ACT) of 250 seconds is maintained with heparin. After the procedure, again, overall status permitting, patients are prescribed a daily regimen of aspirin 325 mg for a minimum of 1 year and clopidogrel 75 mg for a minimum of 2 to 4 weeks.

Conclusion

New techniques in interventional neuroradiology offer the potential to substantially reduce the morbidity and mortality associated with neurovascular trauma. Only occasionally are endovascular procedures considered

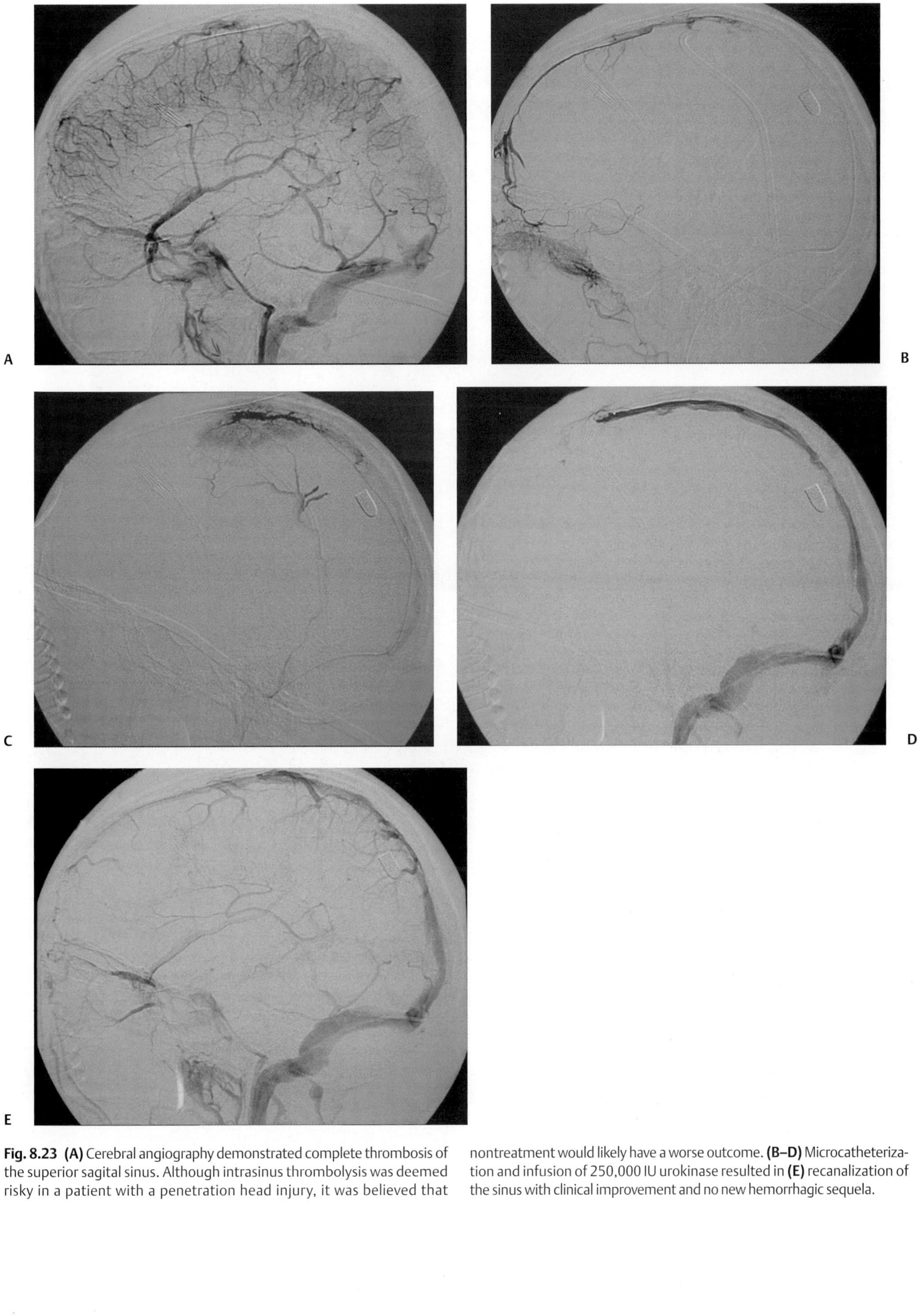

Fig. 8.23 **(A)** Cerebral angiography demonstrated complete thrombosis of the superior sagital sinus. Although intrasinus thrombolysis was deemed risky in a patient with a penetration head injury, it was believed that nontreatment would likely have a worse outcome. **(B–D)** Microcatheterization and infusion of 250,000 IU urokinase resulted in **(E)** recanalization of the sinus with clinical improvement and no new hemorrhagic sequela.

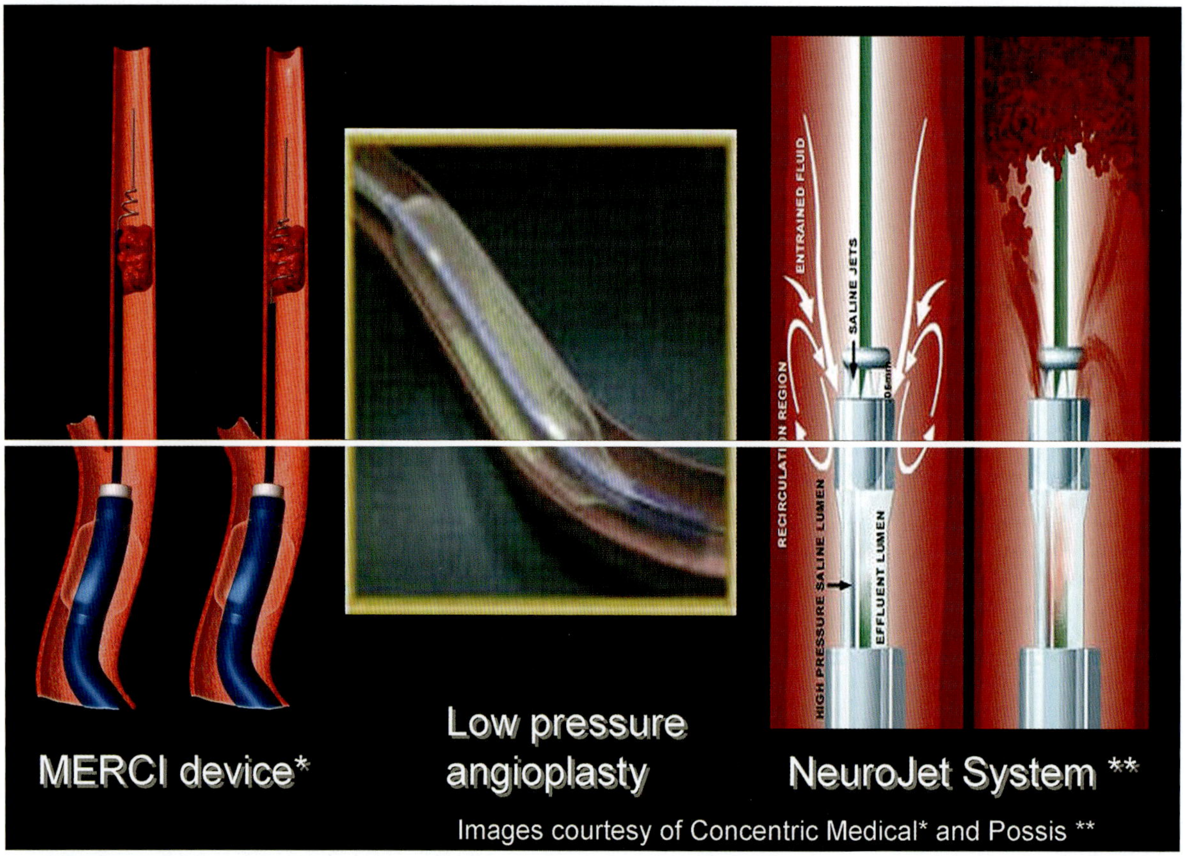

Fig. 8.24 Mechanical thrombectomy. (Images courtesy of Concentric Medical and Possis.)

A-C

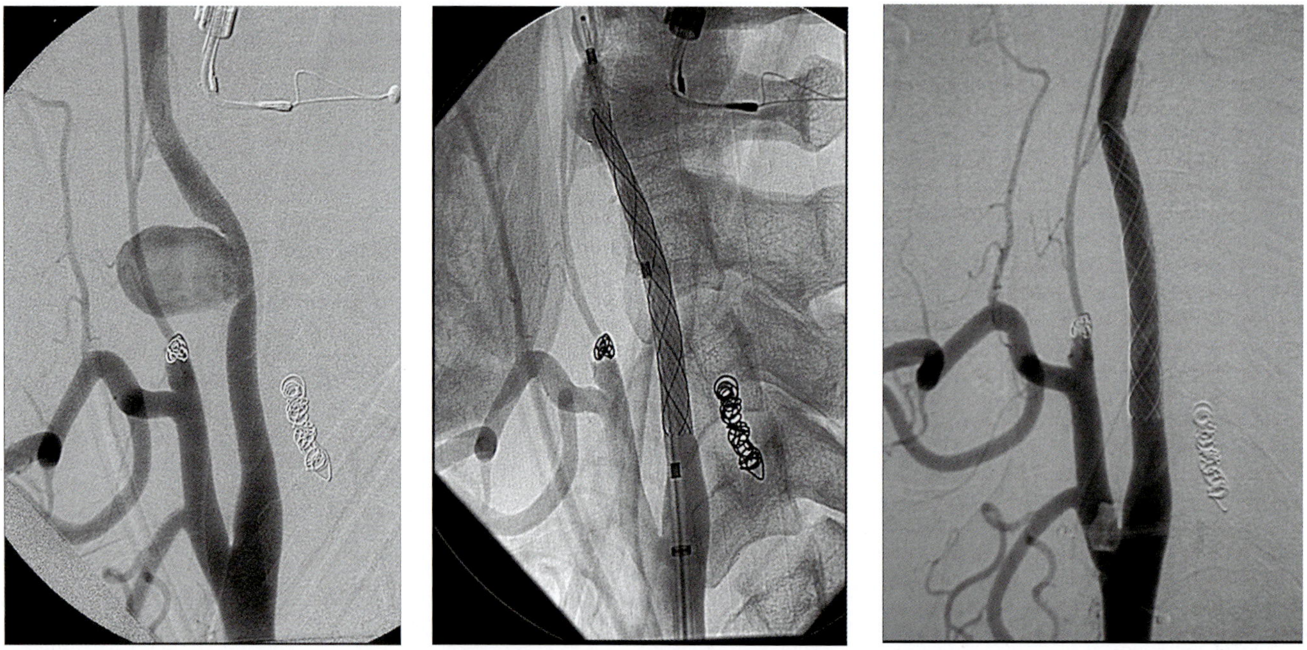

Fig. 8.25 **(A)** Patient with a zone 2 gunshot wound to the neck resulting in transection of the internal maxillary and vertebral arteries and a pseudoaneurysm of the midcervical internal carotid artery. The internal maxillary and vertebral arteries were coil embolized with fibered platinum microcoils. **(B,C)** The internal carotid artery was reconstructed with a covered Wallgraft stent with elimination of the pseudoaneurysm and preservation of antegrade internal carotid arterial flow **(C)**.

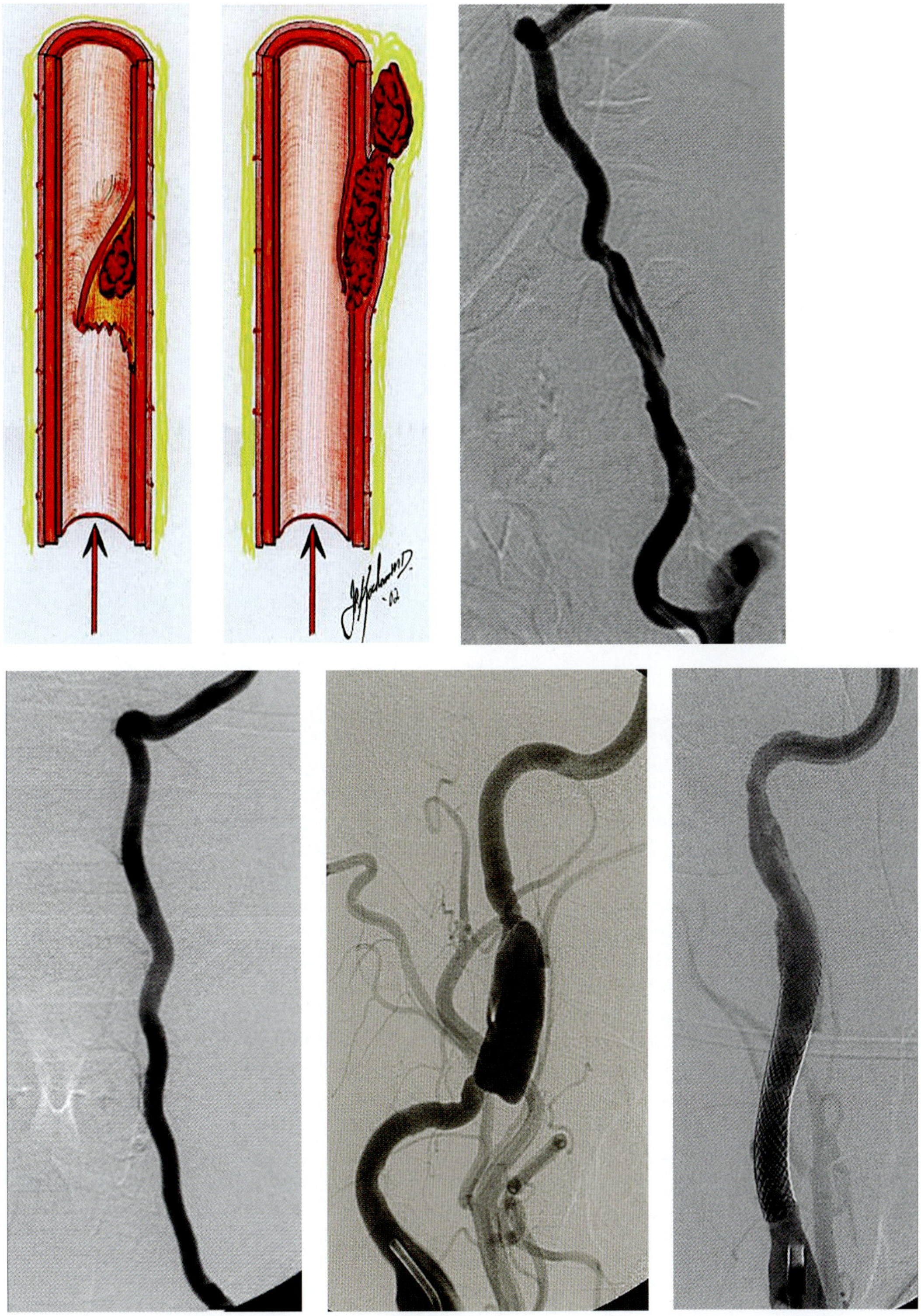

A-C

D-F

Fig. 8.26 Arterial dissection. **(A)** Subintimal dissection with reduction in luminal diameter and subintimal thrombus formation. **(B)** Subadventitial dissection without luminal narrowing and with extraluminal hemorrhage and thrombus formation, for example, pseudoaneurysm. **(C,D)** An intimal dissection **(C)** before and **(D)** after low pressure angioplasty over 2 minutes. **(E,F)** An example of a subadventitial dissection **(E)** before and **(F)** after reconstruction with a Wallstent.

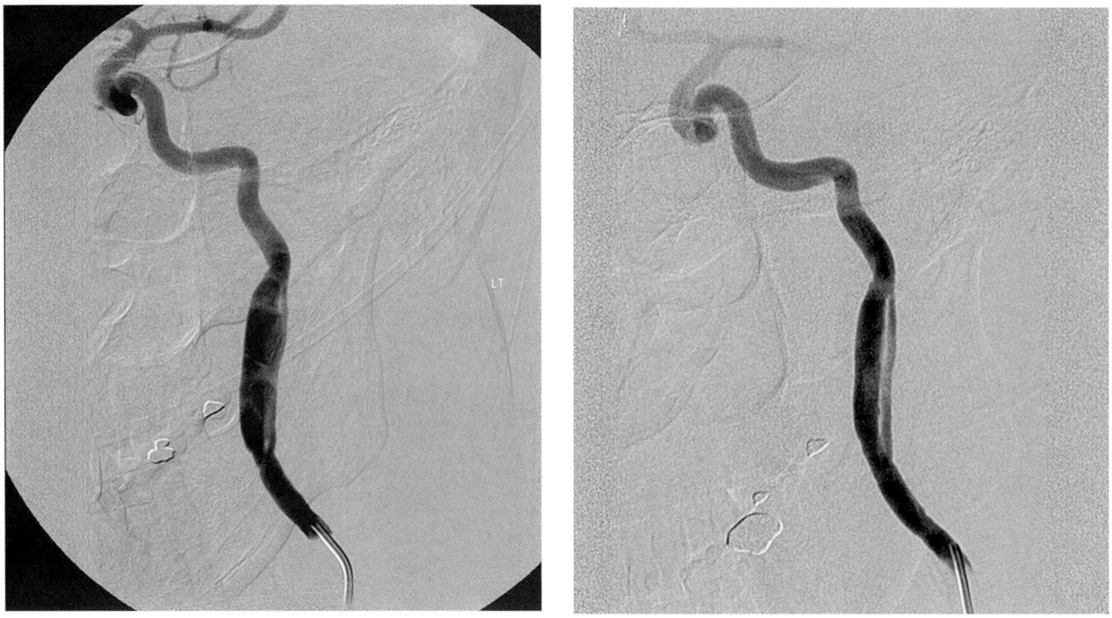

Fig. 8.27 **(A)** Subadventitial dissection. **(B)** Spontaneous healing after 2 weeks of heparin therapy. A residual dual lumen is of no clinical concern.

definitive treatments. In most cases these will be trauma patients. In these instances, the criteria for accepting patients for definitive endovascular therapy include the following: (1) the patient is not considered a surgical candidate because of poor baseline health; (2) previous surgery failed or the lesion is surgically inaccessible; and (3) the lesion is of a type and in a location where the risk of surgical morbidity and mortality is greater than that associated with endovascular treatment.

These procedures pose many risks, and the complications can be devastating. Whereas the majority of risk is accepted during the procedure itself, the delayed risks of thromboembolic sequelae persist over the ensuing 24 hours. For that reason, intensive postprocedural management in a trauma or neuro-ICU setting is essential. Increasing experience and ongoing improvements in delivery systems and embolic materials will continue to reduce the risks to the patient and to facilitate subsequent surgical management.

Cerebral revascularization is a relatively new science with the potential to offer substantial benefit to a large segment of the population, whom, to date, have not had substantial hope for the emergent restoration of cerebral blood flow and neurological function after an acute stroke. Angioplasty and stenting represent a form of secondary stroke prevention, for example, by treating the underlying causes of thromboembolic stroke before a second, possibly more devastating stroke occurs. Thrombolytic therapy and angioplasty are the only tertiary preventive measures currently available to treat and reverse an acute stroke in evolution. The most important factor affecting the successful outcomes of these therapies is the early recognition of an ischemic neurological event. The earlier a neurological deficit is identified, the greater the anticipated benefit from therapy.

The clinician must clearly understand that embolotherapy and cerebral revascularization are not innocuous procedures. There are many potential risks and the complications can be devastating. Nonetheless, interventional neuroradiological procedures can be of enormous benefit in the management of the acutely traumatized patient.

References

1. Connors JJ, Wojak JC. Interventional Neuroradiology: Strategies and Practical Techniques. Philadelphia, Pa: WB Saunders; 1999
2. Kochan JP. Current practice and technique in interventional neuroradiology. eMedicine Journal, topic 906, October 8, 2006, Volume 7, Number 10
3. Lasjaunias P, Berenstein A. Surgical Neuroangiography. Vols. 1–5. Berlin: Springer Verlag; 1992
4. Vinuela F, Halbach VV, Dion JE. Interventional Neuroradiology: Endovascular Therapy of the Central Nervous System. New York: Raven; 1992

5. Ferguson RD, Ferguson JG, Lee LI. Endovascular revascularization therapy in cerebral athero-occlusive disease: angioplasty and stents, systemic and local thrombolysis. Neurosurg Clin N Am 1994;5(3):511–527
6. Ferguson RD, Lee LI, Connors JJ. Angioplasty in the extracranial and intracranial vasculature. Semin Intervent Radiol 1994;11:64–82
7. Kochan JP. Cerebral revascularization. eMedicine Journal, topic 763, August 9, 2002, Volume 3, Number 8, updated February, 2006
8. Tyagi R, Narayan RK, Testaiuti M, et al. Direct thrombolysis in acute cerebral venous thrombosis Toronto, Canada. Abstracts of the AANS/CNS Section on Cerebrovascular Neurosurgery, April, 2001
9. Connors JJ, Wojak JC. Emergency endovascular treatment of stroke. J La State Med Soc 1996;148(11):490–497
10. Kochan JP, Kanamalla US. Carotid artery dissection. eMedicine Journal, topic 132, February 2, 2006, Volume 7, Number 2
11. Lee AH, Kochan JP, Akhtar N, Boyko OB. An overview of penetrating trauma to the head Philadelphia, Pa. Abstracts of the 36th Annual Meeting of the American Society of Neuroradiology, 1998

III Management

9 Mild Brain Injury

Vincent J. Miele and Julian E. Bailes

Although considered a nonsurgical condition, mild brain injury (MBI) is a condition frequently confronted by neurosurgeons. It has many names, including mild head injury (MHI), mild traumatic brain injury (MTBI), and concussion. These injuries, though once considered transient alterations of function that resulted in no permanent structural or functional effects, are now known to cause damage to the brain that can, in some cases, lead to long-term cognitive sequelae, depression, and dementia.[1,2]

Despite being one of the most common of neurological injuries, some of the most dramatic aspects of MBI are not fully understood. Why does it possess amnesic properties? How, when an abrupt loss of consciousness occurs, can such a seemingly profound paralysis of neuronal function occur so abruptly, last so transiently, and recover so spontaneously?

For many physicians, even those who specialize in MBI, this area is confusing due to the paucity of scientific evidence available to support much of the clinical decision making faced in practice. This lack of objective information is due largely to problems with ambiguous definitions of concussion, inconsistent criteria when selecting patients to study, variability of injury mechanisms and locations, and differing means of measuring cognitive function. This chapter is divided into three sections and will provide some guidance to the diagnosis, management, and study of this complex category of brain injury. In the first section, we explore the definition and grading of MBI and discuss the biomechanics, neuroanatomy, and neuropathology of the condition. In the second section, we detail currently utilized methods of examination, from structural imaging to functional testing. In the third section, we deal with the clinical management of MBI.

Definition

Our understanding of MBI is constrained due to the multitude of definitions in use as a result of our evolving appreciation of the disorder. Despite the frequency of MBI, there is no uniform agreement regarding the nature of the illness, and discrepant criteria are utilized by various disciplines for diagnosis. As stated earlier, the condition has many names, including MHI, MTBI, and concussion. Historically, MBI had been defined as "a traumatically induced, transient alteration of neurological function without macroscopic or microscopic abnormality in the brain or long term sequelae."[3] The condition was thought to be completely reversible and closely associated with a brief loss of consciousness. This traditional definition has sustained several modifications as our understanding of MBI has grown.

The belief that MBI is always completely reversible and has no long-term consequences has been dismissed. Patients often have persistent symptoms and subtle neuropsychological deficits, particularly affecting memory. Immunostaining studies of patients who suffered an MBI with an antibody to amyloid precursor protein, a marker of fast axonal transport, have revealed multifocal axonal injury,[4] and objective changes can be appreciated on structural imaging and functional assessment. MBI often occurs without an associated loss of consciousness.

Armed with this new information, an international symposium was held in 2001 and a consensus definition of MBI proposed as "a complex pathophysiological process affecting the brain, induced by traumatic biomechanical forces, with several common features that incorporate clinical, pathological, and biomechanical injury constructs that may be used in defining the nature of a concussive head injury." These features are listed in **Table 9.1**.[5,6] This

Table 9.1 Features of Mild Brain Injury (Concussion)

- Caused by a direct blow to the head, face, neck, or elsewhere on the body with an "impulsive" force transmitted to the head
- Typically results in the rapid onset of short-lived impairment of neurological function that resolves spontaneously
- May result in neuropathological changes, but the acute clinical symptoms largely reflect a functional disturbance rather than structural injury
- Results in a graded set of clinical syndromes that may or may not involve loss of consciousness; resolution of the clinical and cognitive symptoms typically follows a sequential course
- Typically associated with grossly normal structural neuroimaging studies

Sources: Data from McCrory P, Johnston K, Meeuwisse W, et al. Summary and agreement statement of the 2nd International Conference on Concussion in Sport, Prague 2004. Br J Sports Med 2005;39(4):196–204; and Aubry M, Cantu R, Dvorak J, et al. Summary and agreement statement of the 1st International Symposium on Concussion in Sport, Vienna 2001. Clin J Sport Med 2002;12(1):6–11.

definition was revisited at a second international symposium in Prague in 2004 and no changes were made beyond noting that in some cases postconcussive symptoms may be prolonged or persistent.[5]

The Centers for Disease Control and Prevention (CDC) Mild Traumatic Injury Workgroup conceptually defined MTBI as "an injury to the head as a result of blunt trauma or acceleration or deceleration forces that result in one or more of the following conditions: (1) Any period of observed or self-reported transient confusion, disorientation, impaired consciousness, dysfunction of memory around the time of injury, or loss of consciousness lasting less than 30 minutes. (2) Observed signs of neurological or neuropsychological dysfunction, headache, dizziness, irritability, fatigue or poor concentration."[7]

The current literature reflects general agreement regarding the variables defining MBI. These variables include admission Glasgow Coma Scale (GCS) score,[3] length of unconsciousness, absence of focal neurological findings, and length of posttraumatic amnesia (PTA). Most investigators have included the following criteria in their definition of MBI: admission GCS score of 13 through 15, loss of consciousness of <20 minutes, absence of focal neurological deficits, and PTA of <24 hours.[8]

A persistent methodological criticism of the currently used definition of MBI is that it assumes reasonable homogeneity in injury severity among patients meeting these criteria. To date, few studies have substantiated this assumption. In fact, concerns have been expressed regarding the potential heterogeneity in pathophysiology among patients with GCS scores ranging from 13 to 15.[9] Evidence of such a relationship necessitates further classification and grading of injury severity within the MBI category, promoting a more accurate understanding of prognosis and recovery. Additionally, states such as alertness are often determined by subjective criteria that may be interpreted differently by clinicians.[10] More objective measurement tools such as the Galveston orientation and amnesia test[11] and the Reaction Level Scale 85[12] merit further examination.

Epidemiology

Perhaps the most agreed-upon aspect of MBI is that it is one of the most common neurological disorders; in fact, its national prevalence is exceeded only by migraine headache.[13] It has been estimated over 500,000 patients require hospital treatment for MBI each year in the United States, representing 80% of all patients admitted to the hospital for head injury. An additional 200,000 Americans with MBI are treated each year in hospital outpatient settings or physicians' offices[14] and there is no question that the condition is significantly underdiagnosed.[15] The number of persons who receive medical care with an undiagnosed MBI or who sustain an MBI but do not seek care is not known.

The highest incidence of MBI is among persons 15 to 24 years of age and 75 years and older, with an additional less striking peak in incidence in children ages 5 and younger.[15] Males are about twice as likely as females to experience an MBI.[16] MBI is most commonly the result of motor vehicle accidents, violence, and sports/recreational activities.[17] Unfortunately, MBI is becoming an important issue for returning soldiers from the Iraq and Afghanistan wars.[18,19] Although penetrating brain injuries are more readily identified, explosion or blast effect is the leading cause of MBI among active duty military personnel in war zones.[19,20] Rescue workers and victims of terrorism-related attacks[21,22] are also at risk of sustaining an MBI. Additionally, in the U.S. prison population, as many as 87% of incarcerated persons report a history of head injury.[23,24]

Concussions represent as many as 300,000 sport-related injuries annually in the United States.[25] This incidence is certainly underreported because athletes may not recognize that they have sustained a concussion. Although sports- and recreation-related injuries account for 3% of hospitalized persons with TBI, ~90% of sports-related TBIs are mild and may go unreported, thus leading to a lower actual incidence rate of sports-related TBI. Per sport-related activity, studies of high school athletes show the rate of concussions per 1000 exposures as follows: football (0.59 for boys), wrestling (0.25 for boys), soccer (0.18 for boys, 0.23 for girls), field hockey (0.09 for girls), and basketball (0.11 for boys, 0.16 for girls). Nonorganized sports such as skiing and bicycling also result in a substantial number of MBIs.[26]

The epidemiology of mild TBI is still not fully understood, but it is encouraging that the CDC now receives data on TBI-related emergency department visits.[16] Notably, at least 33% of all patients across GCS scores had a positive blood–alcohol level (BAL). This finding demonstrates the ongoing association of head injury and substance use, and further research is needed to clarify the impact of these substances on both admission GCS scores and outcome.[27]

Classification/Grading Scales

Many classification schemes and grading scales have been devised to categorize and help understand MBI. Current grading systems represent the expert opinion of clinicians and researchers; yet, no class I scientific basis exists for any of the systems. It is recommended to be familiar with one grading system and use it consistently, even though it may not be scientifically validated. The most commonly used systems employ three measures of injury: Glasgow

Coma Scale (GCS), presence/length of loss of consciousness (LOC), and length of PTA.

The GCS was created to assess more severe forms of brain injury and is used immediately after a trauma to reflect the level of arousal based on the patient's motor, verbal, and eye responses. The severity of injury is then stratified into mild, moderate, and severe. Mild brain injury corresponds to a GCS score of 13 to 15, moderate corresponds to a score of 9 to 12, and severe injury corresponds to a score of 3 to 8.[3] By itself, GCS classification of MBI (GCS 13 to 15) has long been recognized as having a tremendous amount of clinicopathological heterogeneity.[3,27] In addition, many patients are oriented by the time they are first assessed and therefore score at the top of the GCS. Serious problems thus arise in applying GCS to the assessment of MBI.

An extended version of the Glasgow Coma Scale (GCS-E) has been devised that defines a set of behavioral landmarks fixing the duration of PTA and codes an additional digit that follows the GCS score (**Table 9.2**).[28] The GCS is thus scored in the universally accepted fashion, whereas the amnesia score adds an additional dimension to better define MBI.[28] Administration times of the amnesia scale are widely spaced because regular cueing of PTA may encode memories that would not otherwise be present. Thus, though the amnesia scale is administered as soon as possible after the patient's arrival in the emergency department, the second administration is no sooner than 24 hours after trauma, and the third no sooner than one week after trauma. If there is a fourth administration, it is usually performed in an outpatient setting.[28] Use of the GCS-E for assessment of PTA duration revealed that longer lengths of amnesia following mild TBI were associated with a greater incidence of dizziness, depression, and cognitive impairments during the first weeks after injury. Results suggest that the GCS-E is a useful tool for the prediction of symptoms associated with mild TBI.[29]

LOC is also often used in quantifying the severity of MBI, with LOC of no more than 20 to 30 minutes defined as mild TBI and LOC between 30 minutes and 6 hours moderate TBI, and loss of consciousness of greater than 6 hours is considered severe TBI.[8] Importantly, a patient does not have to suffer an LOC to have suffered an MBI—a misconception that has resulted in the missed diagnosis of MBI in an untold number of patients. Additionally, recent studies suggest that although LOC is perhaps the most dramatic sign of MBI, it may not be a good predictor of short- or long-term neurological functioning, which makes its inclusion in evaluation of head injury severity more controversial.[30]

The last tool commonly used as a surrogate measure of injury severity is the presence and length of retrograde and anterograde PTA.[31] The clinical hallmark of diffuse brain injury is retrograde PTA, which begins with and includes the trauma. Retrograde PTA usually lasts for a period of minutes that shrinks later to seconds. Because of this recovery, estimated length of retrograde PTA varies with the time of measurement after the injury and is poorly reflective of injury severity.

Table 9.2 Amnesia Scale Portion of the Glasgow Coma Scale-Extended (GCS-E)

In applying the GCS-E, the GCS is first scored in the usual way. The amnesia scale is then applied, and the amnesia score entered after a colon so that it will not be mistaken for a decimal with a numeric value. Thus, a patient with a GCS of 15 and with no posttraumatic amnesia (PTA) would have a GCS-E score of 15:7 and a patient with a GCS of 13 and amnesia of more than I hour would be scored 13:5.

Score	
7	No amnesia: client can remember impact, can remember falling and striking a solid surface, etc.
6	Amnesia for 30 minutes or less: client regained consciousness while still in vehicle, in street at scene of incident, etc.
5	Amnesia of 1/2 h to 3 h: remembers being loaded into ambulance, in ambulance on way to hospital, arriving at emergency room, admission to ward, etc.
4	Amnesia of 3 to 24 h: determine duration by content of the first memory, which will be of an event in the ward or of a hospital procedure
3	Amnesia of 1 to 7 d
2	Amnesia of 8 to 30 d
1	Amnesia of 31 to 90 d
0	Amnesia >3 mo
X	Cannot be scored, e.g., can speak but responses are inappropriate or unintelligible, cannot speak because unconscious, intubated, facial fractures, etc.

Source: Data from Nell V, Yates DW, Kruger J. An extended Glasgow Coma Scale (GCS-E) with enhanced sensitivity to mild brain injury. Arch Phys Med Rehabil 2000;81(5):614–617.

Table 9.3 Return to Play (RTP) Guidelines following Mild Traumatic Brain Injury

System	Concussion Grade	Signs/Symptoms	1st Concussion	2nd Concussion	3rd Concussion
American Academy of Neurology	I (Mild)	Transient confusion; no LOC; symptoms or abnormalities resolve in <15 min	Remove from game; may RTP if abnormalities or symptoms clear within 15 min	Terminate game; may RTP after 1 wk without symptoms at rest and with exercise	
	II (Moderate)	Transient confusion; no LOC; symptoms or abnormalities last over 15 min	Terminate game; may RTP after 1 wk asymptomatic at rest and with exertion	Terminate game; may RTP after at least 2 wk asymptomatic at rest and with exertion; withdraw from play for the rest of the season if any CT/MRI abnormalities	
	III (Severe)	Any LOC, either brief (s) or prolonged (min)	Terminate game; transport to hospital if unconscious or if there is evidence of neurological abnormality; if concussion is brief(s), may RTP in 1 wk if no symptoms at rest and with exertion; if concussion is prolonged (mo), RTP in 2 wk if no symptoms	Terminate game; may RTP after minimum of 1 mo asymptomatic; withdraw from play for the rest of the season if any CT/MRI abnormalities	
Colorado Medical Society	I (Mild)	Confusion without amnesia; no LOC	May RTP if without symptoms for at least 20 min	Terminate game/practice; may RTP if asymptomatic for at least 1 wk	Withdraw from play for remainder of season; or may RTP in 3 mo if asymptomatic
	II (Moderate)	Confusion with amnesia; no LOC	Terminate game/practice; may RTP if asymptomatic for at least 1 wk	Consider withdrawing from play for remainder of season; may RTP in 1 mo if asymptomatic	Withdraw from play for remainder of season; may RTP next season if asymptomatic
	III (Severe)	LOC	Terminate game/practice and transport to hospital; may RTP in 1 mo, after 2 consecutive asymptomatic weeks	Withdraw from play for remainder of season; may RTP next season if asymptomatic	Withdraw from play for remainder of season; strongly discourage return to contact sports

(Continued)

Anterograde PTA, defined as the interval between injury and return of continuous recall, is more valuable than retrograde PTA as a measure of injury severity. Unlike retrograde PTA in which there is impaired retrieval, anterograde PTA does not shrink later because the memory dysfunction is not of retrieval but of encoding. On examination, a patient with anterograde PTA usually appears confused but is able to participate in activities such as sporting events. From the patient's perspective, the duration of anterograde PTA cannot be differentiated from any time spent unconscious. As mentioned above, because clinical outcome of milder injuries tends to correlate better with PTA than GCS, an extended Glasgow Coma Scale (GCS-E) has been created that combines an amnesia score with the traditional GCS criteria.[28]

Defining the severity of concussion has been extremely important in the management of athletes with respect to return to play following MBI. This has led to extensive discussion on the grading of such injuries (**Table 9.3**).[32–34] In 1991, return to competition guidelines were created by

Table 9.3 *(Continued)*

System	Concussion Grade	Signs/Symptoms	1st Concussion	2nd Concussion	3rd Concussion
Cantu	I (Mild)	No LOC; PTA of less than 30 min duration	May RTP if asymptomatic for 1 wk; terminate season if CT/MRI abnormalities	RTP in 2 wk if asymptomatic at the time for 1 wk	Withdraw from play for remainder of season; may RTP next season if asymptomatic
	II (Moderate)	LOC less than 5 min in duration or posttraumatic amnesia longer than 30 min but <24 h in duration	RTP after asymptomatic for 2 wk; terminate season if CT/MRI abnormalities	Withdraw athlete for a minimum of 1 mo; may RTP if asymptomatic for 1 wk; consider withdrawing from play for the remainder of season	Withdraw athlete from play for remainder of season; may RTP next season if asymptomatic
	III (Severe)	LOC for >5 min or posttraumatic amnesia for >24 h	Withdraw for minimum of 1 mo; may then RTP if asymptomatic 1 wk	Withdraw from play for remainder of season; may RTP next season if asymptomatic	Consider no further contact sports

Sources: Data from Practice parameter: the management of concussion in sports (summary statement). Report of the Quality Standards Subcommittee. Neurology 1997;48(3):581–585; Colorado Medical Society School and Sports Medicine Committee. Guidelines for the management of concussion in sports. Colo Med 1990;87:4; and Cantu RC. Return to play guidelines after a head injury. Clin Sports Med 1998;17(1):45–60. Refer to specific source for detailed recommendation.

Abbreviations: CT, computed tomography; LOC, loss of consciousness; min, minutes; mo, months; MRI, magnetic resonance imaging; PTA, posttraumatic amnesia; RTP, return to play.

the Colorado Medical Society (CMS) that established three grades of concussion.[33] These were reviewed and endorsed by several professional organizations, including the American Academy of Pediatrics, the American Academy of Sports Medicine, and the American College of Surgeons Committee on Trauma.[35,36] Partially as a result of a feeling among the experts that there was limited scientific data on which to construct medical practice parameters, the guidelines were modified in 1997.[35,37] The desire for a broader consensus of expert opinion resulted in the involvement of the Quality Standards Subcommittee of the American Academy of Neurology. The American Academy of Neurology guidelines were reviewed by several expert organizations including the American Association of Neurological Surgeons, American College of Emergency Physicians, American Academy of Pediatricians, American Academy of Family Physicians, National Athletic Trainers Association, and the American Academy of Neurology.[35]

In 2001, a symposium on concussion in sports was held in Vienna, Austria, to provide recommendations for the improvement of safety and health of athletes who suffer concussive injuries.[6] A second symposium was held in 2004 in Prague, Czech Republic, to revise and update the Vienna consensus recommendations.[5] One of the outcomes of these meetings was an attempt to simplify the classification of MBI by using the categories of either simple or complex to manage the condition versus the numerous grading systems. Simple concussions were defined as an MBI that progressively resolves without complication over 7 to 10 days. Notably, the occurrence of LOC for a short period (less than 1 minute) would not exclude classification in this group. Complex concussions were those from which an athlete suffers persistent symptoms (with or without exertion), specific sequelae (such as concussive convulsions), prolonged loss of consciousness (more than 1 minute), or prolonged cognitive impairment after the injury.[6] This group may also include athletes who suffer multiple concussions over time or where repeated concussions occur with progressively less impact force and require more aggressive management. Despite the plethora of available systems for grading MBI, no system has gained universal acceptance, and the development of validated injury severity scales continues in the published literature.

Biomechanics of Mild Brain Injury

The first step in understanding the biomechanics of MBI is to identify the types of traumatic forces affecting the brain. They can be rotational or linear, compressive or inertial. Forces can be caused by either impact or impulse.[38] Forces transmitted by the former are the result of blows that directly strike the head. The latter, on the other hand, is the result of a force that sets the head in motion without directly striking it, such as a blast injury or sudden deceleration following an automobile accident. Brain injury without head contact has been shown experimentally in comatose nonhuman primates[39] and in harnessed pilots crashing in military aircraft in which the rapidly decelerated cranium may never contact a solid object, yet the brain is irreversibly damaged.[40]

Regardless of how they are delivered, these forces result in inertial (or accelerative) loading and have two main components. The first is linear or translational acceleration/deceleration and is defined as movement of the head in a straight line through its center of gravity. An example of this type of force would be a straight blow to the face.[41] The second is angular or rotational acceleration/deceleration. This type of force occurs when the head is accelerated tangentially and moves through an arc around its center of gravity. A blow to the chin at an angle is an example of this type of acceleration. Although it is possible to separate these two types of forces in the laboratory, in vivo they coexist and their individual contributions to MBI are unknown. It has been demonstrated in vitro with primate head injury models that it is the angular component of force that is primarily responsible for LOC.[42] Linear forces, on the other hand, resulted in focal contusions and hemorrhage but no LOC.

Application of inertial loading via translational or rotational acceleration has at least four consequences[38]:

1. Impact between the surface of the brain and the skull due to rotatory inertial loading of the head
2. Traction on brain stem neurons due to forceful movement of the hemispheres
3. Depression of the skull bone associated with deformation of the underlying brain tissue and the propagation of intracranial pressure waves
4. Acceleration of the head about the axis of the neck

Several theories exist as to how the combination of these forces results in MBI (see section on MBI Theory)

Discussion of the biomechanics of MBI would not be complete without examining the effects of kinetic energy transfer. Why is it much harder to produce a concussion in an animal model when the head is fixed versus free[43]? The principles and behavior of kinetic energy must be considered when answering this question. When the head is not mobile or is in contact with another surface, the kinetic energy will flow through the cranium and into the object that it is in contact with.[38,43] This explains why a victim of an assault who keeps his head still by maintaining it in contact with the ground or a wall is unlikely to lose consciousness; the energy is transferred through the cranium to the object it is in contact with leaving the brain unharmed.[38] This information can be used to an athlete's advantage. A player involved in contact sports can minimize the effects of an impact by tensing the muscles of the neck before the collision occurs. This results in decreased head mobility and increases dispersion of the kinetic energy received from the cranium to the rest of the body.[44] Conversely, not tensing the neck muscles before an impact because it was not anticipated has been demonstrated to increase the risk of MBI.[45] Based on this information the importance of neck strengthening in boxers and football players becomes obvious.

All types of MBI involve the rapid transfer of kinetic energy that requires either absorption or release by the head and brain. Two types of brain injury are the result of this transfer of energy: accelerative and compressive, which have somewhat different mechanisms of action.[43] The brain has gelatinous and viscoelastic properties and is relatively incompressible but readily distortable.[46] Compressive trauma results when there is minimal movement of the head, and the majority of brain injury is the result of a transient increase in intracranial pressure (ICP) due to changes in skull volume caused by its momentary distortion.[47] Although compressive trauma causes waves of increased ICP to pass through the brain, accelerative trauma causes more of a distortion or twisting phenomenon and is more associated with LOC. This type of injury has been seen in video recordings of the swirling and gliding motion of the brain's surface following accelerative trauma captured in animal models.[48]

Newton's Law states that force is the product of mass and acceleration. A slow sustained crushing impact will injure and damage the skull and brain but will not induce a concussion. Kinetic energy must be transferred and expended rapidly. Conversely, a projectile of small mass such as a high velocity bullet may penetrate skull and brain but also will not induce MBI because the mass of the bullet is too small to impart the necessary kinetic energy to the head.[49] It follows, therefore, that if the head is struck by a somewhat larger object, but one that is traveling at a lower speed, MBI may now ensue, even though the overall force was the same in both conditions.

Recent data obtained by finite element (FE) modeling based on professional football head-to-head field collisions has found that rotational acceleration produced maximum shear stress.[50] No significant relationship was found between translational acceleration and shear stress. A 6-year investigation of National Football League (NFL) players demonstrated that those most susceptible to concussion were quarterbacks, wide receivers, and defensive backs who received a facemask impact at an oblique angle.[51] In hockey, concussion is also commonly associated with an eccentric blow to the head, a strike to the face or jaw, or a hit directed to the chin.[52] In taekwon-do, concussion is primarily due to a round-house kick (i.e., angular kick) to the temporal region of the head.[53]

Mild Brain Injury Theory

One of the most fascinating aspects of MBI is the dramatic, but transient, LOC that occurs in some patients. Five prominent theories of concussion, the vascular, reticular, centripetal, pontine cholinergic, and convulsive hypotheses are summarized, and supportive evidence is assessed in this section (**Table 9.4**).[38]

The Vascular Hypothesis

The vascular hypothesis states that the loss of consciousness and other functions following concussion are due to a brief episode of cerebral ischemia or, as sometimes described, cerebral anemia. It is one of the oldest theories of concussion and relies on a mechanism such as vasospasm or vasoparalysis, reflex stimulation, expulsion of the blood from the capillaries, and most commonly, obstruction or arrest of cerebral blood flow (CBF) following compression of the brain.[38] This could be caused by the transient increase in ICP following a blow to the head. The main problem with this theory is that membrane potential and therefore neuronal function can be preserved for some time despite a cessation in its blood supply.[54] Thus, the immediate LOC that can occur with head trauma is not sufficiently explained. In addition, if ischemic processes did underlie the pathophysiology of concussion, then there should invariably be evidence of deficient energy production. It has been shown in animal models that a concussive state could be maintained without any marked exhaustion in energy reserves.[55] Although it is one of the oldest concussion theories, it is now considered obsolete and discredited. Nonetheless, some of the side effects of concussion including amnesia could be partially attributed to cerebral ischemia.

The Reticular Hypothesis

The reticular theory has been the most accepted explanation for the pathophysiology of concussion for the past 50 years. By the middle of the 20th century, significant evidence existed to implicate the brain stem as the principal site of concussion. It contains systems that if affected could explain many of the symptoms associated with MBI, including those controlling blood pressure, heart rate, cerebral blood flow, various reflexes including the righting reflex that depends upon the integration of many brain stem nuclei, equilibrium, nausea and emesis, muscle flaccidity and

Table 9.4 Concussion Theories

- The vascular hypothesis
    - Symptomatology secondary to brief episode of cerebral ischemia
    - Obstruction or arrest of cerebral blood flow following compression of the brain
    - One of the oldest theories
    - Now considered obsolete and somewhat discredited
- The reticular hypothesis
    - Concussive force temporarily disturbs activity within the brain stem including the reticular activating system
    - Most accepted explanation for the pathophysiology of concussion for the past 50 years
- The centripetal hypothesis
    - Rotational forces produce shearing strains that disconnect nerve fibers in a centripetal fashion
    - Disconnection of nerve fibers is only functional, and thus reversible if force is small
    - As forces increase, strains penetrate deeper into the brain, and the nerve fiber disconnections may become structural instead of functional, and thus irreversible
    - Suggests that MBI is on the lesser side of the same spectrum as diffuse axonal injury
- The pontine cholinergic system hypothesis
    - Forces activate an inhibitory cholinergic system located within the dorsal pontine tegmentum that suppresses a variety of behavioral responses
    - Similar to the reticular theory except that concussion is associated with activation of a depressive or inhibitory system
- The convulsive hypothesis
    - Trauma results in functional deafferentation of the cortex as a consequence of diffuse mechanically induced depolarization and synchronized discharge of cortical neurons
    - One of the few theories that does not center on the reticular activating system

pupil dilation. What could not be explained by attributing concussion to the brain stem was the sudden LOC that often occurs with MBI. This missing link was found with the discovery of the reticular activating system (RAS), which extends diffusely all the way up through the midbrain (mesencephalon). Once this center of consciousness in the brain stem was added to the theory, an explanation was in hand that described the majority of MBI sequelae. The basis of the hypothesis is that a concussive force temporarily paralyzes, disturbs, or depresses the activity of the polysynaptic pathways within the brain stem including the RAS. This leads to stupor or coma. Once these pathways become operational again, the cortex can then be reactivated and control can be regained over the inhibitory mechanisms of the medial thalamus. A spontaneous return of awareness and responsiveness would then occur.[38]

Although the reticular hypothesis does provide a straightforward explanation not only for the loss of consciousness but also for the miscellaneous motor and autonomic symptoms that may occur following MBI, it does have limitations. Electroencephalographic (EEG) findings after MBI are not explainable by this theory. The RAS normally exercises inhibitory control over the pacemaker functions of the medial thalamus. If it becomes temporarily deactivated, then the medial thalamic nuclei would be free to coordinate and synchronize slower high-amplitude cortical rhythms. In this case, if a concussive injury temporarily incapacitates the RAS, then the EEG recorded from the cortex would predictably be of a relatively low-frequency high-voltage type, which is not the case in these individuals.[38] In addition, although RAS dysfunction could explain the associated muscle flaccidity and reflex paralysis that follow cerebral concussion, it does not explain the initial convulsive movements often observed in humans and animals. Traumatic amnesia is not well explained by this theory.

The Centripetal Hypothesis

The centripetal theory states that sudden rotational forces set up shearing strains and stresses within the brain immediately upon mechanical loading that disconnect nerve fibers in a basically centripetal fashion.[42] When the force and its resultant mechanical loading are relatively small, the disconnection of nerve fibers is only functional, and thus reversible. It is also confined to the superficial layers of the brain. As the mechanical load increases, shearing and tensile strains penetrate deeper into the brain, and the nerve fiber disconnections may become structural instead of functional and thus irreversible. In other words, MBI is actually "a graded set of clinical syndromes following head injury wherein increasing severity of disturbance in level and content of consciousness is caused by mechanically induced strains affecting the brain in a centripetal sequence of disruptive effect on function and structure. The effects of this sequence always begin at the surfaces of the brain in the mild cases and extend inwards to affect the diencephalic–mesencephalic core at the most severe levels of trauma."[42] This theory suggests that MBI is on the lesser side of the same spectrum as diffuse axonal injury. This theory is quite elegant in its explanation of the symptoms of MBI and their reversibility. If the head trauma is mild, only the subcortex or diencephalon is disconnected from the cortex, which would cause confusion and amnesia but no LOC. If the force is stronger, the less vulnerable mesencephalon could be disconnected from the cortex and would result in LOC. Similarly, disconnection of the brain stem and RAS by a very powerful force would result in LOC and paralysis. The strength of the blow would also determine if the disconnections are functional or structural, which would establish whether the condition is transient or permanent. This theory predicts that LOC would always have associated damage to the more peripheral cortex and subcortex. This theory is considered an extension of the reticular theory, and the mechanism of LOC in both is disruption of the RAS.

The weakness of this theory is that it suggests that only severe head injury results in LOC, which clinically does not appear to be the case. Patients that suffer MBI and should only have peripheral dysfunction often experience nausea, vomiting, and headache that would be more consistent with brain stem injury. In addition, the theory does not explain the convulsive movements that may accompany the acute trauma.

The Pontine Cholinergic System Hypothesis

The pontine cholinergic theory states that the forces associated with MBI activate an inhibitory cholinergic system located within the dorsal pontine tegmentum. This area is loaded with cholinoceptive and cholinergic cells and pathways and its activation suppresses a variety of behavioral responses thought to be indicative of traumatic LOC. The pontine cholinergic theory is very similar to the reticular theory except that in the former concussion is associated with activation of a depressive or inhibitory system. As stated above, the reticular theory is based on depression of an activating system. Both of the theories base the causative dysfunction within the brain stem. Injecting the cholinergic agonist carbachol into the same brain stem regions of a large number of awake animals appeared to substantiate this theory when the animals began displaying behavioral symptoms of concussion similar to those produced by a fluid percussion device within several minutes.[56] Other studies have strengthened the association between acetylcholine (Ach) and the symptoms of concussion.[57,58] Although this theory has waned in popularity recently, its lasting value may be to have redrawn attention to the likelihood that the mechanism of action of concussion may initially involve a state of intense cerebral excitation rather than depressed neuronal activity.[38]

The Convulsive Hypothesis

The convulsive theory of MBI is one of the few theories that does not center on the reticular activating system. Proponents of the theory state that since the symptoms of concussion bear a strong resemblance to those of a generalized epileptic seizure, then it is a reasonable assumption that similar pathobiological processes underlie them both. Both conditions exhibit a near instantaneous LOC, which typically lasts for no more than a few minutes. Following this, a common period of drowsiness, disorientation, and lethargy of varying length occurs.

In this theory, the energy transferred to the brain by trauma results in functional deafferentation of the cortex as a consequence of diffuse mechanically induced depolarization and synchronized discharge of cortical neurons.[38] This theory is supported by several findings. It has been demonstrated that evoked potentials (EPs) and EEGs recorded acutely following concussive trauma are similar to those obtained following the induction of a state of generalized seizure activity.[38] The convulsive theory is readily compatible with neurophysiologic MBI data and can explain traumatic amnesia, autonomic disturbances, and the miscellaneous collection of symptoms of the postconcussion syndrome more adequately than any of its rivals.[38] Additionally, symptoms of minor concussion such as transient amnesia or confusion are often strikingly similar to the effects of petit mal seizures.

Neuropathology of Mild Brain Injury

MBI may result in a mixture of transient and permanent damage to cellular systems that can be observed via neuropathological examination in some cases. Most of these findings can be placed on a spectrum between very mild injury and diffuse axonal injury. Diffuse axonal injury is one of the most important types of brain damage that can occur after MBI and may cause significant learning and memory dysfunction. Because disruption of axonal transport results in amyloid precursor protein (APP) accumulation, APP has been used as a sensitive marker of axonal injury. Because mortality is extremely low with MBI, examination of tissue is mainly performed on appropriate animal models. Examinations were performed on the brains of patients that suffered MBI and died of other causes.[59] In this population, even in so-called minor head injury, anatomic damage to the brain was observed on histopathologic study of sectioned brain tissue. The earliest detectable lesions were found 15 hours after injury and include microglial cell proliferation, petechial hemorrhages, and other signs of diffuse axonal injury (DAI).[59] Previous clinical findings have shown a strong correlation between axonal injury and cognitive dysfunction.[60]

Diffuse damage to the individual cells of the brain has also been shown to occur with sparing of surrounding brain parenchymal and vascular elements. The types of cells damaged with acceleration/deceleration injuries are typically large myelinated cells that decussate and those transferring information to and from cortex. Additionally, disruption of the neuronal cytoskeleton is often present. The degradation or loss of microtubule-associated protein (MAP2) serves as a reliable marker of damage to the neuronal cytoarchitecture. Because MAP2 plays an important role in neurite extension and neural plasticity, its disruption could contribute to the development of cognitive dysfunction after TBI.

One of the biggest contributions of neuropathology to the understanding of MBI is in the analysis and development of concussion theories. There is a large amount of neuropathological data supporting the reticular theory.[10] Specifically, hemorrhagic lesions, alterations in neuronal structure, axonal degeneration, depletion in cell count, and other cytological and morphological changes may be observed, either in the brain stem generally, or more specifically within the reticular substance. These findings suggest that damage to the brain stem and RAS occur in MBI; nevertheless, they do not give insight into the cause of this injury. In addition, many of these structural changes typically do not become apparent until hours, days, or weeks after the trauma, and thus cannot easily account for the acute symptoms of MBI, although they could conceivably be involved in the more long-term sequelae.

Even without observable morphological brain damage, MTBI patients frequently suffer from cognitive deficits, emotional difficulties, and behavioral disturbances. The pathological mechanisms underlying these functional impairments and the recovery process are not fully understood, and it is still unclear what, if any, role organic injury plays in the pathogenesis of MBI. Some mechanisms have been thought to represent the actual substrate of concussion. Alternately, they may be just a form of neuropathological epiphenomena.

Effects of Mild Brain Injury

Short-Term Effects

Posttraumatic Loss of Consciousness

A sudden temporary LOC is one of the most dramatic occurrences associated with MBI. Maintenance of awareness is dependent upon complex interactions between the brain stem, thalamus, hypothalamus, and cortex; a transient interruption of this function can lead to a period of unconsciousness.[10] LOC is known to occur from insult to the brain stem reticular formation. It also occurs following diffuse bilateral impairment of cortical activity even if brain stem reticular formation function is preserved.[10] Several theories exist (discussed above) that try to explain the relationship between the transfer of force to the brain and this disruption of function. It has been postulated that the same type of pathophysiological processes that are responsible for the loss of consciousness in an epileptic attack are similarly involved in the loss of consciousness after a concussive injury. Two main theories exist as to why a generalized epileptic seizure such as grand mal will produce a brief loss of consciousness and responsiveness. The centrencephalon theory is that the LOC ensues when abnormal electrical discharges either invade or arise intrinsically within the pathways and nuclei of the brain stem and thalamic RAS. This transiently inactivates the RAS, preventing it from performing its normal role in the maintenance of wakefulness or control of level of arousal. This conception of the pathophysiology of unconsciousness is not much different from that of the reticular theory of concussion mentioned earlier in this chapter. In contrast, the cortico–cortical and cortico–reticular theory states that hypersynchronous cortical epileptiform activity totally blocks reception of sensory signals thereby functionally deafferentating the cortex and rendering the brain insensible and unresponsive. In this theory, the brain stem and RAS do not play a significant role in LOC.

Importantly, an acute MBI is thought to have a biphasic effect on the brain, consisting of an initial (or ictal) period followed by a longer-lasting depressive one.[61] This would be apparent at both behavioral and neuronal levels. Therefore, the duration of the lack of awareness and insensibility that are collectively labeled as unconsciousness is most appropriately considered the sum of both the ictal and immediate postictal phases.[62]

Traumatic Amnesia

The most significant effect of MBI besides LOC is traumatic amnesia. There appears to be an intimate link between amnesia and MBI so much so that if a patient claims no memory loss, it has been suggested that MBI has not occurred.[63] This amnesia may be retrograde or anterograde. Pretraumatic or retrograde amnesia refers to loss of memory for events which transpired just prior to the concussion. Posttraumatic or anterograde amnesia applies to loss of memory for events after consciousness has been regained. When attempting to use memory loss to evaluate the severity of MBI, several concepts must be kept in mind. First, retrograde amnesia often progressively shrinks during the posttraumatic recovery.[64] Second, the length of the anterograde amnesia has been found to be a generally accurate guide to the severity of the head trauma.[64] As described earlier, the retrograde and anterograde components of learning will be affected in a similar fashion in a generalized seizure and an MBI. Interestingly, patients that receive electroconvulsive therapy also often experience similar amnesia.[65] All of these insults to the brain possess potent amnestic properties when dealing with a newly acquired memory. One of the great advantages of the convulsive theory of MBI is that it can deal more readily and adequately with the loss or impairment of recent short-term memory.

Posttraumatic Convulsive Movements

A variety of acute motor phenomena, for example, tonic posturing or convulsive movements, may accompany a concussion. These are thought to be the result of direct excitation of the descending motor centers of the brain stem reticular formation by neuronal discharges originating in the cortex and subcortex.[38] This excitation is then propagated down the somatic motor pathways of both the pyramidal and extrapyramidal tracts. These convulsive movements may also be facilitated by the temporary loss of control by subcortical inhibitory centers. Although dramatic, these clinical features are generally benign and require no specific management beyond the standard treatment for the underlying concussive injury.

Posttraumatic Autonomic Disturbances

Numerous minor autonomic disturbances are associated with MBI. These include respiratory arrest or apnea; abolition of various reflex functions including corneal, pupillary, and withdrawal responses; relatively prompt flaccidity of the musculature with the patient collapsing into a heap; ephemeral convulsive spasms; irregularities of heart rate including both bradycardia and tachycardia; alterations in CBF; and fluctuations in blood pressure.[38] Because these abnormalities may also be seen following an epileptic seizure, the convulsive theory of MBI readily explains these dysfunctions. These abnormalities are somewhat variable and inconsistent. This may be because hyperstimulation of the autonomic nuclei will result in activation of both the sympathetic and the parasympathetic components of the autonomic nervous system. Because the operation of these two subdivisions is generally antagonistic, their overall interaction or balance would most likely determine the degree and type of autonomic abnormality. Some of the discrepancies in changes in autonomic function, especially with cardiovascular activity, could also be secondary to the biphasic nature of the convulsive process.

Miscellaneous Short-Term Effects

Numerous symptoms including headache, nausea, dizziness, vomiting, fatigue, restlessness, irritability, and confusion may all be commonly experienced by the MBI patient.[38] Other frequently cited symptoms include reduced information processing, diminished learning and memory, and hypersensitivity to stimuli.

Sports-Related MBI and Sideline Concussion Assessment Tool

The diagnosis of sports-related MBI is often made during the competition on the sideline or at ringside and includes evaluation of clinical symptoms, physical signs, cognitive impairment, and/or loss of consciousness. A tool that can be used to readily assess this population is the sideline concussion assessment tool (SCAT) (**Fig. 9.1**).[5] Brief neuropsychological testing that assesses attention and memory function has been shown to be both practical and effective. Such tests include the Maddock's questions[66] and the Standardized Assessment of Concussion.[67] It is important to note that abbreviated testing paradigms are designed to rapidly evaluate a patient on the sideline or at ringside. They are not intended to replace comprehensive neuropsychological testing, which is sensitive enough to detect subtle deficits that may exist beyond the acute episode. They should also not be used as a stand-alone tool for the ongoing management of MBI.[38] The appearance of symptoms may be delayed several hours after a trauma, and standard orientation questions, such as time, place, person, have been shown to be unreliable in the sporting situation when compared with memory assessment.[38,66,67] In sport-related MBI, studies investigating short-term neuropsychological deficits generally show a return to normal performance within 1 week after the concussion.[68–70]

Long-Term Effects

At one time, MBI was thought to be a transient injury with a temporary fluctuation in consciousness that fully resolves over a matter of days. This long-held belief in the transient nature and rapid resolution of symptoms is misleading: symptom resolution is likely not indicative of injury resolution. Even when patients appear to be asymptomatic, combined postural and EEG findings suggest persistent functional deficits.[71]

Recent evidence suggests that there are long-lasting residual disabilities from MBI that are often overlooked using current research methodology.[71] In fact, there is a growing body of knowledge indicating long-lasting functional deficits and associated brain dysfunctions that may persist up to 10 years postinjury, and it has been estimated that as many as 40% of concussed athletes will develop postconcussion symptoms, such as headaches, drowsiness, dizziness, irritability, and sleep disorders.[72] Neuropsychological deficits, such as memory problems and difficulty concentrating, may also develop and affect a person's ability to perform daily activities and return to work.

An additional concern is the effect of MBI on new health problems associated with the aging process. Dementia pugilistica in boxers results from repetitive head injury and leads to chronic disability.[73] Moderate and severe head injury is associated with a 1.5 times increased risk of depression,[74] and a 2.3 and 4.5 times increased risk of Alzheimer disease[75]; it is likely that MBI could similarly increase the risk of these abnormalities.[1,2,76]

Testing for Mild Brain Injury

Structural Imaging

Clinical decision making in head injury is often dependent on imaging findings. Although structural imaging was previously only sufficient to screen out life-threatening focal lesions, its role in MBI is increasing with newer techniques. In addition, an increased reliance on functional imaging techniques such as evoked or event-related potentials may improve the detection of diffuse damage that affects normal function in cellular systems.

Plain Radiographs

Although not as popular in the United States, plain skull radiograph screening for patients with MBI is widely practiced in Europe. They are mainly employed to determine the patient's risk of a more serious injury, such as an intracranial hemorrhage (ICH), and are often a part of inclusion guidelines for computed tomography (CT) imaging. The presence of skull fractures on plain radiographs is associated with a higher rate of intracranial pathology. Importantly, this does not work in the reverse, i.e., the absence of skull fractures does not eliminate the risk for significant intracranial injury. Additionally, in helmeted contact sports that have a significant incidence of MBI, skull fractures are rare.

Computed Tomography

CT imaging's ability to exclude more serious injuries makes it the most commonly utilized radiographic modality in patients with MBI. The greatest immediate risk to a patient with MBI, an intracranial hematoma, is a potentially fatal complication that is often not apparent until clinical deterioration has occurred and recovery is endangered.[77,78] CT is the most reliable diagnostic study to rule out ICH, and its availability has increased in recent

This tool represents a standardized method of evaluating people after concussion in sport. This Tool has been produced as part of the Summary and Agreement Statement of the Second International Symposium on Concussion in Sport, Prague 2004

Sports concussion is defined as a complex pathophysiological process affecting the brain, induced by traumatic biomechanical forces. Several common features that incorporate clinical, pathological and biomechanical injury constructs that may be utilized in defining the nature of a concussive head injury include:

1. Concussion may be caused either by a direct blow to the head, face, neck or elsewhere on the body with an 'impulsive' force transmitted to the head.
2. Concussion typically results in the rapid onset of short-lived impairment of neurological function that resolves spontaneously.
3. Concussion may result in neuropathological changes but the acute clinical symptoms largely reflect a functional disturbance rather than structural injury.
4. Concussion results in a graded set of clinical syndromes that may or may not involve loss of consciousness. Resolution of the clinical and cognitive symptoms typically follows a sequential course.
5. Concussion is typically associated with grossly normal structural neuroimaging studies.

Post Concussion Symptoms

Ask the athlete to score themselves based on how they feel now. It is recognized that a low score may be normal for some athletes, but clinical judgment should be exercised to determine if a change in symptoms has occurred following the suspected concussion event.

It should be recognized that the reporting of symptoms may not be entirely reliable. This may be due to the effects of a concussion or because the athlete's passionate desire to return to competition outweighs their natural inclination to give an honest response.

If possible, ask someone who knows the athlete well about changes in affect, personality, behavior, etc.

Remember, concussion should be suspected in the presence of ANY ONE or more of the following:

- Symptoms (such as headache), or
- Signs (such as loss of consciousness), or
- Memory problems

Any athlete with a suspected concussion should be monitored for deterioration (i.e., should not be left alone) and should not drive a motor vehicle.

For more information see the "Summary and Agreement Statement of the Second International Symposium on Concussion in Sport" in the April, 2005 edition of the Clinical Journal of Sport Medicine (vol 15), British Journal of Sports Medicine (vol 39), Neurosurgery (vol 59) and the Physician and Sportsmedicine (vol 33). This tool may be copied for distribution to teams, groups and organizations. ©2005 Concussion in Sport Group

IIHF

The SCAT Card

(Sport Concussion Assessment Tool)

Athlete Information

What is a concussion? A concussion is a disturbance in the function of the brain caused by a direct or indirect force to the head. It results in a variety of symptoms (like those listed below) and may, or may not, involve memory problems or loss of consciousness.

How do you feel? You should score yourself on the following symptoms, based on how you feel now.

Post Concussion Symptom Scale

	None		Moderate			Severe	
Headache	0	1	2	3	4	5	6
"Pressure in head"	0	1	2	3	4	5	6
Neck Pain	0	1	2	3	4	5	6
Balance problems or dizzy	0	1	2	3	4	5	6
Nausea or vomiting	0	1	2	3	4	5	6
Vision problems	0	1	2	3	4	5	6
Hearing problems / ringing	0	1	2	3	4	5	6
"Don't feel right"	0	1	2	3	4	5	6
Feeling "dinged" or "dazed"	0	1	2	3	4	5	6
Confusion	0	1	2	3	4	5	6
Feeling slowed down	0	1	2	3	4	5	6
Feeling like "in a fog"	0	1	2	3	4	5	6
Drowsiness	0	1	2	3	4	5	6
Fatigue or low energy	0	1	2	3	4	5	6
More emotional than usual	0	1	2	3	4	5	6
Irritability	0	1	2	3	4	5	6
Difficulty concentrating	0	1	2	3	4	5	6
Difficulty remembering	0	1	2	3	4	5	6
(follow up symptoms only)							
Sadness	0	1	2	3	4	5	6
Nervous or Anxious	0	1	2	3	4	5	6
Trouble falling asleep	0	1	2	3	4	5	6
Sleeping more than usual	0	1	2	3	4	5	6
Sensitivity to light	0	1	2	3	4	5	6
Sensitivity to noise	0	1	2	3	4	5	6
Other: ______________	0	1	2	3	4	5	6

What should I do?

Any athlete suspected of having a concussion should be removed from play, and then seek medical evaluation.

Signs to watch for:

Problems could arise over the first 24-48 hours. You should not be left alone and must go to a hospital at once if you:

- Have a headache that gets worse
- Are very drowsy or can't be awakened (woken up)
- Can't recognize people or places
- Have repeated vomiting
- Behave unusually or seem confused; are very irritable
- Have seizures (arms and legs jerk uncontrollably)
- Have weak or numb arms or legs
- Are unsteady on your feet; have slurred speech

Remember, it is better to be safe. **Consult your doctor after a suspected concussion.**

What can I expect?

Concussion typically results in the rapid onset of short-lived impairment that resolves spontaneously over time. You can expect that you will be told to rest until you are fully recovered (that means resting your body and your mind). Then, your doctor will likely advise that you go through a gradual increase in exercise over several days (or longer) before returning to sport.

Fig. 9.1 Sport concussion assessment tool (SCAT).[5]

years to the point that essentially no trauma center or community hospital is without a CT scanner.

Although CT scans have been widely available for almost 3 decades and their utility in brain-injured patients is undeniable, there is of yet no consensus on inclusion criteria for their use in MBI. In an attempt to reduce the number of CT scans ordered, while preserving sensitivity for detecting intracranial lesions, various imaging guidelines have been proposed. One of the most thoroughly validated is the Canadian CT Head Rule (**Table 9.5**)[79]; however, several evidence-based guidelines have been introduced for patients with MBI, and recent analyses and validation studies suggest they can be applied cost effectively.[80,81] Most of these guidelines have indications for CT imaging that include prolonged disturbance of conscious state, GCS less than 15, focal neurological deficit, signs or symptoms of increased ICP, worsening symptoms, seizures related to trauma, or possessing factors considered to be high risk (suspected open, basilar, or depressed skull fracture, multiple episodes of vomiting, and age >65 years). It has also been suggested that any athlete with loss of consciousness (grade 3 concussion) should have a CT scan.

One of the arguments against the routine use of CT imaging in MBI patients is the concern about excessive cost. However, a cost-effectiveness model published in 2006 concluded that the liberal use of CT scanning in mild TBI appears justified,[82] mainly because the adverse outcome of an intracranial hematoma is so costly that it more than balances the expense of CT scans. Numerous American studies support the notion that the relatively high cost of the scan is outweighed by treatment costs saved by its ability to accurately diagnose occult intracranial lesions and allow additional cost savings in some cases by allowing patients whose CT scan does not show any abnormalities to be discharged safely from the emergency department. An additional argument against the routine use of CT imaging in the MBI population is the very small risk of cancer after radiation exposure.[83]

Another barrier to CT imaging, and in fact the majority of current imaging techniques, is that it is difficult to perform in uncooperative small children and adults influenced by drugs/alcohol or who are disorientated due to their injury. Complicating the latter scenario is that commonly used clinical parameters may fail to predict intracranial injury in patients influenced by drugs/alcohol.[84] This is becoming less of an issue with the newer generation of rapid acquisition scanners. An important tenet in the management of this population of patients is that conscious patients should usually not be sedated to make imaging possible.

Magnetic Resonance Imaging

Magnetic resonance imaging (MRI) is not routinely used in the evaluation of MBI patients despite its greater sensitivity and specificity in comparison with CT. One of the reasons for this is that in most cases, there is no correlation between abnormal findings on MRI and either postconcussive symptoms or long-term outcome.[85] Newer sequencing modalities such as gradient echo, perfusion, and diffusion weighted imaging, have greater sensitivity for structural abnormalities, but the lack of published studies as well as the absence of preinjury neuroimaging data currently limits their usefulness in clinical management. In addition, the predictive value of various MRI abnormalities that may be incidentally discovered has not been established. MRI is the study of choice for patients with prolonged symptoms (>7 days) or for late change in neurological signs or symptoms.

Table 9.5 Canadian Computed Tomography Head Rule

- CT Head Rule is only required for application in patients with minor head injuries who have any one of the following:
- High risk (for neurologic intervention)
  - GCS score <15 at 2 h after injury
  - Suspected open or depressed skull fracture
  - Any sign of basal skull fracture (hemotympanum, "raccoon" eyes, cerebrospinal fluid otorrhea/rhinorrhea, Battle's sign)
  - Vomiting ≥two episodes
  - Age ≥65 y
- Medium risk (for brain injury on CT)
  - Amnesia before impact >30 min
  - Dangerous mechanism (pedestrian struck by motor vehicle, occupant ejected from motor vehicle, fall from height >3 feet or five stairs)

Source: Data from Stiell IG, Wells GA, Vandemheen K, et al. The Canadian CT Head Rule for patients with minor head injury. Lancet 2001;357(9266):1391–1396.

Note: Minor head injury is defined as witnessed loss of consciousness, definite amnesia, or witnessed disorientation in a patient with a GCS of 13 to 15.

Abbreviations: CT, computed tomography; GCS, Glasgow Coma Score.

CT imaging is usually the study of choice to detect blood; however, delayed or slowly developing bleeds may be easier to detect on MRI, and gradient echo sequences are better at detecting hemorrhagic change.[85] Diffusion weighted imaging has been shown to identify shearing injuries not evident on T2-weighted/fluid attenuated inversion recovery (FLAIR) or gradient echo sequences[86] and diffusion tensor imaging examines the integrity of the white matter tracts by measuring the degree and direction of water diffusion, providing a potential marker for white matter injury.[87]

T2-weighted sequences, particularly FLAIR, are more sensitive to traumatic lesions. An increased frequency of enlarged, high-convexity Virchow-Robin spaces (VRSs) has been identified in several neurological diseases. MRI has been used to show this abnormality in MBI, suggesting it as a radiological marker of mild head injury that is readily detectable on T2-weighted images. Because their number does not vary with time from injury, VRSs probably reflect early and permanent brain changes. VRSs are not directly associated with neurocognitive findings, suggesting that they may be a result of a shear-strain injury.[88]

Functional Imaging

Although it has been established that MBI usually results in some structural damage to the brain, conventional imaging techniques such as plain radiographs, CT, or MRI have difficulty reliably detecting these abnormalities because of the diffuse nature of these injuries. Functional neuroimaging techniques that examine the metabolic and physiological state of the brain may be the answer to this conundrum. Current functional techniques include positron emission tomography (PET), single photon emission computed tomography (SPECT), and functional magnetic resonance imaging (fMRI). Although these functional modalities are still early in development, they have shown promise in MBI: studies of MBI patients based on resting metabolic measurements using PET and SPECT have shown perfusion deficits that extend beyond any structural damage shown by CT or MRI.[89,90] The most commonly reported finding is frontal cerebral hypometabolism and decreased blood flow.

A disadvantage of PET and SPECT imaging is that a radioactive tracer is required, which greatly limits their clinical application. fMRI, on the other hand, does not require exposure to any radioactive substance, and recent studies have also confirmed the potential of fMRI to provide information regarding neural function during task performance following MBI.[89,91]

Positron Emission Tomography/Single Photon Emission Computed Tomography

A well-defined triphasic pattern of the cerebral metabolic rate of glucose has been identified in head-injured patients and is seemingly stereotypic across a broad range and severity of injury types. There is initially a brief period of hyperglycolysis followed by a relatively prolonged period of metabolic depression. This second period typically lasts several hours and is associated with persistent neurological deficits as long as the metabolic depression is present. This "metabolic depression" phase[92] appears to have physiological consequences because neurobehavioral deficits persist during this period. The third phase is the recovery of metabolic function that parallels the rate of recovery of behavioral function.[93] This temporal pattern of recovery may be taken advantage of to evaluate the injury by both positron emission tomography (PET) and single-photon emission computerized tomography (SPECT), which rely mainly on measuring resting metabolic rates in MBI.

SPECT imaging identifies abnormalities following MBI in over 50% of patients with normal CT scans.[94] The most commonly reported finding in this population is frontal hypometabolism or a decrease in frontal cerebral blood flow. Studies utilizing fluorodeoxyglucose (FDG) PET and SPECT have demonstrated frontal and/or temporal hypometabolism following MBI at rest and during working memory tasks.[95,96] The association between hypoperfusion seen on acute SPECT and brain atrophy after 6 months suggests the possibility of secondary ischemic brain damage, which has been hypothesized to correlate with decreased memory function.[97]

A commonality between experimental and clinical studies appears to be a "floor effect" of metabolic reduction following TBI. During the first month of injury, a similar degree of global cerebral metabolic rate of glucose reduction is found irrespective of the initial GCS.[92,93] This could explain why FDG-PET analysis of the pooled global cerebral metabolic rate of glucose demonstrates that the intermediate metabolic reduction phase begins to resolve ~21 to 30 days following injury, regardless of injury severity.[98]

PET studies have provided evidence that even mild TBI may result in continuing brain behavioral deficits. These imaging modalities can help elucidate dysfunctional brain circuitry in neurobehavioral disorders, and specific brain areas may correlate with deficits in daily neurobehavioral functioning and neuropsychological test findings.[99] PET studies in patients with MBI, after correlating the results with neuropsychological testing and continuing behavioral dysfunction, found that abnormal local cerebral metabolic rates were most prominent in the midtemporal, anterior cingulate, precuneus, anterior temporal, frontal white, and corpus callosum brain regions. These imaging abnormalities have been correlated statistically with overall clinical complaints, most specifically with inconsistent attention/concentration and overall neuropsychological test results. Despite these findings, no consistent correlation is found between neuropsychological deficits and regional abnormalities seen on PET scans.[99]

One of the remaining uncertainties in the clinical utility of PET and SPECT is the unanswered question of whether metabolic changes are uncoupled from functional recovery following TBI. For example, the level of consciousness at the time of a PET scan does not always correlate with the global cerebral metabolic rate of glucose during the metabolic reduction phase.[93] Although FDG PET imaging demonstrates that the period of metabolic reduction following both mild and severe TBI typically persists several weeks, the extent of recovery, in terms of cerebral metabolism and functional disability, may coincide temporally, but not quantitatively based on the methods used.[98] The etiologies of the cerebral metabolic rate of glucose reduction in MBI is certainly multifactorial given the complex nature of TBI; simplification of this fundamental pathobiological state following head injury should be performed with caution.

Several applications of PET and SPECT for MBI have been suggested. It has been shown that within the first 7 days following a sensorimotor cortical lesion, neuronal injury can be exaggerated by increased use of the affected limb.[100] The question then arises as to whether patients with MBI and persistent abnormalities on PET or SPECT are at an increased vulnerability to a second insult. This unknown has even led to the suggestion that early neurorehabilitation could be detrimental.[98] The period of metabolic depression that can be identified by these studies may also be a potential window for pharmacological intervention. Finally, these modalities allow the studying of other physiologic consequences of TBI, including the investigation of molecular processes occurring at the DNA level.

Functional Magnetic Resonance Imaging

Functional magnetic resonance imaging (fMRI) is well suited to detect functional abnormalities associated with concussion because it provides task-specific information about neural function and can be tailored to an individual's specific and most prevalent complaints. This modality is also sensitive to deficits related to the dynamic aspects of neural function that may be evident only under conditions of cognitive load or information processing. The lack of radiation also makes obtaining preinjury baseline examinations in at-risk populations such as athletes more acceptable.

Because fMRI does not rely on radioactive isotopes, multiple sessions can be performed on a single subject within a short period, which is another advantage fMRI has over other brain imaging techniques, such as PET and SPECT. This ability has increased in importance now that recent neuropsychological investigations have demonstrated the importance of employing prospective methods and the detection of between-session differences within a single subject.[68,101] This multiple measurement within-subject approach allows individuals to act as their own control, thereby lessening the need for large normative databases. It also will be more sensitive in identifying pathologic changes within an individual that may be small relative to the typically large between-subject variability observed when physiologic data from larger subpopulations are combined.

An example of the utility of this method of analysis using fMRI was demonstrated with a small group of collegiate football players at risk for concussion. This group was studied using a minimal test battery before the start of the football season and then again if one of the group suffered a concussion. Control players not receiving a concussion were examined again at the conclusion of the season. The study found that although performance was unchanged compared with baseline measures, brain activation was more widespread following concussion compared with both preinjury levels and uninjured subjects during the performance of various memory and sensorimotor tasks. The motor sequencing tasks were the most sensitive to concussion.[91] These results were consistent with cognitive-load induced recruitment of neural resources and that in cases of mild concussions in which little if any decrement in performance is observed: compensation in the neural network recruited during cognitive engagement seems to be required to maintain preinjury performance levels.[102] Abnormal patterns of activation following mild head injury have been reported in previous functional imaging studies using different versions of working memory tasks.[95,102] For example, an fMRI study performed in 2001 reported that mild head injury subjects showed disproportionately high increases in activation compared with a control group in response to moderate working memory processing loads. The abnormal increase in activation was lateralized to the right hemisphere, including the right dorsolateral prefrontal cortex.[102]

A second fMRI study evaluated working memory in adult athletes who had sustained a concussion (1 to 14 months prior to study) and were experiencing postconcussive symptoms.[89] Athletes with concussions had less task-related activation in the middorsolateral prefrontal cortex (important for working memory) than comparison subjects, and there was an inverse correlation between right dorsolateral prefrontal cortex activation and severity of symptoms. In addition, concussed athletes had widespread activations in areas not activated in comparison subjects. Importantly, none of the symptomatic athletes had evidence of axonal injury on structural MRI.[103] These studies provide the framework for the possible clinical utility of fMRI in concussive injury.

Magnetic Resonance Spectroscopy

Using technologies similar to MRI, magnetic resonance spectroscopy (MRS) is capable of detecting microscopic injuries by analyzing intracellular metabolic status. It does this by detecting signals from individual solutes in the body's tissues rather than just tissue water and lipid as in routine MRI. It is well suited to evaluating MBI for several reasons. It is noninvasive, does not utilize radioactive isotopes, and has the ability to quantify many of the metabolites sensitive to hypoxia/ischemia, energy dysfunction, neuronal injury, membrane turnover, and inflammation that have been shown to be associated with brain injury.[104] Evidence of widespread metabolic changes following MBI in regions that appear normal on diagnostic MRI has been reported.[105]

For example, *N*-acetylaspartate (NAA) is a marker of neuronal integrity that is believed to represent diffuse axonal injury or metabolic depression. It has been shown to be reduced in normal-appearing occipital and frontal regions of patients following TBI and is quantifiable by MRS.[104] Concentrations of NAA have been shown to remain low following TBI and are somewhat predictive of cognitive outcomes.[106] Associations have also been made between brain injury and creatine, phosphocreatine, choline, lactate, myoinositol, glutamine, glutamate, adenosine triphosphate (ATP), and inorganic phosphates.[104]

The ability of MRS to detect alterations in high energy phosphates allows it to reflect some of the energy abnormalities that occur following MBI; it could potentially be used to follow recovery of the neural tissue. MRS acquired several days after TBI in the pediatric population has been shown to improve prognostic ability and may provide valuable information for early treatment and intervention planning.[107] Because MRS can be easily implemented on standard MRI scanners and the benefits mentioned above, it may serve an increasing role in the management of MBI.

Magnetic Source Imaging/Magnetoencephalography

Magnetic source imaging (MSI) is a new approach to evaluation of MBI. This modality integrates anatomic data from MRI with electrophysiology data from magnetoencephalography (MEG). MEG allows tracking of real-time brain activity without distortions by differences in conductivity between the brain, skull, and scalp. It does this by measuring the neuromagnetic field of the dendrites organized parallel to the skull surface in a fashion similar to an EEG that measures the potential gradients of dendrites perpendicular to the skull surface.[108] MRI and resting EEG have been compared with resting MSI in postconcussive subjects versus controls: MSI detected more patients with postconcussive symptoms than either EEG or MRI alone. In addition, all patients with abnormal EEG or MRI also had abnormal MSI.[109]

Functional Testing

Electroencephalogram

The study of EEG in severe brain injury has been ongoing for the past 50 years, largely because it represents a more primary and direct measure of cerebral function than secondary indices such as ICP and cerebral blood flow. It provides a noninvasive neurophysiologic correlate of the subject's level of arousal or consciousness. The patterns that appear can complement and at times be more sensitive than traditional clinical evaluation. In fact, EEG assessment has been shown to be more successful than other established neurological investigations in predicting the prognosis for patient survival in some studies.[110] Its usefulness in evaluating patient that have suffered severe traumatic brain injury has led to its use in MBI.

The earliest attempt to quantify the effects of experimental concussion on the EEG was made in 1941 on animal models.[63,111] The result was an immediate generalized loss of amplitude in the EEG with the higher frequencies being the most vulnerable to the concussive blow. In some instances, the suppression of the EEG was so marked as to appear isoelectric. During the recovery phase, slow delta waves appeared in the record. By the end of this period, the EEG rhythms began to return to an approximate baseline pattern. Restoration of reflex activity coincided only roughly with these posttraumatic changes in the EEG. The EEG findings, especially the near instant decrease in cerebral activity, were interpreted as evidence for the theory that the pathophysiological basis of concussion consisted of a brief direct traumatic disruption of neural function.[63] However, a careful analysis of the EEG studies makes it seem more likely that concussion is accompanied by an initial state of excitation rather than inhibition or paralysis of cerebral function. This indicates that the concussive blow must trigger a brief period of intense generalized neuronal discharge.

Numerous studies have demonstrated abnormal EEG patterns in concussed individuals.[112] These abnormalities have been shown despite the fact that conventional MRI and CT scans are unable to detect any cortical damage.[38,112] These changes are thought to be the result of reduced local excitation and synchronization of active generators. This results in reduced EEG amplitude.[71]

EEG findings have been used to explain the reduced functional capabilities, such as postural instability, often observed in athletes following concussive injury.[113] Studies utilizing EEG patterns in isolation and during postural tasks in asymptomatic MBI patients versus controls found an overall decrease in EEG power amplitude across spectrum (δ, θ, α, α2, β, and β2) in MBI subjects, an effect most prominent during standing postures.[71] Importantly, the principle difference between groups in these studies were observed in the higher frequency bands of α2, β, and β2, suggesting that these changes in the EEG were related to the chronic consequences of MBI more than to the acute effects of concussive injury.[38,71,110,114]

Evoked Potentials and Event-Related Potentials

The evaluation of MBI utilizing evoked potentials (EPs) and event-related potentials (ERPs) has been performed with promising results. Both of these testing methods represent the averaged EEG signal in response to a given stimulus. However, EPs are thought to represent processing in the primary sensory pathways, whereas ERPs are more associated with cognitive processes.

Somatosensory EPs (SEPs), first recorded in the 1870s, are bioelectrical responses that are deliberately extracted by feeding a stimulus into the nervous system. The amplitude of these recordings is dwarfed by the higher amplitude voltage of an EEG, and it was not until after World War II that it became possible to make noninvasive recordings from skull or scalp locations. This was accomplished using an electromechanical averager. In signal averaging, unlike the randomly distributed EEG, an EP would always be time-locked to the onset of the sensory stimulus. Thus, the background activity may be cancelled out by summing and averaging multiple responses. The extraction of EPs via signal averaging was made more practical by computer advances in the 1950s, which allowed for the widespread use of EPs for both clinical and experimental purposes.

The earliest reports of SEP evaluation in MBI were in 1956; in 1973, both the EEG and the SEP were simultaneously recording in the chimpanzee.[115] Surprisingly, although the EEG was relatively unaltered by the head injury, there were quite pronounced changes in the SEP. Specifically, a standard concussive blow seemed to transiently abolish the early components of the SEP and a more powerful blow caused the total eradication of all the SEP components. The persistence of this abnormality correlated strongly with the duration of the period of unconsciousness. A less powerful blow that simply stunned the animal produced an overall reduction in amplitude without loss of components. The general principle appeared to be that the greater the concussive force, the greater the distortion to the SEP waveform.

Auditory-evoked potentials such as the brain stem auditory evoked potential (BAEP) and the middle-latency auditory evoked potential (MAEP) have shown abnormalities in the function of the primary auditory pathways following MBI experimentally. The BAEP is a series of early high frequency wavelets arising mostly in the eighth nerve and the auditory brain stem and is commonly used as a marker of brain stem function. In fact, the BAEP has become one of the leading clinical tools for the assessment of peripheral auditory dysfunction and brain stem integrity. Numerous studies have investigated the effects of MBI on the interpeak latencies of the BAEP.[116,117] Although the results have been mixed, it appears that between 11 and 27% of individuals tested showed evidence of significantly increased interpeak latencies, representing a disruption of brain stem function following MBI. Increased I–III interpeak intervals and reduced amplitude of BAEPs have also been recorded in boxers.[118]

MAEP generators are less well known than BAEPs. However, the origins of later components (Pa, Nb, and Pb) of the response have been postulated to be near the auditory cortex with peaks No, Po, and Na originating from subcortical structures. MAEP has been demonstrated to be useful in the determination of functional deficits. Specifically, Na and Pa amplitudes have been shown to be lower and Pa latencies were significantly longer in patients compared with controls.[119]

As mentioned earlier, ERPs represent an averaged EEG signal that is recorded after presenting stimuli related to a specific level of information processing. It consists of a variety of components named according to their polarity (P, positive; N, negative) and their latency (e.g., N1 is the first negative component to appear after the presentation of a stimulus). Each component is associated with a specific level of information processing. This modality has the ability to access cognitive and intentional processing by analyzing, in particular, a P3 wave that is recorded over the central and parietal electrodes. Cognitive event-related potentials (ERPs) seem to be sensitive in the evaluation of concussion effects by allowing the detection of attention and information processing deficits.[120]

The best-known paradigm among the tasks used in ERP is the oddball paradigm, which consists of the presentation of two categories of stimuli having different probabilities of occurrence (frequent and rare stimuli).[121] The appearance of the rare stimulus commonly elicits a strong, positive P3 wave (representing cognitive and attentional processing) over the central and parietal electrodes at 300 to 600 milliseconds after the stimulus presentation. Earlier components, such as N1, reflect automatic information processing. P3 wave reflects the amount of attentional resource allocated in a task or the degree and quality of information processing.[122] Its latency, on the other hand, is associated with the stimulus classification speed. Thus, in patients with attentional deficit and hyperactive disorder, a reduced P3 is common.

As with the majority of testing, ERPs were first evaluated in patients with severe injuries who demonstrated a slow down in cortical responses as reflected by a delayed P3 component, often accompanied by longer response time.[120] The results were more ambiguous with MBI. Several studies reported a prolonged P3 latency,[123] whereas others[124] showed similar P3 latencies in MBI patients and controls. This latency is thought to be related to the patient's information processing speed because it reflects the moment when the stimulus is being evaluated and categorized. It has been suggested that ERP techniques may be more sensitive than standardized or computerized neuropsychological testing.[125]

ERP testing has been performed in the evaluation of athletes thought to have suffered MBI. Concussed athletes demonstrated a significant reduction in the amplitude of the P3 component, which was related to the severity of postconcussive symptoms.[126] ERP measurement has also been used to compare the effects of concussion on attention in athletes. Longer reaction times were exhibited by symptomatic athletes compared with asymptomatic ones and there was an inverse relationship between severity of postconcussion symptoms and P3 component amplitude.[124] These findings provide strong evidence that concussive symptomatology affects attentional capacities. Long-term effects of repeat concussions have also been evaluated using ERP in the athlete. Hockey players who sustained three or more concussions displayed a prolonged P3 latency in visual ERP in comparison with athletes who had no concussion history.[127]

Biochemical Markers

A neurochemical cascade occurs following MBI that causes many changes at the cellular level. This cascade results in several serum markers of brain injury that may be helpful in the diagnosis and management of MBI.[128] This complex cascade begins with axonal stretching and injury of the neuronal membrane that results in an increase in extracellular potassium. This can cause depolarization of the neurons and release of excitatory neurotransmitters. This "neurotransmitter storm," as it has been called, is followed by a suppressed state diffused throughout the brain. During this time, membrane pumps are activated and there is an increase in glucose utilization. At this stage of the cascade, there is also an increased production and accumulation of lactate, which may increase the neural tissues' susceptibility to further insult.[129] Following MBI, there is also a transient decrease in cerebral blood flow and an activation of *N*-methyl-D-aspartate (NMDA) receptors. Oxidative metabolism is impaired secondary to these changes as well as an influx of calcium into the cell with accumulation in the mitochondria. The result is a degree of energy failure and microtubule breakdown. Energy production is further impaired by decreases in magnesium. Several additional changes occur. There is a decrease in inhibitory neurotransmitters such as gamma-aminobutyric acid (GABA) that can decrease the seizure threshold, and a loss of forebrain cholinergic neurons resulting in impaired neurotransmission with possible learning and memory difficulties.[129]

The use of these serum markers of brain injury to diagnose and assess intracranial injury has been extensively studied in the adult population, and to a lesser extent in children. It has been hypothesized that after release from brain tissue, these chemicals pass into the CSF and serum through the blood–brain barrier, which becomes transiently more permeable following the insult. The presence of these biochemical markers can be measured from hours to days after they are released into the CSF or serum and numerous studies have shown that their presence after TBI is a sensitive and specific indicator of injury and outcome.[130]

Several biochemical markers have been linked to MTBI (**Table 9.6**). These include S100 proteins, neuron-specific enolase (NSE), and cleaved tau protein (CTP). Two of the markers that appear to have the most potential in MBI; protein S100B and neuron-specific enolase (NSE) can be measured using a rapid enzyme-linked immunosorbent assay (ELISA) that requires less than 250 μL of serum.[131]

Protein S100B is one of the most researched of the known markers. It is the major low affinity calcium binding protein in astrocytes, and studies suggest that it is a marker of astrocyte injury or death. Its physiologic function is not entirely understood, but recent studies suggest that released protein S100B inhibits synaptic plasticity by binding to receptors on neurons.[132] The serum half-life of protein S100B is 112 minutes, and as a result, increases after TBI are rapid and transient. In adults, serum protein S100B concentrations drawn within 6 hours of head injury are powerful predictors of intracranial pathology and

Table 9.6 Characteristics of Several Biochemical Markers

Biochemical Marker	Location	Serum Half-Life	Sensitivity to Hemolysis
Neuron-specific enolase (NSE)	Neurons, platelets, red blood cells	24 h	Yes
S100B	Astrocytes, bone marrow, fat	112 min	No
Myelin-basic protein (MBP)	Myelin	12 h	No

Source: Data from Berger RP, Kochanek PM, Pierce MC. Biochemical markers of brain injury: could they be used as diagnostic adjuncts in cases of inflicted traumatic brain injury? Child Abuse Negl 2004;28(7):739–754.

outcome.[133] It has long been established as a good identifier of primary and secondary brain damage and stroke and has been found to correlate with an unfavorable short-term outcome in MBI. Previous research in adults has shown that an increase in serum protein S100B can be more sensitive to brain injury than a CT scan.[134] Some recent research has suggested that there may be extracranial sources of protein S100B,[135] though the validity of the methods in these studies has been a topic of debate.

NSE is a glycolytic enzyme that is localized primarily in the cytoplasm of neurons. Multiple studies have found it to be measurable in the serum after TBI of all severities and a marker of neuronal death.[136] Increases in the concentration of this substance in the CSF and serum have also been observed in adults with a variety of nontraumatic neurological conditions including Creutzfeldt-Jakob disease, Parkinson disease, cervical spondylosis, and hypoxia.[137] Importantly, NSE is present in erythrocytes and platelets, as well as neurons. Thus, only nonhemolyzed samples can be analyzed. In addition, NSE has a long (20-hour) half-life, which likely explains why serum levels of NSE often do not correspond to the amount of TBI.

Myelin-basic protein (MBP) is one of the two most abundant proteins in myelin in the central nervous system (CNS) and may be useful as a marker of MBI. Although studies of MBP concentrations after TBI are limited, the literature indicates that increases in serum MBP are specific for ICH and severe TBI. Serum MBP has a very long half-life; concentrations peak ~72 hours after injury and can remain increased for up to 2 weeks after TBI.[138] This prolonged presence in the serum may be an advantage as a screening tool for MBI in asymptomatic individuals in whom serum NSE and protein S100B concentrations are no longer detectable. Because the concentration of MBP peaks later than either NSE or protein S100B, it may be used to assist in determining the timing of injury if used in a panel with these other markers.

The brain-specific fraction of creatinine phosphokinase (CPK-BB) has also been given some attention as a potential marker of MBI. Although it might have some utility in determining MBI, it has lost favor for several reasons. The sensitivity and specificity of CPK-BB has been found to be inadequate for use as an indicator of TBI.[139] It is also hard to measure because its increase is rapid and very transient and measurement requires gel electrophoresis that is time consuming. In addition, testing requires a substantial amount of blood (3 mL) compared with other potential markers of MBI.

Other markers are being evaluated. Glial fibrillary acidic protein (GFAP) levels in peripheral blood have been studied extensively in severe TBI, which can raise its serum concentration by up to 4.6-fold. It has been found to correlate significantly with the injury severity score and CT findings and is higher in patients who had a poor outcome 6 months postinjury than in those who had good outcomes.[140] CTP has been found to be increased in patients with MBI and may prove helpful in identifying patients in this population.[141]

Although the identification of these individual markers of MBI is an exciting step toward improved management of these patients, significantly more research needs to be performed before these markers can be used in a clinical setting. A better understanding of how the markers sensitivity and specificity is altered by the severity of injury is needed. In addition, the occurrence of false-positive and false-negative test results needs to be further evaluated. It is possible that nontraumatic neurological insults can release several of these markers. For example, seizures are a common presenting symptom in general as well as with MBI and it is therefore essential to understand whether seizures in the absence of traumatic injury cause an increase in the biomarkers of interest. Causes of false-negatives, such as the fluid resuscitation of a trauma patient must also be identified.[131]

No single biochemical marker has yet been accepted as a reliable test for MBI or has predicted outcomes consistently. A panel of markers may be needed because the brain contains many different types of cells, each of which has a different threshold for injury as well as different sensitivities to various types of injury. Such a panel would include markers for glial cell injury as well as markers that are sensitive to direct trauma, hypoxia, and inflammation. The use of such a panel would also likely provide insight into the timing of injury. Although significant additional research still needs to be done, it appears that serum biomarkers may ultimately allow clinicians following MBI a powerful new diagnostic tool.

Genetic Testing

With the completion of the human genome map, our understanding of the influence of molecular biology on an individual's susceptibility to injury is expanding. Currently, more than 900 genetic tests are available and many could have applications in MBI. The most well-known susceptibility gene is apolipoprotein E epsilon4 (APOE e4).

APOE is important for lipoprotein transport and cholesterol homeostasis by promoting the recognition and catabolism of APOE-containing lipoproteins (e.g., βVLDL, very low-density lipoprotein, intermediate-density lipoprotein, HDL) by the lipoprotein receptors LDLR, the E/α2M receptor LRP1, gp330/megalin, and the VLDL receptor. It is synthesized predominantly by astrocytes and microglia and thus highly expressed in the brain. The APOE gene, located on chromosome 19, occurs in three common allelic forms, APOE e2, e3, and e4.[142] Several studies have linked the APOE e4 allele to poor outcomes following TBI.[143]

Attention was first focused on this gene when it was linked to late-onset familial and sporadic Alzheimer disease. The neuropathological similarities between chronic traumatic brain injury (CTBI) and Alzheimer disease led to the discovery of the possible link between sports-related brain injury and APOE e4. CTBI is a worrisome complication of contact/collision sports during which the participant sustains repetitive blows to the head of variable force. In 1997, a study was performed on 30 boxers revealing that those with the APOE e4 gene and high exposure to the sport were at an increased risk of neurological dysfunction versus those without the gene. The study also found that all of the boxers that developed severe neurological impairment possessed the APOE e4 allele.[144] The association between this gene and a higher risk of CTBI was strengthened by a second study performed in 1997 in a nonboxing population of neurotrauma patients.[145]

The pathophysiological mechanism for this association may be that β-amyloid is deposited in the brain after head trauma to a greater extent in individuals with the e4 allele. The allele may also affect the efficiency of neuronal repair, which is suggested by the poorer outgrowth of neurites observed in cell cultures containing APOE e4.[146] APOE e4-related alterations in the neuronal cytoskeleton, increased susceptibility to reactive oxygen species in association with APOE e4, and altered intracerebral cholesterol trafficking are other mechanisms proposed to be the cause of increased susceptibility to the athlete with the APOE e4 gene.[142]

The link between APOE e4 and CTBI is not universally accepted. Most studies relating to MBI in sports have had a relatively small population of subjects, and this has been a major criticism. In addition, studies have relied on brief cognitive assessments or coarse measures of global functioning, thereby limiting their conclusions. Other prospective studies on the role of APOE e4 allele in mild to moderate brain injury with more detailed evaluation of neuropsychiatric outcome found no association between the presence of the APOE e4 allele and poor outcome across all measures.

The relationship between this gene and an increased risk of CTBI has major implications. Should all athletes in contact/collision sports be tested for APOE e4 as a part of a preparticipation physical; and should those found to be positive be banned from participation? The genetic profile of an athlete could be useful in determining if the participant is predisposed to a particular injury. If this information is known before participation, the athlete could be properly counseled concerning risks, advised of special techniques and equipment to minimize risk, and given alternative sporting activities.

Management of Mild Brain Injury

Initial Management

Increased interest in MBI has led to a plethora of articles addressing the management of this condition. With such a large amount of information available, the use of evidence-based guidelines is becoming preferred to achieve improved care for MBI patients. In general, the primary goal of management of the acute phase of MBI is to identify surgical lesions using screening devices (neurological examination, prolonged observation, radiological examination). A study of the quality of head injury care in 41 hospitals in the United States showed that most of the preventable mortality was due to late diagnoses of deterioration in patients who initially appeared to have suffered only minor injuries.[147] Thus, at this stage of injury, management should focus on the risk of development of an acute traumatic intracranial hematoma and on prevention of persistent postconcussion symptoms. The literature generally supports the use of CT scanning for all cases of MBI in which at least one of the following is present: loss of consciousness, PTA, or confusion/impaired alertness. Obviously, patients who exhibit a decline in neurological status, pupillary dilatation, or focal neurological deficit not explained by systemic sources, require urgent imaging and possibly neurosurgical consultation.

One of the foundations for the use of MBI guidelines is the stratification of patients into groups based on perceived severity of injury. The Head Injury Severity Scale (HISS)[148] is often recommended for this task (**Table 9.7**). In the case of MBI, only the first two groups of this scale, minimal and mild, are pertinent. For the minimal injury group, hospital admission is not necessary nor is imaging, unless additional risk factors are present. In the mild injury group, CT imaging is usually recommended. If imaging is negative and the patient has no additional risk factors, they also may be

Table 9.7 Head Injury Severity Scale (HISS)

HISS Category	Clinical Characteristics
Minimal	GCS = 15, no LOC
Mild	GCS = 14–15, brief LOC or amnesia (<5 min), impaired alertness or memory
Moderate	GCS = 9–13, or LOC (≥5 min)
Severe	GCS <9

Source: Data from Stein SC, Spettell C. The Head Injury Severity Scale (HISS): a practical classification of closed-head injury. Brain Inj 1995;9(5):437–444.

Abbreviation: GCS, Glasgow Coma Scale; LOC, loss of consciousness.

discharged with appropriate head injury observation instructions. Risk factors including therapeutic anticoagulation or hemophilia, radiographically demonstrated skull fracture, clinical signs of a depressed skull fracture, posttraumatic seizures, shunt-treated hydrocephalus, or multiple injuries should result in both CT imaging and admission for observation. Overnight (i.e., $\geq$12 hours) observation is recommended in the moderate injury group and in cases classified as mild in the unusual circumstance that CT scanning is unavailable.[149] Similar recommendations are supported by the Western Trauma Association Multicenter Study in which 2,766 isolated head injury patients with initial GCS of 13 to 15 were reviewed.[150] Using groupings based on GCS, in patients with a GCS of 15, no neurological or cognitive abnormalities, and a normal brain CT, including absence of skull fracture, it is reasonable to discharge them home with a reliable adult.

Patients that are admitted for surveillance should be strictly observed with a standardized examination objectifying the level of consciousness, pupillary responses, blood pressure, and pulse rate. Examination should be performed every 15 minutes the first 2 hours after admission and thereafter every hour until at least 12 hours after injury.[149] Deterioration during this period of observation is defined as a reduction of the GCS score of $\geq$2 points and/or the development of focal neurological deficits. In cases of deterioration during observation, immediate imaging should be performed.[149]

Another recent recommendation for the management of MBI has divided the condition into two groups, simple and complex, based more on the persistence of symptomatology versus the acute manifestations of the injury. The majority of patients that suffer MBI is in the simple category. They recover in 48 to 72 hours, even with detailed neuropsychological testing, and are headache free within 2 to 4 weeks of the injury. The complex group, on the other hand, encompasses individuals that suffer persistent symptoms. These recommendations are based on experience in the athlete.

In the case of simple concussion, an individual should not be placed in a situation in which they may receive an additional head trauma until completely asymptomatic. Formal neuropsychological screening does not commonly play a role in these injuries; they can often be managed by primary care physicians or by certified athletic trainers working under medical supervision.[151] In sports, the cornerstone of management is rest until all symptoms resolve and then a gradual increase in exertion before return to play.

Individuals that suffer complex concussions require more in-depth management including in some cases formal neuropsychological testing. This population is most appropriately managed by physicians with specific expertise in head injury.

Neuropsychological Management

Despite historically being considered a minor injury, individuals who sustain an MBI often exhibit abnormal neuropsychological profiles, such as deficits in working memory, attention, information processing speed, and more generally, in executive function, known to be linked to the frontal lobe.[68] Neuropsychological testing in the acute setting has been suggested to identify patients at high risk for prolonged cognitive deficits and is rapidly becoming a mainstay in the management of MBI. It has repeatedly demonstrated its value both experimentally and in clinical application and it is recommended that neuropsychological testing be one of the cornerstones of management in complex MBI. It is somewhat less important in the evaluation of simple injuries. One meta-analysis of the relevant literature conducted to determine the impact of MTBI across nine cognitive domains showed that the overall effect of MBI on neuropsychological functioning was moderate. The acute effects ($<$3 months postinjury) were greatest for delayed memory and fluency and no residual neuropsychological impairment by 3 months postinjury were observed.[152] Another meta-analysis established a relationship between MBI and small reductions in cognitive functioning in individuals assessed more than 3 months postinjury.[153]

One of the biggest obstacles to its use in MBI is the questionable need for baseline data. Although this is easily accomplished in the athletic population, few individuals not involved in sports have any need for this preinjury information. These missing data are becoming less important, however, with recent studies of computerized testing suggesting that performance variability may be a key measure for acute concussion diagnosis even in the absence of a baseline.

Computerized testing has several other benefits. The inherent difficulties with most neuropsychological testing are the determination of normal ranges, the sensitivity and specificity of tests, and the effect of practice or learning on test results. Infinitely variable test paradigms are now available with computerized testing, which may overcome some of these concerns.[154] Computerized testing also may solve the logistical problem of many practitioners who do not have a neuropsychologist available; the test may be self-administered and in some cases may even be Web-based.[155] Serial follow-up examinations are also made more practical. A drawback to computerized testing is its increased cost and lack of validation. A comparison between abbreviated formal neuropsychological testing programs and computerized neuropsychological programs performed in 2006 found the estimated cost for abbreviated formal testing to be between $22 and $27 per athlete and between $669 and $677 per athlete for computerized testing.[156]

Detailed neuropsychological testing is employed more often at the professional level and in the management of athletes with MTBI. Both the National Hockey League (NHL) and NFL, along with many college teams, are now utilizing limited neuropsychological testing to document possible prolonged effects of MBI and to assist the clinician in determining return to play and possible retirement issues. It should usually not be performed while the player is symptomatic because it adds nothing to return-to-play decisions, and it may interfere with the testing process by allowing practice effects to confound the results. In certain cases, however, serial follow-up after the injury is valuable, both as a means to encourage athlete compliance and for comparison purposes. When evaluating an athlete's performance, it is usually best to compare results with the individual's previous tests. It has been shown that cognitive recovery may precede or follow clinical symptom resolution, suggesting that the assessment of cognitive function should be an important component in any return to play protocol.[113] One of the inherent problems with neuropsychological testing in athletics is the observation that players may return to baseline while still symptomatic. Most importantly, neuropsychological assessment should not be used as the sole basis of a return-to-play decision, but rather be seen as additional information to be used in clinical decision making.

Pharmacological Management

The pharmacological management of MBI is not given significant attention in most management strategies largely because of the paucity of evidence-based research in this area. Presently, it could be employed in the management of specific symptoms experienced by the patient such as headache, insomnia, or lethargy. Recent advances in the understanding of the pathophysiology of MBI could also increase the utility of pharmacological treatment with the goal of limiting injury at the cellular level and shortening recovery. Although many of the treatments discussed have been studied mainly in severe brain injury, their possible utility for MBI in the near future warrants their mention.[164] It must be emphasized, however, that the MBI population may be more likely to experience detrimental side effects from these therapies than uninjured people, and appropriate vigilance should be maintained when they are employed.

The usefulness of corticosteroids in head trauma is undetermined, with experimental studies demonstrating both benefits and drawbacks.[165] Although their use in MBI is based mainly on their ability to stabilize lysosomal membranes and reduce tissue edema, some steroid compounds also inhibit lipid peroxidation. These include the lazeroids or 21-amino steroids, which could have a protective effect following MBI. For example, tirilazad mesylate has been shown to improve behavioral recovery in mice.[166] Another therapy that has been proposed in TBI to decrease posttraumatic inflammatory complications is the use of hypothermia. However, when instituted immediately following injury, this modality reduces the posttraumatic increase in interleukin-1 β-mediated nerve growth factor production, which can inhibit the nervous system's intrinsic repair mechanism. Both phase 1 and phase 2 trials have been performed and suggest that short (<48 hours) periods of moderate (32 to 33°C) hypothermia are well tolerated and provide limited evidence of a beneficial effect on the outcome following moderate to severe TBI.[167]

Some nutrients such as vitamin C and E may play a role in improving outcome following MBI. The administration of free radical scavengers and antioxidants before injury has provided some protection in various models of CNS trauma where free radicals are generated. The routine use of these compounds has been somewhat dampened, however, by several large epidemiological studies of antioxidant use for cardiovascular disease; they showed that antioxidant therapy was associated with an increase in cancer incidence.[168,169] Other nutritional supplements, such as creatine, have been anticipated to be of benefit in severe TBI.[170] Conversely, hyperbaric oxygen therapy has also been proposed as a potential treatment for MBI. However, it may also have a potentially harmful effect on the injured brain by supplying oxygen for free radical reactions that result in iron-catalyzed lipid peroxidation. The benefits of the delivery of high concentrations of oxygen under pressure are thought to be secondary to cerebral vasoconstriction, improvement in glucose metabolism, and reduction of cerebral edema. Although randomized studies have demonstrated an improved mortality rate with hyperbaric therapy in severe brain injuries, no long-term improvements in functional outcomes have been observed.[171,172]

Arachidonic acid has been a target of treatment for MBI because its metabolism can produce toxic breakdown products such as thromboxanes, peptidyl leukotrienes, and free radicals that may exacerbate the traumatic injury. Although no specific trials of cyclooxygenase inhibitors such as ibuprofen and mixed cyclooxygenase-lipoxygenase inhibitors have been done in MBI, improved outcomes have been observed in animal models of spinal cord injury.[173] Various cytokines and anion transport inhibitors have also been proposed to disrupt the cellular cascade following MBI.[174–176]

For over 50 years, we have known that cholinergic antagonists such as scopolamine can reduce the behavioral deficits following moderate to severe brain injury. This knowledge, combined with the well-documented sympatho-adrenal response following TBI, has given strength to the theory that blocking this response pharmacologically by drugs that modify monoamine function could improve outcomes.[177] This has led to a randomized trial of such therapy. Unfortunately, it was terminated prematurely because of unacceptable psychomimetic side effects.[174] It has also been observed in animal models that increases in the extracellular levels of glutamate and aspartate correlate with the severity of brain injury. Drugs that counteract these changes such as NMDA (*N*-methyl-D-aspartate) antagonists, AMPA (alpha-amino-3-hydroxy-5-methyl-4-isoaxolepropionate) antagonists, and magnesium have bestowed a protective benefit to treated animals. Likewise, there have been limited human studies demonstrating a benefit to these therapies.[178]

The use of antagonists of calcium channels and opiate receptors could have some beneficial effect in MBI. Although the entry of calcium through voltage-dependent channels may contribute to secondary brain injury, several randomized trials of various agents have failed to demonstrate any protective benefit. One novel calcium channel agent, (S)-emopamil, has been shown to be beneficial in experimental injury.[179] The release of endogenous opioids can cause secondary damage to the brain following traumatic injury. In particular, the kappa opioid receptor or its isoforms may be significant in the variation of these injuries, and a reevaluation of data from randomized trials of spinal cord injury suggest a benefit from the opioid receptor antagonist naloxone.[180] Because of its ability to antagonize many of the actions of endogenous opioids, thyrotrophin-releasing hormone (TRH) was initially used in the treatment of acute spinal cord injury. The protective effects of this compound have been found to be dose related and present even if administration is delayed up to 24 hours.[181] This agent is also thought to have an effect on platelet function, leukotriene activation, and excitatory amino acid release.

The brain relies on several neurotrophic factors to recover from injury. The infusion of intracerebral nerve growth factor during the acute phase of experimental head injury has been shown to provide a beneficial effect and is thought to be related to its ability to attenuate traumatically induced apoptotic cell death.[182] The proto-oncogene Bcl-2 promotes the regeneration of severed CNS axons in the mammalian CNS similar to the actions of brain-derived neurotrophic factor. These effects are likely the result of extracellular signaling pathways that are involved in both neuronal survival and axon elongation.[183] Insulin-like growth factor-1 has also been evaluated for the treatment of moderate to severe head injury in a phase II safety and efficacy trial.[184]

Risk Factors for Repeat Injury

Several factors increase an individual's risk of repeat, as well as more severe, MBI. Because athletes are much more likely than the general population to suffer multiple injuries, most of the data on this subject is based on findings in contact sports. For example, a National Collegiate Athletic Association (NCAA) study found that college football players with a history of concussion are more likely to have future concussive injuries with a 7- to 10-day window of increased susceptibility and that repetitive concussions may be associated with slower recovery of neurological function.[157] An epidemiologic study of collegiate and high school football players found that players who sustain one concussion are 3 times more likely to sustain a second one in the same season.[158] It is also well accepted that exposure to repeated MBI over time, as in boxing or soccer, can result in severe cognitive impairment.[127,159]

In boxing and to a lesser extent other contact sports, a large number of brain injuries occur because of fatigue. Early in the bout, the fresh participant has an increased ability to maintain good balance, block and slip punches, and move with a punch when struck (decreasing the amount of force transmitted to the brain). As the match progresses, the fatigued fighter loses this defensive ability and is more vulnerable to head trauma.[160]

The age of an individual may play a role in recovery as well as severity of injury. Although this is certainly not the rule, a prolonged course of recovery in high school as compared with college athletes has been reported, with a significant memory impairment present up to 7 days after injury in high school athletes, but for only 1 day at the college level.[161,162] Conversely, elderly patients (aged 60 years and older) have been demonstrated to have an increased mortality after isolated brain injury.[163] The elderly also often develop an increase in subdural potential space secondary to the natural atrophy of the brain that occurs with age, which could affect the normal buffering of impacts.[160]

Because CSF provides some shock-absorption for the brain, then a brain surface deprived of its normal concentration of shock-absorbing CSF might be more vulnerable to injury. This could be the case in an individual who is dehydrated. Dehydration in athletes can result from the loss of fluids from perspiration as a game or match progresses, or intentionally prior to participation to meet a weight requirement.[160] Another factor might be the relative distribution of CSF based on whether the head is in motion or is at rest when the concussive blow is struck.[44] Other risk factors for sports-related MBI include not wearing mouth guards, poorly fitting helmets, and genetic predisposition.

Postconcussion Syndrome

After suffering an MBI, ~50 to 80% of patients often report a constellation of physical, cognitive, and emotional/behavioral symptoms for days or weeks (**Table 9.8**).[38,185,186] These include persistent recurrent headaches, memory impairment, irritability, and inability to concentrate. Although the

Table 9.8 Symptoms Associated with Postconcussion Syndrome (PCS)

Persistent recurrent headaches	Sensitivity to light and noise	Generalized loss of well-being
Ataxia dizziness	Loss of libido	Attention problems
Generalized fatigue	Memory impairment	Inability to concentrate
Irritability	Apathy	Anxiety
Depression	Change in personality	Vertigo
Difficulty with sleep Insomnia	Giddiness	Visual disturbances
Aggression	Deterioration in work performance	Loss of social skills
Lack of judgment	Inability to sustain effort	Difficulties in recalling material

Sources: Data from Albright JP, McAuley E, Martin RK, Crowley ET, Foster DT. Head and neck injuries in college football: an eight-year analysis. Am J Sports Med 1985;13(3):147–152; Alves W. Natural history of post-concussive signs and symptoms. Phys Med Rehabil Clin N Am 1993;6:21–32; and Gouvier WD, Cubic B, Jones G, Brantley P, Cutlip Q. Postconcussion symptoms and daily stress in normal and head-injured college populations. Arch Clin Neuropsychol 1992;7(3):193–211.

transient occurrence of these symptoms may be a part of the normal recovery process and not a complication, as many as 50% of patients report symptoms for up to 3 months, and 10 to 15% report symptoms for more than a year after injury.[187] In general, when symptoms persist for over a month, the condition is known as postconcussion syndrome (PCS). When the symptoms continue for more than 3 months, it is called persistent PCS with resultant permanent disability. Other commonly used terms for the condition are chronic brain syndrome and posttraumatic syndrome.

Although this condition has been recognized for centuries, the term *postconcussion syndrome* was first used in 1934 to describe the "subjective posttraumatic syndrome... due directly to the blow on the head."[188] It has been a controversial subject, largely based on the incongruity between cases of persisting and sometimes severe disability versus initially mild head trauma from which most patients rapidly recover.[187] The debate over the existence of the syndrome began in the 1860s with the increased amount of railway travel and its associated head injuries due to the high incidence of sudden stops and collisions. As the condition became better recognized, researchers theorized that the posttraumatic disorders resulting from these injuries occurred from mechanical damage to the brain and spinal cord. Without diagnostic imaging, however, these theories were difficult to substantiate.

Concurrently, the increasing influence of psychiatrists such as Freud and Charcot promoted interest in the psychological components of the disorder. In addition, social changes such as legislation providing for worker's compensation increased the focus on nonorganic causes of disability, and over the next century the sentiment in both the scientific community and the public was clearly biased against any organic explanation for PCS. The advent of diagnostic imaging modalities in the 1960s such as CT, MRI, and PET have not significantly clarified the condition because such scans have shown only slight, diffuse abnormalities in a small number of cases. Recently, neuropsychological testing has added weight to the belief that PCS does reflect some kind of residual organic damage; most investigators now believe that a variety of premorbid, injury-related, and postmorbid neuropathological and psychological factors contribute to the development of PCS following MBI.[189]

At the extreme, PCS can be quite severe, with the most dramatic long-term presentation including dementia pugilistica associated with boxing. Even in less severe cases, however, selective attention testing has been demonstrated to be negatively affected in concussed patients with PCS compared with concussed patients without PCS at 6 months postinjury.[190] Thus, these symptoms may identify a subgroup of patients at subsequent increased risk for prolonged cognitive deficits as a result of their injury.[191] The severity of MBI does not necessarily predict the occurrence of PCS. Likewise, the number of concussions has not been a strong predictor of these symptoms. No biomarker has consistently demonstrated the ability to predict PCS after MTBI. A combination of clinical factors in conjunction with biochemical markers may be necessary to develop a comprehensive decision rule that more accurately predicts PCS after MTBI.

Although many organic factors contribute to the condition of PCS, some psychological factors are now believed to explain, in part, the persistence of these complaints.[192] Numerous psychological models have attempted to explain the development and persistence of symptoms, the main component of which is expectation.[193] The expectation-as-etiology model predicts that vague, everyday complaints present before a brain injury are incorrectly attributed to the brain injury, in line with preinjury expectations. This may result in selective attention to symptoms that are congruent with, and support these expectations. This symptom focus thus enhances symptom complaints after injury and reduces retrospective ratings of symptoms before the injury.[193]

The interaction between psychological and biological factors has been termed the coping hypothesis.[194] This hypothesis theorizes that in cases of persistent PCS, there may be a mild underlying physical change to the brain following injury. However, the effects of this damage are magnified by an adverse psychological reaction to the injury. Two broad categories for PCS symptoms have been suggested.[195] Type I is benign and has a good prognosis for recovery and adjustment. Type II represents a group of patients with persistent PCS symptoms. Many never completely recover, do not return to work, and have multiple subjective symptoms without substantial clinical neurological findings. This has been attributed to a "maladaptation resulting from the stress of their injury."[195] The newer quantitative EEGs, or brain mapping with increased sensitivity from computer analysis, may provide greater insights into the relationship between organic and nonorganic causes of PCS.

Malignant Hyperemia (Second Impact Syndrome)

In 1984, the death of a college football player seemed to have resulted from a second seemingly minor blow to the head. At the time it was hypothesized that this fatality was the result of "a repeat blow to an already compliance-compromised brain which precipitated a catastrophic increase in intracranial pressure, perhaps through a loss of vasomotor tone."[196] The term *vascular congestion* syndrome was coined in 1991 following the death of a 17-year-old high school football player from an uncontrollable increase in ICP.[197] Both of these deaths are thought to have been the result of what is now known as second impact syndrome (SIS). SIS is defined as a fatal uncontrollable increase in ICP secondary to diffuse brain swelling, which occurs after a blow to the head is incurred before recovery from a previous blow to the head.[37] The occurrence, phenomena, and pathology of SIS are debated and not universally agreed upon. Significant controversy exists over the validity of this condition due to problems with documentation of the initial event, persistent symptoms, and severity of the second impact.

The pathophysiology of SIS is thought to involve a loss of autoregulation of the brain's blood supply, edema, and uncontrolled intracranial hypertension. This loss of autoregulation leads to vascular engorgement within the cranium, which, in turn, markedly increases ICP and leads to a syndrome of uncal herniation, cerebellar herniation, or both. Animal research has shown that vascular engorgement in the brain after a mild head injury may be difficult, if not impossible, to control in this "double impact" setting. The usual time from second impact to uncontrollable edema is rapid, taking 2 to 5 minutes.[73] There have been 21 reported cases of this condition,[198] which is most often seen in boxing, football, and ice hockey. In most cases, male adolescents or young adults are affected.

Typically, the athlete experiences some degree of post-concussion symptoms after the first head injury. These may include visual, motor, or sensory changes and difficulty with cognitive and memory processes. Before these symptoms resolve, which may take days or weeks, the athlete returns to competition and receives a second blow to the head. The second blow may be minor, perhaps only involving a blow to the chest that jerks the athlete's head and indirectly imparts accelerative forces to the brain. Affected athletes may seem stunned, but usually do not lose consciousness and often complete the play. They usually remain on their feet for 15 seconds to a minute or so, but seem dazed, similar to a grade I concussion without LOC. Often, affected athletes remain on the playing field or walk off under their own power. What happens in the next few moments to several minutes sets this syndrome apart from a concussion or subdural hematoma. Usually, within seconds to minutes of the second impact, the athlete who is conscious yet stunned precipitously collapses to the ground and becomes comatose, with rapidly dilating pupils, loss of eye movement, and evidence of respiratory failure.

The condition is associated with a 50% mortality and nearly 100% morbidity rate.[73] It is important to understand this condition when making return-to-play decisions following a head injury in an athlete. Any athlete still symptomatic from a previous head injury should not be allowed to return to full practice or participation in a contact or collision sport.

Sports-Related Head Injury

Participation in sports carries an inherent risk of injury to the athlete. In the spectrum of sports-related injuries, those to the nervous system have the most potential for significant morbidity and mortality. In fact, head and neck injuries account for up to 70% of traumatic deaths and 20% of permanent disability in athletes[199,200] and have been described in virtually every sport from boxing to golf. Athletes that suffer catastrophic injuries to the head or spinal cord are usually easy to identify, as are those that develop an immediate neurological deficit. More challenging is the diagnosis of an injury with minimal initial symptomatology.

Differentiation between minor and serious injuries is the foundation of management of the athlete. It is estimated that 750,000 Americans suffer injuries annually in recreational activities, with 82,000 (9.1%) sustaining some form of head injury. The frequency of all sports-related

MBIs has been estimated to be up to 300,000 annually in the United States.[201] Head injuries are more common in sports than spinal injuries.

The incidence and severity of head injury and its impact on the player's role in the game vary greatly with the sport involved. Athletic endeavors should be considered according to the nature of the play and participants in terms of types of sporting events and the motivations of the players involved. The most useful classification is that of recreational and nonorganized sports versus organized, sanctioned sports. The former have little formal structure, fewer rules, no refereed officials, less use of protective equipment, and participation by a wide variety of people under a variable set of conditions. In contrast, organized sporting events have structure regarding training, rules and their enforcement, specialized equipment, and physicians and athletic trainers dedicated to the care of those who are injured.

American football, ice hockey, and boxing are commonly referred to when discussing sports-related head injury because of the frequent and obvious violent contact. Over 1.5 million people participate in football (i.e., recreational, high school, collegiate, and professional) annually and the estimated annual incidence of MBIs is 4 to 20%.[73]

Nevertheless, head injuries are commonly observed in sporting activities considered less violent. The United States Consumer Product Safety Commission reported in 1990 that four of the top five sports that cause head injury requiring hospitalization are not the traditional "collision" games. These were basketball, bicycling, baseball, and playground activities (football was the only collision sport to break the top five).[202] Equestrian sports account for ~46,000 emergency room visits annually, with nearly 20% involving the head or neck and 70% of deaths related to head injuries.[203,204] Approximately seven fatalities occur annually related to skateboard injuries with 90% involving severe injury to the head.[205] Recreational and commuter bicyclists have between 1,000 and 1,300 fatalities each year, and the majority are the result of brain injury.[206–208] Although sports such as gymnastics and cheerleading have traditionally been responsible for the highest number of head injuries in the female athlete,[209] women are now crossing into previously male-dominated sports such as boxing and an increasing number of serious head injuries are being incurred in contact/collision sports.[210]

Head injuries occur at one of the highest rates in downhill skiing and often occur as a result of collisions with trees and boulders, as well as other skiers.[211–213] Other recreational sports that are considered to be a high risk for head injury include snowboarding, hang-gliding, skydiving, mountaineering, and race-car driving.[73] The head often initiates the impact in football, and the involved activities are usually blocking or tackling. It is estimated that 250,000 MBIs occur annually in high school football alone.[202,214] Twenty percent of all high school football players suffer a concussion annually and an average of eight fatalities occur secondary to head injuries during participation in the sport every year.[202,215]

Concussions are by far the most common type of sports-related head injury. They account for approximately three-fourths of all head injuries in this population. The recognition in the early 1980s that MBI exists as an important clinical entity began to pave the way for an increased appreciation of concussion in sports. In the 1990s, there was an increased focus on defining and categorizing the athlete with MBI. Evidence suggested that concussion may be more common and serious than previously believed,[26,37,216,217] and the long-term sequelae of repetitive head trauma may be far from benign. In contrast to earlier attitudes, when being concussed was considered an acceptable occurrence for a contact athlete, new evidence has provided proof that ongoing cerebral dysfunction often persists.[218] The concept of MBI or concussion has evolved in recent years, aided in great part by the application of formal neuropsychological and cognitive studies and by studies of patients involved in vehicular accidents and other significant trauma.

Many characteristics and nuances of the sports-related MBI population make diagnosis and treatment difficult. For example, athletes are the only group of patients who routinely and often fervently ask to be returned to play, thus subjecting themselves to further head impact.[73] That may result in subclinical head injury. Although a single episode of MBI seems to be well tolerated overall in the majority of athletes, long-term mental status morbidity is associated with two or more episodes of concussion.[68] Advances in the fields of diagnostic neuroradiology, neurobiology, neuropsychology, and sports medicine now provide the neurosurgeon with more accurate and objective methods of analyzing this population of patients.[73]

There has been no universal agreement on the definition and grading of concussion in sports, and attempts at classification have tended to focus on the presence or absence of a period of LOC and amnesia. However, concussion may present with any combination of the following signs and symptoms: a feeling of being stunned or seeing bright lights, a very brief LOC (seconds), lightheadedness, vertigo, loss of balance, headaches, cognitive and memory dysfunction, tinnitus, blurred vision, difficulty concentrating, lethargy, fatigue, personality changes, inability to perform daily activities, sleep disturbance, and motor or sensory symptoms. Numerous classification systems exist for grading the severity of concussion. Although there is little evidence-based support for any of the systems as most have been developed through clinical experience, three are in widespread use. These are the Cantu,[34] Colorado Medical Society,[219] and

American Society of Neurology systems,[32] which also have associated return-to-play guidelines (**Table 9.3**).

Evidence-Based Guidelines for Return to Sports after Mild Brain Injury

MBI is a common injury that poses difficulty with patient management, particularly when consideration for return to competition is necessary. Recent research has better defined the epidemiological issues related to sports injuries involving the CNS and has also led to classification and management paradigms that help guide decisions regarding athletes' return to play.

Currently, numerous concussion classification schemes with associated return to play guidelines exist. These are based on class II and III literature, as well as expert opinion. In 1991, return-to-competition guidelines were created by the Colorado Medical Society (CMS).[33] These were reviewed and endorsed by several professional organizations, including the American Academy of Pediatrics, the American Academy of Sports Medicine, and the American College of Surgeons Committee on Trauma.[32,36] Because of limited scientific data on which to construct medical practice parameters, the guidelines were modified in 1997.[32,37] The desire for a broader consensus of expert opinion resulted in the involvement of the Quality Standards Subcommittee of the American Academy of Neurology. To aid in creating more evidence-based guidelines, this group performed a literature review from 1966 to 1996 and modified the guidelines based on these data (class II and III) and a consensus of experts[220] (class III). No class I studies were available. The American Academy of Neurology guidelines were reviewed by several expert organizations, including the American Association of Neurological Surgeons, American College of Emergency Physicians, American Academy of Pediatricians, American Academy of Family Physicians, National Athletic Trainers Association, and American Academy of Neurology.[32] The evidence supports classifying the currently accepted guidelines for return to play following an MBI as level II recommendations because only limited data exists comparing individual return to play guidelines and outcomes.

A player's return to contact sports following a head injury is dependent on several variables. The severity of the injury, residual neurological deficits, and previous injuries must be taken into account. A complication in performing outcome studies for return to play guidelines is that there has been no universally accepted definition of a concussion. This muddies the evaluation of epidemiologic data in the literature substantially. MBI may be defined by the duration of LOC, retrograde/PTA, or duration of neurological/neuropsychological abnormalities.

Potential issues that affect return-to-play decisions in the patient that has suffered an MBI include the risk of SIS, increased vulnerability to repeat head injury, and the potential for long-term cumulative effects. Any athlete that is symptomatic should be excluded from contact sports.

Several studies have demonstrated that a premature return to play can increase adverse outcomes from the initial injury, as well as increase the player's risk for repeat injuries.[44,221] Nonetheless, no class I studies are available to confirm or refute this. It has been demonstrated that the risk of sustaining a concussion is 4 to 6 times greater in football players who have suffered previous head injuries (class III).[202]

Neuropsychological testing is important in recognizing the extent of injury and following its evolution. Even mild abnormalities indicate persistent and ongoing adverse effects of previous head injuries. Several authors suggest neuropsychological assessment of the head-injured athlete before return to contact sports is allowed. A controlled, prospective study[222] (class I) examined outcomes in football players suffering MTBI using standardized neuropsychological testing. The study found that the vast majority of football-related head injuries were mild and that the majority of the affected athletes had reversal of their deficits within 5 days. All had resolution of neuropsychological testing abnormalities within 10 days. A second study[223] reported similar findings in patients suffering MTBI that were not sports related (class I).

With regard to MTBI, we recommend adherence to the current guidelines for return to play constructed by the American Association of Neurologists, the Colorado Medical Society, or Cantu[34] (**Table 9.3**). We know of no evidence to date comparing player outcomes based on which system is used. Because of the potential (and unknown incidence) of catastrophic outcomes in this population, to err on the side of conservative management cannot be faulted. We also agree with the recommendation of Cantu[34] suggesting that three grade I concussions, two to three grade II concussions, or one to two grade III concussions are the limit for withdrawal of an athlete from competition for the season.

The modern evidence that is currently available supports the use of the return-to-play guidelines for MTBI listed in **Table 9.3** as a level II recommendation. No evidence is available demonstrating superior outcomes using one particular guideline.

Prevention of Mild Brain Injury

Despite the many advances in diagnosis and management of MBI, the ability to treat or reduce the effects of this condition is limited. As with other traumatic injuries, the greatest impact can be made by prevention. Education of the public with an emphasis on high-risk groups such as male adolescents and athletes would likely have the maximum effect. In addition, health care providers must be educated about the detection of MBI and its management. Ways to educate these populations include Web-based resources, educational videos, and international outreach programs.

One of the best opportunities to effect improvements in MBI occurrence is in organized sports. For example, rule changes barring spearing in football and teaching football players not to lead with their head have significantly reduced the frequency of head injuries. The American Medical Association's Committee on Medical Aspects of Sports organized a conference in 1962, which addressed head protection in athletes.[73] This meeting led to a greater understanding of the need to determine patterns of injury to reduce morbidity in this population. In November 2001, the 1st International Symposium on Concussion in Sport was held in Vienna, Austria, to provide recommendations for the improvement of safety and health of athletes who suffer MBI in ice hockey, football (soccer), and other sports.[6] The 2nd International Symposium on Concussion in Sport was organized by the same group and held in Prague, Czech Republic, in November 2004.[5]

Participants in unorganized sports must also be addressed. Although helmets have been shown to clearly reduce the risk of head injury in recreational bicycling, their usage can be significantly increased in this activity.

An important concept that requires constant review is the upgrading of protective equipment. The use of such "improved" protective equipment can result in the adoption of more dangerous playing techniques, which can cause a paradoxical increase in injury rates. This is a particular concern in child and adolescent athletes in whom head injury rates are often higher than in adult athletes.

Conclusion

The notion that MBI is truly "mild" and completely reversible, in recent years has been replaced with the realization that these injuries often lead to permanent sequelae. As a result, the public and medical practitioners have become more aware of the necessity for accurate and consistent methods of diagnosis and management. The numerous new tools available to evaluate the condition such as fMRI and neuropsychological testing have also sparked increased interest in MBI. Although this increase in attention has led to numerous advances in the understanding of this injury, it has also led to an overwhelming number of varying definitions and guidelines. In this chapter, we have endeavored to integrate and clarify some of the more accepted theories and management strategies that can be used to further advance our understanding of the condition.

References

1. Guskiewicz KM, Marshall SW, Bailes J, et al. Association between recurrent concussion and late-life cognitive impairment in retired professional football players. Neurosurgery 2005;57(4):719–726 discussion 719–726
2. Omalu BI, DeKosky ST, Minster RL, Kamboh MI, Hamilton RL, Wecht CH. Chronic traumatic encephalopathy in a National Football League player. Neurosurgery 2005;57(1):128–134 discussion 128–134
3. Teasdale G, Jennett B. Assessment of coma and impaired consciousness: a practical scale. Lancet 1974;2(7872):81–84
4. Blumbergs PC, Scott G, Manavis J, Wainwright H, Simpson DA, McLean AJ. Staining of amyloid precursor protein to study axonal damage in mild head injury. Lancet 1994;344(8929):1055–1056
5. McCrory P, Johnston K, Meeuwisse W, et al. Summary and agreement statement of the 2nd International Conference on Concussion in Sport, Prague 2004. Br J Sports Med 2005;39(4):196–204
6. Aubry M, Cantu R, Dvorak J, et al. Summary and agreement statement of the 1st International Symposium on Concussion in Sport, Vienna 2001. Clin J Sport Med 2002;12(1):6–11
7. Gerberding J, Binder S. Report to Congress on Mild Traumatic Brain Injury in the United States: Steps to Prevent a Serious Public Health Problem. Atlanta, GA: Centers for Disease Control and Prevention; 2003
8. Ruff RM, Jurica P. In search of a unified definition for mild traumatic brain injury. Brain Inj 1999;13(12):943–952
9. Williams DH, Levin HS, Eisenberg HM. Mild head injury classification. Neurosurgery 1990;27(3):422–428
10. Plum F, Posner JB. The Diagnosis of Stupor and Coma. (3rd ed.) Philadelphia: F.A. Davis; 1980
11. Levin HS, O'Donnell VM, Grossman RG. The Galveston Orientation and Amnesia Test: a practical scale to assess cognition after head injury. J Nerv Ment Dis 1979;167(11):675–684
12. Starmark JE, Stalhammar D, Holmgren E, Rosander B. A comparison of the Glasgow Coma Scale and the Reaction Level Scale (RLS85). J Neurosurg 1988;69(5):699–706
13. Alexander MP. Mild traumatic brain injury: pathophysiology, natural history, and clinical management. Neurology 1995;45(7): 1253–1260
14. Finkelstein E, Corso P, Miller T. The Incidence and Economic Burden of Injuries in the United States. New York: Oxford University; 2006
15. Rehabilitation of persons with traumatic brain injury. NIH Consens Statement 1998;16(1):1–41
16. Langlois J, Rutland-Brown W, Thomas K. Traumatic Brain Injury in the United States: Emergency Department Visits, Hospitalizations, and Deaths. Atlanta, GA: Centers for Disease Control and Prevention; 2004
17. Carr AM, Bailes JE, Helmkamp JC, Rosen CL, Miele VJ. Neurological injury and death in all-terrain vehicle crashes in West Virginia: a 10-year retrospective review. Neurosurgery 2004;54(4):861–866 discussion 866–867
18. Okie S. Traumatic brain injury in the war zone. N Engl J Med 2005; 352(20):2043–2047
19. Scott S, Vanderploeg R, Belager H, Scholten J. Blast injuries: evaluating and treating the postacute sequelae. Federal Practitioner 2005; 22(1):67–75
20. Warden D. Military TBI during the Iraq and Afghanistan wars. J Head Trauma Rehabil 2006;21(5):398–402
21. Mallonee S, Shariat S, Stennies G, Waxweiler R, Hogan D, Jordan F. Physical injuries and fatalities resulting from the Oklahoma City bombing. JAMA 1996;276(5):382–387
22. Centers for Disease Control and Prevention (CDC). Injuries and illnesses among New York City Fire Department rescue workers after

responding to the World Trade Center attacks. MMWR Morb Mortal Wkly Rep 2002;51(special issue):1–5
23. Morrell R, Merbitz C, Jain S, Jain S. Traumatic brain injury in prisoners. J Offender Rehabil 1998;27(3–4):1–8
24. Slaughter B, Fann JR, Ehde D. Traumatic brain injury in a county jail population: prevalence, neuropsychological functioning and psychiatric disorders. Brain Inj 2003;17(9):731–741
25. Thurman DJ, Branche CM, Sniezek JE. The epidemiology of sports-related traumatic brain injuries in the United States: recent developments. J Head Trauma Rehabil 1998;13(2):1–8
26. Powell JW, Barber-Foss KD. Traumatic brain injury in high school athletes. JAMA 1999;282(10):958–963
27. Culotta VP, Sementilli ME, Gerold K, Watts CC. Clinicopathological heterogeneity in the classification of mild head injury. Neurosurgery 1996;38(2):245–250
28. Nell V, Yates DW, Kruger J. An extended Glasgow Coma Scale (GCS-E) with enhanced sensitivity to mild brain injury. Arch Phys Med Rehabil 2000;81(5):614–617
29. Drake AI, McDonald EC, Magnus NE, Gray N, Gottshall K. Utility of Glasgow Coma Scale-Extended in symptom prediction following mild traumatic brain injury. Brain Inj 2006;20(5):469–475
30. Lovell MR, Iverson GL, Collins MW, McKeag D, Maroon JC. Does loss of consciousness predict neuropsychological decrements after concussion? Clin J Sport Med 1999;9(4):193–198
31. Cantu RC. Posttraumatic retrograde and anterograde amnesia: pathophysiology and implications in grading and safe return to play. J Athl Train 2001;36(3):244–248
32. Practice parameter: the management of concussion in sports (summary statement). Report of the Quality Standards Subcommittee. Neurology 1997;48(3):581–585
33. Colorado Medical Society School and Sports Medicine Committee. Guidelines for the management of concussion in sports. Colo Med 1990;87:4
34. Cantu RC. Return to play guidelines after a head injury. Clin Sports Med 1998;17(1):45–60
35. The management of concussion in sports (practice parameter). Report of the Quality Standards Subcommittee. Neurology 1997;48: 581–585
36. Albright JP, McAuley E, Martin RK, Crowley ET, Foster DT. Head and neck injuries in college football: an eight-year analysis. Am J Sports Med 1985;13(3):147–152
37. Kelly JP, Rosenberg JH. Diagnosis and management of concussion in sports. Neurology 1997;48(3):575–580
38. Shaw NA. The neurophysiology of concussion. Prog Neurobiol 2002;67(4):281–344
39. Jane JA, Steward O, Gennarelli T. Axonal degeneration induced by experimental noninvasive minor head injury. J Neurosurg 1985;62(1):96–100
40. Bullock J. Injury and cell function. In: Reilly P, Bullock R, eds. Head Injury. London: Chapman & Hall; 1997:121–141
41. Unterharnscheidt FJ. Injuries due to boxing and other sports. In: Vinken PJ, Bruyn GW, Braakman R, eds. Handbook of Clinical Neurology. Vol 23. Amsterdam: North-Holland; 1975:527–593
42. Ommaya AK, Gennarelli TA. Cerebral concussion and traumatic unconsciousness: correlation of experimental and clinical observations of blunt head injuries. Brain 1974;97(4):633–654
43. Denny-Brown D, Russell WR. Experimental cerebral concussion. J Physiol 1940;99(1):153
44. Cantu RC. Cerebral concussion in sport: management and prevention. Sports Med 1992;14(1):64–74
45. Viano DC, Pellman EJ. Concussion in professional football: biomechanics of the striking player–part 8. Neurosurgery 2005;56(2):266–280 discussion 266–280
46. Holbourn AHS. Mechanics of head injuries. Lancet 1943;2:438–441
47. Scott WW. Physiology of concussion. Arch Neurol Psychiatry 1940;43:270–283
48. Pudenz RH, Shelden CH. The lucite calvarium: a method for direct observation of the brain, II: Cranial trauma and brain movement. J Neurosurg 1946;3:487–505
49. Gurdjian ES, Lissner HR, Webster JE, Latimer FR, Haddad BF. Studies on experimental concussion: relation of physiologic effect to time duration of intracranial pressure increase at impact. Neurology 1954;4(9):674–681
50. Zhang L, Yang KH, King AI. A proposed injury threshold for mild traumatic brain injury. J Biomech Eng 2004;126(2):226–236
51. Pellman EJ, Viano DC, Tucker AM, Casson IR. Concussion in professional football: location and direction of helmet impacts—Part 2. Neurosurgery 2003;53(6):1328–1340, discussion 1340–1321
52. Biasca N, Wirth S, Tegner Y. The avoidability of head and neck injuries in ice hockey: an historical review. Br J Sports Med 2002;36: 410–427
53. Roh JO, Watkinson EJ. Video analysis of blows to the head and face at the 1999 World Taekwondo Championships. J Sports Med Phys Fitness 2002;42(3):348–353
54. Ward AA Jr. Physiological basis of concussion. J Neurosurg 1958; 15(2):129–134
55. Nilsson B, Ponten U. Experimental head injury in the rat, II: Regional brain energy metabolism in concussive trauma. J Neurosurg 1977; 47(2):252–261
56. Katayama Y, DeWitt DS, Becker DP, Hayes RL. Behavioral evidence for a cholinoceptive pontine inhibitory area: descending control of spinal motor output and sensory input. Brain Res 1984;296(2): 241–262
57. Saija A, Hayes RL, Lyeth BG, Dixon CE, Yamamoto T, Robinson SE. The effect of concussive head injury on central cholinergic neurons. Brain Res 1988;452(1–2):303–311
58. Lyeth BG, Dixon CE, Hamm RJ, et al. Effects of anticholinergic treatment on transient behavioral suppression and physiological responses following concussive brain injury to the rat. Brain Res 1988;448(1): 88–97
59. Oppenheimer DR. Microscopic lesions in the brain following head injury. J Neurol Neurosurg Psychiatry 1968;31(4):299–306
60. Gentleman SM, Roberts GW, Gennarelli TA, et al. Axonal injury: a universal consequence of fatal closed head injury? Acta Neuropathol 1995;89(6):537–543
61. Walker AE, Kollros JJ, Case TJ. The physiological basis of concussion. J Neurosurg 1944;1:103–116
62. Gloor P. Generalized epilepsy with bilateral synchronous spike and wave discharge: new findings concerning its physiological mechanisms. Electroencephalogr Clin Neurophysiol Suppl 1978; (34): 245–249
63. Denny-Brown D. Cerebral concussion. Physiol Rev 1945;25:296–325
64. Russell WR. Amnesia following head injuries. Lancet 1935;2:762–763
65. Abrams MT, Doheny KF, Mazzocco MM, et al. Cognitive, behavioral, and neuroanatomical assessment of two unrelated male children expressing FRAXE. Am J Med Genet 1997;74(1):73–81
66. Maddocks DL, Dicker GD, Saling MM. The assessment of orientation following concussion in athletes. Clin J Sport Med 1995;5(1):32–35
67. McCrea M, Kelly JP, Kluge J, Ackley B, Randolph C. Standardized assessment of concussion in football players. Neurology 1997;48(3):586–588
68. Collins MW, Grindel SH, Lovell MR, et al. Relationship between concussion and neuropsychological performance in college football players. JAMA 1999;282(10):964–970
69. Echemendia RJ, Cantu RC. Return to play following sports-related mild traumatic brain injury: the role for neuropsychology. Appl Neuropsychol 2003;10(1):48–55
70. Echemendia RJ, Julian LJ. Mild traumatic brain injury in sports: neuropsychology's contribution to a developing field. Neuropsychol Rev 2001;11(2):69–88
71. Thompson J, Sebastianelli W, Slobounov S. EEG and postural correlates of mild traumatic brain injury in athletes. Neurosci Lett 2005;377(3): 158–163
72. Ingebrigtsen T, Waterloo K, Marup-Jensen S, Attner E, Romner B. Quantification of post-concussion symptoms 3 months after minor head injury in 100 consecutive patients. J Neurol 1998;245(9):609–612
73. Bailes JE, Cantu RC. Head injury in athletes. Neurosurgery 2001; 48(1): 26–45, discussion 45–26

74. Holsinger T, Steffens DC, Phillips C, et al. Head injury in early adulthood and the lifetime risk of depression. Arch Gen Psychiatry 2002;59(1):17–22
75. Plassman BL, Havlik RJ, Steffens DC, et al. Documented head injury in early adulthood and risk of Alzheimer's disease and other dementias. Neurology 2000;55(8):1158–1166
76. Guskiewicz KM, Marshall SW, Bailes J, et al: Recurrent concussion and risk of depression in retired professional football players. Med Sci Sports Exerc 2007;39:903
77. Miller JD, Murray LS, Teasdale GM. Development of a traumatic intracranial hematoma after a "minor" head injury. Neurosurgery 1990;27(5):669–673, discussion 673
78. Servadei F, Vergoni G, Staffa G, et al. Extradural haematomas: how many deaths can be avoided? Protocol for early detection of haematoma in minor head injuries. Acta Neurochir (Wien) 1995; 133(1–2):50–55
79. Stiell IG, Wells GA, Vandemheen K, et al. The Canadian CT Head Rule for patients with minor head injury. Lancet 2001;357(9266):1391–1396
80. Smits M, Dippel DW, de Haan GG, et al. External validation of the Canadian CT Head Rule and the New Orleans Criteria for CT scanning in patients with minor head injury. JAMA 2005;294(12):1519–1525
81. Ibanez J, Arikan F, Pedraza S, et al. Reliability of clinical guidelines in the detection of patients at risk following mild head injury: results of a prospective study. J Neurosurg 2004;100(5):825–834
82. Stein SC, Burnett MG, Glick HA. Indications for CT scanning in mild traumatic brain injury: a cost-effectiveness study. J Trauma 2006; 61(3):558–566
83. Brenner D, Elliston C, Hall E, Berdon W. Estimated risks of radiation-induced fatal cancer from pediatric CT. AJR Am J Roentgenol 2001; 176(2):289–296
84. Cook LS, Levitt MA, Simon B, Williams VL. Identification of ethanol-intoxicated patients with minor head trauma requiring computed tomography scans. Acad Emerg Med 1994;1(3):227–234
85. Hughes DG, Jackson A, Mason DL, Berry E, Hollis S, Yates DW. Abnormalities on magnetic resonance imaging seen acutely following mild traumatic brain injury: correlation with neuropsychological tests and delayed recovery. Neuroradiology 2004;46(7):550–558
86. Huisman TA, Sorensen A, Hergan K. Diffusion-weighted imaging for the evaluation of diffuse axonal injury in closed head injury. J Comput Assist Tomogr 2003;27:5–11
87. Huisman TA, Schwamm L, Schaefer P. Diffusion tensor imaging as potential biomarker of white matter injury in diffuse axonal injury. AJNR Am J Neuroradiol 2004;25:370–376
88. Inglese M, Grossman RI, Diller L, et al. Clinical significance of dilated Virchow-Robin spaces in mild traumatic brain injury. Brain Inj 2006;20(1):15–21
89. Chen JK, Johnston KM, Frey S, Petrides M, Worsley K, Ptito A. Functional abnormalities in symptomatic concussed athletes: an fMRI study. Neuroimage 2004;22(1):68–82
90. Jansen HM, van der Naalt J, van Zomeren AH, et al. Cobalt-55 positron emission tomography in traumatic brain injury: a pilot study. J Neurol Neurosurg Psychiatry 1996;60(2):221–224
91. Jantzen KJ, Anderson B, Steinberg FL, Kelso JA. A prospective functional MR imaging study of mild traumatic brain injury in college football players. AJNR Am J Neuroradiol 2004;25(5):738–745
92. Yoshino A, Hovda DA, Kawamata T, Katayama Y, Becker DP. Dynamic changes in local cerebral glucose utilization following cerebral conclusion in rats: evidence of a hyper- and subsequent hypometabolic state. Brain Res 1991;561(1):106–119
93. Bergsneider M, Hovda DA, Lee SM, et al. Dissociation of cerebral glucose metabolism and level of consciousness during the period of metabolic depression following human traumatic brain injury. J Neurotrauma 2000;17(5):389–401
94. Abdel-Dayem HM, Abu-Judeh H, Kumar M, et al. SPECT brain perfusion abnormalities in mild or moderate traumatic brain injury. Clin Nucl Med 1998;23(5):309–317
95. Chen SH, Kareken DA, Fastenau PS, Trexler LE, Hutchins GD. A study of persistent post-concussion symptoms in mild head trauma using positron emission tomography. J Neurol Neurosurg Psychiatry 2003; 74(3):326–332
96. Umile EM, Sandel ME, Alavi A, Terry CM, Plotkin RC. Dynamic imaging in mild traumatic brain injury: support for the theory of medial temporal vulnerability. Arch Phys Med Rehabil 2002;83(11):1506–1513
97. Hofman PA, Stapert SZ, van Kroonenburgh MJ, Jolles J, de Kruijk J, Wilmink JT. MR imaging, single-photon emission CT, and neurocognitive performance after mild traumatic brain injury. AJNR Am J Neuroradiol 2001;22(3):441–449
98. Bergsneider M, Hovda DA, McArthur DL, et al. Metabolic recovery following human traumatic brain injury based on FDG-PET: time course and relationship to neurological disability. J Head Trauma Rehabil 2001;16(2):135–148
99. Gross H, Kling A, Henry G, Herndon C, Lavretsky H. Local cerebral glucose metabolism in patients with long-term behavioral and cognitive deficits following mild traumatic brain injury. J Neuropsychiatry Clin Neurosci 1996;8(3):324–334
100. Kozlowski DA, James DC, Schallert T. Use-dependent exaggeration of neuronal injury after unilateral sensorimotor cortex lesions. J Neurosci 1996;16(15):4776–4786
101. Lovell MR, Collins MW. Neuropsychological assessment of the college football player. J Head Trauma Rehabil 1998;13(2):9–26
102. McAllister TW, Sparling MB, Flashman LA, Guerin SJ, Mamourian AC, Saykin AJ. Differential working memory load effects after mild traumatic brain injury. Neuroimage 2001;14(5):1004–1012
103. Easdon C, Levine B, O'Connor C. Neural activity associated with response inhibition following traumatic brain injury: an event-related fMRI investigation. Brain Cogn 2004;54:136–138
104. Brooks WM, Friedman SD, Gasparovic C. Magnetic resonance spectroscopy in traumatic brain injury. J Head Trauma Rehabil 2001; 16(2):149–164
105. Govindaraju V, Gauger GE, Manley GT, Ebel A, Meeker M, Maudsley AA. Volumetric proton spectroscopic imaging of mild traumatic brain injury. AJNR Am J Neuroradiol 2004;25(5):730–737
106. Hunter JV, Thornton RJ, Wang ZJ, et al. Late proton MR spectroscopy in children after traumatic brain injury: correlation with cognitive outcomes. AJNR Am J Neuroradiol 2005;26(3):482–488
107. Babikian T, Freier MC, Ashwal S, Riggs ML, Burley T, Holshouser BA. MR spectroscopy: predicting long-term neuropsychological outcome following pediatric TBI. J Magn Reson Imaging 2006;24(4):801–811
108. Wheless JW, Castillo E, Maggio V. Magnetoencephalography (MEG) and magnetic source imaging (MSI). Neurologist 2004;10:138–153
109. Lewine JD, Davis JT, Sloan JH, Kodituwakku PW, Orrison WW Jr. Neuromagnetic assessment of pathophysiologic brain activity induced by minor head trauma. AJNR Am J Neuroradiol 1999;20(5):857–866
110. Thatcher RW, Cantor D, McAlaster R, Geisler F, Krause P. Comprehensive predictions of outcome in closed head-injured patients: the development of prognostic equations. Ann N Y Acad Sci 1991;620:82–101
111. Williams D, Denny-Brown D. Cerebral electrical changes in experimental concussion. Brain 1941;64:223–238
112. Thatcher RW, Biver C, Gomez JF, et al. Estimation of the EEG power spectrum using MRI T(2) relaxation time in traumatic brain injury. Clin Neurophysiol 2001;112(9):1729–1745
113. Bleiberg J, Cernich AN, Cameron K, et al. Duration of cognitive impairment after sports concussion. Neurosurgery 2004;54(5):1073–1078 discussion 1078–1080
114. Thatcher RW, Biver C, McAlaster R, Salazar A. Biophysical linkage between MRI and EEG coherence in closed head injury. Neuroimage 1998;8(4):307–326
115. Ommaya AK, Corrao P, Letcher FS. Head injury in the chimpanzee, I: Biodynamics of traumatic unconsciousness. J Neurosurg 1973; 39(2):152–166
116. Schoenhuber R, Gentilini M. Auditory brain stem responses in the prognosis of late postconcussional symptoms and neuropsychological dysfunction after minor head injury. Neurosurgery 1986;19(4):532–534
117. Rizzo PA, Pierelli F, Pozzessere G, Floris R, Morocutti C. Subjective posttraumatic syndrome: a comparison of visual and brain stem auditory evoked responses. Neuropsychobiology 1983;9(2–3):78–82

118. Haglund Y, Persson HE. Does Swedish amateur boxing lead to chronic brain damage? III: A retrospective clinical neurophysiological study. Acta Neurol Scand 1990;82(6):353–360
119. Drake ME Jr, Weate SJ, Newell SA. Auditory evoked potentials in postconcussive syndrome. Electromyogr Clin Neurophysiol 1996;36(8): 457–462
120. Gaetz M, Weinberg H. Electrophysiological indices of persistent postconcussion symptoms. Brain Inj 2000;14(9):815–832
121. Picton TW. The P300 wave of the human event-related potential. J Clin Neurophysiol 1992;9(4):456–479
122. Kramer AF, Strayer DL. Assessing the development of automatic processing: an application of dual-task and event-related brain potential methodologies. Biol Psychol 1988;26(1–3):231–267
123. Pratap-Chand R, Sinniah M, Salem FA. Cognitive evoked potential (P300): a metric for cerebral concussion. Acta Neurol Scand 1988;78(3):185–189
124. Lavoie ME, Dupuis F, Johnston KM, Leclerc S, Lassonde M. Visual p300 effects beyond symptoms in concussed college athletes. J Clin Exp Neuropsychol 2004;26(1):55–73
125. Gosselin N, Theriault M, Leclerc S, Montplaisir J, Lassonde M. Neurophysiological anomalies in symptomatic and asymptomatic concussed athletes. Neurosurgery 2006;58(6):1151–1161, discussion 1151–1161
126. Dupuis F, Johnston KM, Lavoie M, Lepore F, Lassonde M. Concussions in athletes produce brain dysfunction as revealed by event-related potentials. Neuroreport 2000;11(18):4087–4092
127. Gaetz M, Goodman D, Weinberg H. Electrophysiological evidence for the cumulative effects of concussion. Brain Inj 2000;14(12): 1077–1088
128. Otto M, Holthusen S, Bahn E, et al. Boxing and running lead to a rise in serum levels of S-100B protein. Int J Sports Med 2000;21(8):551–555
129. Giza CC, Hovda DA. The neurometabolic cascade of concussion. J Athl Train 2001;36(3):228–235
130. Ingebrigtsen T, Waterloo K, Jacobsen EA, Langbakk B, Romner B. Traumatic brain damage in minor head injury: relation of serum S-100 protein measurements to magnetic resonance imaging and neurobehavioral outcome. Neurosurgery 1999;45(3):468–475 discussion 475–466
131. Berger RP, Kochanek PM, Pierce MC. Biochemical markers of brain injury: could they be used as diagnostic adjuncts in cases of inflicted traumatic brain injury? Child Abuse Negl 2004;28(7):739–754
132. Nishiyama H, Knopfel T, Endo S, Itohara S. Glial protein S100B modulates long-term neuronal synaptic plasticity. Proc Natl Acad Sci U S A 2002;99(6):4037–4042
133. Raabe A, Grolms C, Sorge O, Zimmermann M, Seifert V. Serum S-100B protein in severe head injury. Neurosurgery 1999;45(3):477–483
134. Spinella PC, Dominguez T, Drott HR, et al. S-100beta protein-serum levels in healthy children and its association with outcome in pediatric traumatic brain injury. Crit Care Med 2003;31(3):939–945
135. Anderson RE, Hansson LO, Nilsson O, Dijlai-Merzoug R, Settergren G. High serum S100B levels for trauma patients without head injuries. Neurosurgery 2001;48(6):1255–1258, discussion 1258–1260
136. Ross SA, Cunningham RT, Johnston CF, Rowlands BJ. Neuron-specific enolase as an aid to outcome prediction in head injury. Br J Neurosurg 1996;10(5):471–476
137. Mokuno K, Kato K, Kawai K, Matsuoka Y, Yanagi T, Sobue I. Neuron-specific enolase and S-100 protein levels in cerebrospinal fluid of patients with various neurological diseases. J Neurol Sci 1983;60(3): 443–451
138. Thomas DG, Palfreyman JW, Ratcliffe JG. Serum-myelin-basic-protein assay in diagnosis and prognosis of patients with head injury. Lancet 1978;1(8056):113–115
139. Ingebrigtsen T, Romner B. Biochemical serum markers for brain damage: a short review with emphasis on clinical utility in mild head injury. Restor Neurol Neurosci 2003;21(3–4):171–176
140. Vos PE, Lamers KJ, Hendriks JC, et al. Glial and neuronal proteins in serum predict outcome after severe traumatic brain injury. Neurology 2004;62(8):1303–1310
141. Bulut M, Koksal O, Dogan S, et al. Tau protein as a serum marker of brain damage in mild traumatic brain injury: preliminary results. Adv Ther 2006;23(1):12–22
142. Kutner KC, Erlanger DM, Tsai J, Jordan B, Relkin NR. Lower cognitive performance of older football players possessing apolipoprotein E epsilon4. Neurosurgery 2000;47(3):651–657, discussion 657–658
143. Friedman G, Froom P, Sazbon L, et al. Apolipoprotein E-epsilon4 genotype predicts a poor outcome in survivors of traumatic brain injury. Neurology 1999;52(2):244–248
144. Jordan BD, Relkin NR, Ravdin LD, Jacobs AR, Bennett A, Gandy S. Apolipoprotein E epsilon4 associated with chronic traumatic brain injury in boxing. JAMA 1997;278(2):136–140
145. Teasdale GM, Nicoll JA, Murray G, Fiddes M. Association of apolipoprotein E polymorphism with outcome after head injury. Lancet 1997;350(9084):1069–1071
146. Pitas RE, Ji ZS, Weisgraber KH, Mahley RW. Role of apolipoprotein E in modulating neurite outgrowth: potential effect of intracellular apolipoprotein E. Biochem Soc Trans 1998;26(2):257–262
147. Klauber MR, Marshall LF, Luerssen TG, Frankowski R, Tabaddor K, Eisenberg HM. Determinants of head injury mortality: importance of the low risk patient. Neurosurgery 1989;24(1):31–36
148. Stein SC, Spettell C. The Head Injury Severity Scale (HISS): a practical classification of closed-head injury. Brain Inj 1995;9(5):437–444
149. Ingebrigtsen T, Romner B, Kock-Jensen C. Scandinavian guidelines for initial management of minimal, mild, and moderate head injuries. The Scandinavian Neurotrauma Committee. J Trauma 2000;48(4):760–766
150. Shackford SR, Wald SL, Ross SE, et al. The clinical utility of computed tomographic scanning and neurologic examination in the management of patients with minor head injuries. J Trauma 1992;33(3):385–394
151. Guskiewicz KM, Bruce SL, Cantu RC, et al. Recommendations on management of sport-related concussion: summary of the National Athletic Trainers' Association position statement. Neurosurgery 2004;55(4):891–895 discussion 896
152. Belanger HG, Curtiss G, Demery JA, Lebowitz BK, Vanderploeg RD. Factors moderating neuropsychological outcomes following mild traumatic brain injury: a meta-analysis. J Int Neuropsychol Soc 2005;11(3):215–227
153. Frencham KA, Fox AM, Maybery MT. Neuropsychological studies of mild traumatic brain injury: a meta-analytic review of research since 1995. J Clin Exp Neuropsychol 2005;27(3):334–351
154. Grindel SH, Lovell MR, Collins MW. The assessment of sport-related concussion: the evidence behind neuropsychological testing and management. Clin J Sport Med 2001;11(3):134–143
155. Collie A, Darby D, Maruff P. Computerised cognitive assessment of athletes with sports related head injury. Br J Sports Med 2001; 35(5):297–302
156. Grindel SH. The use, abuse, and future of neuropsychologic testing in mild traumatic brain injury. Curr Sports Med Rep 2006;5(1): 9–14
157. Guskiewicz KM, McCrea M, Marshall SW, et al. Cumulative effects associated with recurrent concussion in collegiate football players: the NCAA Concussion Study. JAMA 2003;290(19):2549–2555
158. Guskiewicz KM, Weaver NL, Padua DA, Garrett WE Jr. Epidemiology of concussion in collegiate and high school football players. Am J Sports Med 2000;28(5):643–650
159. Collins MW, Lovell MR, Iverson GL, Cantu RC, Maroon JC, Field M. Cumulative effects of concussion in high school athletes. Neurosurgery 2002;51(5):1175–1179, discussion 1180–1171
160. Miele VJ, Bailes JE, Voelker JL. Boxing and the neurosurgeon. Clin Neurosurg 2002;49:396–406
161. Lovell MR, Collins MW, Iverson GL, et al. Recovery from mild concussion in high school athletes. J Neurosurg 2003;98(2):296–301
162. Field M, Collins MW, Lovell MR, Maroon J. Does age play a role in recovery from sports-related concussion? A comparison of high school and collegiate athletes. J Pediatr 2003;142(5):546–553
163. Mosenthal AC, Livingston DH, Lavery RF, et al. The effect of age on functional outcome in mild traumatic brain injury: 6-month report of a prospective multicenter trial. J Trauma 2004;56(5):1042–1048

164. McCrory P. Should we treat concussion pharmacologically? The need for evidence based pharmacological treatment for the concussed athlete. Br J Sports Med 2002;36(1):3–5
165. Braughler JM, Hall ED. "High-dose" methylprednisolone and CNS injury. J Neurosurg 1986;64(6):985–986
166. Hall ED, Yonkers PA, McCall JM, Braughler JM. Effects of the 21-aminosteroid U74006F on experimental head injury in mice. J Neurosurg 1988;68(3):456–461
167. Goss JR, Styren SD, Miller PD, et al. Hypothermia attenuates the normal increase in interleukin 1 beta RNA and nerve growth factor following traumatic brain injury in the rat. J Neurotrauma 1995;12(2): 159–167
168. Clifton GL, Lyeth BG, Jenkins LW, Taft WC, DeLorenzo RJ, Hayes RL. Effect of D, alpha-tocopheryl succinate and polyethylene glycol on performance tests after fluid percussion brain injury. J Neurotrauma 1989;6(2):71–81
169. Yoshida S, Busto R, Ginsberg MD, et al. Compression-induced brain edema: modification by prior depletion and supplementation of vitamin E. Neurology 1983;33(2):166–172
170. Sullivan PG, Geiger JD, Mattson MP, Scheff SW. Dietary supplement creatine protects against traumatic brain injury. Ann Neurol 2000;48(5):723–729
171. Rockswold SB, Rockswold GL, Vargo JM, et al. Effects of hyperbaric oxygenation therapy on cerebral metabolism and intracranial pressure in severely brain injured patients. J Neurosurg 2001;94(3):403–411
172. Rockswold GL, Ford SE, Anderson DC, Bergman TA, Sherman RE. Results of a prospective randomized trial for treatment of severely brain-injured patients with hyperbaric oxygen. J Neurosurg 1992; 76(6):929–934
173. Hallenbeck JM, Jacobs TP, Faden AI. Combined PGI2, indomethacin, and heparin improves neurological recovery after spinal trauma in cats. J Neurosurg 1983;58(5):749–754
174. McIntosh TK. Novel pharmacologic therapies in the treatment of experimental traumatic brain injury: a review. J Neurotrauma 1993; 10(3):215–261
175. Kimelberg HK, Cragoe EJ Jr, Nelson LR, et al. Improved recovery from a traumatic-hypoxic brain injury in cats by intracisternal injection of an anion transport inhibitor. Cent Nerv Syst Trauma 1987;4(1):3–14
176. Faden AI. Comparison of single and combination drug treatment strategies in experimental brain trauma. J Neurotrauma 1993;10(2):91–100
177. Ward A Jr. Atropine in the treatment of closed head injury. J Neurosurg 1950;7(5):398–402
178. Nilsson P, Hillered L, Ponten U, Ungerstedt U. Changes in cortical extracellular levels of energy-related metabolites and amino acids following concussive brain injury in rats. J Cereb Blood Flow Metab 1990;10(5):631–637
179. Okiyama K, Rosenkrantz TS, Smith DH, Gennarelli TA, McIntosh TK. (S)-emopamil attenuates acute reduction in regional cerebral blood flow following experimental brain injury. J Neurotrauma 1994;11(1): 83–95
180. Bracken MB, Holford TR. Effects of timing of methylprednisolone or naloxone administration on recovery of segmental and long-tract neurological function in NASCIS 2. J Neurosurg 1993;79(4):500–507
181. Faden AI, Jacobs TP, Smith MT. Thyrotropin-releasing hormone in experimental spinal injury: dose response and late treatment. Neurology 1984;34(10):1280–1284
182. Sinson G, Perri BR, Trojanowski JQ, Flamm ES, McIntosh TK. Improvement of cognitive deficits and decreased cholinergic neuronal cell loss and apoptotic cell death following neurotrophin infusion after experimental traumatic brain injury. J Neurosurg 1997;86(3):511–518
183. Chen DF, Schneider GE, Martinou JC, Tonegawa S. Bcl-2 promotes regeneration of severed axons in mammalian CNS. Nature 1997; 385(6615):434–439
184. Hatton J, Rapp RP, Kudsk KA, et al. Intravenous insulin-like growth factor-I (IGF-I) in moderate-to-severe head injury: a phase II safety and efficacy trial. J Neurosurg 1997;86(5):779–786
185. Alves W. Natural history of post-concussive signs and symptoms. Phys Med Rehabil Clin N Am 1993;6:21–32
186. Gouvier WD, Cubic B, Jones G, Brantley P, Cutlip Q. Postconcussion symptoms and daily stress in normal and head-injured college populations. Arch Clin Neuropsychol 1992;7(3):193–211
187. Binder LM, Rohling ML, Larrabee J. A review of mild head trauma, I: Meta-analytic review of neuropsychological studies. J Clin Exp Neuropsychol 1997;19(3):421–431
188. Strauss I, Savitsky N. Head injury: neurologic and psychiatric aspects. Arch Neurol Psychiatry 1934;31:893–955
189. Ryan LM, Warden DL. Post concussion syndrome. Int Rev Psychiatry 2003;15(4):310–316
190. Bohnen N, Jolles J, Twijnstra A. Neuropsychological deficits in patients with persistent symptoms six months after mild head injury. Neurosurgery 1992;30(5):692–695, discussion 695–696
191. Cushman JG, Agarwal N, Fabian TC, et al. Practice management guidelines for the management of mild traumatic brain injury: the EAST practice management guidelines work group. J Trauma 2001; 51(5):1016–1026
192. Jacobson RR. The post-concussional syndrome: physiogenesis, psychogenesis and malingering: an integrative model. J Psychosom Res 1995;39(6):675–693
193. Hahn RA. The nocebo phenomenon: concept, evidence, and implications for public health. Prev Med 1997;26(5 Pt 1):607–611
194. vanZomeren A, Brouwer W, Deelman B. Attentional deficits: the riddles of selectivity, speed, and alertness. In: Brooks N, ed. Closed Head Injury: Psychological, Social and Family Consequences. Oxford: Oxford University Press; 1984:74–107
195. Bernad P. Closed head injury (CHI) types I and II with post concussion syndrome (PCS). Clin Electroencephalogr 1988;19:174–175
196. Saunders RL, Harbaugh RE. The second impact in catastrophic contact-sports head trauma. JAMA 1984;252(4):538–539
197. Kelly JP, Nichols JS, Filley CM, Lillehei KO, Rubinstein D, Kleinschmidt-DeMasters BK. Concussion in sports: guidelines for the prevention of catastrophic outcome. JAMA 1991;266(20):2867–2869
198. Cantu RC. Second-impact syndrome. Clin Sports Med 1998;17(1):37–44
199. Van Camp SP, Bloor CM, Mueller FO, Cantu RC, Olson HG. Nontraumatic sports death in high school and college athletes. Med Sci Sports Exerc 1995;27(5):641–647
200. Mueller FO. Fatalities from head and cervical spine injuries occurring in tackle football: 50 years' experience. Clin Sports Med 1998;17(1): 169–182
201. Center for Disease Control. Sports-Related Recurrent Brain Injuries. United States. MMWR Weekly March 14, 1997;46(10):224–227
202. Gerberich SG, Priest JD, Boen JR, Straub CP, Maxwell RE. Concussion incidences and severity in secondary school varsity football players. Am J Public Health 1983;73(12):1370–1375
203. Barone GW, Rodgers BM. Pediatric equestrian injuries: a 14-year review. J Trauma 1989;29(2):245–247
204. Ingemarson H, Grevsten S, Thoren L. Lethal horse-riding injuries. J Trauma 1989;29(1):25–30
205. Retsky J, Jaffe D, Christoffel K. Skateboarding injuries in children: a second wave. Am J Dis Child 1991;145(2):188–192
206. Sacks JJ, Holmgreen P, Smith SM, Sosin DM. Bicycle-associated head injuries and deaths in the United States from 1984 through 1988. How many are preventable? JAMA 1991;266(21):3016–3018
207. Waters EA. Should pedal cyclists wear helmets? A comparison of head injuries sustained by pedal cyclists and motorcyclists in road traffic accidents. Injury 1986;17(6):372–375
208. Weiss BD. Bicycle-related head injuries. Clin Sports Med 1994; 13(1):99–112
209. Miele V, Bailes JE. Neurological injuries in miscellaneous sports. In: Bailes JED, A., ed. Neurological Injuries in Athletes. Lebanon, NH: AANS; 2000:181–251
210. Miele VJ, Carson L, Carr A, Bailes JE. Acute chronic subdural hematoma in a female boxer: a case report. Med Sci Sports Exerc 2004;36(11):1852–1855
211. Friermood TG, Messner DG, Brugman JL, Brennan R. Save the trees: a comparative review of skier-tree collisions. J Orthop Trauma 1994; 8(2):116–118

212. Harris JB. Head injuries in skiers and snowboarders. Can J Neurol Sci 2002;29(3):293, author reply 293
213. Sahlin Y. Alpine skiing injuries. Br J Sports Med 1989;23(4):241–244
214. Wilberger JE. Minor head injuries in American football: prevention of long term sequelae. Sports Med 1993;15(5):338–343
215. Torg JS, Quedenfeld TC, Burstein A, Spealman A, Nichols C III. National football head and neck injury registry: report on cervical quadriplegia, 1971 to 1975. Am J Sports Med 1979;7(2):127–132
216. Jordan SE, Green GA, Galanty HL, Mandelbaum BR, Jabour BA. Acute and chronic brain injury in United States National Team soccer players. Am J Sports Med 1996;24(2):205–210
217. Matser EJ, Kessels AG, Lezak MD, Jordan BD, Troost J. Neuropsychological impairment in amateur soccer players. JAMA 1999;282(10): 971–973
218. Lovell MR. The relevance of neuropsychologic testing for sports-related head injuries. Curr Sports Med Rep 2002;1(1):7–11
219. Fick DS. Management of concussion in collision sports: guidelines for the sidelines. Postgrad Med 1995;97(2):53–56, 59–60
220. Kelly JP, Rosenberg JH. The development of guidelines for the management of concussion in sports. J Head Trauma Rehabil 1998; 13(2): 53–65
221. Cantu RC. Head and spine injuries in the young athlete. Clin Sports Med 1988;7(3):459–472
222. Macciocchi SN, Barth JT, Alves W, Rimel RW, Jane JA. Neuropsychological functioning and recovery after mild head injury in collegiate athletes. Neurosurgery 1996;39(3):510–514
223. Levin HS, Mattis S, Ruff RM, et al. Neurobehavioral outcome following minor head injury: a three-center study. J Neurosurg 1987; 66(2):234–243

10 Moderate Brain Injury

Shelly D. Timmons and John S. Winestone

Moderate traumatic brain injury (TBI), commonly characterized as presenting with Glasgow Coma Scale (GCS) scores from 9 through 12, is an uncommon entity, on which little specific research has been conducted. This is likely due to the infrequency with which moderate TBI occurs relative to more severe injuries and milder injuries. Difficulty with determination of the incidence is compounded by the increasing frequency with which patients are intubated and sedated prior to arrival at the hospital emergency department (ED). Because of the potential for profound functional impairment after moderate TBI, patients must be aggressively treated, with early diagnosis and neurosurgical consultation, serial examinations (physical and radiographic), evacuation of mass lesions, control of intracranial pressure (ICP), and prevention of secondary insults. Maximization of outcomes depends not only on these principles of treatment but upon further refinements in our understanding of post-TBI functional impairments and the development of sensitive metrics with which to assess outcomes in this special patient population.

Definition

Since the original description of the Glasgow Coma Scale (GCS) in 1974,[1] moderate TBI has commonly been defined as patients presenting with TBI and a postresuscitation GCS score of 9 to 12. Some authors, however, have broadened the category in both directions, suggesting that moderate TBI also encompasses patients presenting with GCS 13, as these patients frequently have mass lesions and/or experience neurological deterioration.[2] Others have included those TBI patients with GCS scores as low as 6, theorizing that these less severely injured patients may have more in common physiologically with GCS 9 to 12 patients.[3] These authors also suggested the existence of a dichotomy among moderate TBI patients, separating them into those with GCS 9 to 10 and GCS 11 to 12.

There are 65 possible GCS scores between 9 and 12, inclusive. Some of these do not occur in actuality, e.g., a person with decerebrate posturing who is fully awake and oriented with normal speech. Subtracting those out, there are still 53 possibilities for presentation in this category of injury (**Table 10.1**).

The initial GCS score may also be "artificially" low because of noncentral nervous system (CNS) pathology, such as organ injury producing hypotension and cerebral hypoperfusion or because of intoxication. Elevated serum alcohol levels often contribute to an artificially low GCS score (as high as 73% of moderate TBI patients in ED in one study[4] and 24 to 51% of hospitalized TBI patients in another[5]) (**Table 10.2**). This places moderate TBI patients in the severe TBI category or mild TBI patients in the moderate TBI category, when in fact they have less threatening CNS pathology. Alternatively, patients may deteriorate rapidly due to evolving intracranial pathology, especially progression of intraparenchymal hemorrhages (IPHs) or contusions.

Table 10.1 Possible Glasgow Coma Scale Scores in Moderate Traumatic Brain Injury

Eye (1–4)	Motor (1–6)	Verbal (1–5)	Total (9–12)	Description of Examination
1	6	2	9	Not opening eyes
				Following commands
				Moaning
1	5	3	9	Not opening eyes
				Localizing
				Incomprehensible speech
1	4	4	9	Not opening eyes
				Withdrawing
				Confused speech
1	3	5	9	Not opening eyes
				Decorticate
				Normal speech, oriented

Table 10.1 *(Continued)*

Eye (1–4)	Motor (1–6)	Verbal (1–5)	Total (9–12)	Description of Examination
2	6	1	9	Opening eyes to pain Following commands No speech
2	6	1-I	9-I	Opening eyes to pain Following commands No speech—Intubated
2	5	2	9	Opening eyes to pain Localizing Moaning
2	4	3	9	Opening eyes to pain Withdrawing Incomprehensible speech
2	3	4	9	Opening eyes to pain Decorticate Confused speech
2	2	5	9	Opening eyes to pain Decerebrate Normal speech, oriented
3	5	1	9	Opening eyes to voice Localizing No speech
3	5	1-I	9-I	Opening eyes to voice Localizing No speech—intubated
3	4	2	9	Opening eyes to voice Withdrawing Moaning
3	3	3	9	Opening eyes to voice Decorticate Incomprehensible speech
3	2	4	9	Opening eyes to voice Decerebrate Confused speech
3	1	5	9	Opening eyes to voice No motor Normal speech, oriented
4	4	1	9	Opening eyes spontaneously Withdrawing No speech
4	4	1-I	9-I	Opening eyes spontaneously Withdrawing No speech—intubated

(Continued on Page 210)

Table 10.1 *(Continued)*

Eye (1–4)	Motor (1–6)	Verbal (1–5)	Total (9–12)	Description of Examination
4	3	2	9	Opening eyes spontaneously Decorticate Moaning
4	2	3	9	Opening eyes spontaneously Decerebrate Incomprehensible speech
4	1	4	9	Opening eyes spontaneously No motor Confused speech
1	6	3	10	Not opening eyes Following commands Incomprehensible speech
1	5	4	10	Not opening eyes Localizing Confused speech
1	4	5	10	Not opening eyes Withdrawing Normal speech, oriented
2	6	2	10	Opening eyes to pain Following commands Moaning
2	5	3	10	Opening eyes to pain Localizing Incomprehensible speech
2	4	4	10	Opening eyes to pain Withdrawing Confused speech
2	3	5	10	Opening eyes to pain Decorticate Normal speech, oriented
3	6	1	10	Opening eyes to voice Following commands No speech
3	6	1-I	10-I	Opening eyes to voice Following commands No speech—intubated
3	5	2	10	Opening eyes to voice Localizing Moaning
3	4	3	10	Opening eyes to voice Withdrawing Incomprehensible speech

Table 10.1 *(Continued)*

Eye (1–4)	Motor (1–6)	Verbal (1–5)	Total (9–12)	Description of Examination
3	3	4	10	Opening eyes to voice Decorticate Confused speech
3	2	5	10	Opening eyes to voice Decerebrate Normal speech, oriented
4	5	1	10	Opening eyes spontaneously Localizing No speech
4	5	1-I	10-I	Opening eyes spontaneously Localizing No speech—intubated
4	4	2	10	Opening eyes spontaneously Withdrawing Moaning
4	3	3	10	Opening eyes spontaneously Decorticate Incomprehensible speech
4	2	4	10	Opening eyes spontaneously Decerebrate Confused speech
4	1	5	10	Opening eyes spontaneously No motor Normal speech, oriented
1	6	4	11	Not opening eyes Following commands Confused speech
1	5	5	11	Not opening eyes Localizing Normal speech, oriented
2	6	3	11	Opening eyes to pain Following commands Incomprehensible speech
2	5	4	11	Opening eyes to pain Localizing Confused speech
2	4	5	11	Opening eyes to pain Withdrawing Normal speech, oriented
3	6	2	11	Opening eyes to voice Following commands Moaning

(Continued on Page 212)

Table 10.1 *(Continued)*

Eye (1–4)	Motor (1–6)	Verbal (1–5)	Total (9–12)	Description of Examination
3	5	3	11	Opening eyes to voice Localizing Incomprehensible speech
3	4	4	11	Opening eyes to voice Withdrawing Confused speech
3	3	5	11	Opening eyes to voice Decorticate Normal speech, oriented
4	6	1	11	Opening eyes spontaneously Following commands No speech
4	6	1-I	11-I	Opening eyes spontaneously Following commands No speech—intubated
4	5	2	11	Opening eyes spontaneously Localizing Moaning
4	4	3	11	Opening eyes spontaneously Withdrawing Incomprehensible speech
4	3	4	11	Opening eyes spontaneously Decorticate Confused speech
4	2	5	11	Opening eyes spontaneously Decerebrate Normal speech, oriented
1	6	5	12	Not opening eyes Following commands Normal speech, oriented
2	6	4	12	Opening eyes to pain Following commands Confused speech
2	5	5	12	Opening eyes to pain Localizing Normal speech, oriented
3	6	3	12	Opening eyes to voice Following commands Incomprehensible speech
3	5	4	12	Opening eyes to voice Localizing Confused speech

Table 10.1 *(Continued)*

Eye (1–4)	Motor (1–6)	Verbal (1–5)	Total (9–12)	Description of Examination
3	4	5	12	Opening eyes to voice Withdrawing Normal speech, oriented
4	6	2	12	Opening eyes spontaneously Following commands Moaning
4	5	3	12	Opening eyes spontaneously Localizing Incomprehensible speech
4	4	4	12	Opening eyes spontaneously Withdrawing Confused speech
4	3	5	12	Opening eyes spontaneously Decorticate Normal speech, oriented

The combination of intoxication and intracranial lesions may be particularly worrisome. In one series, nearly half of the moderate TBI patients harboring elevated alcohol levels (105 of 220) had a contusion or hematoma.[6] This subpopulation of moderate TBI patients is potentially at higher risk due to the masking of the signs and symptoms of deterioration by the depressant effects of alcohol.

Finally, measures taken for purposes of patient stabilization and transportation may alter the presenting GCS score. See the discussion below.

Epidemiology

Estimates on the incidence of moderate brain injury indicate that it is the least frequent form of TBI (with mild being the most common). Moderate TBI comprises an estimated 4 to 28% of all TBIs and affects a predominantly younger male group.[2–4,7,8] For hospitalized patients, proportions of TBI patients with moderate injury are likewise small. In Europe, for example, one meta-analysis reported the ratios of mild:moderate:severe at 22:1.5:1.[5] In an American study of children admitted to hospital, 12% had moderate TBI, 30% had severe TBI, and 58% had mild TBI.

Interestingly, in Rimel et al's series,[4] half as many moderate TBI patients were students and twice as many were intoxicated, compared with mild TBI patients. Lower education level, previous work history characterized by unemployment, history of alcohol abuse, and previous brain injuries have all been cited as predisposing factors for moderate TBI. In contrast to studies in severe TBI, an association with the presence of the apolipoprotein E epsilon4 APOE (e4) allele in mild and moderately brain-injured patients and outcome has not been shown.[9] However, this has not been extensively studied, and there was a broad range of pathology in the single group studied thus far.

Table 10.2 Moderate Traumatic Brain Injury: Clinical Findings

- Exam abnormalities with GCS <12: 87%
- Intoxication: 24–73%
- Early posttraumatic seizures (moderate & severe): 4–25%
- Late posttraumatic seizures (moderate & severe): 9–42%
- Transient adrenal insufficiency (moderate & severe): ~1/2

Abbreviations: GCS, Glasgow Coma Scale.

Diagnosis

Assessing an accurate GCS score in the face of field treatment, triage, and transportation practices favoring increased utilization of intubation, pharmacological paralysis, and/or sedation may make it difficult to distinguish moderate from mild TBI and may make moderate TBI appear as severe. Therefore, field GCS is an increasingly important measure for determining severity of injury. Field GCS values in nonintubated patients are predictive of admission GCS and are also highly predictive of outcome, as is the difference between field and admission GCS scores in individual patients.[10] The prehospital GCS is therefore an important determinant of early hospital diagnostic testing and treatment. As there is emerging evidence linking rapidity of response in the field (e.g., field intubation and aeromedical transport) to outcome from both moderate and severe TBI,[11] the field GCS score is highlighted as an important predicate for decision-making in the prehospital arena.

Patients must be carefully monitored with serial neurological examinations. Those who improve may have supportive measures such as mechanical ventilation rapidly weaned. However, it should be noted that despite the sometimes rapid return of eye opening and speech, many moderate TBI patients exhibit delayed ability to consistently follow motor commands.[12] This can result in longer periods of necessary hospital observation and can interfere with rehabilitation strategies. Conversely, those patients who deteriorate must be reinvestigated.

The first report on moderate head injury patients as defined by the GCS demonstrated a high rate of intracranial surgery or ICP monitoring.[4] About a third of these patients had space-occupying lesions, but not all patients had computed tomography (CT) scans because this was early in the CT era. In a more modern era, high rates of positive findings (40%), intracranial lesions (31%), and necessary neurosurgical intervention (8%)[2] also support the recommendation that CT scans should be done as soon as possible after arrival at hospital and completion of neurosurgical consultation (**Table 10.3**). As in other forms of TBI, skull lesions are not predictive of intracranial pathology.[2] About a third of moderate TBI patients will experience progression of radiological abnormalities on serial CT scanning, so follow-up is recommended at 12 to 24 hours for patients who do not improve to GCS >12, or immediately for those who deteriorate.

Magnetic resonance imaging (MRI) is also a useful tool in this population, demonstrating more lesions than CT (44% more in one older study of moderate TBI patients[12]). In another study, 80% of admitted patients with mild or moderate TBI had MRI abnormalities.[13] Correlation of the size of frontal and temporal lesions has been associated with decreased neuropsychological functioning of the frontal and temporal lobes, respectively, making this imaging modality useful for outcomes prediction.[12]

Table 10.3 Radiographic Findings for Moderate Traumatic Brain Injury

- Positive CT findings: 40%
- Intracranial lesions on CT: 31%
- Positive MRI findings: 80%
- Progression of radiographic abnormalities: 32%

Abbreviations: CT, computed tomography; MRI, magnetic resonance imaging.

Management

Prehospital

Prior to arrival at the hospital, advanced trauma life support (ATLS) protocols should be followed, with primary attention being given to the "ABCs" (airway, breathing and circulation) (**Table 10.2**). This is imperative to prevent hypoxemia (SaO_2 <90 mm Hg) and hypotension (systolic blood pressure [SBP] <90 mm Hg), both of which have been shown to adversely affect outcomes after TBI.[14]

Although intubation is usually required in severe brain injury, it may or may not be required in moderate brain injury (29% in one study[15]). The airway must be protected, but the verbal component of the GCS is lost with intubation, and the neurological exam may be compromised by sedatives and/or paralytics needed for intubation, ventilation, and patient safety during transportation and workup. Moderate brain injury patients may not meet clear criteria for intubation initially, but 10 to 20% of patients have a depressed level of consciousness that further deteriorates over time[6] and may require later intubation.

Acute Care

After hemodynamic stabilization and a thorough neurological and physical examination have been performed, a CT scan of the head is performed to evaluate for intracranial pathology if the history or physical reveals cranial trauma, neurological deficit, or loss or depression of consciousness (**Table 10.5**). The European Brain Injury Consortium (EBIC) demonstrated abnormalities in 87% of those with a GCS <12 (**Table 10.2**).[16] Another series found that in patients with a GCS of 9 to 13, 40% of CTs

Table 10.4 Principles of Management: Prehospital

- ATLS protocol
  - Intubation as needed
- Rapid transport to hospital with the following:
  - Critical care capabilities
  - 24/7 CT capabilities
  - Neurosurgical expertise
  - 24/7 OR available

Abbreviations: ATLS, advanced trauma life support; CT, computed tomography; OR, operating room.

Table 10.5 Principles of Management: Acute Care

- ATLS Protocol
  - Avoid hypoxemia
  - Avoid hypotension
- Rapid CT scanning
- Toxicology and alcohol screening tests
- Serial neurological examinations
- Admission to Critical Care Unit
- Neurosurgical consultation
- Follow-up CT scan
  - Lack of improvement to GCS >12
  - Mass lesion
- Consider intracranial pressure monitoring
  - Nonevacuated mass lesions
  - Unobtainable neurological examination
- Surgical evacuation of mass lesions
- Other surgery as indicated
- Nutritional support
- DVT prophylaxis
- Seizure prophylaxis
  - GCS <10
  - Contusion/IPH
  - EDH/SDH
  - Depressed skull fracture
  - Penetrating injury
  - Seizure <24 h after injury
- Pituitary screening examinations

Abbreviations: ATLS, advanced trauma life support; CT, computed tomography; DVT, deep vein thrombosis; IPH, intraparenchymal hemorrhage; EDH, epidural hematoma; GCS, Glasgow Coma Scale; MRI, magnetic resonance imaging; SDH, subdural hematoma.

were abnormal on initial presentation, 32% had radiographic deterioration, and 8% required surgery.[2] If the initial CT is negative, a follow-up CT scan should be done if the patient does not improve to GCS >12 within 12 to 24 hours.

Investigation with laboratory studies to evaluate toxic and metabolic causes of depressed consciousness, including complete metabolic profile, urinalysis, and screening for alcohol and other drugs should be done upon admission. Frequent (hourly) neurological examinations should be employed from the time of admission. It may be necessary to periodically hold or reverse sedation and/or paralytics to obtain an accurate GCS score. Patients should be admitted to a critical care unit, and neurosurgical consultations obtained immediately. Moderate TBI patients should not be treated in institutions without neurosurgical coverage available because of the high incidence of surgical lesions and deterioration.

If the patient deteriorates, immediate CT scanning, intubation (if not previously done), ICP monitoring, and subsequent medical or surgical treatment of ICP elevation may be needed. Mass lesions associated with elevated ICP should be evacuated according to guidelines discussed elsewhere in this text (Chapter 13).

ICP monitoring is recommended in moderate TBI patients with intracranial mass lesions that warrant careful monitoring in the judgment of the neurosurgeon.[14] This may include patients with nonevacuated mass lesions in whom a neurological examination will not be obtainable for a prolonged period, e.g., due to need for general anesthesia for emergency nonneurosurgical procedures or patients who require sedation for respiratory assistance. Also, patients undergoing treatment that could contribute to elevation of ICP, such as prolonged positive end expiratory pressure support on a ventilator, may be ICP-monitoring candidates. Coagulopathy may require correction prior to placement of an intraparenchymal ICP monitor or ventriculostomy catheter.

Nutritional supplementation may be required. Oral intake may be possible, but decreased due to lethargy, nausea, vomiting, or alterations in appetite. Increased nutritional demand is common in the moderate brain injury population. A calorie count is recommended if the patient is taking food orally, and sometimes aggressive enteral support is needed to provide supranormal caloric intake for patients with decreased consciousness or increased metabolic requirements.[17] Furthermore, infectious complications may be reduced in moderate TBI patients treated with enteral or parenteral nutrition early.

Prophylaxis against deep venous thrombosis (DVT) should be employed early in the hospitalization until the patient becomes physically active and/or ambulatory.

The incidence of early posttraumatic seizures (<7 days after injury) is estimated at between 4 and 25% for civilian brain injuries, and late seizures occur in 9 to 42% (**Table 10.2.**).[14] One week of prophylaxis against early seizures in the form of carbamazepine or phenytoin is recommended for patients at high risk, which includes TBI patients with GCS <10, contusion or intraparenchymal hemorrhage (IPH), extraaxial (subdural or epidural) hematoma, depressed skull fracture, penetrating injury, or seizure within 24 hours of injury.[14]

Screening for hypopituitarism is recommended, especially because deficits may contribute to post-TBI sequelae such as fatigue, cognitive disruption, and physical complaints. One study demonstrated that approximately half of a cohort with moderate and severe TBI had at least transient adrenal insufficiency (**Table 10.2**). Factors increasing the likelihood of adrenal insufficiency in this group included greater severity of injury, younger age, early ischemia, and use of etomidate and metabolic suppressants such as propofol and pentobarbital.[18] In the same study, lower cortisol levels were associated with lower blood pressures and higher vasopressor use, suggesting the need for monitoring levels in ventilated and sedated TBI patients, especially those on high-dose metabolic suppressants. Other studies have shown the following predictors of hypopituitarism after TBI: cranial fractures, cerebral injury on imaging, prolonged loss of consciousness, GCS <10, diffuse cerebral edema on initial CT, and hypotension or hypoxia.[19–22] Endocrinology follow-up over time is important because post-TBI hypopituitarism may resolve.[23–27]

Postacute Care

Moderate TBI patients may benefit from postacute-care inpatient or outpatient rehabilitation services (**Table 10.6**). One study demonstrated that the severity of brain injury was not associated with the likelihood of utilizing rehabilitation services but was associated with intensity of services rendered, with many mild and moderate TBI patients gravitating to conventional physical therapy instead of cognitive services.[28] Unfortunately, moderate TBI patients may not receive therapies that would enhance their functional outcomes. One researcher, who explored different forms of rehabilitation in a nonrandomized controlled trial, noted increased productivity in those who had comprehensive neuropsychological rehabilitation programs as opposed to conventional rehabilitation.[29] Patients should be steered to maximal rehabilitation resources to aid in their recovery.

Outcomes

Moderate head injury patients have highly variable outcomes. The majority of moderate TBI patients survive[2,15] but may return to a very different life with significant impairment. Moderate brain injury survivors may suffer from cognitive or behavioral impairments that disrupt relationships, employment, or psychological well-being.

In Rimel et al's seminal study,[4] only 38% of moderate TBI subjects had good outcomes on the Glasgow Outcome Scale (GOS), compared with 75% good outcomes in mild TBI subjects. Even those moderate TBI patients who had good outcomes had significant post-TBI symptomatology, including headache (93%), memory difficulties (90%), and problems performing activities of daily living (87%), and only 7% were asymptomatic (**Table 10.7**). All

Table 10.6 Principles of Management: Rehabilitation

- Comprehensive neuropsychological rehabilitation
  - Cognitive therapy
  - Speech therapy
  - Swallowing therapy
  - Occupational therapy
  - Physical therapy
  - Vocational rehabilitation
- Follow-up neuropsychological and functional testing
  - Cognitive measures
    - Memory
    - Attention
    - Concentration
    - Visual processing
    - Auditory processing
    - Spatial processing
    - Information processing speed
    - Intelligence
    - Flexibility
    - Insight
    - Judgment
    - Motivation
    - Organization/planning
    - Executive functions
  - Psychomotor assessments
    - Dexterity
    - Functional motor impairment
  - Speech
    - Expressive
    - Receptive
    - Motor
  - Affective measures
    - Depression
    - Anxiety
  - Behavior
    - Impulsivity
    - Disinhibition
    - Agitation/combativeness/aggression
  - Social integration
    - Communication
    - Home management
    - Leisure activities
    - Community involvement
    - Return to work
  - Functional measures
    - Functional endurance
    - Functional independence
    - Transportation
  - Driving assessment

Table 10.7 Outcomes (Pre-CT Era) of Moderate Traumatic Brain Injury

- Good outcomes (GOS): 38%
- Asymptomatic: 7%
- Patients with good outcomes
  - Headache: 93%
  - Memory difficulties: 90%
  - Problems with activities of daily living: 87%
  - Neuropsychological deficits: 100%

Abbreviations: CT, computed tomography; GOS, Glasgow Outcome Scale.

subjects demonstrated neuropsychological deficits on all tests employed. As opposed to mild TBI, where premorbid characteristics predicted return to work, return to work in moderate TBIs was predicted by injury severity, e.g., duration of coma, CT diagnoses, and discharge GCS score (**Table 10.8**). Coupled with acute subdural hematoma, moderate TBI resulted in no good recoveries in this series, and 65% were dead or severely disabled (**Table 10.9**). In a later series of 447 patients with GCS 9 to 13,[2] 60% had a good outcome as defined by the GOS at 6 months, whereas 26% were moderately disabled, 7% were vegetative, and 7% were dead (**Table 10.10**). This patient series underwent more frequent CT scanning and had a significant surgical intervention rate, which may account for the improvement in outcomes overall.

Poon et al[30] conducted a prospective longitudinal study of moderate and severe TBI patients and found three independent prognostic factors that were statistically significant: age, GCS, and baseline functional independence measure (FIM) at the time of admission to rehabilitation (**Table 10.11**).

Subjective symptomatology in the absence of physical findings or changes in outward appearance may make it difficult for patients to reintegrate into their premorbid activities or to obtain the assistance they need, or for family and friends to appreciate the extent of their problems (**Table 10.12**). Aggression,[31] fatigue,[32] and posttraumatic headache[33] often plague those who survive moderate TBI, interfering with their social function. Posttraumatic headaches are usually frontal, daily (at least initially), show no correlation with injury severity, demographic characteristics, or affective state, and most abate by 6 months postinjury.[33] Likewise, fatigue among complicated mild, moderate, and severe TBI patients is not related to the severity of the injury.[32]

Table 10.8 Predictors of Return to Work of Moderate Traumatic Brain Injury

- Duration of coma
- CT diagnoses
- Discharge Glasgow Coma Scale
- Not premorbid characteristics

Abbreviations: CT, computed tomography.

Table 10.9 Outcomes of Moderate Traumatic Brain Injury and Acute Subdural Hematoma

- Good recoveries: 0
- Dead or disabled: 65%

Community integration questionnaires may be used to measure social functioning, but for moderately and severely injured patients, there are differences between study participants and their proxies answering the same questions, as opposed to those with mild TBI, who had good agreement with the answers given by their proxies.[34] This suggests that more severely injured patients may lack insight into their problems, and the input of significant others, parents, and children should be sought in regard to the survivors' social functioning.

As evidence emerges regarding reliability of various psychometrics in assessing cognitive outcomes, it is increasingly clear that moderate TBI survivors are prone to significant deficits that may not be apparent at first blush. In an early study by Clifton et al,[35] four neuropsychological measurements (controlled oral word association, grooved pegboard, Trailmaking Part B, and Rey–Osterrieth Complex Figure Delayed Recall tests) best predicted GOS, especially the grooved pegboard test, which measures manual dexterity, among other parameters. Functions requiring interhemispheric and intrahemispheric processing, such as verbal and visual fluency, verbal memory, and speed of visual and tactile information processing, were significantly impaired in another study of moderate and severe TBI.[36]

Table 10.10 Outcomes (CT Era) of Moderate Traumatic Brain Injury

- Good outcome GOS: 60%
  - Good
  - Mildly disabled
- Moderately disabled GOS: 26%
- Vegetative: 7%
- Dead: 7%

Abbreviations: CT, computed tomography; GOS, Glasgow Outcome Scale.

Table 10.11 Prognostic Factors for Moderate Traumatic Brain Injury

- Age
- Glasgow Coma Scale
- Baseline FIM at rehab admission

Abbreviations: FIM, functional independence measure.

Table 10.13 Especially Vulnerable Populations for Moderate Traumatic Brain Injury

- Infants
- Older children
- Older adults

A recent set of novel studies[37,38] sought to demonstrate the effects of TBI severity on functional outcome and to describe the causal pathways. They found that TBI severity has indirect (not direct) effects on functional outcome. Psychological and physical complaints were neither predicted by severity nor predictive of function. Severity did not have direct effects on behavior problems, although behavior problems directly affected functional outcome. Conversely, memory capabilities were predicted by TBI severity but did not significantly predict functional outcome. Finally, information processing speed was predicted by severity and was also predictive of functional outcome.

Special populations deserve special mention (**Table 10.13**). Children and older adults sustaining moderate TBI have unique impairments affecting their function. Children are particularly susceptible to behavioral problems due to their developmental stage. In children, there is evidence that the age of injury is less predictive of outcome than the severity of injury,[39] except that infants with moderate TBI fared worse than older children with moderate TBI in their investigation. The same group showed that behavioral function was not related to severity, and that children with behavioral impairment showed little recovery over time.[40] Behavior significantly affected family burden, as did severity and overall functional impairment.[41] Children coming from positions of lower socioeconomic status and having lower preinjury adaptive abilities were at the worst risk of behavioral problems postinjury (**Table 10.14**).[42] Less than 10% of moderate TBI children ever had clinically significant behavioral symptoms, but when they did, they were stable over time (6 to 30 months).[41]

Table 10.12 Behavioral and Cognitive Problems with Moderate Traumatic Brain Injury

- Aggression
- Fatigue
- Lack of insight
- Manual dexterity problems
- Verbal fluency
- Visual fluency
- Verbal memory
- Speed of visual and tactile information processing

Initial memory and educational performance problems were demonstrated in children with moderate TBI that improved with time, as opposed to persistent global problems in children suffering severe TBI. Adaptive abilities correlated with severity of injury.[41]

Health-related quality of life (HRQOL) assessments are being increasingly utilized as one means of assessing outcome vis-à-vis the patient's and patient's family's perceptions of the impact of injury or illness. For children sustaining moderate or severe TBI in one series, several aspects of the HRQOL, including physical, emotional, social, school, psychosocial, and cognitive functions, were negatively affected by the injury without improvement over time.[43]

Older adult patients may be particularly susceptible to cognitive dysfunction after moderate traumatic brain injury, even more so than after mild or severe TBI.[44] This project defined moderate TBI as GCS 9 to 12, posttraumatic amnesia duration less than one week, or mild TBI with an intracranial complication such as a contusion. Survivors in this study suffered from impairments in information processing speed, verbal memory, language, and decision-making ability. Cognitive decline and decreased ability to perform activities of daily living also characterized these individuals as a result of these specific impairments.

Conclusions

Moderate TBI resembles severe TBI in its pathophysiologic underpinnings and propensity for poor outcomes. Given their relatively good starting point, however, this population may benefit most from the application of higher intensity resources for prehospital transport and treatment, acute care, and rehabilitation services. In the face of rapid treatment, close monitoring, and aggressive therapeutic approaches, moderate TBI patients have potential for good functional outcomes, despite the degree of injury.

Table 10.14 Risk Factors for Behavior Problems in Children with Moderate Traumatic Brain Injury

- Lower socioeconomic status
- Lower preinjury adaptive abilities

References

1. Teasdale G, Jennett B. Assessment of coma and impaired consciousness: a practical scale. Lancet 1974;2:81–83
2. Stein SC, Ross SE. Moderate head injury: a guide to initial management. J Neurosurg 1992;77:562–564
3. Colohan AR, Oyesiku NM. Moderate head injury: an overview. J Neurotrauma 1992;9(Suppl 1):S259–S264
4. Rimel RW, Giordani B, Barth JT, et al. Moderate head injury: completing the clinical spectrum of brain trauma. Neurosurgery 1982;11:344–351
5. Tagliaferri F, Compagnone C, Korsic M, et al. A systematic review of brain injury epidemiology in Europe. Acta Neurochir (Wien) 2006;148:255–268
6. Stein SC. Outcome from moderate head injury. In: Narayan RK, Wilberger JE, Povlishok JT. Neurotrauma. New York: McGraw-Hill; 1996:755–766
7. Hooper SR, Alexander J, Moore D, et al. Caregiver reports of common symptoms in children following a traumatic brain injury. NeuroRehabilitation 2004;19:175–189
8. Von Wild KRH, Wenzlaff P. TBI Study Council. Quality management in traumatic brain injury (TBI): lessons from the prospective study in 6,800 patients after acute TBI in respect of neurorehabilitation. Acta Neurochir Suppl (Wien) 2005;93:15–25
9. Chamelian L, Reis M, Feinstein A. Six-month recovery from mild to moderate traumatic brain injury: the role of the APOE-ε4 allele. Brain 2004;127:2621–2628
10. Davis DP, Serrano JA, Vilke GM, et al. The predictive value of field versus arrival Glasgow coma scale score and TRISS calculations in moderate-to-severe traumatic brain injury. J Trauma 2006;60(5):985–990
11. Davis DP, Peay J, Serrano JA, et al. The impact of aeromedical response to patients with moderate to severe traumatic brain injury. Ann Emerg Med 2005;46(2):115–122
12. Levin HS, Amparo E, Eisenberg HM, et al. Magnetic resonance imaging and computerized tomography in relation to the neurobehavioral sequelae of mild and moderate head injuries. J Neurosurg 1987;66:706–713
13. Levin HS, Williams DH, Eisenberg HM, et al. Serial MRI and neurobehavioural findings after mild to moderate closed head injury. J Neurol Neurosurg Psychiatry 1992;55(4):255–262
14. Brain Trauma Foundation. The American Association of Neurological Surgeons. The Joint Section on Neurotrauma and Critical Care. Prognosis and management of severe traumatic brain injury. J Neurotrauma 2000;17:S6–S7
15. Bulger EM, Copass MK, Sabath DR, et al. The use of neuromuscular blocking agents to facilitate prehospital intubation does not impair outcome after traumatic brain injury. J Trauma 2005;58(4):718–724
16. Murray GD, Teasdale GM, Braakman R, et al. The European Brain Injury Consortium Survey of Head Injuries. Acta Neurochir (Wien) 1999;141(3):223–236
17. Timmons SD. How soon should patients receive nutrition? How much, which formulation, and by which route? In: Valadka AB, Andrews BT, eds. Neurotrauma: Evidence-Based Answers to Common Questions. New York: Thieme; 2005:91–96
18. Cohan P, Wang C, McArthur DL, et al. Acute secondary adrenal insufficiency after traumatic brain injury: a prospective study. Crit Care Med 2005;33(10):2358–2366
19. Benvenga S, Campenni A, Roggeri R, et al. Hypopituitarism secondary to head trauma. J Clin Endocrinol Metab 2000;85(4):1353–1361
20. Dimopoulou I, Tsagarakis S, Theodorakipoulou M, et al. Endocrine abnormalities in critical care patients with moderate-to-severe head trauma: incidence, pattern and predisposing factors. Intensive Care Med 2004;30:1051–1057
21. Edwards OM, Clark JDA. Post-traumatic hypopituitarism: six cases and a review of the literature. Medicine 1986;65:281–290
22. Kelly DF, Gaw Gonzalo IT, Cohan P, et al. Hypopituitarism following traumatic brain injury and aneurysmal subarachnoid hemorrhage: a preliminary report. J Neurosurg 2000;93(5):743–752
23. Aimaretti G, Ambrosio MR, Di Somma C, et al. Traumatic brain injury and subarachnoid haemorrhage are conditions at high risk for hypopituitarism: screening study at 3 months after brain injury. Clin Endocrinol (Oxf) 2004;61:320–326
24. Aimaretti G, Ambrosio MR, Di Somma C, et al. Residual pituitary function after brain injury-induced hypopituitarism: a prospective 12-month study. J Clin Endocrinol Metab 2005;90(11):6085–6092
25. Agha A, Rogers B, Mylotte D, et al. Neuroendocrine dysfunction in the acute phase of traumatic brain injury. Clin Endocrinol (Oxf) 2004;60:584–591
26. Bondanelli M, de Marinis L, Ambrosio MR, et al. Occurrence of pituitary dysfunction following traumatic brain injury. J Neurotrauma 2004;21(6):685–696
27. Estes SM, Urban RJ. Hormonal replacement in patients with brain injury-induced hypopituitarism: who, when, and how to treat? Pituitary 2005;8:267–270
28. Phillips VL, Greenspan AI, Stringer AY, et al. Severity of injury and service utilization following traumatic brain injury: the first 3 months. J Head Trauma Rehabil 2004;19(3):217–225
29. Sarajuuri JM, Kaipio M-L, Koskinen SK, et al. Outcome of a comprehensive neurorehabilitation program for patients with traumatic brain injury. Arch Phys Med Rehabil 2005;86:2296–2302
30. Poon WS, Zhu XL, Ng SCP, Wong GKC. Predicting one year clinical outcome in traumatic brain injury (TBI) at the beginning of rehabilitation. Acta Neurochir Suppl (Wien) 2005;93:207–208
31. Baguley IJ, Cooper J, Felmingham K. Aggressive behavior following traumatic brain injury: how common is common? J Head Trauma Rehabil 2006;21(1):45–56
32. Borgaro SR, Baker J, Wethe JV, et al. Subjective reports of fatigue during early recovery from traumatic brain injury. J Head Trauma Rehabil 2005;20(5):416–425
33. Walker WC, Seel RT, Curtiss G, Warden DL. Headache after moderate and severe traumatic brain injury: a longitudinal analysis. Arch Phys Med Rehabil 2005;86:1793–1800
34. Dawson DR, Markowitz M, Stuss DT. Community integration status 4 years after traumatic brain injury: participant-proxy agreement. J Head Trauma Rehabil 2005;20(5):426–435
35. Clifton GL, Kreutzer JS, Choi SC, et al. Relationship between Glasgow outcome scale and neuropsychological measures after brain injury. Neurosurgery 1993;33(1):34–39
36. Mathias JL, Bigler ED, Jones NR, et al. Neuropsychological and information processing performance and its relationship to white matter changes following moderate and severe traumatic brain injury: a preliminary study. Appl Neuropsychol 2004;11(3):134–152
37. Rassovsky Y, Satz P, Alfano MS, et al. Functional outcome in TBI, I: Neuropsychological, emotional, and behavioral mediators. J Clin Exp Neuropsychol 2006;28(4):567–580
38. Rassovsky Y, Satz P, Alfano MS, et al. Functional outcome in TBI, II: Verbal memory and information processing speed mediators. J Clin Exp Neuropsychol 2006;28(4):581–591
39. Anderson V, Catroppa C, Morse S, et al. Functional plasticity or vulnerability after early brain injury? Pediatrics 2005;116:1374–1382
40. Anderson VA, Catroppa C, Haritou F, et al. Identifying factors contributing to child and family outcome 30 months after traumatic brain injury in children. J Neurol Neurosurg Psychiatry 2005;76:401–408
41. Anderson VA, Catroppa C, Dudgeon P, et al. Understanding predictors of functional recovery and outcome 30 months following early childhood head injury. Neuropsychology 2006;20(1):42–57
42. Anderson VA, Morse SA, Catroppa C, et al. Thirty month outcome from early childhood head injury: a prospective analysis of neurobehavioural recovery. Brain 2004;127:2608–2620
43. McCarthy ML, MacKenzie EJ, Durbin DR, et al. Health-related quality of life during the first year after traumatic brain injury. Arch Pediatr Adolesc Med 2006;160:252–260
44. Rapoport MJ, Herrmann N, Shammi P, et al. Outcome after traumatic brain injury sustained in older adulthood: a one-year longitudinal study. Am J Geriatr Psychiatry 2006;14(5):456–465

11 Severe Brain Injury

Joshua E. Heller and Andrew I. R. Maas

The proper and timely management of severe brain injury is essential to increase survivability and recovery after a head trauma.[1] Affording these critical patients the opportunity for the best possible outcome, return of function and a meaningful life, should be the principle goals of all health care professionals involved in the care of traumatic brain injury (TBI) victims, and success has the potential for a tremendous socioeconomic effect. As discussed in previous chapters, TBI is the leading cause of death among children and young adults in the United States and is an enormous public health problem worldwide.[2,3]

In the United States, the Centers for Disease Control and Prevention (Atlanta, GA) estimates the annual incidence of TBI at 1.5 million. There are ~52,000 deaths from TBI annually, and 80 to 90,000 patients surviving with long-term disability.[4,5] The cost of TBI in 2006 is estimated at over 60 billion dollars per year.[6] In Europe, there are ~1.6 million head injuries treated per year, with an annual mortality rate of ~66,000.[3] In low-income countries the incidence of TBI is increasing exponentially as motorization expands. In this chapter we will review the diagnosis and management of severe brain injury with special attention to the guidelines developed by the Brain Trauma Foundation (BTF) and the European Brain Injury Consortium (EBIC).[7,8] The operative management of brain injury will be discussed in Chapter 13.

Classification

As discussed in Chapter 6, common approaches to classification of the severity of brain injury are based on clinical severity as assessed by the Glasgow Coma Scale (GCS), as well as on structural damage, based upon intracranial diagnosis as determined by diagnostic imaging, i.e., computed tomography.[9] When Teasdale and Jennett described the GCS as a "practical scale" for assessing the level of consciousness in 1974, it was a tool to help standardize communication regarding severity of brain injury and level of coma (**Table 11.1**).[10] The GCS quickly evolved into the universally accepted way to classify severity of head injury and is commonly used to help guide management as well as to estimate prognosis. For assessment of severity in individual patients, the three components of the GCS (eye, motor, and verbal scales) should be reported separately. For purposes of classification, the sum score of these components may be calculated (3 to 15). A postresuscitation sum GCS score of 8 or less corresponds to a severe brain injury.

The Head Injury Severity Scale described by Stein further subcategorizes severe injury into severe and critical groups owing to the extremely grave prognosis for patients with the two lowest possible scores. A postresuscitation GCS score of 5 to 8 corresponds to a "severe brain injury" and a score of 3 to 4 represents "critical brain injury" (**Table 11.2**).[9]

Table 11.1 The Glasgow Coma Scale

Eye opening	4 – Eyes open spontaneously
	3 – Eyes open to voice
	2 – Eyes open to painful stimulus only
	1 – Eyes closed despite noxious stimuli
Motor response	6 – Follows verbal commands
	5 – Localizes painful stimulus
	4 – Withdraws extremity from painful stimulus
	3 – Abnormal flexion posturing (decorticate)
	2 – Abnormal extension posturing (decerebrate)
	1 – No movement of extremities
Verbal response	5 – Oriented (person, place, and time)
	4 – Disoriented but conversant
	3 – Inappropriate words
	2 – Incomprehensible sounds
	1 – No verbal response

Source: Teasdale G, Jennett B. Assessment of coma and impaired consciousness: a practical scale. Lancet 1974;2(7872):81–84

Notes: The Glasgow Coma Scale (GCS) is calculated by adding the *best* score obtained in each category. Assessment of the best motor score is based on the response of the arms.

Examples: A patient who has his eyes open, follows commands, and is conversant and oriented would be given the maximum score $E_4M_6V_5 = 15$. A patient who opens his eyes to a painful stimulus, localizes with pain across the midline, and who only makes incomprehensible sounds has a GCS of $E_2M_5V_2 = 9$. A patient who shows no response despite adequate painful stimulus obtains the minimal score $E_1M_1V_1 = 3$.

GCS should be annotated to indicate significant confounding factors: T—signifies an intubated patient; S—patient that is sedated; P—patient that is chemically paralyzed. For example, a patient who is intubated but has his eyes open and is able to follow commands is a GCS $E_4M_6V_1 = 11T$.

The best score for each response should be documented and communicated in the format demonstrated above.

Table 11.2 Classification of Head Injury Severity

Classification	GCS Score	Other Symptoms
Minimal	15	No loss of consciousness No amnesia
Mild	14 or 15 with	Brief loss of consciousness or amnesia or impaired alertness or memory
Moderate	9 – 13 or	Loss of consciousness ≥ 5 minutes or Focal neurological deficit
Severe	5 – 8	
Critical	3 – 4	

Source: Narayan RK, Wilberger JE, Povlishock JT. Neurotrauma. New York: McGraw-Hill Health Professionals Division; 1996: xxiv, 1558

Abbreviation: GCS, Glasgow Coma Scale.

Table 11.3 Marshall CT Classification

Diffuse injury I	No visible pathology seen on CT scan
Diffuse injury II	Cisterns are present with MLS 0–5 mm and/or: Lesion densities present No high- or mixed-density lesion >25 mL May include bone fragments and foreign bodies
Diffuse injury III (swelling)	Cisterns are compressed or absent with MLS 0–5 mm and No high- or mixed-density lesion >25 mL
Diffuse injury IV (shift)	MLS >5 mm and No high- or mixed-density lesion >25 mL
Evacuated mass lesion	Any lesion surgically evacuated
Nonevacuated mass lesion	High- or mixed-density lesion >25 mL, not surgically evacuated

Abbreviation: CT, computed tomography; MLS, midline shift.

There are clearly limitations and obstacles in classifying brain injury purely based upon the physical examination. Examination findings are often obscured in the acute setting by confounding factors such as intoxication, medical sedation, and paralysis, and in some instances, by spinal cord injury. Notably, the current policy of early sedation and intubation has decreased the prognostic value of the GCS or its motor score for classifying the clinical severity of injury.[11–14] The assessment of structural damage is not influenced by these confounders. Morphologic diagnosis (see also Chapter 7) is often differentiated into focal and diffuse injury patterns.[15] Focal injuries consist mainly of intracranial hemorrhages and contusions, whereas diffuse injuries include concussions, diffuse axonal injury (DAI), or as is often the case in severe brain injury, a combination pattern of multiple injuries in multiple locations.

In 1991, Marshall and colleagues introduced a classification system based on computed tomography (CT) findings. This system grouped patients with TBI into six groups based upon multiple CT characteristics.[16] In this classification system, patients are differentiated based on the presence or absence of a focal mass lesion, and diffuse injuries are subdivided into four groups based on CT signs of increased intracranial pressure (ICP), i.e., compression of basal cisterns and midline shift (**Table 11.3**).

A general limitation of radiological classification is that, although TBI is a dynamic process, the radiological examination on which classification is based constitutes only a momentary picture. Early CT examinations may greatly underestimate the full extent of structural damage. As in the classification of clinical severity (GCS), radiological classification has also been used for prognostic purposes.

In a 2005 study, Maas et al evaluated the predictive power of the Marshall system in a cohort of 2,249 patients. Although they found the system to have strong predictive power, it was demonstrated that "greater discrimination" can be obtained if the individual CT characteristics that underlie the Marshall system, plus several additional parameters (such as presence of traumatic subarachnoid hemorrhage [tSAH], or intraventricular hemorrhage [IVH]) are included in the prognostic model. Thus, they recommend the use of individual characteristics of the CT rather than the Marshall CT classification system in determining prognosis.[17]

In 1975 Jennett and Bond introduced the Glasgow Outcome Scale (GOS) for standardized assessment of outcome following injury and recovery (**Table 11.4**).[18] This scale along with others is often used to determine the effectiveness of therapeutic options and is thus most helpful in brain injury research. A common procedure is to dichotomize the 5-point GOS into two categories: unfavorable and favorable. Unfavorable outcome includes

Table 11.4 The Glasgow Outcome Scale

1	*Death*
2	*Persistent vegetative state*: Patients who remain unresponsive and speechless for weeks to months
3	*Severe disability (conscious but disabled)*: Patients who are dependent for daily support by reason of mental or physical disability, usually a combination of both
4	*Moderate disability (disabled but independent)*: Independent insofar as daily life is concerned. Patients can travel by public transportation and work in a sheltered environment. Disabilities include varying degrees of dysphasia, hemiparesis, or ataxia, as well as intellectual and memory deficits and personality changes.
5	*Good recovery*: Resumption of normal life. Can have minor neurological or psychological deficits. Social outcome should be included in the assessment.

Source: Jennett B, Bond M. Assessment of outcome after severe brain damage. Lancet 1975;1(7905):480–484.

Table 11.5 The Extended Glasgow Outcome Scale

1	Death
2	Vegetative state
3	Lower severe disability
4	Upper severe disability
5	Lower moderate disability
6	Upper moderate disability
7	Lower good recovery
8	Upper good recovery

Source: Maas AI, Marmarou A, Murray GD, Teasdale SG, Steyerberg EW. Prognosis and clinical trial design in traumatic brain injury: the IMPACT study. J Neurotrauma 2007;24(2):232–238

the categories death, vegetative state, and severe disability; favorable outcome includes the categories moderate disability and good recovery. These procedures of dichotomization, however, decreased the sensitivity of the GOS to detect treatment effects and may be considered clinically inappropriate.[19] It is very possible that the sensitivity of trials may be increased by better exploiting the ordinal nature of the GOS and by relating the outcome obtained in individual patients to their initial prognostic risk, rather than applying a standardized dichotomization irrespective of severity.[20] The GOS has been criticized for lack of sensitivity; therefore, the 8-point extended GOS (GOSE) has been introduced to increase the sensitivity of assessment. The use of a structured interview is advocated to obtain more consistency in outcome (**Table 11.5**).[21] By definition, outcome after TBI is multifactorial, and it should be emphasized that the GOS is only a global measure. Various trials in TBI have included different measures for outcome (Barthel Index, Neuropsychological Tests, Quality of Life), but to our knowledge, only one has attempted to combine these into a multifactorial scale.[22]

Mechanism of Injury and Pathophysiology

Little can be done to reverse primary brain injury, the damage to the brain occurring at the moment of impact. Only prevention through public health programs focusing on education (bicycle and ski/snowboarding helmets) and possibly legislation (i.e., motorcycle helmets) can help lower the incidence and potentially the severity of primary brain injury.[23,24] Current therapeutic approaches focus mainly on the prevention and limitation of secondary brain damage.

It is widely accepted that the primary injury, most often through impact, spawns a chain of events that leads to ongoing cellular damage known as secondary brain injury. It is here, at the biochemical level, where physicians may be able to intervene pharmacologically. Basic research has identified many compounds with potential neuroprotective effects.[25–39] Unfortunately, no phase III clinical trials to date have yielded any agents proven to work in the general population. Although clinical trials have yet to yield a proven agent, the potential for neuroprotection in TBI is tremendous and we should not be discouraged by recent failures obtained up until now.[40–42]

In addition to intrinsic pathophysiologic processes, secondary damage may be initiated and exacerbated by secondary systemic and intracranial insults.[43,44] Secondary insults to the brain lead to decreased cellular oxygen delivery and metabolism causing ischemia and further brain cell death. The most well-recognized reversible secondary insults are hypotension, hypoxia, and raised ICP through mass lesion. It is our goal as health care providers and neurosurgeons to stop ongoing brain damage by preventing secondary insults and thus giving the damaged brain the optimal milieu for recovery.

Early Prognostic Factors in Severe Traumatic Brain Injury

In 2000, the BTF published the first revision of the guidelines for management of severe brain injury. Included in this publication was a section on early indicators of prognosis in severe brain injury. It reviewed the literature and evaluated several factors shown by class I and II evidence to have positive predictive value for predicting prognosis. In 2007, results of extensive prognostic analysis of individual data from 8,686 patients enrolled in 11 different studies were published by the IMPACT investigators.[19,45–54] Taken together, the evidence-based analysis conducted by the BTF and the meta-analysis of the IMPACT investigators provide strong evidence in support of predictors in TBI. The BTF guidelines focus on the GCS, age, pupillary reactivity, hypotension, and CT scan characteristics. The IMPACT studies also highlight the importance of laboratory examinations as predictors, and report multivariate analyses on the relative predictive value of parameters.

Glasgow Coma Scale

The initial GCS score, obtained following hemodynamic resuscitation, has been shown to be predictive of outcome in severe TBI, with the lowest scores fairing worse. The motor score in particular has proven to be the most reliable individual component of the GCS in terms of prognostic value. The painful stimulus used to obtain this score in a comatose patient should be standard and consistent. Supraorbital and nail bed pressure are acceptable means of producing painful stimuli; however, supraorbital pressure has been shown to have the least interobserver variation among experienced investigators. It is important to remember to use caution in patients suspected of having facial fractures.

When considering initial GCS in terms of prediction of outcome "the two most important problems are the reliability of the initial measurement and its lack of precision for prediction of good outcome if the initial GCS score is low." If the initial GCS score is reliably obtained, and not tainted by prehospital medications or intubation, approximately 20% of the patients with the worst initial GCS score will survive, and 8 to10% will have a functional survival (GOS 4 to 5).[55]

In 2006, Davis et al evaluated the predictive value of field (fGCS) versus arrival GCS (aGCS) score. Although in general they found a positive correlation between fGCS and aGCS, their study demonstrated that a decrease of 2 or more points between fGCS and aGCS is highly predictive of mortality and the need for neurosurgical procedures.[56] The IMPACT studies found a consistent strong association between the motor score and the 6-month GOS in particular across all studies (odds ratio [OR] = 1.74 to 7.48). The eye and verbal components were also strongly associated with the GOS. This study also found a significant change in motor score from prehospital direct to study hospital enrollment and from the first in hospital to study enrollment scores. It is consequently recommended that the study hospital enrollment GCS be used for prognostic purposes.

Age

Age is one of the strongest independent predictors of outcome in TBI. Increasing age is related to poorer outcome. Many studies have focused on analyzing threshold values and various studies have documented threshold values, varying from 30 to 60 years of age. The IMPACT studies, however, unequivocally demonstrated that the relation between age and outcome is a continuous relationship and holds across different points of dichotomization for the GOS. This relationship can be well approximated by a linear function, which may be considered more appropriate and informative than the stepwise categorical approach adopted in previous studies. The adverse effect of increasing age on outcome in TBI cannot be fully explained by the increased frequency of systemic disease and intracerebral hematoma in older patients.[2]

Pupillary Diameter and Light Reflex

Pupillary diameter and the pupilloconstrictor reflex are two parameters in brain injury that have been studied in relation to prognosis. There is class I evidence to support that bilateral fixed (no constriction to bright light) and dilated (>4 mm) pupils have a >70% positive predictive value for poor outcome (GOS 1 and 2).[57] The BTF made the following recommendations:

- Pupillary light reflex for each eye should be used as a prognostic factor.
- The duration of pupillary dilatation and fixation should be documented.
- A pupillary size greater than 4 mm is recommended as the measure for a dilated pupil.
- A fixed pupil should be defined as no constrictor response to bright light.
- Right or left distinction should be made when the pupils are asymmetric.
- Hypotension and hypoxia should be corrected before assessing pupils for prognosis.
- Direct orbital trauma should be excluded.
- Pupils should be reassessed after surgical evacuation of intracranial hematomas.

The IMPACT studies further confirmed the strong relation between pupillary abnormalities and outcome. The odds ratio for death with no reactive pupils was approximately 3 times as great as one reactive pupil. The prognostic strength of pupil reactivity in predicting outcome was more robust than the GCS or motor score when assessed over time of injury to study hospital admission.

Hypotension

Hypotension is one of the five most powerful predictors of outcome in TBI,[58] the others being age, intracranial (CT) diagnosis, pupillary diameter and reactivity, and postresuscitation GCS score. Hypotension is defined as systolic blood pressure <90 mm Hg, and data from the Traumatic Coma Data Bank (TCDB) have demonstrated that a single hypotensive episode is associated with a doubling of mortality and a significant increase in morbidity. Hypotension has been shown to be statistically independent of other major factors, including age, hypoxia, and the presence or absence of severe trauma to other organ systems. In addition, the positive predictive value for poor outcome increases to 79% when hypotension is combined with hypoxia. Hypotension and hypoxia, unlike the other predictors of outcome, can be modified by changes in health care practice, i.e., prevention through aggressive resuscitation after TBI.

Computed Tomographic Scan Features

As mentioned previously, CT scan features can be used to gauge prognosis in severe TBI. Abnormalities on the initial CT are identified in ~90% of patients with severe head injury, and demonstrated pathology on CT is associated with a worse prognosis. In patients in whom the initial CT is negative, prognosis is often related to the severity of associated extracranial traumatic injuries. A negative head CT does not rule out increased intracranial pressure, and ~40% of patients with initially negative scans develop significant, identifiable pathology.

As alluded to earlier, CT characteristics that have been shown to have prognostic value in TBI are status of the basal cisterns (open versus compressed or absent), presence of midline shift (>5 mm), presence and quantity of tSAH, and presence of a mass lesion.

There have been several models developed to help predict outcome and risk of morbidity and mortality from TBI based upon the above factors and patient characteristics. Risk assessment in TBI is important because it can help "inform relatives of realistic expectations, support clinical decision making and resource allocation, and classify patients according to prognostic risk." In 2006, Hukkelhoven et al evaluated the validity of several of these models and found that external validation varied widely and calibration was relatively poor. They therefore recommend using caution in basing clinical decisions on such models.[59]

Management of Severe Brain Injury

Prehospital Management

In the majority of cases, the first opportunity to assess and treat severe brain injury, prevent secondary insults, and ultimately affect outcome belongs to emergency medical technicians and paramedics working in the Emergency Medical Service (EMS). The proper prehospital management of severe brain injury has become a very important public health topic in recent years, given its potentially tremendous impact on outcome from TBI. In 2000 the BTF, with the support of the U.S. Department of Transportation, released "The Guidelines for Prehospital Management of Traumatic Brain Injury." These guidelines emphasized the importance of the EMS assessment and the potential implications of their treatment decisions. The guidelines were formulated based upon evidence-based medicine and a thorough review of the literature.[60]

Emergency Medical Service Assessment

EMS assessment should follow prehospital trauma life support guidelines focusing initially on airway, breathing, and circulation. In TBI, maintaining oxygenation and perfusion (blood pressure) is of paramount importance to prevent secondary brain damage. Accurate documentation of the neurological status (GCS, pupils, focal deficits) is essential to be able to detect any subsequent change.

Emergency Medical Service Treatment

Airway, Ventilation, and Oxygenation

Hypoxemia is a strong independent predictor of poor outcome and thus it should be corrected rapidly with supplemental oxygen when detected. Continuous pulse oximetry is strongly recommended to avoid a delay in diagnosis of this potentially avoidable source of secondary brain insult. If hypoxemia is present and not able to be corrected with supplemental oxygen it is the opinion of most surgeons that establishing a secure airway in the field should be attempted.[61] The preferred method of establishing an airway is through endotracheal intubation (ETI).

Severe brain-injured patients are often unable to adequately maintain a patent airway. There have been several studies looking at the pros and cons of intubation in the field by EMS personnel as a way to prevent secondary insults by hypoxia and potentially aspiration. These studies often yielded conflicting results. ETI in the field is typically associated with improved oxygen saturation following the establishment of a secure airway. However, studies that investigated continuous measurement of pulse oximetry during intubation by paramedics revealed transient hypoxemia. The San Diego Rapid Sequence Intubation (RSI) trial demonstrated that although paramedics are able to perform RSI successfully in most instances, these patients had poorer outcome when matched to historical controls not intubated in the field.[62] Intubation especially in instances when pharmacological agents are required to relax protective reflexes (cough, gag) may not reduce hypoxemia and aspiration. There is evidence, however, that aspiration probably occurs at the time of injury in severe TBI.

The Brain Trauma Foundation Guidelines for Prehospital Management of Traumatic Brain Injury guidelines determined that in field endotracheal intubation is an option-level recommendation. The decision to intubate should be based upon the patient's pulse oximeter saturation, level of consciousness as based on the GCS, and the experience of emergency personnel, and potentially by distance to the hospital.

Fluid Resuscitation

Hypotension systolic blood pressure (SBP) < 90 mm Hg in adults is associated with a doubling of mortality in severe brain injury. The goal of fluid resuscitation in the prehospital setting is to avoid hypotension and to maintain cardiac output, cerebral blood flow (CBF), and tissue perfusion thus avoiding secondary insult. The most commonly used fluids are isotonic crystalloid solutions, i.e., normal saline and lactated Ringer. Recently, there has been renewed interest in the use of hypertonic saline (HTS) as the initial resuscitation fluid in TBI. Although several studies have shown some promising results, data available at the time of the publication of the guidelines were not strong enough to recommend its routine use.

In 2004, a prospective, randomized, double-blind study was published in the *Journal of the American Medical Association (JAMA)*, in which 229 patients with severe TBI (GCS <9) and hypotension (SBP <100 mm Hg) were given either HTS or conventional fluid (lactated Ringer) resuscitation en route to the hospital. This study used 7.5% saline at a bolus dose of 250 mL. The goal of the study was to determine if the use of HTS in the prehospital setting had any effect on long-term outcome as measured by neurological function (GOS at 6 months). Although there was no demonstrable difference in neurological outcome among survivors of TBI at 6 months in both groups (GOS 5), the HTS group had slightly higher survivability 55% versus 47% in the control group ($p = 0.32$). In addition, patients treated with HTS tended to have lower intracranial pressure (ICP) upon initial measurement in the hospital ($p = 0.08$), although this difference did not reach statistical significance. The study had several limitations including relatively long average transport times to the hospital (that may have allowed for larger volumes of conventional resuscitation fluid), a low patient number (229), and a low power (80%) to detect a 1-grade GOS change.[63]

Brain-Targeted Therapy

In instances where patients are showing signs of neurological decline (loss of 2 points below 8 on GCS) and potentially demonstrating cerebral herniation (decerebrate posturing, dilated nonreactive pupils) the paramedics may elect to use some brain-targeted therapies. Although there is no evidence to support specific guidelines for management, therapies such as hyperventilation remain an option for EMS. Hyperventilation 20 bpm in adults, 30 bpm in children, and 35 to 40 bpm in infants less than 1 year of age is the first-line therapy to be used by paramedics if a patient demonstrates signs of impending herniation. It is important for neurological status to be checked frequently and hyperventilation to be discontinued should the patient no longer require it. Hyperventilation leads to cerebral vasoconstriction and thus reduced CBF thereby exacerbating cerebral ischemia and injury.

Mannitol is an effective drug for reduction of ICP. In the prehospital setting, its use cannot be recommended because of its potential to cause precipitous drops in blood pressure, especially in underresuscitated patients. Hypertonic saline, on the other hand, has been shown to have similar ICP lowering effect without the problems related to blood pressure reduction, and its use is therefore an option.

Medications to help facilitate transport, such as sedatives and paralytic agents, can also be used to keep often combative patients at bay and thus protected from injuring themselves. These medications may have the added benefit of lowering ICP. It is important to be cautious to avoid drops in blood pressure as well as loss of protective reflexes that may predispose patients to aspiration.

Although hypoglycemia is a potentially reversible cause of coma, the prophylactic administration of dextrose to patients with TBI who are comatose is not routinely recommended as hyperglycemia may have a potentially deleterious effect. Prehospital measurement of glucose has been demonstrated to be accurate, especially when a venous sample is tested.[64] The blood glucose should be measured by EMS personnel and dextrose given to those patients who are severely hypoglycemic. In the absence of blood glucose level, dextrose can be given prophylactically in those instances where clinical suspicion of hypoglycemia is high.

Transportation Decisions

Class II evidence supports the recommendation that all regions have an organized trauma system through which EMS personnel follow a protocol that dictates the transport of patients recognized to have severe brain injury directly to a center that can provide the maximum level of care. That center must have the ability to provide immediate CT scanning, prompt neurosurgical care, and the ability to monitor ICP and treat ICP elevations. In the United States, the adoption of this guideline has resulted in significant decreased mortality from TBI. It is well recognized that hospital transfer of patients delays neurosurgical consultation and potential intervention and thus can contribute to worse outcomes.

The European system differs somewhat from that of the United States in that neurotrauma resources in Europe are routinely concentrated in dedicated centers. When a brain-injured patient in Europe presents to a regional care facility that is not fully equipped to handle the gravity of his or her injuries, the patient must be rapidly and safely transported to a neurotrauma center. It is important that the patient be adequately resuscitated and that appropriate measures are taken to prevent secondary brain insults before the transfer occurs. The urge to rush the transfer of the patient without beginning adequate resuscitation measures should be resisted as this has been shown to have deleterious effects. As in the United States, patients should only be transferred once it is safe to do so. In cases of severe TBI the patient needs to be intubated, sedated, and volume resuscitated. Proper monitoring should always be used (electrocardiogram [EKG], pulse oximetry, end tidal CO_2, etc.) when transferring patients (**Fig. 11.1**).

Initial Trauma Management

The hospital management of a severely brain injured patient begins with the ABCs (airway, breathing, circulation). In

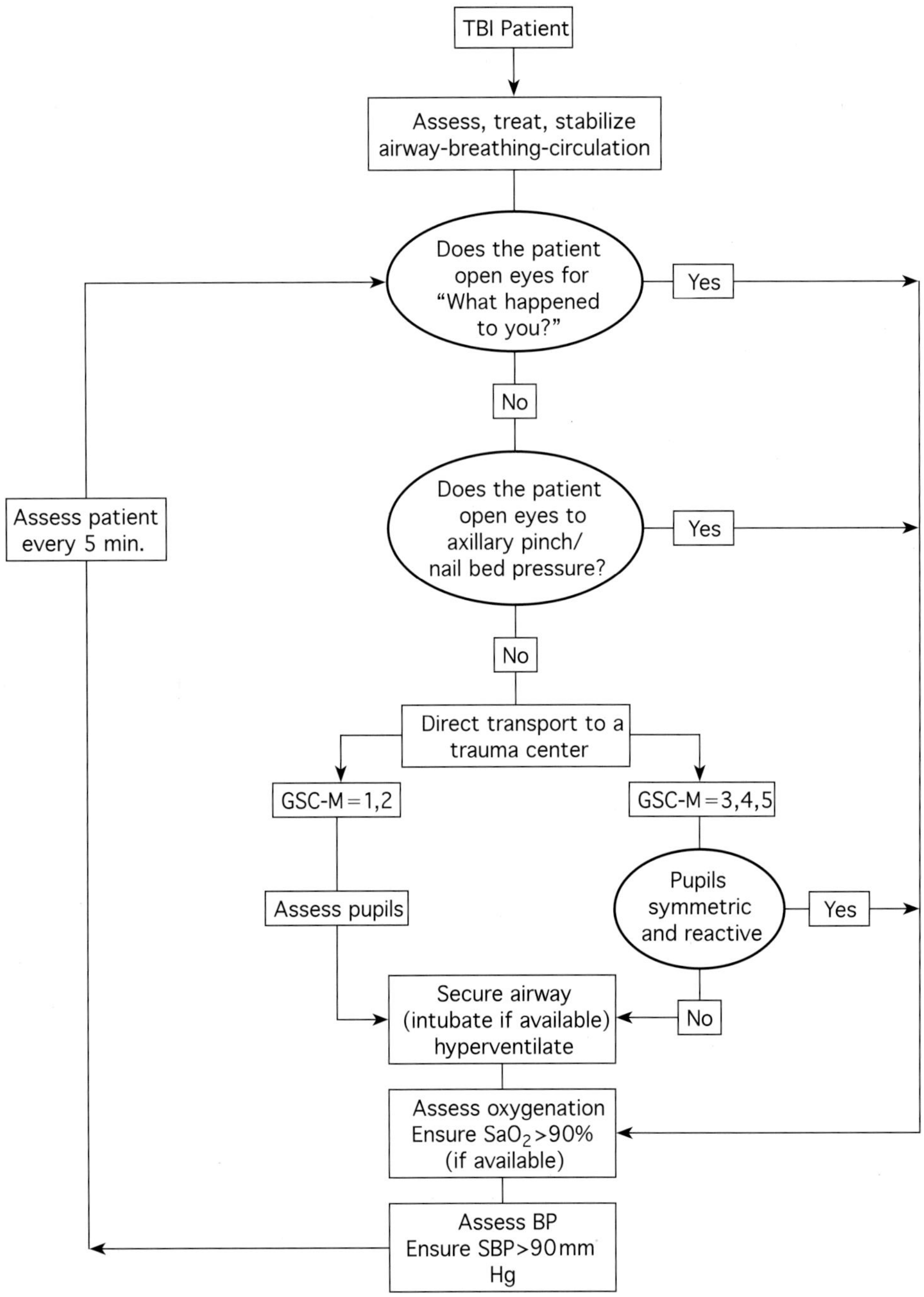

Fig. 11.1 Algorithm for prehospital assessment and treatment of traumatic brain injury (TBI). (From Brain Trauma Foundation. Guidelines for Prehospital Management of Traumatic Brain Injury. New York: Brain Trauma Foundation; 2000 Reprinted with permission. BP, blood pressure; SaO_2, oxygen saturation; SBP, systolic blood pressure.)

the United States, as in most countries across the world, the standards set forth by the American College of Surgeons Committee on Trauma: Advanced Trauma Life Support (ATLS) are followed. The "trauma team" typically consists of surgeons, emergency room physicians, nurses, respiratory therapists, and other hospital staff, and works to quickly identify and treat life-threatening injuries. The team employs a strategy best suited for the institution. In trauma-heavy centers, a horizontal approach is often taken where multiple physicians work simultaneously to help speed-up the evaluation process.

Primary Survey: The ABCDEs

Table 11.6 provides an at-a-glance guide to the ABCDEs.

Table 11.6 ABCDEs

- Airway maintenance with cervical spine protection
- Breathing and ventilation
- Circulation with hemorrhage control
- Disability
- Exposure and environmental control

Airway Maintenance with Cervical Spine Protection

Of utmost importance is the evaluation and establishment of a patent airway. All severe TBI patients and most moderate TBI patients should have a definitive airway (endotracheal intubation) established as soon as possible to prevent hypoxia. These critically ill patients by definition are felt to have too depressed a level of consciousness to adequately protect their airway and thus are at risk for aspiration and hypoxia. The presence of hypoxia has been shown to be an independent predictor of poor outcome, and a definitive airway is the first step in its prevention.

Patients with severe brain injury often have associated facial injuries, including fractures. Care must therefore be taken when intubating the patient or placing gastric tubes so as not to perpetuate injury or cause iatrogenic damage. Although intracranial placement of tubes is an extremely rare occurrence, it has been described, and the CT images obtained afterward are chilling.

Endotracheal rapid-sequence intubation with the physician's direct visualization of the vocal cords with the assistance of a rigid laryngoscope is therefore currently the preferred method of establishing an airway. It is also extremely important to remember the associated incidence of cervical spine fractures with severe TBI. Care should be taken to prevent excessive movement of the cervical spine. Stabilization devices, i.e., c-collars, should be used in all trauma patients. It is imperative to maintain manual inline stabilization of the c-spine whenever the collar is removed and while the airway is being established to prevent potential iatrogenic injury.

Individual patient characteristics and the need for inline stabilization of the cervical spine can make intubation of the patient using a standard laryngoscope extremely difficult. Recently, a new tool that may help make the intubation procedure safer and easier has become more widely available. A video-assisted intubation device such as the angulated video-intubating laryngoscope (AVIL) GlideScope (Verathon, Bothell, WA) or intubating lighted stylet Lightwand or Trachlight (Laerdal Medical AS, Toronto, Canada) affords its user dramatic visualization of the vocal cords without the need to extend the neck. The view that these devices provide can be superior to direct laryngoscopy, and the intubating procedure has been demonstrated to be quick and safe even in the hands of relatively inexperienced users.[65–67] These new devices may prove to be superior to standard laryngoscopes in trauma.

Breathing and Ventilation

The second portion of the trauma evaluation involves inspection of the respiratory system to ensure adequate gas exchange. Ventilation is evaluated through auscultation of the lungs and inspection of the chest wall, and through continuous measurement of pulse oxymetry and if possible end-tidal CO_2. The goal of this portion of the trauma evaluation is the prevention of hypoxia through adequate ventilation. Chest injuries such as tension pneumothorax and sucking chest wounds require immediate treatment and should never be missed.

Circulation with Hemorrhage Control

Hypotension like hypoxia is an independent predictor of poor outcome in TBI. The third portion of the trauma examination is the evaluation of the circulatory system. "Hemorrhage is the predominant cause of postinjury deaths that are preventable by rapid treatment in the hospital setting."[68] Hypotension following injury is considered hypovolemic until proven otherwise. Level of consciousness, skin color, and pulse are used to evaluate the circulatory system quickly. Blood pressure is measured and hypotension prevented through adequate volume resuscitation with warmed isotonic or hypertonic solutions. (Hypotonic intravenous fluids can precipitate cerebral edema and should be avoided in neurotrauma.) External hemorrhage is identified and controlled through direct pressure on the wound or through pneumatic splinting devices.

All trauma patients should have two large bore (16 gauge or larger) peripheral intravenous (IV) catheters placed to allow for rapid infusion of fluid. Standard laboratories including blood count, coagulation, and chemistry profiles along with blood type and cross-match should be drawn at the time of placement of the lines. All women of childbearing age should have β-hCG (beta-human chorionic gonadotropin) checked to rule out pregnancy. Individualized laboratory tests such as alcohol level, drug screens, and antiepileptic levels should be checked in the appropriate patient. A Foley catheter should be placed in all severe TBI patients as urine output can help determine fluid status, as well as allow for measurement of diuresis following mannitol therapy.

Disability

This portion of the primary survey includes a quick yet thorough trauma neurological examination. This is obviously of utmost importance in suspected brain injury and spinal cord injury. The patient's level of consciousness through determination of GCS score as well as pupillary diameter and response to light should be evaluated and recorded. Strength, sensation, deep tendon reflexes, and rectal tone should be tested if possible, especially in those patients suspected of having a spinal cord injury. Spine tenderness should be accessed if possible while maintaining spinal precautions (log roll only). A rigid cervical collar such as a Philadelphia collar or Miami-J collar should be secured if not already done so by EMS personnel. In instances where severity of injury and distracting traumatic injuries precludes the team's ability to perform a thorough neurological examination, simple notation of the patient's level of consciousness (GCS or AVPU [alert, response to verbal stimuli, response to painful stimuli, unconscious]) and whether the patient was able to move his or her extremities prior to intervention is important. A more thorough neurological exam in trauma patients not suspected of having neurological injury is often deferred until a more detailed secondary survey can be performed.

The GCS score as discussed earlier is the preferred way to communicate level of consciousness in TBI. It is easily determined, reproducible by competent observers, and conveys a lot of information, including potential prognosis. However, some traumatologists still use the American College of Surgeons' accepted AVPU method to communicate level of arousal.[68]

In addition to the GCS score, the pupillary exam is of utmost importance. The presence of a dilated pupil in a comatose trauma victim can alert the team to the presence of an intracranial mass lesion and thus expedite neurosurgical evaluation (**Table 11.7**).

Exposure and Environmental Control

The final portion of the primary survey includes a head to toe evaluation of the patient while maintaining spinal precautions. All clothes should be removed from the patient with the help of trauma shears. It is very important not to miss a potentially life-threatening injury because a more obviously injured body part distracts you. After adequate exposure is obtained, it is important not to leave the patient vulnerable to the environment; blankets should be used to keep the patient warm and prevent hypothermia.

Table 11.7 AVPU Level of Consciousness Assessment

- Alert
- Responds to verbal stimuli
- Responds to painful stimuli
- Unconscious

The Secondary Survey

Once the ABCDEs are complete and appropriate interventions to stabilize the patient initiated, the secondary survey begins. The secondary survey, as the name implies, includes a more thorough history and physical exam and careful reassessment of the patient. Information regarding the circumstances that led up to the injury, the patient's premorbid condition, as well as any confounding factors such as antiplatelet or anticoagulation medications, drugs, alcohol, etc., can be very useful and help tailor management.

The patient with severe brain injury will not be able to answer these questions, so history will rely upon family members, witnesses, paramedics, etc. In most institutions, information gathering begins as soon as the patient is brought through the doors. Again, the team can often work in parallel to most efficiently gather information. The most important aspect of the secondary survey is careful reassessment. If a deterioration in the patient's condition occurs, the team must step back, determine the reason, and initiate appropriate therapy. When a problem occurs, always return to the ABCDEs.

Radiographic Assessment (Establishing an Intracranial Diagnosis)

The role of the primary survey is to quickly identify life-threatening injuries and begin interventions to stabilize the patient and prevent secondary brain insults. The primary survey should be followed by the secondary survey and radiographic assessment to establish the intracranial diagnosis.

As discussed in Chapter 7, computed tomography (CT) is the gold standard test in traumatic brain injury. Modern CT has the ability to both quickly and reliably evaluate intracranial injury in trauma. A noncontrast CT scan of the head is a very sensitive test for detecting blood in the epidural, subdural, subarachnoid, intraparenchymal, and intraventricular spaces, as well as in detecting calvarial fractures. CT can also be used to determine the status of the cisterns and fluid spaces of the brain and thus is useful in the evaluation of diffuse injuries. A CT head scan should be the first scan obtained in those patients suspected of having TBI and should always be done prior to the use of intravenous contrast.

In patients with severe TBI, other CT-based testing can be helpful. The advent of CT angiography (CTA) allows for the diagnosis of vascular injury and abnormalities in a quick and noninvasive way. For instance, CTA can help guide surgical decisions and make surgery safer in patients with a parenchymal hemorrhage by first ruling out, or in, an underlying aneurysm or arterial venous malformation

(AVM). CT perfusion (CTP) may also prove to be helpful in trauma, especially in those patients where the CT appearance does not correlate with their poor neurologic condition.

The advent of new multidetector CT scanners has improved the resolution, speed, and ease of obtaining scans. CT assessment of the cervical spine with sagittal and coronal reconstructions is quick and easy; it is a more sensitive alternative to plain radiographs for evaluation of the cervical spine in trauma. The scan is not influenced by patient characteristics such as body habitus and limb injuries, and it does not rely on a "shoulder pull" for obtaining an adequate study as a lateral radiograph often does.

More specialized and time-consuming testing such as magnetic resonance imaging (MRI) or cerebral angiography is rarely indicated. Please refer to Chapter 7 for a more detailed review of imaging in brain injury (**Fig. 11.2**).[69]

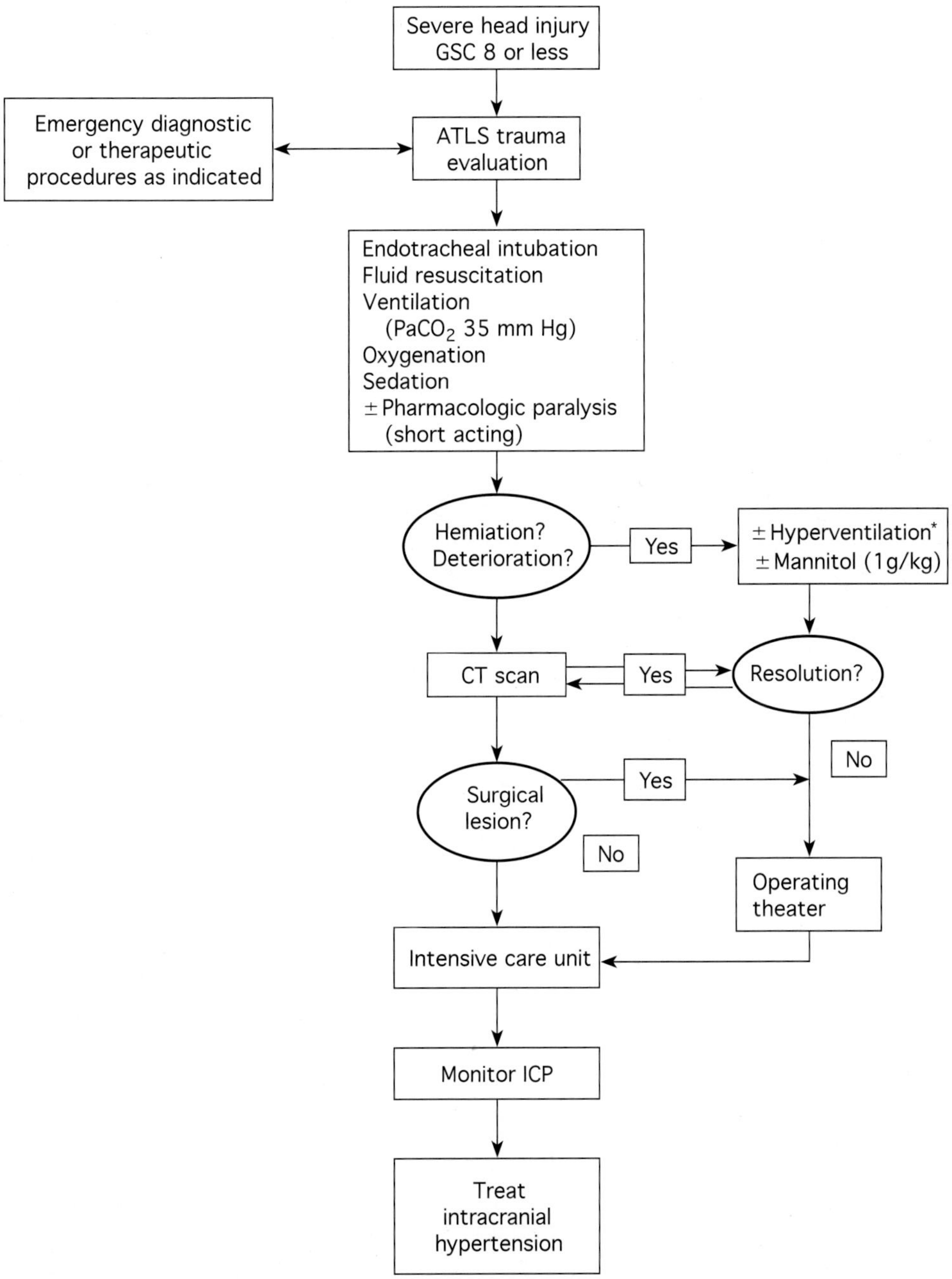

Fig. 11.2 Initial management of a severe head injury. *Only in the presence of signs of herniation or progressive neurological deterioration not attributable to extracranial fractures. (From The Brain Trauma Foundation. The American Association of Neurological Surgeons. The Joint Section on Neurotrauma and Critical Care. Initial management. J Neurotrauma 2000;17(6-7): 463-469). ATLS, Advanced Trauma Life Support; CT, computed tomographic; ICP, intracranial pressure; $PaCO_2$, partial pressure of carbon dioxide.

Table 11.8 Guidelines for the Surgical Management of Traumatic Brain Injury

	Indication for Surgery	Timing	Method
Epidural hematoma	EDH >30 cm^3 *Operative evacuation regardless of GCS* EDH <30 cm^3 *and* <15 mm thickness *and* <5 mm MLS in a patient with GCS >8 *without* focal deficit Can be managed *nonoperatively* with serial CT and close neurological observation in a neurosurgical center	Acute EDH in coma (GCS <9) with anisocoria; should undergo surgical evacuation as soon as possible	Craniotomy
Subdural hematoma	Acute SDH >10 mm thickness *or* >5 mm MLS *Operative evacuation regardless of GCS* *All* patients with acute SDH in coma (GCS <9) should undergo ICP monitoring A comatose patient (GCS<9) with SDH <10 mm thick and <5 mm MLS *Operative decompression* if the GCS score decreased by 2 or more points from time of injury and hospital admission and/or the patient presents with asymmetric or fixed and dilated pupils and/or the ICP >20 mm Hg	Acute SDH and indication for surgery should undergo surgical evacuation as soon as possible	Craniotomy or Craniectomy plus duraplasty
Parenchymal lesions	Parenchymal mass lesion and signs of progressive neurological deterioration referable to the lesion, medically refractory intracranial hypertension or signs of mass effect on CT *Operative decompression/evacuation* Patients with GCS 6–8 with frontal or temporal contusions >20 cm^3 in volume and MLS ≥5 mm and/or cisternal compression on CT or any lesion >50 cm^3 *Operative decompression/evacuation* Patients with parenchymal mass lesion and *no* signs of neurological compromise, with controlled ICP and no signs of mass effect on CT Can be managed nonoperatively with intensive monitoring and serial imaging	Surgery as soon as possible of focal lesions if indicated Decompressive craniectomy within 48 h if refractory ICP	Craniotomy and evacuation of mass lesion for those patients with focal lesions if indicated Bifrontal craniectomy for patients with diffuse, medically refractory cerebral edema and ICH Decompressive procedures for those with clinical or radiographic impending herniation
Posterior fossa mass lesions	Posterior fossa mass lesion with *mass effect** on CT or neurological dysfunction or deterioration referable to the lesion *Operative intervention* Patients with lesion and no significant mass effect or signs of neurological dysfunction Can be managed nonoperatively with close observation and serial imaging	Surgical Intervention as soon as possible if indicated Patients with posterior fossa lesions can deteriorate rapidly and thus worsen prognosis.	*Suboccipital craniectomy* and evacuation of lesion
Depressed cranial fractures	Open (compound) cranial fractures depressed greater than the thickness of the cranium *Operative intervention* to prevent infection Open (compound) cranial fractures with depression <1 mm and *no* clinical or radiographic evidence of dural penetration, significant intracranial hematoma, frontal sinus involvement, gross cosmetic deformity, wound infection, pneumocephalus, or gross wound contamination Can be managed nonoperatively Closed (simple) depressed cranial fractures Can be managed nonoperatively	Early surgical intervention if indicated to reduce chance of infection	Elevation and debridement Primary bony fragment replacement is an option if no evidence of infection at time of surgery *Antibiotics* are recommended for all open fractures.

Source: Bullock MR, Chesnut R, Ghajar J, Gordon D, Hartl R, Newell DW, et al: Guidelines for the Surgical Management of Traumatic Brain Injury. Neurosurgery 58:S1-60; discussion Si-iv, 2006

*Mass effect = distortion, dislocation, or obliteration of the fourth ventricle; compression or loss of visualization of the basal cisterns, or the presence of obstructive hydrocephalus.

Abbreviations: CT, computed tomography; EDH, epidural hematoma; GCS, Glasgow Coma Scale; ICH, intracranial hematoma; ICP, intracranial pressure; MLS, midline shift; SDH, subdural hematoma.

Neurosurgical Assessment and Intervention

Neurosurgical assessment should begin as soon as possible after injury, preferably on admission to the emergency department. In severe brain injury, the patient's initial CT scan in addition to his or her neurological examination findings is used to guide appropriate management and operative decisions. Focal injuries such as epidural hematomas, subdural hematomas, depressed skull fractures, and some parenchymal hemorrhages, as well as some diffuse injuries with evidence of increased intracranial pressure, e.g., compression of the basal cisterns and midline shift (MLS), may require emergent surgical intervention to provide the patient the best chance for survival and functional recovery. The guidelines for the surgical management of TBI were released in a supplement to the journal *Neurosurgery* in March 2006 and will be discussed in more detail in Chapter 13, Scientific Surgical Management. In the appropriate patient, the next step after a CT scan is operative decompression with the goal of relieving ICP elevation and restoring normal cerebral perfusion to salvageable brain tissue (**Table 11.8**).

For those patients who do not yet require surgery, the neurosurgical nonoperative management of severe brain injury begins at this stage. Further management of these critically ill patients should occur either in a dedicated Neurosurgical Intensive Care Unit, or in a Surgical Intensive Care Unit equipped to take care of these patients' special needs. The choice of where these patients go and who ultimately is responsible for their care depends on the institution. The presence of other traumatic injuries and the need for nonneurosurgical procedures can also influence this decision. Regardless, patients with severe TBI, GCS <8, can be considered some of the most critically ill in the hospital, and the quality of how they are managed will affect outcome.

Intensive Care Unit Management and the Prevention of Secondary Insults

The Guidelines for the Management of Severe Brain Injury, initially released by the Brain Trauma Foundation (BTF) in 1995, revised in 2000, 2003, and 2007, along with the European Brain Injury Consortium (EBIC) guidelines released in 1997, help dictate how to best care for patients with severe TBI. The common theme of these guidelines, as mentioned earlier, is the prevention of secondary insults, halting further brain tissue damage, and providing the optimal milieu for recovery. The BTF guidelines are evidence-based recommendations formulated on review of available studies. Each recommendation is given weight based on the quality of the studies available. In the new guidelines the recommendation is categorized as either level I, II, or III based upon the class of evidence in the studies that each recommendation is based upon. The level corresponds to and replaces the previous categories of recommendations: I = standard, II = guideline, and III = option.

As one can imagine, ethical considerations limit the ability to perform randomized prospective studies on certain aspects of patient care, and thus the lack of evidence affects the power in most of these recommendations. The paucity of level I recommendations therefore demonstrates the need for further research in TBI. In contrast to the BTF, the EBIC guidelines were developed based on consensus and expert opinion.

In the following sections we will discuss the management guidelines set by the BTF and the EBIC in regard to the initial management of severe brain injury. The new BTF guidelines published in 2007 address issues such as deep venous thrombosis (DVT) prophylaxis, infection prophylaxis, and nutrition. These subjects will be discussed in more detail in later chapters on intensive care unit (ICU) care and nutrition.

Blood Pressure and Oxygenation

As mentioned earlier, blood pressure and oxygenation are strong predictors of morbidity and mortality following severe brain injury. Although ethical considerations limit prospective randomized studies evaluating effects of hypotension and hypoxia there is good evidence that episodes of hypotension defined as SBP < 90 mm Hg and hypoxia defined as PaO_2 < 60 mm Hg or SaO_2 < 90% can have profound effect on outcome.

The recommendation currently (level II) is to monitor blood pressure and avoid hypotension (SBP < 90 mm Hg).[7] The IMPACT studies, however, show that there is no obvious threshold effect for systolic blood pressure of 90 mm, or indeed at any other value.[48] The relation between blood pressure and outcome is continuous with both lower and higher values of blood pressure being associated with poorer outcome. Although this observation does not lead directly to strong recommendations regarding the management of low blood pressure, it suggests that, although a systolic blood pressure of 90 mm Hg may be considered an absolute minimum, higher values may be preferred. The EBIC guidelines recommend achieving and maintaining a systolic blood pressure of 120 mm Hg as soon as possible.[8] Again, the BTF recommendations are based on evidence in the literature that has consistently demonstrated that a single recorded episode of hypotension <90 mm Hg is one of the five most powerful indicators of outcome from severe TBI. This definition of hypotension is based on statistical norms in adults, and drops in blood pressure below this value correlate with increased morbidity and doubling of mortality as demonstrated by cases in the Traumatic Coma Data Bank (TCDB).[44]

The end point of blood pressure resuscitation has yet to be established by prospective studies. Blood pressure influences cerebral perfusion pressure (CPP) and thus affects outcome. It can be inferred that by maintaining blood pressure at higher values and thus increasing CPP one can improve outcome. To date, there have been no prospective randomized studies in the literature to support this; thus, the BTF recommendation sets only a number to avoid and not the goal of therapy such as that given by the EBIC.

In regard to oxygenation, the recommendation of the BTF (level III) is to continuously monitor oxygenation and to avoid hypoxemia as defined by a $PaO_2 < 60$ mm Hg or $SaO_2 < 90\%$. This recommendation is based on studies in which there was an increase in mortality with observed drops in oxygenation below these critical levels. The EBIC recommends adjusting ventilation to achieve $PaCO_2$ 30 to 35 mm Hg, $PaO_2 > 75$ mm Hg, and $SaO_2 > 95\%$.

Indications for Intracranial Pressure Monitoring

It is well known that patients with severe TBI are at risk for intracranial hypertension (ICH). ICH and reduction of CPP < 50 mm Hg have been shown to correlate with worse outcomes following injury. The current BTF recommendations for ICP monitoring (level II) are to "monitor all salvageable patients with severe TBI (GCS 3 to 8 after resuscitation) and an abnormal CT scan." An abnormal CT constitutes one that demonstrates hematomas, contusions, swelling, herniation, or compressed basal cisterns. In addition, ICP monitoring may be indicated (level III) in patients with a normal CT scan if two or more of the following are noted on admission: age over 40 years, motor posturing (unilateral or bilateral), or SBP <90 mm Hg. There are several choices in ICP monitoring technology (please refer to Chapter 5); however, the current recommendation supports a ventricular catheter connected to an external strain gauge as the most accurate, reliable, and low-cost method of monitoring ICP. The ventricular catheter has the added benefit of being a means through which to lower ICP to normal levels through cerebrospinal fluid (CSF) diversion. External ventricular drain (EVD) placement can therefore be both diagnostic and therapeutic. Other monitoring technologies remain an option for individual patients. For instance, it may be nearly impossible to place an EVD catheter safely in a patient with severely compressed ventricles. A fiberoptic monitor may be a safer choice in that instance. Please see Chapters 4 and 5 for further discussion on this topic.

Intracranial Pressure Thresholds

The normal ICP range in adults is roughly 5 to 15 mm Hg. When ICP is elevated cerebral perfusion is reduced. Reduction in cerebral perfusion leads to secondary injury by reducing brain tissue oxygenation. The measure of cerebral perfusion, the CPP is calculated by subtracting the ICP from the mean arterial pressure (MAP). To have a continuous CPP recording one must continuously measure both ICP and blood pressure. Reduction of CPP below 50 mm Hg is associated with poorer outcomes. Given that CPP is determined by ICP and MAP, one can thus influence this value by adjustments in either of these parameters, i.e., by raising the MAP or lowering the ICP.

$$CPP = MAP - ICP$$

At ICP values greater than normal, the brain becomes at risk for herniation and thus a worse outcome. Therefore, a recommendation for an ICP limit above which treatment should be initiated needed to be established. The current guidelines to determine this threshold are based on a review of the literature. Although an absolute value or "herniation pressure" over which herniation occurs has yet to be established, treatment should be initiated for ICP >20 mm Hg (level II). In determining how best to treat the patient, a combination of factors should be considered (level III). The ICP values along with the clinical picture and CT head scan appearance all play a role. Herniation can occur in situations with ICP values <20 mm Hg (i.e., a large epidural hematoma). Thus, it is imperative to promptly address the patient who develops a blown pupil with CT evidence of a mass lesion regardless of the ICP. The EBIC did not establish a set point over which ICP should be treated; however, the consensus was that ICP maintained over 20 to 25 mm Hg should be treated, especially in the earlier stages following TBI. They pointed out, however, that before initiating ICP-directed therapies such as sedation, CSF drainage, osmotic therapy, etc., it is necessary to check for monitor malfunction and remediable extracranial disorders.

Cerebral Perfusion Pressure Thresholds

In addition to setting a guideline for ICP management, the BTF set out to establish a recommendation in regard to CPP optimization. CPP affects perfusion as it relates to cerebral blood flow. As we know, the brain has the ability to maintain blood flow and thus perfusion tissue over a large pressure range. This control is known as cerebral autoregulation. In brain injury, the brain's autoregulation ability is impaired. It has been proposed that through elevating MAP and thus CPP through volume expansion and the use of hemodynamic agents such as dopamine and epinephrine one can achieve better outcomes. This theory has been tested in several series and although it is evident that CPP should be maintained above a minimum of 50 mm Hg (level III), systemic negative effects such as adult respiratory stress syndrome (ARDS) occur more frequently in patients in whom CPP has been maintained at artificially high values >70 mm Hg (level II). Patients with ARDS had, on average, higher ICP values that were often refractory to treatment, and these patients had worse outcomes.

The current recommendation therefore is not to artificially maintain CPP at higher levels (>70 mm Hg) with volume expansion and hemodynamic pressor agents due to the risk of systemic toxicity and ARDS (level II). CPP values <50 mm Hg should be avoided as this correlates with ischemia and worse outcomes (level III). The target CPP to maintain is thus in the range of 50 to 70 mm Hg (level III). It has been proposed that the goal of therapy should be to maintain CPP >60 to avoid drops below 50. Those with intact autoregulation can tolerate CPP values >70 mm Hg (level III). The EBIC recommendation to maintain CPP 60 to 70 mm Hg is in agreement with these BTF findings.

Hyperosmolar Therapy

When ICP is >20 mm Hg and is refractory to first-line control efforts such as CSF diversion, increasing the head of bed to 30 degrees,[70] and ventilatory control maintaining PCO_2 ~35 mm Hg, hyperosmolar agents can be used to lower ICP. Mannitol and HTS are two hyperosmolar agents commonly used in clinical practice for ICP control.

Mannitol has been used over the past 3 decades and has beneficial effects on ICP, CPP, CBF, brain metabolism, and short-term neurological outcome from TBI. Although the mechanism of action of mannitol has been studied extensively, its ICP lowering effect in humans is not entirely understood. Its effect appears to be two-fold. Initially, mannitol acts as a rheologic agent by expanding the plasma volume, lowering the hematocrit, and allowing for greater deformation of erythrocytes. This effect causes both a reduction in ICP in addition to an increase in CBF. Mannitol also acts as an osmotic agent acting to pull fluid from swollen cells and thus lower ICP by reducing cerebral edema.

The ICP-lowering effect of mannitol decreases with continued use, and bolus dosing appears to be superior to continuous infusion, although to date there are no good studies in humans to recommend the optimal dosing regimen. Doses of mannitol 0.25 to 1 g/kg have classically been used with good success in reducing ICP. A 2007 study showed that bolus dose (infusion over 20 minutes) of 0.5 mg/kg of mannitol was effective in reducing ICP up to 30 mm Hg without sacrificing cerebral oxygenation.[71]

Mannitol can cause renal failure, and its use should be limited if serum osmolality exceeds 320 mOSm. Mannitol also can precipitate a drop in blood pressure and thus lower CPP. Its use prior to placement of an ICP monitoring device and adequate volume resuscitation should therefore be limited. In select instances where the patient is exhibiting signs of herniation and or neurological deterioration not attributable to other causes, its use can be advocated (level III).

HTS can also be used to lower ICP. Unlike mannitol, HTS does not cause drops in blood pressure and its use initially in trauma may therefore be safer than mannitol. HTS is felt to reduce ICP through osmotic mobilization of cerebral water content across an intact blood–brain barrier. In addition, HTS is felt to have a potential neuroprotective effect by reducing leukocyte adhesion in a traumatized brain. HTS may thus limit a deleterious inflammatory response. The optimal dosage and schedule for HTS administration has yet to be established. Several recent case series have alluded to a beneficial effect of bolus administration of high dose 7.2 to 10% HTS in patients with intracranial hypertension refractory to mannitol therapy. Currently, HTS use in severe TBI is a level III recommendation. In our institution, we use 7.5% HTS 2 mL/kg bolus for control of ICP.

Hyperventilation

The ICP-lowering effect of aggressive hyperventilation $PaCO_2 < 25$ mm Hg has been utilized in the treatment of intracranial hypertension and TBI for decades. The mechanism of action through which ICP reduction is achieved has been demonstrated to be cerebral vasoconstriction. Cerebral vasoconstriction reduces CBF and thus the delivery of oxygen to the brain. In TBI cerebral perfusion is already reduced, and this additional reduction in CBF can lead to brain tissue ischemia. Poorer outcomes have been demonstrated in patients in whom prophylactic hyperventilation was used for ICP management. Prophylactic hyperventilation therefore is not recommended by the BTF guidelines (level II).

When a patient is in a crisis and herniation is eminent, however, hyperventilation can be used as a temporizing measure for the reduction of ICP (level III). It is preferable to avoid hyperventilation during the first 24 hours following TBI as this is the time during which CBF is often already critically reduced (level III). If hyperventilation is used, technologies to measure brain oxygen delivery such as jugular venous oxygen saturation (SJO_2) or brain tissue oxygen partial pressure ($BtpO_2$) may prove to be of benefit.

Hypothermia Therapy

There has been some recent evidence that prophylactic hypothermia 32 to 35°C may have a beneficial effect in regard to favorable outcome (GOS scores) compared with normothermic controls when used in TBI (level III). A reduction in mortality, however, has not been statistically identified. There may be a greater mortality risk reduction when target temperatures are maintained for >48 hours. The use of prophylactic hypothermia in TBI is therefore an option, and more research is needed to increase the strength of this recommendation.

Anesthetics, Analgesics, and Sedatives

The use of agents such as morphine, midazolam, and propofol in the management of ICP in the neurology intensive care unit (NICU) has become more common in recent years. These agents act to lower ICP by reducing agitation and pain, lowering blood pressure, and allowing for greater compliance with mechanical ventilation. Propofol is an anesthetic that has both sedative and hypnotic features; it is rapid in onset and has a relatively short duration of action. It can be turned off for neurological examinations and has thus gained tremendous popularity in the management of these patients. In addition, propofol lowers cerebral metabolism, and thus oxygen utilization in the brain, and is felt to be neuroprotective. Propofol use is not without risk, however, and sustained high-dose propofol has been associated with significant morbidity and mortality. Propofol infusion syndrome is associated with "hyperkalemia, hepatomegaly, lipemia, metabolic acidosis, myocardial failure, rhabdomyolysis and renal failure resulting in death." [72]Caution must be exerted with its sustained use, especially at higher doses. The use of propofol in TBI is a level III recommendation. Neither propofol nor the other sedatives and analgesics have been shown to reduce mortality or improve outcome.

Barbiturates such as pentobarbital have been used in the management of ICP for decades. These agents both lower ICP and cerebral metabolism and are felt to be neuroprotective. Their use is associated with negative systemic effects such as hypotension and potential cardiac complications. Patients on barbiturates have a higher incidence of infections and are prone to pneumonia, decubitus ulcers, as well as DVT. Because the patient is essentially under general anesthesia, the gut cannot be utilized for nutrition and these patients must receive a parenteral alternative.

There have been several studies designed to look at the potential benefit of using pentobarbital in ICP management. They found that prophylactic use of pentobarbital leads to increased mortality and worse outcomes. The prophylactic use of pentobarbital is not recommended by the BTF. For patients whose ICP is refractory to surgical and maximal medical management, pentobarbital can be used as a last effort. It is essential for these patients to be hemodynamically stable prior to and during burst suppression. Invasive cardiac monitoring such as Swan–Ganz catheterization can be helpful in optimization.

Antiseizure Prophylaxis

Seizures following TBI (PTS) can be classified as either early (occurring within 1 week of injury) or late (occurring after 7 days). The prophylactic use of antiepileptic for both of these conditions has been evaluated in the literature. The benefit of seizure prophylaxis following trauma needed to be weighed against the potentially deleterious systemic side effects of these medications. It has been demonstrated that routine use of phenytoin reduces the incidence of early PTS with little risk of medication side effect. Its use for a 1-week duration following trauma is therefore recommended by the BTF (level II). Interestingly, early PTS has not been proven to be associated with worse outcomes. Most neurosurgeons feel that a reduction in the incidence of early PTS is beneficial because it prevents ICP spikes and potentially other deleterious consequences of seizure activity.

$$\text{Phenytoin Loading Dose} = \frac{10 - 20\ \text{mg}}{\text{kg IV}}$$

It is cautioned that bolus doses of antiepileptic medications can precipitate hypotension. Phenytoin should be given only after adequate volume resuscitation. Alternatively, use fosphenytoin for bolus dose (1:1 equivalent dosing).

Phenytoin Maintenance Dose: 100 mg orally
or intravenously every 8 hours
(Adjust to maintain plasma level of 10 to 20 μg/mL)

Sustained antiepileptic use beyond 1 week is associated with a significantly higher incidence of drug side effects. In addition, use even at therapeutic levels was not associated with reduction in the rate of late PTS. Use of phenytoin (or another antiepileptic) beyond 1 week is thus not recommended (level II) unless the patient develops epilepsy.[73,74]

Steroids

The only level I recommendation of the BTF guidelines for management of severe brain injury is that steroids are contraindicated. This recommendation was made as a result of the need to halt an international multicenter trial evaluating the potential benefit of methylprednisolone in patients with TBI. The CRASH (corticosteroid randomization after significant head injury) trial was stopped after interim data from over 5 years of enrollment demonstrated an increased risk of death within 2 weeks (21% versus 18%, relative risk [RR] = 1.18) in the steroid group ($p = 0.0001$).[75]

Despite the evidence from the CRASH trial some investigators are still evaluating the potential neuroprotective effects of different forms of steroids in TBI in the animal model.[26]

Effect of BTF Guidelines

There have been several studies evaluating the effect of the implementation of the BTF guidelines in the United States and the EBIC guidelines in Europe in regard to mortality and outcome following severe TBI. Bulger et al in 2002 published a retrospective evaluation of severe TBI management and outcome in the United States, and found a significantly lower mortality rate (27% versus 45%, $p = 0.01$) at institutions that treated severe TBI aggressively.[76] The review included 640 patients at 34 centers over an 8-month period in the late 1990s. At that time, there was still considerable variation in aggressiveness of care and adherence to the guidelines at the different centers. The difference in mortality rate helps emphasize the importance of aggressive management. In a similar review in Croatia, Vukic et al found a significant reduction in mortality (30% versus 44%) and an improvement in outcome following implementation of the BTF guidelines.[2]

In 2005, Patel and colleagues reviewed the status of outcome from severe head injury in the UK where patients often do not present to a facility with onsite neurosurgical care. They found that the mortality rate was 10 times higher for patients with head injury versus those without who presented to and were cared for at these nonneurosurgical centers.[77] Transfer of care in the UK and elsewhere in Europe is often restricted to patients with the presence of a surgical mass lesion. Their review emphasizes the need for aggressive management and potentially for the centralization of care and direct transport to that centralized care for all patients with TBI.

References

1. Biffl WL, Harrington DT, Majercik SD, Starring J, Cioffi WG. The evolution of trauma care at a level I trauma center. J Am Coll Surg 2005; 200(6):922–929
2. Vukic M, Negovetic L, Kovac D, Ghajar J, Glavic Z, Gopcevic A. The effect of implementation of guidelines for the management of severe head injury on patient treatment and outcome. Acta Neurochir (Wien) 1999;141(11):1203–1208
3. Berg J, Tagliaferri F, Servadei F. Cost of trauma in Europe. Eur J Neurol 2005;12(Suppl 1):85–90
4. Corso P, Finkelstein E, Miller T, Fiebelkorn I, Zaloshnja E. Incidence and lifetime costs of injuries in the United States. Inj Prev 2006;12(4): 212–218
5. Thurman DJ, Alverson C, Dunn KA, Guerrero J, Sniezek JE. Traumatic brain injury in the United States: a public health perspective. J Head Trauma Rehabil 1999;14(6):602–615
6. Finkelstein E, Corso PS, Miller TR. The Incidence and Economic Burden of Injuries in the United States. New York: Oxford University Press; 2006
7. Guidelines for the management of severe head injury. Brain Trauma Foundation, American Association of Neurological Surgeons, Joint Section on Neurotrauma and Critical Care. J Neurotrauma 1996;13(11): 641–734
8. Maas AI, Dearden M, Teasdale GM, et al. EBIC-guidelines for management of severe head injury in adults. European Brain Injury Consortium. Acta Neurochir (Wien) 1997;139(4):286–294
9. Narayan RK, Wilberger JE, Povlishock JT. Neurotrauma. New York: McGraw-Hill Health Professions Division; 1996: xxiv, 1558
10. Teasdale G, Jennett B. Assessment of coma and impaired consciousness: a practical scale. Lancet 1974;2(7872):81–84
11. Buechler CM, Blostein PA, Koestner A, Hurt K, Schaars M, McKernan J. Variation among trauma centers' calculation of Glasgow Coma Scale score: results of a national survey. J Trauma 1998;45(3): 429–432
12. Moskopp D, Stahle C, Wassmann H. Problems of the Glasgow Coma Scale with early intubated patients. Neurosurg Rev 1995;18(4): 253–257
13. Stocchetti N, Pagan F, Calappi E, et al. Inaccurate early assessment of neurological severity in head injury. J Neurotrauma 2004;21(9): 1131–1140
14. Balestreri M, Czosnyka M, Chatfield DA, et al. Predictive value of Glasgow Coma Scale after brain trauma: change in trend over the past ten years. J Neurol Neurosurg Psychiatry 2004;75(1):161–162
15. Gennarelli TA, Spielman GM, Langfitt TW, et al. Influence of the type of intracranial lesion on outcome from severe head injury. J Neurosurg 1982;56(1):26–32
16. Marshall L, Marshall SB, Klauber MR, et al. A new classification of head injury based on computerized tomography. J Neurosurg 1992;9(Suppl 1):S287–S292
17. Maas AI, Hukkelhoven CW, Marshall LF, Steyerberg EW. Prediction of outcome in traumatic brain injury with computed tomographic characteristics: a comparison between the computed tomographic classification and combinations of computed tomographic predictors. Neurosurgery 2005;57(6):1173–1182
18. Jennett B, Bond M. Assessment of outcome after severe brain damage. Lancet 1975;1(7905):480–484
19. Maas AI, Marmarou A, Murray GD, Teasdale SG, Steyerberg EW. Prognosis and clinical trial design in traumatic brain injury: the IMPACT study. J Neurotrauma 2007;24(2):232–238
20. Murray GD, Barer D, Choi S, et al. Design and analysis of phase III trials with ordered outcome scales: the concept of the sliding dichotomy. J Neurotrauma 2005;22(5):511–517
21. Wilson JT, Pettigrew LE, Teasdale GM. Structured interviews for the Glasgow Outcome Scale and the extended Glasgow Outcome Scale: guidelines for their use. J Neurotrauma 1998;15(8):573–585
22. Temkin NR, Anderson GD, Winn HR, et al. Magnesium sulfate for neuroprotection after traumatic brain injury: a randomised controlled trial. Lancet Neurol 2007;6(1):29–38
23. Robinson DL. Bicycle helmet legislation: can we reach a consensus? Accid Anal Prev 2007;39(1):86–93
24. Xiang H, Kelleher K, Shields BJ, Brown KJ, Smith GA. Skiing- and snowboarding-related injuries treated in U.S. emergency departments, 2002. J Trauma 2005;58(1):112–118

25. Lee LL, Galo E, Lyeth BG, Muizelaar JP, Berman RF. Neuroprotection in the rat lateral fluid percussion model of traumatic brain injury by SNX-185, an N-type voltage-gated calcium channel blocker. Exp Neurol 2004;190(1):70–78
26. Yang JT, Lee TH, Weng HH, et al. Dexamethasone enhances NT-3 expression in rat hippocampus after traumatic brain injury. Exp Neurol 2005;192(2):437–443
27. Prins ML, Fujima LS, Hovda DA. Age-dependent reduction of cortical contusion volume by ketones after traumatic brain injury. J Neurosci Res 2005;82(3):413–420
28. Di Giovanni S, Movsesyan V, Ahmed F, et al. Cell cycle inhibition provides neuroprotection and reduces glial proliferation and scar formation after traumatic brain injury. Proc Natl Acad Sci U S A 2005; 102(23):8333–8338
29. Bye N, Habgood MD, Callaway JK, et al. Transient neuroprotection by minocycline following traumatic brain injury is associated with attenuated microglial activation but no changes in cell apoptosis or neutrophil infiltration. Exp Neurol 2007;204(1):220–233
30. Hoane MR, Gilbert DR, Holland MA, Pierce JL. Nicotinamide reduces acute cortical neuronal death and edema in the traumatically injured brain. Neurosci Lett 2006;408(1):35–39
31. VanLandingham JW, Cutler SM, Virmani S, et al. The enantiomer of progesterone acts as a molecular neuroprotectant after traumatic brain injury. Neuropharmacology 2006;51(6):1078–1085
32. Sakellaris G, Kotsiou M, Tamiolaki M, et al. Prevention of complications related to traumatic brain injury in children and adolescents with creatine administration: an open label randomized pilot study. J Trauma 2006;61(2):322–329
33. Thornton E, Vink R, Blumbergs PC, Van Den Heuvel C. Soluble amyloid precursor protein alpha reduces neuronal injury and improves functional outcome following diffuse traumatic brain injury in rats. Brain Res 2006;1094(1):38–46
34. Royo NC, Conte V, Saatman KE, et al. Hippocampal vulnerability following traumatic brain injury: a potential role for neurotrophin-4/5 in pyramidal cell neuroprotection. Eur J Neurosci 2006;23(5): 1089–1102
35. Statler KD, Alexander H, Vagni V, et al. Isoflurane exerts neuroprotective actions at or near the time of severe traumatic brain injury. Brain Res 2006;1076(1):216–224
36. Serbest G, Horwitz J, Jost M, Barbee K. Mechanisms of cell death and neuroprotection by poloxamer 188 after mechanical trauma. FASEB J 2006;20(2):308–310
37. Wu A, Ying Z, Gomez-Pinilla F. Dietary curcumin counteracts the outcome of traumatic brain injury on oxidative stress, synaptic plasticity, and cognition. Exp Neurol 2006;197(2):309–317
38. Zohar O, Getslev V, Miller AL, Schreiber S, Pick CG. Morphine protects for head trauma induced cognitive deficits in mice. Neurosci Lett 2006;394(3):239–242
39. Alves OL, Doyle AJ, Clausen T, Gilman C, Bullock R. Evaluation of topiramate neuroprotective effect in severe TBI using microdialysis. Ann N Y Acad Sci 2003;993:25–34
40. Tolias CM, Bullock MR. Critical appraisal of neuroprotection trials in head injury: what have we learned? NeuroRx 2004;1(1):71–79
41. Maas AI. Neuroprotective agents in traumatic brain injury. Expert Opin Investig Drugs 2001;10(4):753–767
42. Maas AI, Steyerberg EW, Murray GD, et al. Why have recent trials of neuroprotective agents in head injury failed to show convincing efficacy? A pragmatic analysis and theoretical considerations. Neurosurgery 1999;44(6):1286–1298
43. Engel DC, Slemmer JE, Vlug AS, Maas AI, Weber JT. Combined effects of mechanical and ischemic injury to cortical cells: secondary ischemia increases damage and decreases effects of neuroprotective agents. Neuropharmacology 2005;49(7):985–995
44. Chesnut RM, Marshall LF, Klauber MR, et al. The role of secondary brain injury in determining outcome from severe head injury. J Trauma 1993;34(2):216–222
45. Murray GD, Butcher I, McHugh GS, et al. Multivariable prognostic analysis in traumatic brain injury: results from the IMPACT study. J Neurotrauma 2007;24(2):329–337
46. Van Beek JG, Mushkudiani NA, Steyerberg EW, et al. Prognostic value of admission laboratory parameters in traumatic brain injury: results from the IMPACT study. J Neurotrauma 2007;24(2):315–328
47. Butcher I, McHugh GS, Lu J, et al. Prognostic value of cause of injury in traumatic brain injury: results from the IMPACT study. J Neurotrauma 2007;24(2):281–286
48. Butcher I, Maas AI, Lu J, et al. Prognostic value of admission blood pressure in traumatic brain injury: results from the IMPACT study. J Neurotrauma 2007;24(2):294–302
49. Mushkudiani NA, Engel DC, Steyerberg EW, et al. Prognostic value of demographic characteristics in traumatic brain injury: results from the IMPACT study. J Neurotrauma 2007;24(2):259–269
50. Marmarou A, Lu J, Butcher I, et al. Prognostic value of the Glasgow Coma Scale and pupil reactivity in traumatic brain injury assessed prehospital and on enrollment: an IMPACT analysis. J Neurotrauma 2007; 24(2):270–280
51. Maas AI, Steyerberg EW, Butcher I, et al. Prognostic value of computerized tomography scan characteristics in traumatic brain injury: results from the IMPACT study. J Neurotrauma 2007;24(2):303–314
52. McHugh GS, Engel DC, Butcher I, et al. Prognostic value of secondary insults in traumatic brain injury: results from the IMPACT study. J Neurotrauma 2007;24(2):287–293
53. McHugh GS, Butcher I, Steyerberg EW, et al. Statistical approaches to the univariate prognostic analysis of the IMPACT database on traumatic brain injury. J Neurotrauma 2007;24(2):251–258
54. Marmarou A, Lu J, Butcher I, et al. IMPACT database of traumatic brain injury: design and description. J Neurotrauma 2007;24(2):239–250
55. The Brain Trauma Foundation. The American Association of Neurological Surgeons. The Joint Section on Neurotrauma and Critical Care. Glasgow Coma Scale score. J Neurotrauma 2000;17(6–7):563–571
56. Davis DP, Serrano JA, Vilke GM, et al. The predictive value of field versus arrival Glasgow Coma Scale score and TRISS calculations in moderate-to-severe traumatic brain injury. J Trauma 2006;60(5):985–990
57. The Brain Trauma Foundation. The American Association of Neurological Surgeons. The Joint Section on Neurotrauma and Critical Care. Pupillary diameter and light reflex. J Neurotrauma 2000;17(6–7):583–590
58. The Brain Trauma Foundation. The American Association of Neurological Surgeons. The Joint Section on Neurotrauma and Critical Care. Hypotension. J Neurotrauma 2000;17(6–7):591–595
59. Hukkelhoven CW, Rampen AJ, Maas AI, et al. Some prognostic models for traumatic brain injury were not valid. J Clin Epidemiol 2006;59(2): 132–143
60. Brain Trauma Foundation. Guidelines for Prehospital Management of Traumatic Brain Injury. New York: Brain Trauma Foundation; 2000
61. Salomone JP, Ustin JS, McSwain NE Jr, Feliciano DV. Opinions of trauma practitioners regarding prehospital interventions for critically injured patients. J Trauma 2005;58(3):509–515
62. Davis DP, Hoyt DB, Ochs M, et al. The effect of paramedic rapid sequence intubation on outcome in patients with severe traumatic brain injury. J Trauma 2003;54(3):444–453
63. Cooper DJ, Myles PS, McDermott FT, et al; HTS Study Investigators. Prehospital hypertonic saline resuscitation of patients with hypotension and severe traumatic brain injury: a randomized controlled trial. JAMA 2004;291(11):1350–1357
64. Holstein A, Kühne D, Elsing HG, et al. Practicality and accuracy of prehospital rapid venous blood glucose determination. Am J Emerg Med 2000;18(6):690–694
65. Lai HY, Chen IH, Chen A, Hwang FY, Lee Y. The use of the GlideScope for tracheal intubation in patients with ankylosing spondylitis. Br J Anaesth 2006;97(3):419–422
66. Biro P, Weiss M. Comparison of two video-assisted techniques for the difficult intubation. Acta Anaesthesiol Scand 2001;45(6):761–765
67. Weiss M, Hartmann K, Fischer JE, Gerber AC. Use of angulated video-intubation laryngoscope in children undergoing manual in-line neck stabilization. Br J Anaesth 2001;87(3):453–458
68. American College of Surgeons. Advanced Trauma Life Support for Doctors: Student Course Manual. Chicago, IL: American College of Surgeons; 1997

69. The Brain Trauma Foundation. The American Association of Neurological Surgeons. The Joint Section on Neurotrauma and Critical Care. Initial management. J Neurotrauma 2000;17(6–7): 463–469
70. Feldman Z, Kanter MJ, Robertson CS, et al. Effect of head elevation on intracranial pressure, cerebral perfusion pressure, and cerebral blood flow in head-injured patients. J Neurosurg 1992;76(2): 207–211
71. Sakowitz OW, Stover JF, Sarrafzadeh AS, Unterberg AW, Kiening KL. Effects of mannitol bolus administration on intracranial pressure, cerebral extracellular metabolites, and tissue oxygenation in severely head-injured patients. J Trauma 2007;62(2):292–298
72. Bratton SL, Chestnut RM, Ghajar J, McConnell Hammond FF, Harris OA, Hartl R, et al: Guidelines for the management of severe traumatic brain injury. J Neurotrauma 2007; 24 Suppl 1:S1–106
73. The Brain Trauma Foundation. The American Association of Neurological Surgeons. The Joint Section on Neurotrauma and Critical Care. Role of antiseizure prophylaxis following head injury. J Neurotrauma 2000;17(6–7):549–553
74. Chang BS, Lowenstein DH. Practice parameter: antiepileptic drug prophylaxis in severe traumatic brain injury: report of the Quality Standards Subcommittee of the American Academy of Neurology. Neurology 2003;60(1):10–16
75. Edwards P, Arango M, Balica L, Cottingham R, El-Sayed H, Farrell B, et al: Final results of MRC CRASH, a randomised placebo-controlled trial of intravenous corticosteroid in adults with head injury-outcomes at 6 months. Lancet 2005; 365:1957–1959
76. Bulger EM, Nathens AB, Rivara FP, Moore M, MacKenzie EJ, Jurkovich GJ ; Brain Trauma Foundation. Management of severe head injury: institutional variations in care and effect on outcome. Crit Care Med 2002;30(8):1870–1876
77. Patel HC, Bouamra O, Woodford M, King AT, Yates DW, Lecky FE; Trauma Audit and Research Network. Trends in head injury outcome from 1989 to 2003 and the effect of neurosurgical care: an observational study. Lancet 2005;366(9496):1538–1544

12 Wartime Penetrating Injuries

Rocco A. Armonda, Randy S. Bell, Samuel Critides, and Alexander H. Vo

Historical Background

The current treatment of penetrating brain injury in military conflict has evolved from the principles established at the end of World War I (WWI) by Dr. Harvey Cushing.[1] Since that time, the strategy of radical debridement utilized in World Wars I and II,[2] the Korean War,[4] the Vietnam War, and the Iran–Iraq War[5] has been followed by an approach of conservative debridement during the Israeli-Lebanon conflict of the 1980s.[6] During Operation Iraqi Freedom (OIF), a method of early radical decompression through the use of hemicraniectomy with conservative debridement and duraplasty has been applied to blast-induced penetrating brain injuries. Although a formal analysis of all casualties is not complete, the immediate impression is that early decompression results in increased survivability and neurological improvement.[7] Ultimately, long-term follow-up will be necessary to determine if early decompression actually improves functional outcome (see **Fig. 12.1**).

The multitude of head injuries associated with trench warfare in WWI challenged early neurosurgeons unlike any prior civil-military conflict.[8] The field of neurosurgery was in its infancy and was unprepared for the complexities of these injuries. Cushing's observations and reports were instrumental during this time in establishing guidelines for treatments. He noted that decreased infection rates limited the major cause of mortality at the time.[1] However, due to the lack of axial imaging and delays in the evacuation process, few operations were actually performed for immediate "life-saving" interventions. Despite these obstacles, Dr. Cushing developed a process of radical debridement of the scalp and skull and irrigation of the track with a catheter, attempting to remove all foreign bodies. This was then followed by a watertight scalp closure without drains. The application of these techniques in a well-equipped center, usually remote from the front, was preferable in his mind to the "frontline" surgery that risked overwhelming infectious morbidity. His classification of penetrating injuries provided the foundation for the concept of limiting secondary injury and promoting eventual reconstruction (**Table 12.1**).

These concepts evolved with improved training and technology during WWII. In a summary of procedures from WWII, Dr. Donald Matson clearly outlined the purpose of far-forward neurosurgery.[9] The tenets of those lessons still hold true in today's interventions and are summarized as follows: (1) the immediate saving of life (hematoma evacuation, brain stem decompression), (2) the prevention of infection, (3) the preservation of the nervous function, and (4) the restoration of anatomic structure.[9] He also attributed the success of medical care in WWII to forward neurosurgical care with specialized equipment, rapid evacuation of casualties to these hospitals permitting early surgery, availability of blood in large amounts in the forward area, and the universal application of antibiotics. The application of these lessons in the current conflict will be the focus of this chapter (**Table 12.2**).

Over the past 5.5 years, our experience has included the treatment of nearly 200 severe, penetrating brain injuries. This population includes a total of 38 patients with severe, traumatic vasospasm, 40 patients with

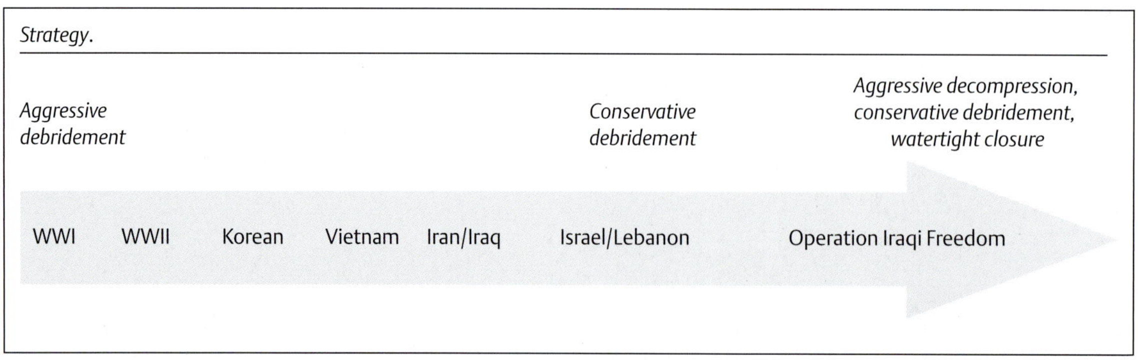

Fig. 12.1 Evolution of neurosurgical approach to wartime penetrating brain injury.

The views presented are the professional opinions of the authors and do not represent the views of the Department of Defense, Department of the Army, or Department of the Navy.

Table 12.1 Cushing's Classification of Penetrating Brain Injury (1918)[1]

Grade	Description	No. of WWI Cases	% Mortality
I	Scalp lacerations with intact skull	22	4.5
II	Wounds with skull fractures/intact dura/ ± depression	54	9.2
III	Wounds with depressed skull fracture/dural laceration	18	11.8
IV	Wounds (guttering type) with in-driven fragments, usually protruding brain	25	24
V	Penetrating wound, lodged projectile, brain usually protruding	41	36.6
VI	Wounds penetrating ventricles with either (a) bone fragments or (b) projectiles	a)14 b)16	a)42.8 b)100
VII	Wounds involving orbitonasal or auropetrosal region with extruding brain	15	73.3
VIII	Perforating wounds, cerebral injury severe	5	80
IX	Craniocerebral injury with massive skull fracture	10	50

traumatic aneurysms, and well over 100 patients who have received decompressive hemicraniectomy. The addition of routine cerebral angiography and transcranial Doppler ultrasonography (US) has augmented patient care. A specific review of our population has revealed that 30% of patients presenting with an initial Glasgow Coma Scale (GCS) of 3 to 5 have good functional outcomes; 60% of patients with GCS >5 have good functional outcomes.

Missiles and Mechanisms of Wartime Penetrating Injuries

The effect of penetrating trauma to the nervous system is dependent on multiple factors (**Fig. 12.2**). As seen in recent conflicts, the incidence of survivable missile injuries (i.e., AK-47 round) to the brain remains low. Recent engagements have identified the use of even higher velocity rounds with longer metal jackets and higher muzzle velocities (i.e., AK-74), which are used as a sniper's weapon of choice. The majority of these wounds is still fatal. This is related to the high likelihood of perforation, global cranial vault disruption, and high cavitation pressures. However, the majority of injuries during Operation Iraqi Freedom have been from roadside "IEDs" or improvised explosive devices. These include vehicle-borne delivery systems commonly referred to as either "car bombs" or "suicide bombers." These munitions are variable in their design and delivery of injury. The injuries are dependent on the explosive that is used, the distance from the explosion, the shape of the projectile, and lastly the viscoelastic properties of the impacted tissue. Such projectiles are propelled by enormous blast-overpressure forces, which may account for the injury force beyond the flying projectiles or the terminal impact. Syndromes of central nervous system (CNS) dysfunction associated with blast injuries have been identified and classified since WWII.[10] During the explosion of such devices, flying projectiles include the materials used to make the bomb (primary projectile) and additional materials (i.e., nails and other metallic objects, rocks, glass, body parts) packed around the device by the enemy (secondary projectiles). These fragments, although traveling with lower terminal velocity compared with the sniper's round, inflict significant destruction due to their abnormal size, shape, and porosity.

Unlike the previously discussed metal fragments, nonmetallic fragments may lead to delayed abscess formation and secondary sepsis. In the case of a vehicle-borne IED (VBIED), the metal from the auto can act as a secondary projectile (**Fig. 12.3**). Debris from surrounding buildings

Table 12.2 Matson's Tenets

Matson's Tenets[9]	Current Application
I. Save life	Application of ATLS/ACLS/far forward homeostasis and hemicraniectomy
II. Prevent infection	Watertight dural closure
III. Preserve nervous system function	Prevention of secondary neurologic injury through advanced neurocritical and neurointerventional care (i.e., meningitis, seizures, stroke)
IV. Restore anatomic function	Restore anatomic protection and contour (i.e., cranioplasty)

Abbreviations: ACLS, advanced cardiac life support; ATLS, advanced trauma life support.

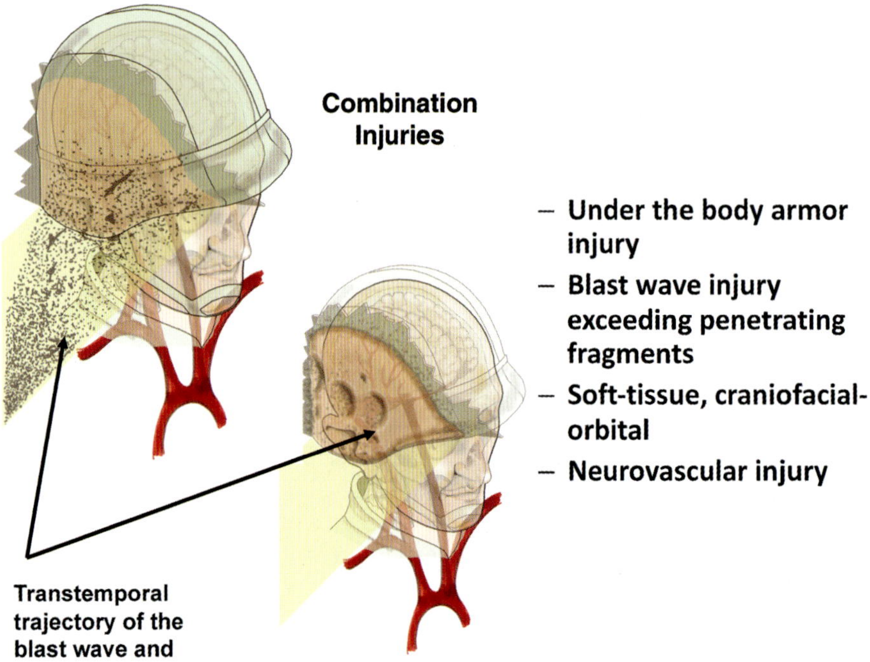

Fig. 12.2 The effect of penetrating trauma to the nervous system is dependent on multiple factors. Four injury patterns are described. Under the body armor injury occurs when the inner portion of the armor delaminates and impacts the underlying scalp, skull, and brain. This creates a piston-like high-energy impact that reverberates through the cerebral tissue and cranial vault. The propelling blast waves exceed the visual identified fragments and lead to remote injuries in the cerebral tissue and surrounding structures. Those structures with immediate and delayed injury (within 2 weeks of impact) include a selective vulnerability of the cerebral conducting arteries. This includes traumatic pseudoaneurysm typically perpendicular to the fragment track, and large conducting vessel injuries at the skull base and circle of Willis. In particular, the supraclinoid carotid artery, where it is fixed at the distal dural ring, has the highest incidence of delayed vasospasm.

in the form of glass or stone can also be propelled and penetrate the calvarium (**Fig. 12.4**). Some of the most lethal of these "antipersonnel" devices include the use of small spherical bolts (**Fig. 12.5**). Reported by the Israelis to have significant lethality when penetrating the cranial vault, these small round fragments have been noted to cause well-delineated anatomic damage as well as minor deficits.[11] In one case, the Israelis identified acute hydrocephalus when the fourth ventricle was occluded by a spherical bolt. In cases in which the cranial base or sylvian or interhemispheric fissure has been penetrated, these fragments can rupture major vessels, create pseudoaneurysms, or even lodge into the venous sinuses. During the initial assessment of patients with metallic and

A

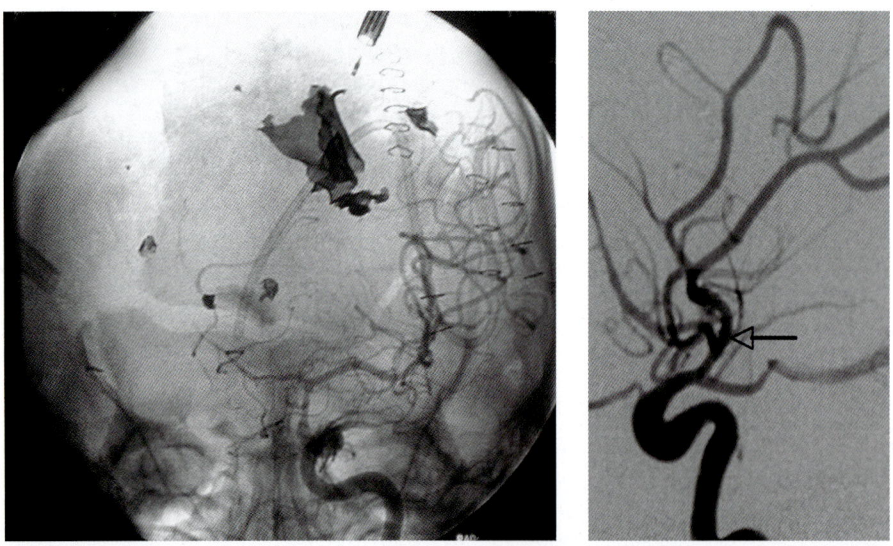

B

Fig. 12.3 **(A)** This patient initially presented with a Glasgow Coma Scale score of 3 with severe burns and scalp tissue loss with a large penetrating fragment from a car bomb crossing the midline above the diencephalon into the interhemispheric fissure. He underwent an immediate right hemicraniectomy, evacuation of a subdural hematoma, and placement of a ventriculostomy. **(B)** He developed delayed severe bilateral vasospasm (*black arrow*) treated with

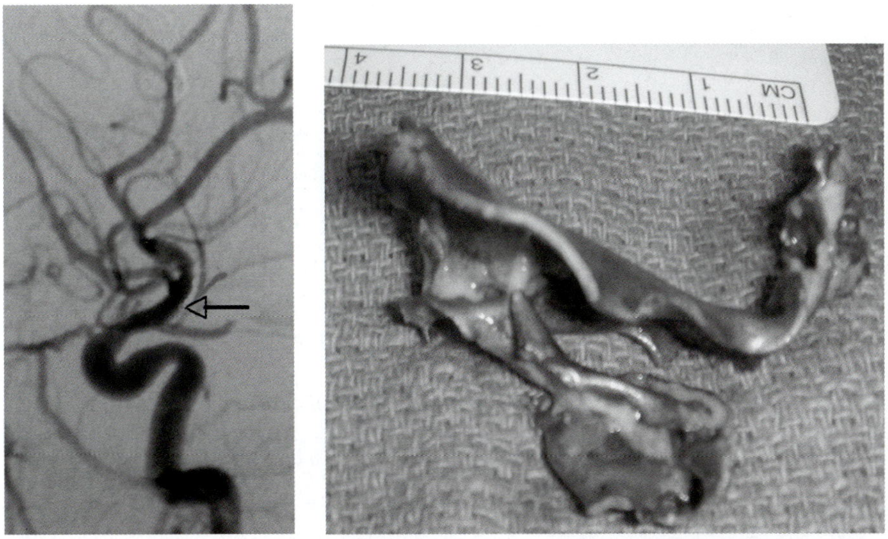

Fig. 12.3 *(Continued)* **(C)** microballoon angioplasty and nicardipine (*black arrow*). **(D)** He was taken back to the operating room for removal of the large metal fragment measuring ~4 cm. He underwent a cranioplasty with tissue expanders previously placed, yet required a latissum dorsi flap due to tissue breakdown. At 36 months postinjury, he is ambulating independently, effectively communicating, and feeding himself.

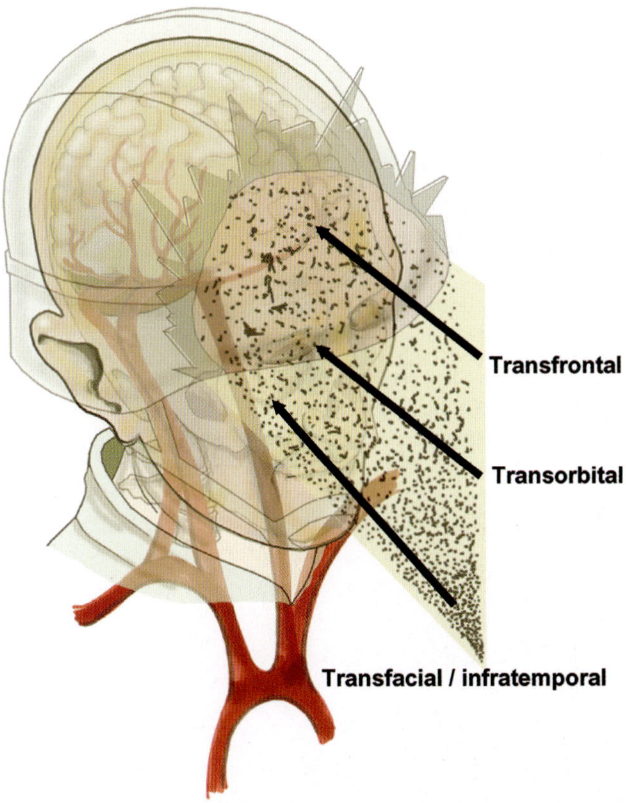

Fig. 12.4 Debris surrounding the explosion is propelled as secondary fragments. In a vehicle or building this occurs in the form of twisted metal, glass, or roadside stones and can penetrate the calvarium via the orbit and midface. In a frontal direction significant anatomic disruption results to the anterior skull base, orbit, midface, airway, and bilateral frontal lobes as well as the anterior cerebral artery complex in the interhemispheric fissure. The soft tissue, supporting bony framework, and anatomic continuity are lost from the skull base to the orbit and infratemporal fossa.

nonmetallic foreign body penetration, the question of removal must be considered and may be influenced by multiple variables. Ventricular or paraventricular location of such metallic or nonmetallic porous material has been associated with delayed infections and late neurological deterioration.[12] Overall, if there is evidence of fragment movement, contact with the cerebrospinal fluid (CSF) within either a cisternal or ventricular location, or location adjacent to a vascular structure, it may be advisable to remove the foreign body (**Table 12.3**). The exception may be interhemispheric bone fragments without vessel abnormality. Regardless of approach, the fragments should be followed radiographically to assess for any evidence of delayed movement or abscess formation. This conservative approach is acceptable because reoperation to remove fragments has not been shown to reduce the seizure rate or the incidence of late infections but has increased the neurological morbidity.[6,13]

Management of Wartime Penetrating Injuries

Initial Resuscitation

The application of Matson's tenets begins at the point of injury. Combat medical personnel are faced with multiple challenges, not least of which is resuscitating the patient while under enemy fire. Unlike the civilian environment, the care of the military casualty is often hindered by the ongoing threat to the unit. Medical teams are specifically targeted by the enemy to discourage, demoralize, and

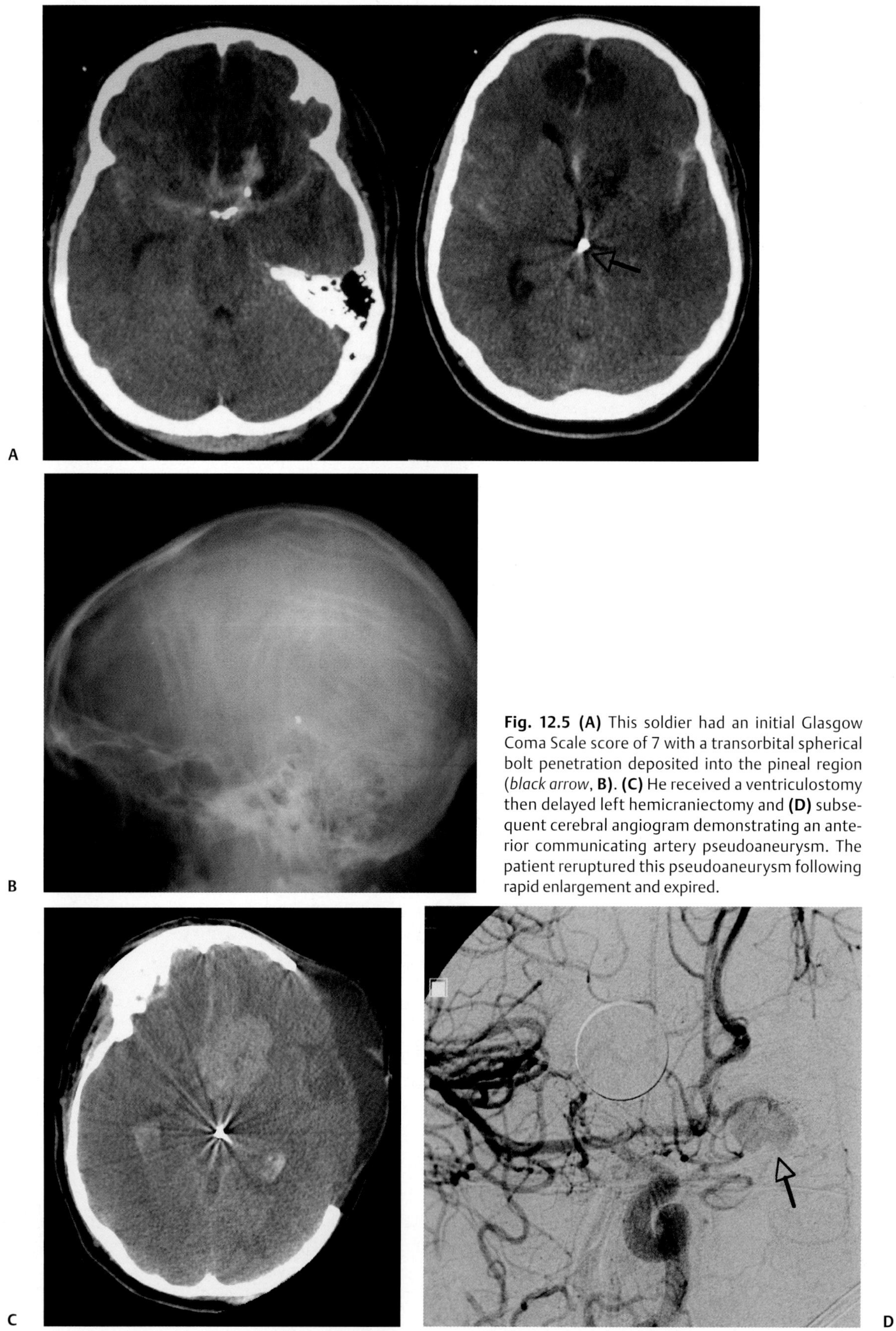

Fig. 12.5 **(A)** This soldier had an initial Glasgow Coma Scale score of 7 with a transorbital spherical bolt penetration deposited into the pineal region (*black arrow*, **B**). **(C)** He received a ventriculostomy then delayed left hemicraniectomy and **(D)** subsequent cerebral angiogram demonstrating an anterior communicating artery pseudoaneurysm. The patient reruptured this pseudoaneurysm following rapid enlargement and expired.

Table 12.3 Criteria for Removal of Intracranial Fragment

- Movement of fragment
- Abscess formation
- Vessel compression or contact
- Porous material in contact with cerebrospinal fluid (i.e., rock, wood)

deter the unit's combat effectiveness. Therefore, a concept of removing the casualty from the "kill-zone" is essential prior to focused resuscitation. In a direct firefight, the medic's first priority may be to return fire in an attempt to suppress the enemy before evacuating the casualty. Because most of the injuries during OIF have occurred from unmanned roadside bombs (i.e., IEDs), the medical plan is typically adjusted. Unlike civilian trauma and previous military conflicts, immediate evacuation from the "kill box" is of the utmost importance. After mobilization to a safer area, initial resuscitation and medical evacuation to the next level of care are conducted.

Early airway and hemorrhage control combined with rapid evacuation is the first stage in the resuscitation of a casualty with severe neurotrauma. Direct transport to neurosurgeons located in the combat support hospital (CSH) has allowed immediate intervention, leading to improved survivability. The exact magnitude of increased survival is difficult to evaluate because, with such rapid evacuations, a higher proportion of expectant wounds are seen by the neurosurgeon than in prior conflicts.

Far Forward Neuroimaging and Neurosurgery

The challenges of complex, severe military penetrating brain injury (PBI) are addressed by the coordinated efforts of physicians, nurses, and technicians at the CSH. In the United States military medical model, the CSH is the first location where both neurosurgery and computerized tomography (CT) scanning are available. After the initial airway, breathing, and circulation have been managed, a hemodynamically stable patient must undergo appropriate imaging. At this stage, it is imperative that no unnecessary delay prevents appropriate cranial decompression for a life-threatening lesion. Occasionally, life-threatening extracranial bleeding must first be treated. Multiple options exist with the most practical and efficient including simultaneous cranial/corporeal intervention or delayed imaging after hemodynamic stability has been achieved. Delayed neuroimaging is used when faced with a closed injury, a neurologically stable patient, or patients undergoing prolonged extracranial procedures without the benefit of an immediate postoperative examination.

The approach to the severely brain injured patient has evolved throughout the current conflict. Because of the long transport flights that must occur, the practice has changed to include wide decompressive hemicraniectomy with subsequent duraplasty and watertight closure as early as possible. The thought is that the decompression may mitigate or reduce incidence of secondary neurological deficits that occur from malignant intracranial hypertension. Nevertheless, as in civilian neurotrauma, most cranial interventions will include early postoperative imaging and intracranial pressure (ICP) monitoring where appropriate.

Medical Evacuation

The medical evacuation of the severely injured soldier or marine to the United States currently involves a stop in Germany and includes over 7,200 miles of travel. The medical hazards of this trip must be taken into consideration and include the effects of delayed cerebral edema, hydrocephalus, or hemorrhage, which may occur during transfers or flight. To address these issues, critical care air transport teams have been instrumental in the strategic evacuations of patients from Baghdad to Germany and beyond. Management of elevated ICP, hypoxia, and hypotension is their primary focus; each team consists of a physician, nurse, and respiratory technician and is rarely supplemented with a neurosurgeon or neurologist. Out of over 21,000 casualties, over 500 intubated neurotrauma patients have been transported in this fashion. Additional operational challenges include enemy activity, weather, and airframe function.

Description of Injuries

Patterns of penetrating trauma in both civilian and military have been classically described based on the fragment path. The key element is the unseen force propelling the fragment. Rarely is this force completely characterized in a bomb blast. Typically, all that is seen are the fragments, spall, or retained overlying clothing driven into the cranial vault. A complete physical examination allows the ability to identify points of foreign body entry or exit. The most commonly missed region of fragment entry includes the retroauricular and suboccipital regions. Fragment entries from these sites are particularly hazardous, with the increased risk of vascular, cranial nerve, or brain stem injury.

Perforating

These injuries typically carry the worst prognosis, especially when associated with high-velocity injuries or when the injuries cross the midline or are transhemispheric. In a large series of civilian gunshot wound (GSW), the lateral penetrating injury had a poorer outcome compared with anteroposterior injuries. Lateral perforation wounds typically have the poorest outcomes. Despite early emergent surgery, functional survivability is rare among these combat casualties. The high-energy force propelling the missile or fragments through the cranial vault creates an immense deforming force. In some cases, this force is so powerful it can deform the entire cranial vault and can be typically seen with injuries from AK-47 rounds (**Fig. 12.6**). The high muzzle velocity can create perforating injuries that will transfer enough injury to "burst" the cranial vault. Such expansive forces will ovalize the skull, resulting in fractured plates of the cranial vault. The centripetal forces explode outward creating deformation of the cranial cavity. Patients with this type of injury may initially present awake, moving spontaneously, and sometimes talking. Invariably, however, many will do poorly despite aggressive surgical intervention. Despite hemicraniectomy and bifrontal decompression, the degree of neuronal disruption rarely leads to functional

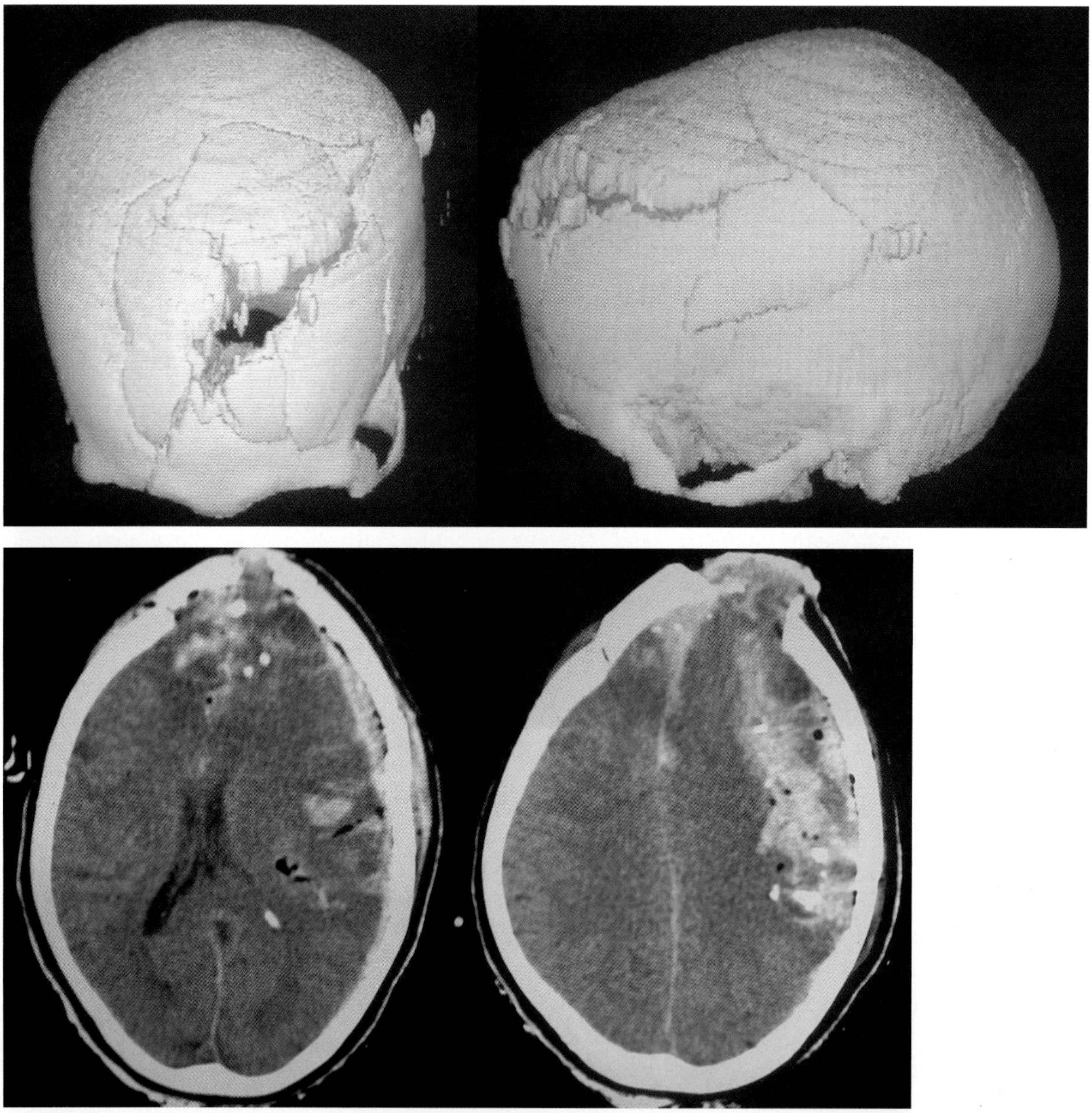

A

B

Fig. 12.6 (A) This civilian victim of a suspected AK-47 perforating round was without body armor and was evacuated to the combat support hospital within 20 minutes of her injury localizing on examination with open, herniating brain through a complex scalp defect. **(B)** Computed tomography demonstrated evidence of global deformity with "bursting pattern" of an expansile skull fracture deforming the skull shape **(A)**. Patient underwent left hemicraniectomy, repair of the anterior aspect of the sagittal sinus, duraplasty, and placement of a monitor. Patient later deteriorated from a coagulopathy on post-operative day (pod) #4.

survival. In some cases, rapid decompression may lead to an associated hypotension especially in hypovolemic patients whose blood pressure will typically drop during decompression. Communicating with your anesthesiologist will allow appropriate anticipation of this response.

Penetrating

The most lethal of the penetrating injuries include those through the central region of the brain, referred to as the zona fatalis (**Fig. 12.7**). This region includes the suprasellar area comprising the third ventricle, hypothalamus, and thalamus. As in civilian wounds, the mortality is near 100%, with functional survival $<2\%$ from wartime wounds in the region. Trajectories that pass through this region with a significant force may disrupt the midline vascular structures, including the anterior communicating artery and the deep venous system, and can result in significant intraventricular hemorrhage. The greatest damage, however, comes from the cavitation track or direct damage to the surrounding reticular activating system, the hypothalamus, and the thalamus. Patients who survive these injuries are typically in a persistent vegetative state. A characteristic sign seen

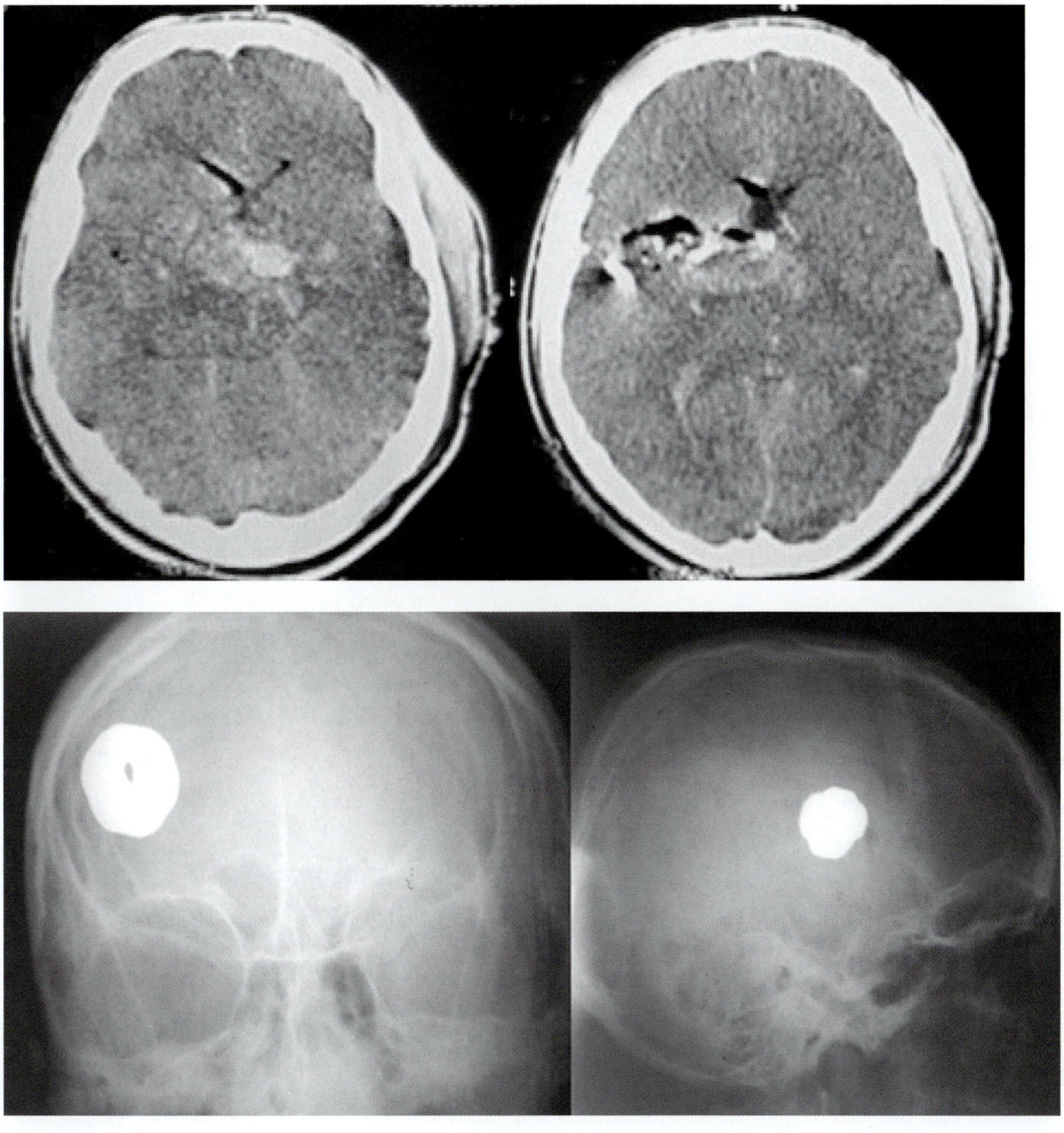

A

B

Fig. 12.7 (A, B) Soldier struck by an improvised explosive device (IED) explosion with a flying hexagonal nut coursing from the left temporal region through the diencephalon bilaterally and into the contralateral right frontal region. On examination, he was initially localizing at the scene then deteriorated to extensor posturing at 30 minutes without a focal new hematoma. He expired within 4 hours of his injury after a conservative course.

Table 12.4 Complications of Wartime Penetrating Brain Injury

Time	Type of Complications	Treatment
0–24 h	ICP increased	Hemicraniectomy
	Hematoma	Evacuation/coagulation correction
	Ischemia	Decompression/ID occlusion
	Anatomic defect	Anatomic closure
	Hypoxia	Airway/pulmonary correction
	Hypotension	Overt or occult EBL
		PRBC/FFP/PLTS vs. whole blood vs. hypotonic saline
24–48 h	ICP increased	Hemicraniectomy
	Hematoma	Evacuation/coagulation correction
	Hydrocephalus	Ventriculostomy
	Edema	Decompression
	Seizure	Antiepileptics/cEEG monitoring
72 h–1st wk	Edema	Medical/surgical decompression
	ICH (Contusion)	Correct coagulopathy
	Hydrocephalus	Ventriculostomy
	CSF leak	Repair/CSF diversion
	Ischemia	Medical/endovascular Tx
	Pseudoaneurysm	Surgical/endovascular Tx
	Seizures	Antiepileptics/cEEG monitoring
2–3rd wk	Infections	R/O abcess, CSF infection
	Vasospasm	TCDs, PbO_2, cEEG, CBF monitoring with combined HHH versus angioplasty
	Pseudoaneurysm	Endovascular versus microsurgery
	Seizures	Antiepileptics
	Delayed hydrocephalus	VP shunt (low-pressure consider use of programmable valve)
1–6 mo	Infection	R/O abscess, meningitis
	Low-pressure hydrocephalus	VP shunt (programmable valve)
	Syndrome of trephine	Reconstructive cranioplasty
	Seizures	Antiepileptics
	Cranioplasty complications	
	Temporalis atrophy	Resuspension/implant/fat graft
	Infection	Prosthesis removal
	Hydrocephalus	VP shunt
	Epidural/subgaleal	Drainage
	Hygroma/hematoma ICH	Evacuation
	Scalp necrosis	Free-flap

Abbreviations: CBF, cerebral blod flow; cEEG, continuous electroencephalogram; CSF, cerebrospinal fluid; EBL, estimated blood loss; FFP, fresh frozen plasma; ICP, intracranial pressure; ICH, intracranial hematoma; HHH, hypervolemic, hypertensive, hyperdynamic; PLTS, platelets; PRBC, packed red blood cells; R/O, rule out; TCD, transcranial doppler; Tx, treatment; VP, ventriculoperitoneal.

in civilian injuries, and occasionally in lower-caliber wartime injuries, is the "tram-track" sign. This represents the cavitation tract and is associated with significant energy transfer, significant edema, and poor outcome. This outcome is commonly repeated in the transhemispheric, transventricular wound. Multiple hemisphere injury and crossing the midline at the level of the corpus callosum or below portends a high mortality and poor functional outcome.[14] As stated earlier, these missile tracts have been associated with pseudoaneurysms. Typically occurring perpendicular to the long axis of the tract, they are associated with ischemia or delayed rupture if not appropriately treated. The M1 segment is particularly vulnerable in some of these paths. Deeply embedded metals are not classically retrieved unless they are in the ventricular system, in motion, compressing a large vascular structure, creating hydrocephalus, or associated with a delayed abscess. Again, the early use of radical hemicraniectomy with duraplasty has allowed a higher survival and earlier, improved functional outcome in this population than previously predicted. In many of these cases, a majority may have presented initially talking before massive edema, shift, and cerebral dysfunction occurred. The patients typically have a poorer examination after the first 48 to 72 hours, usually due to delayed cerebral edema or hydrocephalus. In selected cases, delayed blast-induced vasospasm may occur, although this is typically seen after the first week.

Injury Patterns and Management

Complex cranial–facial injuries are typical in the OIF conflict. Comparable to WWI trench-warfare, the head and neck is a region of selective vulnerability. Injuries that bridge the craniocervical junction, associated orbitofacial injuries, and injuries to the neck have been particularly challenging to treat. Cranial-basal injuries have a tendency to have a higher association with neurovascular injuries with a profound risk for delayed stroke and death. Additionally, this region is also associated with a high rate of CSF leaks, fistulae, and infections. The disruption of the cranial base with communication with the orbit, pharynx, and infratemporal fossa may be associated with cranial nerve injuries, blindness, and globe disruption. Avoiding associated complications begins with a high index of suspicion followed by an aggressive role for neuroangiography, meningitis monitoring, and cranial nerve evaluation (**Table 12.4**).

Orbitofacial Injuries

Orbitofacial injuries in this conflict are highly associated with neurovascular injuries, CSF leakage, and death[15] (**Fig. 12.5**). Biomechanical studies of penetrating trauma to the maxilla and mandible have demonstrated significant force transmission to the brain. In particular, the pressure waves in the brain were greatest when Chinese M193 or M56 military bullets were used in animal models compared with 1.03 grain spheres at 1,400 m/s or at 800 m/s.[16] Transorbital intracranial entry risks injury to the internal carotid, cavernous sinus, anterior communicating artery complex, optic nerve, and cranial nerves II to VI (**Fig. 12.8**). This is most common when the medial aspect of the orbit is penetrated. Diffuse intracranial air associated with a transorbital injury strongly increases irreversible brain stem injury, transorbital cerebral herniation, and increases the risk of death. Disruption of the orbital roof can create a communication with the intracranial cavity, leading to associated CSF leaks, encephalocele, intracranial abscesses, or delayed orbital reconstruction difficulties. In extreme blast cases, the maxillary sinus, orbit, and anterior cranial vault will all communicate through a traumatic disruption, exposing the brain to the sinus mucosa. In such cases, it is usually necessary to re-create surgically the cranial base, orbit, and maxillary sinus to protect the brain and obtain a cosmetically acceptable result. The use of titanium mesh fixation for the anterior skull base floor in theater has allowed subsequent surgeons to then use that foundation to keep the cerebral-orbital spaces separate. This closure is reinforced with pericranium (when available), fascia lata, temporalis fascia, fat, and occasionally split-thickness skull bone graft.

Surgical Considerations

The overall management goals include acute decompression and hemorrhage control. This is typically accomplished with a bifrontal craniotomy or craniectomy. In cases with disruption of the anterior cranial floor and frontal sinus with obvious risk for CSF leakage, a sinus exenteration, skull base reconstruction with watertight dural closure is usually performed. In restricted situations such as those akin to combat conditions involving mass casualties, lack of imaging, and lack of ophthalmology support, a limited procedure may be initially performed. This includes epidural hematoma evacuation followed by transfer to another neurosurgeon within 24 hours for a more definitive anterior skull base reconstruction. This was the case during the attack on the United Nations headquarters in Baghdad where over 150 casualties arrived at the combat support hospital and 30 underwent open surgeries. Half of these required cranial or cervical surgery to remove glass embedded within the cranial vault, face, orbit, or neck. The possible array of penetrating fragments includes glass, rocks, metal, and occasionally the fragments of the suicide bomber. Plain films and the

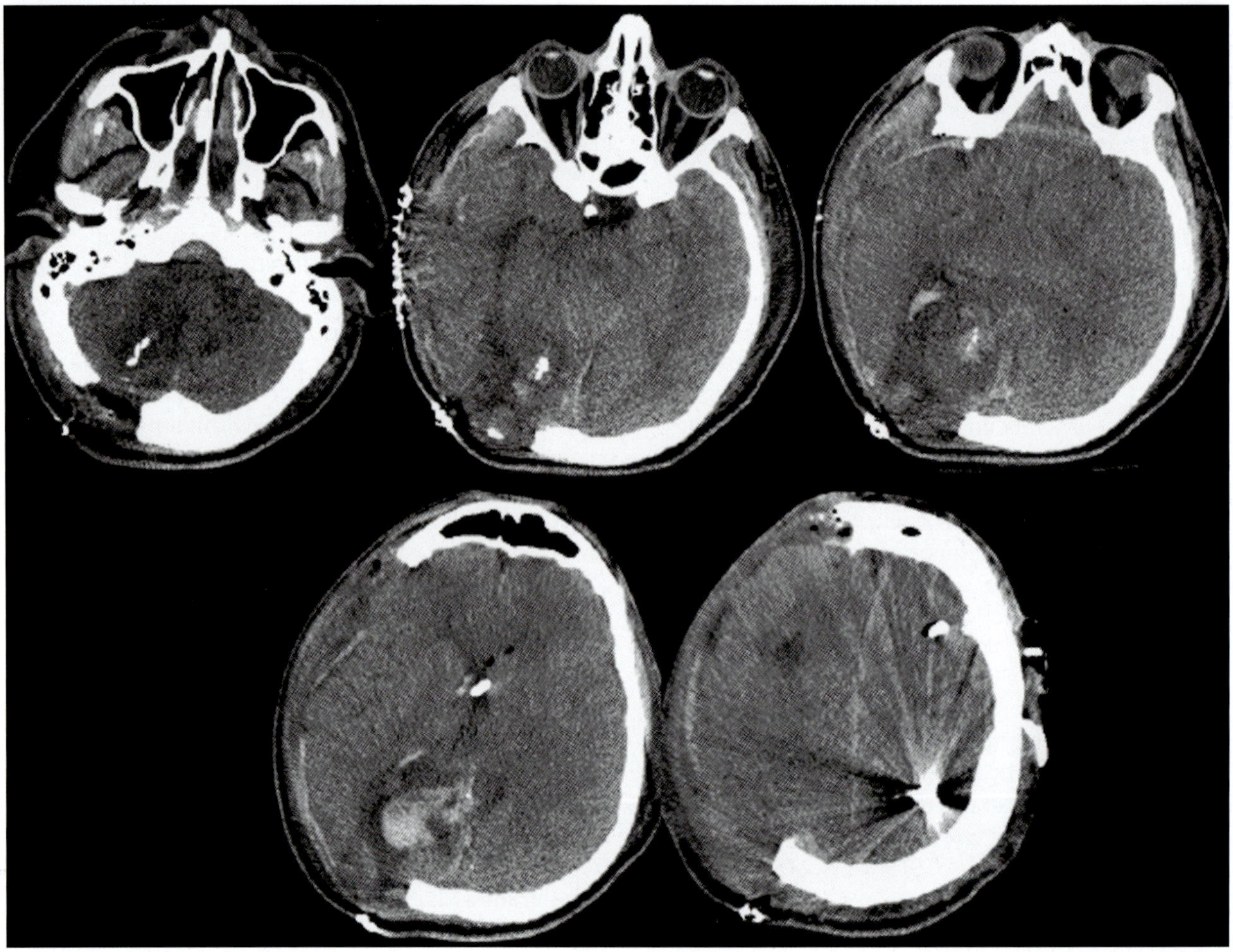

Fig. 12.8 This patient had an initial Glasgow Coma Scale score of 3 with a penetrating right suboccipital fragment passing transtentorially into the occipital lobe on the left, then into the right occipital parietal junction. The patient underwent a suboccipital craniectomy, right hemicraniectomy, transverse sinus ligation preserving the vein of Labbé, and placement of a ventriculostomy. He demonstrated delayed recurrent severe bilateral internal carotid artery, middle cerebral artery vasospasm requiring microballoon angioplasty and nicardipine. His examination improved with following commands, speaking spontaneously, and moving all four extremities. He demonstrated delayed hydrocephalus requiring a ventriculoperitoneal shunt.

physical examination are particularly helpful in understanding the global distribution of the fragments, the path of injury, and the best surgical approach. Unlike metal, an attempt is made early to remove glass, depressed bone over air sinus, clothing, body armor, and rocks from the cranial vault. However, deeply embedded fragments are not pursued unless there is documented delayed movement or vascular compromise. This is in keeping with avoidance of secondary injury through missile tract exploration.

Transtemporal Injuries

Those injuries that penetrate the frontotemporal region of the cranial cavity may include underlying injury to the frontotemporal lobes, internal carotid and middle cerebral arteries, and lateral ventricles with intraventricular hemorrhage (**Fig. 12.9**). Additionally, those associated with a significant force to the skull base may destroy the petrous bone; petrous carotid artery; facial, auditory, and trigeminal nerves as well as the lateral orbit and optic nerve. This can lead to CSF leaks, pseudoaneurysms, blindness, loss of usable hearing, and facial paralysis.

Surgical Considerations

Injuries in the region of the lateral skull base should include proximal exposure and control of the cervical carotid artery and its branches. In cases of intractable epistaxis, endovascular methods are preferred to obtain proximal control but may not be possible in an austere environment. Reconstruction of the petrous carotid artery is particularly challenging in a combat environment. Multiple constraints include the lack of intraoperative angiography, the absence of a high-definition operating microscope and microinstruments, the reduced availability of grafts due to extremity injuries, and most critically, the presence of a swollen, edematous, and hemorrhagic brain. In some cases, it may be more reasonable to perform a proximal and distal supraclinoid internal carotid artery (ICA) ligation to prevent a thromboembolic middle cerebral artery (MCA) stroke.

Laterally displaced entrance wounds may create a significant amount of soft tissue loss. This will challenge both the initial closure as well as the delayed reconstruction. In an attempt to preserve the known vascular pedicles, it may be preferable to base a curvilinear incision behind the ear to the anterior forehead (**Fig. 12.10**). The superior temporal artery will play an important role in scalp viability with a large hemicraniectomy flap.

Preservation of the vein of Labbé and viable MCA branches is an important part of the surgical decompression. Adequate bone removal insures that venous compromise from swelling at the bone edge will not occur. Following dural opening, a careful examination of the sylvian and cortical MCA branches should take place because the branches of the middle cerebral artery most

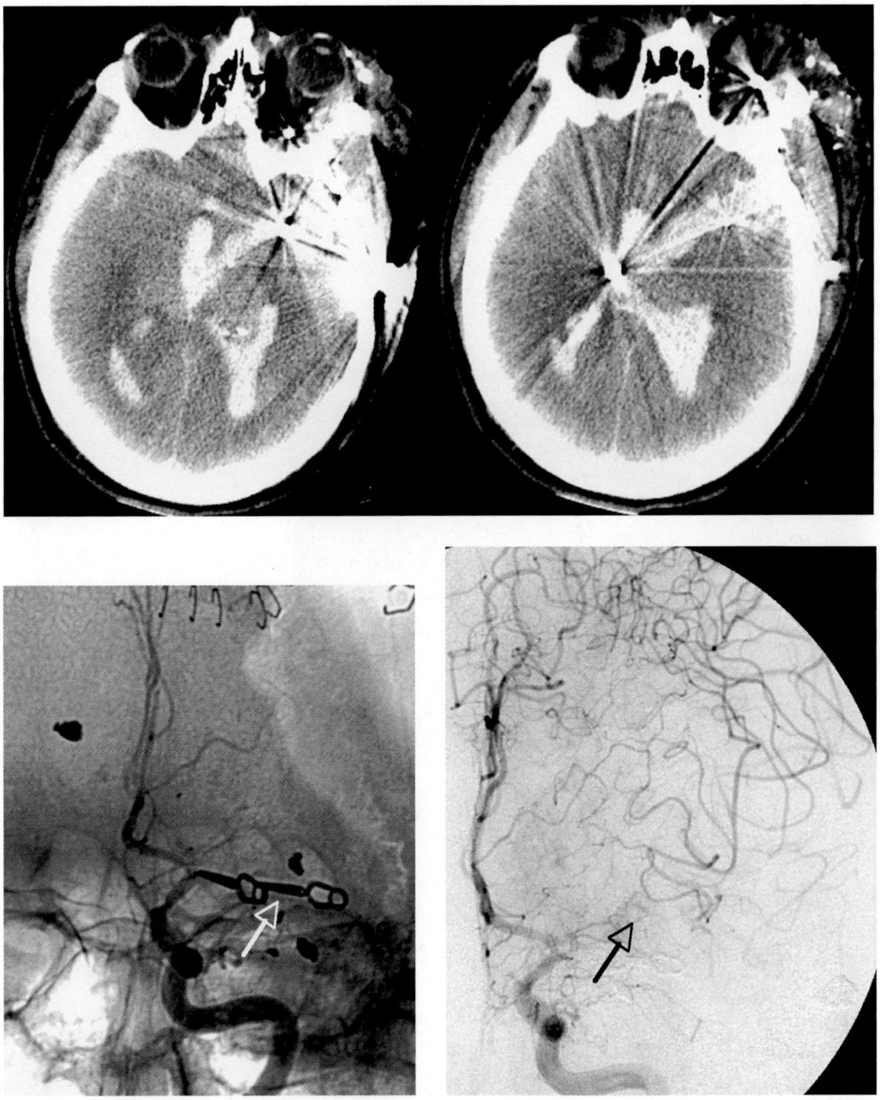

A B C

Fig. 12.9 (A) This soldier presented with a Glasgow Coma Scale score of 3 with a lateral temporal penetrating fragment coursing through the sylvian fissure, central diencephalon bilaterally, and third ventricle with significant SAH, IVH, and temporal lobe hematoma. He underwent a left hemicraniectomy, clipping of a transected left middle cerebral artery **(B**; *white arrow*, **C**; *black arrow***)**, evacuation of the temporal lobe hematoma, and placement of a ventriculostomy **(B, C)**. The postoperative course was complicated by posterior circulation delayed severe vasospasm requiring microballoon angioplasty and intraarterial nicardipine 1.

(Continued on page 250)

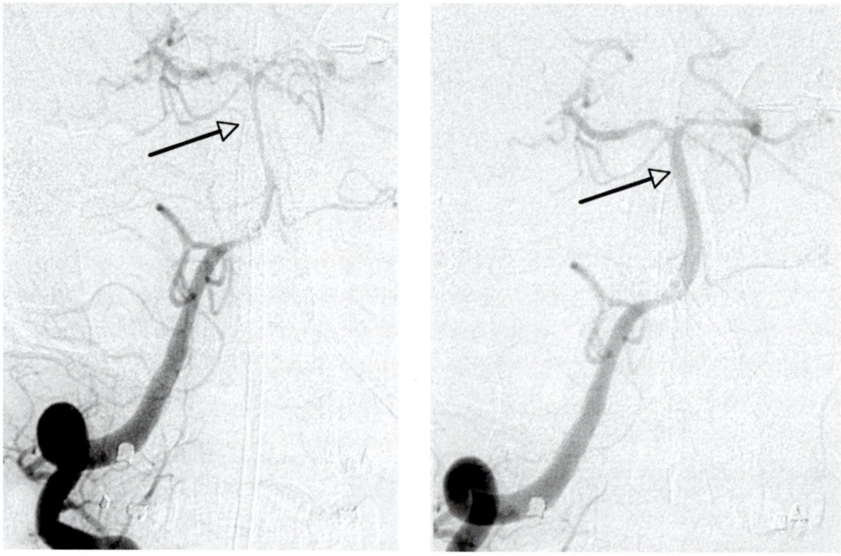

D E

Fig. 12.9 *(Continued)* **(D, E)**. Delayed cranioplasty was performed at 6 months and required ventriculoperitoneal shunting for delayed hydrocephalus. The patient's best examination at 8 months remains minimally reactive localizing, but the patient is noncommunicative with a right hemiplegia.

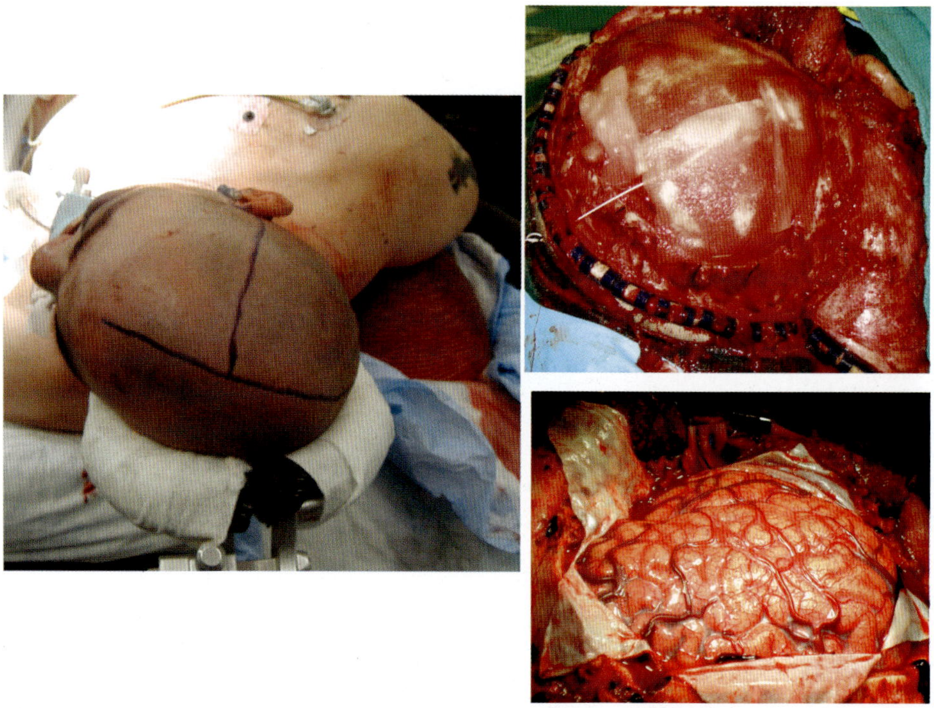

A B C

Fig. 12.10 **(A)** Alternative hemicraniectomy incision with midline curvilinear incision with vertical bisecting incision to the root of the zygoma. Originally described by Dr. Ludwig Kempe at the Walter Reed Army Medical Center during procedures for hemispherectomy and reintroduced in the current conflict by Major Jon Martin, MD, while serving in Balad, Iraq, in spring 2007 [Kempe, L. Operative Neurosurgery Vol 1. New York: Springer Verlag; 1968; 180–189]. Brain is covered by synthetic dura after placement of an ipsilateral intracranial pressure monitor, tunneled at the midline, a large 7fr subgaleal drain is then placed before closing the scalp **(B, C)**.

commonly injured include those in the distal cortical surface or lateral fissure. Typically, pseudoaneurysms are perpendicular to the fragment path in the zone of cavitation adjacent to the track and, if encountered, should be excluded from the normal circulation. Suspicion for traumatic aneurysms should arise when a sylvian fissure hematoma, focal parenchymal blood (i.e., gyrus rectus hematoma), or a hematoma remote from the fragment are present.

Delayed complications from injuries in this region include CSF leaks, pseudoaneurysm rupture, thromboembolic strokes, and flap necrosis associated with devascularization (**Table 12.4**). Commonly, CSF leaks include a disruption of the petrous skull base with underlying low-pressure hydrocephalus. In the presence of a hemicraniectomy, a distended flap may lead to CSF egress through the disrupted petrous ridge, subgaleal space, and possibly through the wound. In an effort to decrease this occurrence, we routinely place ventriculostomies to decompress the hemicraniectomy flap and afford another pathway for CSF egress while the disrupted skull base is sealing. Except in extreme cases with multiple ventriculostomies, we have avoided the routine use of early lumbar drainage due to concerns with cranial spinal pressure dissociation, meningitis, and lumbar overdrainage.

Pseudoaneurysm management has challenged current practice patterns during the current conflict. More pseudoaneurysms have been detected and treated in the first 2 years of this war than in the entire 10 years of the Iran–Iraq conflict.[3,17] Unfortunately, early in the conflict, delayed rupture resulted in death, coma, progressive paralysis, and near-fatal cardiac arrest from epistaxis in patients demonstrating early recovery from their initial neurological injury. This observation has prompted a concerted effort toward early detection and treatment. An aggressive screening process composed of early CT and cerebral angiography performed upon arrival to a stateside hospital by an experienced neurointerventionalist is now our standard of care. CT angiography (CTA) alone has been inadequate secondary to technical limitations stemming from metal artifacts, poor timing of the contrast bolus with venous contamination, and contrast diverted from stenosed conductance vessels. The criteria for a screening angiogram are outlined in **Table 12.5**. If the pseudoaneurysm is associated with a well-defined neck and is endovascularly accessible, the preference at our institution is early exclusion with either coils or stent-assisted coiling. In cases with distal pericallosal or MCA aneurysms, early microsurgery is the preferred treatment. The recurrence rate for endovascularly treated aneurysms approaches 30% in the senior author's series and requires close follow-up (**Fig. 12.11**). Repeat angiography at 3 months followed by either repeat endovascular treatment or open microsurgery has been the current strategy.

Suboccipital or Occipital Injuries

These injuries can be some of the most lethal due to the extent of injury to the brain stem, venous sinuses, and multiple intracranial compartments. Low-velocity fragments or high-velocity missiles that pass from the posterior fossa into the supratentorial compartment may create a path of injury that includes as many as three cerebral compartments (i.e., the ipsilateral cerebellum, occipital-temporal lobe, and contralateral parietal-occipital lobes) (**Fig. 12.8**). Additional injuries to the cervical spinal cord, vertebrobasilar circulation, and cranial nerves are possible. In one specific case in our series, an extracranial, suboccipital fragment resulted in a proximal posterior inferior cerebellar artery (PICA) traumatic aneurysm that subsequently ruptured.

Table 12.5 Evolution of Criteria for Intracranial Angiography following Penetrating Injury

Iran–Iraq War*	Operation Iraqi Freedom†
Penetrating injury through pterion, orbit, posterior fossa	Previous criteria plus:
Penetrating fragment with intracranial hematoma	Known cerebral artery sacrifice and/or pseudoaneurysm at the time of initial exploration
	Known cerebral artery sacrifice and/or pseudoaneurysm at the time of initial exploration
	Blast-induced penetrating injury with GCS <8
	TCD evidence of posttraumatic vasospasm
	Spontaneous decrease in $PBrO_2$

Source: Data from *Aarabi B. Traumatic aneurysms of brain due to high velocity missile head wounds. Neurosurgery 1988;22(6 Pt 1):1056–1063 and †Armonda RA, Bell RS, Vo AH, et al. Wartime traumatic cerebral vasospasm. Recent reviews of combat casualties. Neurosurgery 2006 Dec: 59: 1215–1225. Discussion 1225.

Abbreviations: GCS, Glasgow Coma Scale, $PBrO_2$, partial pressure brain tissue oxygen; TCD, transcranial doppler.

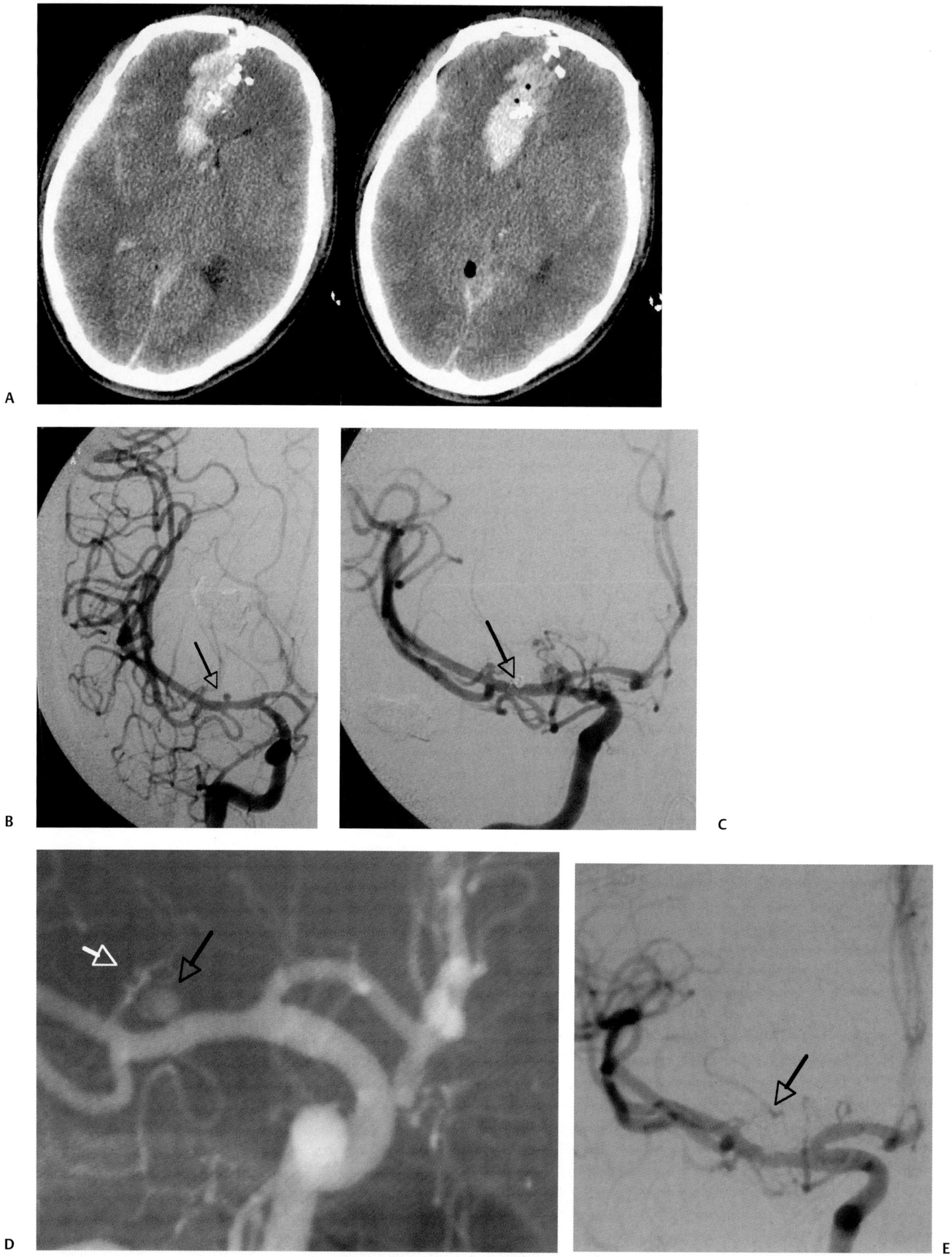
A
B
C
D
E

Surgical Considerations

Operative exposure, decompression, and homeostasis are all challenging in this area. The incision should allow exposure above and below the transverse-sigmoid sinus and allow decompression of the supratentorial hemisphere. A large C-shaped incision based on the mastoid to the subocciput to the midline forehead may provide the greatest needed exposure. Vascular injuries may include both major arterial and venous structures. The vertebral artery is typically prone to injury just proximal to the sulcus arteriosus and between C2–C3. The venous sinuses and the torcula are particularly vulnerable to spreading bone fractures that may displace the underlying bone through the outer wall of the venous sinus. In the subocciput, a "guttering" wound as described by Cushing can result in disruption of the jugular foramen with bony fracture through the jugular bulb and a delayed venous epidural hematoma of the posterior fossa. Homeostasis around the venous sinus can be obtained with the use of multiple strategies including muscle and dural elevation, sinus ligation, and oversewing with an attempt to preserve the sinus when possible, especially if dominant and including the vein of Labbé or the torcular. Additional hemostatic agents such as fibrillary Surgicel (Johnson & Johnson, New Brunswick, NJ) combined with Gelfoam (Pfizer, Inc., New York, NY), Surgicel, and cottonoid patties can be used.

Vertex or Parietal Entrance

Due to modern body armor, these are the most infrequent types of injuries seen in the current conflict. When occurring, they are usually associated with a delamination of the underlying body armor with a secondary skull fracture and rarely any metallic penetration of the cranial vault. The kinetic energy of the missile or fragment is transmitted from the helmet to the skull to the underlying brain. These injuries are associated with a range of scalp, bone, dural, and diffuse brain injuries. In extreme life-threatening cases, there is a gaping stellate scalp laceration, open-depressed skull fracture, and herniating brain from the defect. The CT scan may demonstrate significant bony fragments propelled deep into the brain. In some cases, the bony fragments act as secondary projectiles tearing through brain tissue creating secondary hematomas. When these bony fragments are propelled with such tremendous force, they can also create pseudoaneurysms in their path with disruption of the interhemispheric branches of the callosomarginal and pericallosal vessels. Occasionally, these forces are displaced over a venous sinus; techniques for exposing, securing, and repairing the sinus should be employed as well as precautions to avoid inadvertent air-emboli. The use of bilateral exposures allows the neurosurgeon to have the ability to adequately expose the longitudinal sinus, decompress both hemispheres, and control bleeding from either side of the falx cerebri. A coronal incision also helps facilitate wound closure and if necessary releases of scalp tension with partial-thickness scalp incisions, which can be skin-grafted and allow the primary wound to heal without tension.

Conclusion

The neurosurgical care of the penetrating brain-injury patient has evolved significantly since World War I. In early conflicts, a penetrating brain injury usually resulted in mortality. Today, we have seen an unprecedented functional survival from even the most severe penetrating injuries. A combination of factors has led to this outcome: the use of technologically advanced body armor, far forward brain stem decompression, and rapid strategic evacuation of patients to specialized and sophisticated neurocritical care. The lessons learned from our experience and from the conflicts that have preceded Operation Iraqi Freedom stress that patient selection for aggressive interventions is critical in maximizing outcome and avoiding vegetative survival (i.e., intervention in the setting of bihemispheric midbrain perforation may not be advisable). Additionally, the anticipation of late complications like pseudoaneurysm rupture, delayed stroke from vasospasm, and hydrocephalus in viable survivors could be the difference between vegetation or good functional recovery.

Fig. 12.11 **(A)** This soldier was struck by an improvised explosive device with penetrating fragments coursing from the forehead transhemispherically from the frontal pole to the occipital lobe. Patient was initially awake, then deteriorated to localizing with contralateral hemiparesis. In theater, patient underwent a bifrontal craniotomy, frontal sinus exenteration, dural repair with placement of a ventriculostomy. Despite a trajectory above the sylvian fissure, he developed a low-density in the anterior aspect of the head of the caudate. **(B)** A cerebral angiogram demonstrated evidence of a traumatic middle cerebral artery pseudoaneurysm (*black arrow*) and subsequent delayed severe vasospasm. **(C)** This was initially treated with endosaccular coiling and angioplasty. **(D)** Eight weeks later the aneurysm recurred (*black arrow*) with coil compaction (*white arrow*) and was **(E)** then microsurgically clipped. At 6 months, he has returned to normal activity without any deficits.

References

1. Cushing H. A series of wounds involving the brain and its enveloping structures. Br J Surg 1918;5:558–684
2. Eden K. Mobile neurosurgery in warfare, experiences in the Eighth Army's Campaign in Cyrenaica, Tripolitania, and Tunisia. Lancet 1943;2:689–692
3. Aarabi B. Traumatic aneurysms of brain due to high velocity missile head wounds. Neurosurgery 1988;22(6 Pt 1):1056–1063
4. Meirowsky AM. Penetrating wounds of the brain. In: JB Costes, ed. Neurological Surgery of Trauma. Washington, DC: Office of the Surgeon General, Department of the Army; 1965:103–136
5. Carey ME, Young H, Mathis JL, Forsythe J. A bacteriologic study of craniocerebral missile wounds from Vietnam. J Neurosurg 1971;34:145–154
6. Brandvold B, Levy L, Feinsod M, George E. Penetrating craniocerebral injuries in the Israeli involvement in the Lebanese conflict, 1982–1985: an analysis of a less aggressive approach. J Neurosurg 1990;72:15–21
7. Bell R, Vo A, Porter C, et al. Wartime neurovascular injuries: review of the effectiveness of early, aggressive, endovascular management in the setting of blast-related cerebral vasospasm. Neurosurgery 2006;59(2): 455–456
8. Simpson DA, David D. The genesis of craniomaxillofacial surgery. ANZ J Surg 2004;74:71–77
9. Matson D. The management of acute craniocerebral injuries due to missiles. In: Spurling G, Woodhall B, eds. Surgery in WWII: Neurosurgery Vol 1. Washington, DC: Office of the Surgeon General, Department of the Army; 1958
10. Cramer F. Blast concussion and cerebral injuries due to explosion waves. In: Spurling G, Woodhall B, eds. Surgery in WWII: Neurosurgery Vol 1. Washington, DC: Office of the Surgeon General, Department of the Army; 1958
11. Roth J, Mayo A, Elran H, Razon N, Kluger Y. Brain injuries caused by spherical bolts. J Neurosurg 2005;102:864–869
12. Rosenwasser RH, Andrews W, Jimenez F. Penetrating craniocerebral trauma. Surg Clin North Am 1991;71:305–316
13. Amirjamshidi A, Abbassioun K, Rahmat H. Minimal debridement or simple wound closure as the only surgical treatment in war victims with low-velocity penetrating head injuries: indications and management protocol based upon more than 8 years follow-up of 99 cases from Iran-Iraq conflict. Surg Neurol 2003;60(2):105–110, discussion 10–1
14. Aldrich EF, Eisenberg HM, Saydjari C, et al. Predictors of mortality in severely head-injured patients with civilian gunshot wounds: a report from the NIH Traumatic Coma Data Bank. Surg Neurol 1992;38(6):418–423
15. Dillon JD Jr, Meirowsky A. Facio-orbito-cranial missile wounds. Surg Neurol 1975;4:515–518
16. Tan Y, Zhou S, Jiang H. Biomechanical changes in the head associated with penetrating injuries of the maxilla and mandible: an experimental investigation. J Oral Maxillofac Surg 2002;60(5):552–556
17. Amirjamshidi A, Rahmat H, Abbassioun K. Traumatic aneurysms and arteriovenous fistulas of intracranial vessels associated with penetrating head injuries occurring during war: principles and pitfalls in diagnosis and management: a survey of 31 cases and review of the literature. J Neurosurg 1996;84(5):769–780

13 Scientific Surgical Management

Randall M. Chesnut

Background and Overview

During the early stages of evolution of our present approach to traumatic brain injury (TBI), surgery was the only intervention that we had to offer, outside of simple medical observation of the TBI patient. One consequence of this was a protracted period wherein *nonsurgical* TBI was considered *nontreatable* TBI, and patients without mass lesions were triaged differently from those with patently surgical disease. More recently, the importance of nonoperative management in determining outcome has become increasingly recognized, with an associated burgeoning of interest and involvement from emergency medicine physicians, trauma surgeons, and intensivists. Presently, as we realize that probably over 90% of TBI care is nonoperative, TBI management has necessarily become a team effort, integrally incorporating both surgeons and nonsurgeons.

Unfortunately, the momentum of this internecine swing, coupled with resource issues linked to shortages in neurosurgical coverage, has led some to suggest that neurosurgeons are not *conditiae sine qua non* to trauma care in general and TBI care in particular.[1] Not only does such posturing ignore the seminal and continuing, fundamental contributions of the specialty of neurosurgery to TBI management, but it also denies the critical and burgeoning role for the integral involvement of physicians dedicated to and capable of optimal management of posttraumatic intracranial pathology in all of its forms. As reflected below in options for the surgical management of contusions and the entire concept of early decompression for intracranial hypertension, surgery should not be viewed as the final option in treating TBI. By definition, this requires the active involvement of a neurosurgeon in TBI management; someone for whom the decision to operate is constantly an option rather than an admission of defeat. In this light, this section on the surgical management of TBI should be viewed as fundamental to overall treatment, rather than a section of interest only to surgical neurologists.

Certain overall concepts are relevant to any discussion of surgery, including the issues of indications for surgery, the timing of the intervention, and the techniques used. Indications can be absolute (life-saving surgery, damage control) or relative (e.g., surgery as an alternative to other treatment modalities). In general, physical manifestations of intracranial hypertension and herniation (such as anisocoria or motor posturing, computed tomography [CT] evidence of cisternal compression or midline shift, or deterioration of monitored physiological parameters such as intracranial pressure [ICP]) are strong indications for intervention; whether such intervention is surgical will depend on the underlying pathology.

In any area of trauma, life-saving surgery should be performed as soon as possible; this would intuitively extend to TBI, where the concept of "time is brain" reflects the uniquely powerful influence of morbidity over mortality in recovery. Unfortunately, the timing of surgery does not easily lend itself to controlled trials, making it difficult to quote hard data when interacting with physicians and health care systems that are less ready to take a patient to theater. Although there are no data supporting an argument for benefit of delaying emergent or urgent neurosurgical intervention in isolated TBI, extracranial injuries can strongly influence such decisions on an individual patient basis. The timing issue becomes even more difficult when the surgical intervention is not do-or-die.

For many years, the surgical management of TBI has been based on anecdotal practice and "clinical intuition." Such logic leads to the assumption that an intracranial mass lesion in a brain trauma patient with neurological compromise should be evacuated. Anecdotal practice suggests that this evacuation should be done as soon as possible by craniotomy. As evidence-based medicine comes to the fore in the face of increasing social, economic, legal, and even ethical queries into the form and substance of medical practice, however, almost everything that we do becomes open to question. Thus, the need for evidence-reports arises to codify the state of knowledge on medical topics and evidence-based practice guidelines to assist in optimizing management.

One of the most common inquiries to the original authors of the Guidelines for the Management of Severe Traumatic Brain Injury[2] (all of whom were neurosurgeons) was why there were no guidelines for surgical management. The definitive response to this appeared in *Neurosurgery* in 2006 as the "Guidelines for the Surgical Management of Traumatic Brain Injury."[3]

The formulation of these guidelines used the same evidence-based medicine approach that we had employed in drawing up the previously published guidelines for acute

TBI management in adults[2] and in the pediatric population,[4] for penetrating trauma,[5] and for prehospital TBI care.[6] The details of this process are outlined in detail in introductory sections in all of these publications and will not be fully covered here. Briefly, five surgical topics were covered, comprising acute epidural hematomas, acute subdural hematomas, traumatic parenchymal lesions, posterior fossa mass lesions, and depressed skull fractures. For each of these topics, we performed a thorough search of the available English literature back to 1975 (e.g., for the era of CT use in TBI), including a broad electronic search augmented by pearling. Using explicit, evidence-based medicine methodology, we classified each relevant retrieved article according to its scientific rigor using a 3-point scale (class I–III). Based on the scientific quality of the articles germane to each topic, we generated practice parameters. The highest level of practice recommendations are practice *standards*, which were based on class I evidence and reflect a high degree of clinical certainty. Practice *guidelines* were based on class II evidence and reflect a moderate degree of clinical certainty. Practice *options* were based on class III evidence and reflect unclear clinical certainty. Every step has been explicitly documented in the publication, and all involved literature is summarized in evidentiary tables published with the guidelines (**Table 13.1**).

For the purpose of this chapter, surgical sections have also been incorporated from the Guidelines for the Acute Medical Management of Severe Traumatic Brain Injury in Infants, Children, and Adolescents[4] (i.e., the chapter on surgical treatment of intracranial hypertension) and from the Guidelines for the Management of Penetrating Brain Injury[5] (i.e., the chapters on surgical management of penetrating brain injury and on the management of cerebrospinal fluid leaks). All chapters reflect the same rigor summarized above.

In the end, there were no class I or II studies and, consequently, there are no practice standards or guidelines in these documents. Although practice recommendations were generated for each of the topics, it is critical to bear in mind their level of evidentiary support. A brief discussion of the implications of practice options and medical decision making in the absence of class I or II literature follows the presentation of the guidelines in this chapter.

The goal of this section is to outline the evidentiary basis for the surgical management of TBI. The vast majority of what we do (and will continue to do for some time in the future) is based on our own personal experiences, what we have learned in our training and during other educational ventures, and our interpretation of the literature to which we have been exposed, all superimposed on our gestalt of an individual clinical situation. The purpose of this chapter will be to present a rigorous and unbiased, evidence-based synopsis of the literature to assist in clinical decision making. Unless otherwise indicated (vide infra), this information will not vary from that presented in the evidence reports cited. Individual discussions that are not reflected in these evidence reports are contained within each following subsection entitled, Outside of the Evidence Report. These sections are designed merely to assist in incorporating the evidentiary recommendations into actual practice. Although technical aspects of surgery can profoundly influence its efficacy, a discussion of techniques is beyond the scope of this discussion. Only the most general relevant aspects will be mentioned here.

The Decision to Operate

Obviously, the performance of every surgical intervention is predicated on a decision to operate. Such a decision reflects not only the physiologic and anatomic indications (as discussed herein), but also the even more difficult issues of salvageability and quality of life. The surgeon is frequently asked to make early prognostic judgments by family and loved ones to couch a decision on operative management in view of (often incomplete) information on the wishes of the patient or the legal next of kin. As such, optimizing one's understanding of prognostic variables is every bit as critical as the information contained in this chapter. For evidence reports on prognostication in TBI, the reader is referred to sections on prognosis in the Guidelines for the Management of Severe Head Injury[2] and the Guidelines for the Management of Penetrating Brain Injury.[5]

Table 13.1 Classification of Evidence–Based Medical Literature

Class I	Practice standards	Highest level of practice recommendations Reflects high degree of clinical certainty Recommendation at level of treatment standard should strongly influence one's practice
Class II	Practice guidelines	Reflects moderate degree of clinical certainty Recommendation at level of treatment standard should strongly influence one's practice—physician may deem it nonrelevant in individual situations
Class III	Practice options	Reflects unclear clinical certainty No mandate to follow such recommendations as the treatment has unclear clinical efficacy and has not been proven superior to alternative therapies

Recommendations for Future Research

Finally, one of the most often overlooked, but critically important aspects of any evidence report are the recommendations for future research. At the point of finishing the exhaustive and detailed review of the entire body of literature on a topic that is necessary to write such a report, the authors are intimately familiar with the shortcomings of the literature as it stands and with the general form of investigations that would ally such shortcomings. As we are presently in the process of updating all of the TBI evidence reports, we are noting that the majority of the deficiencies extant during the original reports continue to plague the updating process. To lessen the likelihood that this will continue in the future, recommendations for future research from the evidence reports are summarized at the end of each subsection in this chapter.

Incorporating Evidence-Based Medicine into Clinical Practice

There is a continuing proliferation of literature in every aspect of medicine. The widely ranging quality of published reports does not necessarily allow the reader to count on the editorial process to ensure that publication represents scientific rigor in study design, execution, or analysis. Unfortunately, evaluating the literature for such qualities is not a simple process, requiring specific training and time to perform adequately. In addition, the proliferation of educational offerings of often uncontrolled (or even intentionally biased) quality further complicates the picture. How often do we hear quoted unpublished abstracts from meetings or even Web pages when discussing medical treatment? It is true that not adapting one's treatment in the face of solid class I evidence that is relevant to one's patient population is an error. It is also true, however, that altering one's practice based on information of marginal or unclear scientific rigor is unwise. Outside of exceptional circumstances, we do not have unbiased, independent, long-term, validated follow-up data on all of our patients, corrected for risk-adjustment using valid, multivariate statistics. As such, our experience is only anecdote and the plural of *anecdote* is not *evidence*. Therefore, a concise, rigorous, unbiased, and comprehensive summary of the literature (as presented in a properly conducted evidence report) should be a very valuable asset to the practicing physician.

One frequent objection to evidence-based medicine is that it represents an intrusion into the autonomy of an *individual* physician's treatment of an *individual* patient (i.e., the *practice* of medicine). In truth, given the present state of the literature, evidence reports almost never mandate a certain form of treatment, due to the rarity of well-designed and performed class I studies. Much of the basis of this objection arises from ignoring the level of the practice recommendations as they reflect the class of the underlying evidence. A recommendation at the level of a treatment standard *should* strongly influence one's practice. A recommendation at the level of a treatment guideline should also influence one's practice in that it should be considered to probably be the best treatment in the majority of clinical situations relevant to the recommendation. In an individual instance, however, the physician may deem it nonrelevant or incorrect (**Table 13.1**). If their reasoning is clear or documented, there should be no issue with proceeding differently.

For the situation of a recommendation at the level of a treatment option, the recommended treatment is, by definition, of unclear clinical significance, in that it has not been proven efficacious or shown superior to competing treatment modalities in rigorous trials. As such, there is absolutely no mandate to follow such recommendations (even though they were considered by the evidence-report authors to be perhaps the most reasonable out of a group of similar choices). Rather than an intrusion, an evidence report should be seen as a service to the physician, facilitating (but rarely controlling) clinical decision-making in light of the available evidence.

How, then, is one to practice in the face of a vast preponderance of class III evidence and treatment options? Obviously, the practice of medicine must go on, despite the often-marginal status of the literature. Treatment decisions must be made anyway. As such, the value of realizing the class III nature of the evidence lies in understanding the less-than-solid nature of the support for a given clinical decision and proceeding accordingly. Decisions made based on literature of this quality must not be felt definitive; rather, the clinician should rely on a degree of skepticism, manifest as diligent follow-up, to allow timely alterations in treatment paradigms when the initially chosen option proves ineffective. It is facilitating the understanding that one is proceeding on uncertain ground that is the real clinical value of evidence reports and evidence-based treatment recommendations that are comprised of only treatment options. More than telling one what to do, they serve as a warning that there are no guarantees at that level of evidentiary support, and that attentiveness and caution are prudent.

Finally, of course, treatment recommendations with lower levels of scientific support are a call for improved research, both to researchers and to funding institutions. In that light, the Recommendations for Future Research sections in evidence reports should be taken very seriously. The most disappointing aspect of the process of renewing an evidence report is finding the same shortcomings and errors in the body of literature that has followed the dissemination of the initial publication.

Table 13.2 Epidural Hematoma (EDH)

Origin	Implications
Fracture-related disruption of middle meningeal artery	Area of temporal bone—likely to rapidly and continually expand
Nonarterial EDH	Area of temporal bone—management influenced by high risk due to clots and inability to differentiate low and high pressure lesions
Venous EDH	Causes: Rupture of veins bridging dura mater and extracranial sinuses Lacerated cerebral venous sinus (e.g., transverse or sagittal sinus) Likely to expand—no reliable imaging to assist this prediction
Skull fracture bleeding	Small—frequently do not expand in absence of sinus damage or coagulopathy

Epidural Hematomas

Epidural hematomas develop between the dura mater and the inner table of the skull (**Table 13.2**). They may originate from arterial or venous hemorrhage or from bleeding fractured bone. The classic (and one of the most lethal) epidural hematomas arise from fracture-related disruption of the middle meningeal artery, which is closely applied and adherent to the thin bone of the temporal skull. Expanding under arterial pressure, it is likely to rapidly and continually expand. Nonarterial epidural hematomas may occur in the same region, but the high risk afforded by clots of arterial origin and our inability to easily differentiate low- versus high-pressure lesions has always strongly influenced the management of epidural collections in the lateral temporal area.

Venous epidural hematomas may occur due to rupture of veins bridging between the dura mater and extracranial sinuses (e.g., the sphenopalatine sinus at the temporal tip) or when a lacerated cerebral venous sinus such as the transverse or sagittal sinus bleeds into this space. These are lower pressure hematomas and less likely to expand, but there are no reliable imaging signs that can be used to assist in such prediction. Ergo, these lesions should also be considered dangerous. Epidural collections arising solely from skull fracture bleeding are most often small and most frequently do not expand in the absence of damage to an adjacent sinus or coagulopathy. Nevertheless, nonoperative management based on anticipated stability should be supported by serial imaging.

The classic lucid interval (which actually occurs in only a minority of epidural hematomas) results when the patient recovers from a brief loss of consciousness related to the blow per se and deteriorates later due to rising ICP and mass effect. The morbidity of epidural hematomas arises from compression of the underlying brain. They are not usually associated with underlying parenchymal damage, so that early diagnosis and intervention should be highly successful. Morbidity and mortality directly reflect the level of consciousness at the time of surgery, with mortality ranging from 0% for patients conscious throughout, through 27% with the classic lucid internal, to over 50% for patients who never regain consciousness. This has produced an aggregate mortality with aggressive surgical management of around 9%.[7]

The Guidelines for the Surgical Management of Traumatic Brain Injury were able to identify nothing more definitive than class III evidence regarding the indications for surgery for epidural hematomas.[3] As such, they only provided treatment recommendations at the option level. These recommendations are presented in **Table 13.3**.

As with most intracranial lesions, data on surgical indicators in epidural hematomas are highly confounded because a subset of study patients will have undergone surgery based on criteria that are often inconsistent or obscure. The guidelines were therefore based on analyses of studies describing (1) factors associated with good or poor outcome in patients treated surgically, and (2) outcome in those patients initially selected for nonoperative management, including features associated with delayed surgery.

Patient selection bias in studies of operative management was analyzed by Servadei et al.[8] Factors found significant by regression analysis were midline shift of > 5 mm

Table 13.3 Class III (Practice Options) Evidence Regarding the Indications for Surgery for Epidural Hematomas

Indications for surgery	An EDH >30 cc should be surgically evacuated regardless of the patient's GCS score. An EDH <30 cc and with <15-mm thickness and with <5-mm midline shift in patients with a GCS score >8 without focal deficit can be managed nonoperatively with serial CT scanning and close neurological observation in a neurosurgical center.
Timing	It is strongly recommended that patients with an acute EDH in coma (GCS score <9) with anisocoria undergo surgical evacuation as soon as possible.
Methods	There are insufficient data to support one surgical treatment method. However, craniotomy provides a more complete evacuation of the hematoma.

Abbreviations: EDH, epidural hematoma; CT, computed tomography; GCS, Glasgow Coma Scale.

Table 13.4 Patient Outcomes of Surgical Treatment

Predictors of Good Outcomes	Predictors of Poor Outcomes
No signs of transtentorial herniation (e.g., abnormal pupillary reactivity, motor posturing)	Pupillary abnormality
Minimal duration of such signs when present	Lower Glasgow Coma Scale (GCS) or GCS motor subscale score
Higher admission GCS scores	Large hematomas Midline shift >10 mm Compression or elimination of basal cisterns Presence of other intracranial lesions

or clot thickness of >15 mm. A pediatric study using similar modeling statistics found the same two parameters, plus hematoma volume, to be predictive of surgery (although they did not provide suggested threshold values).[9]

Predictors of good outcome in the group of patients treated surgically (**Table 13.4**) include the absence of signs of transtentorial herniation (e.g., abnormal pupillary reactivity and motor posturing), minimal duration of such signs when present, and higher admission Glasgow Coma Scale (GCS) scores.[10] Predictors of poor outcome following surgery include pupillary abnormality, lower GCS or GCS motor subscale score, large hematomas, midline shift >10 mm, compression or elimination of the basal cisterns, or delay in surgery, as well as the presence of other intracranial lesions.[11–13] Because patients with these factors were treated surgically, their relevance to surgical decision making is limited to suggesting that their presence should inhibit the consideration of nonoperative management and strongly support clot evacuation with all possible speed.

Reports on patients managed without surgery manifest a patient selection bias tending toward those with minimal mass effect on the basal cisterns or midline, thickness <12 to 20 cm, higher GCS scores (not comatose; generally >12), and lesion volume <30 cc.[8–11,14,15] There is also a strong bias against nonoperative management of patients with lesions in the middle cranial fossa. There are no studies of nonoperative management of patients in coma. Predictors of good outcome in this select group of patients treated nonoperatively include the absence of signs of transtentorial herniation (e.g., normal pupillary reactivity and no motor posturing), no or minimal midline shift, clot thickness <15 mm, and visible basal cisterns.[10,11,14,15]

Chen et al analyzed a group of 14 patients who failed nonoperative management and underwent delayed surgery.[11] Factors statistically associated with such a course were epidural hematoma volume >30 cc, clot thickness >15 mm, or >5 mm of midline shift on the initial CT scan. In their study of 111 patients, all achieved favorable outcome, so their indicators for the decision to operate may be conservative.

The timing of surgery has not been found to be critical when all patients with epidural hematomas are studied in aggregate. Delay to surgery has been found to covary with mortality for patients with pupillary abnormalities or motor signs of herniation[12,16,17] and with mortality and morbidity for patients in coma.[18] These data support the emergent status of hematoma evacuation in patients with epidural hematomas who are neurologically compromised.

Outside of the Evidence Report

Given the ease and safety of surgical evacuation of pure epidural hematomas, many believe surgery to often be the conservative (i.e., safest and most sure) method of management of such lesions.[19] Obviously, it is desirable to avoid surgery when unnecessary. On the other hand, considerations such as having a patient deteriorate under observation and the need to delay other necessary procedures to allow clinical observation of the level of consciousness may prompt operative management even in some cases felt amenable to nonsurgical treatment. Clearly, when observation and serial imaging are the chosen course, the patient must be admitted to an intensive care unit (ICU; where frequent neurological checks will be reliably performed) and the imaging schedule must be clearly defined and confirmed at the time of admission. Lapses in either can have devastating results.

The guidelines do not deal with epidural hematomas that are diagnosed late or received at an institution with neurosurgical capabilities with significant delay. Such circumstances sometimes afford a window of observation and a set of serial CT images that demonstrate lack of progression over a time window that would otherwise not have existed. At present, surgical decision making in such instances must be made on a one-by-one basis, without literature guidance.

Drainage of Epidural Hematomas by Nonneurosurgeons

Most likely due to the importance of expediency in the evacuation of epidural hematomas in the neurologically compromised patient, studies that involve relatively short transport times (e.g., under ~3 to 4 hours) strongly support direct admission to and management at neurotrauma centers.[20,21] Unfortunately, for reasons such as distance, lack of transport vehicles, weather, etc., direct admissions or even rapid transfers to neurotrauma centers are not always possible. As such, there is much interest as to the efficacy of surgical management of epidural hematomas by nonneurosurgeons at remote institutions.

Wester compared patients with epidural hematomas evacuated at a university hospital neurosurgical center versus those treated at local centers by general surgeons or orthopaedic trauma surgeons.[22] He reported a longer time to decompression, generally inadequate technique, and increased morbidity and mortality in those patients undergoing surgery outside of the university setting. Unfortunately, details of pre- and postoperative neurological examinations and imaging studies and the precise reasons that led to the surgery being done in lieu of transfer were not available on all patients. These authors felt that such an approach was an ineffective anachronism due to the modern ability to transfer these patients very rapidly to neurosurgical centers in Norway.

In contrast, Rinker et al reported a case series suggesting notable benefit from bur hole/craniectomy drainage at remote institutions in Montana, performed by nonneurosurgeons who had previously undergone training in the procedure.[23] A neurosurgeon was consulted prior to each procedure for approval and guidance, was available for consultation during the operation, and accepted the patient in transfer following the emergent procedure. Outcomes were very satisfactory, there were no significant complications, and it was calculated that the operations were consummated in less time than it would have taken to deliver the patient to the regional trauma center emergency department. Notable differences between the Rinker and Wester studies were the detailed training of the nonneurological surgeons in the techniques, the inclusion of the neurosurgeon in the process by telephone, and longer transport times in the former report.

These studies would suggest that careful planning, training, and communication in anticipation of insurmountable delays in transferring patients with acute epidural hematomas to neurotrauma centers can allow temporizing, life-saving decompressions to be performed by nonneurosurgeons under controlled circumstances with beneficial results. Significant preparation appears necessary and the issue of how to maintain competence in such procedures by nonneurosurgeons remains open.

Basic Surgical Management of an Epidural Hematoma

The focal nature of epidural hematomas allows a more directed craniotomy. When not related to bleeding from an artery or a large venous sinus, evacuation can generally be safely accomplished through a limited incision and a small flap. Of course, the approach should be more expansive (or expandable) when access to structures such as the sagittal or transverse sinus or the foramen spinosum are anticipated as possibly necessary. A single bur hole is often all that is necessary to allow craniotomy, as the dura is already stripped from the inner table of the skull. (This same fact makes bur holes by nonneurosurgeons much safer in the presence of epidural clots.) During evacuation of the clot, the surgeon should search for any bleeding sources and manage them definitively. The bone flap can generally be replaced. Tack-up sutures should be used to eliminate any dead space, particularly when fracture bleeding is possible. A drain should be left in the epidural space.

Recommendations for Future Research

The Guidelines for the Surgical Management of Traumatic Brain Injury[3] stressed several areas felt particularly in need of future research in this area, including

- Class I or II outcome studies to determine indications for and efficacy of surgical evacuation of epidural hematomas, allowing for statistical risk adjustment
- Indications for and efficacy of evacuation of epidural hematomas by nonneurosurgeons at remote locations where transfer prior to decompression may be a less desirable option. Such studies should involve identification of at-risk centers and candidate surgeons, adequate training, available real-time consultation with a neurosurgeon, and optimal postdecompressive transfer and management arrangements.

Subdural Hematomas

Subdural hematoma is the most common trauma-related surgical intracranial mass lesion (**Table 13.5**). Sixty-six to 80% present in coma, and pupillary abnormalities are present in one third to one half.[13,24–26] The mechanism of injury is most commonly traffic accidents in adults 18 to 40 years of age, switching to falls for those over 65.[27]

A subdural hematoma lies between the brain and the dura mater. The most frequent etiologies include rupture of vessels (generally veins) bridging the subdural space or bleeding from parenchymal injuries, contusions and intracerebral hematomas being the most common.[25,26] Although acute subdural hematomas may occur in isolation, even lacking associated subarachnoid blood,[28] they are most frequently associated with underlying damage to the brain substance. Indeed, generally the subdural hematoma per se is not responsible for the outcome, but rather the damage to the brain substance. As such, although evacuation of an expanding subdural hematoma may be lifesaving in controlling ICP, it is not so definitive as evacuation of an epidural hematoma in achieving good outcome. Mortality

Table 13.5 Subdural Hematoma (SDH) Characteristics

Most common trauma-related surgical intracranial mass lesion
66–80% present in comatose state
33–50% present with pupillary abnormalities
Mechanism of injury:
Commonly road traffic accidents in those between 18–40 years of age
Falls in those 65 and older
Lesion location: lies between brain and dura mater
Most common etiologies:
Rupture of vessels bridging subdural space
Bleeding from parenchymal injuries (most common = contusions, intracerebral hematomas)
SDH is not solely responsible for adverse outcomes, but rather damage to the brain substance is more important—that is why evacuation is not as definitive as in epidural hematoma.
Mortality: remains as high as 52–60%

continues to remain as high as 52 to 60% in patients with subdural hematomas requiring surgery.[29–31]

The Guidelines for the Surgical Management of Traumatic Brain Injury were able to identify nothing more definitive than class III evidence regarding the indications for surgery for subdural hematomas.[3] As such, they only provided treatment recommendations at the option level. These recommendations are presented in **Table 13.6**.

Table 13.6 Class III (Practice Options) Evidence regarding the Indications for Surgery for Subdural Hematomas

Indications for surgery	An acute subdural hematoma with a thickness >10 mm or midline shift >5 mm on CT should be surgically evacuated, regardless of the patient's GCS score.
	All patients with acute subdural hematoma in coma (GCS score <9) should undergo intracranial pressure monitoring.
	A comatose patient (GCS score <9) with a subdural hematoma <10-mm thickness and midline shift < 5 mm should undergo surgical evacuation of the lesion if any of the following are true:
	The GCS score decreased between the time of injury and hospital admission by 2 or more points.
	The patient presents with asymmetric or fixed and dilated pupils.
	The intracranial pressure exceeds 20 mm Hg.
Timing	In patients with acute subdural hematoma and indications for surgery, surgical evacuation should be done as soon as possible
Methods	f surgical evacuation of an acute SDH in a comatose patient (GCS <9) is indicated, it should be done using a craniotomy with or without bone flap removal and duraplasty.

Abbreviations: CT, computed tomography; GCS, Glasgow Coma Scale, SDH, subdural hematoma.

Several factors have been correlated with outcome from subdural hematoma, including age, status, course of the GCS score, pupillary status, acute and chronic comorbidities, and CT imaging findings (including midline shift, compression of the basal cisterns, hematoma thickness, and presence of other intracranial lesions such as contusions or subarachnoid hemorrhage). Unfortunately, it is difficult to separate signs of correctable pathology from simple markers of injury severity and to then determine which such findings are best treated surgically. Although of interest, studies that determine indications for surgery in a post hoc fashion are of limited utility because they are confounded by generally indistinct clinical judgment factors and lack the required solid linkage between the surgical decision and improved outcome. As such, we lack strong evidence regarding the efficacy of surgery for those more badly injured patients with subdural hematomas that meet generally accepted but scientifically unfounded "mandates" for operative management. We have somewhat better evidence on patients who present in better condition.

Several studies address nonoperative management of subdural hematomas. Unfortunately, the criteria for selection of such patients are not explicit in these series although they all exclude patients with GCS scores at the lower end of the spectrum. These series have suggested that midline shift >5 mm or hematoma thickness >10 mm are associated with a need for delayed evacuation (although the delay was as long as 14 days in these reports).[32,33]

Servadei et al tested a protocol for nonoperative management of comatose patients with subdural hematomas.[34] Candidates had hematomas <10-mm thick and <5 mm of midline shift, showed no neurological deterioration, and underwent ICP monitoring. In this series, two of 15 candidate patients required surgery for intracranial hypertension and evolving intracerebral lesions. Two-thirds of the nonoperative group achieved good outcome.

The guidelines analyzed the evidence on the adverse association between advancing age, but were unable to find evidence that there is a strong age-sensitive interaction with surgical versus nonsurgical management, outside of questions of salvageability. These data do suggest that such considerations are relevant with respect to vigorous medical or surgical treatment in patients over 65 years of age.[27,30,35,36]

There are no controlled studies on the timing of surgery and outcome. All relevant studies are retrospective and have difficulty with controlling for confounding variables such as systemic hypotension and associated intracranial pathology. Studies on the interval between injury and surgery are somewhat mixed; most support a positive relationship, but some find no difference or even a negative correlation. More relevant are the reports on the interval between neurological deterioration or signs of herniation and operative intervention, which support a correlation between early surgery and improved outcome.[17,18] Based on synthesis of such class III evidence, the treatment option suggests that those patients selected for surgery should have their subdural hematoma evacuated as soon as possible.

Regarding the issue of surgical technique, there is one study that suggests that bur hole drainage of acute subdural hematomas in patients with low GCS scores is associated with increased mortality and poorer recovery.[29] Another study found increased mortality in patients who underwent decompressive craniotomy versus craniotomy with or without duraplasty but was unable to adequately control for confounding due to injury severity variables.[30] At an option level, the evidence report supported evacuation by craniotomy but did not otherwise specify procedural details.

Outside of the Evidence Report

Intracranial Pressure Monitoring

The indications for emergent evacuation are CT or clinical evidence of significant mass effect. Particularly because there is most commonly damage to the underlying brain, a small subdural hematoma does not eliminate the possibility of intracranial hypertension, so liberal use of ICP monitoring should be considered.

Noncomatose patients with small subdural hematomas and no evidence of herniation or neurological deterioration may be considered for nonoperative management. If such is selected, the patient must be kept under close clinical observation in an ICU setting with serial imaging to prove lack of expansion of the clot. ICP monitoring may also be considered in such patients, despite their higher level of consciousness.

Damage Control Surgery

In concept, evacuation of an acute subdural hematoma is a neurosurgical form of damage control surgery. It is frequently performed in the setting of polytrauma, where other systemic injuries are present and sometimes incompletely evaluated, the immediate course of the brain injury (e.g., likelihood of lesion evolution, swelling, etc.) is undetermined, there may be complicating factors such as coagulopathy or hemodynamic instability, and the patient would optimally be in ICU rather than theater. As such, the goals are to minimize or eliminate the acutely life-threatening neurosurgical issues in an expeditious fashion, without exposing the patient to undue risks. Viewed as such, there is much to be said for a large skin flap and generous craniotomy to allow for unforeseen circumstances such as remote sources of hemorrhage or malignant brain swelling. Should it be decided to leave the bone flap out, a large area of decompression is desirable. Large exposures also allow clot evacuation under direct vision. One of the principles of damage control surgery is to just do what is necessary rather than "be a hero." Leaving a bit of remote subdural blood is certainly preferable to tearing a frontal or parietal bridging vessel under the edge of the flap and then having to spend 15 to 20 minutes cleaning up the bleeding. Consistent with the damage control philosophy, it is also reasonable to leave out the flap in patients who appear to be actively swelling during surgery, will poorly tolerate intense ICP treatment, or will need other early surgical procedures for extracranial injuries.

Recommendations for Future Research

The Guidelines for the Surgical Management of Traumatic Brain Injury[3] stressed several areas in particular need of future research in this area, including the following:

- Class I or II outcome studies of the efficacy of surgical evacuation of subdural hematomas of sufficient power to allow for stratification with multivariate modeling of confounding variables. Such studies should allow addressing indications for and timing of surgery and should allow identification of groups that do and do not benefit from operative management, either versus medical management or as the natural history of their disease (e.g., in the aged patient).

Parenchymal Lesions

Intraparenchymal lesions may be focal or nonfocal (**Table 13.7**). Focal lesions include contusions, lacerations, hematomas, and infarctions. Nonfocal lesions include edema, disseminated swelling, and diffuse (axonal) injury. Such lesions may occur in isolation; more commonly, however, they appear in combination with

Table 13.7 Intraparenchymal Lesions

Focal	Nonfocal
Contusions	Edema
Lacerations	Disseminated swelling
Herniations	Diffuse axonal injury
Infarctions	

Table 13.8 Factors Correlated with Intracranial Hypertension or Neurological Deterioration

Physical Factors	Extracranial Factors
Type of lesion	Age
Location	Glasgow coma score
Volume	Hypotension
Presence of subarachnoid blood	Pupillary response
Cisternal compression	Brain stem reflexes
Midline shift	Coagulopathy
Surrounding edema	Presence and course of intracranial (IC) hypertension

other intracranial lesions. They may be apparent and stable from initial presentation, evolve over time, or appear in a delayed fashion. A subclass of hematomas that appear later has been termed delayed traumatic intracerebral hematoma (DTICH).

There are a large number of factors that have been correlated with intracranial hypertension or neurological deterioration in the face of intraparenchymal lesions (**Table 13.8**). Physical factors include type of lesion, location, volume, presence of subarachnoid blood, cisternal compression, midline shift, and surrounding edema. Several extracranial factors also correlate with outcome for patients with parenchymal lesions, including age, GCS, hypotension, pupillary responses, brain stem reflexes, coagulopathy, and presence and course of intracranial hypertension.

It was the goal of this evidence report to identify a subset of these factors the surgical management of which independently improves patient outcome or forestalls subsequent deterioration. It is the very question of the exact efficacy of surgery directed at specific indicators that is the main impediment to strong evidentiary statements in this area. There are no prospective studies on this topic; those studies that attempt to address this issue in a retrospective fashion lack explicit, comprehensive risk adjustment in their analyses.[37,38] As such, the practice parameters remain at the level of treatment options, based primarily on the ability of surgery to lower intracranial hypertension and the adverse influence on outcome of neurological deterioration prior to operative intervention.

The Guidelines for the Surgical Management of Traumatic Brain Injury were able to identify nothing more definitive than class III evidence regarding the indications for surgery for parenchymal lesions.[3] As such, they only provided treatment recommendations at the option level. These recommendations are presented in **Table 13.9**. The Guidelines for the Acute Medical Management of Severe Traumatic Brain Injury in Infants, Children, and Adolescents were able to identify nothing more definitive than class III evidence regarding the indications for surgery for parenchymal lesions.[4] As such, they only provided treatment recommendations at the option level. These recommendations are presented in **Table 13.10**.

Traumatic intraparenchymal lesions have long been a bastion of nonoperative management. Only recently has the concept of surgical management become a topic of general discussion and continues to engender significant controversy (**Table 13.11**). Despite the assumed value of decreasing mass effect arising from intracerebral hematomas (and, to a lesser extent, contusions), the frequent lack of clear lesion margins and the perceived surgical risk to surrounding, potentially salvageable brain drive the arguments that the outcome will not be improved by surgery. In light of this reasoning, simply demonstrating mass effect or correlating various anatomic and clinical parameters with patient deterioration or

Table 13.9 Class III (Practice Options) Evidence Regarding the Indications for Surgery for Intraparenchymal Lesions

Indications for surgery	Patients with parenchymal mass lesions and signs of progressive neurological deterioration referable to the lesion, medically refractory intracranial hypertension, or signs of mass effect on CT scan should be treated operatively.
	Patients with GCS score 6–8 with frontal or temporal contusions >20 cc in volume with midline shift 5 mm and/or cisternal compression on CT scan, and patients with any lesion >50 cc in volume should be treated operatively.
	Patients with parenchymal mass lesions who do not show evidence for neurological compromise, have controlled intracranial pressure, and no significant signs of mass effect on CT scan may be managed nonoperatively with intensive monitoring and serial imaging.
Timing and methods	Craniotomy with evacuation of mass lesion is recommended for those patients with focal lesions and the surgical indications listed above.
	Bifrontal decompressive craniectomy within 48 hours of injury is a treatment option for patients with diffuse, medically refractory posttraumatic cerebral edema and resultant intracranial hypertension.
	Decompressive procedures, including subtemporal decompression, temporal lobectomy, and hemispheric decompressive craniectomy, are treatment options for patients with refractory intracranial hypertension and diffuse parenchymal injury with clinical and radiographic evidence for impending transtentorial herniation.

Abbreviations: CT, computed tomography; GCS, Glasgow Coma Scale.

Table 13.10 Class III (Practice Options) Evidence regarding the Indications for Surgery for Intraparenchymal Lesions in Infants, Children, and Adolescents

- Decompressive craniectomy should be considered in pediatric patients with severe TBI, diffuse cerebral swelling, and intracranial hypertension refractory to intensive medical management.
- Decompressive craniectomy should be considered in the treatment of severe TBI and medically refractory intracranial hypertension in infants and young children with abusive head trauma.
- Decompressive craniectomy may be particularly appropriate in children with severe TBI and refractory intracranial hypertension who have a potentially recoverable brain injury. Decompressive craniectomy appears to be less effective in patients who have experienced extensive secondary brain insults. Patients who experience a secondary deterioration on the GCS and/or evolving cerebral herniation syndrome within the first 48 h after injury may represent a favorable group. Patients with an unimproved GCS of 3 may represent an unfavorable group.

Abbreviations: GCS, Glasgow Coma Scale; TBI, traumatic brain injury.

poor outcome does not directly support the efficacy of surgery. In the absence of controlled trials, we are left with attempts to retrospectively analyze the influence of surgery on outcome using multivariate analysis to adjust for confounding variables. At present, we have produced only class III evidence on this topic.

In general, the decision to perform surgery has been based on current medical data and the perceived risk of subsequent deterioration as estimated by the neurosurgeon. The primary data reported as valuable in such decision making include the size and location of the lesions, CT indicators of mass effect, degree and course of ICP, and status of the neurological examination with particular attention to progressive deterioration.[37–40] Although ICP is a critical component of this list, a sizable percentage of patients may demonstrate late deterioration without intracranial hypertension.[39] The issue then becomes whether patients with poor GCS scores, who are deteriorating or who are felt at risk of deterioration, will benefit from surgery.

Table 13.11 Surgical Management of Intraparenchymal Lesions

- Only recently has surgical management been discussed and remains controversial
  - Advantages: value of decreased mass effect arising from intracranial hematomas
  - Disadvantages: lack of clear lesion margins and risk to surrounding brain
- Decision to perform surgery rests on judgment of surgeon – must consider different variables:
  - Lesion size and location
  - Computed tomography indicators of mass effect
  - Degree and ease of management of intracranial hypertension
  - Status of neurological exam (paying close attention to progressive deterioration)

In a population of 202 patients with traumatic intracerebral hematomas, Choksey et al covaried craniotomy against a large spectrum of confounding variables.[37] Their logistic regression model found craniotomy to improve outcome with significant interactions with GCS score and hematoma volume >16 cc.

Mathiesen et al retrospectively analyzed 218 patients with isolated intracerebral lesions from the prospectively collected HIT-2 database.[40] They found that the groups that benefited from surgery were (1) patients with mass lesions >50 cc; (2) patients with lesions >20 cc with radiological signs of mass effect (compression of basal cisterns or midlines shift ≥5 mm); (3) patients with temporal contusions and radiological signs of mass effect. In these patients, neurological deterioration prior to surgery worsened recovery, supporting early surgery.

Katayama et al retrospectively constructed a small case-control study (using historical controls) to study the influence of surgery on patients with frontal lobe contusions and medically intractable intracranial hypertension.[38] They reported that surgical evacuation of the contusions was associated with a 22% mortality versus an 88% mortality in the nonsurgical group.

Delayed Traumatic Intracerebral Hematomas

Delayed traumatic intracerebral hematomas (DTICH) is most generally used to describe lesions appearing in an area of the brain previously demonstrated to be normal on CT imaging.[41,42] Most DTICH lesions appear within 48 to 72 hours[43,44] in patients with initially abnormal CT scans.[42,44] Factors associated with DTICH include secondary systemic insults, coagulopathy, and decompressive craniotomy.[45,46] Outside of DTICH alone, over 50% of patients with severe TBI will show evolution of their intracranial lesions over time, further stressing the importance of serial imaging.[47] There is no literature specifically germane to the role of surgery in managing DTICH.

Surgical Management of Nonfocal Intraparenchymal Lesions

Outside of evacuating a large, isolated intracerebral hematoma, the surgical management of nonfocal intraparenchymal lesions or diffuse swelling constitutes the performance of decompressive craniotomy. The logic behind this operation is to decrease the ICP and improve the compliance of the brain by decreasing the constraints on its ability to expand. That such obtains has been demonstrated intraoperatively for both removal of the bone flap and opening of the dura.[48,49] Comparison of ICP courses prior to and following such surgery has reinforced the efficacy of such a procedure in treating intracranial hypertension and reduced compliance.[48,50–52]

The literature on this topic generally supports decompression for refractory intracranial hypertension but uniformly lacks clear, prospectively tested selection criteria or internal controls.[50,53–55] Guerra prospectively studied an explicit treatment protocol defining ICP treatment and the triggers for decompression for refractory intracranial hypertension.[53] They reported favorable results for decompression. Unfortunately, their only controls were published results from studies of alternative treatments.

Polin et al[57] performed a retrospective case-control study of decompressive craniectomy for refractory intracranial hypertension in patients with Diffuse Injury III[56] patterns on CT. They gathered their controls from the Traumatic Coma Data Bank dataset, matching them for age, gender, and admission GCS score as well as maximum ICP during operationally defined preoperative and postoperative periods (defined according to a posited operative time of 48 hours after injury). They reported significantly better mortality and morbidity figures for the surgery group, particularly if the preoperative ICP maximum was <40 mm Hg and surgery was performed at ≤48 hours from injury.

In keeping with the lack of class I or II evidence on this topic and ongoing concerns regarding quality of life in those patients "rescued" by decompressive craniectomy, the recommendations in the Guidelines for the Surgical Management of Traumatic Brain Injury are very limited. They support the consideration of decompressive craniectomy as a treatment option for medically refractory intracranial hypertension, performed in an expeditious fashion. Relative indications for such surgery were not felt sufficiently well defined to warrant specification. More definitive guidelines will hopefully be obtained following completion of the two ongoing randomized controlled trials (RCTs) on this topic (RESCUEicp[58] and DECRA[59] trials).

The Guidelines for the Acute Medical Management of Severe Traumatic Brain Injury in Infants, Children, and Adolescents also addressed the issue of decompressive craniectomy.[4] Two class III pediatric studies were unique to these guidelines. Cho et al performed a prospective, case control study of medical therapy with or without early decompression for children with abusive brain injury.[60] Surgery was associated with decreased mortality and improved outcome. Taylor et al reported the results of a prospective RCT of decompression versus no surgery in 27 pediatric TBI patients with refractory intracranial hypertension.[61] Decompression consisted of bilateral temporal decompressions with no or minimal durotomy. They reported a strong, but nonsignificant trend toward improved ICP and better 6-month outcome for the surgery group. Although this was a prospective RCT, it was classified as class III evidence due to sample size and concerns regarding generalizability.

The recommendations in the Guidelines for the Acute Medical Management of Severe Traumatic Brain Injury in Infants, Children, and Adolescents[4] are similar to those of the Guidelines for the Surgical Management of TBI,[3] consisting of option-level support for considering decompressive craniectomy in the setting of medically refractory intracranial hypertension. Notably, they did extend these recommendations to cover brain injury due to abuse. Reflecting their analysis of the pediatric literature, they attempted to offer some guidelines for patient selection. They suggested that patients with GCS >3, who do not have devastating primary injuries and in whom early evolving secondary injuries appear to be strong determinants of potential recovery, constitute the most favorable candidates. They also stressed expeditious decompression when craniectomy is chosen.

Outside of the Evidence Report

Although efficacy remains without solid proof and the indications are not clearly defined, the Guidelines for the Surgical Management of Traumatic Brain Injury support the inclusion of surgical intervention into our armamentarium for managing traumatic parenchymal injuries. Because many of the suggested indications involve degrees of failure of ICP control or the progression of neurological deficits, it is important that (1) such patients be closely observed in a setting where reliable, repeated testing will be performed, with serial imaging at least until progression of neurological status, lesion size, or edema can be ruled out; and (2) ICP monitoring be considered when suspicious intraparenchymal lesions are present, including in patients who may be considered to have moderate or even mild TBI. In addition, given the evidence that delayed surgery is less effective, surgical decompression should not simply be relegated to the role of a last-ditch effort (**Table 13.12**). The potential use of decompressive craniectomy should be considered in light of frequent reevaluation of any difficult patient's course and response to treatment, with concomitant consideration of confounding extracranial variables (such as preexisting comorbidities or other injuries). Medical refractoriness of ICP control may arise not only from failure of all nonoperative measures, but also from issues such as a patient not being medically capable of tolerating such measures or when such treatments collide with interventions aimed at other serious issues. Obviously, this requires close involvement of the neurosurgical department in all aspects of the care of such patients.

Table 13.12 Indications for Decompressive Craniotomy

Indications
Intractable intracranial hypertension
Anticipated intractability of intracranial hypertension (e.g., steady or rapidly rising therapeutic intensity level)
Unfavorable risk:benefit ratio for nonoperative second-tier ICP treatments (e.g., barbiturate use in patient with pneumonia or unstable blood pressure)
Need to rapidly and definitively obviate the need for further ICP treatment (e.g., patient with intracranial hypertension who is developing ARDS)

Abbreviations: ARDS, adult respiratory stress syndrome; ICP, intracranial pressure.

In the absence of a specific literature, DTICH should probably be managed using the same set of indicators employed in surgical decision making for acute intraparenchymal lesions.

Surgical Techniques in Decompressive Craniectomy

The goal of decompressive craniectomy is to violate the basic principle of the Monro–Kellie Doctrine by expanding the space for the brain forcibly. To this end, removal of large bone flaps and leaving the dura widely open (with or without duraplasty) will be most effective (**Table 13.13**). Large openings will avoid the tissue damage and venous congestion that can occur with smaller craniectomies in the face of vigorous brain swelling. A large variety of techniques have been discussed, but there is very little basis for their objective comparison. There are several factors that might influence the surgical approach. Unilateral swelling is often best treated by a large, unilateral decompression. Diffuse, bifrontal, or bitemporal mass effect is better treated by bilateral frontal (or pan-frontal) techniques. Because these are generally sick patients, the surgeon must consider how much surgical time, blood loss, and tissue manipulation the patient can safely tolerate. One should consider how large an area is felt to need decompression (although the hazards of small decompressive flaps are well known). The impact of the decompression on postoperative management may also be germane. Some surgeons merely "float" the bone flap, rather than remove it. We tend to remove bilateral frontotemporoparietal flaps, leaving a thin strip of bone over the sagittal sinus to assist in monitor placement and postoperative helmet wear. Unfortunately, although uncommon, catastrophic injuries have occurred from fairly minor traumas to these patients prior to cranioplasty.

Table 13.13 Surgical Techniques in Decompressive Craniectomy

Technique	Comment
Removal of large bone flaps, leaving dura widely open	Most effective technique—avoids brain fungation and facilitates venous drainage
Unilateral decompression	Most effective for unilateral swelling
Bilateral frontal techniques	Most effective for diffuse, bifrontal, or bitemporal mass effect—need to consider surgical time, blood loss, and tissue manipulation tolerances of the patient
Management after decompression	Reassess intracranial pressure, cerebral blood flow, and metabolism, compliance postsurgery, and altered physiology (i.e., absent static autoregulation)

Although the goal of the surgery is to eliminate the need for further ICP treatment, intracranial hypertension does not always fully resolve following decompression. Because the physiology has now been altered, reassessment of ICP, cerebral blood flow and metabolism, and compliance are often critical to determine the need for and proper course of management after decompression. For instance, we have found that static autoregulation is generally absent after such operations, which may lead to hyperemic intracranial hypertension that may or may not need treating.

Recommendations for Future Research

The Guidelines for the Surgical Management of Traumatic Brain Injury[3] or The Guidelines for the Acute Medical Management of Severe Traumatic Brain Injury in Infants, Children, and Adolescents[4] stressed several areas felt particularly in need of future research in this area, including the following (**Table 13.14**):

- Class I or II outcome studies on the role of surgical management of intracerebral contusions and hematomas, compared with medical management of ICP and perfusion:metabolism matching
- Class I or II outcome studies of the safety and efficacy of decompressive craniotomy in the adult and pediatric populations, allowing for appropriate and valid risk adjustment. It is hoped that the ongoing RESCUEicp[58] and DECRA[59] trials will be of use in addressing this research need.
- Statistically solid investigations into the role of decompressive operations as treatment options earlier than the occurrence of medically refractory intracranial hypertension.
- Studies to identify physiologic indications for evacuation of intraparenchymal lesions or decompressive craniectomy, such as ICP course, pattern and value of the therapeutic intensity level, brain tissue oxygen saturation level, etc.

Table 13.14 Recommendations for Future Research in the Surgical Management of Parenchymal Lesions

Class I or II outcome studies on the role of surgical management of intracerebral contusions and hematomas, compared with medical management of intracranial pressure (ICP) and perfusion:metabolism matching
Class I or II outcome studies of the safety and efficacy of decompressive craniotomy in the adult and pediatric populations, allowing for appropriate and valid risk adjustment. It is hoped that the ongoing RESCUEicp[58] and DECRA[59] trials will be of use in addressing this research need.
Statistically solid investigations into the role of decompressive operations as treatment options earlier than the occurrence of medically refractory intracranial hypertension
Studies to identify physiologic indications for evacuation of intraparenchymal lesions or decompressive craniectomy, such as ICP course, pattern, and value of the therapeutic intensity level, brain tissue oxygen saturation level, etc.
Studies to evaluate the optimal surgical approaches to decompressive craniectomy

- Studies to evaluate the optimal surgical approaches to decompressive craniectomy

Table 13.15 Depressed Skull Fractures

Role	Skull fracture is the strongest predicator of intraparenchymal injury—the utility of this correlation has changed with the recent evolution and common use of computed tomography (CT).
Closed, nondisplaced fractures	Treated nonsurgically
Open fractures	Associated with overlying laceration that penetrates galea aponeurotica
	Accounts for the majority of depressed skull fractures
	Infection rate ~5–11%
	Epilepsy in ~15%
	Mortality in ~19%
Goals of treatment	Cosmesis
	Minimizing posttraumatic neurological deficits and epilepsy
	Avoiding infection (critical)—use of antibiotic is effective
Evolution of treatment	Traditionally all treated surgically—modern approach considers nonsurgical treatment with use of CT

Depressed Skull Fractures

A fracture of the skull is a strong, perhaps the strongest, predictor of intraparenchymal injury,[62–64] although the ascendant role of CT in evaluating patients with TBI now generally renders this correlation to historical interest (**Table 13.15**). Uncomplicated, nondisplaced, closed fractures are not treated surgically. The majority of depressed skull fractures are open[65,66] and are associated with infection rates of 5 to 11%,[67–69] associated epilepsy in up to 15%,[65,70] and mortality as high as 19%.[69,71] The goals of treatment are focused on cosmesis, minimizing the likelihood of posttraumatic neurological deficits and epilepsy, and avoidance of infection. Traditionally, compound fractures were treated surgically, whereas indications for operative management for all fractures have been depression beyond the inner table of the skull, presumably to minimize posttraumatic deficits or seizure disorders. Extenuating factors, such as facial sinus involvement or the presence of an underlying surgical mass lesion may separately determine the necessity of surgery. In general, the routine approach to depressed skull fractures arose from studies performed prior to the CT era, which established a strong correlation between penetration of the skull and neurological and epileptic disorders as well as between such disorders and infectious complication of compound injuries.[65,67,70] The Guidelines for the Surgical Management of TBI focused on studies from the post-CT era.

In these discussions, a fracture is defined as open (compound) if is associated with an overlying laceration that penetrates the galea aponeurotica.

The Guidelines for the Surgical Management of Traumatic Brain Injury were able to identify nothing more definitive than class III evidence regarding the indications for surgery for depressed skull fractures.[3] As such, they only provided treatment recommendations at the option level. These recommendations are presented in (**Table 13.16**).

All of the studies upon which these guidelines were based are class III, so the variables examined were not manipulated. As such, parameters such as "depression >1 cm" are more serendipitous than scientifically determined. Elevation of depressed bone does not appear critical in altering the incidence of posttraumatic epilepsy in simple, depressed skull fractures.[72]

Avoidance of infection is critical. Expeditious wound management and the use of antibiotics appear very effective in preventing infection in open wounds, obviating routine elevation and débridement.[69,71] When surgery is performed reasonably promptly, the incidence of infection does not appear to be increased by primary replacement of bone fragments,[66,73,74] even in the presence of obvious contamination.[74]

Unfortunately, the retrospective nature of these reports leaves the proper definition of "prompt surgery" and "contamination" somewhat unclear. In general, however, this evidence report greatly liberalizes the management

Table 13.16 Class III (Practice Options) Evidence regarding the Indications for Surgery for Depressed Skull Fractures

Indications for surgery	Patients with open (compound) skull fractures depressed greater than the thickness of the skull should undergo operative intervention to prevent infection.
	Patients with open (compound) depressed skull fractures may be treated nonoperatively if there is no clinical or radiographic evidence of dural penetration, significant intracranial hematoma, depression >1 cm, frontal sinus involvement, gross cosmetic deformity, wound infection, pneumocephalus, or gross wound contamination.
	Nonoperative management of closed (simple) depressed skull fractures is a treatment option.
Timing	Early operation is recommended to reduce the incidence of infection.
Methods	Elevation and débridement is recommended as the surgical method of choice.
	Primary bone fragment replacement is a surgical option in the absence of wound infection at the time of surgery.
	All management strategies for open (compound) depressed fractures should include antibiotics.

of depressed fractures in general and compound fractures in particular, in contrast to "traditional" management, eliminating a primary surgery in many patients and a secondary cranioplasty in most.

Outside of the Evidence Report

Of all of the sections in the Guidelines for the Surgical Management of Traumatic Brain Injury, this one questions the most generally accepted tenets of treatment, including the necessity of routine operative management of open, depressed skull fractures. It should be kept in mind, however, that the literature base remains at class III. Until more rigorous data are available, application of the recommendations contained herein should be accompanied by diligence in ensuring optimal outcome in individual patients through follow-up and serial imaging. In particular, it is important to avoid infectious complications.

Recommendations for Future Research

The Guidelines for the Surgical Management of Traumatic Brain Injury[3] stressed several areas in particular need of future research in this area, including the following:

- Well-designed, prospective studies or RCTs of surgical technique to examine issues such as bone fragment replacement versus removal, dural laceration repair, the removal of metal fragments, etc., with respect to outcome variables such as incidence of infection, incidence of epilepsy, need for reoperation, surgical complications, etc., in addition to outcome.

Posterior Fossa Mass Lesions

Posterior fossa lesions represent a minority of traumatic mass lesions but are problematic due to their treacherous nature and our lack of adequate monitoring technology applicable to this intracranial compartment (**Table 13.17**). As opposed to the situation with supratentorial lesions, mass effect in the posterior fossa frequently presents with precipitous, often permanent neurological deterioration, due to the small compartment volume and the direct proximity of the brain stem. As such, early and more subtle signs of deterioration such as increasing headache or increasing somnolence cannot be reliably used to determine the need for surgical intervention, as they more frequently can for the supratentorial compartment. In the absence of the ability to measure ICP or tissue oxygen tension in the posterior fossa, we are left with anatomic markers as virtually our sole tools.

The Guidelines for the Surgical Management of Traumatic Brain Injury were able to identify nothing more definitive than class III evidence regarding the indications for surgery for posterior fossa mass lesions.[3] As such, they only provided treatment recommendations at the option level. These recommendations are presented in (**Table 13.18**).

This literature consists entirely of class III studies, all of which involve retrospectively collected data. Because the vast majority of acute posterior fossa lesions are epidural hematomas, most studies deal exclusively with these lesions. In addition, the majority of publications deal with attempting to identify factors associated with neurological deterioration (requiring surgery) or death. Difficulty with adequately controlling the contribution of confounding variables such as presenting GCS and associated supratentorial lesions greatly weakened all outcome analyses.

Table 13.17 Posterior Fossa Mass Lesions

Role	Accounts for a minority of traumatic mass lesions
Problematic	Due to treacherous nature and lack of adequate monitoring technology
Often presents with	Precipitous, often permanent neurological deterioration
	Increasing headache
	Increasing somnolence
	Computed tomography evidence of associated hydrocephalus

Table 13.18 Class III (Practice Options) Evidence Regarding the Indications for Surgery for Posterior Fossa Mass Lesions

Indications for surgery	Patients with mass effect on computed tomography (CT) scan or with neurological dysfunction or deterioration referable to the lesion should undergo operative intervention. Mass effect on CT scan is defined as distortion, dislocation, or obliteration of the fourth ventricle, compression or loss of visualization of the basal cisterns, or the presence of obstructive hydrocephalus.
	Patients with lesions and no significant mass effect on CT scan and without signs of neurological dysfunction may be managed by close observation and serial imaging.
Timing	In patients with indications for surgical intervention, evacuation should be performed as soon as possible because these patients can deteriorate rapidly, thus worsening their prognosis.
Methods	Suboccipital craniectomy is the predominant method reported for evacuation of posterior fossa mass lesions and is therefore recommended.

As noted above, the recommendations for surgical intervention are based on findings consistent with mass effect on CT imaging. For epidural hematomas, qualitative findings, such as the presence of hydrocephalus or deformation of the fourth ventricle, appear to correlate with improved outcome with surgery.[75–78] Although no quantitative definition of surgical mass effect is uniformly available, mass volume >10 cc, thickness >15 mm, and shift >5 mm are reasonably representative of parameters applicable to acute epidural hematomas.[76–78] Surgical indicators for subdural hematomas or intraparenchymal lesions are even less clear due to a distinct dearth of studies, but hematoma diameter >3 cm, obscuration of the fourth ventricle, or hydrocephalus has been suggested.[79,80] Qualitatively, mass effect on the fourth ventricle or the basal cisterns, or obstructive hydrocephalus is a fairly consistent surgical indicator across all lesions.

Bozbuga et al presented the results of a treatment protocol for epidural hematomas where surgery was predicated on any signs of mass effect and all patients without mass effect were managed nonoperatively.[75] Notably, all nonoperatively managed patients had GCS ≥14. No patient required delayed decompression. All patients treated without surgery did well. Due to confounding variables, a comparison of outcomes between the two groups was not valuable. This study suggests that epidural hematomas without mass effect in patients with very good levels of consciousness can be safely managed without surgery. The available literature supports surgical management of the rest of these lesions prior to neurological deterioration.

Outside of the Evidence Report

For epidural hematomas, the procedure is fairly straightforward in the absence of involvement of major venous sinuses. Evacuation of the hematoma and control of any encountered sources should be definitive. Whenever sinus involvement is suspected, resources for rapid, large-volume transfusion should be made available, and exposure should allow access to all aspects of the venous structure whenever possible. Obviously, it is desirable to maintain patency of such sinuses, but this is not always possible. In relatively stable cases, preoperative vascular imaging (e.g., CT venography) can be useful for planning.

Acute decompression of a posterior fossa subdural or intraparenchymal mass lesion is an instance of neurosurgical damage control. Mass effect on the fourth ventricle and brain stem must be removed and prevented from recurring. There is no literature to guide estimation of the risk of lesion evolution or edema progression in the posterior fossa, so generous decompression and duraplasty are generally recommended. This is true even more so than in the supratentorial space, as we have no reliable methods or parameters for measuring and treating posterior fossa compartmental pressures. Frank hematomas that are large or readily accessible can be removed, but this, in itself, does not usually afford sufficient decompression in the acute setting. Removal of normal cerebellar tissue for decompressive purposes is not recommended.

Consideration should be given to placement of an external ventricular drain prior to, during, or following surgery based on the presence of ventriculomegaly or perception of compression of cerebrospinal fluid (CSF) outflow tracts.

Recommendations for Future Research

The Guidelines for the Surgical Management of Traumatic Brain Injury[3] stressed several areas in particular need of future research in this area, including the following:

- Class I or II outcome studies on posterior fossa mass lesions to determine the efficacy of and indications for surgical management. Studied indicators should include neurological status and course, CT evidence of mass effect (with or without frank hematoma)

Penetrating Brain Injury

Penetrating brain injury comprises the gamut from bullet wounds through shrapnel or other foreign objects, civilian or military settings, intentional-interpersonal, self-inflicted,

Table 13.19 Penetrating Brain Injury

Includes	Bullet wounds, shrapnel, stab injuries, etc.; intentional-interpersonal, self-inflicted or accidental circumstances, in civilian or military settings
Case mortality	Approximately 94%
Civilian vs. military setting mortality rates	Military = 16–25%
	Civilian = 54–61%
	Variation due to differences in transport logistics and triage, as well as physics and circumstances of injuries
Decision to operate based on	Clinical course
	Status of entry (and exit) wounds
	Presence of hematoma (mass effect)
	Presence of herniation
	Intracranial pressure
	Prognostic impressions and quality-of-life issues
Wound management	Simple wounds—irrigated and closed at bedside
	Complex wounds—more formal surgical approach, stressing the importance of watertight closure of healthy tissue
Infection control	Coverage with broad spectrum antibiotics in all patients
	Avoidance or elimination of cerebrospinal fluid leakage
Vascular injury	Angiographic study recommended, particularly when vascular injury is suspected (e.g., wound trajectory through or near sylvian fissure, supraclinoid carotid, cavernous sinus, or major venous sinus, substantial and otherwise unexplained subarachnoid hemorrhage, or delayed hematoma)

or accidental circumstances, etc. (**Table 13.19**). The case mortality of penetrating brain injuries is estimated at 94% by the Centers for Disease Control and Prevention (Atlanta, GA).[81] Presentation of such patients to treatment facilities represents a subpopulation selected by factors such as natural history and triage. Mortality in modern military settings appears to be in the range of 16 to 25%,[82,83] whereas mortality in patients surviving to hospital in civilian settings appears to be in the range of 54 to 61%,[84,85] the difference, in part, due to differences in transport logistics and triage.

Military and civilian injuries differ significantly in terms of projectile type and velocity, associated injuries, prehospital triage and transport, and so on. Nevertheless, the literature bases complement each other, and recommendations within the Guidelines for the Management of Penetrating Brain Injury did not differentiate between the two sources.[5] As such, the literature discussion herein will combine them.

As with nonpenetrating brain injuries, the decision to operate is profoundly influenced by prognostic impressions regarding mortality and quality-of-life issues. Prognosis in penetrating injuries remains inexact, and a discussion of such is outside the scope of this chapter. The Guidelines for the Management of Penetrating Brain Injury present an evidence report on prognosis to which the reader is referred.[5]

The Guidelines for the Management of Penetrating Brain Injury were able to identify nothing more definitive than class III evidence regarding the indications for surgery.[5] As such, they only provided treatment recommendations at the option level. These recommendations are presented in (**Table 13.20**).

Although the issue of limited débridement was addressed in civilian literature prior to military studies, the largest and best controlled studies come from the latter. There are no controlled trials in this area, although some large studies are able to use multivariate statistics to achieve reasonable risk adjustment.[86] The U.S. military command policy in place through the Vietnam conflict mandated aggressive removal of all intracranial bone or metal fragments, including reexploration if necessary.[87,88] Publications from non-U.S. conflicts, where wound management was felt paramount and aggressive débridement of foreign material was not routine,[86,89,90] report morbidity and mortality rates that are very comparable to those from U.S. studies. CT-era civilian studies appear to corroborate the efficacy of limited débridement in the nonmilitary setting although their numbers are much smaller.[84,85,91] The appeal of abandoning routine complete débridement is further enhanced by reports of significant associated complication rates, particularly for repeated surgery.[88,92]

One of the arguments for aggressive débridement has been to decrease the incidence of epilepsy. Relevant to this issue, the largest and best controlled study is that by

Table 13.20 Class III (Practice Options) Evidence Regarding the Indications for Surgery for Penetrating Brain Injury

- Treatment of small entrance bullet wounds to the head with local wound care and closure in patients whose scalp is not devitalized and have no "significant" intracranial pathologic findings is recommended. (Note: The term *significant* has yet to be clearly defined. However, the volume and location of the brain injury, evidence of mass effect, e.g., displacement of the midline 5 mm or compression of basilar cisterns from edema or hematoma, and the patient's clinical condition all pertain to significance.)
- Treatment of more extensive wounds with nonviable scalp, bone, or dura with more extensive débridement before primary closure or grafting to secure a watertight wound is recommended. In patients with significant fragmentation of the skull, débridement of the cranial wound with either craniectomy or craniotomy is recommended.
- In the presence of significant mass effect, débridement of necrotic brain tissue and safely accessible bone fragments is recommended. Evacuation of intracranial hematomas with significant mass effect is recommended.
- In the absence of significant mass effect, surgical débridement of the missile track in the brain is not recommended based on class III evidence that outcomes are not measurably worse in patients who do not have aggressive débridement. Routine surgical removal of fragments lodged distant from the entry site and reoperation solely to remove retained bone or missile fragments are not recommended.
- Repair of an open-air sinus injury with watertight closure of the dura is recommended. Clinical circumstances dictate the timing of the repair. Any repairs requiring duraplasty can be at the discretion of the surgeon as to material used for closure.
- Surgical correction is recommended for cerebrospinal fluid (CSF) leaks that do not close spontaneously, or are refractory to temporary CSF diversion. During the primary surgery, every effort should be made to close the dura and prevent CSF leaks.

Salazar et al on 421 patients from the Vietnam Head Injury Study.[93] Among other covarying factors, they found that the incidence of posttraumatic epilepsy was associated with retained metal fragments but not with retained bone. These correlations were corroborated in a smaller and less well-controlled study using a population treated with less aggressive débridement.[83] The Guidelines for the Management of Penetrating Brain Injury interpreted these studies as supporting the abandonment of routine complete débridement of bone fragments.[5] Whether there is a role for attempting to selectively remove all metal fragments (without causing further tissue injury) for the expressed purpose of decreasing the incidence of late seizures has not been studied and remains quite unclear.

Given the very strong correlation between CSF leaks, infection, and morbidity and mortality,[94] the Guidelines for the Management of Penetrating Brain Injury recommended aggressive attempts to avoid such leaks.[5] It is noted that not all of them occur at entry or exit wounds, some appearing clinically associated with fracture sites, etc.[94] There were no recommendations as to surgical management techniques.

Regarding the issue of timing of surgery, these guidelines determined the available literature inadequate to support evidence-based recommendations.[5] It was suggested that surgery be performed as soon as the indications for operation are recognized.

Civilian studies of both adult and pediatric patients, including the incorporation of limited wound management approaches in applicable patients, have included the surgical evacuation of intracranial hematomas associated with and felt to be contributing to mass effect or intracranial hypertension.[84,85,91] No studies were large enough to assess the independent contribution of such hematoma removal to improved survival, so the recommendation contained in the penetrating brain injury guidelines is a treatment option to evacuate hematomas with significant mass effect (where significant is not defined) in patients deemed salvageable.[5]

Outside of the Evidence Report

Once a penetrating brain injury patient has been deemed salvageable, a decision to operate is based on the clinical course, status of the entry (and exit, where present) wounds, whether there is a hematoma responsible for mass effect, herniation, or intracranial hypertension, and the ICP. Early initiation of ICP monitoring is supported at an option level in these guidelines.[5] As coagulopathy and lesion progression is common in these patients, repeated CT imaging should be considered.

Simple wounds can be irrigated and closed at the bedside. More complex wounds may require the same in theater. Wound care will require a more formal surgical approach when there is significant wound devitalization or tissue loss, brain or CSF is apparent in the wound, or the bone is too depressed or badly comminuted. The importance of avoiding a CSF leak cannot be overstressed, emphasizing the necessity of watertight closure. The scalp wound should be managed such that viable tissue is approximated without tension.

The occurrence of a traumatic aneurysm or arteriovenous fistula should be investigated by CT angiography or conventional angiography.[5] This is particularly true when the trajectory involves the circle of Willis or the sylvian fissure or there is a large intracerebral hematoma.

The danger and gravity of intracranial infection in penetrating injury to the brain warrant antibiotic coverage. The Guidelines for the Management of Penetrating Brain Injury recommend the routine use of broad spectrum antibiotics in these cases to cover the wide range of organisms that may be involved.[5] There is insufficient evidence to allow recommendations regarding either the specific antibiotics or the duration of treatment.

Recommendations for Future Research

The Guidelines for the Management of Penetrating Brain Injury[5] stressed several areas in particular need of future research in this area (**Tables 13.21**), including the following:

- Outcome studies of limited versus radical débridement of penetrating brain wounds, designed to allow statistical control for variables such as type of injury, admission GCS score, and timing of surgery
- Outcome studies designed to determine which intracranial mass lesions should be evacuated

Table 13.21 Recommendations for Future Research in the Surgical Management of Penetrating Brain Injuries

- Outcome studies of limited versus radical débridement of penetrating brain wounds, designed to allow statistical control for variables such as type of injury, admission Glasgow Coma Scale score, and timing of surgery
- Outcome studies designed to determine which intracranial mass lesions should be evacuated

References

1 Moore EE, Maier RV, Hoyt DB, Jurkovich GJ, Trunkey DD. Acute care surgery: J Am Coll Surg 2006;202(4):698–701
2. Bullock R, Chesnut R, Clifton G, et al. Guidelines for the Management of Severe Head Injury. J Neurotrauma 1996;13(11):639–734
3. Bullock MR, Chesnut R, Ghajar J, et al. Guidelines for the Surgical Management of Traumatic Brain Injury. Neurosurgery 2006;58(3, Suppl): S1–S60
4. Adelson PD, Bratton SL, Carney NA, et al. Guidelines for the Acute Medical Management of Severe Traumatic Brain Injury in Infants, Children, and Adolescents. Pediatr Crit Care Med 2003;4(3, Suppl):S72–S75
5. Aarabi B, Alden TD, Chesnut RMD, et al. Guidelines for the Management of Penetrating Brain Injury. J Trauma 2001;51(2, Suppl):S1–S86
6. Gabriel EJ, Ghajar J, Jagoda A, Pons PT, Scalea T, Walters BC. Guidelines for prehospital management of traumatic brain injury. J Neurotrauma 2002;19(1):111–174
7. Marshall LF, Gautille T, Klauber MR, et al. The outcome of severe head injury. J Neurosurg 1991;75:S28–S36
8. Servadei F, Faccani G, Roccella P, et al. Asymptomatic extradural haematomas: results of a multicenter study of 158 cases in minor head injury. Acta Neurochir (Wien) 1989;96(1–2):39–45
9. Bejjani GK, Donahue DJ, Rusin J, Broemeling LD. Radiological and clinical criteria for the management of epidural hematomas in children. Pediatr Neurosurg 1996;25(6):302–308
10. Bezircioglu H, Ersahin Y, Demircivi F, Yurt I, Donertas K, Tektas S. Nonoperative treatment of acute extradural hematomas: analysis of 80 cases. J Trauma 1996;41(4):696–698
11. Chen TY, Wong CW, Chang CN, et al. The expectant treatment of "asymptomatic" supratentorial epidural hematomas. Neurosurgery 1993;32(2):176–179, discussion 179
12. Lee EJ, Hung YC, Wang LC, Chung KC, Chen HH. Factors influencing the functional outcome of patients with acute epidural hematomas: analysis of 200 patients undergoing surgery. J Trauma 1998;45(5):946–952
13. van den Brink WA, Zwienenberg M, Zandee SM, van der Meer L, Maas AI, Avezaat CJ. The prognostic importance of the volume of traumatic epidural and subdural haematomas revisited. Acta Neurochir (Wien) 1999;141(5):509–514
14. Bullock R, Smith RM, van Dellen JR. Nonoperative management of extradural hematoma. Neurosurgery 1985;16(5):602–606
15. Cucciniello B, Martellotta N, Nigro D, Citro E. Conservative management of extradural haematomas. Acta Neurochir (Wien) 1993;120(1–2):47–52
16. Cohen JE, Montero A, Israel ZH. Prognosis and clinical relevance of anisocoria-craniotomy latency for epidural hematoma in comatose patients. J Trauma 1996;41(1):120–122
17. Sakas DE, Bullock MR, Teasdale GM. One-year outcome following craniotomy for traumatic hematoma in patients with fixed dilated pupils. J Neurosurg 1995;82(6):961–965
18. Haselsberger K, Pucher R, Auer LM. Prognosis after acute subdural or epidural haemorrhage. Acta Neurochir (Wien) 1988;90(3–4):111–116
19. Pickard JD, Bailey S, Sanderson H, Rees M, Garfield JS. Steps towards cost-benefit analysis of regional neurosurgical care. BMJ 1990;301(6753): 629–635 [see comments]
20. Bricolo AP, Pasut LM. Extradural hematoma: toward zero mortality: a prospective study. Neurosurgery 1984;14(1):8–12
21. Poon WS, Li AK. Comparison of management outcome of primary and secondary referred patients with traumatic extradural haematoma in a neurosurgical unit. Injury 1991;22(4):323–325
22. Wester K. Decompressive surgery for "pure" epidural hematomas: does neurosurgical expertise improve the outcome? Neurosurgery 1999;44(3):495–500, discussion 500–492
23. Rinker CF, McMurry FG, Groeneweg VR, Bahnson FF, Banks KL, Gannon DM. Emergency craniotomy in a rural level III trauma center. J Trauma 1998;44(6):984–989, discussion 989–990
24. Dent DL, Croce MA, Menke PG, et al. Prognostic factors after acute subdural hematoma. J Trauma 1995;39(1):36–42, discussion 42–33
25. Massaro F, Lanotte M, Faccani G, Triolo C. One hundred and twenty-seven cases of acute subdural haematoma operated on: correlation between CT scan findings and outcome. Acta Neurochir (Wien) 1996; 138(2):185–191
26. Servadei F, Nasi MT, Giuliani G, et al. CT prognostic factors in acute subdural haematomas: the value of the 'worst' CT scan. Br J Neurosurg 2000;14(2):110–116
27. Howard MA III, Gross AS, Dacey RG Jr, Winn HR. Acute subdural hematomas: an age-dependent clinical entity. J Neurosurg 1989;71(6): 858–863
28. Domenicucci M, Strzelecki JW, Delfini R. Acute posttraumatic subdural hematomas: "intradural" computed tomographic appearance as a favorable prognostic factor. Neurosurgery 1998;42(1):51–55
29. Hatashita S, Koga N, Hosaka Y, Takagi S. Acute subdural hematoma: severity of injury, surgical intervention, and mortality. Neurol Med Chir (Tokyo) 1993;33(1):13–18
30. Koc RK, Akdemir H, Oktem IS, Meral M, Menku A. Acute subdural hematoma: outcome and outcome prediction. Neurosurg Rev 1997; 20(4):239–244
31. Zumkeller M, Behrmann R, Heissler HE, Dietz H. Computed tomographic criteria and survival rate for patients with acute subdural hematoma. Neurosurgery 1996;39(4):708–712, discussion 712–703
32. Mathew P, Oluoch-Olunya DL, Condon BR, Bullock R. Acute subdural haematoma in the conscious patient: outcome with initial non-operative management. Acta Neurochir (Wien) 1993;121(3–4):100–108
33. Wong CW. Criteria for conservative treatment of supratentorial acute subdural haematomas. Acta Neurochir (Wien) 1995;135(1–2):38–43
34. Servadei F, Nasi MT, Cremonini AM, Giuliani G, Cenni P, Nanni A. Importance of a reliable admission Glasgow Coma Scale score for determining the need for evacuation of posttraumatic subdural hematomas: a prospective study of 65 patients. J Trauma 1998;44(5): 868–873

35. Jamjoom A. Justification for evacuating acute subdural haematomas in patients above the age of 75 years. Injury 1992;23(8):518–520
36. Wilberger JE Jr, Harris M, Diamond DL. Acute subdural hematoma: morbidity, mortality, and operative timing. J Neurosurg 1991;74(2):212–218
37. Choksey M, Crockard HA, Sandilands M. Acute traumatic intracerebral haematomas: determinants of outcome in a retrospective series of 202 cases. Br J Neurosurg 1993;7(6):611–622
38. Katayama Y, Tsubokawa T, Miyazaki S, Kawamata T, Yoshino A. Oedema fluid formation within contused brain tissue as a cause of medically uncontrollable elevation of intracranial pressure: the role of surgical therapy. Acta Neurochir Suppl (Wien) 1990;51:308–310
39. Bullock R, Golek J, Blake G. Traumatic intracerebral hematoma: which patients should undergo surgical evacuation? CT scan features and ICP monitoring as a basis for decision making. Surg Neurol 1989;32(3):181–187
40. Mathiesen T, Kakarieka A, Edner G. Traumatic intracerebral lesions without extracerebral haematoma in 218 patients. Acta Neurochir (Wien) 1995;137(3–4):155–163, discussion 163
41. Bollinger O. Uber traumatische spät-apoplexie: ein beitrag zur lehre von der hirnerschaütterung. Internationale beiträge zur wissenschaftlichen medicine Festschrift Rudolph Virchow Berlin. Hirchwald. 1891;2:457–470
42. Gentleman D, Nath F, Macpherson P. Diagnosis and management of delayed traumatic intracerebral haematomas. Br J Neurosurg 1989;3(3):367–372
43. Sprick C, Bettag M, Bock WJ. Delayed traumatic intracranial hematomas: clinical study of seven years. Neurosurg Rev 1989;12(Suppl 1):228–230
44. Tseng SH. Delayed traumatic intracerebral hemorrhage: a study of prognostic factors. J Formos Med Assoc 1992;91(6):585–589
45. Gudeman SK, Kishore PR, Miller JD, Girevendulis AK, Lipper MH, Becker DP. The genesis and significance of delayed traumatic intracerebral hematoma. Neurosurgery 1979;5(3):309–313
46. Kaufman HH, Moake JL, Olson JD, et al. Delayed and recurrent intracranial hematomas related to disseminated intravascular clotting and fibrinolysis in head injury. Neurosurgery 1980;7(5):445–449
47. Lobato RD, Gomez PA, Alday R, et al. Sequential computerized tomography changes and related final outcome in severe head injury patients. Acta Neurochir (Wien) 1997;139(5):385–391
48. Hase U, Reulen HJ, Meinig G, Schurmann K. The influence of the decompressive operation on the intracranial pressure and the pressure-volume relation in patients with severe head injuries. Acta Neurochir (Wien) 1978;45(1–2):1–13
49. Yoo DS, Kim DS, Cho KS, Huh PW, Park CK, Kang JK. Ventricular pressure monitoring during bilateral decompression with dural expansion. J Neurosurg 1999;91(6):953–959
50. Gower DJ, Lee KS, McWhorter JM. Role of subtemporal decompression in severe closed head injury. Neurosurgery 1988;23(4):417–422
51. Munch E, Horn P, Schurer L, Piepgras A, Paul T, Schmiedek P. Management of severe traumatic brain injury by decompressive craniectomy. Neurosurgery 2000;47(2):315–322, discussion 322–313
52. Whitfield PC, Patel H, Hutchinson PJ, et al. Bifrontal decompressive craniectomy in the management of posttraumatic intracranial hypertension. Br J Neurosurg 2001;15(6):500–507
53. Guerra WK, Gaab MR, Dietz H, Mueller JU, Piek J, Fritsch MJ. Surgical decompression for traumatic brain swelling: indications and results. J Neurosurg 1999;90(2):187–196
54. Kunze E, Meixensberger J, Janka M, Sorensen N, Roosen K. Decompressive craniectomy in patients with uncontrollable intracranial hypertension. Acta Neurochir Suppl (Wien) 1998;71:16–18
55. Yamaki T, Hirakawa K, Ueguchi T, Tenjin H, Kuboyama T, Nakagawa Y. Chronological evaluation of acute traumatic intracerebral haematoma. Acta Neurochir (Wien) 1990;103(3–4):112–115
56. Marshall LF, Bowers-Marshall S, Klauber MR, et al. A new classification of head injury based on computerized tomography. J Neurosurg 1991;75(Suppl):S14–S20
57. Polin RS, Shaffrey ME, Bogaev CA, et al. Decompressive bifrontal craniectomy in the treatment of severe refractory posttraumatic cerebral edema. Neurosurgery 1997;41(1):84–92, discussion 92–84
58. Hutchinson PJ, Corteen E, Czosnyka M, et al. Decompressive craniectomy in traumatic brain injury: the randomized multicenter RESCUEicp study (*www.RESCUEicp.com*). Acta Neurochir Suppl (Wien) 2006;96:17–20
59. Rosenfeld JV, Cooper DJ, Kossmann T, Murray L, Kaye AH. Decompressive craniectomy. J Neurosurg 2007;106(1):195–196, author reply 197
60. Cho DY, Wang YC, Chi CS. Decompressive craniotomy for acute shaken/impact baby syndrome. Pediatr Neurosurg 1995;23(4):192–198
61. Taylor A, Butt W, Rosenfeld J, et al. A randomized trial of very early decompressive craniectomy in children with traumatic brain injury and sustained intracranial hypertension. Childs Nerv Syst 2001;17(3):154–162
62. Chan KH, Mann KS, Yue CP, Fan YW, Cheung M. The significance of skull fracture in acute traumatic intracranial hematomas in adolescents: a prospective study. J Neurosurg 1990;72(2):189–194
63. Hung CC, Chiu WT, Lee LS, Lin LS, Shih CJ. Risk factors predicting surgically significant intracranial hematomas in patients with head injuries. J Formos Med Assoc 1996;95(4):294–297
64. Servadei F, Ciucci G, Pagano F, et al. Skull fracture as a risk factor of intracranial complications in minor head injuries: a prospective CT study in a series of 98 adult patients. J Neurol Neurosurg Psychiatry 1988;51(4):526–528
65. Braakman R. Depressed skull fracture: data, treatment, and follow-up in 225 consecutive cases. J Neurol Neurosurg Psychiatry 1972;35(3):395–402
66. Wylen EL, Willis BK, Nanda A. Infection rate with replacement of bone fragment in compound depressed skull fractures. Surg Neurol 1999;51(4):452–457
67. Jennett B, Miller JD. Infection after depressed fracture of skull. Implications for management of nonmissile injuries. J Neurosurg 1972;36(3):333–339
68. Mendelow AD, Campbell D, Tsementzis SA, et al. Prophylactic antimicrobial management of compound depressed skull fracture. J R Coll Surg Edinb 1983;28(2):80–83
69. van den Heever CM, van der Merwe DJ. Management of depressed skull fractures: selective conservative management of nonmissile injuries. J Neurosurg 1989;71(2):186–190
70. Jennett B, Miller JD, Braakman R. Epilepsy after monmissile depressed skull fracture. J Neurosurg 1974;41(2):208–216
71. Heary RF, Hunt CD, Krieger AJ, Schulder M, Vaid C. Nonsurgical treatment of compound depressed skull fractures. J Trauma 1993;35(3):441–447
72. Steinbok P, Flodmark O, Martens D, Germann ET. Management of simple depressed skull fractures in children. J Neurosurg 1987;66(4):506–510
73. Adeloye A, Shokunbi MT. Immediate bone replacement in compound depressed skull fractures. Cent Afr J Med 1993;39(4):70–73
74. Blankenship JB, Chadduck WM, Boop FA. Repair of compound-depressed skull fractures in children with replacement of bone fragments. Pediatr Neurosurg 1990;16(6):297–300
75. Bozbuga M, Izgi N, Polat G, Gurel I. Posterior fossa epidural hematomas: observations on a series of 73 cases. Neurosurg Rev 1999;22(1):34–40
76. Karasawa H, Furuya H, Naito H, Sugiyama K, Ueno J, Kin H. Acute hydrocephalus in posterior fossa injury. J Neurosurg 1997;86(4):629–632
77. Otsuka S, Nakatsu S, Matsumoto S, et al. Study on cases with posterior fossa epidural hematoma: clinical features and indications for operation. Neurol Med Chir (Tokyo) 1990;30(1):24–28
78. Tsai FY, Teal JS, Itabashi HH, Huprich JE, Hieshima GB, Segall HD. Computed tomography of posterior fossa trauma. J Comput Assist Tomogr 1980;4(3):291–305
79. d'Avella D, Servadei F, Scerrati M, et al. Traumatic intracerebellar hemorrhage: clinicoradiological analysis of 81 patients. Neurosurgery 2002;50(1):16–25, discussion 25–17
80. Pozzati E, Grossi C, Padovani R. Traumatic intracerebellar hematomas. J Neurosurg 1982;56(5):691–694
81. Center for Disease Control. Surveillance data on traumatic brain injury. MMWR Morb Mortal Wkly Rep 1997;46:8–11

82. Aarabi B. Surgical outcome in 435 patients who sustained missile head wounds during the Iran-Iraq War. Neurosurgery 1990;27(5):692–695, discussion 695
83. Brandvold B, Levi L, Feinsod M, George ED. Penetrating craniocerebral injuries in the Israeli involvement in the Lebanese conflict, 1982–85. J Neurosurg 1990;72:15–21
84. Shoung HM, Sichez JP, Pertuiset B. The early prognosis of craniocerebral gunshot wounds in civilian practice as an aid to the choice of treatment. Acta Neurochir (Wien) 1985;74:27–30
85. Suddaby L, Weir B, Forsyth C. The management of.22 caliber gunshot wounds of the brain: a review of 49 cases. Can J Neurol Sci 1987;14:268–272
86. Aarabi B, Taghipour M, Alibaii E, Kamgarpour A. Central nervous system infections after military missile head wounds. Neurosurgery 1998;42(3):500–507, discussion 507–509
87. Carey ME, Young HR, Rish BL, Mathis JL. Follow-up study of 103 American soldiers who sustained a brain wound in Vietnam. J Neurosurg 1974;41:542–549
88. Hammon WM. Analysis of 2187 consecutive penetrating wounds of the brain from Vietnam. J Neurosurg 1971;34:127–131
89. Levi L, Borovich B, Guilburd JN, et al. Wartime neurosurgical experience in Lebanon, 1982–85, I: Penetrating craniocerebral injuries. Isr J Med Sci 1990;26(10):548–554
90. Taha JM, Saba MI, Brown JA. Missile injuries to the brain treated by simple wound closure: results of a protocol during the Lebanese Conflict. Neurosurgery 1991;29:380–383
91. Sarnaik AP, Kopec J, Moylan P, Alvarez D, Canady A. Role of aggressive intracranial pressure control in management of pediatric craniocerebral gunshot wounds with unfavorable features. J Trauma 1989;29:1434–1437
92. Carey ME, Young HR, Mathis JL. The neurosurgical treatment of craniocerebral missile wounds in Vietnam. Surg Gynecol Obstet 1972;135:386–390
93. Salazar AM, Jabbari B, Vance SC, Grafman J, Amin D, Dillon JD. Epilepsy after penetrating head injury, I: Clinical correlates: a report of the Vietnam Head Injury Study. Neurology 1985;35(10):1406–1414
94. Nagib MG, Rockswold GL, Sherman RS, Lagaard MW. Civilian gunshot wounds to the brain: prognosis and management. Neurosurgery 1986;18(5):533–537

14 Pediatric Brain Injury

John Ragheb and Ryan S. Trombly

Pediatric traumatic brain injury is a significant cause of morbidity and mortality throughout the developed world. Severe brain injuries often leave children with significant, overt, lifelong deficits. Although the vast majority of head injuries are described as "mild" these injuries may still lead to subtle yet profound learning difficulties and behavioral problems that affect the child and the child's social milieu. The financial and societal costs of childhood traumatic injuries on the families, health care system, and society as a whole are astronomical. Injuries among children and adolescents in 2000 were estimated to result in a total $34.6 billion in lifetime costs, in addition to depriving the world of the child's potential contributions to society.[1]

Epidemiology

Traumatic injuries are the leading cause of death in children, exceeding all other causes combined in those under 18 years of age. Head injuries are quite common and responsible for a significant proportion of illnesses affecting children in their early years of life (**Table 14.1**). Approximately 475,000 children less than 14 years of age sustain a traumatic brain injury (TBI) every year.[2] Most of these are evaluated and sent home or never seek medical attention; however, TBI results in 37,000 admissions and 2,685 deaths each year. Although children less than 4 years old have the highest rate of emergency room visits, adolescents have a higher rate of admission. The mortality rates from traumatic injuries are highest in children less than 4 years of age and those 15 to 19 years of age. Although falls may account for the majority of TBI (39%), the precise mechanisms of injury leading to TBI vary with age. In infants, inflicted injuries remain the leading cause of TBI resulting in hospitalization and death. The median age of inflicted TBI is ~3 months.[3,4] The precise incidence of inflicted injuries remains uncertain as 2.6% of maternal caregivers admit to shaking a child at some stage as a method for enforcing discipline. With increasing age, the incidence of inflicted injuries declines as falls and transportation-related accidents become an increasing problem. A recent report from California found that 21 of 100,000 children suffered injuries as occupants of a motor vehicle; 28 of 100,000 were pedestrians struck by motor vehicles.[5] TBIs result in direct medical and indirect costs related to lost productivity and potential, which may reach an estimated $60 billion in the United States.[6]

Table 14.1 Epidemiology of Pediatric Traumatic Brain Injury (TBI)

- TBIs are common in children, estimated at 200/100,000 per year. Most are mild.
- Mortality is highest in infants and teens.
- Most children that die from a traumatic injury die with or because of their brain injury.

The majority of TBIs in children are mild. The annual incidence is likely to be greater than 200 per 100,000 children. Although there is no standard definition of mild TBI, the majority of studies refer to the Glasgow Coma Scale (GCS) score of 13 to 15 or an injury to the head with a posttraumatic amnesia of less than 30 minutes. Although less than 1% of mild TBI may require neurosurgical intervention, the subsequent cognitive and behavioral symptoms may be significant. The cognitive and behavioral consequences of mild TBI on the developing child are poorly understood and incompletely characterized and, when present, may take some time to resolve.

Classification of Pediatric Head Injury

Injuries to the central nervous system have been characterized as primary and secondary injuries.[7] The primary injury represents the immediate effects of impact and dissipation of energy within the neuraxis. These injuries include direct neuronal and glial disruption, laceration of the brain, shearing of axons, and vascular injuries. Although the primary injury is complete in the matter of a few milliseconds, there is strong evidence that a whole host of secondary factors can augment the extent of ultimate neurological injury. These include hypoxia, hypotension, systemic trauma, fluid and electrolyte disturbances, infections, etc. At the neuronal level, this translates into release of free radicals and neuronal death. Although the primary effects of injury cannot be reversed, the control of systemic factors can theoretically reduce the extent of further injury.

Pediatric TBI can be classified as focal if the injury is localized anatomically, clinically, and by imaging, or diffuse if the injury is widespread, multilobar. In addition, a host of secondary factors can aggravate the primary brain injury (**Table 14.2**).

Table 14.2 Classification of Pediatric Head Injury

- Diffuse
  - Diffuse axonal injury
  - Diffuse brain swelling
- Focal
  - Contusion/hematoma
  - Brain laceration
  - Extraaxial hemorrhage
    - Epidural hematoma
    - Subdural hematoma
    - Subarachnoid hematoma
- Secondary factors
  - Brain swelling
  - Brain shift/herniation
  - Seizures
  - Hemodynamic factors
    - Hypotension
    - Hypoxia
  - Metabolic disturbances
    - Hyponatremia
    - Hyperthermia
    - Hypercapnia
    - Acidosis

Focal Injuries

Focal injuries include contusions, lacerations, and intraparenchymal hematomas that result in localized damage (**Table 14.3**). This can then lead to an increasing mass resulting in brain shift and distortions with its secondary consequences. These direct or "coup" injuries are most often related to the bony prominences in the cranial vault such as the sphenoidal ridge, temporal base, orbital roof, rigid falx, or underlying fracture sites. Contrecoup injuries occur more frequently in the older children and are the result of the brain striking the skull opposite the point of impact.

Table 14.3 Pediatric Focal Injuries and Hemorrhage

- Epidural hematomas are common in children and many do not require evacuation. On occasion, these hematomas may become very large and result in anemia, potentially requiring transfusion prior to or during surgery.
- Subdural hematomas are less common in children than adults, and are often related to high-velocity injuries or abusive head injury.
- Massive diffuse hemispheric brain swelling in children can occur associated with relatively small subdural hemorrhages, abusive head injury, or the second impact syndrome.

Extradural Hematoma

Extradural hematomas are nearly always associated with an overlying fracture. The majority of these hematomas are located in the temporal and parietal regions. Posterior fossa epidural hematomas comprise 25 to 40% of all lesions in the posterior fossa and are relatively common in children (**Fig. 14.1**). Although small hematomas may be observed if the patient is fully conscious, the majority of posterior fossa hematomas are evacuated. Whereas small epidural hematomas will require no intervention, these hematomas may become quite large in infants and young children. Therefore, close observation of small hematomas is essential. Large hematomas that require surgical evacuation may occasionally result in anemia; therefore, it is vital to have blood available in the operating room for emergent transfusion. Young infants often may be in shock with the loss of blood into the epidural space and, hence, require transfusion at the start of the operation.

Subdural Hematoma

Subdural hematomas may be located in the posterior fossa or the supratentorial space. The posterior fossa subdural hematomas are located adjacent to the tentorium and often resolve spontaneously. Supratentorial subdural hematomas may be large, cause substantial midline shifts,

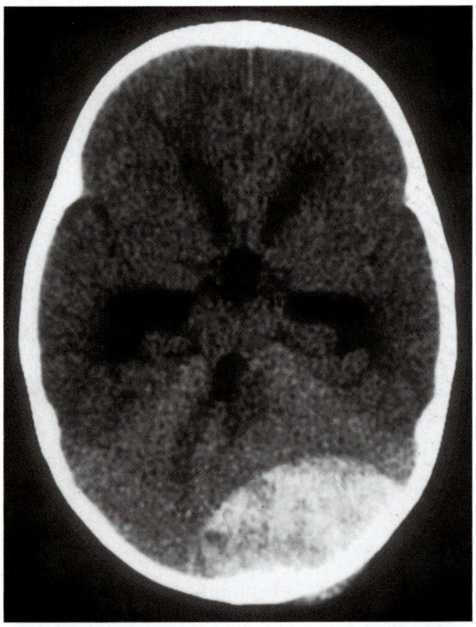

Fig. 14.1 This axial computed tomography (CT) image of a child shows a large epidural hematoma with acute hydrocephalus caused by a fall from the trunk of a moving vehicle. This child's fracture crossed the transverse sinus and therefore requires a craniotomy both above and below the sinus to evacuate the clot safely and control the transverse sinus injury.

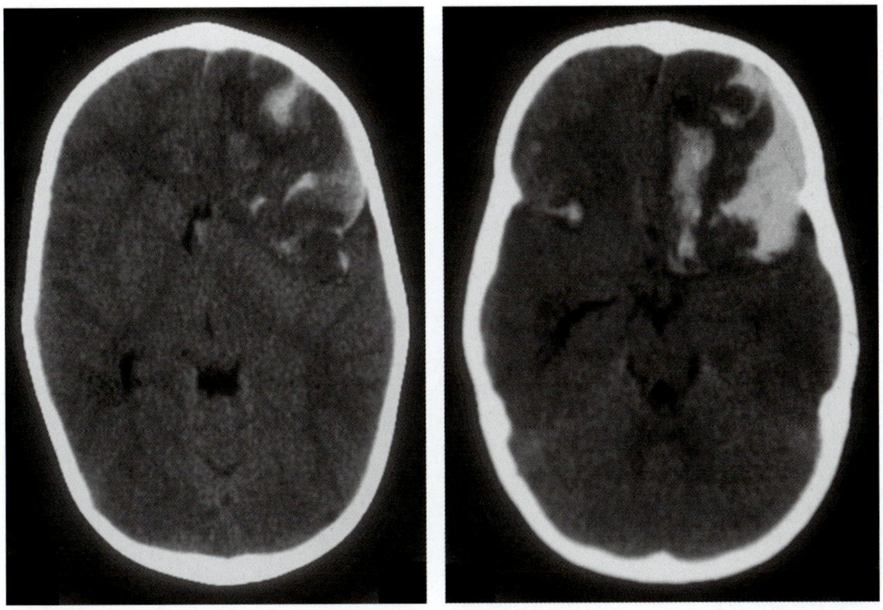

Fig. 14.2 (A,B) Axial computed tomography (CT) images of a toddler that fell climbing out of the crib on to a tile floor. Note the basal frontal hemorrhagic contusion and intracerebral hematoma in the left frontal lobe and the small contrecoup contusion at the opposite pterion. She did not have any evidence of coagulopathy and her contusion resolved without the need for evacuation of the hematoma.

and may be associated with cerebral contusion or laceration. These are evacuated and may also require removal of the devitalized brain. Subdural hemorrhages are significantly less common in children than in adults and, when present, are usually the results of high velocity injuries or nonaccidental trauma.

Intracerebral Hematoma

Intracerebral hematomas are frequently caused by acceleration/deceleration injuries and occur most commonly in the basifrontal and basitemporal regions. Some of these may be in the deep parenchyma of the brain. The majority can be treated conservatively; however, those with significant mass effect or shift may require evacuation if clinically indicated (**Fig. 14.2**).

Diffuse Injuries

Diffuse brain injuries are characterized by generalized disturbance of neuronal function in the setting of an admission computed tomography (CT) scan that is normal or with minimal abnormality. Diffuse injuries have a wide spectrum of severity and occur as a result of energy distribution throughout the entire brain. The pathological substrate of this injury is thought to lie in the shearing of the axons at the gray–white junction, corpus callosum, and the brain stem (**Fig. 14.3**).[8] These injuries are the result of angular acceleration/deceleration with the extent of injury proportional to the energy dissipated or the angular velocity of the brain. The clinical presentation depends on the extent of axonal dysfunction or disruption and can range from a minor concussion to severe diffuse axonal injury with profound and prolonged impairment of neurological function. The patients may decerebrate, have abnormal gaze palsy, pupillary changes, and autonomic disturbances. The radiological findings may range from normal to multiple deep white matter, corpus callosum, and brain stem hematomas. These changes are best appreciated on magnetic resonance imaging (MRI) of the brain.

Diffuse Brain Swelling

Diffuse brain swelling is a reactive posttraumatic phenomenon characterized by raised intracranial pressure due to a marked increase in cerebral blood volume. This phenomenon was first described by Bruce et al in 1981.[9] They showed that delayed deterioration after a lucid interval was often associated with a global increase in cerebral blood flow suggesting vascular engorgement and an increase in cerebral blood volume. Muizellaar et al[10] showed impaired autoregulatory capacity in 41% of children with severe TBI. However, these findings have been disputed by other authors.[11] Recently, Vavilala et al[12] once again showed that autoregulation can be impaired in children with severe TBI who do not have a focal hematoma. Overall, it does seem to suggest that children with diffuse brain swelling tend to have a poorer outcome than adults. The exact pathophysiology of this entity is poorly understood

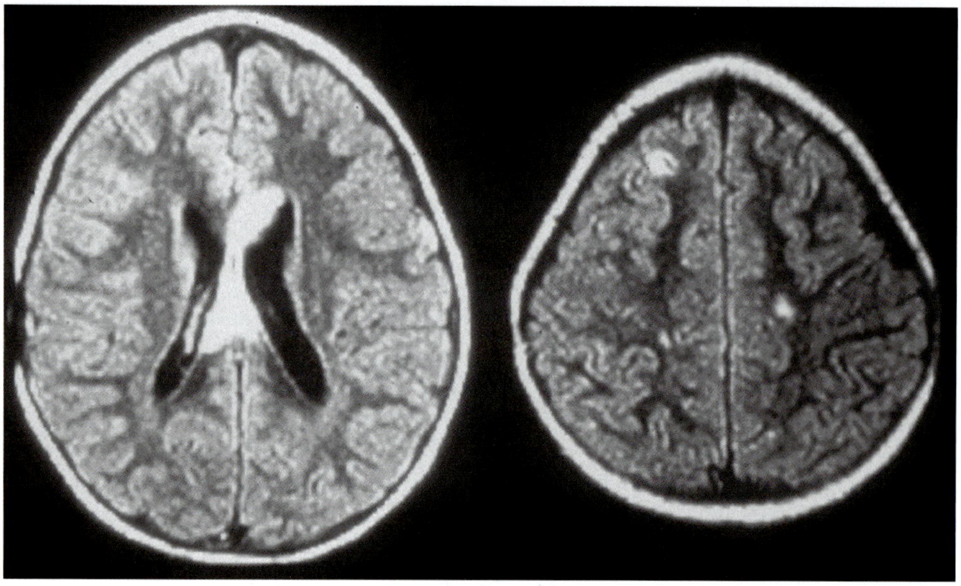

Fig. 14.3 Axial fluid attenuated inversion recovery magnetic resonance image of a child that suffered a severe traumatic brain injury in a motor vehicle crash. Note the areas of bright signal in the corpus callosum and at the gray–white matter junction.

and may be driven by hyponatremia, hyperemia, hypoxia, ischemia, loss of blood-flow autoregulation, or hyperglycolysis. Whatever the underlying cause, it can be a major cause of serious deterioration after a minor head injury. Aggressive control of intracranial pressure (ICP) results in a good neurological outcome. Infants and young children are uniquely susceptible to diffuse hemispheric swelling. This is occasionally associated with thin subdural hemorrhage, particularly in the setting of nonaccidental injury.

Nonaccidental Trauma

Nonaccidental head injury, inflicted, or abusive head injury and shaken-baby syndrome, are all terms that are used to describe head injuries in the setting of child abuse, which is recognized now as a major health care problem (**Table 14.4**). Most victims are children less than 3 years of age and many present with a host of other medical problems and injuries. These include axial and appendicular skeletal injuries of varying age and severity, and soft tissue injuries in various stages of severity and duration. These children may often be malnourished and have poor hygiene. Caffey[13,14] described the presence of acute subdural hemorrhage, which was often characterized by interhemispheric, subarachnoid and retinal hemorrhages, and epiphyseal injuries in children and coined the term *shaken baby syndrome.* This was suspected to result from rotational forces on the brain tearing subdural vessels. These rotational forces are accentuated with the large head pivoting on the small neck and body of an infant. These children present with an altered mental status, which may vary from irritable to unresponsive. The history offered is often incongruous with the severity of the clinical picture. The neurological examination reflects the severity of the injury. Seizures are seen in a large number of these children. Funduscopic examinations are mandatory and often show retinal hemorrhages. Computed tomographic studies often show subdural and subarachnoid hemorrhages. The brain parenchyma may be edematous with loss of gray–white differentiation or show extensive low attenuation suggesting associated ischemia of the brain. The management of these children is aimed at stabilizing the hemodynamic status, controlling raised intracranial pressure, utilizing anticonvulsant medications, and avoiding metabolic disturbances as the injured brain recovers. The prognosis is often directly related to the neurological examination at presentation. Federal and state laws mandate that suspected cases be reported to the appropriate authorities.

Table 14.4 Pediatric Nonaccidental Head Injury

Abusive head injury must be suspected whenever the history is inconsistent with the clinical or imaging findings.
Workup should include a thorough search for other injuries and referral to the appropriate investigative authorities.

Skull Fractures

Skull fractures are common injuries in children, particularly uncomplicated linear fractures (**Table 14.5**). Most of these are not associated with intracranial bleeding; yet they may be associated with extradural and/or intracerebral hematomas depending on the extent of the initial insult.

Table 14.5 Pediatric Skull Fractures

- Linear skull fractures are common findings after falls in children. Children with uncomplicated skull fractures that can be clinically and reliably observed at home do not require hospital admission.
- Many minor depressed fractures, particularly ping-pong type fractures in infants, do not require operative intervention and will remodel spontaneously.
- Fractures with a suspected dural laceration must be explored to avoid the subsequent development of a leptomeningeal cyst.

Fractures crossing venous sinuses require special caution during repair as these are more often associated with extradural hematomas. The majority of linear fractures in young children are caused by falls. These are extremely common in toddlers and infants as they learn to stand, walk, and explore their surroundings. Although CT scanning is the test of choice to identify intracranial hemorrhage and fracture, occasionally axially oriented fractures may be missed. These can be detected on a careful inspection of the CT scan scout image. The vast majority of linear skull fractures require no treatment and heal without sequelae. Uncomplicated linear fractures may not require admission to the hospital if the child has a normal neurological examination, no intracranial injury, and a home situation where the child can be reliably observed for any deterioration in mental status. All other children are best monitored in the hospital. Specific care should be given to rule out the possibility of child abuse in young infants and toddlers. The real issue with skull fractures is not the injury to the cranial vault itself, but the potential underlying neurological injury that governs the management and recovery from head injury.

Depressed Skull Fracture

Depressed skull fractures are relatively common in children and account for ~10% of all skull fractures.[15] Closed depressed fractures usually do not require any surgical intervention unless associated with a suspected dural laceration or when present in locations of cosmetic importance (**Fig. 14.4**). A unique variant of depressed fracture seen in infants is the ping-pong or pond fracture. These are usually a consequence of malpositioned forceps during delivery or short-distance falls. Most depressed fractures are small and remodel over time under the influence of the underlying developing brain; however, some may be large and require surgical intervention (**Fig. 14.5**). A small bur hole at the edge of the fracture and elevation of the fracture can be accomplished with a Penfield elevator. Compound depressed fractures with an overlying scalp laceration may require débridement if the wound is grossly contaminated or a dural laceration is suspected. The fracture fragments may be returned to the site after débridement if the contamination is limited, therefore avoiding the need for a future cranioplasty.

Growing Skull Fracture

A growing skull fracture, also known as a leptomeningeal cyst, is a unique, but rare complication. It is usually seen with skull fractures in young children,[16,17] but can be seen

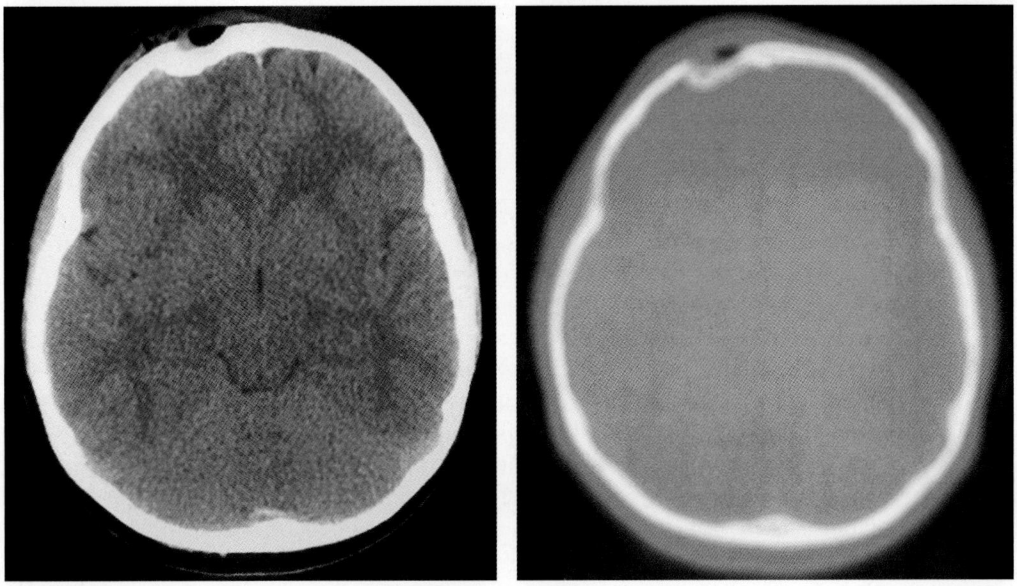

A B

Fig. 14.4 (A,B) Small depressed fracture in a child caused by an errant golf club as seen on axial computed tomography (CT), soft tissue and bone windows. The overlying laceration was cleansed and closed in the emergency department and the fracture was above the hair line. This fracture will remodel without the need for surgical intervention.

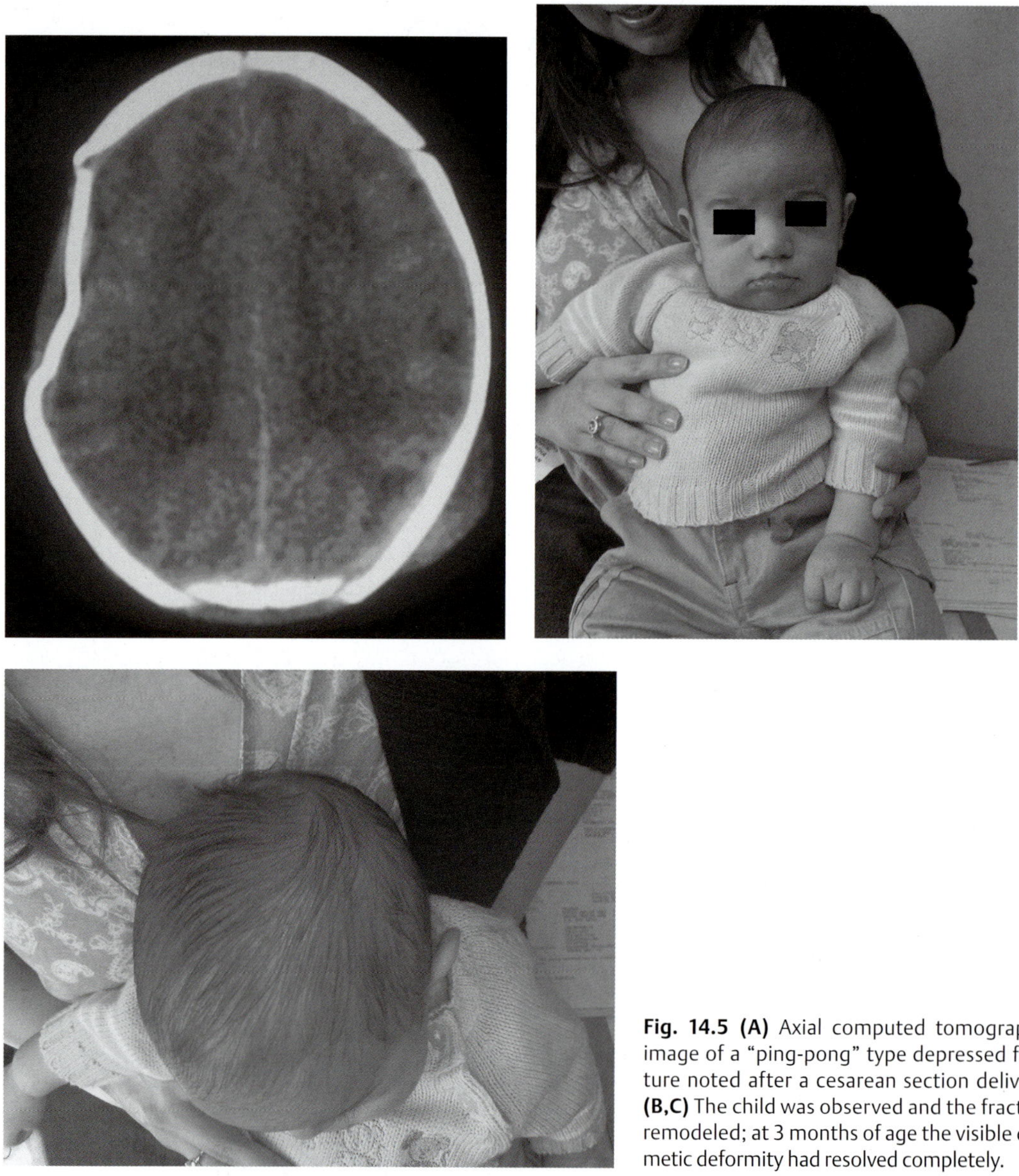

A B C

Fig. 14.5 (A) Axial computed tomographic image of a "ping-pong" type depressed fracture noted after a cesarean section delivery. **(B,C)** The child was observed and the fracture remodeled; at 3 months of age the visible cosmetic deformity had resolved completely.

at any age. Linear or complex fractures that are associated with an underlying dural laceration and brain injury are the essential precursor of a growing skull fracture (**Fig. 14.6**). The fracture edges are often split by the energy of the injury. The pulsations of the brain allow the brain to herniate through the dural tear. Gradually, over weeks and months, the fractured edges are further eroded becoming wide and smooth. The brain pulsations along the edges of the dura and bone can cause progressive injury to the adjacent cortex. These fractures are often located in the parietal region, but may be present in the occipital region, posterior fossa, or the roof of the orbit. Driven by the growing brain and/or the normal cerebral pulsation, the brain herniates through the fracture and dural defect, widening both defects over time (**Fig. 14.7**). The dural defect often becomes much wider than the bone defect. These children present with a focal, pulsatile swelling, which consists of cerebrospinal fluid (CSF) and the herniating brain (i.e., the leptomeningeal cyst), as well as progressive neurological deficit and seizures. The diagnosis can be easily confirmed with a CT scan or MRI. The treatment consists of a wide craniotomy, dural repair after minimal resection of gliotic, herniated brain, and cranioplasty. A cranioplasty should be performed with autologous bone whenever possible to allow for continued skull growth and prosthetic materials should always be avoided. Associated hydrocephalus may require CSF diversion, but CSF shunting should never be used as a primary method of treatment for a growing skull fracture.

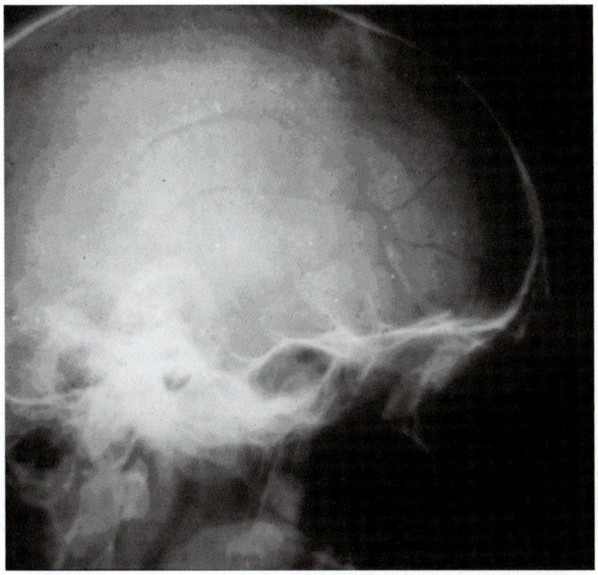

Fig. 14.6 Complex stellate fractures as seen on this lateral plain radiograph are commonly associated with an underlying dural and brain injury.

Basilar Skull Fracture

Basilar skull fractures account for 15 to 19% of skull fractures in children.[18–20] Although the frontal and sphenoid sinus may not be pneumatized in children less than 5 years of age, a CSF leak may occur via the anterior cranial base or petrous bone through the nose or ear. This stops spontaneously in nearly all children. The head should be kept elevated and any straining or vigorous manipulation of the ear or nose to remove clotted blood should be avoided. An examination of the middle ear and hearing evaluation should be delayed for a few weeks until the CSF leak has abated. There is no role for prophylactic antibiotics to prevent meningitis as their use may increase the risk of unusual or drug resistant organisms. Basilar skull fractures (**Fig. 14.8**) may be associated with injury to the middle ear, carotid artery, venous sinuses, and cranial nerves as they exit the foramina.

Management of Raised Intracranial Pressure

Neurosurgical care of the brain-injured pediatric patient is aimed at treating significant intracranial hematomas and preventing secondary insults to the injured brain. Treatment is directed at controlling ICP and maintaining adequate cerebral perfusion pressure (CPP). General principles include avoidance of fever and hypoxemia, maintenance of normal ventilation, adequate jugular venous outflow, and adequate sedation and analgesia. ICP monitoring is indicated in children with GCS scores of 8 or below or whenever there is a suspicion of raised ICP and the clinical exam cannot be used to monitor the child. Many methods of monitoring ICP are available. Those methods that require fixation of a threaded "bolt" into the skull cannot be used in infants. Otherwise, the techniques, indications, and methods are comparable to that in adults (**Table 14.6**). We prefer monitoring ICP with a ventricular catheter, which allows not only monitoring ICP, but helps in controlling ICP by providing CSF drainage.

A

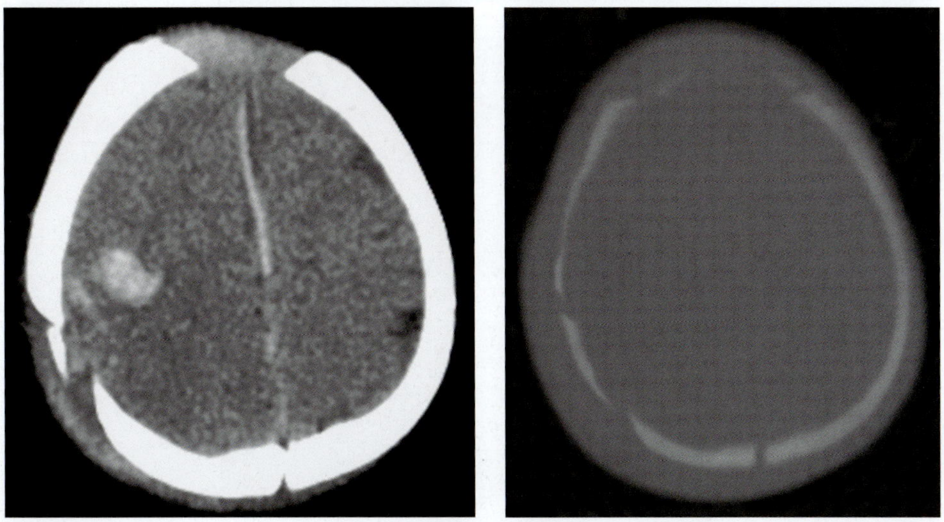

B

Fig. 14.7 Axial, soft tissue, and bone window computed tomographic (CT) images of an infant that suffered an inflicted head injury. She was discharged into the foster care system and did not return for several months after the injury. **(A,B)** Upon her return she was noted to have a soft swelling of the right scalp and a left hemiparesis. Her CT scan, scout, brain, and bone window images reveal widening of her parietal fracture, bone erosion, and underlying encephalomalacia.

(Continued on page 282)

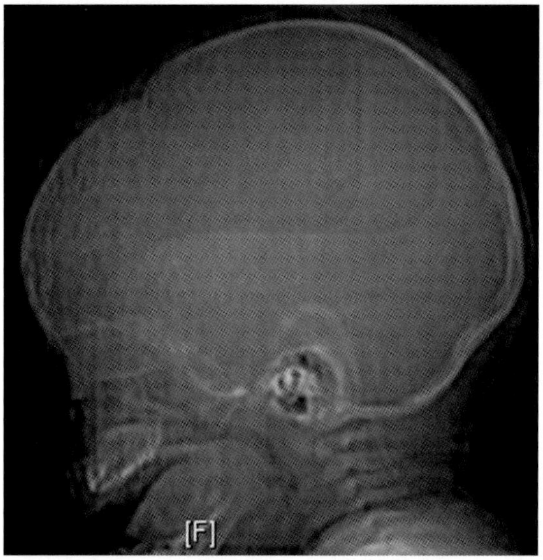

C

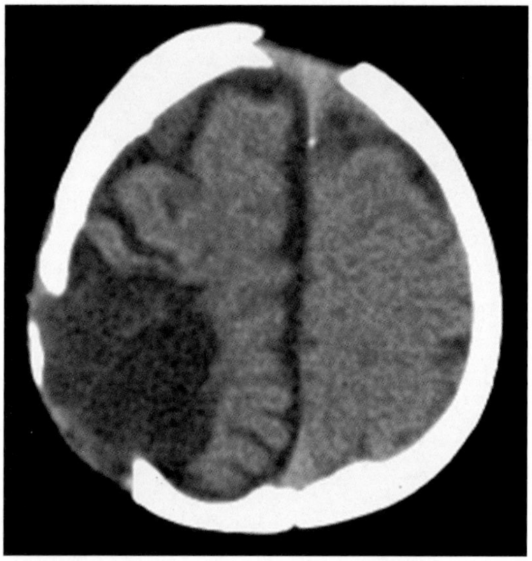

D

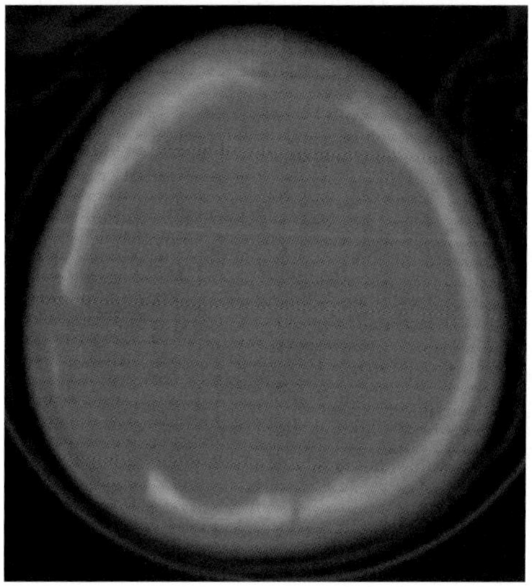

E

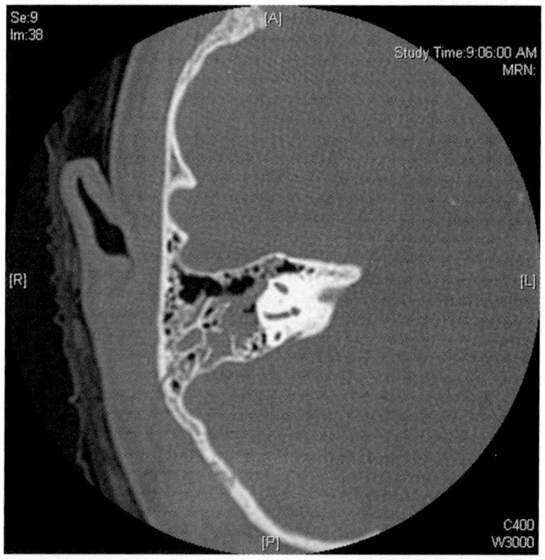

F

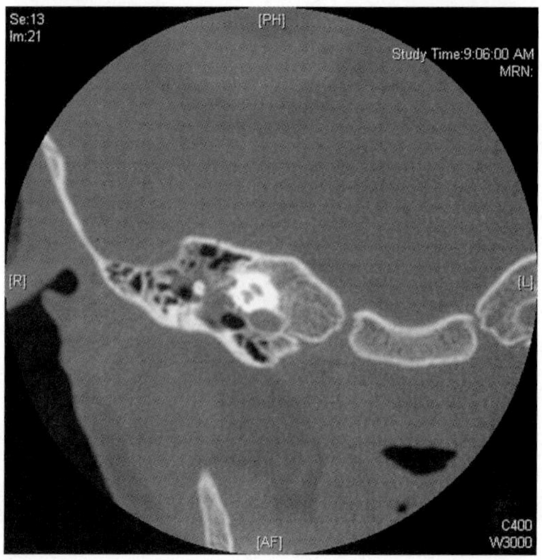

G

Fig. 14.7 *(Continued)* **(C–E)** Axial and coronal CT images of a child that fell from a shopping cart and suffered a longitudinal fracture of the right petrous bone. **(F,G)**

Table 14.6 Intracranial Pressure Management in Children

- Management of raised ICP as per the Pediatric TBI Guidelines in **Fig. 14.9**
- Critical thresholds for raised ICP and CPP must be age appropriate.
- Decompressive craniectomy may improve survival and outcome after severe TBI when performed as soon as medical management fails to control ICP
- Meticulous maintenance of physiologic homeostasis, seizure prevention, and avoidance of hyperthermia and infection will avoid many of the secondary injuries that can affect outcome after TBI.
- Seizures after TBI are more common in children < 2 years old with a GCS score <9. Seizure prophylaxis is indicated to prevent early posttraumatic seizures in select children during the first week after injury.

Abbreviations: CPP, cerebral perfusion pressure; GCS, Glasgow Coma Scale; ICP, intracranial pressure; TBI, traumatic brain injury.

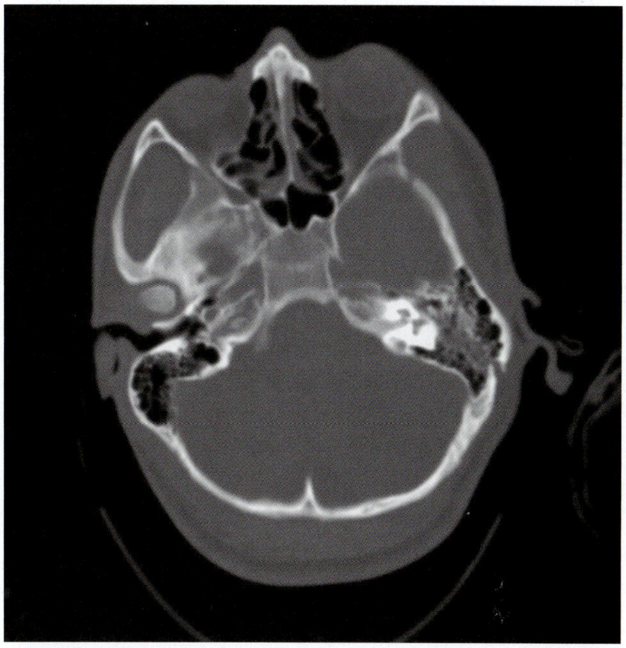

Fig. 14.8 A longitudinal fracture through the left petrous bone going toward the carotid canal.

If ICP remains elevated despite these measures, the possibility of a new intracranial mass lesion must always be considered. Beyond these interventions lie the possibilities of managing raised ICP with hyperosmolar therapy, hyperventilation, barbiturates, hypothermia, and decompressive craniotomy. As described in the Pediatric Traumatic Head Injury Guidelines, a rational incremental approach in a "tiered" fashion, which escalates therapy based on ICP, response to treatment, and the risks of the intervention, standardizes care, reduces mortality, and improves outcome (**Fig. 14.9**).[21] Although this exhaustive review of the pediatric TBI literature reached no standards per se and few recommendations, many options for management were identified. There exists a wide range of treatment strategies for the care of the severely head-injured child. The decision whether to monitor ICP and the method is provider dependent. The many treatment options used to control elevated ICP make comparisons between regimens difficult, and make it impossible to proclaim uniform standards. As recently as 2001, a survey of all pediatric intensive care units in the United Kingdom found a wide discrepancy between its centers, with variable use of barbiturates, mannitol, hypothermia, and hyperventilation. There was no significant difference between the treatment of pediatric and adult head injury.

Hyperosmolar Therapy

Elevated ICP can be treated with hyperosmolar therapy when conservative measures such as positioning, sedation, and CSF drainage prove inadequate. What constitutes a child's threshold for ICP above which treatment is necessary has not been rigorously defined. In general, the goal is to keep ICP < 20 cm of H_20, <18 in patients younger than 6 years old and <15 in those less then 24 months. Many different hyperosmolar agents have been used in the past; currently the most prevalent agents are mannitol and hypertonic saline. It is unclear what agent is superior, and most likely the differences are negligible provided that ICP is well controlled and euvolemia is maintained throughout treatment.

Mannitol has been the agent of choice in hyperosmolar therapy since the 1970s. Good clinical results were obtained over a wide range of mannitol dosages (0.25 g/kg to 1.5 g/kg), provided that ICP was well controlled and euvolemia was maintained. One group demonstrated that smaller doses of mannitol have equal efficacy, but fewer side effects.[22] The use of hypertonic saline became a point of interest in the 1980s when trauma researchers who had used hypertonic saline to resuscitate burn patients or patients in shock noticed a significant benefit in patients with head injury. A subgroup analysis from a prospective, randomized, multicenter trial of prehospital resuscitation of trauma patients noticed a survival rate of 34% in patients who received hypertonic saline compared with 12% in patients who received lactated Ringer (LR) solution.[23]

Although the majority of the studies are based on adult subjects, other studies have documented similar efficacy in the use of hypertonic saline in the immediate and early acute period of resuscitation after head trauma in children. Simma et al[24] randomized 35 head-injured children with GCS scores <8 into two arms, one to receive lactated LR solution for resuscitation and the other receiving 2% hypertonic saline. Although survival and outcomes were

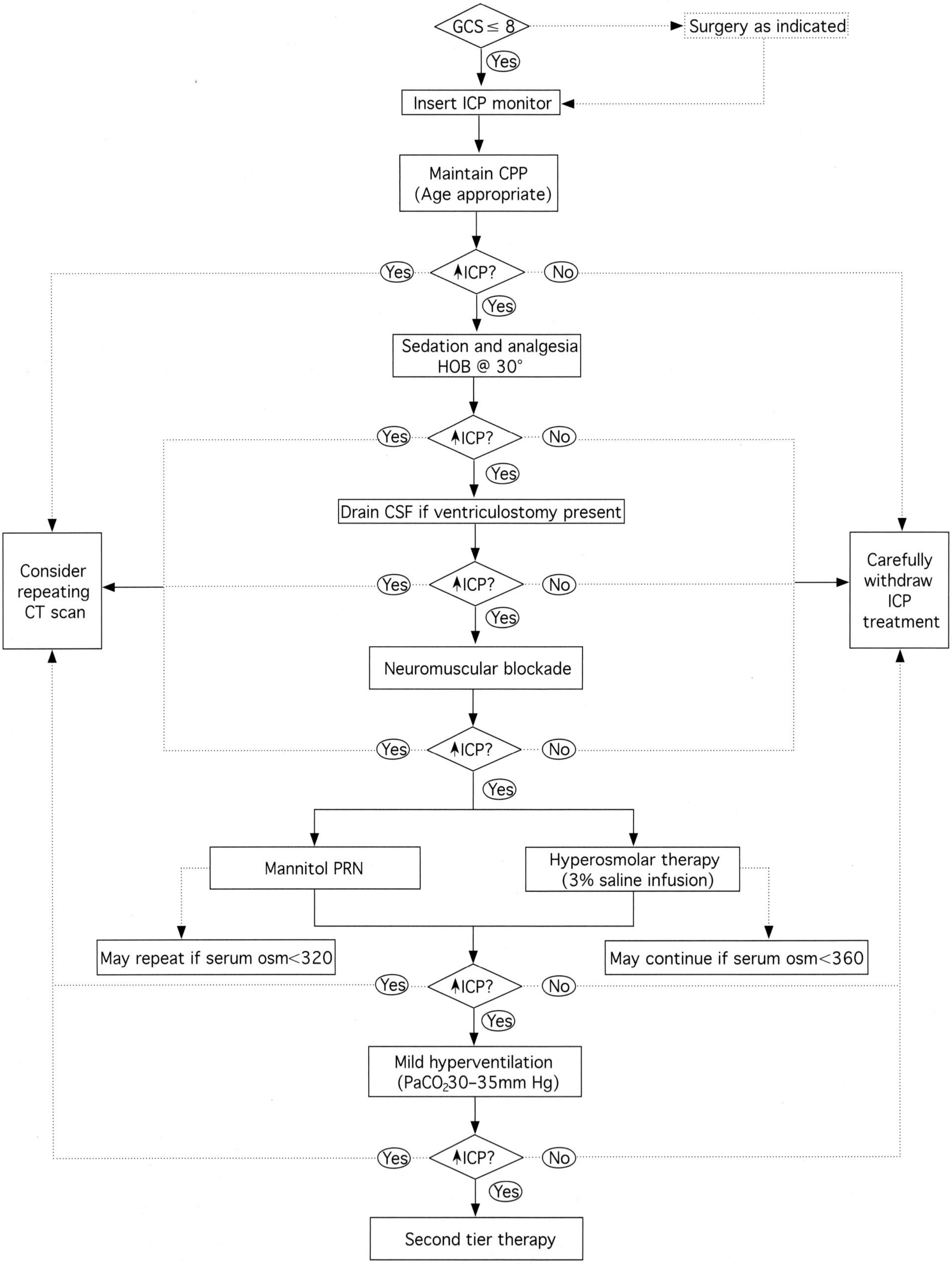

A

Fig. 14.9 (A) First-tier therapy for pediatric traumatic brain injury. GCS, Glasgow Coma Scale; ICP, intracranial pressure; CPP, cerebral perfusion pressure; HOB, head of bed; CSF, cerebrospinal fluid; CT, computed tomography; PRN, as needed.

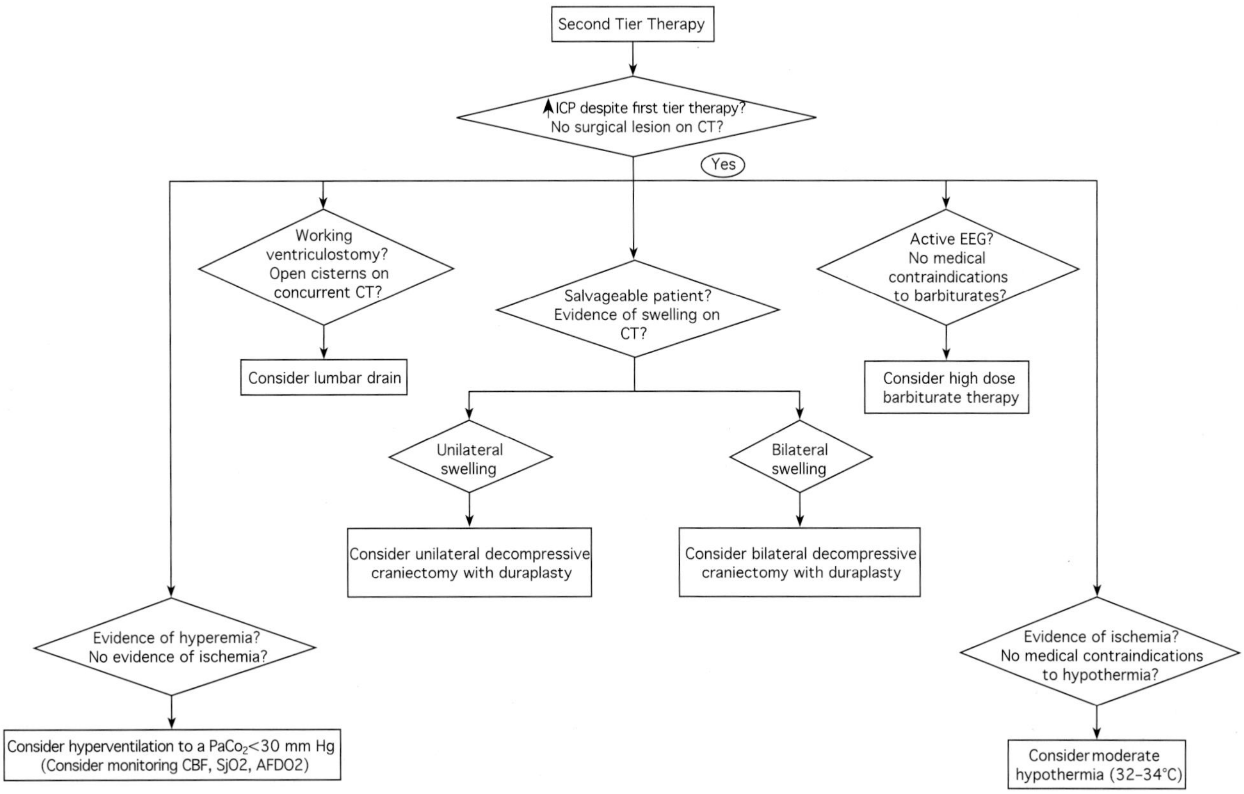

B

Fig. 14.9 *(Continued)* **(B)** Second-tier therapy. Tx, treatment; ICP, intracranial pressure; CT, computed tomography; EEG, electroencephalogram; CBF, cerebral blood flow; $PaCO_2$, carbon dioxide in arterial blood; SjO2, jugular venous oxygen saturation; AJDO2, arteriojugular venous difference in oxygen content.

similar in the two groups, the group receiving LR as resuscitation fluid required more interventions, developed adult respiratory stress syndrome (ARDS) more often, and had longer intensive care unit (ICU) stays when compared with the group treated with hypertonic saline. The use of hypertonic saline now extends beyond the phase of initial resuscitation after trauma. It has been shown to control elevated ICP after trauma, and many researchers feel it has a very safe side effect profile. Hypertonic saline helps to replete the intravascular volume and augments cardiovascular performance; furthermore, it avoids the risks of renal failure, hypokalemia, hypotension, and rebound intracranial hypertension associated with mannitol. Studies on cerebral blood flow have suggested that hypertonic saline increases capillary diameter by shrinking endothelial cells, and similar shrinkage of red blood cells increases their deformability; the end result is an increase in cerebral blood flow. Beyond acting as an osmotic agent, hypertonic saline also stimulates the release of atrial natriuretic factor (ANP) and counteracts the effect of the vasoconstrictor endothelin.[25] Hypertonic saline also elevates arterial pressure and exerts a rheologic plasma expansion, which results in a reduction in blood viscosity and increase in cerebral blood flow.[26] A meta-analysis of the literature between 1965 and 1999 revealed a lack of uniformity between concentrations and volumes of hypertonic saline administered, and small patient populations. Nevertheless, a trend was noted toward a definite reduction in ICP and few, if any adverse effects, in patients treated with hypertonic saline.[27]

There is no consensus on the ideal concentration of hypertonic saline needed to provide the best clinical response. An animal study from 1993 showed that the use of 7% hypertonic saline controlled ICP as well as mannitol.[28] Since that time, several human studies have corroborated its safety and efficacy in humans suffering from intracranial hypertension. Vialet et al[29] randomized patients with head trauma and persistent coma to receive isovolume infusions of 7.5% hypertonic saline or 20% mannitol whenever ICP was sustained above 25 mm Hg. The study showed that patients treated with hypertonic saline had fewer episodes per day (7 vs. 13) of elevated intracranial pressure, and the daily duration of elevated ICP was far shorter (67 vs. 131 minutes). The osmolality of the hypertonic saline was more than twice that of the mannitol administered in this study. A more recent study made a direct comparison between isoosmolar administrations of mannitol and 7.5% hypertonic saline/6% dextran solution. The study randomized each patient who required treatment of elevated ICP to receive boluses of mannitol followed by hypertonic saline, or vice versa, in an effort to compare the effects of saline and mannitol within the same patient. After enrolling nine patients, the study concluded that hypertonic saline was more often effective in lowering ICP into the goal range, and its duration of effect was significantly longer (148 minutes vs. 90 minutes). The equiosmolar infusions of mannitol or hypertonic saline allowed direct comparison of their efficacies as hyperosmolar agents. Although it is more expensive than mannitol, hypertonic saline/dextran is more efficacious and requires fewer interventions.[30]

There is evidence that hypertonic saline can be used to control elevated ICP in cases refractory to all other interventions. Horn et al[31] presented a retrospective review of 10 consecutive patients with elevated ICP despite adequate sedation, paralysis, hyperventilation, barbiturate coma, and mannitol given 0.35 g/kg every 4 hours. The researchers demonstrated that bolus infusions of 7.5% hypertonic saline could still achieve control of ICP despite the failure of all other interventions. During treatment, serum sodium and serum osmolality were carefully controlled. Based on these results the authors favored the use of hypertonic saline for primary hyperosmolar therapy.

When hyperosmolar therapy is indicated our approach is to use mannitol initially in intermittent doses of 0.25 to 1.0 g/kg repeated every 4 to 6 hours as needed to control ICP. Adequate hydration with isotonic fluids to maintain euvolemia and close monitoring to keep the serum osmolarity ≤320 (mg/dL) is essential. When this fails, we then proceed to 3% NaCl at 0.1 to 1.0 cc/kg/h until ICP is controlled or the serum sodium reaches 165 to 170.

Decompressive Craniectomy

Decompressive craniectomy provides another option for the control of refractory ICP when first- and second-tier therapies fail. As with hyperosmolar therapy, the literature regarding decompressive craniectomy is difficult to assess because thresholds of treatment and treatment interventions differ widely. Surgical treatment of elevated intracranial pressure dates back to the days of Dandy and Cushing. In the early 1970s, a bifrontal craniectomy was used in a series of 50 head-injured patients with a survival rate of 22%. The authors employed this drastic intervention only in patients who were comatose, apneic, decerebrate, or had dilated pupils unilaterally or bilaterally. Among their survivors many were described as neurologically normal and returned to work and school.[32] A similar study performed a few years later reported a higher survival rate, but found worse neurological recoveries.[33] The salvage of head-injured patients in a coma with brain stem dysfunction has a high failure rate, and a high cost associated with each failure. It is often wondered if these procedures help severely injured patients avoid early death but survive in a vegetative state.

Polin et al[34] reported some promising results with decompressive craniectomy for control of ICP. They presented a series of 35 patients with elevated ICP despite hyperventilation, mannitol, sedation, and paralysis that underwent bifrontal craniectomy. These patients were compared with matched controls from the Traumatic Coma Data Bank (TCDB). The rate of recovery with moderate disability was 37%, and 44% in pediatric patients. ICP was lowered in all patients after surgery, and was lower than the ICP of the matched controls. The authors stressed that decompression was most effective when performed early and was not effective in patients with sustained ICP >40 or if the GCS score was 3. Although this study did not employ barbiturates or CSF drainage to help control ICP, despite the bias of comparing selected patients to historical controls, it suggests that decompressive craniectomy has a definite role in selected patients with severe head injury and elevated ICP. Guerra et al[35] demonstrated similarly promising results. From 1977 to 1997, 57 patients underwent decompressive craniectomy (31 unilateral and 26 bilateral) after a standard medical regimen failed to control ICP. Ten percent of patients remained in a vegetative state; 10% survived with a permanent neurological deficit, and 58% achieved social rehabilitation. The authors advocated decompressive craniectomy for a selected subgroup of trauma patients when applied early for the control of refractory ICP.[35]

Hypothermia

Hypothermia offers another possible treatment in the care of the head-injured patient. Although it has been studied extensively in laboratory models of TBI, ischemia, and stroke and found to be beneficial, the human data supporting its use is mixed and its use is controversial. Conversely, it is generally agreed that hyperthermia should be avoided at all costs. Laboratory studies using moderate hypothermia in mature and immature animals, trials of hypothermia in neonates with hypoxic-ischemic injury, and phase II studies in adults for 24 to 48 hours after TBI have supported the safety and efficacy of hypothermia.[36–38] Marion et al[36] conducted a randomized prospective study between normothermia and hypothermia among all patients between the ages of 16 and 75 with an admission GCS scores of 3 to 7, unless hypotension, hypoxia, or prolonged rescue excluded the patients. Moderate hypothermia between 32°C and 33°C was achieved with cold saline gastric lavage and cooling blankets and was maintained for 24 hours. The patient was then rewarmed slowly. The results showed that ICP was lower in the hypothermia group, especially in the first 36 hours after injury, and at early follow-up there was a trend toward better outcome in the patients treated with hypothermia. Fifty percent of the patients had a good outcome or moderate disability, as compared with 25% of matched controls from the Traumatic Coma Data Bank.[36] The long-term follow-up of these results showed that hypothermia hastened the neurological recovery of patients with initial GCS scores of 5 to 7 and imparted a trend toward improved outcome at 12 months; no significant differences were noted among patients with initial GCS scores of 3 or 4.[37] Shiozaki et al[38] reported similar encouraging results in controlling raised ICP with mild hypothermia. Clifton et al[39] reported a 15% improvement in outcome at 6 months in patients treated with moderate hypothermia for 48 hours. However, these initial results were not supported by the National Acute Brain Injury Study: Hypothermia.[40] They studied 392 patients 16 to 65 years of age and concluded that hypothermia was not effective in improving outcome in patients with severe head injury; 57% of patients in either group had a poor outcome. Secondary analysis showed that the outcome was better among patients who were younger than 45, were hypothermic at admission, and were treated with hypothermia. All these studies investigated adults more than 16 years of age. Children are believed to have unique pathophysiological mechanisms and sequelae following head injury[41]; hence, they may have a more favorable response to hypothermia as has been demonstrated in neonates treated with hypothermia for hypoxic-ischemic insults.[42,43] In one of the earliest reports in the use of hypothermia in children, Gruszkiewicz et al[44] suggested that hypothermia improved the prognosis among severely head-injured children. Among 191 children with severe head injuries, 42 presented with signs of brain stem injury: decerebrate rigidity, pupillary disturbances, and irregular breathing. These patients were cooled to between 31°C and 36°C for 1 to 16 days, during which time adequate sedation was maintained, mannitol was administered, and serial lumbar punctures were performed. Treatment was continued until decerebrate rigidity cleared and respirations normalized. Twenty-two died in the immediate hospitalization and 20 survived, with the majority able to attend regular classes in school, often with a need for special tutoring. In a multicenter phase II clinical trial, Adelson et al[45] demonstrated that moderate hypothermia in children with severe TBI was safe. Although there was no statistical difference in the mean ICP when compared with children who were not treated with hypothermia, there was a decrease in the mean hourly ICP and reduction in the number of times when the ICP and was greater than 20 mm Hg thus indicating an improvement in the overall severity of ICP. This effect was also seen in children who were cooled later (after 6 hours). Although there was a trend toward a higher risk of arrhythmias (sinus tachycardia that was managed with hydration), there was no significant difference in risk of coagulopathy, infections, or secondary hematomas. There was a trend toward rebound elevation of ICP during the rewarming period. Overall these studies suggest that hypothermia may help control the ICP in children with severe TBI. Questions remain unanswered with regard to the duration of treatment needed and the speed of rewarming. These questions will hopefully be answered by the ongoing phase III multicenter trial of moderate hypothermia for children with severe TBI.

Postraumatic Seizures

Postraumatic seizures are a common complication of pediatric TBI. Postraumatic epilepsy (PTE), defined as recurrent spontaneous seizures, develops in 10 to 20% of children with severe TBI and is often difficult to treat.[3,46] Early posttraumatic seizures usually occur in the first week after TBI, whereas PTE usually presents after the first week. Seizures may occur at the time of impact with rapid return to normal mental status and absence of intracranial abnormality. Seizures that occur immediately around the time of injury, also called impact seizures, are seen more often in children, particularly in infants. The overall incidence of posttraumatic seizure of any type regardless of the severity of injury is 5.5 to 21%. The majority of these seizures occur during the initial 24 hours after TBI. The incidence of posttraumatic seizures increases with the severity of injury and inversely with age. Posttraumatic seizures have been observed in 2 to 6% of children with mild TBI, 12 to 27% with moderate TBI, and 23 to 35% of those with severe TBI.[47,48] Posttraumatic seizures are also 2.5 times more likely in children younger than 2 years of age as compared with children 3 to 12 years.[49] Posttraumatic seizures are more frequent in children with nonaccidental TBI, with reported rates of 48 to 65% as compared with 15 to 17% in accidental TBI.[50] The occurrence of PTE also increases the longer children are followed after TBI. Five years after TBI, the cumulative probability of PTE was 0.7% for mild, 1.2% for moderate, and 10% for severe TBI. In contrast, 30 years later the cumulative probability increases to 2.1% for mild, 4.2% for moderate, and 16.7% for severe TBI.[51,52] Children commonly receive empiric treatment with antiseizure prophylaxis after an acute trauma based on the belief that they have a lower seizure threshold than adults. Nevertheless, a randomized double-blind trial found that patients treated with phenytoin had a 12% rate of late seizures compared with a 6% rate of late seizures in patients receiving placebo. This incidence of late posttraumatic epilepsy in children was slightly lower than the adult rate.[53] A retrospective chart review of pediatric blunt head injury patients between 1988 and 1990 found that among 194 patients, 18 suffered from posttraumatic seizures, and 14 patients had seizures occur within 24 hours of injury. The study found that initial GCS was the most reliable predictor of posttraumatic epilepsy: 38.7% of patients with GCS scores of 3 to 8 had seizures, whereas only 3.8% of patients with GCS scores of 9 to 15 had convulsions. Based on the preference of the treating physician, some patients in the GCS 3 to 8 group in this retrospective review received phenytoin: treated patients dropped their rate of seizures from 53% to 15%.[54] The authors supported the use of phenytoin for the prevention of early posttraumatic seizures.

Another retrospective review of pediatric trauma patients reached similar conclusions. A review of pediatric patients treated for head injury between 1980 and 1986 in Chicago found the incidence of posttraumatic seizures to be 9.8%, with 95% of these episodes occurring within the first 24 hours after injury. Those patients with diffuse cerebral edema, GCS scores between 3 and 8, and acute subdural hematoma were significantly more likely to develop seizures: a seizure rate of 35% prevailed in this group, compared with a rate of 5% in patients with minor head injury.[48] Age did not affect the incidence of seizures in this study.

So, a relevant question is whether prophylactic antiseizure medicines are beneficial, especially among the subgroup of severely injured children. Two studies shed light on this matter.[53,55] Between 1976 and 1979, 245 patients were randomized between phenytoin and placebo for the control of early seizures after blunt or penetrating head injury. Patients were included only if they were felt to have a 10% or greater chance of having a seizure. Five patients on phenytoin and four patients on placebo had early seizures, and the authors did not feel that prophylaxis was justified based on these results.[53] On the contrary, a significant reduction in early seizures was found in a study that spanned 4 years and included 586 patients treated for head injury in Seattle, Washington. These patients were randomized to placebo or phenytoin and the treatment was continued for up to 1 year after injury. The rate of early seizures was only 3.6% in the phenytoin group; it was significantly worse (14.2%) in the placebo group. The difference in rate of late seizures was not significant; in fact, the phenytoin group had a higher rate of seizures (21.5%) compared with the placebo group (15.7%). The authors concluded that phenytoin is indicated in reducing the rate of early seizures.[55]

Prevention of Head Injury

Traumatic brain injury carries a significant risk of mortality and a potential lifetime of morbidity that may preclude living a productive and emotionally satisfying life. Although a tremendous amount of work has been done on treating the consequences of primary brain injury and limiting the secondary factors that may aggravate the degree of neurological insult, the primary prevention of brain injury would logically have the most impact in reducing the degree of neurological morbidity and mortality. Many organizations like Think First, National Safe Kids campaign, and the Program for Playground Safety are involved in raising awareness of TBI and injury prevention. Simple steps, such as the use of helmets while skating and biking as well as the use of safety seats and seat belts, have gone a long way to reduce the extent and severity of injuries. These programs need our support, and discussion of injury awareness and prevention should be part of medical practice.

There has been a great interest in the consequences of minor head injury resulting in concussion. Multiple studies have suggested that a second concussion significantly affects the recovery of neurological function as compared with after the initial concussion. It is important that young athletes in school not be allowed to continue to play after a concussion. Children may suffer symptoms such as difficulty in concentration or memory, poor reasoning, headaches, excessive tiredness, or emotional lability. The time before they can be allowed to return can vary and should be determined based on a documented return to their preinjury status and complete resolution of all posttraumatic symptoms.

Summary

Head injuries of all grades of severity can have a profound effect on the developing brain. Although the management principles relating to the management of intracranial masses following head injury are not any different from adults, certain age-related differences are present. These include diffuse brain swelling, impaired cerebral autoregulation, reduced seizure threshold, nonaccidental injuries, and the increased susceptibility of the developing brain, among others. Careful attention to control the influence of systemic factors including hypoxia, hypotension, ICP, CPP, and the use of anticonvulsants can help prevent secondary injury. Further research in hypothermia, measures to control free radicals, improvement in functional and metabolic imaging of the injured brain will help in preventing secondary injury and improve outcome.

References

1. Finkelstein EC, Corso PS, Miller TR. The Incidence and Economic Burden of Injuries in the United States. New York: Oxford University Press; 2006
2. Langlois J, Rutland-Brown W, Thomas K. Traumatic Brain Injury in the United States: Emergency Department Visits, Hospitalizations and Deaths. Atlanta, GA: Centers for Disease Control and Prevention, National Center for Injury Prevention and Control; 2004
3. Barlow KM, Spowart JJ, Minns RA. Early posttraumatic seizures in non-accidental head injury: relation to outcome. Dev Med Child Neurol 2000;42(9):591–594
4. Keenan HT, Runyan DK, Marshall SW, Nocera MA, Merten DF, Sinal SH. A population-based study of inflicted traumatic brain injury in young children. JAMA 2003;290(5):621–626
5. Agran PF, Winn D, Anderson C, Trent R, Walton-Haynes L. Rates of pediatric and adolescent injuries by year of age. Pediatrics 2001; 108(3):E45
6. Traumatic Brain Injury. In: Control NCfIPa, ed; 2007
7. Miller JD, Sweet RC, Narayan R, Becker DP. Early insults to the injured brain. JAMA 1978;240(5):439–442
8. Adams JH, Graham DI, Murray LS, Scott G. Diffuse axonal injury due to nonmissile head injury in humans: an analysis of 45 cases. Ann Neurol 1982;12(6):557–563
9. Bruce DA, Alavi A, Bilaniuk L, Dolinskas C, Obrist W, Uzzell B. Diffuse cerebral swelling following head injuries in children: the syndrome of "malignant brain edema". J Neurosurg 1981;54(2):170–178
10. Muizelaar JP, Ward JD, Marmarou A, Newlon PG, Wachi A. Cerebral blood flow and metabolism in severely head-injured children II: Autoregulation. J Neurosurg 1989;71(1):72–76
11. Sharples PM, Matthews DS, Eyre JA. Cerebral blood flow and metabolism in children with severe head injuries II: Cerebrovascular resistance and its determinants. J Neurol Neurosurg Psychiatry 1995; 58(2):153–159
12. Vavilala MS, Muangman S, Tontisirin N, et al. Impaired cerebral autoregulation and 6-month outcome in children with severe traumatic brain injury: preliminary findings. Dev Neurosci 2006; 28(4–5):348–353
13. Caffey J. On the theory and practice of shaking infants: its potential residual effects of permanent brain damage and mental retardation. Am J Dis Child 1972;124(2):161–169
14. Caffey J. The whiplash shaken infant syndrome: manual shaking by the extremities with whiplash-induced intracranial and intraocular bleedings, linked with residual permanent brain damage and mental retardation. Pediatrics 1974;54(4):396–403
15. Ersahin Y, Mutluer S, Mirzai H, Palali I. Pediatric depressed skull fractures: analysis of 530 cases. Childs Nerv Syst 1996;12(6):323–331
16. Gupta SK, Reddy NM, Khosla VK, et al. Growing skull fractures: a clinical study of 41 patients. Acta Neurochir (Wien) 1997;139(10):928–932
17. Muhonen MG, Piper JG, Menezes AH. Pathogenesis and treatment of growing skull fractures. Surg Neurol 1995;43(4):367–372, discussion 372–363
18. Dagi TF, Meyer FB, Poletti CA. The incidence and prevention of meningitis after basilar skull fracture. Am J Emerg Med 1983;1(3):295–298
19. Liu-Shindo M, Hawkins DB. Basilar skull fractures in children. Int J Pediatr Otorhinolaryngol 1989;17(2):109–117
20. Koonsman M, Dunn E, Hughes K, Kendrick B, Moody J. How much monitoring is needed for basilar skull fractures? Am J Surg 1992; 164(5):487–490
21. Adelson PD, Bratton SL, Carney NA, et al. Guidelines for the acute medical management of severe traumatic brain injury in infants, children, and adolescents. Chapter 17. Critical pathway for the treatment of established intracranial hypertension in pediatric traumatic brain injury. Pediatr Crit Care Med 2003;4(3, Suppl):S65–S67
22. Marshall LF, Smith RW, Rauscher LA, Shapiro HM. Mannitol dose requirements in brain-injured patients. J Neurosurg 1978;48(2):169–172
23. Vassar MJ, Fischer RP, O'Brien PE, et al. A multicenter trial for resuscitation of injured patients with 7.5% sodium chloride: the effect of added dextran 70. The Multicenter Group for the Study of Hypertonic Saline in Trauma Patients. Arch Surg 1993;128(9):1003–1011, discussion 1011–1003
24. Simma B, Burger R, Falk M, Sacher P, Fanconi S. A prospective, randomized, and controlled study of fluid management in children with severe head injury: lactated Ringer's solution versus hypertonic saline. Crit Care Med 1998;26(7):1265–1270
25. Boldt J, Knothe C, Zickmann B, Hammermann H, Stertmann WA, Hempelmann G. Volume loading with hypertonic saline solution: endocrinologic and circulatory responses. J Cardiothorac Vasc Anesth 1994;8(3):317–323
26. Doyle JA, Davis DP, Hoyt DB. The use of hypertonic saline in the treatment of traumatic brain injury. J Trauma 2001;50(2):367–383
27. Qureshi AI, Suarez JI. Use of hypertonic saline solutions in treatment of cerebral edema and intracranial hypertension. Crit Care Med 2000; 28(9):3301–3313
28. Matteucci MJ, Wisner DH, Gunther RA, Woolley DE. Effects of hypertonic and isotonic fluid infusion on the flash evoked potential in rats: hemorrhage, resuscitation, and hypernatremia. J Trauma 1993; 34(1):1–7
29. Vialet R, Albanese J, Thomachot L, et al. Isovolume hypertonic solutes (sodium chloride or mannitol) in the treatment of refractory posttraumatic intracranial hypertension: 2 mL/kg 7.5% saline is more effective than 2 mL/kg 20% mannitol. Crit Care Med 2003;31(6):1683–1687
30. Battison C, Andrews PJ, Graham C, Petty T. Randomized, controlled trial on the effect of a 20% mannitol solution and a 7.5% saline/6% dextran solution on increased intracranial pressure after brain injury. Crit Care Med 2005;33(1):196–202, discussion 257–198
31. Horn P, Munch E, Vajkoczy P, et al. Hypertonic saline solution for control of elevated intracranial pressure in patients with exhausted response to mannitol and barbiturates. Neurol Res 1999;21(8):758–764
32. Kjellberg RN, Prieto A Jr. Bifrontal decompressive craniotomy for massive cerebral edema. J Neurosurg 1971;34(4):488–493
33. Venes JL, Collins WF. Bifrontal decompressive craniectomy in the management of head trauma. J Neurosurg 1975;42(4):429–433
34. Polin RS, Shaffrey ME, Bogaev CA, et al. Decompressive bifrontal craniectomy in the treatment of severe refractory posttraumatic cerebral edema. Neurosurgery 1997;41(1):84–92, discussion 92–84
35. Guerra WK, Gaab MR, Dietz H, Mueller JU, Piek J, Fritsch MJ. Surgical decompression for traumatic brain swelling: indications and results. J Neurosurg 1999;90(2):187–196
36. Marion DW, Obrist WD, Carlier PM, Penrod LE, Darby JM. The use of moderate therapeutic hypothermia for patients with severe head injuries: a preliminary report. J Neurosurg 1993;79(3):354–362
37. Marion DW, Penrod LE, Kelsey SF, et al. Treatment of traumatic brain injury with moderate hypothermia. N Engl J Med 1997;336(8):540–546
38. Shiozaki T, Sugimoto H, Taneda M, et al. Effect of mild hypothermia on uncontrollable intracranial hypertension after severe head injury. J Neurosurg 1993;79(3):363–368
39. Clifton GL, Allen S, Barrodale P, et al. A phase II study of moderate hypothermia in severe brain injury. J Neurotrauma 1993;10(3):263–271, discussion 273
40. Clifton GL, Miller ER, Choi SC, et al. Lack of effect of induction of hypothermia after acute brain injury. N Engl J Med 2001;344(8):556–563
41. Aldrich EF, Eisenberg HM, Saydjari C, et al. Diffuse brain swelling in severely head-injured children: a report from the NIH Traumatic Coma Data Bank. J Neurosurg 1992;76(3):450–454
42. Gunn AJ. Cerebral hypothermia for prevention of brain injury following perinatal asphyxia. Curr Opin Pediatr 2000;12(2):111–115
43. Gunn AJ, Gluckman PD, Gunn TR. Selective head cooling in newborn infants after perinatal asphyxia: a safety study. Pediatrics 1998;102(4 Pt 1):885–892
44. Gruszkiewicz J, Doron Y, Peyser E. Recovery from severe craniocerebral injury with brain stem lesions in childhood. Surg Neurol 1973;1(4): 197–201
45. Adelson PD, Ragheb J, Kanev P, et al. Phase II clinical trial of moderate hypothermia after severe traumatic brain injury in children. Neurosurgery 2005;56(4):740–754, discussion 740–754

46. Appleton RE. Seizure-related injuries in children with newly diagnosed and untreated epilepsy. Epilepsia 2002;43(7):764–767
47. Chiaretti A, De Benedictis R, Polidori G, Piastra M, Iannelli A, Di Rocco C. Early post-traumatic seizures in children with head injury. Childs Nerv Syst 2000;16(12):862–866
48. Hahn YS, Fuchs S, Flannery AM, Barthel MJ, McLone DG. Factors influencing posttraumatic seizures in children. Neurosurgery 1988;22(5): 864–867
49. Ratan SK, Kulshreshtha R, Pandey RM. Predictors of posttraumatic convulsions in head-injured children. Pediatr Neurosurg 1999;30(3):127–131
50. Keenan HT, Runyan DK, Marshall SW, Nocera MA, Merten DF. A population-based comparison of clinical and outcome characteristics of young children with serious inflicted and noninflicted traumatic brain injury. Pediatrics 2004;114(3):633–639
51. Annegers JF, Hauser WA, Coan SP, Rocca WA. A population-based study of seizures after traumatic brain injuries. N Engl J Med 1998;338(1): 20–24
52. Frey LC. Epidemiology of posttraumatic epilepsy: a critical review. Epilepsia 2003;44(Suppl 10):11–17
53. Young B, Rapp RP, Norton JA, Haack D, Walsh JW. Failure of prophylactically administered phenytoin to prevent post-traumatic seizures in children. Childs Brain 1983;10(3):185–192
54. Lewis RJ, Yee L, Inkelis SH, Gilmore D. Clinical predictors of posttraumatic seizures in children with head trauma. Ann Emerg Med 1993;22(7):1114–1118
55. Temkin NR, Dikmen SS, Wilensky AJ, Keihm J, Chabal S, Winn HR. A randomized, double-blind study of phenytoin for the prevention of post-traumatic seizures. N Engl J Med 1990;323(8):497–502

IV Critical Care

15 Neurological Critical Care

Opeolu M. Adeoye and Lori A. Shutter

The goal of neurocritical care in the management of central nervous system (CNS) injured patients is to prevent and/or minimize secondary CNS injury while optimizing physiological parameters that are frequently deranged in critically ill patients. To this end, the neurointensivist must deal not only with the unique consequences of the injured CNS but also the pulmonary, cardiac, infectious, and other complications that commonly occur in the intensive care unit (ICU). These potential complications during ICU care of traumatic brain injury (TBI) are discussed in detail in the following chapters. The goal of this chapter is to provide a general overview and approach to the ICU management of severe TBI. In addition, we will review some neurological syndromes that frequently occur in critically ill patients, regardless of the primary injury.

In particular, we will discuss (1) the initial evaluation of the TBI patient with special attention to airway, breathing, and circulation (ABCs), with attention paid to the evidence for striving to avoid hypoxia or hypotension; (2) the management of intracranial hypertension and cerebral edema; (3) hypothermia in TBI; (4) prevention of common complications of ICU care like infections and venous thrombosis; and (5) the occurrence and treatment of neurological complications such as seizures, pituitary dysfunction, cranial nerve injury, behavioral abnormalities, neuropathy, and myopathy in critical illness.

Initial Evaluation of the Traumatic Brain-Injured Patient

By the time the majority of TBI patients arrive in the ICU, they would have been evaluated in the emergency department (ED) and had some basic interventions performed. Nonetheless, it is prudent upon ICU arrival to reassess the patient and review the history, imaging, and laboratory results. In this regard, one always begins with assessment of the ABCs. Patient transport is fraught with potential complications as patients are often hurriedly moved to the ICU in elevators too small to easily accommodate the patient and care providers. As such, intubated patients need to be assessed for tube placement, oxygenation, and ventilation; nonintubated patients need to have their airway reassessed for continued ability to protect and maintain an adequate airway. Repeat vital signs should be performed promptly upon ICU arrival, with a focus on immediate management of any hypoxia or hypotension. Communication between ED and ICU medical care teams is key to ensure important factors in the patient's condition are passed on to the in-hospital staff. For instance, if the ED or prehospital intubation was difficult on a patient, this needs to be communicated clearly to the ICU team, who will be making extubation or tracheostomy decisions during the ICU stay. Also, isolated hypoxic or hypotensive events are frequently not well documented in the medical records and may have profound influence on patients' ultimate outcomes. TBI patients also frequently have other nonobvious injuries as a consequence of the mechanism of trauma.

A comprehensive evaluation by the ED and trauma team including a detailed examination along with computed tomography (CT) images of the chest, abdomen, and pelvis may be necessary in patients with an unreliable examination secondary to TBI. Cervical spine evaluation by plain x-rays or CT may also need to be performed, with spinal stability maintained until the patient can be clinically cleared. Long bone injuries may also occur and the patient should be assessed for this possibility. Finally, seemingly innocuous findings during the early assessment may in fact complicate subsequent hospital course. For instance, occult lacerations that are not irrigated and repaired early on, or repaired lacerations with sutures that need to be removed may serve as a source of infection during the hospital stay. The ICU team needs to recognize and address such issues. Altogether, the initial evaluation of the TBI patient on ICU arrival consists of careful attention to the ABCs, a detailed history and physical examination encompassing communication with previous caretakers, and a thorough review of images and laboratory results already obtained prior to ICU arrival.

Managing Hypoxia and Hypotension

Prolonged hypoxia and hypotension in any field of medicine clearly have adverse consequences; thus, no randomized controlled trial assessing the impact of these events on patient outcomes will ever be performed for obvious ethical reasons. Isolated episodes of hypoxia or hypotension, however, are not uncommon in the care of critically ill patients and may occur during endotracheal intubation or procedural sedation or as a consequence of the primary injury or illness. The adverse impact of these secondary insults on outcome after TBI has been recognized over the past 30 years, and even a single episode of hypoxia or hypotension is to be avoided as suggested by multiple studies.[1–5]

In a seminal article from 1978, Miller et al reported on a prospective cohort of 100 consecutive patients with severe TBI. Adverse events evaluated in that study included hypotension, hypoxia, anemia, and hypercarbia, each of which was found to be associated with increased morbidity and mortality. Hypotension in that study was defined as an isolated episode of systolic blood pressure (SBP) less than 95 mm Hg. Unfortunately, hypotension was not analyzed independently of the other factors, and further work had to be done to clarify the impact of the individual factors on TBI patient outcomes.[1]

Definitive information was gained through a prehospital prospective study of 717 consecutive TBI patients by Chesnut et al. They evaluated the effect of hypotension on TBI outcomes and found that it was an independent predictor of poor outcome. In addition, a single documented episode of hypotension was sufficient to double mortality and increase morbidity. The study also found that patients with correction of hypotension prior to ED arrival did better than those who were still hypotensive on ED arrival.[2] In a prospective, randomized, double-blind, multicenter trial of 7.5% hypertonic saline (HTS) as a prehospital resuscitative fluid in trauma patients, Vassar et al reported that raising the blood pressure in hypotensive severe TBI patients improved outcomes in proportion to the efficacy of resuscitation.[3] These findings underscore the importance of optimizing the prehospital, ED, and ICU care of the TBI patient as each may have a profound impact of patients' outcomes. Unfortunately, hypotension and hypoxia are not uncommon early in the course of the severe TBI patient's care. In a cohort study of 50 TBI patients transported by helicopter, hypoxia (defined as SaO_2 <90%) occurred in 55% of cases; hypotension (defined as SBP <90 mm Hg) occurred in 24% of cases. Both clinical factors exerted a negative impact on outcome.[4] Finally, in a study of 107 TBI patients, early episodes of hypotension, but not hypoxia, were found to predict mortality, with odds ratios increasing from 2.1 to 8.1 with repeat episodes of hypotension.[5]

In summary, both hypotension and hypoxia adversely impact patient outcomes following TBI. Prevention and correction of early episodes of hypoxia or hypotension need to occur in the prehospital or ED setting; nevertheless, care must be taken during the ICU or hospital stay to quickly and aggressively avoid repeat episodes of hypoxia and hypotension given the adverse consequences that these entail.

Managing Intracranial Hypertension

Refractory intracranial hypertension is the most concerning consequence of severe TBI, as persistently high intracranial pressure (ICP) may lead to compromised cerebral perfusion pressure (CPP), decreased cerebral blood flow (CBF), ischemia, brain herniation, and death. The goal of ICP management is to maintain global and regional CBF to meet the metabolic needs of the injured brain while preventing secondary brain injury due to poor perfusion. To achieve this, historically clinicians focused on a so-called vertical approach whereby the goals were to optimize ICP, sometimes compromising other factors that affect the injured brain. Alternatively, a school of thought aimed at optimizing CPP developed. We will discuss both of these approaches, then offer the contemporary approach that comprises a more "horizontal" management of elevated ICP.

ICP elevation has been recognized to complicate care of TBI patients for decades. A retrospective study published in 1979 found that 100 consecutive patients managed to maintain a goal ICP <15 mm Hg had better outcomes compared with other published reports at the time with less-aggressive ICP control goals.[6] Narayan et al subsequently performed a retrospective analysis of 207 consecutive severe TBI patients managed with a goal ICP of <20 mm Hg.[7] Patients whose ICP remained <20 mm Hg were found to have improved outcomes compared with those in which ICP could not be successfully controlled. These two studies raise an obvious question: What should the ICP goal be in clinical practice? In an analysis of 428 patients undergoing ICP monitoring, logistic regression was utilized to determine predictors of poor outcomes. A threshold value of 20 mm Hg was found to best correlate with 6-month outcomes.[8] Classically, maintaining this target ICP of 20 mm Hg has been the teaching, but various investigators suggest different targets for ICP treatment, and recent reports question targeting ICP in isolation.

In an observational study of 291 patients, Chambers et al sought to determine ICP and CPP thresholds associated with outcome using receiver operating characteristic (ROC) curves.[9] When ICP values were above 10 mm Hg, the sensitivity of ICP for predicting poor outcome increased; however, at 30 mm Hg, the sensitivity of ICP for predicting outcome was only 61%.[9] In a prospective trial of 27 patients managed such that ICP goal was either 20 or 25 mm Hg, while CPP was maintained above 70 mm Hg and jugular venous oxygen saturation (SjO_2) was maintained above 54%, no difference in outcome was found between the 20 and 25 mm Hg groups.[10] These reports suggest that a "one-size-fits-all" approach to severe TBI patients may be inadequate, and different thresholds need to be considered for the individual patient. Just as many researchers have targeted ICP in isolation, others have focused on CPP-guided treatment.

In a study of 34 patients with severe TBI, CPP was aggressively maintained at greater than 70 mm Hg using volume expansion, flat patient positioning, and catecholamine infusions as necessary. Overall mortality was 21%, but mortality ascribed to uncontrolled ICP was 8%.[11] This was the first report to suggest CPP-guided therapy may have advantages over ICP-guided therapy. However, this case series of 34 patients was not randomized, and although it significantly impacted on clinical practice for many years subsequent studies have questioned CPP-guided therapy. Maintaining CPP >70 mm Hg in severe TBI has been associated with an increased incidence of adult respiratory distress syndrome (ARDS) without any evidence of improved functional outcomes.[12,13] Some investigators have assessed the impact of various CPP thresholds on outcome after TBI. In a case series, Young et al reported good outcomes in patients managed with goal CPP >60 mm Hg, even though those patients had ICPs occasionally as high as 40 mm Hg.[14] In a review of their experience over 12 years, a group in Taiwan found that patients with a modified CPP goal of 60 mm Hg had fewer complications and better outcomes than did patients managed primarily with ICP targeted or CPP >70 mm Hg targeted therapy.[15] In a retrospective analysis of 429 severe TBI patients, mortality was found to dramatically increase for patients with ICP >20 mm Hg or CPP <55 mm Hg; excessive CPP (>95 mm Hg) was also associated with poorer outcomes.[16] The 2007 Guidelines for Management of Severe Traumatic Brain Injury from the Brain Trauma Foundation (BTF) and the American Association of Neurological Surgeons (AANS) has reviewed these studies and subsequently recommended that CPP be maintained in the 50 to 70 mm Hg range while keeping ICP below 20 mm Hg.[17]

Many factors that have different underlying pathophysiology may contribute to ICP elevations. Using a systematic approach that progresses in level of intensity from "low tech" to "high tech," the clinician should address ICP elevation that follows a 'horizontal' algorithm to address specific problems. If the underlying problem contributing to ICP elevation can be identified and fixed, the patient may not require particularly aggressive measures. For instance, the reading on the ICP monitor may be elevated because the patient's head is turned to the side, and simply straightening the neck to increase venous drainage may resolve the ICP issues. In addition, elevating the head of the bed and ensuring this elevation is in the 30- to 45-degree range may have the same effect. ICP may be elevated secondary to agitation, hypoxia, and/or pain and these issues must be identified and addressed. Other factors that may contribute to ICP elevation that are not so easily fixed include outflow obstruction (perhaps from intraventricular blood), mass lesion, ischemia, and/or cerebral edema. Obstruction may be treated by placement of an intraventricular catheter with occasional cerebrospinal fluid (CSF) drainage as needed; ischemia may be addressed by increasing CBF through blood pressure augmentation, hyperemia may be treated with vasoconstrictors, and mass lesions may be surgically removed.

The management of cerebral edema and osmotic therapy will be addressed individually.

The multifactorial aspect of intracranial hypertension suggests that issues need to be addressed individually, or horizontally, rather than vertically or in a hierarchical pattern (**Fig. 15.1**).

Cerebral Edema and Osmotic Therapy Using Mannitol or Hypertonic Saline

Cerebral edema is classically described as "vasogenic" or "cytotoxic/cellular." Vasogenic edema is thought to be due to disruption of the blood–brain barrier (BBB) causing extracellular water accumulation. Cytotoxic edema is thought to reflect sustained intracellular water accumulation as a consequence of cell death. The mechanism of cerebral edema after TBI has generally been poorly understood. Historically, it has been thought to be primarily vasogenic. However, recent magnetic resonance imaging (MRI) studies suggest that edema after TBI is, in fact, primarily cellular.[18] Recent advances in the basic sciences have also identified a family of cell wall proteins known as aquaporins, which are thought to be extremely important in the regulation of cerebral water diffusion.[19,20] Although these are promising areas of future targeted intervention for prevention and treatment of cerebral edema, current management generally follows some basic principles.

Osmotic therapy has been used in the treatment of cerebral mass effect and intracranial hypertension since the 1960s and remains the mainstay of therapy to date. The ideal osmotic agent would remain in the intravascular space and not cross the BBB, thereby drawing intracellular and extracellular water into the vascular space and reducing cerebral edema. Mannitol has historically been the most commonly used osmotic agent for treatment of edema and elevated ICP in neurocritical care. Several studies have shown that mannitol decreases ICP in TBI patients,[21] but unfortunately there has never been a randomized study showing that mannitol improves outcome after TBI. Due to certain consequences of mannitol therapy that will be discussed below, HTS has become an alternative to mannitol

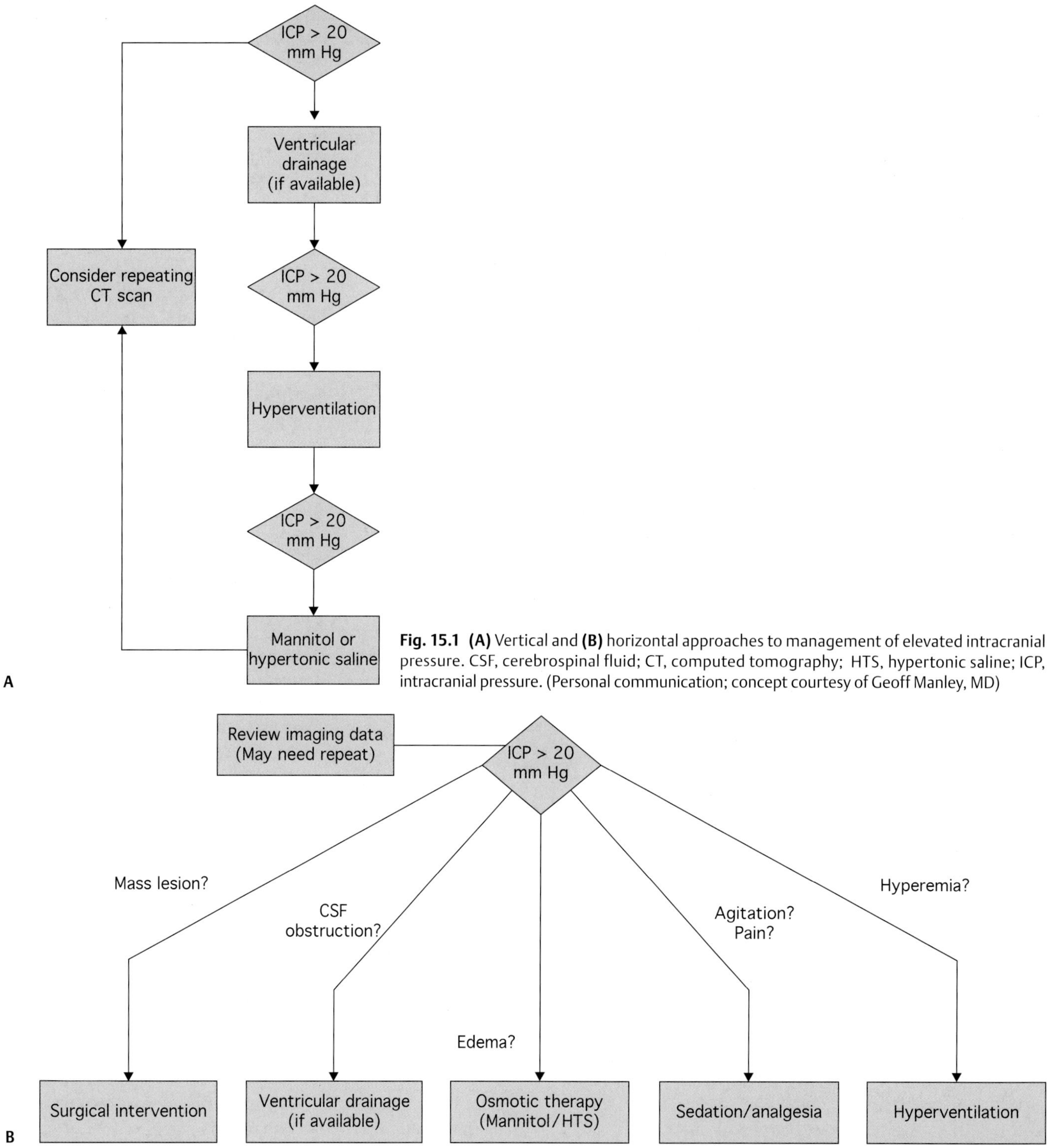

Fig. 15.1 (A) Vertical and **(B)** horizontal approaches to management of elevated intracranial pressure. CSF, cerebrospinal fluid; CT, computed tomography; HTS, hypertonic saline; ICP, intracranial pressure. (Personal communication; concept courtesy of Geoff Manley, MD)

for treatment of edema and ICP elevation after TBI and other neurological emergencies.[22] First, we will review the available evidence for mannitol use in TBI, then discuss potential advantages of HTS over mannitol, and finally, offer recommendations for clinical practice.

Mannitol has been shown to be effective in lowering ICP in TBI.[21,23–25] The potential advantages of mannitol as the preferred osmotic agent include its relative impermeability to the intact BBB, its lowering effect on blood viscosity thereby decreasing mechanical resistance,[26] and

Table 15.1 Comparison of Hypertonic Saline and Mannitol

Parameter	Hypertonic Saline	Mannitol
Volume	Volume expander	Initially expands, but causes diuresis/hypotension
Serum osmolality	Increased	Increased
Crossing blood–brain barrier	Less likely	More likely
Impact on ICP	Similar reduction	Similar reduction
Impact on CPP	Maintains CPP	May reduce CPP due to hypotension/diuresis
Immunomodulation	May decrease inflammation	No significant effect

Abbreviations: ICP, intracranial pressure; CPP, cerebral perfusion pressure.

ready availability and prolonged experience with its use. However, mannitol does have some adverse effects that are concerning in TBI patients. Mannitol readily crosses the injured BBB and accumulates in the brain, potentially drawing water back into the brain and causing "rebound" intracranial hypertension.[27] It is also excreted unchanged in the urine and, while initially a volume expander, may then cause a profound diuresis, potentially leading to hypotension and decreased CPP that may lead to secondary injury in the TBI patient.[28] HTS may have some advantages with regard to these potential adverse effects of mannitol. Thus, HTS is gaining increasing favor for use in the management of cerebral edema and intracranial hypertension.

HTS was initially studied as a resuscitative fluid in hypotensive trauma victims.[29] Although no benefit to 7.5% HTS was determined for all patients in that study, a subgroup analysis found improved outcomes in patients with TBI.[30] Subsequent studies focused on treatment of elevated ICP and edema in TBI with promising results.[21] The theoretical advantages of HTS over mannitol include the fact that hypertonic saline is less permeable to the intact BBB than mannitol, it acts as a sustained volume expander without the subsequent diuresis, and it may have favorable immunomodulatory properties that decrease inflammation.[22] In addition, Vialet et al have shown that HTS is effective in lowering ICP in cases that were refractory to mannitol therapy.[31] Unfortunately, this study of only 20 patients is the largest of limited head-to-head comparisons of mannitol and HTS for the management of elevated ICP, and it did not compare equiosmolar doses of the two agents. Also, different HTS studies have used various concentrations ranging from 1.9 to 29% concentration of sodium chloride formulations containing dextran and/or sodium acetate have also been used in the different studies, making direct comparisons difficult. Thus, more studies are needed to determine the optimal osmotic agent for treatment of intracranial hypertension, and the optimal formulation of HTS and method of infusion needs to be clarified.

Summary

In summary, ICP elevation is a serious complication in severe TBI. The approach to management must be systematic and consistent. The individual patient must be taken into account, and higher ICP levels may be tolerated in some patients if CPP is adequate. CPP levels in the 50 to 70 mm Hg range are likely sufficient, and ICP should be maintained below 20 mm Hg. Mannitol or HTS may be used for treatment of elevated ICP as outlined in the algorithm. **Table 15.1** lists characteristics of HTS and mannitol. The neurointensivist must remain vigilant and needs to direct the care of the patient in close collaboration with the neurosurgeon. Although not proven effective, barbiturate coma and decompressive hemicraniectomy should be considered for patients in whom other aggressive medical measures have failed. Management options for ICP control are presented in **Table 15.2**.

Use of Hypothermia in TBI

Hypothermia has been studied as a possible neuroprotective agent for reducing secondary brain injury from various causes over the past 60 years. Its mechanism as a neuroprotectant remains a matter of debate. While hypothermia has been shown to be effective in reducing secondary injury following cardiac arrest,[32,33] no human studies have demonstrated an unequivocal benefit of hypothermia in TBI.

The National Acute Brain Injury Study: Hypothermia (NABIS:H) was a randomized controlled trial to test the effect of induced hypothermia on patients with acute TBI. Two hundred sixty-eight subjects were randomized to cooling to 33°C or maintenance of normothermia at 37°C.[34]

Table 15.2 Options for Management of Intracranial Pressure

Initial Treatment Plan

- Secure airway and provide oxygenation, ventilation, & intravenous fluids during trauma resuscitation
- Maintain SaO_2>90%, SBP > 90%, and $PaCO_2$ 35–40 mm Hg
- Avoid hypotension: Increase MAP to maintain CPP >60 mm Hg
- Obtain CT scan of brain as indicated
- Initiate ICP/ventriculostomy monitoring per indications:
  - GCS ≤8 after initial resuscitation with an abnormal CT on admission (i.e., hematoma, contusion, edema, or compressed basal cisterns) and deemed to have survivable brain injury
  - GCS ≤8 after initial resuscitation in patients with a normal CT and 2 or more of the following: age >40 years, unilateral or bilateral posturing, SBP <90 mm Hg

Standard Admission NICU Goals

- Assure head and neck alignment: Position head of bed at 20–30 degrees (as appropriate for spine status)
- Retape endotracheal tube tape (avoid taping at back of neck)
- Careful monitoring to maintain: SaO_2 >90%, PCO_2 38–44 mm Hg, ICP <25 mm Hg, CPP >60 mm Hg, temperature 36–37C, glucose 80–110 mg/dL
- Ensure sedation and analgesia goals are met
- If ventriculostomy in place, keep clamped to allow continuous ICP monitoring

NICU Interventions for ICP Elevations

Treatment options for unprovoked ICP elevation of >20 mm Hg that persists for more than 5 minutes. Interventions should be initiated based on clinical situation and potential etiology of ICP elevation.

Therapeutic interventions for signs of acute herniation

- Bolus of mannitol (0.25–1.0 g / kg) or 3% NaCl (250 mL). Maintain serum Osmo <320 mOsm/L and euvolemia
- Hyperventilation to $PaCO_2$ <35 mm Hg

Therapeutic interventions for raised ICP

- Increase sedation and analgesia as tolerated (maintain CPP >60 mm Hg)
- If ventriculostomy in place, drain 5–10 mL cerebrospinal fluid
- Maintain CPP >60 mm Hg, use vasopressors as needed
- Mannitol 0.25–1.0 g/kg or 3% NaCl to achieve a goal Na^+ of 145–155 (maintain serum Osmo <320 mOsm/L and euvolemia)
- Mild hyperventilation to $PaCO_2$ of 33–38 mm Hg (maintain $PbtO_2$ >20 mm Hg)
- Hypothermia to temperature of 33–34°C
- Decompressive hemicraniectomy
- Barbiturate coma with EEG monitoring to confirm burst-suppression

Diagnostic interventions

- Consider repeating a brain CT scan to assess for structural lesion
- EEG for possible seizure

Abbreviations: CT, computed tomography; EEG, electroencephalogram; GCS, Glasgow Coma Scale; ICP, intracranial pressure; CPP, cerebral perfusion pressure; MAP, mean arterial pressure; Na^+, sodium; NaCl , sodium chloride; NICU, neuro-intensive care unit; PaO_2, peripheral capillary saturation; $PaCO_2$, carbon dioxide in arterial blood; PCO_2, partial pressure of carbon dioxide; $PbtO_2$, brain tissue oxygenation; SBP, systolic blood pressure.

The trial was negative. The investigators noted from their preclinical work that cooling was most effective when instituted rapidly after injury. Despite this focus, they enrolled subjects up to 6 hours postinjury, and the average time to target temperature was 8.4 ± 3.0 hours. In the quartile of subjects with the most delayed cooling, the average time to target temperature was 12.7 ± 2.5 hours after injury. Interestingly, an unplanned subset analysis of 102 patients who arrived at the hospital with a temperature of 35°C or lower and therefore reached the target temperature very quickly, showed a clinically significant improvement in outcome (Relative Risk [RR] = 0.8, 95% CI = 0.6 to 1.0) that was marginally statistically significant. Subsequently, the National Institutes of Neurological Disorders and Stroke (NINDS) has funded NABIS:H II, a follow-up study that will seek to enroll patients who arrive hypothermic to prospectively verify the subset analysis found in the initial trial. At about the same time as the NABIS:H trial, a very small Japanese trial was performed in which hypothermia was induced more quickly (within 3 to 4 hours of injury) in patients with TBI.[35] The 26 rapidly cooled subjects had significantly better neurological outcomes than normothermic controls.

NABIS:H II is expected to complete enrollment in 2010. In the meantime, ICUs across the country are in fact either inducing hypothermia or aggressively maintaining normothermia in TBI patients. Fever is common in TBI patients admitted to the ICU and is clearly harmful to the injured brain.[36] Maintaining normothermia is likely beneficial and is recommended by the current TBI management guidelines.[17] Unfortunately, there is insufficient evidence at this time to recommend routine hypothermia for severe TBI outside of study protocols.

Managing Nonneurological Issues for TBI Patients in Intensive Care

Severely ill TBI patients are often endotracheally intubated and mechanically ventilated, are chemically sedated and bed-bound during the course of their ICU stay and have nasal or oral feeding tubes, central venous catheters, bladder catheters, rectal pouches, and other invasive monitors to follow their hemodynamic and physiological states. Management of these patients is complex, and the patients are particularly prone to developing any number of complications associated with ICU care. In the next few sections, we will discuss routine ICU care such as ventilator management and nutrition, prevention of infections, and other complications of ICU care such as ventilator-associated pneumonias (VAP), line sepsis and bacteremia, venous thrombosis, bedsores and ulcers, among other things that could seriously complicate patient care and outcomes.

Ventilator Management and Ventilator-Associated Pneumonia in TBI

Respiratory failure is the most common nonneurological organ dysfunction in severe TBI.[37] Despite this, few studies have assessed ventilator management in TBI patients. Recent trials are beginning to focus on respiratory mechanics after TBI and the effect mechanical ventilation may have on outcome. A small prospective trial randomized 21 TBI patients to volume control ventilation and zero positive end-expiratory pressure (ZEEP) versus 8 cm H_2O positive end-expiratory pressure (PEEP).[38] After 5 days of mechanical ventilation, abnormal respiratory mechanics were exhibited by the ZEEP group and appeared to be prevented by moderate levels of PEEP. The impact this may have on patient outcomes remains unknown. In a prospective observational study of 137 isolated TBI patients ventilated for >24 hours, 31% of patients developed acute lung injury (ALI) and ALI was independently predictive of mortality and poor neurological outcomes.[39] At the present time, the best modes of ventilation to optimize respiratory mechanics and minimize risk of ALI in TBI are unknown and warrant clinical trials.

Ventilator-associated pneumonia (VAP) is common and contributes greatly to morbidity and mortality in critically ill patients.[40] Incidence rates of VAP have been estimated at 10 to 25% with mortality rates of 10 to 40%. In addition, hospital lengths of stays and cost are also increased in patients who develop VAP.[40–43] VAP has been characterized as early (<4 days) or late (≥4 days) based on the duration of mechanical ventilation. Early VAP should be treated with antibiotics that cover typical community organisms. Appropriate agents may include a macrolide (e.g., azithromycin) and third-generation cephalosporin (e.g., ceftriaxone). Late VAP, however, should be assumed to be caused by hospital-acquired organisms that carry a higher potential for resistance, as such, a broader antibiotic coverage should be utilized. Empiric gram-positive coverage for methicillin-resistant *Staphylococcus aureus* with vancomycin is appropriate; gram-negative coverage should cover for *Pseudomonas aeruginosa*; some appropriate agents include cefepime, gentamicin, tobramycin, imipenem, and piperacillin/tazobactam. Recommended antibiotic regimens for VAP are listed in **Table 15.3**. Clinicians should become familiar with the biogram of their local facility to guide antibiotic choices. It has been shown that initial broad coverage that is then narrowed after the actual causative organism is identified is a safer and more effective way to treat VAP.[44] Few data are available regarding VAP in TBI patients in particular.

In a prospective observational cohort study of 60 TBI patients with VAP, Zygun et al[45] reported a higher risk of VAP among patients with polytrauma compared with those with isolated TBI. They also reported a longer duration of mechanical ventilation, longer ICU and hospital length of

Table 15.3 Antibiotic Recommendations for Ventilator-Associated Pneumonia (VAP)

VAP <4 days (presumed community-acquired)	VAP ≥4 days (presumed hospital-acquired)
Azithromycin plus third-generation cephalosporin (ceftriaxone/cefotaxime/ceftazidime)	Vancomycin or linezolid for methicillin-resistant *Staphylococcus aureus* plus antipseudomonal agents listed below
Third-generation quinolones (levofloxacin, moxifloxacin)	Aminoglycosides (tobramycin, gentamicin)
Ampicillin-sulbactam	Fourth-generation cephalosporins, e.g., cefepime
Ertapenem	Carbapenems, e.g., imipenem
	Piperacillin-tazobactam

stay (LOS), and more frequent tracheostomies in TBI patients who developed VAP compared with those who did not.[45]

Preventive strategies for VAP have largely focused on minimizing oropharyngeal colonization and decreasing the risk of aspiration of oropharyngeal or gastric contents. In a randomized clinical trial of 86 medical ICU patients, Drakulovic et al compared a semirecumbent or supine bed position and determined the incidence of VAP.[46] Microbiologically confirmed pneumonia occurred in 5% of the semirecumbent group compared with 23% of the supine group, although there was no difference in mortality. No other trial has examined the impact of semirecumbent bed position on VAP incidence to our knowledge. However, this low cost and relatively simple intervention may have a dramatic consequence on patient morbidity and should be practiced routinely. In addition to elevation of the head of the bed, sucralfate has been shown to decrease the risk of VAP compared with the usual H2-blockers used for stress ulcer prophylaxis.[47] As such, sucralfate should be considered for stress ulcer prophylaxis in patients who are low risk for gastrointestinal bleeding. Using the Centers for Disease Control and Prevention (CDC) Guidelines for Prevention of Nosocomial Pneumonia and aggressively auditing staff to ensure compliance, Cocanour et al reported a decrease in VAP rates from 22.3 to 32.7 to 0 and 12.8 infections per 1,000 ventilator days.[48] This demonstrates that prevention of VAP has to be an institutional commitment to achieve meaningful results. Simple things such as elevation of the head of the bed, washing/ sanitizing of hands by health care providers, and appropriate antibiotic coverage once VAP is suspected may reduce patient morbidity, ICU cost, and LOS. Although no randomized trial has been performed, early tracheostomy is also gaining recent favor in TBI management.

Seeking to develop criteria for TBI patients who would require tracheostomy, Gurkin et al[49] performed a retrospective review of all TBI patients in their trauma registry over a 6-year period. Logistic regression analysis was used to identify Glasgow Coma Scale (GCS) score ≤8, injury severity score ≥25, and ventilator days >7 as predictive of requiring tracheostomy. They suggested performing early tracheostomy to decrease morbidity and LOS.[49] Another retrospective review of 55 patients found no difference in mortality, ventilator days, or VAP rates, but found a decrease in ICU LOS in early (<7 days) versus late (>7 days) tracheostomy patients.[50] A prospective randomized trial is warranted. **Table 15.4** lists patient characteristics that may warrant early tracheostomy.

Catheter-Related Infections in TBI

Central venous catheters (CVCs) are frequently used in the ICU to deliver fluids, nutrition, and drugs, and to monitor hemodynamic status. Infection of these catheters is the most frequent complication and is associated with increased morbidity, mortality, and duration of hospital stay. Catheter-related bloodstream infections (CBSIs) are associated with mortality rates of 10 to 20%, prolonged hospitalization, and medical costs of up to $10,000 per hospitalization.[51,52] Unfortunately, patients in the ICU are generally ill enough that CVCs are needed as part of patient care. As such, the emphasis of this discussion is to cover methods of preventing CBSIs in ICU patients.

CVC location has been associated with infectious and thrombotic complications. A randomized trial found that subclavian vein placement of a CVC was associated with lower rates of venous thrombosis and infection compared with femoral location.[53] Although jugular and subclavian locations have not been compared head to head in a trial,

Table 15.4 Patients to Be Considered for Early (<7 Days) Tracheostomy

Glasgow Coma Score: ≤8
Injury Severity Score: ≥25
Anticipated length of mechanical ventilation: >7 days

Sources: Gurkin SA, Parikshak M, Kralovich KA, Horst HM, Agarwal V, Payne N. Indicators for tracheostomy in patients with traumatic brain injury. Am Surg 2002;68:324–328. Ahmed N, Kuo YH. Early versus late tracheostomy in patients with severe traumatic head injury. Surg Infect (Larchmt) 2007;8:343–347.

the available evidence suggests a lower thrombosis and infectious rate in the subclavian location.[54] Antimicrobial impregnated catheters have been studied for prevention of CBSIs. Chlorhexidine and silver sulfadiazine impregnated catheters were reported to lower the rate of CBSIs from 7.6 per 1,000 catheter days to 1.6 per 1,000 catheter days.[55] Minocycline and rifampin-coated catheters are likely even more effective than the chlorhexidine and silver sulfadiazine-coated catheters in preventing CBSIs.[56] However, cost-effectiveness analyses indicate that antimicrobial-coated catheters should be reserved for instances where the infection rates are >2%.[57]

Catheters should be placed under maximal sterile barrier precautions, as this approach has been shown to reduce CBSIs and cost.[58] Chlorhexidine as the skin disinfectant prior to insertion has been shown to be superior to iodine or alcohol for preventing CBSIs.[59] Experienced care providers should either place or closely supervise placement of CVCs because this can decrease the risk of complications. Ultrasound guidance should be utilized when feasible, but may not be particularly useful for placing a subclavian CVC. Catheters should be removed as soon as they are no longer used in the patient's care. There is no evidence for prophylactically changing a catheter after a prescribed period, although the risk of infection does increase after 3 days.[51,52] A suspected CBSI should be investigated with blood cultures from the CVC and from a peripheral site. Although positive cultures do not absolutely confirm a catheter-related bloodstream infection (because colonization of the catheter or contamination during blood draw may cause positive cultures), negative cultures have a 99% negative predictive value and almost certainly rule out the CVC as the source of infection.[60] Initial treatment of a suspected CVC infection should cover both gram-negative and gram-positive organisms. Treatment should then be narrowed or discontinued once an organism is identified or the cultures are negative, respectively.

Venous Thromboembolism Prophylaxis and Treatment in TBI

Venous thrombosis occurs frequently in critically ill patients and may contribute to patient morbidity and poor outcomes by causing pulmonary embolism (PE). An estimated 20% of severe TBI patients will develop deep venous thrombosis (DVT) without prophylaxis.[61] However, distinctions are made about clinically relevant and irrelevant DVTs. It is generally thought that DVTs discovered in the calf veins as part of routine screening do not lead to clinically significant adverse events,[62] but clots in more proximal veins are more likely to cause PE. Pulmonary emboli have been reported to occur in <1% of TBI patients during their hospital stay.[63] However, the potential threat to life and inherent difficulties with anticoagulation in patients with intracranial injury make prevention of venous thromboembolism a priority in the ICU management of severe TBI.

Prevention of thromboembolism may be achieved using either mechanical compression or pharmacologically with heparinoid drugs. No randomized controlled trials have compared these two modalities for DVT prophylaxis in TBI or other cranial pathology for that matter. A prospective observational study evaluated a pneumatic compression device for DVT prophylaxis in 523 neurosurgical patients, 89 of whom had TBI.[64] DVT rates were 0% in TBI and 3.8% in other patients in the study. Another prospective observational study evaluated enoxaparin use within 24 hours of ED arrival in 150 TBI patients. Although DVT rates were only 2%, the study protocol was changed to starting enoxaparin 48 hours after ED arrival due to bleeding requiring craniotomy in two out of 24 patients.[65] Although DVT prophylaxis remains a part of the ICU management of TBI, little evidence is available to guide clinicians. We favor use of pneumatic compression devices upon initial hospital admission and then add prophylactic heparinoids as early as 24 hours after admission once repeat head CT scans have shown stabilization of intracranial hematomas. The current guidelines make grade III recommendations for using pneumatic compression devices and/or heparinoids for DVT prophylaxis, but stated there was insufficient literature evidence to make any recommendation regarding the appropriate timing of heparinoid initiation.[17]

Transfusions in TBI

The concept that maintaining a hematocrit >30% after TBI has little supportive evidence. In a subgroup analysis of 67 patients with moderate to severe TBI from the multicenter, randomized, controlled Transfusion Requirements in the Critical Care (TRICC) trial, no significant differences were found in 30-day mortality, ICU LOS, or hospital LOS between patients with targeted hemoglobin goals of 7 to 9 g/dL compared with those with goal hemoglobin of 10 to 12 g/dL.[66] In contrast, there is now evidence that transfusions can result in immunomodulation and ALI[67,68] and are associated with increased mortality and morbidity in trauma patients.[69] Therefore present management should limit transfusions unless there are clear signs of physiological compromise in volume status, hemodynamic state, electrocardiogram (EKG) findings, cardiovascular disease, or cerebral oxygen tension.

Nutrition in TBI

Few studies on the impact of nutrition on TBI patients specifically are available. In a randomized controlled trial comparing the impact of early parenteral nutrition (within 7 days) versus delayed enteral nutrition (within 2 weeks) in 38 TBI patients, the early parenteral group were found to have improved survival, a positive nitrogen balance, and a higher albumin than the delayed enteral nutrition group. The authors concluded that early total parenteral nutrition had a favorable impact on survival after TBI.[70] However, a subsequent study by the same group in 51 TBI patients found no difference in morbidity or mortality among patients randomized to full enteral or parenteral nutrition within 3 days of injury and suggested that the advantage from the first study may have simply been due to overall malnutrition in the 2-week group.[71] To achieve full nutritional support with a trend toward better 6-month outcomes, the current guidelines recommend initiating nutrition within 72 hours of injury.[17] The route and formulation of nutritional supplementation have also been debatable.

No studies of various formulations of enteral or parenteral nutrition in isolated TBI patients have been published. To maintain adequate nitrogen balance, a >15% protein content is recommended for most enteral formulations in trauma patients.[17] Although branch chain amino acids improve outcomes in septic patients and glutamine supplementation is believed to decrease infection rates,[72] these findings have not been confirmed in TBI patients. With regard to route of feeding, although concerns remain about the possibility of increased risk of aspiration with gastric as opposed to jejunal feeding, no route has been found to be superior to others in terms of meeting nutritional needs, complications, and/or patient outcomes.[17] Lastly, hyperglycemia is well recognized to be associated with worse outcomes in TBI.[73–75] It remains debatable whether hyperglycemia is a marker of disease severity or a causative factor with regard to poor outcomes. The only prospective report on the subject was the subgroup analysis on 63 patients with isolated TBI requiring 3 or more days of mechanical ventilation in the intensive insulin trial by Van den Berghe et al.[76] Patients in the intensive therapy arm had lower mean ($p = 0.003$) and maximum ($p < 0.0001$) ICP compared with controls, achieved optimal CPP with lower vasopressor doses ($p = 0.01$), and had fewer seizures ($p < 0.0001$). No difference in mortality existed between the groups. These findings and any impact in mortality need to be confirmed in a larger prospective study. Current recommendations are to maintain serum glucose below 200 mg/dL.[17]

In summary, general intensive care of TBI commonly involves a variety of factors that may seriously impact on patient outcomes. Special care must be taken to appropriately manage these issues and avoid complications that may compromise general ICU care. Protocols in the ICU provide a systematic approach that minimizes variability in the care provided to the severely ill TBI patient and improves patient outcomes and are recommended by current guidelines.[17]

Neurological Syndromes

Neurological issues that may develop in the severely ill TBI patient and occasionally in any critically ill patient include herniation syndromes, seizures in the critically ill TBI patient, critical illness neuropathy/myopathy, and pituitary dysfunction and electrolyte abnormalities.

Herniation Syndromes

Cerebral herniation can occur after trauma or due to severe cerebral edema in other critically ill patients. The resultant horizontal or vertical displacement of cerebral tissue can lead to compression of vascular structures or cranial nerves, and obstruction of cerebrospinal fluid. This process can produce potentially irreversible pathological changes. Specific herniation syndromes have been described, with the clinical signs generally progressing in a rostrocaudal pattern. Herniation syndromes occur commonly in critical care, and prompt recognition is essential to optimize chances of adequate treatment. **Table 15.5** lists common herniation syndromes.

Falcine or Cingulate Herniation

The lateral displacement of a cerebral hemisphere can force the cingulate cortex under the falx cerebri. This results in compression of the anterior cerebral artery

Table 15.5 Common Herniation Syndromes in the Intensive Care Unit

Syndrome	Clinical Findings
Falcine or cingulated herniation	Lower extremity weakness/sensory loss, impairments of motor planning, apraxia, abulia or akinetic mutism, transcortical motor aphasia, and incontinence
Uncal or tentorial herniation	Dilation of ipsilateral pupil; ipsilateral hemiparesis (Kernohan's notch syndrome)
Central or transtentorial herniation	Decreased responsiveness or unexplained agitation; sixth cranial nerve palsy
Foraminal herniation	Bilateral cranial nerve palsies, depressed respiration, cardiac arrhythmias, brain death

(ACA), the great cerebral vein and surrounding tissues, thus worsening any existing ischemia and edema. Infarction of the ACA region can produce lower extremity weakness and sensory loss, impairments of motor planning, apraxia, abulia or akinetic mutism, transcortical motor aphasia, and incontinence. Compression of the great cerebral vein can obstruct vascular drainage of deep cerebral regions and may increase ICP.

Uncal or Tentorial Herniation

Expanding lesions in the temporal lobe or fossa can displace the hippocampus and uncus of the temporal lobe toward the midline. This process produces the classic signs of deterioration from herniation. The ipsilateral third cranial nerve and posterior cerebral artery (PCA) become trapped between the uncus and tentorial edge. Dilation of the ipsilateral pupil will be the initial clinical finding, and occipital infarction can occur due to compression of the PCA. In addition, the adjacent midbrain is forced against the opposite edge of the tentorium. The resultant compression of the contralateral cerebral peduncle produces a falsely localizing hemiparesis on the *same side* as the mass lesion (Kernohan's notch syndrome).

Central or Transtentorial Herniation

Central herniation of the cerebral hemispheres through the tentorial notch causes downward displacement of the brain stem. The medial perforating branches of the basilar artery are stretched, resulting in impairment of vascular perfusion. Brain stem ischemia produces alterations in the level of consciousness (decreased responsiveness or unexplained agitation). A sixth cranial nerve palsy may develop in response to caudal displacement with compression of the nerve against the petrous ligament.

Foraminal Herniation

Caudal displacement of supratentorial or posterior fossa structures can cause descent of tissues below the foramen magnum. The resultant compression of medullary cardiac and respiratory centers can be life threatening.

Seizures in TBI

Seizures following TBI may occur at the time of injury (immediate), during the first week due to acute complications from the injury (early), or weeks to months after injury in the form of a posttraumatic seizure disorder (delayed). Among all patients with TBI, ~2% develop seizures (defined as any seizure), but this number varies widely depending primarily on the severity of injury. In severe TBI patients, historical data suggest that ~12% develop early seizures.[77,78] Antiepileptic drugs (AEDs) are routinely used for treatment of posttraumatic seizure disorder, but the question that frequently arises clinically is whether or not to prophylactically treat TBI patients with AEDs in the acute period of injury and for how long after injury. Practice patterns vary widely,[79] but recent trials and guidelines provide a guide for clinicians.

In a randomized, double-blind, placebo controlled trial of 404 patients, severe TBI patients were treated for a year with placebo or phenytoin beginning within 24 hours of injury.[80] Serum phenytoin levels were maintained in the therapeutic range. Within 7 days of injury, 3.6% of the patients assigned to phenytoin had seizures, as compared with 14.2% of patients assigned to placebo (risk ratio 0.27, $p < 0.001$). Between day 8 and the end of the first year, 21.5% of the phenytoin group had seizures compared with 15.7% of the placebo group. By the end of year 2, 27.5% of the phenytoin group and 21.1% of the placebo group had seizures. The authors concluded that prophylactic phenytoin has a beneficial effect in reducing seizures only during the first week following severe TBI. Although this study definitely addressed the issue of prophylactic AEDs for clinically apparent seizures, questions remained about the potential of subclinical seizures contributing to morbidity and mortality following severe TBI.

In a prospective observational study of 94 consecutive moderate-to-severe TBI patients monitored with continuous electroencephalogram (cEEG) for the first 14 days after injury, convulsive and nonconvulsive seizures occurred in 22% of patients, with status epilepticus occurring in six patients. More than half of the seizures were nonconvulsive and were diagnosed based on cEEG only. All six patients with status epilepticus died compared with a mortality rate of 24% in the nonseizure group. Seizures occurred despite initiation of AEDs in the ED and maintenance of adequate drug levels.[81]

Current recommendations for seizure prophylaxis following severe TBI are that AEDs should be started early after diagnosis of severe TBI and continued for 7 days, reflective of the studies above.[17] Questions persist as to whether less severe cases of TBI would benefit from AED prophylaxis given the frequency of nonconvulsive seizures in the moderate-to-severe group mentioned above. Larger cEEG studies of TBI patients are warranted to better define patients who may benefit from seizure prophylaxis or who may warrant treatment beyond the currently recommended 7 days.

Critical Illness Polyneuropathy/Myopathy

Critical illness neuropathy/myopathy (CIPNM) is a continuum of a syndrome that in the past decade has been increasingly recognized as a serious consequence of prolonged ICU care. Neuromuscular weakness during ICU stay has traditionally been thought to be due to muscle atrophy or fatigue, but electrophysiologic and muscle biopsy studies suggest a distinct pathophysiology that is generally underrecognized in the ICU setting.

CIPNM is estimated to occur in 25 to 63% of patients who have been mechanically ventilated for 1 week.[82–84] Timing of exam, criteria for CIPNM diagnosis, and primary reason for ICU admission impact the reported occurrence of CIPNM. Clinical features of CIPNM consist predominantly of distal muscle weakness and wasting, worse in the lower extremities. Facial weakness is rarely present. Thus, the development of distal weakness or a decrease in motor responsiveness with obvious facial grimace and decreased deep tendon reflexes should raise suspicion of CIPNM. Thirty percent of patients have isolated motor symptoms, but sensory deficits may occur concurrently.[85] Laboratory tests are not diagnostic, although creatine kinase levels may be mildly elevated. Nerve conduction and electromyography studies show both motor and sensory axonal dysfunction in the upper and lower extremities, although sensory nerve potentials may be normal.[86,87] Nerve and muscle biopsy studies may also be performed. In a prospective study, muscle biopsies were taken from 30 patients who developed CIPNM. Neuropathic changes were found in 37%, myopathic in 40%, and a combination in 23% of the biopsies. Activated leukocytes producing both pro- and antiinflammatory cytokines were found in the skeletal muscle of the CIPNM patients, suggesting an inflammatory component.[88] No uniform diagnostic criteria currently exist for CIPNM, but its potential impact on patient outcomes warrants consideration of the diagnosis in the appropriate patient.

The occurrence of CIPNM as diagnosed by specific electrophysiologic and clinical criteria has been associated with the Acute Physiology, Age and Chronic Health Evaluation (APACHE III) score and the presence of the systemic inflammatory response syndrome (SIRS).[89] In that prospective study of 98 mechanically ventilated patients, 33% developed CIPNM. Sepsis and severity of illness as measured by multiorgan system failure were identified as other risk factors for CIPNM. Limited data are available to assess methods of adequately preventing or treating CIPNM. In the intensive insulin therapy study by Van den Berghe et al, the rate of CIPNM defined by electrodiagnostic testing was reduced from 52 to 29% in the 63 patients with isolated TBI requiring 3 or more days of mechanical ventilation.[76] The antiinflammatory properties of intensive insulin were postulated as potentially explaining this benefit. The prognosis of CIPNM is poorly understood and methods adequately treating the ailment once identified are also lacking at this time. However, in the ICU environment where difficulties may arise with liberation from the ventilator and patient disposition is dependent upon this, recognizing CIPNM may have direct implications for patient care and utilization of resources. The approach toward rehabilitation and expectations of rehabilitation may also be influenced by the recognition of CIPNM. Further study of this entity is warranted.

Pituitary Dysfunction and Electrolyte Abnormalities

The posterior pituitary gland is involved with the regulation of fluid balance. Syndromes from injury to the posterior pituitary are well recognized and usually present early after TBI. They include syndrome of inappropriate antidiuretic hormone secretion (SIADH) and diabetes insipidus (DI). Neuroendocrine abnormalities from anterior pituitary dysfunction may not become apparent until months after brain injury. The anterior pituitary releases several hormones that influence growth, adrenal, reproductive, and thyroid function. Pituitary injury will present with symptoms related to the affected target organ. Growth hormone deficiency may be clinically silent in adults, but delayed bone maturation and stunted growth can develop in children. Low levels of adrenocorticotropin hormone can produce stress-related fatigue, hypotension, fever, and cognitive changes. Loss of hypothalamic dopamine inhibition can produce hyperprolactinemia and associated galactorrhea, anovulation, gynecomastia, and impotence. Hypogonadism results from gonadotropin deficiency and presents with decreased libido, impotence, amenorrhea, and loss of secondary sexual characteristics. Thyroid function regulates metabolism, and any injury to the hypothalamic–pituitary axis can produce hypothyroidism. Symptoms include cognitive slowing, low basal metabolic rate, cold intolerance, fatigue, and anemia. Complete disruption of the hypothalamic–pituitary axis results in panhypopituitarism with dysfunction of all systems.

Risk factors for neuroendocrine dysfunction after brain injury include trauma affecting the frontal lobes, basilar skull fractures, and severe injury with >24 hours of post-traumatic amnesia. Suspicion for anterior pituitary dysfunction should be high in patients with unexplained hypotension, weight loss, fatigue, loss of libido, or depression. The workup should consist of urine and serum osmolality, thyroxine (T4), and T3 uptake tests, serum pooled testosterone (average three samples), thyroid-stimulating hormone, follicle-stimulating hormone, luteinizing hormone, growth hormone, and cortisol levels. An endocrine consult is warranted for patients with abnormal results.

Sodium disturbance is common in the ICU, and normal sodium balance depends on many factors. The renin–angiotensin–aldosterone system maintains renal sodium and water resorption and stimulates thirst. Antidiuretic hormone (ADH) is secreted with increases in osmolality and hypovolemia to decrease renal excretion of free water. TBI can alter the balance of these systems resulting in either hyponatremia or hypernatremia. Hyponatremia is the most common sodium abnormality with a reported overall incidence of 9%.[90] It occurs in response to three different syndromes: the syndrome of inappropriate secretion of antidiuretic hormone (SIADH), cerebral salt wasting (CSW), or psychogenic polydipsia. Because fluid intake is generally monitored in the ICU setting, our discussions will focus on SIADH and CSW.

Syndrome of Inappropriate Antidiuretic Hormone

SIADH is the most common cause of hyponatremia after TBI. The incidence ranges from 2 to 5%, with reports as high as 33% in severe TBI.[91,92] Different mechanisms may prompt ADH release after TBI. These include increased ICP, hypercapnia, hypothalamic dysfunction, alterations in responsiveness of osmoreceptors, and medications. The clinical criteria for SIADH consist of hyponatremia with normovolemia, low serum osmolality, low urine output, high urine sodium, urine osmolality > serum osmolality, and high ADH levels. Treatment is primarily through fluid restriction and the avoidance of hypotonic intravenous (IV) fluids. In more severe or refractory cases, demeclocycline (300 mg every 6 hours), fluorocortisone (0.1 to 0.2 mg a day), HTS (500 cc over several hours), or salt by mouth or gastric tube may be necessary.

Cerebral Salt Wasting

Hyponatremia in the second week after TBI is probably due to CSW.[91] The mechanism is probably related to an increased release of atrial natruretic factor and renal sodium loss. The clinical picture consists of hyponatremia with hypovolemia, high urine output, and normal to increased serum osmolality. A comparison of the clinical findings in SIADH and CSW is reviewed in **Table 15.6**. Daily body weights can help in assessing the patient's volume status. At this time, treatment should focus on hydration and salt supplementation. Currently, conivaptan is an arginine vasopressin antagonist that is being studied in a medical patient population for treatment of hyponatremia in euvolemic and hypervolemic patients.[93] This agent and perhaps others may play a future role in the management of hyponatremia in TBI.

Table 15.6 Comparison of Clinical Findings in Syndrome of Inappropriate Antidiuretic Hormone (SIADH) and Cerebral Salt Wasting (CSW)

Parameter	SIADH	CSW
Serum sodium	Decreased	Decreased
Serum osmolality	Decreased	Normal – increased
Urine sodium	Increased	Increased
Urine output	Decreased	Increased
Volume status	Normovolemia	Hypovolemia
Body weight	Increased	Decreased

Diabetes Insipidus

DI is relatively uncommon after TBI, but can be seen in patients with severe injuries or damage along the hypothalamic–pituitary axis resulting in the inadequate secretion of ADH. The patient will demonstrate hypernatremia with polyuria, polydipsia, hypovolemia, increased serum osmolality, and low urine osmolality. Diagnosis can be made with careful fluid deprivation followed by vasopressin. DI will respond to treatment with pitressin, vasopressin, and fluid supplementation.

Iatrogenic Hypernatremia

The use of mannitol with furosemide or hypertonic saline for ICP management can result in elevations of serum sodium. Insensible fluid loss through an endotracheal tube or tracheostomy, fever or sweating can increase sodium. Phenytoin, captopril, Narcan (DuPont Pharma, Wilmington, DE), and ethanol can inhibit ADH secretion. Enteral tube feedings can have high levels of sodium. Any of these factors can result in iatrogenic hypernatremia. Correction can be accomplished by adjusting fluid and electrolyte intake.

Other Electrolyte Abnormalities

Potassium regulation can be affected after brain injury. Many mechanisms can produce hypokalemia. Aldosterone secretion in response to physical stress leads to an increase in potassium excretion. Hyperventilation produces respiratory alkalosis, which drives potassium intracellular and lowers serum levels. Diet, nausea, vomiting, and medications such as diuretics, mannitol, antibiotics, or corticosteroids may result in hypokalemia. Clinical symptoms of hypokalemia include cardiac conduction abnormalities, weakness, and hyporeflexia. Treatment should focus on resolution of the underlying cause and potassium supplementation. Hyperkalemia usually results from metabolic acidosis, renal failure, or hypoadrenalism. Glucose or insulin administration will increase cellular absorption of potassium.

Hypomagnesemia can result from excessive urinary excretion, alkalosis, sepsis, diuretics, and aminoglycosides. The relationship between magnesium and calcium suggests that hypomagnesemia increases the risk of secondary injury by worsening calcium-related excitotoxicity.

The clinical findings include weakness, tetany, hyperreflexia, and cognitive changes. Either enteral or intravenous supplementation can be used for treatment.

Dysautonomia

Catecholaminergic surges after brain injury can result in a hyperdynamic cardiovascular state with hypertension, tachycardia, and increased cardiac output.[94] Although the hyperdynamic state usually resolves, posttraumatic hypertension may persist. Injuries to the hypothalamic periventricular nucleus can interfere with blood pressure regulation. Injury to the orbitofrontal cortex can disrupt vagal activity and cardiovascular sympathetic tone. Beta-blockers are an effective treatment, and may help control any associated reflex tachycardia. Alpha-adrenergic agonists, calcium channel blockers, and angiotensin-converting enzyme agents can also be used, but vasodilators should be avoided acutely as they potentially can cause hypotension and thus decrease cerebral perfusion.

Hyperthermia should prompt an infectious workup, but in some patients, an infectious source may not be identified or temperature elevations may persist even with adequate antibiotic treatment. Phenytoin allergy is a common cause of fever and rash in this setting. Central fever should also be considered. This can present as mild to moderate fever, or severe and labile fluctuations of temperature may occur. The coordination of thermoregulatory function is accomplished in the hypothalamus, and damage can result in abnormal thermogenic responses. Treatment primarily involves antipyretics and cooling blankets. Propranolol and bromocriptine have reported benefit in the treatment of persistent central fever.[95,96] A recent case series of six patients suggested potential benefit with gabapentin.[97]

In summary, neurological syndromes in the severely ill TBI patient may lead to prolonged ventilatory dependence, increased length of hospital stay, and worse outcomes. Care must be taken to identify and treat these syndromes to optimize the potential for good patient outcomes.

Conclusion

Severely ill TBI patients are a special population requiring particular expertise to appropriately manage. The goal of the neurointensivist in the care of these patients is to prevent secondary brain injury while addressing common issues that afflict critically ill patients. The initial assessment focuses on evaluation of the ABCs and avoidance of hypotension and hypoxia. Subsequently, ICP and CPP must be optimized; infections prevented, or quickly recognized and treated; thromboembolism prevented or recognized and treated; and other complications of ICU care routinely screened for, identified, and treated. The care of these patients is complicated, and institutions should develop protocols to standardize care to avoid lapses in assessment and treatment.

References

1. Miller JD, Sweet RC, Narayan R, Becker DP. Early insults to the injured brain. JAMA 1978;240:439–442
2. Chesnut RM, Marshall LF, Klauber MR, et al. The role of secondary brain injury in determining outcome from severe head injury. J Trauma 1993;34:216–222
3. Vassar MJ, Fischer RP, O'Brien PE, et al. A multicenter trial for resuscitation of injured patients with 7.5% sodium chloride: the effect of added dextran 70. The Multicenter Group for the Study of Hypertonic Saline in Trauma Patients. Arch Surg 1993;128:1003–1011
4. Stocchetti N, Furlan A, Volta F. Hypoxemia and arterial hypotension at the accident scene in head injury. J Trauma 1996;40:764–767
5. Manley G, Knudson M, Morabito D, Damron S, Erickson V, Pitts L. Hypotension, hypoxia, and head injury: frequency, duration, and consequences. Arch Surg 2001;136:1118–1123
6. Marshall LF, Smith R, Shapiro H. The outcome with aggressive treatment in severe head injuries, I: The significance of intracranial pressure monitoring. J Neurosurg 1979;50:20–25
7. Narayan RK, Kishore P, Becker D, et al. Intracranial pressure: to monitor or not to monitor? A review of our experience with head injury. J Neurosurg 1982;56:650–659
8. Marmarou A, Anderson RL, Ward JD, et al. Impact of ICP instability and hypotension on outcome in patients with severe head trauma. J Neurosurg 1991;75:S159–S66
9. Chambers IR, Treadwell L, Mendelow AD. Determination of threshold levels of cerebral perfusion pressure and intracranial pressure in severe head injury by using receiver-operating characteristic curves: an observational study in 291 patients. J Neurosurg 2001;94:412–416
10. Ratanalert S, Phuenpathom N, Saeheng S, Oearsakul T, Sripairojkul B, Hirunpat S. ICP threshold in CPP management of severe head injury patients. Surg Neurol 2004;61:429–435
11. Rosner MJ, Daughton S. Cerebral perfusion pressure management in head injury. J Trauma 1990;30:933–940
12. Contant CF, Valadka AB, Gopinath SP, Hannay HJ, Robertson CS. Adult respiratory distress syndrome: a complication of induced hypertension after severe head injury. J Neurosurg 2001;95:560–568
13. Robertson CS, Valadka AB, Hannay HJ, et al. Prevention of secondary ischemic insults after severe head injury. Crit Care Med 1999;27:2086–2095
14. Young JS, Blow O, Turrentine F, Claridge JA, Schulman A. Is there an upper limit of intracranial pressure in patients with severe head injury if cerebral perfusion pressure is maintained? Neurosurg Focus 2003;15:E2
15. Huang SJ, Hong WC, Han YY, et al. Clinical outcome of severe head injury in different protocol-driven therapies. J Clin Neurosci 2007;14:449–454
16. Balestreri M, Czonsyka M, Hutchinson P, et al. Impact of intracranial pressure and cerebral perfusion pressure on severe disability and mortality after head injury. Neurocrit Care 2006;4:8–13
17. Brain Trauma Foundation and the American Association of Neurological Surgeons. 2007 Guidelines for Management of Severe Traumatic Brain Injury. Available at: www.braintrauma.org. Accessed Sept. 27, 2007
18. Marmarou A, Signoretti S, Fatouros PP, Portella G, Aygok GA, Bullock MR. Predominance of cellular edema in traumatic brain swelling in patients with severe head injuries. J Neurosurg 2006;104:720–730

19. Marmarou A. A review of progress in understanding the pathophysiology and treatment of brain edema. Neurosurg Focus 2007;22:E1
20. Warth A, Simon P, Capper D, et al. Expression pattern of the water channel aquaporin-4 in human gliomas is associated with blood-brain barrier disturbance but not with patient survival. J Neurosci Res 2007;85:1336–1346
21. Roberts I, Schierhout G, Wakai A. Mannitol for acute traumatic brain injury (Cochrane Review). Cochrane Database Syst Rev 2003;2:CD001049
22. Ogden AT, Mayer SA, Connelly ES Jr. Hyperosmolar agents in neurosurgical practice: the evolving role of hypertonic saline. Neurosurgery 2005;57:207–215
23. Allen CH, Ward JD. An evidence-based approach to management of increased intracranial pressure. Crit Care Clin 1998;14:485–495
24. Bullock R. Mannitol and other diuretics in severe neurotrauma. New Horiz 1995;3:448–452
25. Smith HP, Kelly DLJ, McWhorter JM, et al. Comparison of mannitol regimens in patients with severe head injury undergoing intracranial monitoring. J Neurosurg 1986;65:820–824
26. Burke AM, Quest DO, Chien S, Cerri C. The effects of mannitol on blood viscosity. J Neurosurg 1981;55:550–553
27. Fishman RA. Brain edema. N Engl J Med 1975;293:706–711
28. Cloyd JC, Snyder BD, Cleermans B, Bundlie SR, Blomquist CH, Lakatua DJ. Mannitol pharmacokinetics and serum osmolality in dogs and humans. J Pharmacol Exp Ther 1986;236:301–306
29. Mattox KL, Maningas PA, Moore EE, et al. Prehospital hypertonic saline/dextran infusion for post-traumatic hypotension. The U.S.A. Multicenter Trial. Ann Surg 1991;213:482–491
30. Wade C, Grady J, Kramer G. Efficacy of hypertonic saline dextran (HSD) in patients with traumatic hypotension: metaanalysis of individual patient data. Acta Anaesthesiol Scand Suppl 1997;110:77–79
31. Vialet R, Albanese J, Thomachot L, et al. Isovolume hypertonic solutes (sodium chloride or mannitol) in the treatment of refractory posttraumatic intracranial hypertension: 2 mL/kg 7.5% saline is more effective than 2 mL/kg 20% mannitol. Crit Care Med 2003;31:1683–1687
32. Bernard SA, Gray TW, Buist MD, et al. Treatment of comatose survivors of out-of-hospital cardiac arrest with induced hypothermia. N Engl J Med 2002;346:557–563
33. The Hypothermia After Cardiac Arrest Study Group. Mild therapeutic hypothermia to improve the neurologic outcome after cardiac arrest. N Engl J Med 2002;346:549–556
34. Clifton GL, Miller ER, Choi SC, et al. Lack of effect of induction of hypothermia after acute brain injury. N Engl J Med 2001;344:556–563
35. Aibiki M, Maekawa S, Yokono S. Moderate hypothermia improves imbalances of thromboxane A2 and prostaglandin I2 production after traumatic brain injury in humans. Crit Care Med 2000;28:3902–3906
36. Thompson HJ, Tkacs NC, Saatman KE, Raghupathi R, McIntosh TK. Hyperthermia following traumatic brain injury: a critical evaluation. Neurobiol Dis 2003;12:163–173
37. Zygun DA, Kortbeek JB, Fick GH, Laupland KB, Doig CJ. Non-neurologic organ dysfunction in severe traumatic brain injury. Crit Care Med 2005;33:654–660
38. Koutsoukou A, Perraki H, Raftopoulou A, et al. Respiratory mechanics in brain-damaged patients. Intensive Care Med 2006;32:1947–1954
39. Holland MC, Mackersie RC, Morabito D, et al. The development of acute lung injury is associated with worse neurologic outcome in patients with severe traumatic brain injury. J Trauma 2003;55:106–111
40. Ibrahim EH, Tracy L, Hill C, Fraser VJ, Kollef MH. The occurrence of ventilator-associated pneumonia in a community hospital: risk factors and clinical outcomes. Chest 2001;120:555–561
41. George DL, Falk PS, Wunderink RG, et al. Epidemiology of ventilator-acquired pneumonia based on protected bronchoscopic sampling. Am J Respir Crit Care Med 1998;158:1839–1847
42. Chastre J, Fagon JY. Ventilator-associated pneumonia. Am J Respir Crit Care Med 2002;165:867–903
43. Heyland DK, Cook DJ, Griffith L, Keenan SP, Brun-Buisson C. The attributable morbidity and mortality of ventilator-associated pneumonia in the critically ill patient. The Canadian Critical Trials Group. Am J Respir Crit Care Med 1999;159:1249–1256
44. Chastre J, Wolff M, Fagon JY, et al. Comparison of 8 vs 15 days of antibiotic therapy for ventilator-associated pneumonia in adults: a randomized trial. JAMA 2003;290:2588–2598
45. Zygun DA, Zuege DJ, Boiteau PJ, et al. Ventilator-associated pneumonia in severe traumatic brain injury. Neurocrit Care 2006;5:108–114
46. Drakulovic MB, Torres A, Bauer TT, Nicolas JM, Nogué S, Ferrer M. Supine body position as a risk factor for nosocomial pneumonia in mechanically ventilated patients: a randomised trial. Lancet 1999; 354:1851–1858
47. Cook DJ, Reeve BK, Guyatt GH, et al. Stress ulcer prophylaxis in critically ill patients: resolving discordant meta-analyses. JAMA 1996;275: 308–314
48. Cocanour CS, Peninger M, Domonoske BD, et al. Decreasing ventilator-associated pneumonia in a trauma ICU. J Trauma 2006;61:122–129
49. Gurkin SA, Parikshak M, Kralovich KA, Horst HM, Agarwal V, Payne N. Indicators for tracheostomy in patients with traumatic brain injury. Am Surg 2002;68:324–328
50. Ahmed N, Kuo YH. Early versus late tracheostomy in patients with severe traumatic head injury. Surg Infect (Larchmt) 2007;8:343–347
51. Pittet D, Tarara D, Wenzel RP. Nosocomial bloodstream infection in critically ill patients: excess length of stay, extra costs, and attributable mortality. JAMA 1994;271:1598–1601
52. Reed CR, Sessler CN, Glauser FL, Phelan BA. Central venous catheter infections: concepts and controversies. Intensive Care Med 1995;21: 177–183
53. Merrer J, De Jonghe B, Golliot F, et al. Complications of femoral and subclavian venous catheterization in critically ill patients: a randomized controlled trial. JAMA 2001;286:700–707
54. McGee DC, Gould MK. Preventing complications of central venous catheterizations. N Engl J Med 2003;348:1123–1133
55. Maki DG, Stolz SM, Wheeler S, Mermel LA. Prevention of central venous catheter-related bloodstream infection by use of an antiseptic-impregnated catheter: a randomized, controlled trial. Ann Intern Med 1997;127:257–266
56. Darouiche RO, Raad II, Heard SO, et al. A comparison of two antimicrobial-impregnated central venous catheters. Catheter Study Group. N Engl J Med 1999;340:1–8
57. Veenstra DL, Saint S, Sullivan SD. Cost-effectiveness of antiseptic-impregnated central venous catheters for the prevention of catheter-related bloodstream infection. JAMA 1999;282:554–560
58. Raad II, Hohn DC, Gilbreath BJ, et al. Prevention of central venous catheter-related infections by using maximal sterile barrier precautions during insertion. Infect Control Hosp Epidemiol 1994;15: 231–238
59. Maki DG, Ringer M, Alvarado CJ. Prospective randomised trial of povidone-iodine, alcohol, and chlorhexidine for prevention of infection associated with central venous and arterial catheters. Lancet 1991;338:339–343
60. DesJardin JA, Falagas ME, Ruthazer R, et al. Clinical utility of blood cultures drawn from indwelling central venous catheters in hospitalized patients with cancer. Ann Intern Med 1999;131:641–647
61. Kaufman HH, Satterwhite T, McConnell BJ, et al. Deep vein thrombosis and pulmonary embolism in head injured patients. Angiology 1983;34:627–638
62. Buller HR, Agnelli G, Hull RD, Hyers TM, Prins MH, Raskob GE. Antithrombotic therapy for venous thromboembolic disease: the Seventh ACCP Conference on Antithrombotic and Thrombolytic Therapy. Chest 2004;126:401S–428S
63. Page RB, Spott MA, Krishnamurthy S, Taleghani C, Chinchilli VM. Head injury and pulmonary embolism: a retrospective report based on the Pennsylvania Trauma Outcomes study. Neurosurgery 2004;54: 143–148
64. Black PM, Baker MF, Snook CP. Experience with external pneumatic calf compression in neurology and neurosurgery. Neurosurgery 1986;18:440–444
65. Kim J, Gearhart MM, Zurick A, Zuccarello M, James L, Luchette FA. Preliminary report on the safety of herapin for deep venous thrombosis prophylaxis after severe head injury. J Trauma 2002;53:38–42

66. McIntyre LA, Fergusson DA, Hutchison JS, et al. Effect of a liberal versus restrictive transfusion strategy on mortality in patients with moderate to severe head injury. Neurocrit Care 2006;5:4–9
67. Taylor RW, Manganaro L, O'Brien J, Trottier SJ, Parkar N, Veremakis C. Impact of allogenic packed red blood cell transfusion on nosocomial infection rates in the critically ill patient. Crit Care Med 2002;30: 2249–2254
68. Toy P, Lowell C. TRALI–definition, mechanisms, incidence and clinical relevance. Best Pract Res Clin Anaesthesiol 2007;21:183–193
69. Malone DL, Dunne J, Tracy JK, Putnam AT, Scalea TM, Napolitano LM. Blood transfusion, independent of shock severity, is associated with worse outcome in trauma. J Trauma 2003;54:898–905
70. Rapp RP, Young B, Twyman D, et al. The favorable effect of early parenteral feeding on survival in head-injured patients. J Neurosurg 1983;58:906–912
71. Young B, Ott L, Twyman D, et al. The effect of nutritional support on outcome from severe head injury. J Neurosurg 1987;67:668–676
72. Garcia-de-Lorenzo A, Ortiz-Leyba M, Planas JC, et al. Parenteral administration of different amounts of branch-chain amino acids in septic patients: clinical and metabolic aspects. Crit Care Med 1997;25: 418–424
73. Lam AM, Winn HR, Cullen BF, Sundling N. Hyperglycemia and neurological outcome in patients with head injury. J Neurosurg 1991;75: 545–551
74. Young B, Ott L, Dempsey R, Haack D, Tibbs P. Relationship between admission hyperglycemia and neurologic outcome of severely brain-injured patients. Ann Surg 1989;210:466–472
75. Jeremitsky E, Omert LA, Dunham CL, Wilberger J, Rodriguez A. The impact of hyperglycemia on patients with severe brain injury. J Trauma 2005;58:47–50
76. Van den Berghe G, Schoonheydt K, Becx P, Bruyninckx F, Wouters PJ. Insulin therapy protects the central and peripheral nervous system of intensive care patients. Neurology 2005;64:1348–1353
77. Annegers JF, Hauser WA, Coan SP, Rocca WA. A population-based study of seizures after traumatic brain injuries. N Engl J Med 1998;338:20–24
78. Hauser WA. Prevention of post-traumatic epilepsy. N Engl J Med 1990;323:540–542
79. Dauch WA, Schutze M, Guttinger M, Bauer BL. Post-traumatic seizure prevention: results of a survey of 127 neurosurgery clinics. Zentralbl Neurochir 1996;57:190–195
80. Temkin NR, Dikmen SS, Wilensky AJ, Keihm J, Chabal S, Winn HR. A randomized, double-blind study of phenytoin for the prevention of post-traumatic seizures. N Engl J Med 1990;323:497–502
81. Vespa PM, Nuwer MR, Nenov V, et al. Increased incidence and impact of nonconvulsive and convulsive seizures after traumatic brain injury as detected by continuous electroencephalographic monitoring. J Neurosurg 1999;91:750–760
82. Lacomis D, Petrella JT, Giuliani MJ. Causes of neuromuscular weakness in the intensive care unit: a study of ninety-two patients. Muscle Nerve 1998;21:610–617
83. Hund E. Neurological complications of sepsis: critical illness polyneuropathy and myopathy. J Neurol 2001;248:929–934
84. De Jonghe B, Sharshar T, Lefaucheur JP, et al. Paresis acquired in the intensive care unit: a prospective multicenter study. JAMA 2002;288: 2859–2867
85. Coakley JH, Nagendran K, Yarwood GD, Honavar M, Hinds CJ. Patterns of neurophysiological abnormality in prolonged critical illness. Intensive Care Med 1998;24:801–807
86. Coakley JH, Nagendran K, Honavar M, Hinds CJ. Preliminary observations on the neuromuscular abnormalities in patients with organ failure and sepsis. Intensive Care Med 1993;19:323–328
87. Hund E, Genzwurker H, Bohrer H, Jakob H, Thiele R, Hacke W. Predominant involvement of motor fibres in patients with critical illness polyneuropathy. Br J Anaesth 1997;78:274–278
88. De Letter MA, van Doorn PA, Savelkoul HF, et al. Critical illness polyneuropathy and myopathy (CIPNM): evidence for local immune activation by cytokine-expression in the muscle tissue. J Neuroimmunol 2000;106:206–213
89. De Letter MA, Scmitz PI, Visser LH, et al. Risk factors for the development of polyneuropathy and myopathy in critically ill patients. Crit Care Med 2001;29:2281–2286
90. Bacic A, Gluncic I, Gluncic V. Disturbances in plasma sodium in patients with war head injuries. Mil Med 1999;164:214–217
91. Vingerhoets F, de Tribolet N. Hyponatremia hypo-osmolarity in neurosurgical patients. "Appropriate secretion of ADH" and "cerebral salt wasting syndrome." Acta Neurochir (Wien) 1988;91:50–54
92. Doczi T, Tarjanyi J, Huszka E, Kiss J. Syndrome of inappropriate secretion of antidiuretic hormone (SIADH) after head injury. Neurosurgery 1982;10(6 Pt 1):685–688
93. U.S. National Institutes of Health. Available at: www.clinicaltrials.gov. Accessed September 27, 2007
94. Clifton GL, Robertson CS, Grossman RG. Cardiovascular and metabolic responses to severe head injury. Neurosurg Rev 1989;12(Suppl 1): 465–473
95. Meythaler JM, Stinson AM III. Fever of central origin in traumatic brain injury controlled with propranolol. Arch Phys Med Rehabil 1994;75: 816–818
96. Baguley IJ, Cameron ID, Green AM, Slewa-Younan S, Marosszeky JE, Gurka JA. Pharmacological management of dysautonomia following traumatic brain injury. Brain Inj 2004;18:409–417
97. Baguley IJ, Heriseanu RE, Gurka JA, Nordenbo A, Cameron ID. Gabapentin in the management of dysautonomia following severe traumatic brain injury: a case series. J Neurol Neurosurg Psychiatry 2007;78:539–541

16 Pulmonary Critical Care

Ubaldo Martin, Sheila Weaver, and Gerard J. Criner

The primary drivers for the existence of critical care units include patients who require clinical surveillance that is more intensive than can be provided on a normal ward; the need for efficient deployment of specially trained staff to provide this surveillance, along with the sophisticated technology that they manage; and the need to apply solutions to disordered cerebral and systemic physiology.[1]

The progenitors of neurological intensive care units (NICUs) stem from the use of mechanical ventilators to treat polio patients by Ibsen in Copenhagen[2]; the inception of Spalding and Crampton's respiratory ICUs at the Radcliffe Infirmary[3]; the creation of cardiac care units by Killup that provided a model for the application of special technology (continuous electrocardiogram [ECG] monitoring) and focused treatment (lidocaine); and the modern medical-surgical ICU with its capability to monitor cardiac hemodynamics and the postoperative neurosurgical wards that promoted specific neurological examination surveillance by special nurses and the application of intracranial pressure (ICP) monitoring. In all these circumstances, the ability to monitor and treat a physiological change was the impetus to create special units, and its existence became the basis for the establishment of a new medical field, critical care medicine. The first large NICUs were opened in the 1970s in the Massachussetts General and Johns Hopkins Hospitals.[1] The concept of the NICU is relatively young and although responsible for significant advances (fluid management in subarachnoid hemorrhage, treatment of status epilepticus, etc.), there remain significant limitations in multiple areas.

In this chapter we intend to discuss the modern aspects of mechanical ventilation, its application and complications, and its use in special circumstances such as the acute respiratory distress syndrome (ARDS). In the latter portion of this chapter we will elaborate on evidence for some selected ICU practices (glycemic control, sepsis management) that are most applicable to the NICU.

Indications for Intubation and Mechanical Ventilation

The neurosurgical patient may require endotracheal intubation with mechanical ventilation for a variety of reasons. Respiratory compromise in critically ill patients is an immediate concern that requires aggressive airway management and ventilatory management as well as an assessment of the etiology of the respiratory failure.

There are many indications for endotracheal intubation and mechanical ventilation in the neurosurgical patient. However, any patient with a decreased level of mental status that is not sufficient enough to maintain a patent airway, cough, or clearing of secretions is a common indication in the NICU (**Table 16.1**). This impairment may be in the absence of any primarily ventilatory dysfunction.

Table 16.1 Indications for Mechanical Ventilation

Impaired respiratory drive

- Central nervous system injury
- Sedation
- Drug overdose

Impaired respiratory muscle function

- Muscle weakness
    - Neuropathies
    - Myopathies
    - Deconditoning
    - Electrolyte/metabolic abnormalities
- Mechanical disadvantage
    - Dynamic hyperinflation
    - Chest wall deformity

Hypercapneic respiratory failure

- Increased respiratory load
    - Obstructive lung disease (asthma, emphysema)
    - Restrictive lung disease (pulmonary fibrosis, pneumonia, congestive heart failure)
    - Metabolic acidosis
    - Increased carbon dioxide states (obesity hypoventilation, obstructive sleep apnea)

    Secretions

Hypoxic respiratory failure

- Ventilation-perfusion imbalance
- Alveolar hypoventilation
- Diffusion defecit
- Inadequate inspired oxygen
- Sepsis

Generally, a patient with a Glasgow Coma Scale (GCS) score <10 should be considered at high risk for airway compromise; the risk of aspiration increases further with a decreasing GCS score.[4] In patients with a waning mental status, the inability to maintain airway patency is a major concern along with the risk of impending aspiration despite adequate oxygenation. Any patient with decreased respiratory drive as a result of his or her central nervous system (CNS) insult, or an inability to adequately ventilate as a consequence of neurological dysfunction, requires intubation. This type of respiratory failure is referred to as primary "pump" failure. Some patients, however, may develop an increase in respiratory drive (e.g., from fever or increased work of breathing), which may lead to respiratory muscle fatigue necessitating intubation. The presence of hypoxemia, partial pressure of oxygen in the alveoli (PaO_2) <60 mm Hg or worsening hypercapnea partial pressue of carbon dioxide, arterial ($PaCO_2$) >45 mm Hg, especially without evidence of underlying lung disease, may also require mechanical ventilation. Although noninvasive ventilation (NIV) has been widely used in the setting of hypercapnic and hypoxemic respiratory failure, its use is precluded in patients with neurological deficits or inability to protect the airway. NIV is therefore less likely to be a useful tool for the management of acute respiratory failure in the setting of acute neurological injury.

It is helpful when attempting to characterize the etiology of the respiratory failure into "pump failure" or "lung failure." Pump failure relates to conditions that impair the bellows function of respiration. Lung failure is due to conditions that impair gas exchange. Even with preserved lung function, any condition inhibiting the appropriate movement of the chest wall and thoracic cage can result in a disproportionate demand on the muscles of respiration, increasing oxygen demand and resulting in respiratory failure. Likewise, patients who have normal pump function, but who have parenchymal lung disease that impairs oxygenation and removal of carbon dioxide, are also at risk for respiratory failure. Pump failure in the NICU is likely to be more common, secondary to the patient's underlying neurological insult, which can result from decreased CNS output, severe weakness of the respiratory muscles, or neuromuscular disorders (**Table 16.2**).

Table 16.2 Neurological Diseases Causing Pump Failure and Lung Failure

Pump Failure	Lung Failure
Central nervous system	*Intrinsic lung disease*
• Drug overdose	• Asthma
• Stroke	• Chronic obstructive lung disease
• Head trauma	• Bronchitis
Spinal cord, neuromuscular disease	• Pneumonia
	• Pulmonary embolism
• Myasthenia gravis	• Acute respiratory distress syndrome
• Guillan-Barré	
• Polio	• Acute lung injury
• Polymyositis	• Alveolar hemorrhage
• Neuromuscular blocking agents	*Cardiac* • Pulmonary edema
• Critical illness polyneuropathy	• Valvular disease
Chest wall	
• Kyphoscoliosis	
• Flail chest	
Upper airway obstruction	
• Glottic stenosis	
• Paradoxical vocal cord dysfunction	
• Laryngospasm	

Although respiratory failure can be divided into pump and lung function components, multiple components need to be taken into account when evaluating the cause and treatment of respiratory failure. Overall, the respiratory system is divided into: (1) the CNS; (2) the peripheral nervous system; (3) the neuromuscular system; (4) the thorax and pleura; (5) the upper airways; (6) the cardiovascular system; and (7) the lower airways, including the alveoli (**Table 16.3**). Normal respiration relies on the delicate and intricate functioning of all these systems. Malfunction of any one or more of these systems can lead to respiratory failure.

Respiratory failure can also be characterized as hypercapnic or hypoxic respiratory failure. Generally, diseases that are related to pump failure lead to hypercapnic respiratory failure. Those related to lung failure lead to hypoxic respiratory failure. As patients deteriorate clinically, a combination of these entities will ensue.

The purpose of mechanical ventilation in the NICU is frequently supportive, to provide adequate ventilation for the patient until the process that caused respiratory failure

Table 16.3 Components of the Respiratory System That Fail and Cause Respiratory Failure

- Central nervous system
- Peripheral nervous system
- Neuromuscular junction
- Thorax and pleura
- Upper airways
- Cardiovascular systems
- Lower airways and alveoli

resolves. The modes of ventilation as well as technique of weaning from mechanical ventilation will be covered later in this chapter.

Effects of Mechanical Ventilation on Cerebral Perfusion Pressure

Neurosurgical patients who have sustained significant brain injury often require mechanical ventilation for supportive care during the treatment of their neurological insult. The goals and methods of delivering mechanical ventilation have been a topic of debate in the neuroanesthesia and neuro-ICU for more than 40 years.[5] Collectively, these injuries can result in acute changes in blood pressure, blood flow, or inflammation in the brain. As a result of the neurological process, pulmonary complications, such as neurogenic pulmonary edema (NPE), acute lung injury (ALI), and ARDS all account for significant morbidity and mortality in these patients. This chapter will review ventilator management strategies in this patient population.

Pathophysiology

Normal ICP for adults is <10 mm Hg and pressure >20 mm Hg is usually considered a threshold for starting therapy targeted at lowering the pressure. Cerebral perfusion pressure (CPP) is calculated as the difference between the mean arterial pressure (MAP) and the ICP. A CPP of 60 mm Hg is commonly accepted as the minimum before treatment is warranted.[6] The Monro-Kellie doctrine states that any increase in the volume of the cranial contents (e.g., brain, blood, or cerebrospinal fluid) will elevate ICP. If one of these three elements increases in volume, it must occur at the expense of volume of the other two elements. However, as volume increases, compensatory mechanisms are exhausted leading to a rise in ICP (**Fig. 16.1**).[6]

Effect of Positive End-Expiratory Pressure

The use of positive end-expiratory pressure (PEEP) in neurosurgical patients has been the source of controversy, as high PEEP may increase ICP through increasing central venous pressure. Furthermore, decreased right ventricular preload, decreased blood pressure, and subsequent decreased cardiac output from increased thoracic pressure or PEEP may also lead to decreased CPP. There have been many studies with small numbers of patients looking at the effects of PEEP on ICP and cerebral blood flow (CBF). It is felt that high levels of PEEP may be harmful to patients with impaired cerebral autoregulation because these patients may not tolerate the increased intracranial volume

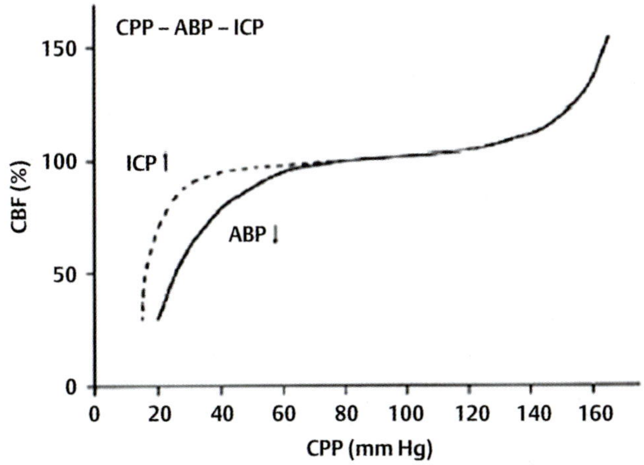

Fig. 16.1 Relationship of cerebral blood flow versus cerebral perfusion pressure. ABP, arterial blood pressure; CPP, cerebral perfusion pressure; ICP, intracranial pressure. (From Miller DJ, Stanek A, Langfitt TW. Concepts of cerebral perfusion pressure and vascular compression during intracranial hypertension. Prog Brain Res 1972;31:411–432.)

if they are already at the upper end of the ICP curve.[7] These factors can potentially result in ischemia and worsening neurological damage. There is a general lack of data on whether changes in ICP and CBF from mechanical ventilation significantly affect clinical outcome.

A recent study by Muench et al[8] described 10 patients who had acute respiratory compromise with anterior circulation aneurysms and Fischer grade 3 hemorrhages. The study predictably demonstrated that with increasing PEEP from 5 to 20 cm H_2O over a 7 day period, CBF and MAP tended to decrease. In addition, ICP tended to increase with increasing levels of PEEP. However, restoring MAP normalized CBF despite the persisting increase in PEEP. Six of 10 patients developed hemodynamically relevant vasospasm on day 7. Subgroup analysis found no differences between patients who developed vasospasm and those who did not. MAP and CBF decreased in unison with increasing PEEP and then normalized with hemodynamic support. Although increasing PEEP had consequences on cerebral perfusion, it did not appear to have clinical relevance.

In a similar study by McGuire et al,[9] a heterogeneous group of patients with severe head injury requiring mechanical ventilation were evaluated for changes in cerebral perfusion and ICPs with varying levels of PEEP. Patients were ventilated with tidal volumes (V_T) between 10 and 15 mL/kg, which are considered high volumes by current recommendations.[10] Patients were exposed to PEEP settings of 0, 5, 10, and 15 cm H_2O in random sequence. These settings were maintained for at least 5 minutes and hemodynamic parameters, ICP, and CPP were recorded. They found no significant changes in ICP or CPP with a PEEP of ≤15 cm H20 in patients with increased ICP (mean 18.8 mm Hg).

Hyperventilation

Hyperventilation is one of the most effective methods available for the rapid reduction of ICP. The CO_2 reactivity of intracerebral vessels is one of the intrinsic biological mechanisms involved in the regulation of CBF. Experimental studies using a pial window technique clearly demonstrated that the action of CO_2 on cerebral vessels is mediated by changes in extracellular fluid pH[11]; molecular CO_2 and bicarbonate ions do not directly affect vasoreactivity on these vessels. Although even a mild traumatic brain injury (TBI) can reduce the ability of cerebral vessels to react to changes in $PaCO_2$, most patients with moderate or severe TBI retain at least some global CO_2 reactivity. As a result, hyperventilation consistently lowers ICP.[12]

Despite the effectiveness of hyperventilation in lowering ICP, use of this treatment modality has fallen out of favor, primarily because of the simultaneous effect on CBF. Current guidelines for the management of TBI recommend avoiding hyperventilation during the first 24 hours after injury, when CBF is generally lowest, and recommend that moderate hyperventilation may be used subsequently, but only as a treatment for an elevated ICP.[13] The effect of a reduction in $PaCO_2$ on CBF in a normal subject is ~3% per mm Hg. Early studies in normal subjects using the Kety Schmidt technique[14] for measuring global CBF demonstrated that reducing PCO_2 from 37 to 19 mm Hg resulted in a decrease in global CBF from 45 to 25 mL/100 g/min.[15,16] Cerebral oxygen extraction was increased, but cerebral oxygen consumption (cerebral metabolic rate of oxygen; $CMRO_2$) remained unchanged. Only when $PaCO_2$ was further reduced to an average value of 10 mm Hg was $CMRO_2$ significantly reduced, suggesting that ischemia may have resulted from the reduction in CBF. Studies in patients with TBI follow this same pattern, with hyperventilation resulting in a consistent decrease in global CBF and increasing global cerebral oxygen extraction, but no reduction in $CMRO_2$ until the very extreme levels of PCO_2 are reached. However, patients with TBI often have areas of brain that are hypoperfused as a result of their brain injury, and these patients may be more vulnerable to regional effects of hyperventilation on CBF. Recent studies using positron emission tomography (PET) show that reduction in $PaCO_2$ to levels of 25 to 30 mm Hg does reduce regional CBF, even in areas of the brain that are hypoperfused at baseline.[17,18] Furthermore, hyperventilation increases the volume of the brain that is marginally perfused, but no significant reduction in regional $CMRO_2$ has been observed at these levels of PCO_2.[17,18] The conclusion of these recent studies seems to be that hyperventilation regularly reduces CBF and increases the proportion of the brain that is critically hypoperfused, but does not result in ischemia at the levels of PCO_2 that are commonly used in clinical practice.

The consequences of these hemodynamic effects of hyperventilation on outcome after severe TBI have been studied multiple times, and there is no consistent neuroprotective effect. One randomized clinical trial has shown an adverse effect of chronic hyperventilation in TBI patients.[19] Experimental studies using cortical injury models demonstrate that hyperventilation for 5 hours after TBI increased hippocampal neuron loss.[20] Complex interactions between autoregulation, the effect of ischemia, and the effect of trauma itself makes comparing data a complex endeavor. Overall, it seems that the effect of hyperventilation is transient and should only be briefly employed in acute situations until more definitive measures are established for the management of edema.

Monitoring in the Neurological Intensive Care Unit

The birth of critical care medicine can be possibly traced to the inception of bedside hemodynamic monitoring using the Swan-Ganz catheter. Despite its controversies, the catheter radically changed monitoring in the unit and made substantial physiological information readily available. Although a discussion of this subject is not within the scope of this chapter, it is important to delineate some of the most important aspects of body function to be monitored in this complex group of patients, including lung mechanics and gas exchange. As expressed earlier, the close interactions with CPP warrant establishing a relationship between lung mechanics and complex multimodal monitoring (CBF monitoring, brain tissue oxygenation, and intracerebral microdialysis) in the NICU.

Peak Airway Pressure

Peak airway pressure or peak inspiratory pressure is the maximal airway pressure recorded at the end of inspiration during positive pressure ventilation in a relaxed patient. It represents the total pressure needed to overcome resistance related to the ventilator circuit, endotracheal tube and airway, in addition to the elastic recoil of the lungs and chest wall (**Fig. 16.2**).

In the completely relaxed patient without airway obstruction or significant resistance from the ventilator circuit, endotracheal tube, or secretions, peak pressure may reflect alveolar pressure. Peak pressure is affected by the resistive properties of the circuit, the endotracheal tube, and the airway; therefore it does not always reflect alveolar pressure. In the presence of small-bore endotracheal tubes, significant airway obstruction, and secretions a large amount of energy is dissipated and high peak pressures do not reflect alveolar pressure and are unlikely

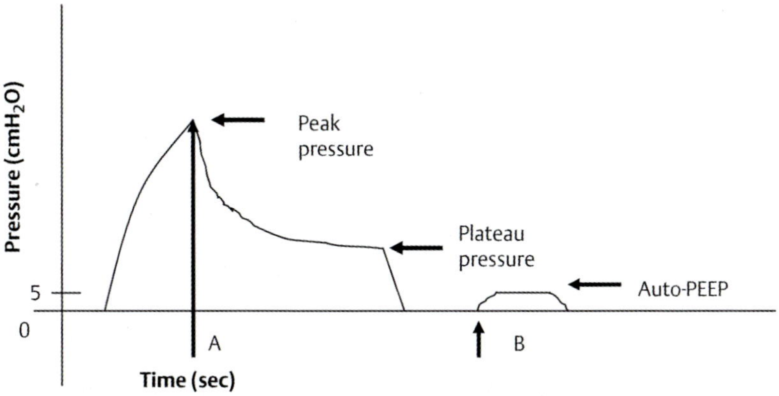

Fig. 16.2 Display of airway pressure versus time. **(A)** Inspiratory pressures. The peak pressure occurs at inspiration; 2 to 5 seconds after inspiratory pressure occlusion, the airway pressures drops to the plateau. The difference between peak and plateau pressures represents the contribution of airway obstruction. **(B)** A rise in expiratory pressure with expiratory airway occlusion at end expiration represents intrinsic peak or auto-PEEP.

to be associated with the development of barotrauma. Increased peak pressures are also observed in patients with increased thoracoabdominal elastic loads, such as the morbidly obese, extremely edematous, or those having massive ascites where these pressures do not result in alveolar rupture. A sudden increment in peak airway pressures should raise the suspicion of pneumothorax, significant bronchospasm, large airway atelectasis, pulmonary edema, or mucous plug formation.

Plateau Pressure

In a relaxed patient receiving assist control ventilation (ACV), applying an inspiratory pause at the end of passive inspiration will result in an immediate drop in airway opening pressure (peak airway pressure; Paw) to a lower value (plateau pressure; Pplat), which is reached after 3 to 5 seconds (**Fig. 16.2**). The difference between Paw and Pplat represents the contribution of the obstructive component. Hence, Pplat reflects lung and chest wall elastance, whereas Paw additionally reflects the resistive properties of the airways during inspiratory flow. High Pplats are seen in patients with diffuse lung diseases, such as ARDS or multilobar pneumonia. High Pplats are also found in patients with morbid obesity or chest wall deformities (e.g., kyphoscoliosis) and reflect decreased chest wall compliance.

Increasing emphasis has been placed on monitoring Pplats in mechanically ventilated patients so as to prevent ventilator-induced lung injury (VILI). In healthy lungs, a transpulmonary pressure of 35 cm H_2O inflates the lungs to total lung capacity. In patients with acute lung injury or pulmonary edema, total lung capacity may be effectively reduced due to alveolar loss or collapse. Therefore, the V_T delivered with each ventilator-assisted breath may overdistend more compliant regions of the lungs. The resultant higher Pplats may lead to alveolar overdistension of more compliant alveolar units. Alveolar overdistention is one of the purported mechanisms resulting in VILI (see below).

Several randomized, controlled trials have evaluated maintaining Pplats below 35 cm H_2O in patients with ARDS, with some studies demonstrating improved survival.[10,21–24] Maintaining Pplats <35 cm H_2O has also been shown to reduce inflammatory markers, and to reduce the incidence of multiple organ failure in patients with ARDS.[24] For ARDS patients with significant elevation of Pplats, pressure control ventilation with or without permissive hypercapnia has been employed to avoid VILI.

Intrinsic Positive End-Expiratory Pressure

At the end of expiration, alveolar and airway pressures equal atmospheric pressure. Intrinsic positive end-expiratory pressure (PEEPi), or auto PEEP, occurs when alveolar pressure exceeds atmospheric pressure at the end of expiration. PEEPi results in an increased intrathoracic pressure and elevated end-expiratory lung volume.[25]

In patients with underlying airflow obstruction secondary to asthma or emphysema, the patient may not be able to completely exhale. In these circumstances, if sufficient expiratory time is not permitted to allow full exhalation, progressive hyperinflation and PEEPi occurs.[26,27]

Increases in intrathoracic pressure may lead to significant hemodynamic consequences, such as decreased venous return and reduced cardiac output. Moreover, dynamic hyperinflation foreshortens the respiratory muscles and places them at mechanical disadvantage, thereby contributing to an increased work of breathing.[26,27]

PEEPi may occur in patients with significant airflow obstruction, in patients ventilated with high V_T and a small-bore endotracheal tube in place, or when the chosen ventilator settings result in an insufficient expiratory time to allow exhalation to the resting end-expiratory lung volume (**Table 16.4**). Under these conditions, patients are unable to completely exhale before the next inspiration begins, leading to progressive air trapping.

Two methods of determining PEEPi have been described. Static PEEPi is measured by occluding the ventilator

Table 16.4 Causes of Elevated Intrinsic PEEP (PEEPi)

- Underlying obstructive airways disease
- High levels of mechanical ventilation
- Small endotracheal tube
- Ventilator settings that provide insufficient expiratory time

expiratory port at the end of exhalation, which causes the pressure in the lungs and the mechanical ventilator to equilibrate; the level of PEEPi can be read from the ventilator's manometer. Modern ventilators will accomplish this in an automated fashion. Dynamic PEEPi is determined by determining the drop in intrathoracic pressure that is required for inspiratory flow to begin.[28]

Compliance

Compliance is defined as volume change per unit of pressure change. If airway pressure is plotted against delivered volume, the slope of the resulting curve (P-V curve) represents compliance (**Fig. 16.3**). The curve is not linear at its extremes; the points at which a plateau is detected are called inflection points. In the curve depicted in **Fig. 16.3**, two inflection points, a lower inflection point (LIP) and an upper inflection point (UIP) can be identified.

Static compliance can be calculated as

$$Ctot = V_T / (Pplat - Total\ PEEP)$$

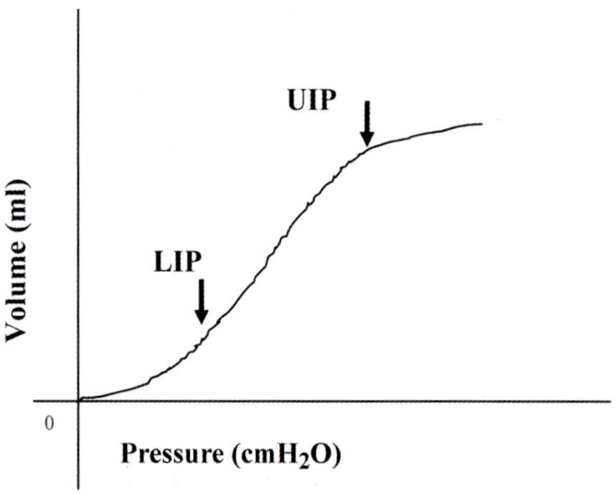

Fig. 16.3 Lung volume versus airway pressure plots. The slope of the lung's pressure–volume curve represents lung compliance. The lower inflection point (LIP) represents the minimal pressure that needs to be generated to displace lung volume. The upper inflection point (UIP) represents the pressure above which further increases in pressure minimally increase lung volume displacement.

where V_T is tidal volume and total PEEP is the sum of extrinsic PEEP and intrinsic PEEP. In a normal person, compliance is ~50 to 80 mL/cm H_2O.

Mechanical Ventilation

Setting the Ventilator

Table 16.5 shows the region components of setting the ventilator.

Fraction of Inspired Oxygen Concentration

The principal means to increase PaO_2 are to raise the fraction of inspired oxygen (FIO_2) concentration and/or to increase the lung volume at which the lungs are being ventilated. If a patient demonstrates appropriate oxygen saturation with a particular level of FIO_2 prior to intubation, a similar FIO_2 can be used as an initial setting; otherwise, it is generally acceptable to initiate ventilatory support with an FIO_2 of 1.0. FIO_2 should be rapidly titrated to minimize the potential for possible O_2 toxicity.

Tidal Volume

A V_T of 10 to 15 mL/kg was traditionally used to ventilate patients, but available data show that these volumes may cause alveolar overdistension and VILI. Current indications suggest using V_T between 6 and 10 mL/kg.[24] This is particularly important in patients with ARDS or severe bronchospasm. It is important to recognize that these new "protective ventilator strategies" may not be applicable in patients with conditions causing decreased chest wall compliance, such as kyphoscoliosis and obesity.

Table 16.5 Setting the Ventilator

- Mode
  - Assist-control ventilation (ACV)
  - Synchronized intermittent mandatory ventilation (SIMV)
  - Pressure support ventilation (PSV)
  - Pressure control ventilation (PCV)
- Fraction of inspired oxygen concentration (FIO_2)
- Tidal volume (V_T)
- Inspiratory flow rate (IFR)
- Respiratory rate (RR)
- Inspiratory:expiratory ratio (I:E ratio)
- Continuous positive airway pressure (CPAP)
- Positive end-expiratory pressure (PEEP)

Inspiratory Flow Rate

The inspiratory flow rate, measured in L/min, determines how fast a V_T is delivered. The inspiratory time (T_I) is a function of V_T and flow rate:

$$T_I = V_T\,(L)/\text{Flow Rate}\,(L/min)$$

The expiratory time (TE) is determined by the inspiratory flow rate and the ventilator's frequency. For a set rate of 10 bpm, the total respiratory cycle time (Ttot) is 6 seconds. The TE can be determined by subtracting the result of equation above from Ttot. The flow rate may be altered during the inspiratory cycle by the use of a specific inspiratory flow pattern. Patterns include rectangular, ascending ramp, descending ramp, and sinusoidal flow patterns.

The relationship between inspiration and expiration is known as the inspiration:expiration (I:E) time ratio. It is clear from this, that inspiratory flow rate should be set taking into account that it will affect T_I and I:E ratio.

Respiratory Rate

Once V_T and FIO_2 have been set, a respiratory rate needs to be set. This has to be done taking into account the patient's actual rate demand, the patient's anticipated ventilatory requirements, and the impact of set respiratory rate on breath timing.

Unless the patient is sedated or paralyzed, respiratory rates below 10 and 15 bpm are poorly tolerated. Neurohumoral feedback from lung edema and inflammation generally results in a rapid, shallow breathing pattern. Additionally, discrepancies between actual and machine set respiratory rates may lead to breathing patterns with an inverse I:E time ratio, which are poorly tolerated.

The machine rate should therefore be set close to the patient's own rate. If the actual rate is so high that effective ventilation cannot be accomplished, sedation and/or paralysis may be required after a careful search for rapidly reversible causes of tachypnea (pain, discomfort, fever, etc.).

Inspiration:Expiration Ratio

The relationship between the time spent on inspiration and the time spent on expiration is called the I:E ratio. The I:E ratio is not set by the operator; it results from altering the different parameters that have been discussed until now. In normal spontaneously breathing subjects, there is abundant time to empty the inspired V_T. In certain pathological states, such as asthma and chronic obstructive pulmonary disease (COPD), the decrement in expiratory flow may require a prolonged time to empty the inspired lung volume. The relationships among V_T, respiratory rate (f), inspiratory flow rate, and I:E ratio are shown in **Fig. 16.4**.

If inspiratory flow is increased and V_T and f remain constant, the inspiratory time will be shortened and the I:E ratio will be decreased (e.g., 1:2 to 1:4) (**Fig. 16.4**). Decreasing inspiratory flow under the same conditions results in the opposite effect.

If V_T is decreased while maintaining a constant inspiratory flow and f, will also shorten the inspiratory time and decrease the I:E ratio (**Fig. 16.4**).

Decreasing f while maintaining V_T and a constant inspiratory flow results in an increase in the duration of the cycle (Ttot); inspiratory time remains the same and expiratory time increases (**Fig. 16.4**).

Basic Modes of Mechanical Ventilation

The mode of mechanical ventilation describes a particular set of characteristics or variables (cycle, trigger, and limit) that define how ventilation is provided.

Assist Control Ventilation

ACV is the most common mode of mechanical ventilation initially applied to patients who present with hypercapnic or hypoxemic respiratory failure. With ACV the physician sets a minimal rate and V_T (or pressure). The patient may trigger the mechanical ventilator at a faster rate, but the set volume (or pressure) will be delivered with each breath. As described above, in the AC mode, the ventilator can be triggered by flow or by pressure. When the ventilator is set to be triggered by pressure, the patient has to generate a certain amount of pressure (usually 1–3 cm H_2O) to open the solenoid valve and receive a ventilator-assisted breath. If the ventilator is set to be triggered by flow, following a patient's inspiratory effort, the ventilator will sense a decrement in the circuit's baseline flow and only then deliver a breath. If the patient has no spontaneous inspiratory efforts, the ventilator will be time triggered based on the set respiratory rate.

The V_T is generally set at 6 to 10 mL/kg. In patients with emphysema, large volumes will be preferentially delivered to the most diseased and compliant areas. As a result, a large proportion of the delivered volume will not participate in gas exchange and will rather contribute to dynamic hyperinflation, intrinsic PEEP, decreased cardiac output, and worsening ventilation/perfusion mismatch. In patients with ARDS, who characteristically present with large regional variations in compliance, large V_T will result in overdistension of the more compliant regions and may contribute to VILI.

Controlled mechanical ventilation (CMV), the predecessor of ACV, delivered mandatory V_T at a set rate independent of the patient's own respiratory cycle. The major disadvantage of CMV is patient discomfort, which

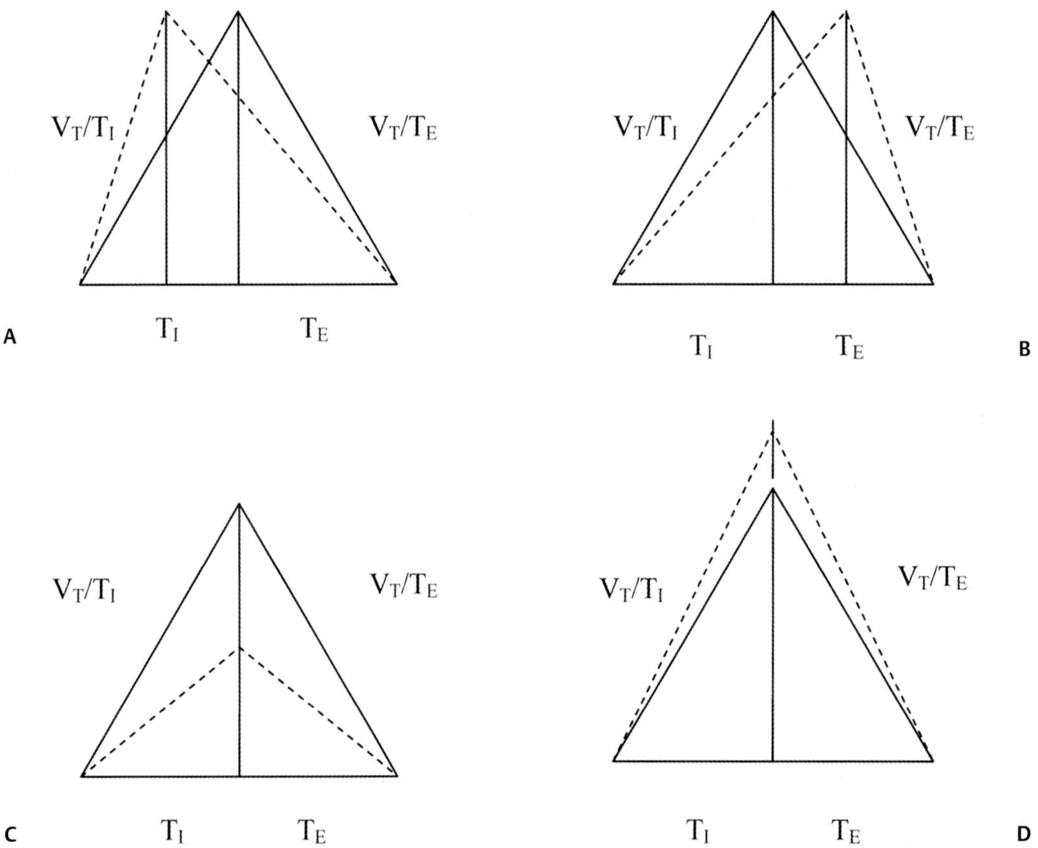

Fig. 16.4 Display of relationships among tidal volume (V_T), respiratory rate (f), inspiratory flow rate (V_T/T_I), expiratory flow rate (V_T/T_E) and the I:E ratio, (T_I) inspiratory time, and (T_E) expiratory time. **(A)** The impact of increasing inspiratory flow rate, if the tidal volume and breathing rate remains constant. An increase in inspiratory flow increases expiratory time. **(B)** The impact of decreasing inspiratory flow rate if tidal and breathing rate an constant. A decrease in inspiratory flow decreases expiratory time. **(C)** The impact of reducing tidal volume while maintaining the same inspiratory flow rate and respiratory rate. **(D)** The impact of an increase in tidal volume with maintenance of the respiratory and inspiratory flow rates.

results from an increase in the work of breathing when mandatory breaths are asynchronous with the patient's own respiratory efforts. Patients are also unable to alter their minute ventilation (V_E) if their clinical situation changes (e.g., an increase in CO_2 or a decrease in pH).

Synchronized Intermittent Mandatory Ventilation

Synchronized intermittent mandatory ventilation (SIMV) is a ventilator mode in which the ventilator mandatory breaths are delivered in synchrony with the patient's inspiratory effort. Breaths are delivered at a set rate and volume. In between mandatory breaths, the patient is allowed to breath spontaneously from a demand valve or a continuous flow of gas. Spontaneous breaths may also be supported with titratable levels of PS or continous positive airway pressure (CPAP). During SIMV, each time cycle is divided into mandatory and spontaneous time periods. If a patient is ordered to have a SIMV rate of 6 bpm, each cycle is 10 seconds. During the initial phase of each cycle, the ventilator, in synchrony with the patient's effort, will provide a preset V_T. If the patient makes no effort during this initial phase, a machine-delivered breath will be given at the beginning of the spontaneous phase to guarantee a backup rate. During the spontaneous phase the patient's inspiratory effort will not trigger a mechanical ventilator breath, and the V_T is determined by the patient's spontaneous effort.

SIMV was originally believed to facilitate weaning by avoiding alkalemia and disuse atrophy, and by gradually reducing the number of ventilator-assisted breaths over time. Conversely, two randomized, controlled trials have clearly shown that SIMV prolongs the weaning process over T-piece or PS weans.

Pressure Support Ventilation

In contrast to ACV, pressure support ventilation (PSV) is a pressure-preset, flow-cycled ventilator mode intended to support spontaneous respiratory efforts. With each inspiratory effort, the patient triggers the ventilator, which maintains the preset pressure level in the inspiratory circuit throughout inspiration.

Pressurization of the inspiratory circuit ends when flow rate decreases at the end of the patient's inspiratory effort. Depending on the ventilator model, the inspiratory cycle ends when flow rate is <5 L/min or when flow rate decreases below 25% of the peak inspiratory flow rate. The inspiratory cycle may also be terminated by an increase in pressure above the preset value, indicating that expiration has begun. There are no set values for the amount of pressure support to be applied, but pressure is generally titrated toward achieving expired V_T >5 to 7 mL/kg, a decrease in respiratory rate (i.e.: ≤35 breaths/min), and a decrement in the patient's work of breathing (i.e., decreased use of accessory inspiratory muscles). The patient retains control of the length and depth of the inspiratory cycle and may influence the percentage of the total support provided by the ventilator and the flow profile on a breath-to-breath basis. V_T are determined by a combination of PSV settings, the patient's effort, and the patient's underlying pulmonary mechanics.

PSV has been successfully used as part of a weaning strategy in patients who have adequate respiratory parameters. PSV may decrease inspiratory workload, but muscle unloading may be variable and is dependant upon underlying respiratory pathophysiology. In patients with COPD, PSV may contribute to an increased work of breathing, as ventilator inflation persists into the patient's neural expiratory phase. This may also result in patient–ventilator asynchrony.

Pressure Control Ventilation

The majority of patients receiving mechanical ventilation within current ICUs are ventilated using various forms of volume-control ventilation; a preset V_T is delivered with each breath. In volume-control ventilation, the volume is held constant while airway pressure varies with changes in airway, lung, or chest wall mechanics. Pressure control ventilation (PCV) is a form of pressure-limited ventilation where airway pressure is held constant, while V_T varies with changes in airway resistance, or lung and chest wall mechanics. As a result, patients may receive variable V_T with each respiratory effort depending on the dynamic changes in the resistive and elastic components of the respiratory system. During PCV, the rate, pressure limit, and inspiratory time are set on the ventilator. Breaths are initiated at a preset rate (time cycled) and gas flows into the patient breathing circuit until the preset pressure is reached. At this point, gas flow is reduced to the minimum flow required to maintain the airway pressure at the preset level until inspiratory time elapses.

PCV has been used in clinical settings where increased Paws (implying increased alveolar pressures) are encountered and feared to predispose the patient to VILI. It has been used in cases of ARDS where fine control of the mean airway pressure is desired, and other modes have failed to adequately ventilate and/or oxygenate the patient. PCV usually results in a higher mean airway pressure than volume-limited ventilation, but allows for lower Paws. Patients treated with PCV must be sedated and/or paralyzed to achieve adequate comfort and effective ventilation.

A randomized, controlled trial compared PCV with volume-controlled ventilation.[29] Both ventilator modes were adjusted to maintain Pplats <35 cm H_2O. The study evidenced an increment in mortality and multiorgan system failure in the volume control group, but by multivariate analysis, the ventilatory modality was not shown to be a predictor for mortality. Although there are theoretical advantages to PCV, the requirements for prolonged sedation and paralysis are worrisome, and the routine adoption of this mode of ventilation is unwarranted at this time.

Continuous Positive Airway Pressure and Positive End-Expiratory Pressure

CPAP is a mode of ventilatory support that is applied to spontaneously breathing patients. During the respiratory cycle, a constant pressure is applied to the airway throughout inspiration and expiration. The level of CPAP is the only variable that is adjusted by the physician.

CPAP is commonly combined with PSV. CPAP may be used with PSV to decrease the amount of respiratory effort required to trigger a ventilator breath. CPAP has been used with PSV or alone in patients weaning from mechanical ventilation to prevent small airway collapse and atelectasis. Noninvasive CPAP delivery is commonly used to treat obstructive sleep apnea and, more recently, it has been used in the management of acute respiratory failure. In the setting of respiratory failure from ARDS or congestive heart failure, decreases in lung compliance may lead to significant alveolar collapse, with an increased alveolar shunt fraction and refractory hypoxemia. Extrinsic PEEP has been used as an adjunctive technique during mechanical ventilation in these patients to prevent alveolar collapse, recruit alveoli, and improve oxygenation by increasing end-expiratory lung volume (EELV) and by decreasing intrapulmonary shunt. In patients with ARDS, selection of extrinsic PEEP can be accomplished in two ways: (1) by titrating extrinsic PEEP up, while carefully following oxygenation and pulmonary mechanics; (2) by setting the extrinsic PEEP above the LIP obtained by constructing a pressure–volume curve (see below). The method chosen to titrate extrinsic PEEP does not appear to have a significant impact on clinical outcome. In a recent study by Pelosi et al[30] a good correlation was observed between clinically guided extrinsic PEEP and that obtained by pressure–volume curve analysis.

The addition of extrinsic PEEP is also helpful in decreasing the patient's respiratory workload while on assisted or supported modes of mechanical ventilation.

Patients with PEEPi must overcome a significant amount of pressure before they can elicit flow from the ventilator. This results in difficult ventilator triggering, delayed breath delivery, increased work of breathing, and patient–ventilator asynchrony. Some authors advocate applying extrinsic PEEP in these circumstances to facilitate triggering. Although the addition of extrinsic PEEP may decrease the workload required to initiate a ventilator breath, it is important to remember that in many instances, hyperinflation and PEEPi are dynamic conditions that are subject to change with therapy. Emphasis should be placed in therapeutic strategies aimed at alleviating bronchospasm and decreasing the I:E ratio.

Extrinsic PEEP, however, has distinct disadvantages. It increases intrathoracic pressure, which may decrease venous return and compromise cardiac output and O_2 delivery. Extrinsic PEEP has the most effect on the compliant regions of the lungs, and overdistention of normal lung units may occur, contributing to the alveolar dead space fraction. Concern exists that extrinsic PEEP, especially at higher levels, may contribute to VILI.[31]

Mechanical Ventilation in Specific Circumstances: ARDS and Neurogenic Pulmonary Edema

Patients with acute neurological disease are at high risk to develop aspiration pneumonia, acute lung injury, ARDS, and neurogenic pulmonary edema (NPE). In the complex setting of brain injury, these entities add a significant comorbidity and complicate prognosis. In this section we will discuss pathophysiological aspects of these entities and their supportive management with mechanical ventilation.

NPE is a potentially life-threatening complication of several acute neurological conditions, including subarachnoid hemorrhage (SAH), intracerebral hemorrhage, head injury, and seizure. A series of 457 patients with SAH reported a 6% incidence of severe NPE.[32] Increased age and a worse clinical grade of SAH were associated with NPE. Hypoxia results from an increase in extravascular lung water (EVLW); the extent of this increase correlates directly with the magnitude of the intrapulmonary shunt and the degree of hypoxia. Analysis of hemodynamic data and measurement of pulmonary edema fluid protein content, both in humans and in animal models, has led to the development of two conflicting theories as to the mechanism of NPE.

Proponents of the hydrostatic mechanism cite the low edema fluid-to-plasma protein ratio and the frequent presence of left ventricular dysfunction to support the concept that pulmonary venous and hence alveolar capillary hypertension are the cause of NPE.[33,34] Conversely, some patients have edema fluid with a high protein level suggesting increased permeability of the alveolar capillary wall. In addition, indices of left ventricular performance (pulmonary artery wedge pressure [PAWP], central venous pressure, and cardiac index) may be normal.[35] Animal models of NPE using intracisternal injection of veratrine have revealed that shortly after the cerebral insult, pulmonary blood volume increases with pronounced rises in pulmonary arterial and left atrial pressures.[36] This is thought to occur due to massively increased sympathetic discharge. The magnitude of the pulmonary hypertension correlated in this model with the increase in EVLW. In humans, pulmonary artery pressures of 110/60 mm Hg have been recorded in acute SAH.[37] The pulmonary edema that results in this situation is clearly hydrostatic in origin, but high pressure can disrupt alveolar capillaries (stress failure), which may subsequently lead to the formation of exudative or high permeability pulmonary edema.[38] Thus, in different patients with NPE, there may be a hydrostatic mechanism, a high permeability mechanism, or a combination of both mechanisms to explain the increase in EVLW.

Whether knowing the precise cause in individual patients is important is a matter of conjecture. As well as being a direct threat to life, the severe hypoxia that results from NPE may worsen the neurological injury. Positive pressure ventilation and the use of high levels of PEEP are frequently required and may worsen cerebral perfusion (and therefore outcome) by reducing cardiac output and by impeding cerebral venous drainage.

A study by Kahn et al[39] looked at the incidence, risk factors, and outcome of patients with acute lung injury with SAH. The study found that in a study group of 170 patients with aneurysmal SAH, 27% met the definition of ALI, and 18% met the definition for ARDS at some point in their ICU hospital stay. Increasing severity of illness, increasing Hunt and Hess grade, severe sepsis, and blood transfusions were all independently associated with developing lung injury. In contrast, ICP and vasospasm were not associated with the development of ALI. One limitation is that this study did not assess left ventricular filling pressures resulting in pulmonary edema from left heart dysfunction. They concluded that ALI is a common complication of SAH and independently associated with worse outcomes. Further studies are needed to assess incidence of ALI and ARDS in brain injury patients along with the effects of prospective lung protective strategies.

Interestingly, in some cases, the prevention of vasospasm after an SAH may result in pulmonary edema. In addition to nimodipine, following an SAH secondary to an aneurysm patients are treated with hyperdynamic therapy. This includes the maintenance of hypertension, hypervolemia, and hemodilution to help prevent vasospasm. This is the so-called triple-H therapy. A systematic review of triple-H therapy for prophylaxis of vasospasm found that there were few well-designed prospective studies.[40] However, because of the induced hypervolemia, pulmonary edema and heart failure are likely consequences.

Current evidence suggests that lung protective ventilation, a combination of low V_T (6 mL/kg of V_T) and low Pplats of ≤30 cm of water will result in decreased mortality. The decrement in mortality may be related to a reduction in further disruption of the alveolar-capillary membrane, a decrement in inflammatory markers, or both.[10,24] There are no studies that directly address mechanical ventilation in patients with acute brain injury, but the two most important issues are the use of PEEP and its effects on CPP, and the effect that therapeutic hypervolemia (e.g., in patients with SAH) could have on the patient's morbidity and mortality. Two studies may indirectly give an idea about these issues. In the first one, researchers randomly assigned 549 patients with ALI and ARDS to receive mechanical ventilation with either lower or higher PEEP levels, which were set according to different tables of predetermined combinations of PEEP and FIO_2.[41] Mean (±SD) PEEP values on days 1 through 4 were 8.3 ± 3.2 cm of water in the lower-PEEP group and 13.2 ± 3.5 cm of water in the higher-PEEP group ($p < 0.001$). The rates of death before hospital discharge were 24.9% and 27.5%, respectively ($p = 0.48$; 95% confidence interval for the difference between groups, −10.0 to 4.7%). From day 1 to day 28, breathing was unassisted for a mean of 14.5 ± 10.4 days in the lower-PEEP group and 13.8 ± 10.6 days in the higher-PEEP group ($p = 0.50$).[41] The results of this trial suggest that in patients with ALI and ARDS clinical outcomes are similar whether lower or higher PEEP levels are used. The level of PEEP applied in these cases is far lower than one would anticipate causing significant changes in CPP. The second trial[42] compared a conservative and a liberal strategy of fluid management using explicit protocols applied for 7 days in 1000 patients with ALI. The primary end point was death at 60 days. The rate of death at 60 days was 25.5% in the conservative-strategy group and 28.4% in the liberal-strategy group ($p = 0.30$; 95% confidence interval for the difference, −2.6 to 8.4%). The mean (±SE) cumulative fluid balance during the first 7 days was −136 ± 491 mL in the conservative-strategy group and 6992 ± 502 mL in the liberal-strategy group ($p < 0.001$). The conservative strategy improved lung function and shortened the duration of mechanical ventilation and intensive care without increasing nonpulmonary-organ failures. Although this study favors the use of a conservative strategy, it also suggests that increased fluids may not necessarily worsen mortality in ARDS.[43] Whether these studies are directly applicable to the NICU scenario is not completely clear, but considering similar pathophysiological mechanisms, low V_T strategies should be strongly considered.

Complications

Ventilator-Associated Pneumonia

Hospital-acquired pneumonia (HAP) generally has a bacterial etiology; it is currently the second most common nosocomial infection in the United States, and it is associated with high mortality and morbidity (**Table 16.6**).[44] The presence of HAP increases hospital length of stay by an average of 7 to 9 days per patient and results in excess costs.[44–46] Although HAP is not a reportable illness, available data suggest that it occurs at a rate of between 5 and 10 cases per 1,000 hospital admissions, with the incidence increasing by as much as six- to 20-fold in mechanically ventilated patients.[44,47–49]

The incidence of ventilator-associated pneumonia (VAP) may be up to two times higher in patients diagnosed by qualitative or semiquantitative sputum cultures compared with quantitative cultures of lower respiratory tract secretions.[44,50]

HAP accounts for up to 25% of all ICU infections and for more than 50% of the antibiotics prescribed.[50] VAP occurs in 9 to 27% of all intubated patients.[44,46] In ICU patients, nearly 90% of episodes of HAP occur during mechanical ventilation.

In mechanically ventilated patients, the incidence increases with duration of ventilation. The risk of VAP is highest early in the course of the hospital stay, and it is estimated to be 3%/day during the first 5 days of ventilation, 2%/day during days 5 to 10 of ventilation, and 1%/day after this.[51] Because most mechanical ventilation is short term, approximately half of all episodes of VAP occur within the first 4 days of mechanical ventilation.

Table 16.6 Complications of Mechanical Ventilation

Ventilator-associated pneumonia

- Occurs in 9–27% of all intubated patients
- Most likely to occur within the first 10 days of ventilation
- Microbiology depends upon temporal occurrence of pneumonia and time of intubation

Ventilator-induced lung injury (VILI) barotrauma

- VILI includes damage to alveolar and surfactant production/function
- *Barotrauma* refers to pneumothorax, pneumomediastinum, and pneumoperitoneum

Time of onset of pneumonia is an important epidemiological variable and risk factor for specific pathogens and outcomes in patients with HAP and VAP. Early-onset HAP and VAP, defined as occurring within the first 4 days of hospitalization, usually carry a better prognosis and are more likely to be caused by antibiotic-sensitive bacteria. Late-onset HAP and VAP (5 days or more) are more likely to be caused by multidrug-resistant (MDR) pathogens, and are associated with increased patient mortality and morbidity. However, patients with early-onset HAP who have received prior antibiotics or who have had prior hospitalization within the past 90 days are at greater risk for colonization and infection with MDR pathogens and should be treated similarly to patients with late-onset HAP or VAP.[52] The crude mortality rate for HAP may be as high as 30 to 70%, but many of these critically ill patients with HAP die of their underlying disease rather than pneumonia. The mortality related to the HAP or "attributable mortality" has been estimated to be between 33 and 50% in several case-matching studies of VAP. Increased mortality rates were associated with bacteremia, especially with *Pseudomonas aeruginosa* or *Acinetobacter* species, medical rather than surgical illness, and treatment with ineffective antibiotic therapy.[53,54]

Prevention

Intubation and mechanical ventilation are significantly associated with HAP[43,46] and should be avoided whenever possible. Although noninvasive mechanical ventilation has been shown to be an interesting alternative for certain patients,[55–58] its use in acute neurological disorders is limited because of the need for patients to be cooperative. Specific strategies have been used to decrease the duration of mechanical ventilation, such as improved methods of sedation and weaning protocols.[59–63] Continuous aspiration of subglottic secretions, through the use of a specially designed endotracheal tube, has significantly reduced the incidence of early-onset VAP in several studies.[64–66]

Placing the patient in a supine position is a significant factor for aspiration and the development of VAP. Several studies have shown the increased incidence of aspiration in the supine position and the decreased likelihood of decreasing the incidence of VAP by placing the patient in a semirecumbent position.[67–70]

Diagnosis

Current guidelines for VAP emphasize the need to establish the presence of pneumonia using clinical and microbiological criteria.[71] The presence of a new or progressive radiological infiltrate, and at least two out of three clinical features (fever >38°C, leukocytosis or leukopenia, or purulent secretions) are the most accurate criteria to start antibiotics.[72] Current guidelines recommend using quantitative cultures, lower respiratory tract secretions obtained by bronchoalveolar lavage (BAL), endotracheal aspirates, or protected specimen brushing.[71]

Treatment

The most important consideration in treating HAP is whether the patient has risk factors for MDR pathogens. The duration of hospitalization is also important factor, and patients hospitalized for more than 4 days are at greater risk for MDR pathogens. The timeliness and adequacy of empiric treatment are extremely important. Because delays in the administration of appropriate therapy have been associated with excess hospital mortality,[73–75] the prompt administration of empiric therapy for patients with VAP is essential. The current American Thoracic Society (ATS) management strategy for patients with VAP is summarized in **Fig. 16.5.**[71] It calls for lower respiratory tract sample acquisition and rapid administration of broad spectrum antibiotics. The decision tree to determine the use of broad spectrum versus limited spectrum antibiotics is summarized in **Fig. 16.6**. Antibiotic use should also be based on local microbiological data. After 2 to 3 days on antibiotics, patients should have a careful reevaluation. If cultures are positive, deescalation of antibiotics should be done to prevent resistance. In patients in whom initial antibiotic therapy is adequate and in whom isolates do not show *Pseudomonas*, the duration of the antibiotic course can be shortened to 7 to 10 days, instead of the traditional 14 to 21 days.[76]

Ventilator-Induced Lung Injury and Barotrauma

The notion of barotrauma was coined some 60 years ago by Macklin and Macklin,[77] but in the past decades it has become increasingly clear that mechanical ventilation can cause injury in multiple ways. In aggregate, multiple studies have established four specific VILI mechanisms, namely: (1) regional overdistension caused by the application of a local stress or pressure that forces cells and tissues to assume shapes and dimensions that they do not assume during unassisted breathing[78]; (2) so-called low-volume injury associated with the repeated recruitment and derecruitment of unstable lung units, which causes the abrasion of the epithelial airspace lining by interfacial forces[79]; (3) the inactivation of surfactant triggered by large alveolar surface area oscillations that stress surfactant adsorption and desorption kinetics and are associated with surfactant aggregate conversion[80]; and (4) interdependence mechanisms that raise cell and tissue stress between neighboring structures with different mechanical properties.[81]

As described earlier in this chapter multiple strategies are currently being adopted to minimize the presence and

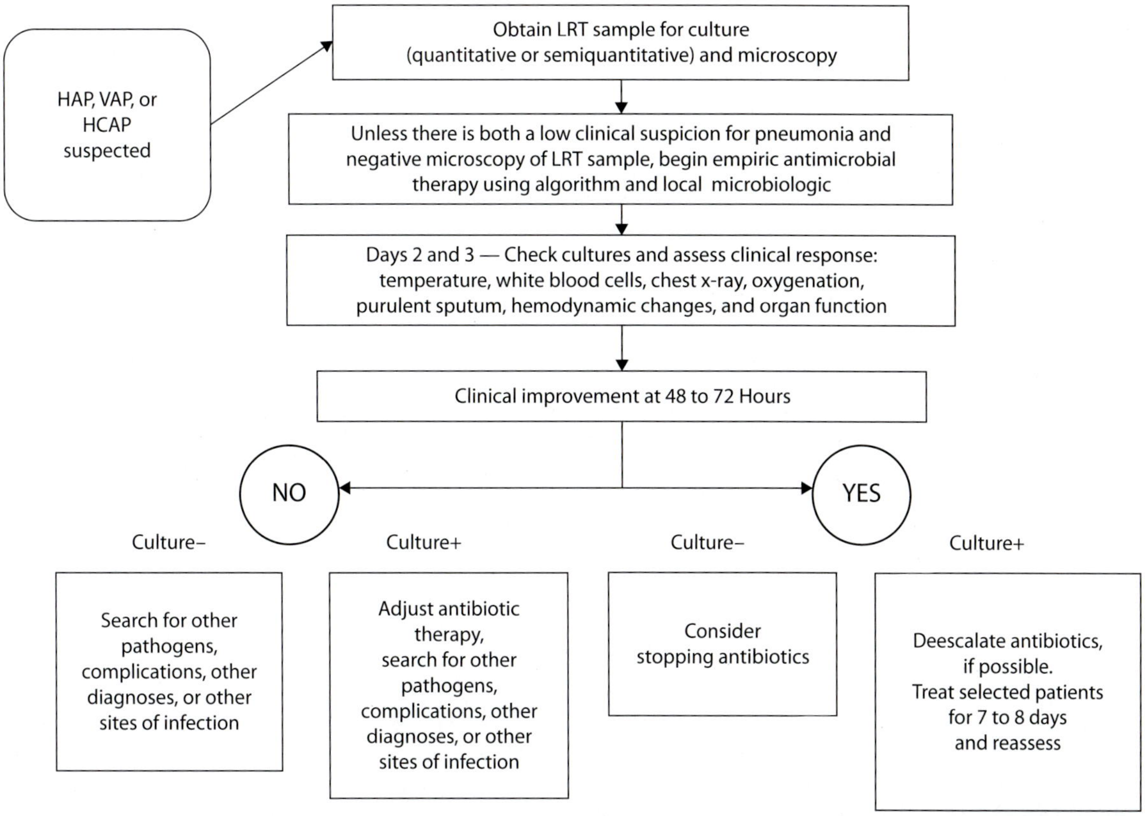

Fig. 16.5 An approach to the diagnosis and management of hospital-acquired or ventilator-acquired pneumonia (HAP or VAP).

perpetuation of VILI in critically ill patients. Lung "protective strategies" of mechanical ventilation using smaller V_T and adequate use of PEEP have been shown to decrease mortality and as well as the expression of inflammatory markers.

Unlike VILI, which involves damage directed at the alveolus and surfactant production/function, barotrauma refers to the presence of pneumothorax, pneumomediastinum, and pneumoperitoneum as consequences of mechanical ventilation. Although certainly significant as a cause of morbidity, at least one study has shown no difference in mortality between patients with ALI who develop barotrauma and those who do not.[82]

Weaning from Mechanical Ventilation

Mechanical ventilation is highly beneficial, but it is also associated with significant complications, such as decreased cardiac output, increased ICP, VAP, and VILI. Weaning patients from mechanical ventilation remains one of the most challenging aspects of intensive care (**Table 16.7**). About 20 to 25% of ventilated patients fail an initial attempt at discontinuing mechanical ventilation and will require more concentrated and prolonged attempts at discontinuing mechanical ventilation (i.e., weaning).[83] For patients requiring prolonged mechanical ventilation, ~40% of the time spent on the ventilator is devoted to the weaning process.[84] This percentage is even higher in patients with specific diseases such as COPD, who may spend up to 60% of their time on mechanical ventilation undergoing active weaning attempts.

Determining the Cause of Respiratory Failure

Before mechanical ventilation can be safely withdrawn, the abnormality precipitating respiratory failure must be identified and must show favorable signs of response to treatment. To identify the physiological cause of respiratory failure, it is useful to separate the causes of respiratory failure into three major categories: (1) hypoxemic respiratory failure, (2) ventilatory pump failure, and (3) psychological factors.

Hypoxemic respiratory failure can be the result of hypoventilation, impaired pulmonary gas exchange, or decreased mixed venous blood oxygen content. The chest radiograph, physical examination, and alveolar-arterial oxygen gradient are useful in distinguishing between intrapulmonary shunting, increased physiological dead

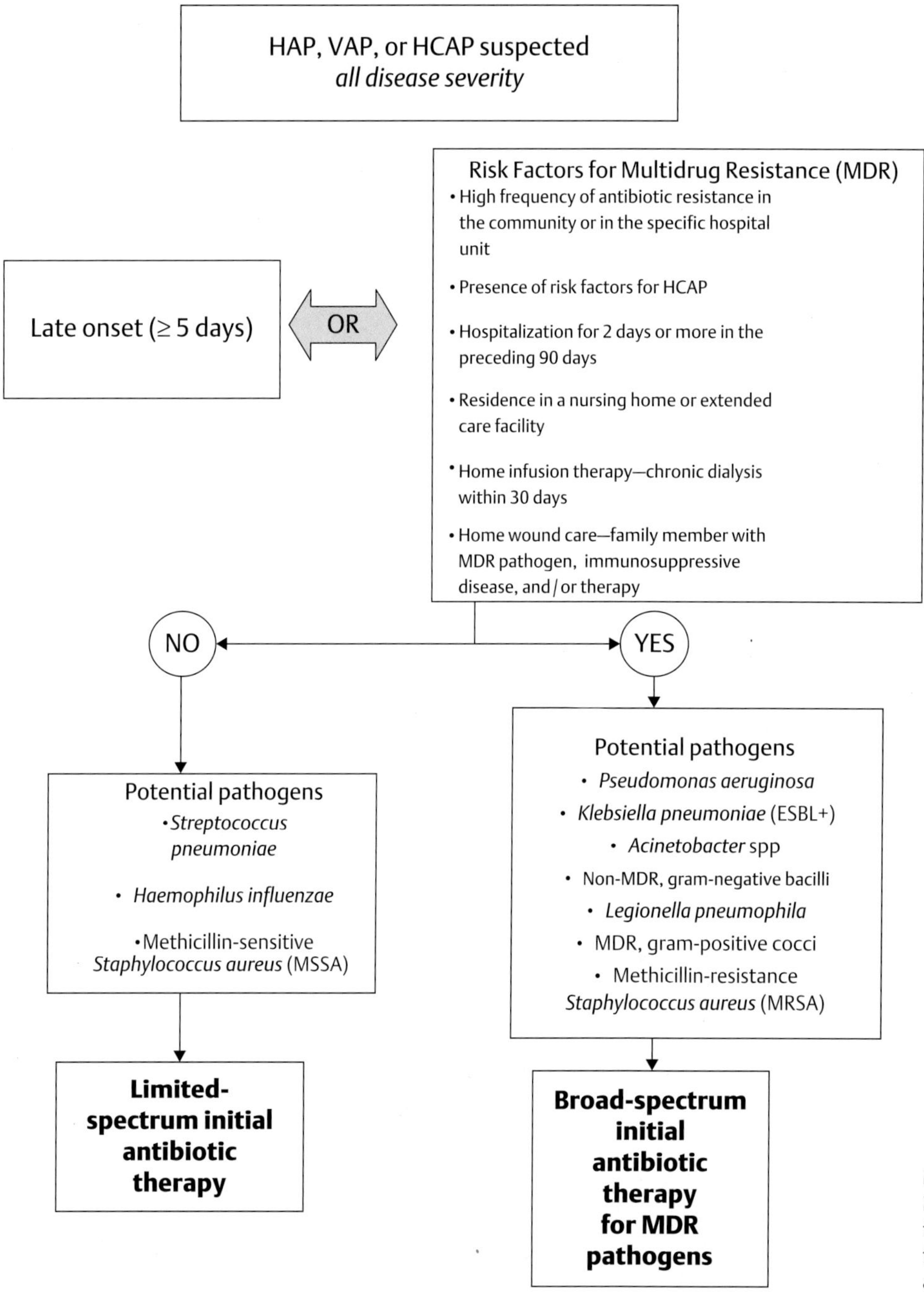

Fig. 16.6 The effects of prior hospitalization or use of antibiotics on bacterial flora and subsequent antibiotic choice for hospital-acquired or ventilator-acquired pneumonia (HAP or VAP).

Table 16.7 Weaning from Mechanical Ventilation

Determine the cause of respiratory failure
• Pump versus lung failure
Bedside predictors of weaning outcome
• Gas exchange
• Ventilatory variables
• Respiratory shallow breathing index
• Spontaneous breathing trial performance

space, and alveolar hypoventilation as possible causes of hypoxemic respiratory failure.

Respiratory pump dysfunction is considered by some authors to be the most common cause of failure to wean from mechanical ventilation. Failure of the respiratory system as a pump may occur whenever respiratory demand exceeds ventilatory pump capacity.

Respiratory pump failure may occur due to an increased ventilatory load (even in patients with normal respiratory pump), resulting from increased dead space;

hypermetabolism due to sepsis and/or fever; increased CO_2 production due to increased carbohydrate load, or inappropriately elevated central respiratory drive. On the other hand, normal or only slightly elevated ventilatory loads may not be sustained by subjects with decreased respiratory pump capacity due to impaired central respiratory drive, phrenic nerve dysfunction, or severe derangements of respiratory muscle function (i.e., underlying neuromuscular disease, electrolyte disturbances).

Abnormalities of central respiratory drive can be seen in patients with structural injury to the CNS, overuse of sedative agents, and metabolic alkalosis. Diaphragm dysfunction can be seen in patients with cold-induced phrenic nerve injury or direct diaphragm injury that may occur during cardiothoracic surgery.[85] Diaphragm dysfunction has also been reported in patients following upper abdominal surgery.

Hyperinflation is frequently overlooked as a cause for failure to wean in patients with acute exacerbation of severe asthma or COPD. Hyperinflation causes a shortening in the diaphragm precontraction length, which causes the diaphragm to work at a disadvantageous portion of its tension-length curve. It also alters the orientation of the diaphragmatic fibers medially inward and decreases the length of the zone of apposition, factors that further lead to a decrease in diaphragm's force-generating capacity.

Other disorders commonly encountered in the ICU that may result in abnormal respiratory muscle function thereby hindering weaning include undernutrition, electrolyte disturbances (hypophosphatemia, hypokalemia, hypocalcemia, hypomagnesemia), and thyroid dysfunction. Additionally, respiratory muscle atrophy has been suggested as a consequence of prolonged mechanical ventilation, when patients make no respiratory efforts. In a study in pigs, 5 days of mechanical ventilation with sedation and complete diaphragm inactivity resulted in disturbed diaphragm contractility and activation, whereas nerve conduction and neuromuscular transmission were not affected.[86] In a study in healthy baboons,[87] 11 days of mechanical ventilation and neuromuscular blockade resulted in nonsignificant changes in hemodynamics, oxygenation, and/or lung function. However, significant impairment in diaphragmatic endurance and strength were seen. Based on these studies, it is likely that prolonged mechanical ventilation by itself impairs diaphragmatic function independent of underlying lung disease, but studies in human subjects are lacking.

When Is the Patient Ready to Be Weaned?

Before a weaning attempt is made certain prerequisites should be met. The most important prerequisite appears to be the resolution or significant improvement in the underlying cause of respiratory failure. Patients should be hemodynamically stable, with minimal or no need for vasopressor agents. The absence of sepsis or hyperthermia should be confirmed. Sedative drugs and neuromuscular blocking agents should be discontinued. Patients should be awake, alert, and able to manage secretions and protect their airway. Significant fluid, electrolyte, and metabolic disorders should be corrected prior to weaning attempts. Adequate gas exchange, marked by a PaO_2 to FIO_2 ratio, FIO_2 requirements $\leq$50%, and PEEP $\leq$5 cm H_2O are all desirable. Adequate respiratory muscle strength needs to be ensured (maximum inspiratory pressure [MIP] or negative inspiratory force $\leq$–25 cm H_2O).[2]

Predictors of Weaning Outcome

Over the past years considerable research has been devoted to finding parameters that accurately predict weaning from mechanical ventilation. Although the adequacy of pulmonary gas exchange has to be assessed before initiating weaning, overall gas exchange variables have poor predictive values.[88] Although adequate arterial oxygenation is essential to initiate weaning, it is clear that the predictive value of this index by itself is insufficient to predict weaning outcome.

The strength and endurance of the respiratory system seem to be a major determinant of weaning outcome. Sahn and Lakshminarayan[89] were among the first to describe the use of simple bedside criteria to assist decisions in discontinuing ventilatory support.

In a study involving 100 patients, these investigators measured resting minute ventilation (MV), maximum voluntary ventilation (MVV; i.e., maximum sustainable ventilation over 15 seconds) and MIP with the aid of a spirometer. Seventy-six patients who had an MV <10 L/min, MIP $\leq$–30 cm H_2O, MVV two times their resting MV, and who were able to complete a 2 hour spontaneous breathing trial via an endotracheal tube were successfully extubated. Seven additional patients who had an MIP $\leq$–25 cm H_2O and a mean MV of 10.2 L/min were able to be extubated despite the fact that they were not able to double their resting MV. By contrast, 17 patients who had an MIP >–22 cm H_2O were not able to be extubated.

However, application of these criteria in subsequent studies did not yield comparable results. When evaluating 47 patients on mechanical ventilation, Tahvanainen et al[90] found that using a MIP greater <–30 cm H_2O as a weaning predictor resulted in a false-negative result in 11 out of 11 patients and a false-positive result in eight out of 23 patients.

The observation of the development of rapid, shallow breathing, the presence of asynchronous or paradoxical thoracoabdominal movements, and marked accessory muscle recruitment during a spontaneous breathing trial, heralding an unsuccessful weaning trial, led to studies examining breathing patterns during weaning.

Yang and Tobin[91] combined measurements of frequency (f) and V_T into the rapid shallow breathing index, f/V_T. They obtained data from 36 patients and noticed that an $f:V_T$ ratio of 105 breaths/min/L best differentiated patients who weaned successfully from those who failed. They subsequently validated the index in 64 patients, comparing it against conventional weaning indexes. An $f:V_T < 105$ predicted a successful weaning trial. The positive and negative predictive values were 0.78 and 0.95, respectively. In patients ventilated for less than 2 weeks an $f:V_T < 105$ predicted successful weaning in ~80% of patients.

Epstein[92] attempted to define the etiology of weaning failure in patients whose $f:V_T$ predicted weaning success. It became evident that the initial respiratory process was the cause for extubation failure in only one out of 14 patients with an $f:V_T < 100$, whereas a new problem, such as heart failure and upper airway obstruction, was the most common cause requiring reintubation.[92] This study confirmed the high positive predictive value of the $f:V_T$ index. It also suggested that this index may be less accurate when it does not reflect the underlying pathophysiological cause of respiratory failure (i.e., heart failure) or when the cause is not present at the time of index measurement (i.e., upper airway obstruction due to laryngeal edema).

In a randomized, prospective trial, Ely et al[93] studied 300 consecutive medical and coronary care unit ventilated patients. The intervention group ($n = 149$) underwent daily screening of respiratory function to identify those patients capable of spontaneous breathing. Patients had to satisfy five criteria to be considered for a spontaneous breathing trial (e.g., $PaO_2:FIO_2 < 200$, PEEP <5 cm H_2O, adequate coughing during suctioning, $f:V_T$ ratio <105, and no need for sedative or vasopressor agents). Intervention patients meeting these criteria underwent a 2 hour T-piece spontaneous breathing trial. Physicians were notified if patients successfully completed the trial. Control patients had daily screening but no other interventions. Patients assigned to the intervention group received mechanical ventilation for a median of 4.5 versus 6 days in the control group ($p = 0.003$). The group assigned to the intervention had a significant reduction in the incidence of self-extubation, reintubation, tracheostomy, and mechanical ventilation >21 days. Additionally, ICU costs were significantly reduced in the intervention group. This emphasizes the need for a specific strategy, which allows for daily screening for patients who are ready to wean.

It is important to recognize that successful weaning from ventilatory support does not ensure that a patient will be successfully extubated. Clinical assessment is important in establishing which patients can be safely extubated. Important factors to be considered include the patient's level of consciousness, which should be adequate, allowing for airway protection, the presence of a gag reflex, and the ability to cough and clear the airway. One of the most difficult aspects to evaluate is upper airway patency. The presence of laryngeal edema can lead to respiratory failure, especially in patients with decreased respiratory reserve. Some investigators advocate the use of the cuff leak test, which consists in establishing the presence of an air leak around the endotracheal tube when the cuff is deflated and the tube is occluded. The presence of an air leak is reassuring and relatively sensitive in predicting a positive outcome from extubation, but the specificity of the test is very low.[94] Despite this, it is clear from most studies that around 80% of patients will be extubated after a spontaneous breathing trial. The remaining 20% will require more concentrated weaning efforts, but the majority will eventually be extubated.

Trials of Spontaneous Breathing

Once patients show an improvement or resolution of the underlying cause of respiratory failure and fulfill the previously mentioned criteria, weaning attempts can be initiated. The abrupt discontinuation of mechanical ventilation through a T-tube system is the simplest method of weaning. Patients who have spent relatively short periods on mechanical ventilation (<7 days), or in whom no problems with the resumption of unassisted breathing is expected, can be placed on a spontaneous breathing trial on a T-tube circuit. Traditionally, patients are placed on a T-tube circuit for 2 hours. If they do not develop signs of respiratory distress, such as nasal flaring, tachypnea, abdominal–rib cage paradoxical movements or tachycardia, arrhythmias, oxygen desaturation, or hypo- or hypertension during this time, they are extubated. If signs of intolerance occur, mechanical ventilation is resumed and weaning attempts are restarted in 24 hours. Approximately 75% of the patients who undergo a T-tube weaning trial will be able to be extubated. The 2 hour duration of the spontaneous breathing trial has recently been challenged. In a study that involved more than 500 patients, patients underwent a traditional 120 minute spontaneous breathing trial versus a 30 minute trial.[95] There was no significant difference within groups in the percentage of patients who were extubated, the percentage of patients who remained extubated at 48 hours, and the in-hospital mortality.

In difficult to wean patients, mechanical ventilation is gradually discontinued. Short trials of spontaneous breathing are followed by periods of rest on the ventilator in the assist-control mode. The duration of the trials is slowly increased; once the patient is able to tolerate 2 hours of spontaneous breathing, the weaning process is completed and the patient can be extubated.

Two randomized, controlled studies[96,97] prospectively compared the efficacy of three different weaning techniques: intermittent mandatory ventilation (IMV), pressure support, and spontaneous breathing trials. Brochard et al[96] found that a significantly greater number of patients could be weaned successfully after 21 days with PSV than with the other methods. This group also reported that weaning time was significantly shorter with pressure support (5.7 days) than with spontaneous breathing trials (8.5 days) or IMV (9.9 days). In contrast, Esteban et al[97] found that a once daily trial of spontaneous breathing led to extubation twice as quickly as PSV and about three times more quickly than IMV. There was no difference between a once daily spontaneous breathing trial and intermittent spontaneous breathing trials (attempted at least twice daily). Some of the differences in these studies are the result of different criteria to assess tolerance to weaning and weaning completion. Esteban's group considered extubation if patients tolerated 5 cm H_2O of pressure support for 2 hours versus 8 cm H_2O in Brochard et al's study. During application of IMV, Esteban et al extubated patients once they were able to tolerate a backup rate of 5 breaths per minute for two hours; in contrast, Brochard's group criteria required patients to tolerate 24 hours at a rate of 4 breaths per minute (a significant ventilatory challenge).

Both studies were similar in concluding that SIMV was less efficient in weaning patients, but differed as to whether PS or T-piece was the superior weaning method. Overall, either PS or T-piece weaning techniques can be successful if patients are properly selected, and either method is appropriately implemented.

A flow diagram incorporating previously discussed approaches to weaning in a stepwise fashion is shown in **Fig. 16.7**.

Prolonged Mechanical Ventilation

Patients likely to be extubated within 2 weeks from the time of intubation can be managed with an endotracheal tube. However, significant patient discomfort, facial injuries that would complicate reintubation, or upper airway edema/obstruction that would complicate reintubation may necessitate early tracheotomy in these patients. Any patient who fails to improve within 1 week or who is expected to need artificial airway management beyond 2 weeks is likely to benefit from a tracheostomy.[98] In a retrospective study, placement of a tracheostomy after >21 days of intubation was associated with a higher rate of failure to wean from mechanical ventilation, longer ICU stay, and higher ICU mortality.[99]

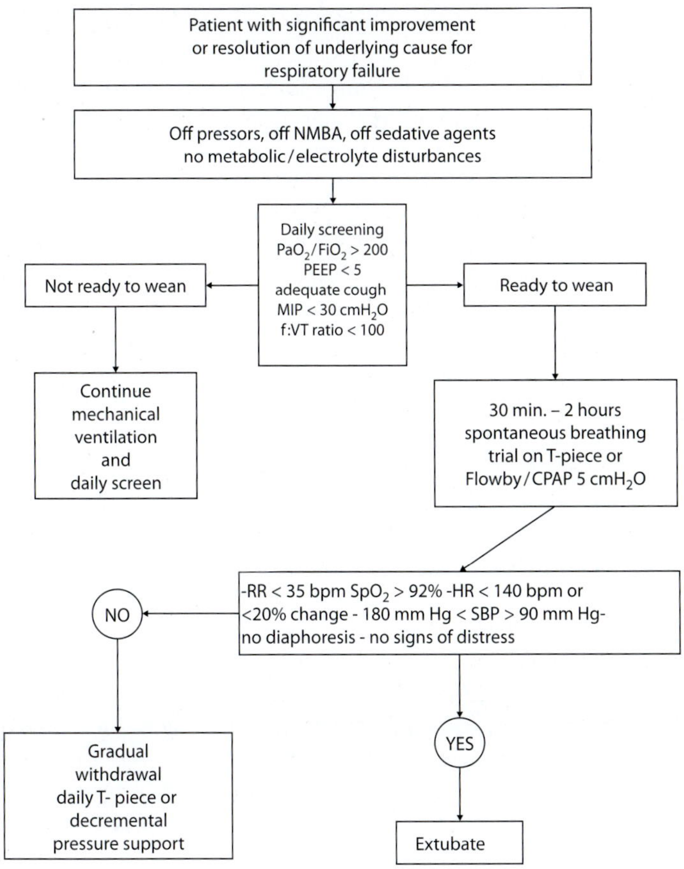

Fig. 16.7 An approach to the evaluation and techniques of weaning in patients receiving mechanical ventilation. CPAP, continuous positive airway pressure; MIP, maximum inspiratory pressure; PEEP, positive end-expiratory pressure.

In patients with an evolving illness such as myasthenic crisis or Guillain-Barré syndrome, it is prudent to wait 14 days before placement of a tracheotomy. This gives the patient time to respond to immunotherapy or to spontaneously recover. About one-third of patients may no longer need intubation and mechanical ventilation after 2 weeks.

Lessons from the Respiratory and the Surgical Intensive Care Unit

A variety of nonpulmonary treatments have been recently recognized as important in improving patient outcome in the ICU (**Table 16.8**).

Blood Transfusions

A landmark prospective randomized trial comparing liberal and conservative "triggers" to transfusion in ICU patients not exhibiting active bleeding and without underlying cardiac disease demonstrated that awaiting a hemoglobin level of 7.0 g/dL as opposed to a level of 9.0 g/dL before initiating transfusion resulted in less transfusion and no adverse effects on outcome.[100] In fact, in those patients who were less severely ill, as judged by low APACHE II (Acute Physiology and Chronic Health Evaluation II) scores, mortality was improved in the "restricted transfusion" group, which was thought to result from immunosuppressive effects of non–leukocyte-depleted red blood cell units with consequent increased risk for infection. Multiple studies have identified exposure to allogeneic blood products as a risk factor for postoperative infection and postoperative pneumonia, and the length of time of blood storage as another factor modulating risk.[101–105] In one prospective, randomized, controled trial the use of leukocyte-depleted red blood cell transfusions resulted in a reduced incidence of postoperative infections, and specifically a reduced incidence of pneumonia in patients undergoing colorectal surgery.[103] Routine red blood cell transfusion should be conducted with a restricted transfusion trigger policy. Whether leukocyte-depleted red blood cell transfusions will further reduce the incidence of pneumonia in broad populations of patients at risk remains to be determined.

Table 16.8 Other Important Management Issues in Pulmonary/Critical Care

Blood transfusions
• Transfusion threshold
• Transfusion related acute lung injury (TRALI)
Hyperglycemia
• Effects of hyperglycemia on infection treatment
• Benefits of rigorous glycemic control with insulin protocols
Sedation management
• Benefits of daily interruption of continuous sedation
Advances in sepsis treatment
• Goal-directed therapy for resuscitation
• Recombinant activated protein C

Insulin Therapy

Van den Berghe et al[106] randomly assigned 1,548 patients admitted to a surgical ICU to receive either intensive intravenous (IV) insulin therapy to keep the blood glucose level between 80 and 110 mg/dL or conventional care, with IV insulin only if the blood glucose level rose above 215 mg/dL and a goal range of 180 to 200 mg/dL. Intensive insulin therapy reduced mortality. The mortality rate in the ICU was 4.6% with intensive insulin therapy versus 8.0% with conventional therapy ($p < 0.04$). In patients who remained in the ICU for more than 5 days, the mortality rate was 10.6% with intensive therapy versus 20.2% with conventional therapy ($p = 0.005$). Intensive insulin therapy also reduced in-hospital mortality. Furthermore, the patients treated with the intensive insulin regimen had fewer episodes of sepsis, shorter length of stay in the ICU, less need for prolonged mechanical ventilation and renal replacement therapy, and a lower incidence of polyneuropathy, a common complication in ICU patients. In a follow-up study[107] in medical ICUs, 1,200 patients who were expected to have a stay of at least 3 days were randomized with concealed allocation to intensive insulin treatment (target blood glucose 80–110 mg/dL) or conventional insulin treatment (target blood glucose 180–200 mg/dL) using an insulin pump. Although the intention was to enroll only patients who would be in the ICU for 3 days or more, only 767 of the 1,200 patients actually stayed that long. There was no difference in in-hospital mortality rates between the two treatment groups as a whole, but there were morbidity benefits: less new renal injury (5.9% vs. 8.9%), earlier weaning from mechanical ventilation, and earlier discharge from the ICU and hospital. In the subgroup of 767 patients who actually spent at least 3 days in the ICU, the in-hospital death rate was lower in the intensive treatment group (43% vs. 52.5%; $p = 0.009$; number needed to treat = 10). On the other hand, among patients staying in the ICU fewer than 3 days, there were more deaths in the intensive treatment group (26.8% vs. 18.7%; $p = 0.05$) Morbidity was also reduced by intensive treatment in the group staying in the ICU fewer than 3 days.

Daily Cessation of Sedation

Kress et al[59] performed a randomized, controlled trial in patients receiving mechanical ventilation in one medical ICU. Sixty patients were enrolled in the control group and 68 in the intervention group. In the intervention group, an investigator interrupted the sedative infusion every day and waited until the patient either woke up and could follow instructions or became uncomfortable or agitated, in which case the infusion was resumed. If the sedative was resumed, half of the previous dose was given and adjusted according to need. The control group had the sedation interrupted only at the discretion of the medical ICU team. Patients in the intervention group had a shorter duration of mechanical ventilation (4.9 days vs. 7.3 days, $p = 0.004$) and a shorter median length of stay in the ICU (6.4 days vs. 9.9 days, $p = 0.02$). They also required less diagnostic testing to assess mental status.

Advances in Sepsis

Perhaps one of the most important aspects of the management of sepsis is the early initiation of aggressive comprehensive treatment. In a study by Rivers et al early goal-directed therapy guided by a modified triple lumen catheter and aiming at improving cardiac output, hemoglobin, and volume status resulted in a reduction in mortality (30.5% in the early goal treatment group vs. 46.5% in the standard therapy group, $p = 0.009$). The Recombinant Human Activated Protein C Worldwide Evaluation in Severe Sepsis (PROWESS) study,[108] a multicenter randomized, controlled trial, showed that the administration of r-APC (also known as drotrecogin alfa [activated] or Xigris [Eli Lilly & Co.]) reduced mortality from severe sepsis or septic shock by 6% compared with placebo.[108,109] Subgroup analyses suggested that survival with r-APC was improved in patients whose APACHE II scores were 25 or greater and who also had dysfunction of two or more organs. Receiving r-APC was also associated with a trend toward an increased risk of bleeding (3.5% vs. 2.0%, $p = 0.06$). In the PROWESS trial, r-APC was started within 24 hours after the criteria for severe sepsis were met.

A second large, randomized, controlled trial[110] that compared the efficacy of r-APC with that of placebo in patients with less severe sepsis (defined as zero or one organ dysfunction) was terminated early, when there appeared to be no mortality benefit for this patient population. This study did not address the timing of administration. Future research efforts exploring the optimal timing for administration of r-APC and other anticoagulants will help determine its role in the earlier stages of severe sepsis and septic shock.

References

1. Ropper AH. The development of the neurologic intensive care unit. Cleve Clin J Med 2004;71:S4–S5
2. Piatt C, Martin UJ, Criner GJ. Mechanical ventilation. In: Criner GJ, ed., D'Alonzo GA, assoc. ed. Critical Care Study Guide. New York: Springer-Verlag; 2002
3. Tobin
4. Adnet F, Baud F. Relation between Glasgow Coma Scale and aspiration pneumonia. Lancet 1996;348:123–124
5. Rossanda M, Vecchi G. Determination of cerebral autoregulatory status and PCO_2 responsiveness. Int Anesthesiol Clin 1979;17:425–438
6. Miller JD, Stanek A, Langfitt TW. Concepts of cerebral perfusion pressure and vascular compression during intracranial hypertension. Prog Brain Res 1972;35:411–432
7. Huseby JS, Luce JM, Cary JM, Pavlin EG, Butler J. Effects of positive end-expiratory pressure on intracranial pressure in dogs with intracranial hypertension. J Neurosurg 1981;55:704–707
8. Muench E, Bauhuf C, Roth H, et al. Effects of positive end-expiratory pressure on regional cerebral blood flow, intracranial pressure, and brain tissue oxygenation. Crit Care Med 2005;33:2367–2372
9. McGuire G, Crossley D, Richards J, Wong D. Effects of varying levels positive end-expiratory pressure on intracranial pressure and cerebral perfusion pressure. Crit Care Med 1997;25:1059–1062
10. Vincent JL, Fink MP, Marini JJ, et al. Intensive care and emergency medicine: progress over the past 25 years. Chest 2006;129:1061–1067
11. Kontos HA, Raper AJ, Patterson JL Jr. Analysis of vasoactivity of local pH, CO_2, and bicarbonate on pial vessels. Stroke 1977;8:358–360
12. Oertel M, Kelly DF, Lee JH, et al. Efficacy of hyperventilation, blood pressure elevation, and metabolic suppression therapy in controlling intracranial pressure after head injury. J Neurosurg 2002;97:1045–1053
13. Dharker SR, Bhargava N. Bilateral epidural haematoma. Acta Neurochir (Wien) 1991;110:29–32
14. Kety SS, Schmidt CF. The nitrous oxide method for the quantitative determination of cerebral blood flow in man: theory, procedure, and normal values. J Clin Invest 1948;27:476–483
15. Wollman H, Smith TC, Stephen GW, Colton ET III, Gleaton HE, Alexander SC. Effects of extremes of respiratory and metabolic alkalosis on cerebral blood flow in man. J Appl Physiol 1968;24:60–65
16. Alexander SC, Smith TC, Strobel G, Stephen GW, Wollman H. Cerebral carbohydrate metabolism of man during respiratory and metabolic alkalosis. J Appl Physiol 1968;24:66–72
17. Coles JP, Minhas PS, Fryer TD, et al. Effect of hyperventilation on cerebral blood flow in traumatic head injury: clinical relevance and monitoring correlates. Crit Care Med 2002;30:1950–1959
18. Diringer MN, Videen TO, Yundt K, et al. Regional cerebrovascular and metabolic effects of hyperventilation after severe traumatic brain injury. J Neurosurg 2002;96:103–108
19. Muizelaar JP, Marmarou A, Ward JD, et al. Adverse effects of prolonged hyperventilation in patients with severe head injury: a randomized clinical trial. J Neurosurg 1991;75:731–739
20. Forbes ML, Clark RS, Dixon CE, et al. Augmented neuronal death in CA3 hippocampus following hyperventilation early after controlled cortical impact. J Neurosurg 1998;88:549–556
21. Amato MB, Barbas CS, Medeiros DM, et al. Effect of a protective-ventilation strategy on mortality in the acute respiratory distress syndrome. N Engl J Med 1998;338:347–354
22. Brochard L, Roudot-Thoraval F. The Collaborative Group on VT Reduction. Tidal volume (VT) reduction in acute respiratory distress syndrome (ARDS): a multicenter randomized study [abstract]. Am J Respir Crit Care Med 1997;155:A505

23. Stewart TEM, Meade O, Granton J, et al. Pressure and volume limited ventilation strategy (PLVS) in patients at high risk for ARDS: results of a multicenter trial. N Engl J Med 1998;338(6):355–361
24. The Acute Respiratory Distress Syndrome Network. Ventilation with lower tidal volumes as compared with traditional tidal volumes for acute lung injury and the acute respiratory distress syndrome. N Engl J Med 2000;342:1301–1308
25. Pepe PE, Marini JJ. Occult positive end-expiratory pressure in mechanically ventilated patients with airflow obstruction. Am Rev Respir Dis 1982;126:166–170
26. Appendini L, Patessio A, Zanaboni S, et al. Physiologic effects of positive end-expiratory pressure and mask pressure support during exacerbations of chronic obstructive pulmonary disease. Am J Respir Crit Care Med 1994;149:1069–1076
27. Ranieri VM, Guiliani R, Cinnella G, et al. Physiologic effects of positive end-expiratory pressure in patients with chronic obstructive pulmonary disease during acute ventilatory failure and controlled mechanical ventilation. Am Rev Respir Dis 1993;147:5–13
28. Jubran A. Monitoring mechanics during mechanical ventilation. Semin Respir Crit Care Med 1999;20:65–79
29. Esteban A, Alía A, Gordo F, et al. Prospective randomized trial comparing pressure-controlled ventilation and volume-controlled ventilation in ARDS. Chest 2000;117:1690–1696
30. Pelosi P, Cadringher P, Bottino N. Sigh in respiratory distress syndrome. Am J Respir Crit Care Med 1999;159:872–880
31. Hubmayr RD. Ventilator induced injury without biotrauma? J Appl Physiol 2005;99:384–385
32. Solenski NJ, Haley EC, Kassel NF, et al. Medical complications of aneurysmal subarachnoid hemorrhage: a report of the multicenter, cooperative aneurysm study. Crit Care Med 1995;23:1007–1017
33. Smith WS, Matthay MA. Evidence for a hydrostatic mechanism in human pulmonary edema. Chest 1997;111:1326–1333
34. Parr MJA, Finfer SR, Morgan MK. Lesson of the week: reversible cardiogenic shock complicating subarachnoid haemorrhage. BMJ 1996;313:681–683
35. Touho H, Karasawa J, Shishido H, Yamada K, Yamazaki Y. Neurogenic pulmonary edema in the acute stage of hemorrhagic cerebrovascular disease. Neurosurgery 1989;25:762–768
36. Maron MB, Holcomb PH, Dawson CA, Rickaby DA, Clough AV, Linehan JH. Edema development and recovery in neurogenic pulmonary oedema. J Appl Physiol 1994;77:1155–1163
37. Wray NP, Nicotra MB. Pathogenesis of neurogenic pulmonary edema. Am Rev Respir Dis 1978;118:783–786
38. West JB, Mathieu-Costello O. Stress failure of pulmonary capillaries: role in lung and heart disease. Lancet 1992;340:762–767
39. Kahn JM, Caldwell EC, Deem S, Newell DW, Heckbert SR, Rubenfeld GD. Acute lung injury in patients with subarachnoid hemorrhage: incidence, risk factors, and outcome. Crit Care Med 2006;34:196–202
40. Treggiari MM, Walder B, Suter PM, Romand JA. Systematic review of the prevention of delayed ischemic neurological deficits with hypertension, hypervolemia, and hemodilution therapy following subarachnoid hemorrhage. J Neurosurg 2003;98(5):978–984
41. Brower RG, Lanken PN, MacIntyre NR, et al. Higher versus lower positive end-expiratory pressures in patients with the acute respiratory distress syndrome. N Engl J Med 2004;351:327–336
42. National Heart Lung and Blood Institute Acute Respiratory Distress Syndrome (ARDS) Clinical Trials Network; Wiedemann HP, Wheeler AP, Bernard GR, et al. Comparison of two fluid-management strategies in acute lung injury. N Engl J Med 2006;354(24):2564–2575
43. Tablan OC, Anderson LJ, Besser R, Bridges C, Hajjeh R, Healthcare Infection Control Practices Advisory Committee, Centers for Disease Control and Prevention. Guidelines for preventing health-care–associated pneumonia, 2003: recommendations of the CDC and the Healthcare Infection Control Practices Advisory Committee. MMWR Recomm Rep 2004;53(RR-3):1–36
44. Chastre J, Fagon JY. Ventilator-associated pneumonia. Am J Respir Crit Care Med 2002;165:867–903
45. Fagon JY, Chastre J, Hance AJ, Montravers P, Novara A, Gibert C. Nosocomial pneumonia in ventilated patients: a cohort study evaluating attributable mortality and hospital stay. Am J Med 1993;94:281–288
46. Rello J, Ollendorf DA, Oster G, et al. Epidemiology and outcomes of ventilator-associated pneumonia in a large US database. Chest 2002;122:2115–2121
47. Celis R, Torres A, Gatell JM, Almela M, Rodriguez-Roisin R, Agusti-Vidal A. Nosocomial pneumonia: a multivariate analysis of risk and prognosis. Chest 1988;93:318–324
48. Bonten MJ, Bergmans DC, Stobberingh EE, et al. Implementation of bronchoscopic techniques in the diagnosis of ventilator-associated pneumonia to reduce antibiotic use. Am J Respir Crit Care Med 1997;156:1820–1824
49. Richards MJ, Edwards JR, Culver DH, Gaynes RP. Nosocomial infections in medical ICUs in the United States: National Nosocomial Infections Surveillance System. Crit Care Med 1999;27:887–892
50. Torres A, Aznar R, Gatell JM, et al. Incidence, risk, and prognosis factors of nosocomial pneumonia in mechanically ventilated patients. Am Rev Respir Dis 1990;142:523–528
51. Cook DJ, Walter SD, Cook RJ, et al. Incidence of and risk factors for ventilator-associated pneumonia in critically ill patients. Ann Intern Med 1998;129:433–440
52. Trouillet JL, Chastre J, Vuagnat A, et al. Ventilator-associated pneumonia caused by potentially drug-resistant bacteria. Am J Respir Crit Care Med 1998;157:531–539
53. Rello J, Ausina V, Ricart M, Castella J, Prats G. Impact of previous antimicrobial therapy on the etiology and outcome of ventilatorassociated pneumonia. Chest 1993;104:1230–1235
54. Heyland DK, Cook DJ, Griffith L, Keenan SP, Brun-Buisson C, Canadian Critical Trials Group. The attributable morbidity and mortality of ventilator-associated pneumonia in the critically ill patient. Am J Respir Crit Care Med 1999;159:1249–1256
55. Nava S, Ambrosino N, Clini E, et al. Noninvasive mechanical ventilation in the weaning of patients with respiratory failure due to chronic obstructive pulmonary disease: a randomized, controlled trial. Ann Intern Med 1998;128:721–728
56. Carlucci A, Richard JC, Wysocki M, Lepage E, Brochard L. Noninvasive versus conventional mechanical ventilation: an epidemiologic survey. Am J Respir Crit Care Med 2001;163:874–880
57. Nourdine K, Combes P, Carton MJ, Beuret P, Cannamela A, Ducreux JC. Does noninvasive ventilation reduce the ICU nosocomial infection risk? A prospective clinical survey. Intensive Care Med 1999;25:567–573
58. Keenan SP. Noninvasive positive pressure ventilation in acute respiratory failure. JAMA 2000;284:2376–2378
59. Kress JP, Pohlman AS, O'Connor MF, Hall JB. Daily interruption of sedative infusions in critically ill patients undergoing mechanical ventilation. N Engl J Med 2000;342:1471–1477
60. Marelich GP, Murin S, Battistella F, Inciardi J, Vierra T, Roby M. Protocol weaning of mechanical ventilation in medical and surgical patients by respiratory care practitioners and nurses: effect on weaning time and incidence of ventilator-associated pneumonia. Chest 2000;118:459–467
61. Needleman J, Buerhaus P, Mattke S, Stewart M, Zelevinsky K. Nursestaffing levels and the quality of care in hospitals. N Engl J Med 2002;346:1715–1722
62. Thorens JB, Kaelin RM, Jolliet P, Chevrolet JC. Influence of the quality of nursing on the duration of weaning from mechanical ventilation in patients with chronic obstructive pulmonary disease. Crit Care Med 1995;23:1807–1815
63. Brook AD, Ahrens TS, Schaiff R, et al. Effect of a nursing-implemented sedation protocol on the duration of mechanical ventilation. Crit Care Med 1999;27:2609–2615

64. Mahul P, Auboyer C, Jospe R, et al. Prevention of nosocomial pneumonia in intubated patients: respective role of mechanical subglottic secretions drainage and stress ulcer prophylaxis. Intensive Care Med 1992;18:20–25
65. Pneumatikos I, Koulouras V, Nathanail C, Goe D, Nakos G. Selective decontamination of subglottic area in mechanically ventilated patients with multiple trauma. Intensive Care Med 2002;28: 432–437
66. Kollef MH, Skubas NJ, Sundt TM. A randomized clinical trial of continuous aspiration of subglottic secretions in cardiac surgery patients. Chest 1999;116:1339–1346
67. Torres A, Serra-Batlles J, Ros E, et al. Pulmonary aspiration of gastric contents in patients receiving mechanical ventilation: the effect of body position. Ann Intern Med 1992;116:540–543
68. Orozco-Levi M, Torres A, Ferrer M, et al. Semirecumbent position protects from pulmonary aspiration but not completely from gastroesophageal reflux in mechanically ventilated patients. Am J Respir Crit Care Med 1995;152:1387–1390
69. Davis K Jr, Johannigman JA, Campbell RS, et al. The acute effects of body position strategies and respiratory therapy in paralyzed patients with acute lung injury. Crit Care 2001;5(2):81–87
70. Drakulovic MB, Torres A, Bauer TT, Nicolas JM, Nogue S, Ferrer M. Supine body position as a risk factor for nosocomial pneumonia in mechanically ventilated patients: a randomised trial. Lancet 1999; 354:1851–1858
71. American Thoracic Society. Guidelines for the management of adults with hopital-acquired, ventilator-associated, and healthcare-associated pneumonia. Am J Respir Crit Care Med 2005;171:388–416
72. Fabregas N, Ewig S, Torres A, et al. Clinical diagnosis of ventilator associated pneumonia revisited: comparative validation using immediate postmortem lung biopsies. Thorax 1999;54:867–873
73. Kollef MH, Sherman G, Ward S, Fraser VJ. Inadequate antimicrobial treatment of infections: a risk factor for hospital mortality among critically ill patients. Chest 1999;115:462–474
74. Iregui M, Ward S, Sherman G, Fraser VJ, Kollef MH. Clinical importance of delays in the initiation of appropriate antibiotic treatment for ventilator-associated pneumonia. Chest 2002;122: 262–268
75. Ibrahim EH, Sherman G, Ward S, Fraser VJ, Kollef MH. The influence of inadequate antimicrobial treatment of bloodstream infections on patient outcomes in the ICU setting. Chest 2000;118: 146–155
76. Chastre J, Wolff M, Fagon JY, et al. Comparison of 8 vs 15 days of antibiotic therapy for ventilator-associated pneumonia in adults: a randomized trial. JAMA 2003;290:2588–2598
77. Macklin MT, Macklin CC. Malignant interstitial emphysema of the lungs and mediastinum as an important occult complication in many respiratory diseases and other conditions: an interpretation of the clinical literature in the light of laboratory experiment. Medicine 1944;23:281–358
78. Vlahakis NE, Hubmayr RD. Cellular stress failure in ventilator injured lungs. Am J Respir Crit Care Med 2005(171):1328–1342. Published ahead of print February 1, 2005 doi:10.1164/rccm.200408-1036SO
79. Muscedere JG, Mullen JB, Gan K, Slutsky AS. Tidal ventilation at low airway pressures can augment lung injury. Am J Respir Crit Care Med 1994;149:1327–1334
80. Veldhuizen RA, Welk B, Harbottle R, et al. Mechanical ventilation of isolated rat lungs changes the structure and biophysical properties of surfactant. J Appl Physiol 2002;92:1169–1175
81. Mead J, Takishima T, Leith D. Stress distribution in lungs: a model of pulmonary elasticity. J Appl Physiol 1970;28:596–608
82. Weg JG, Anzueto A, Balk RA, et al. The relation of pneumothorax and other air leaks to mortality in the acute respiratory distress syndrome. N Engl J Med 1998;338:341–346
83. Krachman SL, Martin UJ, D'Alonzo GE. Weaning from mechanical ventilation: an update. J Am Osteopath Assoc 2001;101:387–390
84. Esteban A, Anzueto A, Alia I, et al. How is mechanical ventilation employed in the intensive care unit? An international utilization review. Am J Respir Crit Care Med 2000;161:1450–1458
85. Katz MG, Katz R, Schachner A, et al. Phrenic nerve injury after coronary artery bypass grafting. Ann Thorac Surg 1998;65:32–35
86. Radell PJ, Remahl S, Nichols DG, Eriksson L. Effects of prolonged mechanical ventilation and inactivity on piglet diaphragm function. Intensive Care Med 2002;28:358–364
87. Anzueto A, Peters JI, Tobin MJ, et al. Effects of prolonged controlled mechanical ventilation on diaphragmatic function in healthy adult baboons. Crit Care Med 1997;25:1187–1190
88. Lessard MR, Brochard L. Weaning from ventilatory support. Clin Chest Med 1996;17(3):475–490
89. Sahn SA, Lakshminarayan S. Bedside criteria for discontinuation of mechanical ventilation. Chest 1973;63:1002–1005
90. Tahvanainen J, Salmenperä M, Nikki P. Extubation criteria after weaning from intermittent mandatory ventilation and continuous positive airway pressure. Crit Care Med 1983;11:702–707
91. Yang KL, Tobin MJ. A prospective study of indexes predicting the outcome of trials of weaning from mechanical ventilation. N Engl J Med 1991;324(21):1445–1450
92. Epstein SK. Etiology of extubation failure and the predictive value of the rapid shallow breathing index. Am J Respir Crit Care Med 1995; 152:545–549
93. Ely EW, Baker AM, Dunagan DP. Effect of duration of mechanical ventilation of identifying patients capable of breathing spontaneously. N Engl J Med 1996;335:1864–1869
94. Fisher MM, Raper RF. The "cuff leak" test for extubation. Anaesthesia 1992;47:10–12
95. Esteban A, Alia I, Tobin MJ. The effect of spontaneous breathing trial duration on outcome of attempts to discontinue mechanical ventilation. Am J Respir Crit Care Med 1999;159:512–518
96. Brochard L, Rauss A, Benito S, et al. Comparison of three methods of gradual withdrawal from ventilatory support during weaning from mechanical ventilation. Am J Respir Crit Care Med 1994;150: 896–903
97. Esteban A, Frutos F, Tobin M, et al. A comparison of four methods of weaning patients from mechanical ventilation. N Engl J Med 1995; 332:345–350
98. Heffner JE. The role of tracheotomy in weaning. Chest 2001;120: 477S–481S
99. Hsu C, Chen K, Chang C. Timing of tracheostomy as a determinant of weaning success in critically ill patients: a retrospective study. Crit Care 2005;9(1):R46–R52
100. Hebert PC, Wells G, Blajchman MA, et al, Transfusion Requirements in Critical Care Investigators, Canadian Critical Care Trials Group. A multicenter, randomized, controlled clinical trial of transfusion requirements in critical care. N Engl J Med 1999;340: 409–417
101. Vamvakas EC, Carven JH. Exposure to allogeneic plasma and risk of postoperative pneumonia and/or wound infection in coronary artery bypass graft surgery. Transfusion 2002;42:107–113
102. Vamvakas EC, Craven JH. Transfusions and postoperative pneumonia in coronary artery bypass graft surgery: effect of the length of storage of transfused red cells. Transfusion 1999;39: 701–710
103. Jensen LS, Kissmeyer-Nielsen P, Wolff B, Qvist N. Randomised comparison of leukocyte depleted versus buffy-coat-poor blood transfusion and complications after colorectal surgery. Lancet 1996;348: 841–845
104. Leal-Noval SR, Marquez-Vacaro JA, Garcia-Curiel A, et al. Nosocomial pneumonia in patients undergoing heart surgery. Crit Care Med 2000;28:935–940
105. Leal-Noval SR, Rincon-Ferrari MD, Garcia-Curiel A, et al. Transfusión of blood components and postoperative infection in patients undergoing cardiac surgery. Chest 2001;119:1461–1468

106. Van den Berghe G, Wouters P, Weekers F, et al. Intensive insulin therapy in the critically ill patients. N Engl J Med 2001;345:1359–1367
107. Van den Berghe G, Wilmer A, Hermans G, et al. Intensive insulin therapy in the medical ICU. N Engl J Med 2006;354:449–461
108. Bernard GR, Vincent JL, Laterre PF, et al. Efficacy and safety of recombinant human activated protein C for severe sepsis. N Engl J Med 2001;344:699–709
109. Bernard GR, Ely EW, Wright TJ, et al. Safety and dose relationship of recombinant human activated protein C for coagulopathy in severe sepsis. Crit Care Med 2001;29:2051–2059
110. Abraham E, Laterre PF, Garg R, et al Administration of drotrecogin alfa. (Activated) in Early Stage Severe Sepsis (ADDRESS) Study Group. Drotrecogin alfa (activated) for adults with severe sepsis and a low risk of death. N Engl J Med 2005;353(13):1332–1341

17 Cardiovascular Critical Care

Mustapha A. Ezzeddine and Adnan I. Qureshi

The relationship between the traumatized brain and the cardiovascular system is complex and multifaceted. Brain trauma can lead to cardiac injury, hypertension, hypotension, and autonomic instability. Initial blood pressure (BP) is an important prognostic indicator in traumatic brain injury (TBI). Subsequent BP management, linked to cerebral perfusion pressure (CPP) management, is a cornerstone of intensive care therapy and may play an important role in controlling secondary brain injury.

Systemic Blood Pressure in TBI

Patients presenting with isolated TBI often present acutely hypertensive. A catecholamine surge occurs as a stress response to the brain trauma, similar to that seen with other types of acute brain injury such as aneurysmal subarachnoid hemorrhage[1] and stroke[2] (**Table 17.1**).

It has long been known than increased intracranial pressure (ICP) can trigger a sympathetically mediated compensatory response, the so-called Cushing's response.[3] This is a hemostatic reflex preserving CPP. It can be abolished by a surgical or pharmacological sympathectomy.[4]

Later work demonstrated that brain trauma alone, without any rise in ICP, also leads to a massive release of epinephrine and norepinephrine in the systemic circulation.[5]

Similar findings were noted in clinical studies, again showing an increase in circulating catecholamines, with concomitant increase in BP.[1,6,7]

Table 17.1 Systemic Blood Pressure in TBI

- Patients with isolated traumatic brain injury (TBI) are acutely hypertensive
- Brain trauma induces a catecholamine surge
- Hypotension and hypoxia are also common with brain injuries; early hypotension appearing more injurious
- Isolated brain injury without any complicating systemic factors can lead to hypotension
- Hypotension might also be mediated by a relative adrenal insufficiency

Hypotension is also common on presentation with TBI. It is often associated with hypoxia and is an independent predictor of poor outcome. In a study from the Traumatic Coma Data Bank involving 717 patients with severe head injury, ~35% suffered from hypotension, which was linked to a 150% increase in mortality.[8] In the pediatric population, BP lower than the 75th percentile of age-appropriate systolic BP was associated with worse outcome in severe TBI, even if systolic blood pressure (SBP) was >90 mm Hg.[9]

Early hypotension appears to be more injurious. Comparing the location of hypotension (field, emergency department, and intensive care unit), Coates at al showed that early hypotension,was a better predictor of poor outcome than delayed hypotension or the use of SBP <90 mm Hg.[10]

Several factors are thought to lead to hypotension in TBI. These include concomitant systemic trauma, acute blood loss, hypoxia, cardiac contusion, myocardial stunning, and endocrine dysfunction.

Isolated brain injury without any complicating systemic factors can lead to hypotension. In one study[11] of a single center, consecutive series of 231 hypotensive blunt trauma patients, hypotension was associated with brain injury alone in 30% of the cases. Other studies have shown similar results.[12]

The frequency appears to be much higher in the pediatric population,[13] with isolated head injury accounting for up to 43% of hypotension in pediatric trauma. Animal studies further support these findings, showing that concomitant TBI in a pig model blunts the cardiovascular response to hemorrhagic shock and can lead to hypotension without any blood loss.[14]

Some reports suggest that hypotension might also be mediated by a relative adrenal insufficiency. In one study, 80 patients with severe TBI underwent serial serum cortisol and adrenocorticotropic hormone measurement.[15] Adrenal insufficiency was detected in about half of the subjects. It occurred more frequently in younger patients, more severe injury, and early ischemic insult. It was also associated with the use of etomidate, propofol, and pentobarbital. Another study involving 29 severe TBI cases requiring vasopressor therapy used a high-dose corticotropin stimulation test to identify adrenal insufficiency.[16] Forty-eight percent of the patients had a hemodynamic response to hydrocortisone replacement therapy. The issue

Table 17.2 Factors That Lead to Hypotension in TBI

- Concomitant systemic trauma
- Acute blood loss

Hypoxia

- Cardiac contusion
- Myocardial stunning
- Endocrine dysfunction
- Blood loss
- Cardiac contusion
- Stunned myocardium

Table 17.3 Brain Injuries and Systemic Blood Pressure

- Patients with ischemic stroke are often hypertensive on admission.
- Increasing levels of acute hypertension have been shown to adversely impact outcomes following cerebrovascular events.
- In ischemic stroke, hypertension control is beneficial in the long term, but might be harmful in the acute phase.
- Hypertension on presentation with ICH may cause hematoma expansion,[33,34] a common occurrence in the first 24 hours after the initial hemorrhage, which is associated with neurological deterioration and poor outcome.[35,36]

Abbreviations: ICH, intracranial hemorrhage.

of steroids replacement in this patient population is further complicated by the results of the CRASH (corticosteroid randomization after significant head injury) Trial, a large randomized controlled trial of placebo versus intravenous (IV) methylprenisolone in the first 48 hours of brain trauma,[17] that showed a slight increase in mortality in patients randomized to steroids (**Table 17.2**).

Lessons from Management of Systemic Blood Pressure in Other Brain Injuries

The mechanisms of brain injury in TBI are complex and include some of the same pathophysiology as acute ischemic stroke, primary intracerebral hemorrhage, and aneurysmal subarachnoid hemorrhage. Thus, BP management strategies in these diseases are of relevance for the traumatized brain.

Patients with ischemic stroke are often hypertensive on admission, with ~80% of patients presenting to an emergency department for signs and symptoms of acute stroke having elevated BP at admission.[2] There is subsequent gradual decline, most prominently in the first 24 to 48 hours following onset. The rate of decline is correlated to the initial stroke severity and ischemic stroke subtypes.[18,19] Elevated cortisol levels in plasma and saliva have been linked to the acute elevation of BP in acute stroke, indicating a stress response.[20] (**Table 17.3**).

The presence and increasing levels of acute hypertension have also been shown to adversely impact outcomes following cerebrovascular events. Recent data from the European Cooperative Acute Stroke Study (ECASS) (a randomized controlled clinical trial comparing fibrinolytic therapy with tissue plasminogen activator with placebo in 620 patients) examined how BP changes, shortly after stroke, influence long-term outcomes.[21] Elevated BP during the first 72 hours after stroke was associated with lower rates of favorable clinical outcomes at 90 days. Reduced variability of BP during 72 hours after hospitalization demonstrated a similar correlation. Other studies have further confirmed the negative impact of BP variability in the acute period on outcome, possibly a reflection of autonomic dysfunction.[22]

The relationship between BP and acute stroke mortality does not appear to be linear, but rather U-shaped. Two large prospective studies have demonstrated increased mortality with lower BP levels (in normotensive or hypotensive ranges).[23,24]

Hypertension at the time of presentation is also a significant risk factor for hemorrhagic transformation[25–27] and may also increase the conversion of hypoperfused regions to frank infarction.[28]

In ischemic stroke, hypertension control, although clearly beneficial in the long term, might be harmful in the acute phase. In a prospective case series of 115 acute stroke patients, SBP reduction was independently associated with a worse clinical outcome.[29] Similar association between diastolic BP reduction was noted among patients with partial anterior circulation infarction in an analysis of the Intravenous Nimodipine West European Stroke Trial (INWEST), an acute stroke trial using an intravenous calcium channel blocker.[30]

Hypertension on presentation with intracranial hemorrhage (ICH) is common[31] and is associated with poor outcome.[32] It is suspected to contribute to hematoma expansion,[33,34] a common occurrence in the first 24 hours after the initial hemorrhage, which is associated with neurological deterioration and poor outcome.[35,36]

It remains unclear whether acute hypertension is a cause of hematoma enlargement or a manifestation of worsening of the initial injury. In the acute phase, as with ischemic stroke, the optimal treatment of hypertension in patients with ICH is not well defined.[33] Elevated BP may promote hematoma expansion; however, lowering BP may worsen perihematoma tissue ischemia.[37] Conflicting data exist regarding the presence of perihematoma ischemia. Some

Table 17.4 Changes in Regional Cerebral Blood Flow and Metabolism following ICH

First stage	Hibernation stage, which comprises hypoperfusion and hypometabolism in the perihematoma region. There is a coupling of metabolism and flow; therefore there is no ischemia. This stage lasts for ~2 days,
Second stage	Exists between 2 and 14 days. Stage of reperfusion, which consists of patchy areas of normal or hyperperfusion in the perihematoma region.
Third stage	The stage of normalization associated with complete recovery of regional cerebral blood flow and metabolism is observed after 14 days.[44]

Abbreviations: ICH, intracranial hemorrhage.

Table 17.5 Cerebral Autoregulation and Blood Pressure

- Under normal physiological conditions, cerebral blood flow is regulated within a narrow range despite changes in the cerebral perfusion pressure (CPP).
- CPP is defined as the difference between mean arterial pressure (MAP) and intracranial pressure (ICP).
- In intact cerebral circulation, the ICP is low (~5 mm Hg), and CPP is therefore approximately equal to MAP.
- Cerebral blood flow does not begin to drop appreciably until the CPP falls below ~50 mm Hg, and it does not increase until CPP exceeds ~150 mm Hg.
- Cerebral autoregulation predominantly occurs at the level of small arteries and arterioles.[47]
- A relatively small degree of systemic blood pressure reduction might pose a significant risk of hypoprefusion and ischemia.[49]

animal experiments have suggested that a transient reduction of blood flow occurs in conjunction with hemorrhage,[38,39] compounded by impairment of autoregulation. However, these findings have been disputed by other investigators.[40,41] A study using diffusion-perfusion magnetic resonance imaging (MRI) of acute ICH patients demonstrated perihemorrhagic hypoperfusion but no ischemia.[42] A smaller study using positron emission tomography in a similar patient population showed no significant reduction in regional cerebral blood flow following moderate reduction in BP in the perihematoma region, suggesting intact autoregulation.[43] Qureshi et al proposed three stages of changes in regional cerebral blood flow and metabolism following ICH. The first stage is the hibernation stage, which comprises hypoperfusion and hypometabolism in the perihematoma region. There is essentially a coupling of metabolism and flow, and thus there is no ischemia. This stage lasts for ~2 days. The second stage that exists between 2 and 14 days is the stage of reperfusion, which consist of patchy areas of normal- or hyperperfusion in the perihematoma region. The stage of normalization associated with complete recovery of regional cerebral blood flow and metabolism is observed after 14 days.[44] (**Table 17.4**).

Cerebral Autoregulation and Blood Pressure

Under normal physiological conditions, cerebral blood flow is regulated within a narrow range despite changes in the CPP, a process that is referred to as cerebral autoregulation.[45,46] The CPP is defined as the difference between mean arterial pressure (MAP) and ICP. In the intact cerebral circulation, the ICP is low (~5 mm Hg), and CPP is therefore approximately equal to MAP. Under these circumstances, cerebral blood flow does not begin to drop appreciably until the CPP falls below ~50 mm Hg, and it does not increase until CPP exceeds ~150 mm Hg. Cerebral autoregulation predominantly occurs at the level of small arteries and arterioles.[47]

Maintaining CPP is a cornerstone of increased ICP management in TBI. Impaired autoregulation is common in brain trauma.[48] Thus, even a relatively small degree of systemic BP reduction might pose a significant risk of hypoprefusion and ischemia.[49] The loss of cerebral perfusion with diminished BP is even further accentuated in patients with increased ICP. The importance of maintaining adequate BP is further emphasized by the negative effects of hypotension,[50] and the high frequency of decreased cerebral perfusion.[51] A randomized trial of 189 TBI patients compared this approach of maintaining CPP >70 mm Hg with an ICP-targeted protocol.[52] Maintaining CPP >70 resulted in fewer episodes of jugular bulb oximetry desaturation but did impact overall outcome.

Conversely, acute hypertension in a patient with impaired cerebral in autoregulation with impairment in the blood–brain barrier, commonly seen in such injuries, might lead to worsening of cerebral edema and ICP. Although well demonstrated in animal experiments,[53] this is not readily demonstrated in clinical studies.[54] Induced hypertension might adversely affect other organs. In a randomized trial of cerebral blood flow–targeted or ICP-targeted therapy, there was a fivefold increase of acute respiratory distress syndrome (ARDS).[52] (**Table 17.5**).

Neurogenic Cardiac Injury

It has been long recognized that myocardial injury can occur as a result of brain injury. As with hypertension, it is thought to be related to the sudden release of catecholamines and subsequent subendocardial ischemia. This has been well demonstrated in TBI, ICH, ischemic stroke,

Table 17.6 Neurogenic Cardiac Injury

- Myocardial injury can occur as a result of acute brain injury; severe abnormalities in heart rate variability are indicators of poor outcome.[67]
- Increased serum levels of cardiac enzymes, creatinine kinase. and troponin are seen in 6 to 45% of these patients.[55–60] Patients with TBI, ICH, and ischemic stroke are especially susceptible to subarachnoid hemorrhage.
- Perfusion studies and coronary angiograms are often normal.
- Ventricular dysfunction is thought to be at least partially reversible.
- β-blockers might provide some cardiac benefits by counteracting the cardiac effects of catecholamines.

Abbreviations: ICH, intracranial hemorrhage; TBI, traumatic brain injury.

and, especially, subarachnoid hemorrhage. Increased serum levels of cardiac enzymes, creatinine kinase, and troponin are seen in 6 to 45% of these patients.[55–60] These elevated enzymes are correlated with a worse neurological injury and increased mortality. On pathological examination, the main finding is contraction band necrosis in the subendocardium, with the myocytes in a state of hypercontraction.[61]

In addition to the presence of elevated cardiac enzymes, cardiac systolic dysfunction has also been noted, in up to 28% of subarachnoid hemorrhage patients.[62,63] Perfusion studies and coronary angiograms are often normal. This ventricular dysfunction is thought to be at least partially reversible, as shown in small case series.[64]

Optimal treatment of this cardiac dysfunction is unclear and must balance the often conflicting needs for maintaining adequate CPP for neurological reasons and for lowering of BP to protect the heart. It has been suggested that β-blockers might provide some cardiac benefits by counteracting the cardiac effects of catecholamines (**Table 17.6**).

Autonomic Dysfunction

Cardiac arrhythmias, electrocardiogram (EKG) changes, and other evidence of autonomic dysfunction have been noted in severe brain injury.[61,65] Some of these occur in conjunction with the above-described neurogenic cardiac injury. Most, however, occur with no evidence of cardiac dysfunction. Experimental and clinical evidence suggests that injury to the insular cortex, hypothalamus, or medulla results in abnormal activity in the autonomic nervous system. The cardiac manifestation of this is on a spectrum, ranging from abnormal heart rate variability only detected by specialized testing, to the so-called sympathetic storms, as well as cardiac arrhythmias.

Table 17.7 Autonomic Dysfunction

- Most autonomic dysfunction occurs with no evidence of cardiac dysfunction.
- Electrocardiogram changes are frequently noted in brain injury. These include ST segment elevation or depression, T wave inversion and QT interval prolongation.
- A wide range of arrhythmias are commonly noted, mostly in the acute phase of the injury.
- Paroxysmal autonomic storms, diencephalic seizures, acute midbrain syndrome, sympathetic storms, and hypothalamic-midbrain dysregulation syndrome all present with cyclic high fever, tachycardia, hypertension, sweating, and tachypnea, with variable motor posturing.[68]
- Paroxysmal autonomic storms usually occur in younger patients, with severe diffuse axonal injury and evidence of brain stem involvement; usually noted in the first week of injury, but might persist weeks or months[71]
- Successful treatment has been reported with benzodiazepines, opiates, β-blockers, bromocriptine, clonidine, and gabapentin.[69,70]

Heart rate variability abnormalities tend to normalize in the subacute period paralleling neurological recovery.[66] It has been suggested that severe abnormalities in heart rate variability are a predictor of poor outcome.[67] EKG changes are frequently noted in brain injury. These include ST segment elevation or depression, T wave inversion, and QT interval prolongation. These findings should prompt a search for other possible causes, such as cardiac injury or metabolic abnormalities, and close cardiac monitoring. A wide range of arrhythmias is commonly noted, most commonly in the acute phase of the injury.

A syndrome of cyclic high fever, tachycardia, hypertension, sweating, and tachypnea, with variable motor posturing, can occur as a manifestation of autonomic dysfunction following brain trauma.[68] This syndrome has been termed *paroxysmal autonomic storms*, *diencephalic seizures*, *acute midbrain syndrome*, *sympathetic storms*, and *hypothalamic-midbrain dysregulation syndrome*, among others. It usually occurs in younger patients with severe diffuse axonal injury and evidence of brain stem involvement. Successful treatment has been reported with benzodiazepines, opiates, β-blockers, bromocriptine, clonidine, and gabapentin.[69,70] It is usually noted in the first week of injury but might persist weeks or months[71] (**Table 17.7**).

Choice of Vasoactive Agents for Blood Pressure Control

A main concern when BP control is required in TBI is choosing an agent that is easily and reliably titratable, to maintain CPP within the desired range. Thus IV antihypertensives

Table 17.8 Intravenous Antihypertensive Medications

Drug	Mechanism of Action	Dose	Onset/Duration	Side Effects
Esmolol	β adrenergic blocker	0.5–1 mg/kg loading dose, followed by 50–300 μg/kg infusion	1 min/10–20 min	Bronchospasm, heart block, bradycardia
Labetalol	Mixed α/β adrenergic blocker	10–80 mg bolus, 2 mg/min infusion, with up titration	2–5 min/2–6 h	Bronchospasm, heart block, bradycardia
Nicardipine	Dihydropyridine calcium channel blocker	2.5–30 mg/h, titrated by 2.5 mg/h every 5 min	5–15 min/4–6 h	Tachycardia
Nitroprusside	Direct-acting arterial and venous vasodilator	0.25–10 μg/kg/min, very potent	Immediate/1–2 min	Thiocyanate toxicity, high potency, potential for increased intracranial pressure, coronary steal
Fenoldopam	Dopamine (DA1) agonist	0.1–0.6 μg/kg/min	5–10 min/10–15 min	Profound hypotension, tachycardia
Enalaprilat	Angiotensin-converting enzyme inhibitor	0.625–5 mg IV q6 h	5–10 min/2–6 h	Hyperkalemia, renal failure, angioedema
Hydralazine	Direct-acting vasodilator	10–20 mg IV, repeated every 6 h	5–15 min/2–6 h	Unpredictable antihypertensive effect, tachycardia
Nitroglycerin	Direct-acting arterial and venous vasodilator	5–100 μg/kg/min	1–5 min/5–10 min	Reflex tachycardia, tolerance, potential for increased intracranial pressure, headache

(**Table 17.8**) are the first line of drugs used, supplemented at a later time with oral drugs if needed. Sodium nitroprusside is a very potent antihypertensive but is to be used with extreme caution in brain injured patients, as it is known to cause cerebral vasodilatation with a concomitant increase in ICP[72] as well to impair cerebral autoregulation. Nicardipine, a short-acting calcium channel blocker, is effective and easily to titrate in most patients. It is to be avoided when tachycardia is an issue. Esmolol is very effective for controlling heart rate but has less prominent antihypertensive effects. No trial has compared these different agents head to head. Comparing data from studies of hypertension treatment in ICH suggests better control using nicardipine drip versus a strategy using labetalol, hydralazine, and nitroprusside.[37,73]

When pharmacologically inducing hypertension to maintain CPP goal, it is important to ascertain adequate cardiac preload and avoid hypovolemia to minimize systemic side effects. A goal of a central venous pressure of 8 to 12 mm Hg is often used. Phenylephrine, a pure α agonist, and norepinephrine, a mixed α/β agonist, are the first-line inotropic agents. When compared with norepinephrine, dopamine was less predictable in inducing hypertension in a randomized trial.[74] If there is evidence of neurogenic myocardial dysfunction, it has been suggested that pure α agonists are ineffective in raising BP.[75] In these circumstances it is preferred to use a drug that would primarily increase cardiac contractility, such as dobutamine (**Table 17.9**). A small case series suggests that milrinone might be more effective than dobutamine in raising BP[76] (**Table 17.10**).

Table 17.9 Vasopressor Drugs

Drug	Inotropic	Chronotropic	Vasoconstriction
Phenylepherine	0	0	+++
Norepinepherine	++	++	+++
Dobutamine	+++	0/+	0/−
Dopamine	+++	+	0/+++
Vasopressin	0/+	0	+++

Neuroprotective Effects of Antihypertensive Medication

In addition to their primary effect of lowering BP, some antihypertensive medications demonstrate neuroprotective properties. It has been recently recognized that the angiotensin II receptor subtype 2 (AT2), is upregulated in the central nervous system (CNS) during cerebral ischemia.[77] Pretreatment with an AT2 antagonist has been reported to protect against ischemia in a rat model of focal ischemia.[78] Angiotensin-converting enzyme (ACE) inhibitors also seem to reduce free radical–induced injury in an animal model of ischemic stroke.[79] In a large clinical trial, despite the clear benefit of ACE inhibitors in reducing the risk of stroke, their effect on BP was minimal, raising the question of potential neuroprotection.[80] A small retrospective study demonstrated that use of ACE

Table 17.10 Choice of Vasoactive Agents*

- Intravenous antihypertensives are the first-line drugs used, supplemented later with oral drugs if needed.
- Sodium nitroprusside is a very potent antihypertensive; use with extreme caution in the brain-injured patient because it can cause cerebral vasodilation.[72]
- Nicardipine, a short-acting calcium channel blocker, is effective and can be easily titrated in most patients.
- Esmolol is very effective for controlling heart rate but has less prominent antihypertensive effects.
- Hypertension treatment in ICH suggests better control using nicardipine drip versus a strategy using labetalol, hydralazine, and nitroprusside.[37,73]
- It is important to ascertain adequate cardiac preload and avoid hypovolemia to minimize systemic side effects.
- It has been suggested that pure α agonists are ineffective in increasing blood pressure in the setting of severe cardiac dysfunction.[75]

*Also see Table 17.1.

Abbreviations: ICH, intracranial hemorrhage.

Table 17.11 Neuroprotective Effects of Antihypertensive Medication

- Angiotensin II receptor subtype 2 (AT2) is upregulated in the CNS during cerebral ischemia.[77]
- ACE inhibitors also seem to minimize free radical–induced injury in animal models of ischemic stroke.[79]
- Intracellular calcium influx is a key event in ischemic cell death; nimodipine, an oral calcium channel blocker, has been shown to improve outcome after subarachnoid hemorrhage[82] (but not traumatic subarachnoid hemorrhage[84]).

Abbreviations: ACE, angiotensin-converting enzyme; CNS, central nervous system.

inhibitors prior to the acute stroke was associated with less severe infarcts.[81]

Intracellular calcium influx is a key event in ischemic cell death. Nimodipine, an oral calcium channel blocker, has been shown to improve outcome after subarachnoid hemorrhage,[82] possibly via a neuroprotective effect.[83] This benefit did not extend to traumatic subarachnoid hemorrhage.[84] In animal studies, other calcium channel blockers have shown a protective effect,[85] but clinical studies remain negative.[86] (**Table 17.11**).

References

1. Dilraj A, Botha JH, Rambiritch V, Miller R, van Dellen JR. Levels of catecholamine in plasma and cerebrospinal fluid in aneurysmal subarachnoid hemorrhage. Neurosurgery 1992;31(1):42–50
2. Leonardi-Bee J, Bath PM, Phillips SJ, Sandercock PA ; IST Collaborative Group. Blood pressure and clinical outcomes in the International Stroke Trial. Stroke 2002;33(5):1315–1320
3. Cushing H. Concerning a definite regulatory mechanism of the vasomotor centre which controls blood pressure during cerebral compression. Bull Johns Hopkins Hosp 1901;12:290–292
4. Roozekrans NT, van Zwieften P. The role of the adrenergic nervous system in the pressor response due to acute elevation of intracranial pressure (Cushing's response): a pharmacological analysis. Arch Int Pharmacodyn Ther 1977;228(1):79–91
5. Rosner MJ, Newsome HH, Becker DP. Mechanical brain injury: the sympathoadrenal response. J Neurosurg 1984;61(1):76–86
6. Clifton GL, Ziegler MG, Grossman RG. Circulating catecholamines and sympathetic activity after head injury. Neurosurgery 1981;8(1):10–14
7. Schulte Esch J, Murday H, Pfeifer G. Haemodynamic changes in patients with severe head injury. Acta Neurochir (Wien) 1980;54(3–4):243–250
8. Chesnut RM, Marshall LF, Klauber MR, et al. The role of secondary brain injury in determining outcome from severe head injury. J Trauma 1993;34(2):216–222
9. Vavilala MS, Bowen A, Lam AM, et al. Blood pressure and outcome after severe pediatric traumatic brain injury. J Trauma 2003;55(6):1039–1044
10. Coates BM, Vavilala MS, Mack CD, et al. Influence of definition and location of hypotension on outcome following severe pediatric traumatic brain injury. Crit Care Med 2005;33(11):2645–2650
11. Mahoney EJ, Biffl WL, Harrington DT, Cioffi WG. Isolated brain injury as a cause of hypotension in the blunt trauma patient. J Trauma 2003;55(6):1065–1069
12. Chesnut RM, Gautille T, Blunt BA, Klauber MR, Marshall LF. Neurogenic hypotension in patients with severe head injuries. J Trauma 1998;44(6):958–963
13. Partrick DA, Bensard DD, Janik JS, Karrer FM. Is hypotension a reliable indicator of blood loss from traumatic injury in children? Am J Surg 2002;184(6):555–559
14. Fulton RL, Flynn WJ, Mancino M, Bowles D, Cryer HM. Brain injury causes loss of cardiovascular response to hemorrhagic shock. J Invest Surg 1993;6(2):117–131
15. Cohan P, Wang C, McArthur DL, et al. Acute secondary adrenal insufficiency after traumatic brain injury: a prospective study. Crit Care Med 2005;33(10):2358–2366
16. Bernard F, Outtrim J, Lynch AG, Menon DK, Matta BF. Hemodynamic steroid responsiveness is predictive of neurological outcome after traumatic brain injury. Neurocrit Care 2006;5(3):176–179

17. Edwards P, Arango M, Balica L, et al. CRASH trial collaborators: final results of MRC CRASH, a randomised placebo-controlled trial of intravenous corticosteroid in adults with head injury-outcomes at 6 months. Lancet 2005;365(9475):1957–1959
18. Christensen H, Meden P, Overgaard K, Boysen G. The course of blood pressure in acute stroke is related to the severity of the neurological deficits. Acta Neurol Scand 2002;106(3):142–147
19. Vemmos KN, Spengos K, Tsivgoulis G, et al. Factors influencing acute blood pressure values in stroke subtypes. J Hum Hypertens 2004; 18(4):253–259
20. Ahmed N, de la Torre B, Wahlgren NG. Salivary cortisol, a biological marker of stress, is positively associated with 24-hour systolic blood pressure in patients with acute ischaemic stroke. Cerebrovasc Dis 2004;18(3):206–213
21. Yong M, Diener HC, Kaste M, Mau J. Characteristics of blood pressure profiles as predictors of long-term outcome after acute ischemic stroke. Stroke 2005;36(12):2619–2625
22. Stead LG, Gilmore RM, Vedula KC, Weaver AL, Decker WW, Brown RD Jr. Impact of acute blood pressure variability on ischemic stroke outcome. Neurology 2006;66(12):1878–1881
23. Okumura K, Ohya Y, Maehara A, Wakugami K, Iseki K, Takishita S. Effects of blood pressure levels on case fatality after acute stroke. J Hypertens 2005;23(6):1217–1223
24. Vemmos KN, Tsivgoulis G, Spengos K, et al. U-shaped relationship between mortality and admission blood pressure in patients with acute stroke. J Intern Med 2004;255(2):257–265
25. Levy DE, Brott TG, Haley EC Jr, et al. Factors related to intracranial hematoma formation in patients receiving tissue-type plasminogen activator for acute ischemic stroke. Stroke 1994;25(2):291–297
26. Panzer RJ, Feibel JH, Barker WH, Griner PF. Predicting the likelihood of hemorrhage in patients with stroke. Arch Intern Med 1985;145(10): 1800–1803
27. Adams HP Jr, del Zoppo G, Alberts MJ, et al; American Heart Association. American Stroke Association Stroke Council; Clinical Cardiology Council; Cardiovascular Radiology and Intervention Council; Atherosclerotic Peripheral Vascular Disease and Quality of Care Outcomes in Research Interdisciplinary Working Groups. Guidelines for the early management of patients with ischemic stroke: a scientific statement from the Stroke Council of the American Stroke Association. Stroke 2003;34(4):1056–1083
28. Ay H, Koroshetz WJ, Vangel M, et al. Conversion of ischemic brain tissue into infarction increases with age. Stroke 2005;36(12):2632–2636
29. Oliveira-Filho J, Silva SC, Trabuco CC, Pedreira BB, Sousa EU, Bacellar A. Detrimental effect of blood pressure reduction in the first 24 hours of acute stroke onset. Neurology 2003;61(8):1047–1051
30. Ahmed N, Nasman P, Wahlgren NG. Effect of intravenous nimodipine on blood pressure and outcome after acute stroke. Stroke 2000; 31(6):1250–1255
31. Wallace JD, Levy LL. Blood pressure after stroke. JAMA 1981;246(19): 2177–2180
32. Fogelholm R, Avikainen S, Murros K. Prognostic value and determinants of first-day mean arterial pressure in spontaneous supratentorial intracerebral hemorrhage. Stroke 1997;28(7):1396–1400
33. Qureshi AI, Tuhrim S, Broderick JP, Batjer HH, Hondo H, Hanley DF. Spontaneous intracerebral hemorrhage. N Engl J Med 2001;344(19): 1450–1460
34. Ohwaki K, Yano E, Nagashima H, Hirata M, Nakagomi T, Tamura A. Blood pressure management in acute intracerebral hemorrhage: relationship between elevated blood pressure and hematoma enlargement. Stroke 2004;35(6):1364–1367
35. Brott T, Broderick J, Kothari R, et al. Early hemorrhage growth in patients with intracerebral hemorrhage. Stroke 1997;28(1):1–5
36. Davis SM, Broderick J, Hennerici M, et al; Recombinant Activated Factor VII Intracerebral Hemorrhage Trial Investigators. Hematoma growth is a determinant of mortality and poor outcome after intracerebral hemorrhage. Neurology 2006;66(8):1175–1181
37. Qureshi AI, Harris-Lane P, Kirmani JF, et al. Treatment of acute hypertension in patients with intracerebral hemorrhage using American Heart Association guidelines. Crit Care Med 2006;34(7): 1975–1980
38. Bullock R, Brock-Utne J, van Dellen J, Blake G. Intracerebral hemorrhage in a primate model: effect on regional cerebral blood flow. Surg Neurol 1988;29(2):101–107
39. Nath FP, Kelly PT, Jenkins A, Mendelow AD, Graham DI, Teasdale GM. Effects of experimental intracerebral hemorrhage on blood flow, capillary permeability, and histochemistry. J Neurosurg 1987;66(4):555–562
40. Qureshi AI, Wilson DA, Hanley DF, Traystman RJ. Pharmacologic reduction of mean arterial pressure does not adversely affect regional cerebral blood flow and intracranial pressure in experimental intracerebral hemorrhage. Crit Care Med 1999;27(5):965–971
41. Qureshi AI, Wilson DA, Hanley DF, Traystman RJ. No evidence for an ischemic penumbra in massive experimental intracerebral hemorrhage. Neurology 1999;52(2):266–272
42. Schellinger PD, Fiebach JB, Hoffmann K, et al. Stroke MRI in intracerebral hemorrhage: is there a perihemorrhagic penumbra? Stroke 2003; 34(7):1674–1679
43. Powers WJ, Zazulia AR, Videen TO, et al. Autoregulation of cerebral blood flow surrounding acute (6 to 22 hours) intracerebral hemorrhage. Neurology 2001;57(1):18–24
44. Qureshi AI, Hanel RA, Kirmani JF, Yahia AM, Hopkins LN. Cerebral blood flow changes associated with intracerebral hemorrhage. Neurosurg Clin N Am 2002;13(3):355–370
45. Beausang-Linder M, Bill A. Cerebral circulation in acute arterial hypertension–protective effects of sympathetic nervous activity. Acta Physiol Scand 1981;111(2):193–199
46. Ngai AC, Winn HR. Modulation of cerebral arteriolar diameter by intraluminal flow and pressure. Circ Res 1995;77(4):832–840
47. Wahl M, Schilling L. Regulation of cerebral blood flow:a brief review. Acta Neurochir Suppl (Wien) 1993;59:3–10
48. Golding EM, Robertson CS, Bryan RM Jr. The consequences of traumatic brain injury on cerebral blood flow and autoregulation: a review. Clin Exp Hypertens 1999;21(4):299–332
49. Rose JC, Mayer SA. Optimizing blood pressure in neurological emergencies. Neurocrit Care 2004;1(3):287–299
50. Chesnut RM, Marshall SB, Piek J, Blunt BA, Klauber MR, Marshall LF. Early and late systemic hypotension as a frequent and fundamental source of cerebral ischemia following severe brain injury in the Traumatic Coma Data Bank. Acta Neurochir Suppl (Wien) 1993;59:121–125
51. Bouma GJ, Muizelaar JP, Stringer WA, Choi SC, Fatouros P, Young HF. Ultra-early evaluation of regional cerebral blood flow in severely head-injured patients using xenon-enhanced computerized tomography. J Neurosurg 1992;77(3):360–368
52. Robertson CS, Valadka AB, Hannay HJ, et al. Prevention of secondary ischemic insults after severe head injury. Crit Care Med 1999;27(10): 2086–2095
53. Yamaguchi S, Kobayashi S, Yamashita K, Kitani M. Pial arterial pressure contribution to early ischemic brain edema. J Cereb Blood Flow Metab 1989;9(5):597–602
54. Bouma GJ, Muizelaar JP. Relationship between cardiac output and cerebral blood flow in patients with intact and with impaired autoregulation. J Neurosurg 1990;73(3):368–374
55. Jensen JK, Atar D, Mickley H. Mechanism of troponin elevations in patients with acute ischemic stroke. Am J Cardiol 2007;99(6):867–870
56. Chalela JA, Ezzeddine MA, Davis L, Warach S. Myocardial injury in acute stroke: a troponin I study. Neurocrit Care 2004;1(3):343–346
57. Urbaniak K, Merchant AI, Amin-Hanjani S, Roitberg B. Cardiac complications after aneurysmal subarachnoid hemorrhage. Surg Neurol 2007;67(1):21–28
58. Banki NM, Kopelnik A, Dae MW, et al. Acute neurocardiogenic injury after subarachnoid hemorrhage. Circulation 2005;112(21):3314–3319
59. Naidech AM, Kreiter KT, Janjua N, et al. Cardiac troponin elevation, cardiovascular morbidity, and outcome after subarachnoid hemorrhage. Circulation 2005;112(18):2851–2856
60. Hays A, Diringer MN. Elevated troponin levels are associated with higher mortality following intracerebral hemorrhage. Neurology 2006;66(9):1330–1334

61. Kopelnik A, Zaroff JG. Neurocardiogenic injury in neurovascular disorders. Crit Care Clin 2006;22(4):733–752, abstract ix–x
62. Kono T, Morita H, Kuroiwa T, Onaka H, Takatsuka H, Fujiwara A. Left ventricular wall motion abnormalities in patients with subarachnoid hemorrhage: neurogenic stunned myocardium. J Am Coll Cardiol 1994;24(3):636–640
63. Lee VH, Connolly HM, Fulgham JR, Manno EM, Brown RD Jr, Wijdicks EF. Tako-tsubo cardiomyopathy in aneurysmal subarachnoid hemorrhage: an underappreciated ventricular dysfunction. J Neurosurg 2006;105(2):264–270
64. Banki N, Kopelnik A, Tung P, et al. Prospective analysis of prevalence, distribution, and rate of recovery of left ventricular systolic dysfunction in patients with subarachnoid hemorrhage. J Neurosurg 2006; 105(1):15–20
65. Wittebole X, Hantson P, Laterre PF, et al. Electrocardiographic changes after head trauma. J Electrocardiol 2005;38(1):77–81
66. Keren O, Yupatov S, Radai MM, et al. Heart rate variability (HRV) of patients with traumatic brain injury (TBI) during the post-insult subacute period. Brain Inj 2005;19(8):605–611
67. Biswas AK, Scott WA, Sommerauer JF, Luckett PM. Heart rate variability after acute traumatic brain injury in children. Crit Care Med 2000;28(12):3907–3912
68. Baguley IJ, Nicholls JL, Felmingham KL, Crooks J, Gurka JA, Wade LD. Dysautonomia after traumatic brain injury: a forgotten syndrome? J Neurol Neurosurg Psychiatry 1999;67(1):39–43
69. Baguley IJ, Cameron ID, Green AM, Slewa-Younan S, Marosszeky JE, Gurka JA. Pharmacological management of dysautonomia following traumatic brain injury. Brain Inj 2004;18(5):409–417
70. Baguley IJ, Heriseanu RE, Gurka JA, Nordenbo A, Cameron ID. Gabapentin in the management of dysautonomia following severe traumatic brain injury: a case series. J Neurol Neurosurg Psychiatry 2007;78(5):539–541
71. Blackman JA, Patrick PD, Buck ML, Rust RS Jr. Paroxysmal autonomic instability with dystonia after brain injury. Arch Neurol 2004; 61(3):321–328
72. Turner JM, Powell D, Gibson RM, McDowall DG. Intracranial pressure changes in neurosurgical patients during hypotension induced with sodium nitroprusside or trimetaphan. Br J Anaesth 1977;49(5):419–425
73. Qureshi AI, Mohammad YM, Yahia AM, et al. A prospective multicenter study to evaluate the feasibility and safety of aggressive antihypertensive treatment in patients with acute intracerebral hemorrhage. J Intensive Care Med 2005;20(1):34–42
74. Steiner LA, Johnston AJ, Czosnyka M, et al. Direct comparison of cerebrovascular effects of norepinephrine and dopamine in head-injured patients. Crit Care Med 2004;32(4):1049–1054
75. Muizelaar JP, Becker DP. Induced hypertension for the treatment of cerebral ischemia after subarachnoid hemorrhage: direct effect on cerebral blood flow. Surg Neurol 1986;25(4):317–325
76. Naidech A, Du Y, Kreiter KT, et al. Dobutamine versus milrinone after subarachnoid hemorrhage. Neurosurgery 2005;56(1):21–27
77. Makino I, Shibata K, Ohgami Y, Fujiwara M, Furukawa T. Transient upregulation of the AT2 receptor mRNA level after global ischemia in the rat brain. Neuropeptides 1996;30(6):596–601
78. Groth W, Blume A, Gohlke P, Unger T, Culman J. Chronic pretreatment with candesartan improves recovery from focal cerebral ischaemia in rats. J Hypertens 2003;21(11):2175–2182
79. Ravati A, Junker V, Kouklei M, Ahlemeyer B, Culmsee C, Krieglstein J. Enalapril and moexipril protect from free radical-induced neuronal damage in vitro and reduce ischemic brain injury in mice and rats. Eur J Pharmacol 1999;373(1):21–33
80. The Heart Outcomes Prevention Evaluation Study. I: Effects of an angiotensin-converting-enzyme inhibitor, ramipril, on cardiovascular events in high-risk patients. N Engl J Med 2000;342(3):145–153
81. Selim M, Savitz S, Linfante I, Caplan L, Schlaug G. Effect of pre-stroke use of ACE inhibitors on ischemic stroke severity. BMC Neurol 2005; 5(1):10
82. Pickard JD, Murray GD, Illingworth R, et al. Effect of oral nimodipine on cerebral infarction and outcome after subarachnoid haemorrhage: British aneurysm nimodipine trial. BMJ 1989;298(6674):636–642
83. Mesis RG, Wang H, Lombard FW, et al. Dissociation between vasospasm and functional improvement in a murine model of subarachnoid hemorrhage. Neurosurg Focus 2006;21(3):E4
84. Vergouwen MD, Vermeulen M, Roos YB. Effect of nimodipine on outcome in patients with traumatic subarachnoid haemorrhage: a systematic review. Lancet Neurol 2006;5(12):1029–1032
85. Clausen T, Bullock R. Medical treatment and neuroprotection in traumatic brain injury. Curr Pharm Des 2001;7(15):1517–1532
86. Langham J, Goldfrad C, Teasdale G, Shaw D, Rowan K. Calcium channel blockers for acute traumatic brain injury. Cochrane Database Syst Rev 2003;(4):CD000565

18 Nutrition

Toshihiko Yanagawa and Rani Nasser

Head injuries may lead to a perturbance of systemic metabolism in the neurosurgery patient. One such complication involves the induction of metabolism; raising the metabolic need of an individual. There may also be a deviation in nitrogen balance during the weeks after an injury. This deviation from homeostatic balance in nitrogen is primarily due to loss of nitrogen from protein. Therefore, compensating for the change in metabolic need as well as supplementing lost nitrogen can assist in patient recovery. Providing adequate nutrition during these critical weeks can improve the prospects of survival and lessen the disability after head injury. Although nutritional support needed to expedite recovery, sometimes nutrition is withheld in cases where gastrointestinal motility is attenuated.

The necessity of nutritional support has been underscored, the next logical step is the standardized implement of an appropriate protocol. Have standards for nutritional support in traumatic brain injury been established? The answer to this question is partially "yes," and partially "no or unclear." The ambiguity is partially due to the vast array of head injuries, which incur uncertainty in standardizing a protocol. Moreover, there are insufficient evidence-based data to support a standardized treatment. Despite these shortcomings, this chapter will attempt to provide some evidence-based guidelines and to report current recommendations for nutritional support.

Pathophysiology and Metabolism

Neurosurgical patients with moderate to severe head injury demonstrate alterations in metabolic responses. These deviations from homeostatic values are manifested in the form of both hypermetabolism and hypercatabolism. Hypermetabolism is the increased energy expenditure and caloric need. Hypercatabolism results in self-directed protein breakdown, as indicated by abnormally high urinary nitrogen excretion and a negative nitrogen balance.

In a study demonstrating hypermetabolism by Clifton et al,[1] the measured resting energy expenditure (REE) of nonsedated head injury patients was elevated to 138% ± 37% compared with the predicted normal basal energy expenditure (BEE). In another study by Robertson et al[2] the correlation between hypermetabolism and severity of head injury was demonstrated in patients with a Glasgow Coma Scale (GCS) score of 4 to 5 who consequently had a high REE, 168% ± 53% of predicted BEE. Furthermore, those patients with a GCS score of 6 to 7 had lower REE, 129% ± 31% of expected values. Moreover, increased body temperatures associated with hypermetabolism were also associated with an increased REE by 45%/C° in patients with a GCS score of 4 to 5 and by 15%/C° in those with a GCS score of 6 to 7. Sedatives, paralyzing agents, and propranolol all decreased REE values. Robertson et al had also shown that the increase in oxygen utilization is associated with an increase in plasma catecholamines.[2] In these studies, extrinsic steroid therapy may have had a role in producing a hypermetabolic response. In the nonsteroid-treated head injury patients, the mean measured REE was 1.4 ± 0.5 times the predicted BEE. This response appeared to be directly caused by the head injury.[3]

In addition to hypermetabolism, the self-consuming metabolic process of hypercatabolism has also been noticed in neurosurgical patients who sustained head injuries. In normal fasting humans, the nitrogen catabolism is 3 to 5 g N/day. In contrast, severely brain injured patients have a nitrogen catabolism rate on the order of 14 to 25 g N/day.[4] In the study by Young et al,[3] despite at least 1.5 g of protein per kg of body weight per day, the mean nitrogen balance was still negative and lasted 3 weeks. Furthermore, the serum albumin levels dropped from a mean of 3.09 ± 0.2 g/dL on admission to 1.98 ± 0.4 within 2 weeks. In addition, there was a marked weight loss (mean: 15.6 ± 5.9 kg). These patients also demonstrated a positive nitrogen (N)-balance of 2.3 g/kg/day of protein. The Brain Trauma Foundation[5] reported that more than 20% of severe head injury patients (GCS score 3–8) have a negative N-balance of more than 30 g/day and almost all of the others have negative N-balances of at least 20 g/day during the first 7 to 10 days after injury. In the absence of adequate nutritional support, the hypercatabolic state rapidly causes the breakdown of a large amount of endogenous protein. Chiolero et al[6] found that N-balance correlated negatively with urinary levels of catecholamines and plasma glucagons. It has been suggested that the severity of hypermetabolism and hypercatabolism

Table 18.1 Nuitritional Assessment of the Head Injured

Energy Requirement	
This demonstrates a method to calculate predicted energy expenditure (PEE) in the absence of indirect calorimetry using the variables sex, height (Ht), body weight (Wt), and age (A)	
PEE (kcal/day) = REE (kcal/day) (resting energy expenditure)	
= basal energy expenditure (BEE) × activity factor × injury factor*	
where BEE (kcal/day) is calculated using the Harris-Benedict equation:	
BEE (male) = 66.47 + 13.75 Wt + 5.0 Ht − 6.76 A	
BEE (female) = 665.1 + 9.56 Wt + 1.85 Ht − 4.68 A	
with weight in kilograms, height in centimeters, and age in years.	
Energy Expended	
MEE (kcal/day) =	3.94 $_{V}O_2$ + 1.11 $_{V}CO_2$ − 2.17 UN
$_{V}O_2$ (mL/min):	Volume of oxygen consumption
$_{V}CO_2$ (mL/min):	Volume of carbon dioxide production
UN (g/day):	Urea nitrogen
RQ =	$_{V}O_2/_{V}CO_2$
Nitrogen Balance Calculation	
The following equations are used to calculate nitrogen balance:	
Nitrogen balance (N-balance) =	N intake (g/day) − N output (g/day)
Nitrogen balance (N-balance) =	Protein (g)/6.25 − urea N (g/day) × 5/4
Nitrogen balance (N-balance) =	Protein (g)/6.25 − (urea N + 4) (g/day)

*Activity factor = 1.2 (confined to bed), 1.3 (out of bed); injury factor = 1.3 (trauma), 1.6 (trauma with steroids), 1.6 (major sepsis), 2.0 (severe burns). The equation and activity factors are quoted from Long et al[7] and were partially revised by the chapter authors.

Abbreviations: BEE, basal energy expenditure; BMR, basic metabolic rate; MEE, measure energy expenditure; PEE, predicted energy expenditure; REE, resting energy expenditure; RQ, respiratory quotient; UN, urea nitrogen.

Note: An RQ of 0.9 to 1.0 indicates carbohydrate oxidation; 0.7 indicates primary lipid oxidation; 0.85 signifies mixed substrate oxidation; and >1.0 indicates lipogenesis.

may be correlated with the magnitude of catecholamine release (**Table 18.1**).[7]

Pathophysiology and Metabolic Consequences

Patients with moderate to severe head injuries usually develop protein-calorie malnutrition. The increased metabolic catabolism results in atrophy of skeletal muscle as well as visceral and circulating proteins that are indicative of the systemic effects of catabolism.[8] Under such circumstances patients are easily prone to multiple organ dysfunctions. Some common complications are systemic dysfunction of the cardiopulmonary, intestinal, and immune systems (**Table 18.2**). Malnutrition is thought to increase the mortality and morbidity rates in head injury patients.

Table 18.2 Consequences of Malnutrition to Head Injury

1. *Metabolic change*
   - Increased body protein utilization = body protein loss
2. *Decreased physical activities*
   - Loss of skeletal muscle protein causes fatigue of respiratory muscles and fall of physical activities.
   - Fatigue of respiratory muscles weakens excretion strength of sputum.
   - Fall of physical activity causes decubitus ulcers.
3. *Immune suppression*
   - Granulocyte (neutrophils): decline of the chemotactic and sterilization activity
   - Lymphocyte: reduction in number of lymphocytes, proliferation to PHA and ConA
   - Macrophage: decline of phagocytosis, supplying of growth factor, opsonization

Table 18.2 *(Continued)*

4. *Delay of wound healing*
   - Disorders of protein synthesis, collagen synthesis, and fibroblast malfunction cause delay of wound healing. Location of wound is easily compromised with infection, and wound infection causes sepsis.
5. *Bacterial translocation*
   - Lack of glutamine intake and long-term fasting cause atrophy of intestinal mucosa.
   - This mucosal atrophy causes bacterial translocation and leads to sepsis.

ConA, concanavalinA; PHA, phytohemaglutinin

Nutritional Therapy for the Brain Injured

Nutritional Assessments

Nutritional assessment is extremely important in the medical intervention and rehabilitation of the neurosurgical patient. Aside from being a very viable preemptive screening tool for high-risk patients, nutritional assessment can be just as valuable in determining certain pharmaceutical thresholds. The nutritional state of the patient should be evaluated precisely and promptly to increase patient survival rate and avoid malnutrition-associated morbidities (see **Table 18.1**).[7]

Energy Requirement and Expenditure

To assess the energy requirement of a patient, the measured energy expenditure (MEE) and respiratory quotient (RQ) values are used to make the assessment. One of the cardinal indicators of metabolism is the consumption of oxygen and the production of carbon dioxide. Indirect calorimetry is a measurement of such above-mentioned values and is performed using the equipment of the Sensor Medics 2900 metabolic cart. In addition, this unit specifically measures the volume, temperature, and partial pressure of expired gases. When the volume of oxygen consumption ($_VO_2$), volume of carbon dioxide production ($_VCO_2$), and urinary nitrogen are measured, the following formula can be utilized to measure the amount of energy expended.[4]

$$\text{MEE (kcal/day)} = 3.94(_VO_2) + 1.11(_VCO_2) - 2.17\text{UN}$$
(Urea Nitrogen) (See **Table 18.1**)

As demonstrated by the above-mentioned formula, the quantifiable energy expenditures are manifested through MEE values. MEE is affected by patient state, such as fever, infection, or the therapy itself. Substances such as barbiturates, steroids, sedative agents, and cardiovascular drugs also affect MEE values. The ratio of MEE:BEE is the magnitude of the stress. In practical settings, nutritional support should be adjusted after obtaining a metabolic profile. Previously published studies provide a range of values of the MEE:BEE ratio that many clinicians use as an indicator: (kcal/kg/day) as 25 to 30 in resting, 25 to 30 in mild stress, 30 to 35 in moderate stress, and 35 to 40 in severe stress state.

Rapid Turnover Proteins

Serum albumin is commonly used in the evaluation of malnutrition. However, in the case of short-term nutrition deficiency, serum albumin does not decrease because it has a half life of around 20 days. Rapid turnover proteins, such as retinol-binding protein (RBP), prealbumin (PA), and transthyretin (TTR) transferrin (TF), synthesized in the liver; all have short half lives. Therefore, rapid turnover proteins are more sensitive to acute changes in calorie and protein intake and should be used as a more precise marker of malnutrition (**Table 18.3**).

Glucose Metabolism

Hyperglycemia appears to result from increased hepatic glucose production rather than decreased glucose utilization. Glucose is synthesized from such sources as lactic acids, pyruvic acids, and amino acid substrates under the influence of increased concentrations of catecholamines, glucagons, and cortisol. Severe hyperglycemia tends to

Table 18.3 Serum Rapid Turnover Protein and Half-life Period

Malnutrition	Albuming/dL	Transferin (mg/dL)	Prealbumin (mg/dL)	TTR (mg/dL)	RBP (mg/dL)	IGF-1 (IU)
Severe	<2.4	<100	<5			
Moderate	2.5–3.0	100–150	6–10			
Mild	3.1–3.4	151–200	11–15			
Normal	3.5–5.3	201–300	16–40		2.7–7.6	0,55–1.4
T ½ (day)	17–23	7–10	1.9		12–14 h	2–8 h

Abbreviations: TTR, transthyretin; RBP, retinol-binding protein; IGF-1, insulin-like growth factor-1. T ½, half life; h, hours correlate with a poor patient outcome. It is generally thought that hyperglycemia causes lactate accumulation or acidosis in the brain.[9] When the blood glucose level exceeds 225 mg/dL, glucose loads must be reduced. Furthermore, insulin administration should be regulated to maintain a blood glucose level under 225 mg/dL.[10]

Fat Metabolism

The oxidation of lipid as an energy substrate is generally increased in trauma patients. Lipid mobilization and turnover are also enhanced in these patients. If serum lipemia is not present, the general principles for lipid administration may be employed. However, if serum lipemia is present and serum triglyceride level exceeds 500 mg/dL, total calories and/or the dose of omega (ω)-6 polyunsaturated fatty acid (PUFA) should be reduced.[10]

Two fat emulsions containing either long-chain triglycerides (LCTs) or a mixture of 50% medium-chain triglycerides (MCTs) and 50% LCTs were compared in 24 head trauma patients over a 10 day period. Cumulative N-balance remained negative (−10 g N/day; i.e., −100 g N/10 days) and comparable in both groups. However, thyroxin-binding PA concentrations increased significantly in patients receiving the MCT-LCT mixture. Calon et al[11] concluded that MCT might have a beneficial effect on visceral protein metabolism after trauma.

Nutritional Recommendations

Tier 1 Recommendations

The initial nutritional recommendation for a patient with moderate to severe head injury is a high-energy, protein-rich regimen. During the nutrient administration, the onset of hyperglycemia should be prevented. Hyperglycemia has been correlated with a poor patient outcome, partially because hyperglycemia has been linked with acidosis (lactate accumulation) of the brain.[9] (See **Tables 18.4** and **18.5**.)[3,12]

Tier 2 Recommendations

Once caloric and protein needs have been defined, other questions remain to be addressed.

- Does the period and degree of hypermetabolism and hypercatabolism jeopardize the patient's recovery from head injury?
- Is it possible to meet the patient's caloric and protein needs with enteral or parenteral feeding during the early posttraumatic period?
- Does early aggressive nutritional support improve the patient's outcome?

As mentioned previously, the nutritional support protocol is not fully standardized. This is partially due to the

Table 18.4 Example of Nutritional Support for the Head Injured

	Young et al, 1985[3]	Wilson et al, 2001[12]
Nutritional Support		
Nonprotein caloric intake (kcal/kg of body weight/day)	40–50	30–35
Protein intake (g/kg/day)	2.0–2.5	2.0–2.5
Lipid (% of nonprotein kcal)	30–50	Not recommended in early stage
Glucose	No more than 7 g/kg/day	Prevent hyperglycemia by carefully regulating insulin
Monitoring		
Nutritional status*	EE and RTP during first 2 weeks	EE and RQ twice weekly
Body weight	At least 3 times/week	
Nitrogen (N) balance (N intake–urea N)	Weekly	Once or twice weekly until adequate nutrition
	Other	
Prevention of gastroesophageal reflux		Keep upright; check gastric residuals
Recommendation	Adequate nutrition	Early adequate nutrition, preferably via enteral

*EE and RQ are measured by indirect calorimetry.

Abbreviations: EE, energy expenditure; RQ, respiratory quotient; RTP, rapid turnover protein.

Table 18.5 Adequate Nutrition Recommendations for the Head Injured

Young et al.[3] proposed the following:

- Administration of 40 to 50 nonprotein kcal/kg body of weight
- Administration of 2.0 to 2.5 g of protein/kg of body weight until nitrogen excretion abates
- Administration of 30 to 50% of nonprotein kcal as lipid
- Administration of no more than 7 g of glucose/kg of body weight/day
- Monitoring of nutritional status using indirect calorimetry, serum level of rapid turnover protein (such as RBP) during first 2 weeks after head injury
- Weight measurement at least 3 times per week
- Weekly nitrogen balance calculation and urinary nitrogen loss calculation by either total nitrogen or urea nitrogen

See also **Table 18.4.**

Abbreviations: RBP, retinol-binding protein.

vast assortment of head injuries; some of which compromise gastrointestinal function. Therefore, nutritional support for acutely head-injured patients is sometimes delayed until satisfactory gastrointestinal functions have returned during the postinjury period.[13–15] In particular, if enteral feeding is provided by a nasogastric (NG) tube, feeding is often delayed until bowel sounds are detected. Total parenteral nutrition (TPN) provides an alternative to conventional enteral (gastric) feeding that can be used in the acute post–head injury period. However, the advantages of TPN may be offset by the occurrence of significant catheter-related complications.

Some benefits to conventional enteral nutrition (EN) may prevent malnutrition, intestinal mucosal atrophy, and preservation of normal gut flora.[16] Early enteral feeding has also been shown to reduce intestinal bacterial translocation.[17] This argument forms the basis of more recent techniques of enteral feeding via the jejunum. On the other hand, enteral feeding could possibly result in aspiration and pneumonia, whereas jejunal feeding may result in peritoneal leakage.

Before second-tier recommendations can be made regarding "parenteral versus enteral nutrition," the relatively common frequency of gastrointestinal dysfunctions in head injury patients should be considered further. Head injury patients with gastrointestinal abnormalities may present with increased gastric residuals. The increased gastric residuals are a result of delayed gastric emptying. Furthermore, prolonged paralytic ileus, abdominal distention aspiration pneumonia, and diarrhea are other corroborating findings that deem a patient intolerant of EN.

In practical settings, NG nutritional administration tends to be chosen because of its ease of delivery and its low cost. Tolerance of enteral feeding is inversely related to increased intracranial pressure and severity of brain injury.[15] The clinician may choose the postpyloric placement or TPN to preempt the possibility of feeding interruption due to gastric residuals. The pursuit of postpyloric enteral feeding is supported by the important concept of maintaining physical function as much as possible. Enteral feedings may be delivered in several forms: endoscopic, percutaneous endoscopic gastrostomy (PEG), PEG with jejeunostomy, and also open jejeunostomy tube placement.[18]

TPN is a classic and reliable route of administration to secure the nutritional requirement of the patient. Currently, nutritional support is performed by combining enteral and parenteral nutrition if necessary. According to practical intervention, implementation of a nutritional support algorithm as a combining example assumed the amount of gastric residuals as an index value[19] (**Fig. 18.1**). (See **Table 18.6.**)[12]

Innovations and Obstacles in Nutritional Therapy for the Brain Injured

Immunonutrients

Attention must also be directed toward immunonutrition, specifically, the modulation of the inflammatory response to injury and infection. This intervention would thereby improve the clinical outcome by modulating such immunonutrient compounds as ω-3 PUFA, glutamine, arginine, S-amino acids, and nucleotides. These are listed in **Table 18.7.**[20] There are also vitamins and other nutrients that may be of specific benefit after brain injury. The immune and metabolic responses to injury are initiated by secretion of proinflammatory cytokines, such as interleukin (IL)-1, IL-6, and tumor necrosis factor α (TNFα). The tissue damage caused by the immune response should be compensated for, to avoid excessive oxidant damage (**Fig. 18.2**).[20] Immune suppression, hyperinflammation, and oxidant damage are areas of interest with feasible prospects of intervention.

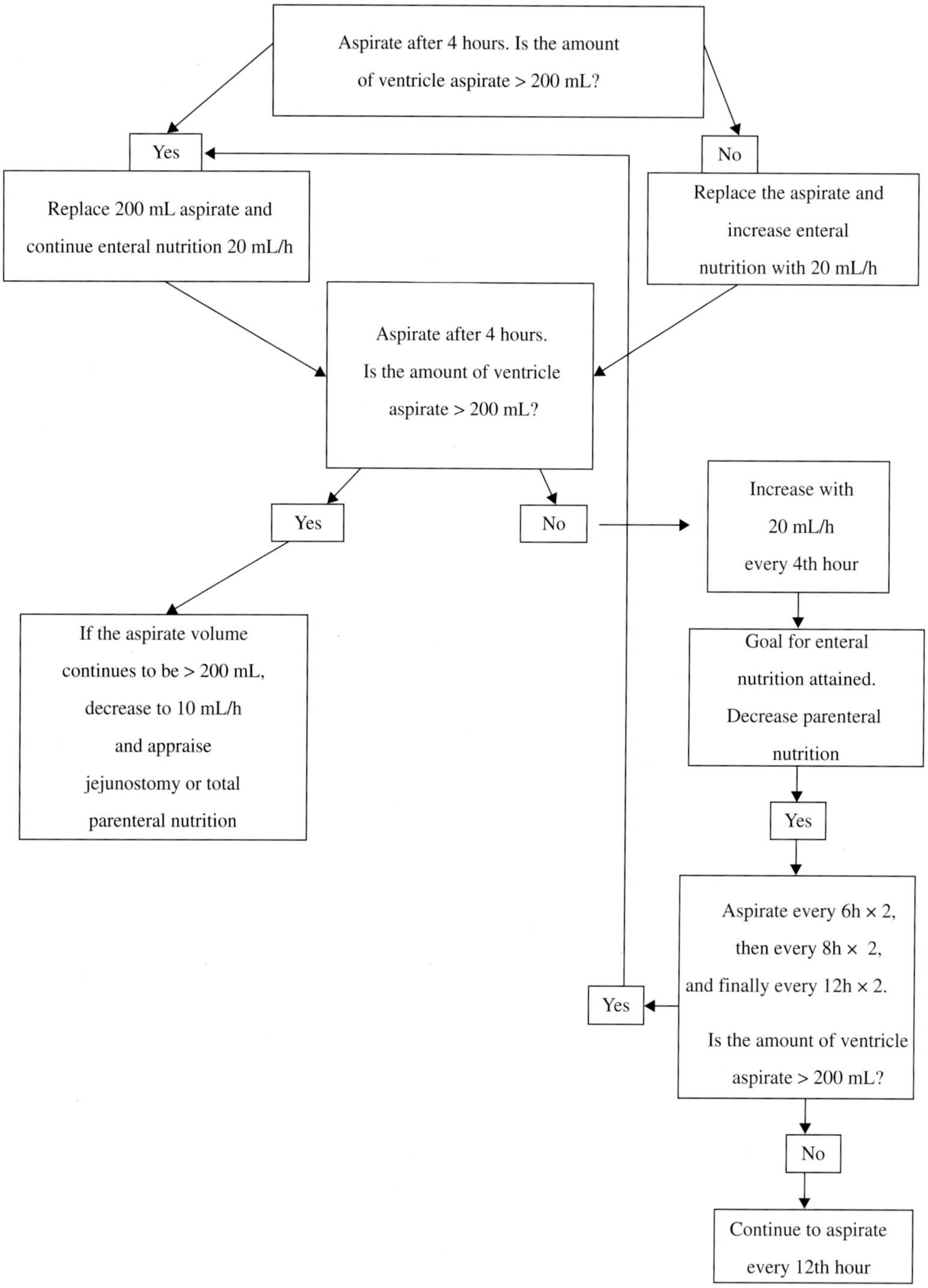

Fig. 18.1 Nutrition support algorithm. (From Woien H, Bjork IT. Nutrition of the critically ill patient and effects of implementing a nutritional support algorithm in ICU. J Clin Nurs 2006;15(2):168–177. Reprinted by permission.)

Vitamin E, ascorbic acid, and glutathione are also incorporated as part of the antioxidant defense. Furthermore, vitamin B6 and riboflavin act as cofactors for the abovementioned defense system.

Although animal model studies suggest that all these components may exert a beneficial effect, randomized, controlled trials using immunonutrition are still limited among studies of head injury patients. Metaanalysis of heterogeneous critically ill patients with burns, sepsis, trauma, and postoperative patients suggests that immunonutrition may not reduce mortality rates. However, a reduction in hospital stay, decreased requirements for ventilation, and lower infection rate are achieved with immunonutrition therapy.[21] Briassoulis et al[22] reported

Table 18.6 Enteral Feeding Recommendations for the Head Injured

Wilson et al[12] made the following recommendations:
• Enteral feeding should begin as soon as the patient is hemodynamically stable
• Nonprotein caloric intake of at least 30–35 kcal/kg/day
• Protein intake of 2.0–2.5 g/kg/day
• Keeping the patients upright and checking residuals (for avoidance of GI reflux, aspiration), gastric feeding, jejunal feeding
• GI tract problem within 3 days; TPN is begun within 24–48 h as to either one or both routes by third or fourth day
• Prevent hyperglycemia by carefully regulating the glucose and insulin intake
• Indirect calormetry to determine respiratory quotient and resting energy expenditure, twice weekly
• To determine N-balance, urinary nitrogen should be measured in 24 h specimens, once or twice weekly until the nutrition is adequate

See also **Table 18.4.**

Note: Although we can almost accept such a practical recommendation, the evidence extracted from systematic review is only "early feeding may reduce mortality and morbidity" (Yanagawa et al, 2000, 2002[26]).

Abbreviations: GI, gastrointestinal; TPN, total parenteral nutrituion.

a randomized, blinded, controlled study among a total of 40 mechanically ventilated children with severe head injury. Patients who were placed on an immune-enhancing diet (supplemented with glutamine, arginine, antioxidants, and omega-3 fatty acid) showed lower IL-8 level and fewer positive gastric cultures. Nosocomial infection, length of stay, length of mechanical ventilation, and survival rate did not differ between the studied groups. In another study,[23] 20 brain injury patients were randomized to receive either an early enteral diet (control) or the same formula with glutamine and probiotics (study group). There were no documented mortalities during the study. Furthermore, the study concluded that the nutrition administered with glutamine and probiotics decreased the infection rate and shortened the stay within the intensive care unit (ICU).

Data pertaining to the interaction between individuals' genotypes during the response to injury and infection would help further the application of immunonutrition in head injury (**Fig. 18.3**).[20]

Insulin-Like Growth Factor 1

Hatton et al[24] reported the effect of insulin-like growth factor 1 (IGF-1) on the catabolic state and clinical outcome of 33 head injury patients. Under aggressive nutritional support, patients were randomized to one of two groups: 17 patients with IGF-1 (treatment group) or 16 patients without IGF-1 (control group). During the 14 day dosing period, the control patients lost weight, whereas the treated patients gained weight despite a significantly higher MEE and lower caloric intake ($p = 0.02$). Furthermore, 15 (88%) treated and 13 (81%) control patients survived the first week. Moreover, there were no deaths pertaining to patients whose serum IGF-1 concentrations were higher than 350 ng/mL. Eight of the 11 treated patients with serum IGF-1 concentrations that were at least 350 ng/mL achieved moderate-to-good outcome scores at 6 months, compared with only one of five patients with lower concentrations ($p < 0.05$). These findings indicate that pharmacological concentrations of IGF-1 may improve clinical outcomes. In addition, nitrogen utilization in

Table 18.7 Immunonutrients and Their Function

Immunonutrients	Function
ω-3 polyunsaturated fatty acids	Act as anti-inflammatory agents, reverse immunosuppression
S amino acids	Enhance antioxidant status via glutathione synthesis
Glutamine	Nutrients for immune cells, improve gut barrier function, act as a precursor for glutathione
Arginine	Substrate for NO synthesis, stimulate growth hormone synthesis, improve helper T cell numbers
Nucleotides	RNA and DNA precursors, improve T cell function

Source: From Grimble RF. Nutritional modulation of immune function. Proc Nutr Soc 2001;60(3):389–397. Reprinted with permission.

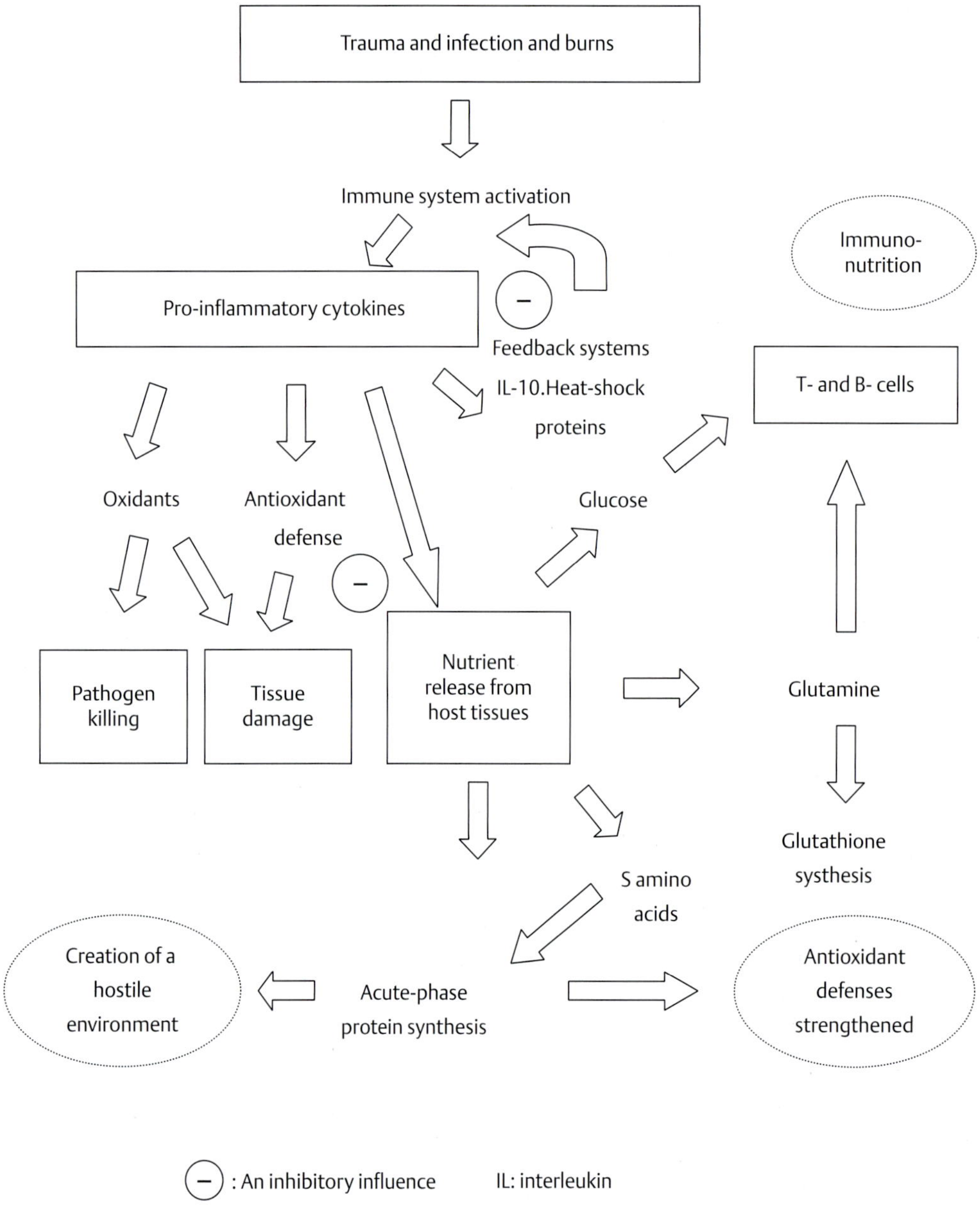

Fig. 18.2 The immune and metabolic response to injury and infection. Minus sign (–) represents an inhibitory influence. IL: interleukin. (From Grimble RF. Nutritional modulation of immune function. Proc Nutr Soc 2001;60(3):389–397. Reprinted by permission.)

patients with moderate-to-severe head injury was also expected to improve.

Zinc

Young et al[25] reported on 68 patients with severe, closed head injury who were enrolled in a prospective, double-blind, randomized, controlled trial of supplemental zinc versus standard zinc therapy. One month after injury, the mortality rates in the standard group and zinc supplement group were 26% and 12%, respectively. Glasgow Coma Scale (GCS) scores of the supplement group exceeded the adjusted mean GCS score of the standard group at day 28. The mean motor GCS score of the supplement group was significantly higher than those of the standard group on days 15 and 21. The mean serum PA and RBP concentrations were significantly higher in the supplement group at 3 weeks after head injury. This study[25] indicated that zinc supplementation during the immediate postinjury period is associated with an improved rate of visceral protein and neurological recovery.

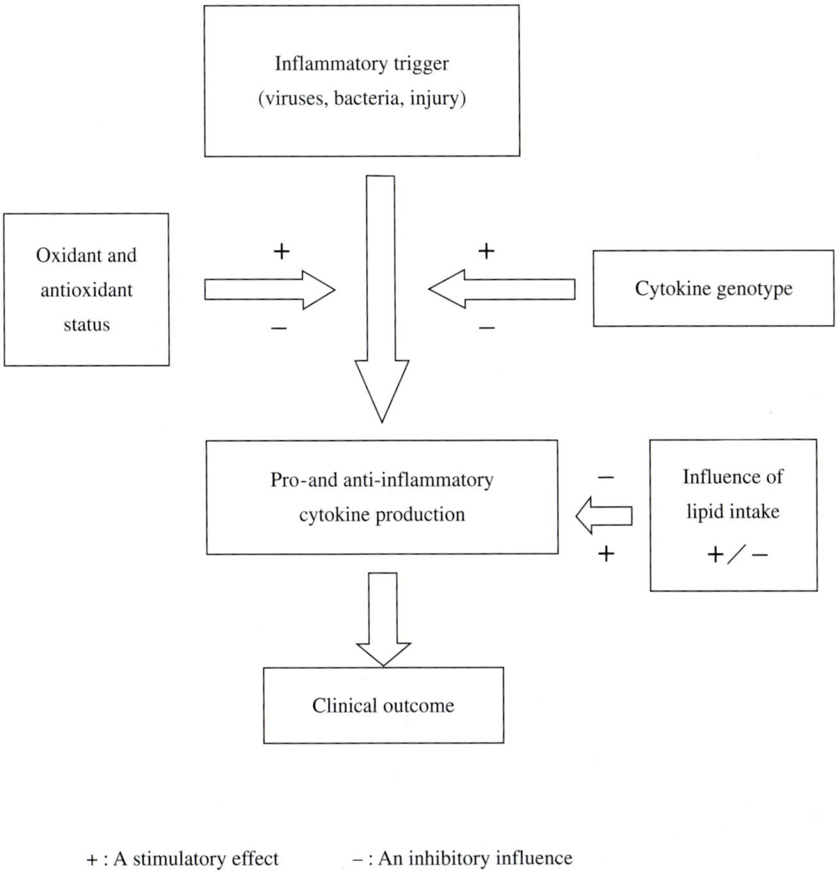

Fig. 18.3 Nutritional and genetic influence on cytokine production and clinical outcome. Plus sign (+) represents a stimulatory effect. Minus sign (–) represents an inhibitory influence. (From Grimble RF. Nutritional modulation of immune function. Proc Nutr Soc 2001;60(3):389–397. Reprinted by permission.)

Tier 3 Recommendations

In the present time, the single conclusion that can be made is that immune-modulated formula seems to be very well tolerated in head injury patients. This is in part due to the few studies available that can potentially resolve ambiguity regarding the benefits of immunonutrients.

Systematic Review of Nutrition of the Head Injured

In the remaining portion of the chapter, some fundamental objectives pertaining to nutrition and the neurosurgical patient are underscored utilizing excerpts from an article by Yanagawa et al regarding nutrition in head injury.[26] References from the article are cited to reinforce and expand on principles regarding the timing and route of nutrition for patients with sustained head injuries.

Background

The relative effectiveness of the different nutritional strategies following head injury has been examined in several randomized, controlled trials. The objective of these trials is to ascertain the optimal timing in nutritional therapy (early versus delayed). In addition, these trials sought to investigate the optimal route (enteral or parenteral) of nutritional supplementation following head injury. The participants in the studies were patients of all ages with acute TBI of any severity. This diverse array of patients includes patients with multiple injuries.

Two forms of intervention were employed during the randomized, controlled trials. The early versus delayed nutritional support as well as the parenteral versus enteral nutritional support were engaged in accumulating data. Mixed nutrition (enteral plus parenteral) were regarded as enteral if the enteral calories exceeded 50% of caloric intake. Furthermore, in the case of enteral feeding, the review also examined the preferred method of delivery; in particular, gastric versus jejunal.

The outcomes were quantified using the Glasgow Outcome Scale.[27] This scale included the following categories: death, persistent vegetative state, severely disabled, moderately disabled, and good recovery. This scale was modified for the purpose of this review so that the scale was dichotomized with death. A persistent vegetative state and severe disability denoted a poor outcome, whereas moderate disability and good recovery denoted a good outcome. The length of hospital stay, as well as the frequency of infection, was also factored into the outcome assessment.

Methods of the Review

One reviewer went through the search results and selected those articles that met the inclusion criteria. Two reviewers independently extracted the following information from each trial: strategy for allocation concealment, number of randomized patients, duration of follow-up, and the number lost to follow-up. The major outcome of the data sought were the numbers of deaths and numbers of patients who were disabled at the end of the study period. Data were also extracted on the incidence of infections. (See **Tables 18.8** and **18.9.**)[28]

The relative risks and 95% confidence intervals for mortality were calculated for each trial. Heterogeneity between trials was tested using a χ-squared test, where p less than or equal to 0.05 was taken to indicate significant heterogeneity. As long as a statistical heterogeneity did not exist, for dichotomous data, relative risk and 95% confidence intervals were calculated using a fixed effects model. A funnel plot to detect publication bias was not attempted as there were too few trials to detect asymmetry.

Results

There were 11 identified randomized, controlled trials that looked at the timing and route of support in head injured patients (**Table 18.10**).[13,20,29] These trials include a total of 534 patients. Seven trials looked at the timing of the nutritional intervention (284 participants), and seven trials looked at the route of nutritional support (222 participants). Three of the trials (Hadley et al 1986,[31] Rapp et al 1983,[13] and Young et al 1987[30]) are in both comparisons as they address early versus late, and parenteral nutrition versus EN.

Table 18.8 Identifying Trials Using Database Searches

	Strategy for identifying trials in CENTRAL and MEDLINE
#1	head injury*
#2	explode "Head-Injuries"/ all subheadings
#3	head trauma
#4	cranial trauma
#5	explode "Brain-Injuries"/ all subheadings
#6	brain injury*
#7	cranial injury*
#8	brain trauma
#9	#1 or #2 or #3 or #4 or #5 or #6 or #7 or #8
#10	enteral
#11	enteral nutrition
#12	enteral feeding
#13	"Enteral-Nutrition"/ all subheadings
#14	parenteral
#15	parenteral feeding
#16	parenteral nutrition
#17	explode "Parenteral-Nutrition"/ all subheadings
#18	#10 or #11 or #12 or #13 or #14 or #15 or #16 or #17
#19	#9 and #18

Source: These terms were combined with an RCT/CCT filter. EMBASE was also searched using the free text terms listed above. Strategies for searching CENTRAL and MEDLINE were developed for this review using MeSH subject terms of SilverPlatterASCII 3.0 WINNSelected Databases. The reference lists of all identified trials and review articles were checked. This search was last updated in March 2002.

The Timing of Support: Early versus Delayed

The timing of the nutritional intervention (early versus late) was looked at in the following trials: Grahm et al 1989[32] (early jejunal feeding versus gastric feeding when bowel sounds returned), Hadley et al 1986[31] (early TPN versus delayed NG enteral feeding), Minard et al 2000[33]

Table 18.9 Allocation of Concealment

C =	The letter C was assigned to the poorest quality and A to the best quality trials in which concealment was inadequate (such as alternation or reference to case record numbers or to dates of birth).
B =	Trials in which the authors either did not report an allocation concealment approach at all or reported an approach that did not fall into category A or C
A =	Trials deemed to have taken adequate measures to conceal allocation (i.e., central randomization; numbered or coded bottles or containers; drugs prepared by the pharmacy; serially numbered, opaque, sealed envelopes; or other description that contained elements convincing of concealment)

Note: Because there is evidence that the quality of allocation concealment particularly affects the results of studies, two reviewers scored this quality on the scale used by Schulz et al[28] as shown above. Where the method used to conceal allocation was not clearly reported, the authors were contacted, if possible, for clarification. Moreover, the scores allocated were compared and differences were resolved.

Table 18.10 Characteristics of the Studies

Study	Participants	Interventions	AC
Borzotta et al, 1994[29]	Fifty-nine patients with head injury (including multiple injuries), 18 to 60 years, GCS score ≤8 persisting over 24 hours. Patients with spinal cord injury, preexisting metabolic disease, renal failure, or inflammatory bowel disease were excluded.	1. TPN; $n = 21$ 2. Jejunal EN; $n = 28$	B
Chiarelli et al, 1996[38]	Twenty-four patients requiring intensive care after major surgery or suffering from severe head injury or major neurological impairment	All patients initially received TPN. After 4 days they were weaned to: 1. Total EN ($n = 12$); or 2. Mixed EN and TPN ($n = 12$). In this group 50% of calories came from EN and 50% from TPN.	B
Grahm et al, 1989[32]	Thirty-two patients with severe head injury and a GCS of ≤10 persisting for 6 hours	1. Early jejunal EN (under fluoroscopic, within 36 hours); $n = 17$ 2. EN (gastric feedings initiated after day 3 or when gastric function returned); $n = 15$	C
Hadley et al, 1986[31]	Forty-five patients with isolated head injury GCS ≤10 at 6 hours postinjuries, age 16–61	Nutritional support within 48 hours as either: 1. TPN (8.5% amino acid, 25% glucose solution, 10% intralipid twice weekly); $n = 24$ 2. EN (nasogastric, isocal HCN [Meade Johnson, Nutritional Division, Evansville, IN]); $n = 21$	C
Minard et al, 2000[33]	Thirty patients with severe head injury as defined by a GCS score >3 and <11 within 6 hours of injury	1. Early feeding via nasogastric tube placed endoscopically, feeding within 60 hours of injury ($n = 12$). 2. Feeding initiated when gastroparesis resolved ($n = 15$). All patients received an immune-enhancing forumla containing supplemental arginine, nucleic acids, fatty acids, and fiber.	B
Nataloni et al, 1999[39]	Thirty patients with head injury who were expected to stay in the ICU for more than 3 days. Patients were excluded if they had diabetes mellitus, renal or hepatic failure, pancreatitis, abdominal surgery, or brain death.	1. EN 2. Parenteral nutrition in all patients feeding was initiated 2 days after ICU admission and continued until ICU discharge.	B
Rapp et al, 1983[13]	Thirty-eight head-injured patients. Patients with severe extracranial injuries that were expected to alter metabolic demands or to delay use of standard enteral nutrition, such as abdominal organ injury, were excluded from the study.	1. TPN; within 48 hours, 42.5 g/L of amino acid, 25% dextrose, 250–500 soybean oil ($n = 20$) 2. Standard EN; nasogastric, Vital (a high nitrogen product) ($n = 18$)	B
Sacks et al, 1995[34]	Nine patients with severe, closed head injury, 18 to 65 years, GCS 3–12 Patients with hepatic dysfunction, hypertriglycemia, infection, or significant intraabdominal injuries were excluded.	1. Early parenteral nutrition at day 1 ($n = 4$) 2. Delayed parenteral nutrition at day 5 ($n = 5$)	C
Suchner et al, 1996[40]	Thirty-four patients with traumatic head injury or spontaneous cerebral lesion undergoing an emergency craniotomy (trauma 13, spontaneous cerebral lesion 21) with a GCS ≤10 (but two exceptions). Patients with hepatic or renal failure, diabetes mellitus, hypermetabolic desease, or malnutrition were excluded.	Initiated on the first postoperative day as either: 1. TPN; glucose 10, 20, 40%; amino acid 10%; lipid 20% (half MCT) ($n = 17$) 2. Total EN; nasogastric, OSMOLITE (Abbott Nutrition, Columbus, OH) an Isotonic balanced diet ($n = 17$)	B
Taylor et al, 1999[35]	Eighty-two patients with severe head injury necessitating mechanical ventilation, best GCS >3, and over 10 years old were included in the trial.	1. Enhanced EN ($n = 41$) 2. Standard EN ($n = 41$) EN was started from day 1 in both groups of patients. In the intervention group (enhanced	C

(Continued on page 350)

Table 18.10 *(Continued)*

Study	Participants	Interventions	AC
	Patients with a gunshot head wound, presence of organ failure, potentially fatal disease pre–head injury, or moribund state immediately post–head injury were excluded.	EN) patients were started at the feed rate that would meet their full estimated requirements from day 1.	
Young et al, 1987[30]	Fifty-one brain injured patients with peak 24 hour GCS score of 4–10	1. TPN within 48 hours ($n = 23$) 2. EN via nasogastric or nasoduodenal routes, Ensure Plus (Abbott Nutrition) or TraumaCal (Meade-Johnson, Evansville, IN) ($n = 28$)	B

Abbreviations: EN, enteral nutrition; GCS, Glasgow Coma Scale; MCT, medium chain triglyceride; TPN, total parenteral nutrition.

(early enteral feeding versus late enteral feeding), Rapp et al 1983[13] (early TPN versus traditional EN), Sacks et al 1995[34] (early TPN versus delayed TPN), Taylor et al 1999[35] (standard EN versus enhanced EN), and Young et al 1987[36] (early TPN versus delayed EN). The Taylor et al study[35] was included in the early versus late comparison as it was felt that the comparison of standard EN versus enhanced EN meant in effect that the patients in the enhanced EN group were getting more enteral feeding sooner than those in the standard EN group. The Young et al study[36] was reported in two articles, one with the first 58 patients and the second with the total 96 patients. However, deaths were only reported in the first article with 58 patients; so this report was used for the purpose of the metaanalysis. The Hausmann et al study[37] was excluded because this trial looked at a combined enteral/parenteral regimen compared with TPN. The combined regimen did not state what percentage of calories was provided by which method. However, it did appear that more than 50% of calories were provided by TPN, which, according to the reviews inclusion criteria, would have classified it as TPN, thereby making the comparison TPN versus TPN.

Of the seven trials addressing the timing of support, data on mortality were obtained for all seven trials (284 participants). The relative risk (RR) for death with early nutritional support was 0.67 (95% CI 0.41–1.07) (**Fig. 18.4A**). Data on disability were available for three of the seven trials (Hadley et al 1986,[31] Rapp et al 1983,[13] Taylor et al 1999[35]). The RR for death or disability at the end of follow-up was 0.75 (0.50–1.11) (**Fig. 18.4B**). One study (Taylor et al 1999)[35] reported a median number of days of hospital stay and one study (Grahm et al 1989)[32] reported the length of stay in the ICU. The study by Minard et al[33] reported median length of stay in the ICU and in the hospital. The data on the incidence of infection were presented in several different ways in different trials and were therefore unable to conform to a metaanalysis. These data are presented in **Table 18.11**.

The Route of Feeding: Parenteral versus Enteral

The route of the nutritional intervention was looked at in the following trials: Borzotta et al [29] (TPN versus jejunal EN), Chiarelli et al[38] (all patients received TPN; then one group weaned to total EN and one group had mixed TPN and EN. Because the enteral calories did not exceed 50% of the total intake, this group was classified as TPN), Hadley et al[31] (TPN versus NG EN), Nataloni et al[39] (EN versus TPN), Rapp et al[13] (TPN versus EN), Suchner et al[40] (TPN versus EN—both started at the same time), and Young et al[36] (TPN versus EN).

Seven trials were found that compared parenteral nutrition versus EN. Because early support often involves parenteral nutrition, three of the seven trials were also included in the previous analyses.

Five of the trials reported mortality (Borzotta et al,[29] Chiarelli et al,[38] Hadley et al,[31] Rapp et al,[13] Young et al[30]), with a total of 207 participants. The RR for mortality at the end of the follow-up period was 0.66 (0.41–1.07) (**Fig. 18.5A**). The RR for death or disability was 0.69 (95% CI 0.40–1.19) from two of the five trials (Hadley et al,[31] Rapp et al[13]) (**Fig. 18.5B**). Two trials (Borzotta et al,[29] Chiarelli et al[38]) reported the length of hospital stay. The data on the length of the hospital stay and infection are presented in **Table 18.12**.

Enteral Nutrition: Jejunal versus Gastric

There was only one trial (Graham et al)[32] in this category. There were no deaths in this trial and the RR is not estimable.

Discussion

This systematic review summarizes the evidence from randomized, controlled trials of nutritional support following head injury.

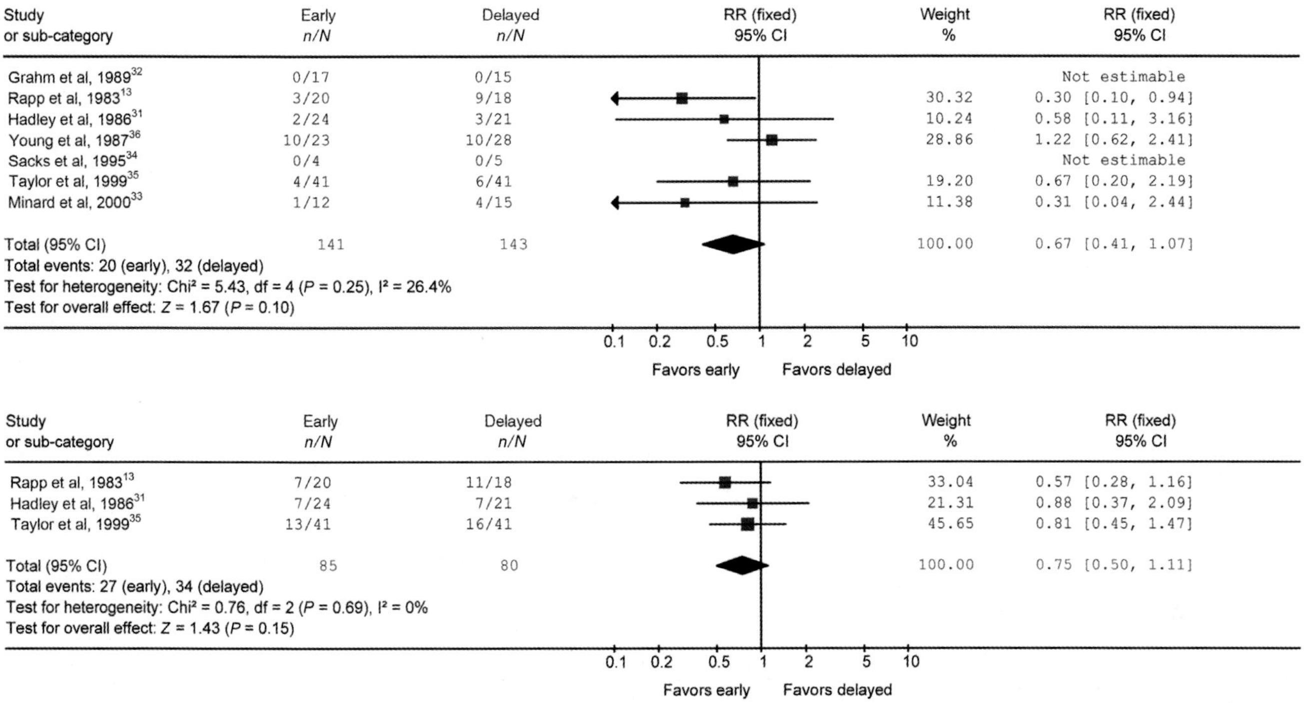

Fig. 18.4 (A) Result of comparison (1) Timing of intervention: early versus delayed. Outcome: mortality at the end of follow-up. **(B)** Result of comparison (2) Timing of intervention: early versus delayed. Outcome: poor outcome at the end of follow-up. CI, confidence interval; RR, relative risk.

Table 18.11 Comparison of Studies for the Timing of Nutritional Support: Early versus Delayed

Study	Outcome	Preferable
Length of Hospital Days		
Grahm et al, 1989[32]	The median length of ICU stay was 7 days (range 4–19 days for the early group and 10 days for the control group).	Early
Minard et al, 2000[33]	The average length of ICU stay was 18.5 days in the early group and 11.3 days in the late group. When deaths were excluded the average length of stay was 19.3 days in the early group and 11.7 days in the late group.	Delayed
Taylor et al, 1999[35]	The early enhanced EN group achieved discharge more quickly (median days to discharge 30 versus 46 for the control group).	Early
Infection		
Grahm et al, 1989[32]	In the early jejunal EN group ($n = 17$) 3 patients had infections (pneumonia, 2; bronchitis, 1). In the delayed EN group ($n = 15$) there was a total of 14 infections reported in 10 patients (3, pneumonia; 10, bronchitis; 1, ventriculitis).	Early
Hadley et al, 1986[31]	In the TPN group ($n = 24$) there was a total of 17 bacterial infections. In the NG group ($n = 21$) there was a total of 15 bacterial infections. These infections occurred in 25 patients; however, it is not reported how many of those patients were in each group. Only the total number of infections for each group is reported.	No judgment
Minard et al, 2000[33]	In the early nutrition group ($n = 12$) 6 patients developed pneumonia and in the late group ($n = 15$) 7 patients developed pneumonia.	No difference
Sacks et al, 1995[34]	In the early TPN group ($n = 4$) 3 patients developed an infection. In the delayed TPN group ($n = 5$) 4 patients developed an infection. This information was obtained on contact with the author.	No difference
Taylor et al, 1999[35]	One patient in each group suffered aspiration pneumonia (confirmed by tracheal aspiration of feed). Pneumonia from all causes occurred in 63% of the delayed group and 44% of the early group.	Early

(Continued on page 352)

Table 18.11 *(Continued)*

Study	Outcome	Preferable
Young et al, 1987[36]	The incidence of infections was recorded as percentages. In the TPN group ($n = 23$), no patients had sepsis, 26.1% got a urinary tract infection, and 26.1% had pneumonia. In the EN group ($n = 28$) 10.7% had sepsis, 25% had a urinary tract infection, and 32.1% had pneumonia. Septicemia was defined by fever, increased WBC count, and positive blood cultures.	Early

Abbreviations: EN, enteral nutrition; ICU, intensive care unit; NG, nasogastric; TNP, total parenteral nutrition; WBC, white blood cell.

Timing of nutritional support is strongly influenced by the type of feeding used. Parenteral nutritional was usually started between 24 and 72 hours of the injury, but most often within 48 hours of the injury. In the case of enteral (NG tube) feeding, nutritional support was typically started much later when bowel sounds could be heard. Bowel sounds were usually detected between 3 and 5 days of injury. Jejunal enteral feeding, however, could be started earlier despite poor gastric emptying. This review addressed the timing and route of nutritional support. There was a trend toward improved survival and reduced disability with early support, but the trials were small and the precision of the point estimates was low.

The pooled results from trials comparing parenteral nutrition and EN suggested a trend toward better outcomes with parenteral nutrition, despite the low precision of the point estimates for mortality. In this comparison, the trials by Hadley et al,[31] Rapp et al,[13] and Young et al[30] used NG tube feeding for the enteral arm of the trial. In which case, the observed effects may be explained by the timing rather than the route of feeding.

If patients are on TPN for a prolonged period of time, catheter-related infection might emerge more often. Two trials[29,30] reported the effect of route of feeding on the incidence of infection of any type. Although there are statistically no differences between TPN and EN, both trials showed a trend toward fewer infections with TPN than with EN. Three trials[29–31] reported the effect of route of feeding on the occurrence of pneumonia, in which, there was a trend toward a reduction in incidence of pneumonia in the TPN group. Young et al[30] pointed out that the lack of adequate nutrient administration during the first week postinjury in the EN group might account for the greater incidence of septic shock in the EN group, rather than in the TPN group.

The focus of many of the trials included in this review was on nutritional outcomes, and many failed to report the effect of the alternative feeding strategies on

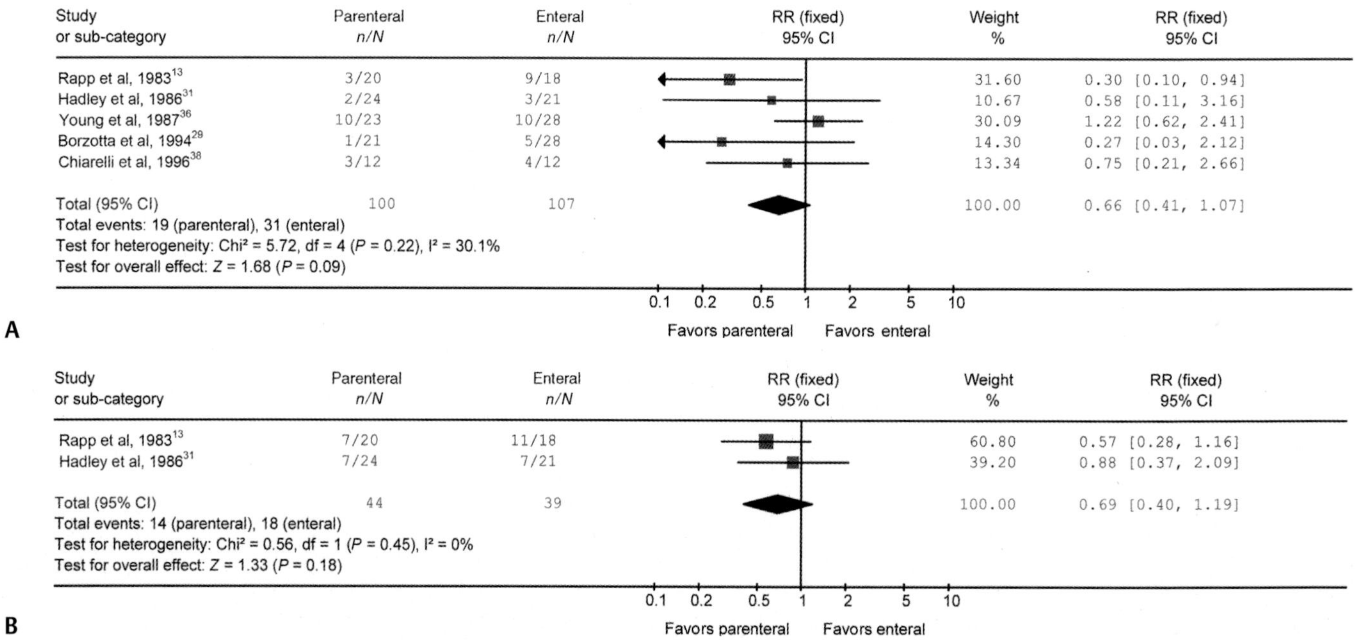

Fig. 18.5 (A) Result of comparison (3) Route of intervention: parenteral versus enteral. Outcome: mortality at the end of follow-up. **(B)** Result of comparison (3) Route of intervention: parenteral versus enteral. Outcome: poor outcome at the end of follow-up. CI, confidence interval; RR, relative risk.

Table 18.12 Comparison of Studies for the Route of Administration of Nutrition: Parenteral versus Enteral

Study	Outcome	Preferable
Length of Hospital Days		
Borzotta et al, 1994[29]	In the TPN group the mean length of hospital stay in days was 39.9 (SD 14) and in the EN group the mean length of stay in days was 39.1 (SD 23.1).	No difference
Chiarelli et al, 1996[38]	The median number of days for hospital stay was given. For the EN group the number was 41 (SD 23) and for the mixed nutrition group the median number of days was 37 (SD 13).	No difference
Infection		
Borzotta et al, 1994[29]	In the TPN group ($n = 21$) there was a total of 39 infections (sinusitis, 6: bronchitis, 6: pneumonia, 9: peritonitis, 1: wound infection, 1: *Clostridium difficile,* 4; UTI, 6; intravascular device, 2; bacteremia, 4). This was a total of 1.86 infections per patient. In the ENT group ($n = 28$), there was a total of 51 infections (meningitis, 2; sinusitis, 3; bronchitis, 6; pneumonia, 15; wound infection, 6; *Clostridium difficile,* 2; UTI, 6; intravascular device, 3; bacteremia, 8). This was a total of 1.89 infections per patient.	No difference*
Chiarelli et al, 1996[38]	In the group weaned to EN ($n = 12$) there were 6 cases of bronchoaspiration, and in the group weaned to a mixture of total EN and PN ($n = 12$) there were 7 cases of bronchoaspiration.	No judgment
Hadley et al, 1986[31]	These are the same data that are in the early versus late comparison.	No judgment
Young et al, 1987[36]	These are the same data that are in the early versus late comparison.	No judgment*

*There was a trend toward a reduction in the incidence of pneumonia in the TPN group.

Abbreviations: EN, enteral nutrition; SD, standard deviation; TPN, total parenteral nutrition; UTI, urinary tract infection.

death and disability. All of the authors of the included trials were contacted in an attempt to obtain any unpublished outcome data, but many of the trialists could not be contacted. Because we were unable to obtain mortality and disability data for all of the included trials, we could not exclude the possibility of bias due to the selective publication of trial outcomes showing stronger treatment effects. Also the length of follow-up varied from 2 weeks to 12 months in those trials that did investigate disability.

It would appear from this review that there have been few trials in nutritional support following head injury, which makes it difficult for the clinician to make an evidence-based decision about the nutritional support in head-injured patients. Overall, the quality of the trials was poor; all of the trials had either inadequate or unclear allocation concealment and most had not attempted to intentionally treat analysis. Indeed, in some of the studies the researchers admitted excluding patients who had died from the final analysis.

Conclusions

The results of this review suggest that early feeding may be associated with fewer infections and a trend toward better outcomes in terms of survival and disability. However, the trials were small and consequently the precision of the point estimates were low. Further trials of nutritional support following head injury are required. These trials should report not only nutritional outcomes but also outcomes such as death, disability, infectious complications, and ICU and hospital lengths of stay. Trials should be structured to be large enough to detect modest but nevertheless clinically important treatment effects.

References

1. Clifton GL, Robertson CS, Grossman RG, Hodge S, Foltz R, Garza C. The metabolic response to severe head injury. J Neurosurg 1984;60(4):687–696
2. Robertson CS, Clifton GL, Grossman RG. Oxygen utilization and cardiovascular function in head-injured patients. Neurosurgery 1984;15(3):307–314
3. Young B, Ott L, Norton J, et al. Metabolic and nutritional sequelae in the non-steroid treated head injury patient. Neurosurgery 1985;17(5):784–791
4. Gadisseux P, Ward JD, Young HF, Becker DP. Nutrition and the neurosurgical patient. J Neurosurg 1984;60(2):219–232
5. Brain Trauma Foundation. Nutritional support of brain-injured patients. J Neurotrauma 1996;13(11):721–729
6. Chiolero R, Schutz Y, Lemarchand T, et al. Hormonal and metabolic changes following severe head injury or noncranial injury. JPEN J Parenter Enteral Nutr 1989;13(1):5–12
7. Long CL, Schaffel N, Geiger JW, Schiller WR, Blakemore WS. Metabolic response to injury and illness: estimation of energy and protein needs

from indirect calorimetry and nitrogen balance. JPEN J Parenter Enteral Nutr 1979;3(6):452–456
8. Wilson RF, Soullier G. The validity of two-hour creatinine clearance studies in critically ill patients. Crit Care Med 1980;8(5):281–284
9. Marie C, Bralet J. Blood glucose level and morphological brain damage following cerebral ischemia. Cerebrovasc Brain Metab Rev 1991;3(1): 29–38
10. Cerra FB, Benitez MR, Blackburn GL, et al. Applied nutrition in ICU patients: a consensus statement of the American College of Chest Physicians. Chest 1997;111(3):769–778
11. Calon B, Pottecher T, Frey A, Ravanello J, Otteni JC, Bach AC. Long-chain versus medium and long-chain triglyceride-based fat emulsion in parental nutrition of severe head trauma patients. Infusions therapie 1990;17(5):246–248
12. Wilson RF, Dente C, Tyburski JG. The nutritional management of patients with head injuries. Neurol Res 2001;23(2–3):121–128
13. Rapp RP, Young DB, Twyman D, et al. The favorable effect of early parenteral feeding on survival in head-injured patients. J Neurosurg 1983;58(6):906–912
14. Ott L, McClain C, Young B. Nutrition and severe brain injury. Nutrition 1989;5(2):75–79
15. Norton JA, Ott LG, McClain C, et al. Intolerance to enteral feeding in the brain-injured patient. J Neurosurg 1988;68(1):62–66
16. Maynard ND, Bihari DJ. Postoperative feeding. BMJ 1991;303(6809): 1007–1008
17. Moore FA, Feliciano DV, Andrassy RJ, et al. Early enteral feeding, compared with parenteral, reduces postoperative septic complications: the results of a meta-analysis. Ann Surg 1992;216(2):172–183
18. Ott L, Annis K, Hatton J, McClain M, Young B. Postpyloric enteral feeding costs for patients with severe head injury: blind placement, endoscopy, and PEG/J versus TPN. J Neurotrauma 1999;16(3):233–242
19. Woien H, Bjork IT. Nutrition of the critically ill patient and effects of implementing a nutritional support algorithm in ICU. J Clin Nurs 2006;15(2):168–177
20. Grimble RF. Nutritional modulation of immune function. Proc Nutr Soc 2001;60(3):389–397
21. Beale RJ, Bryg DJ, Bihari DJ. Related; immunonutrition in the critically ill: a systematic review of clinical outcome. Crit Care Med 1999; 27(12):2799–2805
22. Briassoulis G, Filippou O, Kanariou M, Papassotiriou I, Hatzis T. Temporal nutritional and inflammatory changes in children with severe head injury fed a regular or an immune-enhancing diet: a randomized, controlled trial. Pediatr Crit Care Med 2006;7(1):56–62
23. Falcao de Arruda IS, de Aguilar-Nascimento JE. Benefits of early enteral nutrition with glutamine and probiotics in brain injury patients. linical. Clin Sci (Lond) 2004;106(3):287–292
24. Hatton J, Rapp RP, Kudsk KA, et al. Intravenous insulin-like growth factor-I (IGF-I) in moderate-to-severe head injury: a Phase II safety and efficacy trial. J Neurosurg 1997;86(5):779–786
25. Young B, Ott L, Kasarskis E, et al. Zinc supplementation is associated with improved neurologic recovery rate and visceral protein levels of patients with severe closed head injury. J Neurotrauma 1996;13(1):25–34
26. Yanagawa T, Bunn F, Roberts I, Wentz R, Pierro A. Nutritional support for head-injured patients. Cochrane Database Syst Rev 2000(2): CD001530;2002(3):CD001530
27. Jennett B, Bond M. Assessment of outcome after severe brain damage. Lancet 1975;1(7905):480–484
28. Schulz KF, Chalmers I, Hayes RJ, Altman DG. Empirical evidence of bias: dimensions of methodological quality associated with estimates of treatment effects in controlled trials. JAMA 1995;273(5):408–412
29. Borzotta AP, Pennings J, Papasadero B, et al. Enteral versus parenteral nutrition after severe closed head injury. J Trauma 1994;37(3):459–468
30. Young B, Ott L, Twyman D, et al. The effect of nutritional support on outcome from severe head injury. J Neurosurg 1987;67(5):668–676
31. Hadley MN, Grahm TW, Harrington T, Schiller WR, McDermott MK, Posillico DB. Nutritional support and neurotrauma: a critical review of early nutrition in forty-five acute head injury patients. Neurosurgery 1986;19(3):367–373
32. Grahm TW, Zadrozny DB, Harrington T. The benefits of early jejunal hyperalimentation in the head-injured patient. Neurosurgery 1989;25(5):729–735
33. Minard G, Kudsk K, Melton S, Patton JH, Tolley EA. Early versus delayed feeding with an immune-enhancing diet in patients with severe head injuries. JPEN J Parenter Enteral Nutr 2000;24(3):145–149
34. Sacks GS, Brown RO, Teague D, Dickerson RN, Tolley EA, Kudsk KA. Early nutrition support modifies immune function in patients sustaining severe head injury. JPEN J Parenter Enteral Nutr 1995;19(5): 387–392
35. Taylor SJ, Fettes SB, Jewkes C, Nelson R. Prospective, randomized, controlled trial to determine the effect of early enhanced enteral nutrition on clinical outcome in mechanically ventilated patients suffering head injury. Crit Care Med 1999;27(11):2525–2531
36. Young B, Ott L, Haack D, et al. Effect of total parenteral nutrition upon intracranial pressure in severe head injury. J Neurosurg 1987;67:7 6–80
37. Hausmann D, Mosebach KO, Caspari R, Rommelsheim K. Combined enteral-parenteral nutrition versus total parenteral nutrition in brain-injured patients: a comparative study. Intensive Care Med 1985;11(2): 80–84
38. Chiarelli AG, Ferrarello S, Piccioli A, et al. Total enteral nutrition versus mixed enteral and parenteral nutrition in patients at an intensive care unit. Minerva Anestesiol 1996;62(1–2):1–7
39. Nataloni S, Gentili P, Marini B, et al. Nutritional assessment in head injured patients through the study of rapid turnover visceral proteins. Clin Nutr 1999;18(4):247–251
40. Suchner U, Senftleben U, Eckart T, et al. Enteral versus parenteral nutrition: effect on gastrointestinal function and metabolism. Nutrition 1996;12:13–22

19 Infection

Gregory Mayro, Rafik Samuel, and Bennett Lorber

Although most of the morbidity and mortality that attends traumatic brain injury (TBI) results from the initial trauma, infectious sequelae can have devastating consequences. Indeed, fever itself, regardless of whether it is infectious in origin, is of grave concern in the neurosurgical patient. Elevated body temperature in people who have suffered TBI is a significant predictor of mortality, worse outcome, and extended intensive care unit (ICU) and hospital stays. Consequently, fever deserves diligent attention and appropriate management.[1–3]

Fever, hypoxia, hypotension, acidosis, and elevated intracranial pressure (ICP) from multiple causes, including infection, may be sequelae of TBI. The unpredictability of TBI compels efforts to focus on the prevention and reduction of these potential secondary complications. The spectrum of infections complicating TBI is wide and includes brain abscess, cerebritis, infected intracerebral hematomas, and meningitis as reported in a review by Taha et al[4] of 30 intracranial infections following missile injuries sustained in the Lebanese conflict. In this study, risk factors for infection included extensive brain injury, coma, cerebrospinal fluid (CSF) fistula, inadequate initial debridement or incomplete dural closure, in addition to the trajectory of a missile's path through an air sinus.[4]

We will highlight infectious complications of TBI and will review several common nosocomial infections along with important considerations in the management of fever in the ICU patient (**Table 19.1**).

Subgaleal Abscess

"... even among the walking wounded every scalp wound must be regarded as a potential penetrating lesion of the brain ..."[5]

Lacerations or puncture wounds of the scalp predispose to infections such as cellulitis and, less commonly, subgaleal abscesses by directly inoculating the soft tissue with microbes. Subgaleal abscesses and osteomyelitis remain the most concerning complications of what appears to be superficial trauma. Careful examination of one patient's subgaleal abscess revealed several hairs driven into the periosteum, serving as the nidus for infection.[6] Data on subgaleal abscesses are limited. Goodman et al[6] reported on five cases of subgaleal abscess complicating scalp trauma and noted that the etiology tended to be polymicrobial. Appropriate management requires incision, drainage, and debridement if necessary. Given the polymicrobial nature of these infections, antibiotic coverage should be directed at anaerobic bacteria as well as the more common gram-positive bacteria that are part of the normal skin flora (**Table 19.2**). Though a rare occurrence, subgaleal hematomas resulting from a contusion may subsequently form an abscess[7] and thus require close clinical and radiographic follow-up. Appropriate management of any trauma that causes even minor injury would include appropriate assessment of the need for tetanus prophylaxis.

Table 19.1 Potential Infections Complicating Traumatic Brain Injury

- Wound infection
- Subgaleal abscess
- Cranial osteomyelitis
- Empyema, subdural and extradural
- Brain abscess
- Meningitis

Osteomyelitis

Osteomyelitis is an inflammatory reaction of the bone and bone marrow usually due to bacterial infection. This process may be associated with necrosis and/or new bone formation. It occurs by one of three mechanisms: direct inoculation of pathogens into the bone, bony involvement that follows spread from an adjacent infection (i.e., contiguous osteomyelitis), or hematogenous seeding of the bone. Osteomyelitis may result from the TBI; however, it may follow surgical interventions intended to manage

Table 19.2 Posttraumatic Subgaleal and Brain Abscess: Microbiology and Empirical Antimicrobial Therapy

Common Microbial Pathogens	Empirical Antimicrobial Therapy
Staphylococci (especially *Staphylococcus aureus*), streptococci, gram-negative rods, and anaerobes	Vancomycin + a third-generation cephalosporin*,† +/− metronidazole *or* Vancomycin + meropenem

*Cefotaxime, ceftriaxone

†Use ceftazidime (third-generation) or cefepime (fourth-generation) if *Pseudomonas aeruginosa* is suspected

Table 19.3 Clinical and Laboratory Markers of Cranial Osteomyelitis

- Fever (uncommon)
- Nonhealing or spontaneously draining wound
- Headache
- Local swelling, erythema, or tenderness
- Normal to elevated white blood cell count
- ↑ Erythrocyte sedimentation rate
- ↑ C-reactive protein

the primary injury (e.g., bone resection, bur holes to relieve pressure, halo fixations or other procedures involving pin-tracks or fixation, skin grafts or muscle flaps, etc.). Even seemingly minor trauma or lacerations may cause osteomyelitis as a result of inadequate cleansing and/or wound closure of the initial trauma.[8] Information specifically regarding posttraumatic osteomyelitis of the skull is limited and reflects its low incidence. Most of the information related here reflects what is known about posttraumatic osteomyelitis in general, regardless of the anatomical site. Osteomyelitis risk factors in the setting of an open fracture include the severity of fracture, the degree of bacterial contamination, soft tissue injury severity, and inadequate or delayed (>5 hours) surgical debridement.[9,10] Osteomyelitis may be classified as acute, subacute, or chronic based on the duration of symptoms (<10 days, 10 days to 3 months and >3 months, respectively), but perhaps more clinically relevant is appreciating its potentially indolent presentation. Symptoms may be obvious such as a nonhealing or spontaneously draining wound. However, more subtle signs such as headache, local tenderness, or swelling may occur. Fever is an uncommon finding and, when present, tends to be low grade.[11] The white blood cell count (WBC) may be normal to mildly elevated; the same may be said of the erythrocyte sedimentation rate (ESR).[11] C-reactive protein (CRP) is a more sensitive indicator of inflammation and may be of more diagnostic utility. Both ESR and CRP may be used to track disease activity and/or response to antibiotic therapy (**Table 19.3**). Magnetic resonance imaging (MRI) is a sensitive test to demonstrate osteomyelitis and is the imaging test of choice if there are no contraindications. False-positive MRI findings attributed to postoperative scarring and/or edema have been reported.[12] Computed tomography (CT) may prove definitive in such equivocal situations.

Definitive diagnosis and optimal management of osteomyelitis require pathological and microbiological analysis of bone biopsy specimens taken during debridement of the affected area. Appropriate antibiotic therapy is best determined by susceptibility testing of organisms isolated from bone biopsy specimens. Given the nature of traumatic injury, the microbiology tends to be polymicrobial. Normal skin flora may contaminate the wound in addition to environmental organisms introduced into the wound by the trauma (e.g., shards of metal with rust, soil, etc). Surgical interventions for trauma management broaden the potential microbial etiology to include nosocomial pathogens. The most commonly isolated pathogens are staphylococci or aerobic gram-negative rods[13] (**Table 19.4**).

Management entails adequate debridement of involved bone (craniotomy if necessary) in addition to antimicrobial therapy. In the immediate posttraumatic period, the administration of antibiotics within 6 to 8 hours for open fractures is the standard of care in the United States; prophylactic intravenous antibiotics decreased the incidence of acute or early infection as well as chronic osteomyelitis in a review of patients who had suffered open limb fractures.[14,15] The importance of thorough debridement after the initial injury and during subsequent surgical interventions cannot be overemphasized; no matter the duration of antibiotic administration, poor outcomes may be expected without adequate debridement.[14] Otherwise, assuming a delayed presentation in the patient who

Table 19.4 Posttraumatic and Postneurosurgical* Osteomyelitis: Microbiology and Culture-Directed Antimicrobial Therapy

Predisposing Condition	Common Microbial Pathogens	Antimicrobial Agents
Posttraumatic	*Staphylococcus aureus*	Vancomycin, linezolid, or daptomycin†
	Gram-negative rods	Third-generation cephalosporin‡ or meropenem
	Anaerobic organisms	Metronidazole or meropenem
Postneurosurgical	Methicillin-resistant *S. aureus* (MRSA)	Vancomycin, linezolid, or daptomycin[b]
	Pseudomonas aeruginosa	Third-generation cephalosporin‡ or meropenem

*Microbiology reflects etiology for posttraumatic and postsurgical osteomyelitis in general, not necessarily posttraumatic brain injury.

†Suggested agents presume MRSA isolated.

‡Cefotaxime, ceftriaxone, but can use ceftazidime (third-generation) or cefepime (fourth-generation) if *Pseudomonas aeruginosa* is suspected.

is hemodynamically stable and without evidence of intracranial extension of the infection, empirical antibiotics can be safely withheld until biopsy is performed. Empirical antibiotics in this setting may significantly decrease the culture's yield. After obtaining the specimen (multiple if possible), empirical therapy with vancomycin and cefepime would be sufficient (**Table 19.4**). The duration of antibiotic therapy for osteomyelitis ranges from 4 to 6 weeks after the last debridement. In addition to close clinical follow-up; weekly ESR and CRP levels would assist in monitoring the response to therapy.

Empyema

Another potentially devastating complication of TBI is the development of a subdural or extradural empyema. In one case series, both closed head and penetrating injuries preceded the development of an empyema.[16] Empyemas may result from spread of a contiguous infection (e.g., an otorhinogenic infection, meningitis, a subgaleal abscess or an osteomyelitis that has developed in the vicinity of a prior craniotomy or fracture line), retrograde thrombophlebitis, or, rarely, hematogenous seeding of a subdural hematoma (e.g., septic emboli). However, the neglected or underappreciated scalp wound is more often the explanation for a cranial empyema in the setting of trauma.[16,17]

The distinction between subdural and extradural empyemas is significant. In general, subdural empyemas are more common and more lethal and are considered medical and surgical emergencies. If not urgently drained, subdural empyemas are rapidly fatal, whereas extradural empyemas appear to have a more benign course.[17,18] Subdural empyemas of any cause comprise 15 to 20% of all intracranial infections[19] with mortality rates that range between ~10% and 14%.[16,18,20] For those who survive, 10 to 44% will have permanent neurological sequelae.[19] Though data are limited regarding extradural empyemas, one case series detected a good outcome, as defined by Glasgow outcome score of at least 4 or 5, in 81 of 82 patients with an extradural empyema.[17] Risk factors have not been defined, but presumably inadequate debridement is critical. In a review of 55 posttraumatic empyema cases, 23 patients were described as having "a septic sinus oozing pus at the site of a healed laceration" on presentation.[16] Untreated, empyemas may lead to seizures, osteomyelitis, hydrocephalus, and death.[20] Factors associated with a poor outcome include a delay in recognition and intervention or severe cognitive deficit upon presentation.[21]

Empyemas can present distantly in time from the initial trauma. In two separate case series, patients experienced symptoms for ~19 days (range, 4–60 days) for subdural empyemas[16] and ~10 days (range, 1–49 days) for extradural empyemas prior to presentation.[17] Clinical features can be as subtle as they are menacing with extradural empyemas tending to be less fulminant. The most common symptoms recorded in one case series of posttraumatic patients with subdural empyemas were headache (84%), fever (69%), and neck stiffness (65%).[16] However, subdural empyema presentations can be striking with fevers >39°C, headache, nausea, vomiting, and a rapidly declining mental status.[19] Neurological findings such as depressed levels of consciousness, focal deficits, hemiparesis, and seizures may be found in both types of empyemas but are more common in subdural empyemas.[16,17] Approximately 80% of patients with subdural empyema may also display signs of meningismus.[19] Initial neurological deficits may be reversed with appropriate and swift management[20] (**Table 19.5**).

Table 19.5 Clinical Feature Comparison of Subdural and Extradural Empyemas

Clinical Features	Subdural	Extradural
High-grade fever >39°C	+++	+
Headache, nausea, vomiting	+++	++
Meningismus	+++	+
Rapidly declining mental status	++++	+
Focal neurological findings or seizures	++	+
High mortality rate if untreated	++++	+

++++ Strong correlation

+ Weak correlation

MRI remains the diagnostic test of choice to detect and discern between extradural and subdural empyema and to assess severity. CT is an excellent and expeditious alternative if MRI is not feasible.[16,22] Gram stain and culture analysis of surgically obtained specimens are essential in guiding antimicrobial therapy.

Pathogens implicated in intracranial empyemas include microaerophilic streptococci, anaerobes, and a variety of gram-negative organisms[17,18,23]; infections are often polymicrobial. The organism most commonly isolated in two separate retrospective analyses of cranial empyemas following trauma was *Staphylococcus aureus*[16,17](**Table 19.6**).

Table 19.6 Empyema Microbiology and Empirical Antimicrobial Therapy

Common Microbial Pathogens	Empirical Antibiotic Therapy
Streptococci, staphylococci, gram-negative rods, and anaerobes	Vancomycin + a third-generation cephalosporin[*,†] +/− metronidazole *or* Vancomycin + meropenem

[*]Cefotaxime, ceftriaxone

[†]Use ceftazidime (third-generation) or cefepime (fourth-generation) if *Pseudomonas aeruginosa* is suspected.

Appropriate management entails early recognition, prompt and thorough debridement, and surgical drainage of pus in addition to pathogen-directed parenteral antimicrobial therapy. No randomized, placebo-controlled studies have compared drainage modalities, but data touting the superiority of one modality over the other can be found for both craniotomies[18,20,24–31] and more limited procedures such as bur holes.[21,32–34] In patients with subdural empyemas, Nathoo et al reported that bur hole procedures were associated with increased rates of morbidity and repeat operations.[20] However, in a separate analysis of extradural empyemas, Nathoo et al[17] advocated bur holes or limited craniotomies. From their experience, extradural empyemas tend to be thin, easily drainable, and "never loculated."[17] Whatever method is chosen, ample decompression of the brain and exhaustive drainage of pus will predict the best outcome.[20,35,36] Nathoo et al documented six patients with small extradural empyemas who did not have any signs or symptoms suggestive of infection and were managed successfully without surgical intervention.[17]

Until definitive culture results are known, empirical broad spectrum antibiotics that cover for gram-negative, gram-positive organisms (including methicillin-resistant *S. aureus* [MRSA]) and anaerobes are recommended (**Table 19.6**). Given the gravity of empyemas, particularly subdural empyemas, antibiotics should not be withheld pending acquisition of appropriate specimens for microbiological analysis. There is no ideal duration for antibiotics. After identification of the causative organisms, antibiotics should be continued for a period of time following confirmation of continued clinical improvement and radiographic resolution of the empyema.

Brain Abscess

An abscess, unlike an empyema, is a well circumscribed collection of pus that is essentially walled off from the tissue in which it is encased. Seeding of the brain parenchyma with subsequent abscess formation can occur by hematogenous spread (e.g., bacteremia), by spread from a contiguous focus of infection (e.g., otogenic, paranasal sinus), or by direct inoculation (e.g., trauma, postoperative). Dural penetration or blunt trauma (less common) may lead to the formation of brain abscesses; closed head injury was the initiating event in 10 of 36 patients who developed brain abscess in one case series.[37] Children have developed frontal lobe abscesses following penetrating orbital trauma from pencil tips or wooden toys.[38–40] Abscess is a relatively rare complication of TBI; rates of occurrence range from ~2 to ~3%.[4,41,42] Since the 1970s, mortality rates of brain abscesses in general, have ranged from 0 to 24%; for those who survive, 20 to 70% experience neurological complications.[43] Poor prognostic factors include a short duration of symptoms prior to presentation, and significant changes in or a rapidly declining mental status.[44,45] If left untreated, a brain abscess may result in intraventricular rupture, which carries a mortality >80%.[44] Rapid diagnosis and intervention are essential to a better outcome.

Much like other post-TBI infections, the presentation can be delayed and insidious. One study reported a mean interval of 113 days from the initial trauma to the time of diagnosis,[37] and a case report of an 8-year-old boy detailed his presentation 8 years after the triggering accident.[46] Headache is the most common presenting symptom (~70%), followed by changes in mental status and focal neurological deficits; fever may be present (~50%).[43] Subtle personality changes or bizarre behavior may implicate frontal lobe involvement.[47]

The diagnosis relies heavily on a high degree of suspicion and imaging because the usual laboratory markers of infection (e.g., leukocytosis, elevated ESR) may not be present. CT or MRI will demonstrate the abscess or its beginning stages (i.e., cerebritis), but MRI soft-tissue resolution and imaging detail is superior to CT.[48] Lymphoma, toxoplasmosis, brain metastases, and neurocysticercosis may mimic the appearance of an abscess, especially if there are multiple brain abscesses. Definitive antimicrobial therapy will be guided by culture of specimens obtained through aspiration or craniotomy (**Table 19.2**).

Management involves adequate drainage (by craniotomy or something less invasive) and antimicrobials with good CSF penetration. Although there have been reports of successful treatment with antibiotics alone,[49–52] for abscesses >2.5 cm, one case series found that surgical therapy was essential.[53]

Good antimicrobial CSF penetration is essential to achieve effective therapy. Empirical antibiotic recommendations may be found in **Table 19.2**. If the decision is made to include metronidazole for anaerobic coverage, its neurotoxic side effects (i.e., peripheral neuropathy, seizures, depressed mentation, or somnolence) bear special respect in this patient population, particularly in patients with moderate to severe to liver disease.[44]

The recommended duration of intravenous therapy is at least 6 to 8 weeks assuming clinical improvement and radiological resolution.[43,44,54] Serial imaging every ~2 weeks is essential to verify radiological improvement or to prompt further intervention.[54]

Meningitis

Posttraumatic Meningitis

Unlike community-acquired bacterial meningitis in which the initial event is nasopharyngeal colonization with subsequent mucosal invasion and bacteremia that ultimately seeds the central nervous system, traumatic bacterial meningitis involves a dural tear creating a CSF fistula allowing direct introduction of nasopharyngeal or auditory canal flora into the CSF.[55] Despite the dural violation that often accompanies TBI, posttraumatic meningitis is relatively uncommon, with an incidence that ranges from 0.2 to 17.8%.[55] Meningitis is more frequent following basilar skull fracture with reported incidences from ~9 to ~18%.[56–59] Although it is less common, meningitis has also been reported following closed head injuries or blunt trauma.[60] Basilar and front skull fractures and the presence of a CSF leak are among the most commonly cited risk factors for posttraumatic meningitis.[55–59,61,62] The incidence rises when the CSF leak continues beyond 7 days.[63] Anything that increases the inoculation of pathogens into the CSF fluid, such as an increased ICP (perhaps secondary to cerebral edema or Valsalva-like maneuvers) or a fistula that did not close would increase the risk of meningitis.[64] Though there have been conflicting reports, a metaanalysis failed to find any statistically significant difference in the risk of developing meningitis among patients who had CSF rhinorrhea versus those who had CSF otorrhea.[65]

The time to presentation and the findings on presentation are often muddled by coincident neurological sequelae from the initiating trauma. The interval between the initial injury and presentation of meningitis may range from 2 to 4 weeks.[55,60] Signs and symptoms consistent with meningitis such as fever, headache, altered sensorium, and neck stiffness may not be obtainable because of the patient's level of disability or may reflect the trauma and not necessarily an infection.[57,66] Any change in the mental status of a relatively interactive, posttraumatic patient should serve to alert the clinician. Otorrhea and rhinorrhea, although not always a sign of concurrent meningitis, may herald its development.[55] Glucose-containing nasal secretions are indicative of CSF leakage,[67] but the finding would only prompt further diagnostic testing, and the absence of any glucose would not rule out meningitis.[55]

Diagnosis relies on CSF analysis (cell count, glucose and protein levels) or bacterial visualization on Gram stain or isolation by culture. CSF findings consistent with community-acquired bacterial meningitis are presented in **Table 19.7**, but in the posttraumatic or postneurosurgical patient these may be altered. The yield of Gram stain and culture may be significantly less given the likelihood of prior antimicrobial therapy in these patients.

Causative pathogens reflect the normal flora of the nasopharynx, the paranasal sinuses, and/or the external auditory canal.[65] The most common causative organisms for a given mode of injury (blunt vs. penetrating) and a given setting (posttraumatic, postneurosurgical, and CSF shunt-related) are found in **Table 19.8**. Initial management requires antimicrobial therapy and making efforts to reduce elevated ICP (i.e., elevate the head of bed; administer stool softeners and/or antitussive medication as needed; avoid intratracheal suction, endotracheal intubation, hyperventilation, hyperextension of the neck [impedes the free flow of CSF through the foramen magnum], hyperosmolar agents, and high-dose barbiturates; and employ external ventricular drains or CSF shunts, if necessary).[55] Empirical antimicrobial regimens may be found in **Table 19.8**.

Table 19.7 Cerebrospinal Fluid Findings in Patients with Bacterial Meningitis

Cerebrospinal Fluid Parameter	Typical Finding
Opening pressure	200–500 mm H_2O
White blood cell count	1000–5000/mm^3 (range, <100 to >10,000
% neutrophils	≥80%
Protein	100–500 mg/dL
Glucose	≤40mg/dL
CSF:serum glucose	≤0.4
Gram stain	Positive in 60–90%
Culture	Positive in 70–85%

Source: Adapted from Tunkel AR. Bacterial Meningitis. Philadelphia: Lippincott Williams & Wilkins; 2001.

Abbreviations: CSF, cerebrospinal fluid.

There are no data to indicate the best time for surgical intervention in a patient with a persistent CSF leak but without meningitis. Given the fact that most leaks resolve in ~7 days, some clinicians recommend waiting at least 2 weeks before undertaking surgical repair in a patient without evidence of meningitis.[60] Repeat bouts of meningitis in the posttraumatic patient should raise concern that a dural tear has not healed completely and may require surgical intervention.[64]

Most evidence does not support the use of prophylactic antibiotics for the prevention of meningitis in patients with a basilar skull fracture or a CSF leak. In a Cochrane analysis of five randomized, controlled trials and 17 nonrandomized, controlled trials in patients with a CSF leak that compared nonstandardized antibiotic prophylactic regimens with placebo or with no intervention, there was no significant difference in terms of reducing the incidence of meningitis, all-cause mortality, meningitis-related mortality, or the need for surgical correction.[68] Multiple retrospective studies and metaanalyses have failed to show any benefit of prophylactic antibiotics in the setting of a basilar skull fracture or a CSF leak, or even in those with posttraumatic pneumocephalus.[65,69,70] The

Table 19.8 Recommendations for Empirical Antimicrobial Therapy for Purulent Meningitis

Predisposing Factor	Common Bacterial Pathogens	Antimicrobial Therapy
Basilar skull fracture	*Streptococcus pneumoniae, Haemophilus influenzae*, group A *β*-hemolytic streptococci	Vancomycin + third-generation cephalosporin*
Penetrating head trauma	*Staphylococcus aureus*, coagulase-negative staphylococci (especially *Staphylococcus epidermidis*), aerobic gram-negative rods (including *Pseudomonas aeruginosa*)	Vancomycin + cefepime or ceftazidime or meropenem
Postneurosurgery	Aerobic gram-negative rods (including *P. aeruginosa*), *S. aureus*, coagulase-negative staphylococci (especially *S. epidermidis*)	Vancomycin + cefepime or ceftazidime or meropenem
CSF shunt	Coagulase-negative staphylococci (especially *S. epidermidis*), *S. aureus*, aerobic gram-negative rods (including *P. aeruginosa*), *Propionibactirium acnes*	Vancomycin + cefepime or ceftazidime or meropenem†

Source: Adaptedfrom Tunkel et al. Practice guidelines for the management of bacterial meningitis. Clin Infect Dis 2004;39:1267–1284. Reprinted by permission.

Abbreviation: CSF, cerebrospinal fluid.

*Ceftriaxone or cefotaxime

†In infants and children, vancomycin alone is reasonable unless Gram stains reveal the presence of gram-negative rods.

case for not using prophylactic antibiotics in this setting is made stronger by the finding that CSF leaks may spontaneously resolve 7 to 10 days after fracture.[59,71] Because there was no statistically significant difference in the risk of meningitis between patients who had dural tears repaired acutely and patients whose leaks resolved spontaneously within 7 days of the initial trauma,[57] it seems justifiable to withhold antibiotics and to closely follow the posttraumatic patient with a CSF leak.

Postneurosurgical Meningitis

In the postneurosurgical setting not involving trauma, meningitis is uncommon. In clean neurosurgical procedures with prophylactic antibiotics, the rate of bacterial meningitis ranges from 0.5 to 0.7%, whereas for clean-contaminated procedures the rate ranges from 0.4 to 2.0%.[55] Although CSF leakage remains a risk factor in both the posttraumatic and postneurosurgical setting, the pathophysiology in the latter has more to do with microbial colonization or localized infection in a sinus or at the site of an incision or device (e.g., CSF shunt, EVD, or ICP).[55] In a retrospective analysis of over 6000 patients, excluding cases that were associated with an EVD or CSF shunt, postcraniotomy independent risk factors for bacterial meningitis included the presence of a CSF leak, male sex, surgical duration >4 hours and concomitant surgical incision.[72] Risk factors in the setting of transsphenoidal surgery (in addition to the surgery itself)[73] include postoperative CSF rhinorrhea and radiological evidence of sinusitis.[74]

Recognition of meningitis in the postneurosurgical patient may be difficult because much of the clinical picture may be attributed to surgical or traumatic sequelae.[57,75] Presentation may occur as early as 10 days after surgery.[55] A review of 70 patients with meningitis following neurosurgery failed to show any statistically significant distinguishing features among those having bacterial meningitis, chemical meningitis, or meningitis of indeterminate cause with regard to temperature, fever ≥7 days, headache, vomiting, postoperative seizure, somnolence, confusion, agitation, or nuchal rigidity.[65] Again, fever or subtle changes in behavior or mental status may be the only indications of meningitis.

Diagnosis relies primarily on CSF analysis; however, interpretation can be complicated. Given that these patients have commonly been treated with multiple courses of antibiotics, the yield of routine CSF Gram stains and cultures can be significantly affected; CSF cultures may be negative in up to 70% of cases of bacterial meningitis.[76,77] Additionally, postneurosurgical CSF profiles in bacterial and aseptic (also known as chemical meningitis) are similar.[55] However, some studies have attempted to reveal subtle distinctions. A retrospective analysis of 70 postneurosurgical patients found that a CSF WBC >7500/mL and a CSF glucose level <10 mg/dL were never present in patients with chemical meningitis.[78] A retrospective study of 73 postneurosurgical patients who had undergone a lumbar puncture within 40 days of surgery found that CSF lactate levels ≥4.0 mmol/L, when compared with CSF to blood glucose ratios ≤0.4, had higher sensitivity (88% vs. 77%), specificity (98% vs. 87%), and positive (0.96 vs. 0.77) and negative (0.94 vs.0.87) predictive values for bacterial meningitis.[79] A CSF lactate ≥4.0 mmol/L should prompt consideration of empirical antibiotics in postneurosurgical patients pending culture results.[80]

Causative pathogens are most commonly gram-negative bacteria and staphylococci (**Table 19.8**).[72,80] In one report of gram-negative rod meningitis following neurosurgery, the most common bacteria were *Klebsiella pneumoniae, Enterobacter cloacae,* and *Escherichia coli.*[81]

Definitive treatment would entail antibiotic therapy tailored to the causative pathogen (**Table 19.8**). There are no randomized trials that have determined the best length of treatment. One review of gram-negative bacterial meningitis in the posttraumatic and postneurosurgical setting revealed no treatment failures in patients who received appropriate parenteral antibiotics for 14 days after the last positive culture.[81] In most cases, assuming appropriate clinical response, therapy would be at least 14 to 21 days.

Although it is widely accepted that prophylactic antibiotics in the setting of a craniotomy decreases associated wound infection rates,[82] two retrospective studies did not show a statistically significant decrease in the incidence of meningitis.[72,83] Additional analysis revealed that prophylaxis seemed to select for resistant organisms.[83] Nevertheless, given the increasing incidence of MRSA in the hospital setting, perioperative antibiotic prophylaxis with vancomycin 15 mg/kg given 2 hours prior to craniotomy and once again 12 hours later is justified.

Postoperative external lumbar drainage (ELD) in patients who had transsphenoidal surgery and intraoperative evidence of a CSF to decrease the risk of postneurosurgical meningitis has also been explored. In a prospective, nonrandomized study, ~1.0% (1 out of 70) patients developed meningitis in the ELD-treated. These findings, although provocative, require further study.[84]

Infections Due to CSF Shunts, External Ventricular Drains, and ICP Monitors

TBI sequelae such as cerebral edema, hydrocephalus, hemorrhage, and increased ICP often require diagnostic and therapeutic interventions that carry their own risk of infection. Infections can result from microbial colonization at the time of implantation of CSF shunts, external ventricular drains (EVDs), and ICP monitors (ICPMs).[85] CSF shunts may also become infected by retrograde bacterial invasion from the distal end of the shunt by breakdown of the wound or skin overlying the shunt and by hematogenous seeding.[86] Each aforementioned device is capable of causing meningitis or ventriculitis, but only CSF shunt infection may result in peritonitis, bacteremia, or vascular shunt-related nephritis (estimated to occur in 4 to 14% of patients).[86] The incidence of infection ranges from 0.3 to 39% for CSF shunts[87] and 0 to 22% for EVDs.[86] Data regarding ICPMs are limited, but the rate of infection is presumably very low.

One retrospective study found no evidence of infection in 95 patients who were also receiving continuous antibiotic prophylaxis.[88]

Risk factors for CSF shunt infection include the presence of a postoperative CSF leak, premature birth, intraoperative use of a neuroendoscope, nonsterile handling of the shunt system, low level of neurosurgical experience, and procedure duration.[86,89,90] Risk factors for EVD-related infection include duration of catheterization (>5 days), ventriculostomy irrigation, craniotomy, depressed cranial fracture with CSF leak, intraventricular and subarachnoid hemorrhage, EVD site leakage, drain blockage, and systemic infection.[91–93] The type of drainage, lumbar versus ventricular, was not found to influence the risk of bacterial meningitis.[92] In a retrospective study of 255 patients who had an ICPM, reduced rates of infection were found when employing a subarachnoid screw (7.5%) compared with a subdural cup catheter (14.9%) or a ventriculostomy catheter (21.9%).[94]

Device-related ventriculitis and meningitis may have an indolent presentation characterized most frequently by headache, nausea, lassitude, or changes in mental status.[86] Fever may not be evident, and meningeal signs and symptoms are uncommon.[86] CSF shunt infections, by virtue of their distal placement in the vascular, peritoneal, or pleural space, may present with another constellation of symptoms. A ventriculoatrial shunt infection associated with bacteremia might present with fevers, chills, nausea, and tachycardia. Abdominal pain or bloating may be a clue to a ventriculoperitoneal shunt-related peritonitis.[95] Skin overlying the implanted shunt that appears erythematous, tender, swollen, or that has purulent drainage, may indicate a subcutaneous or deeper infection.

Diagnosis of ventriculitis or meningitis rests primarily on CSF analysis including Gram stain, culture, cell count with differential, and levels of glucose and protein. Direct shunt samples offer a better culture yield (~90%)[96] when compared with specimens obtained via lumbar punctures (58% in VA shunts and 79% in VP shunts).[97] In VA-shunt-related settings, blood cultures should be obtained as they are positive in >90% of cases.[95]

The most common cause of CSF shunt infections is a coagulase-negative staphylococcus (*Staphylococcus epidermidis*), followed by *S. aureus* and then aerobic gram-negative rods.[86,92,98] *S. epidermidis* was also the most common isolate in a prospective study involving ICPMs.[99]

Corynebacterium spp., historically considered contaminants, are increasingly recognized as pathogens in neurosurgical device–related infection[100,101] (**Table 19.8**).

Optimal management requires removal of the infected shunt/EVD/ICPM, appropriate antimicrobial therapy, and continued CSF drainage.[85,86,102,103] Exceptions to this may include isolation of the community-acquired pathogens *Neisseria meningitidis* or *Streptococcus pneumoniae*, coagulase-negative staphylococcal infection,[104,105] a VP shunt infection whose distal portion may be externalized,[86,106] and Ommaya reservoir infections.[107]

The same principles that guide antimicrobial therapy in meningitis, empyema, and abscess apply here; CSF penetration is essential. Low cure rates with antibiotics alone have been attributed to the ability of coagulase-negative staphylococci to adhere to the foreign body and to produce a "slime" that in essence creates a buffer to antibiotics.[108,109] Although no randomized trials have demonstrated the benefit of intraventricular therapy, case reports have suggested the utility of such an approach along with systemic antibiotics in complicated infections[105] (**Table 19.9**).

Initial antimicrobial therapy pending stain and culture results should be vancomycin. Limited data exist to support a standard duration of therapy, but, assuming clinical improvement, continuing appropriate antibiotics for 7 to 10 days after documented culture-negative CSF or after the device has been removed should be adequate.[110]

If transitioning from an EVD to a CSF shunt, or if reimplanting a CSF shunt after treatment for an infection, consultation with an infectious diseases specialist is recommended as the timing of these will rest on the causative pathogen and the duration of ongoing infection, and may entail continued monitoring of CSF drainage, empirical antibiotics, and repeated CSF sampling.[111]

Despite the increased risk associated with catheterization >5 days, a randomized trial of 103 patients demonstrated that routine EVD changes at 5 day intervals did not decrease the risk of EVD-associated infection.[112]

The benefit of continuous antimicrobial therapy for the duration of catheterization has been mixed. In one case series, the rate of infection for patients who received continuous prophylactic antibiotics was virtually identical to those who received periprocedural dosing.[113] A randomized trial of prophylactic antibiotics for the duration of EVD catheterization found a significant reduction in the rates of infection (11% vs. 3%); however, this came at the cost of an increased incidence of resistant organisms.[114] At this point, the evidence would argue against continuous prophylaxis.

Evidence seems to support the use of antibiotic-impregnated ventricular catheters (AIVCs). In one prospective, randomized trial involving 288 patients, EVDs impregnated with minocycline and rifampin were half as likely to become colonized compared with the control catheters (~18% vs. ~37%, respectively, $p < 0.0002$). CSF culture-proved infections were also reduced (~9% in control cohort vs. ~1% in AIVC cohort, $p = 0.002$); however, ~95% of the patients in each group received systemic antibiotics (~13 days in control group vs. ~11 days in AIVC group).[115] Furthermore, a prospective observational study of 139 patients admitted to the neuro-ICU (NICU) determined that the culture-proved infection rate in the AIVC (minocycline/rifampin) group was 0.88%, lending support to the use of AIVC.[116]

A metaanalysis of 36 studies reached no consensus regarding antibiotic prophylaxis for ICPMs and EVDs.[117] A metaanalysis involving CSF shunts found a statistically significant reduction in risk of CSF shunt–related infection (~50%) with the use of antibiotic prophylaxis in settings where the baseline rate of infection was ≥5%.[118]

Because a foreign body is being placed in a sterile space, because of the increasing prevalence of MRSA, and because of the device-related morbidity and costs of these infections, the administration of prophylactic vancomycin 15mg/kg given 2 hours prior to device placement and once again 12 hours later is justified.

Table 19.9 Antimicrobial Agents Administered by the Intraventricular Route*

Antimicrobial Agent	Daily Intraventricular Dose
Vancomycin	5–20 mg†
Gentamicin	1–8 mg
Tobramycin	5–20 mg
Amikacin	5–50 mg‡
Colistin	10 mg[a]
Quinupristin/dalfopristin	2–5 mg
Amphotericin	0.1–0.5 mg§

Source: From Tunkel et al. Practice guidelines for the management of bacterial meningitis. Clin Infect Dis 2004;39:1267–1284. Reprinted by permission.

*There are no specific data that define the exact dose of intraventricular antimicrobial agents that should be used in cerebrospinal fluid shunt infections.

†Most studies have used a 10 to 20 mg dose.

‡Thirty milligrams daily is the usual intraventricular dose.

§Dosage for *Candida* shunt infection.

Fever and Nosocomial Infections

Many neurotrauma patients require central venous catheters, urinary catheters, and prolonged intubation. These invasive procedures put patients at high risk for infections. The most common infections acquired in an ICU setting include ventilator-associated pneumonia, bacteremia, urinary tract infections (UTIs), *Clostridium difficile* diarrhea, and infected decubitus ulcers. Fever in these patients is not always due to infection. Some noninfectious causes of fever include reactions to medications, thromboembolic disease, and transfusion reactions (**Table 19.10**).

Table 19.10 Common Nosocomial Infections in the ICU

- Pneumonia (including ventilator and aspiration pneumonia)
- Bacteremia (including indwelling catheter–related infections)
- Urinary tract infections
- *Clostridium difficile* diarrhea
- Infected decubitus ulcers

Pneumonia

Nosocomial pneumonia or hospital-acquired pneumonia (HAP) is defined as a pneumonia that develops beyond 48 to 72 hours after admission to the hospital.[119] The highest risk of HAP is in those patients who are being supported by mechanical ventilation (VAP), where the risk of infection is up to 7 per 1,000 hospitalizations.[120] In addition, HAP carries a 20 to 50% mortality rate.[121] The most common organisms causing VAP include the gram-negative bacteria and *S. aureus*[122] (**Table 19.11**). It is however; very important to know which organisms are prevalent in your NICU. Multiple risk factors increase the likelihood of HAP or VAP. Those particular to the NICU include intracranial pressure monitoring, and depressed consciousness and age over 70 years.[123]

Diagnosis of VAP may be challenging, and diagnostic criteria usually include a new infiltrate on chest x-ray associated with fever, leukocytosis, and purulent endotracheal secretions. In one study of HAP, <75% of the cases were accurately predicted. For VAP, there is <50% accuracy.[124] The main reasons why these criteria are not more sensitive is that there are many causes of each of the classic predictors of pneumonia that may confound the picture. Bronchoscopy has been used to help make the diagnosis of VAP. Multiple studies have investigated the utility of bronchoalveolar lavage, protected brush sampling, and quantitative measures of bacteria. Based on a consensus review, there are not enough data to determine which technique is best.[119]

Treatment of HAP usually is based on empiric antibiotics with subsequent adjustment after culture results have returned. It has been shown that waiting for results of the cultures before starting antibiotics or choosing incorrect antibiotic coverage is associated with higher mortality than treating broadly initially and deescalating the antibiotics later.[125] Therefore, coverage should include vancomycin or linezolid for MRSA combined with a fourth-generation cephalosporin, carbapenem, fluoroquinolone, or β-lactam/β-lactamase inhibitor to cover gram-negative rods, including *Pseudomonas*. Duration of antibiotic therapy for HAP has been studied, and it appears that 8 days of treatment is as efficacious as 2 weeks. However, those patients with *Pseudomonas* spp. had a higher rate of recurrence in the shorter duration group.[122]

Table 19.11 Nosocomial Pneumonia Pathogens and Recommended Antimicrobial Therapy

Bacteria	Rate (%)*	Recommended Antibiotic†
MRSA	33	Vancomycin or linezolid
Pseudomonas spp	14	Cefepime, carbapenem, ciprofloxacin, or piperacillin/tazobactam
Enteric gram-negative rods‡	24	Cefepime, carbapenem, ciprofloxacin, or piperacillin/tazobactam
Resistant *Acinetobacter* spp		Carbapenem, tigecycline, or colistin

*May vary within each institution

†Susceptibilities vary within each institution.

‡*Escherichia coli*, *Klebsiella* spp, *Enterobacter* spp, etc.

Abbreviations: MRSA, methicillin-resistant *S. aureus*.

Bacteremia

Bacteremia in the ICU setting may complicate central venous or arterial catheters (64%) or may follow dissemination of infection from another site (36%). The most common causes of bloodstream infection are *S. epidermidis*, *S. aureus*, *Enterococcus* spp., and *Candida* spp. The gram-negative rods play a lesser role.[126]

Treatment of bacteremia depends on the specific organism, the duration of the bacteremia, and whether or not the catheter is removed. For coagulase-negative staphylococci, treatment includes vancomycin for 5 to 7 days if the catheter is removed or 14 days if it is not removed. *S. aureus* carries significant risk of disseminated disease. Treatment of *S. aureus* bacteremia requires removal of the catheter and a minimum of 14 days of therapy with vancomycin or if susceptible, nafcillin. If the bacteremia is prolonged, or if the catheter is not removed, treatment should be for 4 weeks unless a transesophageal echocardiogram demonstrates no valvular lesions.[127] Enterococcal bacteremia should be treated with ampicillin if susceptible, vancomycin if ampicillin resistant, or daptomycin or linezolid if vancomycin resistant. The duration of therapy includes 14 days of therapy and removal of the catheter[128] (**Table 19.12**).

Candidemia should be treated with an antifungal agent and removal of the catheter. Patients with candidemia should have an endophthalmologic examination ~2 weeks after the diagnosis of candidemia to check for endophthalmitis.[129]

Gram-negative bacteremia is less common but may be more associated with sepsis. If the patient is unstable, the catheter should be removed immediately and broad

Table 19.12 Line-related Infections in the ICU

Organisms	Rate (%)*	Antibiotics†	Duration‡
Coagulase-negative staphylococci	35.9	Vancomycin, daptomycin, or linezolid	5–7 days
Staphylococcus aureus	16.8	Vancomycin, daptomycin	14 days
Enterococcus	9.8	Vancomycin, daptomycin, or linezolid	14 days
Candida	10.1	Amphotericin B, fluconazole, or an echinocandin	14 days
Pseudomonas	4.7	Cefepime, carbapenem, ciprofloxacin, or piperacillin/tazobactam	14 days
Enteric gram-negative rods	14.5	Ceftriaxone, cefepime, carbapenem, ciprofloxacin, or piperacillin/tazobactam	14 days
Acinetobacter	1.6	Carbapenem, tigecycline, or colistin	14 days

*May vary within each institution.

†Susceptibilities vary within each institution.

‡Duration based on time from documented clearance of bacteremia.

spectrum coverage with a carbapenem and aminoglycoside may be the best choice. In addition to treatment for 14 days with antibiotics and removal of the catheter, gram-negative bacteremias are more likely to be secondary to a cause other than a catheter-associated bacteremia, and other etiologies of bacteremia should be looked for such as UTI, abdominal source, hepatobiliary source, or decubitus ulcers.[128]

In addition to catheter-related bacteremia, two other forms of catheter infections are recognized. Exit site infections present with purulence at the skin site where the catheter exits. Tunnel infections present with pain, tenderness, and erythema over the subcutaneously tunneled part of the catheter. In these cases, the drainage should be cultured and the line may need to be removed. Antibiotic therapy for 10 to 14 days is recommended, with the antimicrobial based on susceptibilities of the organisms that are isolated.[128]

Urinary Tract Infections

UTIs cause upwards of 40% of nosocomial infections. These infections usually do not directly increase mortality. However, if associated with bacteremia, mortality can reach 20%. The major risk factor for UTI is a urinary catheter. The incidence increases with the duration of the catheter at ~5% per day of catheterization. Other risk factors include female sex, long hospital stay, diabetes, and the presence of another site of infection.[130,131]

Diagnosis of UTI includes a urine culture and urinalysis with microscopy. It is important to sample the fluid from the freshly produced urine and not from the urine collection bag. A urinalysis showing 10 or more WBC/mL is predictive of a UTI. With true infection cultured organism numbers are usually10^5 colony forming unit [CFU]/mL; lesser numbers of organisms should cause the diagnosis of UTI to be questioned.[132] The most common causes of UTI are aerobic gram-negative rods, staphylococci, streptococci, enterococci, and yeast.

For treatment of gram-negative bacteria, a fluoroquinolone or fourth-generation cephalosporin usually is appropriate. For a gram-positive organism, vancomycin may be appropriate; however, the likelihood of vancomycin-resistant enterococci may be increased in patients already on antibiotics. In these patients linezolid or daptomycin may be a better initial choice. If funguria is noted, fluconazole may be a good choice for treatment. Duration of treatment usually is 14 days. In addition, removal of the catheter or replacement may be of benefit in reducing the amount of bacteria or yeast and therefore assisting in treatment.[133]

Clostridium difficile Diarrhea

C. difficile is another very commonly acquired nosocomial pathogen. This organism usually colonizes the gastrointestinal tract after the usual colonizing bacteria are killed by antibiotic use. It can then produce a toxin that leads to a profuse watery diarrhea. In-patients are colonized ~20 to 30% of the time; however, symptomatic disease occurs only in 10 to 20% of those colonized. Risk factors for *C. difficile* diarrhea include older age, hospitalization, and antibiotic use.[134]

Symptoms of disease vary from mild watery diarrhea to severe colitis with toxic megacolon. Typically, disease includes diarrhea, fever, leukocytosis, abdominal pain, and fecal leukocytes in the setting of antibiotic use. Recently, there has been an increase in a more virulent strain of *C. difficile* associated with severe colitis and increased mortality.[135]

The best method for diagnosis includes a cytotoxin assay; however, most laboratories use an enzyme immunoassay, which is specific but has a 10% false-negative rate. Because of the false-negative rate, it may be beneficial to repeat the test two to three times. Another way to make a diagnosis includes endoscopy to visualize the typical finding of yellow plaques termed *pseudomembranes*.[134]

Treatment of *C. difficile* includes removal of the offending antibiotic agent, if possible, in addition to administering either oral metronidazole or oral vancomycin. The usual duration of therapy is 10 days. Both agents have similar efficacy rates around 90 to 97%. Intravenous metronidazole is an alternative if the patient cannot tolerate an oral regimen. Improvement is expected within 3 to 5 days. In a patient receiving metronidazole, if improvement does not occur in that time frame, then a switch from metronidazole to vancomycin is indicated. There has been no demonstrable benefit of using the two agents together. There is also no benefit in using metronidazole or vancomycin as prophylactic agents to prevent *C. difficile* diarrhea.[136,137]

Infected Decubitus Ulcers

Patients who are in the ICU for a prolonged period of time may develop pressure ulcers and tissue necrosis. Colonization of these ulcers may occur and can lead to infection of the underlying soft tissue or even bone with resultant cellulitis, abscess formation, osteomyelitis, or disseminated infection. Organisms isolated from superficial cultures may represent colonization and not reflect the true etiology of an infection. Therefore, diagnosis of infection includes a deep wound culture, optimally a surgical debridement culture. It is also be helpful to review the Gram stain to look for evidence of white cells. Antibiotics should be chosen to target the organisms that are isolated. In addition, débridement of all necrotic tissue, drainage of any abscess, and keeping the wound clean are the keys to successful treatment.

Noninfectious Causes of Fever

There are many causes of fever in the ICU that are not due to infections. Some of the most common causes include drug-related fever, thromboembolic disease, neuroleptic malignant syndrome, adrenal insufficiency, thyrotoxicosis, and transfusion reactions. Some sources have claimed that high temperature (>102°F) points to an infectious etiology, but this is not at all a reliable predictor[138] (**Table 19.13**).

Table 19.13 Common Noninfectious Causes of Fever

- Drug-related fever
- Thromboembolic disease
- Adrenal insufficiency
- Delirium tremens
- Neuroleptic malignant syndrome
- Thyrotoxicosis
- Transfusion reactions
- Central fevers

Drug fever is likely the most common noninfectious cause of fever; however, the true incidence is not known. Fever that begins shortly after initiation of a new medication may be a clue to drug fever; however, this is not always a helpful clue because fever due to drug hypersensitivity may develop weeks after initiation of a drug. If other signs of drug allergy are noted, they may suggest drug-related fever. These include peripheral eosinophilia, bone marrow suppression, elevated liver enzymes (phenytoin), rash, or eosinophiluria.

Thromboembolic disease occurs in ~10 to 30% of patients in an ICU.[139] Patients with pulmonary emboli develop low-grade fever ~14% of the time.[140] In a patient with extremely high fever, tachycardia, and hypertension, thyrotoxicosis, delirium tremens, and neuroleptic malignant syndrome should be considered, especially if routine cultures are negative. In patients who have a history of steroid use and a presentation of hypotension, fever, low sodium, and high potassium, adrenal insufficiency should be suspected. This is easily ruled out by an AM cortisol and an adrenocorticotropic hormone (ACTH) stimulation test.[141]

Initial Antibiotics Prescribed for Infection Control in the NICU

Pending definitive culture and susceptibility results, the initial choice of antibiotics in the NICU depends on multiple factors. The most important of these factors is the antibiogram: the types of bacteria isolated in the unit and their antibiotic susceptibilities. Infection causing bacteria in the ICU setting often vary from hospital to hospital and even from one ICU to another within a single hospital. It is important to be familiar with the pathogens responsible for recent infections within your own particular unit to appropriately select initial therapy. In general, gram-positive infections in the ICU are due to *S. aureus*, coagulase-negative staphylococci, enterococci, and streptococci. Empiric antibiotic coverage for these organisms should be vancomycin. However, if the organism isolated is susceptible to a β-lactam (penicillin or cephalosporin), the β-lactam may be better for that infection.

Table 19.14 Antibiotics Used in the ICU

Agent	Typical Dose Given	Bacteria Covered
Vancomycin	1 g IV every 12 hours*	Staphylococci, enterococci, streptococci
Linezolid	600 mg IV or PO every 12 hours	Same as vancomycin plus VRE
Daptomycin†	4 mg/ kg IV daily for skin and soft tissue infections; 6 mg/kg IV daily for bacteremia	Same as linezolid
Metronidazole	500 mg every 6–12 hours‡	Anaerobes and *Clostridium difficile*
Meropenem	1 g IV every 8 hours for serious infections	*Pseudomonas*, enteric gram-negative rods, acinetobacter, streptococci, anaerobes
Imipenem	500 mg IV every 6 hours for serious infections	*Pseudomonas*, enteric gram-negative rods, acinetobacter, streptococci, anaerobes
Cefepime	2 g IV every 8–12 hours for serious infections	*Pseudomonas*, enteric gram-negative rods
Ciprofloxacin	400 mg IV every 12 hours	*Pseudomonas*, enteric gram-negative rods
Piperacillin/tazobactam	3.375 g IV every 6 hours or 4.5 g IV every 8 hours	*Pseudomonas*, enteric gram-negative rods, enterococcus, anaerobes
Tigecycline	100 mg IV first dose, then 50 mg IV every 12 hours	Enteric gram-negative rods, enterococci (including vancomycin-resistant species), staphylococci, streptococcus, anaerobes
Colistin	2.5 mg/kg IV every 12 hours	*Pseudomonas*, enteric gram-negative rods, acinetobacter
Fluconazole	400 mg IV or PO daily for systemic infections	*Candida albicans*, *C. tropicalis*, *C. parapsilosis*, and most *C. glabrata*
Echinocandins§	Depends on agent‖	All *Candida* spp.
Amphotericin B	0.5–1 mg/kg IV daily	Most *Candida* spp.

*For *Clostridium difficile* infection, start with125 mg PO every 6 hours.

†Do not use for pneumonia.

‡For *C. difficile,* start with 500 mg PO every 8 hours.

§Currently available echinocandins are caspofungin, micafungin, and anidulafungin.

‖Caspofungin dose 70 mg followed by 50 mg daily. Micafungin dose is 150 mg daily. Anidulafungin dose is 200 mg followed by 100 mg daily.

Abbreviations: IV, intravenous; PO, per os (by mouth).

The most common gram-negative organisms isolated include the enteric gram-negatives, *Pseudomonas* spp., and *Acinetobacter* spp. In general, carbapenems, aminoglycosides, fourth-generation cephalosporins, fluoroquinolones, betalactam/betalactamase combinations, and newer agents are effective. **Table 19.14** lists the antimicrobials most likely used in the ICU along with their doses and the bacteria that they are active against.

References

1. Jones PA, Andreas PJD, Midgley S, et al. Measuring the burden of secondary insults in head-injured patients during intensive care. J Neurosurg Anesthesiol 1994;6:4–14
2. Diringer MN, Reaven NL, Funk SE, Uman GC. Elevated body temperature independently contributes to increased length of stay in neurological intensive care unit patients. Crit Care Med 2004;32:1489–1495
3. McIlvoy LH. The effect of hypothermia and hyperthermia on acute brain injury. AACN Clin Issues 2005;16:488–500
4. Taha JM, Saba MI, Brown JA. Intracranial infection after missile injuries to the brain: a report of 30 cases from the Lebanese Conflict. Neurosurgery 1991;29:864–868
5. Cushing H. A study of a series of wounds involving the brain and its enveloping structures. Br J Surg 1918;5:558–684
6. Goodman SJ, Cahan L, Chow AW. Subgaleal abscess: a preventable complication of scalp trauma. West J Med 1977;127:169–172
7. Arana E, Vallcanera A, Santamaria JA, Sanguesa C, Cortina H. *Eikenella corrodens* skull infection: a case report with review of the literature. Surg Neurol 1997;47:389–391
8. Phillips NI, Robertson IJA. Osteomyelitis of the skull vault from a human bite. Br J Neurosurg 1997;11:168–169
9. Patzakis MJ, Wilkins J. Factors influencing infection rate in open fracture wounds. Clin Orthop Relat Res 1989;243:36–40
10. Kindsfater K, Jonassen EA. Osteomyelitis in grade II and III open tibia fractures with late debridement. J Orthop Trauma 1995;9:121–127
11. Gross T, Kaim AH, Regazzoni P, Widmer AF. Current concepts in posttraumatic osteomyelitis: a diagnostic challenge with new imaging options. J Trauma 2002;52:1210–1219
12. Ledermann HP, Kaim A, Bongartz G, Steinbrich W. Pitfalls and limitations of magnetic resonance imaging in chronic posttraumatic osteomyelitis. Eur Radiol 2000;10:1815–1823

13. Berbari EF, Steckleberg JM, Osmon DR. Osteomyelitis. In: Mandell GL, Bennett JE, Dolin R, eds. Mandell, Douglas and Bennett's Principle of Infectious Diseases. Philadelphia: Elsevier Churchill Livingstone; 2005:1322–1332
14. Gosselin RA, Roberts I, Gillespie WJ. Antibiotics for preventing infection in open limb fractures. Cochrane Database Syst Rev 2004;1:CD003764
15. Seligson D, Henry SL. Treatment of compound fractures. Am J Surg 1991;161:693–701
16. Nathoo N, Nadhvi S, van Dellen JR. Traumatic cranial empyemas: a review of 55 patients. Br J Neurosurg 2000;14:326–330
17. Nathoo N, Nadvi S, van Dellen JR. Cranial extradural empyema in the era of computed tomography: a review of 82 cases. Neurosurgery 1999;44:748–753
18. Nathoo N, Nadvi S, van Dellen JR, Gouws E. Intracranial subdural empyemas in an era of computed tomography: a review of 699 cases. Neurosurgery 1999;44:529–536
19. Tunkel AR. Subdural empyema, epidural abscess, and suppurative intracranial thrombophlebitis. In: Mandell GL, Bennett JE, Dolin R, eds. Mandell, Douglas and Bennett's Principle of Infectious Diseases. Philadelphia: Elsevier Churchill Livingstone; 2005:1164–1171
20. Nathoo N, Nadvi S, Gouws E, van Dellen JR. Craniotomy improves outcomes for cranial subdural empyemas: computed tomography-era experience with 699 patients. Neurosurgery 2001;49:872–877
21. Mauser HW, Tulleken CAF. Subdural empyema: a review of 48 patients. Clin Neurol Neurosurg 1984;86:255–263
22. Weingarten K, Zimmerman RD, Becker RD, Heuer LA, Haermes AB, Deck MAF. Subdural and epidural empyema: MR imaging. AJR Am J Roentgenol 1989;152:615–621
23. Yoshikawa TT, Chow AW, Guze LB. Role of anaerobic bacteria in subdural empyema: report of four cases and review of 327 cases from English literature. Am J Med 1975;58:99–104
24. Bhandari YS, Sarkari NBS. Subdural empyema: a review of 37 cases. J Neurosurg 1970;32:35–39
25. Bannister G, Williams B, Smith S. Treatment of subdural empyema. J Neurosurg 1981;55:82–88
26. Bradley PJ, Shaw MDM. Subdural empyema management of the primary source. Br J Clin Pract 1984;38:85–88
27. Cowie R, Williams B. Late seizures and morbidity after subdural empyema. J Neurosurg 1983;58:569–573
28. Feuerman T, Wackym PA, Gade GF, Dubrow T. Craniotomy improves outcome in subdural empyema. Surg Neurol 1989;32:105–110
29. Hockley AD, Williams B. Surgical management of subdural empyema. Childs Brain 1983;10:294–300
30. Smith HP, Hendrick B. Subdural empyema and epidural abscess in children. J Neurosurg 1983;58:392–397
31. Williams B. Cerebral abscess. Br J Neurosurg 1990;4:248–251
32. Bok AP, Peter JC. Subdural empyema: burr holes or craniotomy? A retrospective computerized tomography-era analysis of treatment in 90 cases. J Neurosurg 1993;78:574–578
33. Miller ES, Dias PS, Uttley D. Management of subdural empyema: a series of 24 cases. J Neurol Neurosurg Psychiatry 1987;50:1415–1418
34. Shearman CP, Lees PD, Taylor JC. Subdural empyema: a rational management plan—the case against craniotomy. Br J Neurosurg 1987;1:179–183
35. Glass RL. Osteoplastic flap method in the treatment of subdural abscess. J Neurosurg 1947;36:1–9
36. Le Beau J, Creissard P, Harispe L, Redondo A. Surgical treatment of brain abscess and subdural empyema. J Neurosurg 1973;38:198–203
37. Patir R, Sood S, Bhatia R. Post-traumatic brain abscess: experience of 36 patients. Br J Neurosurg 1995;9:29–35
38. Bank DE, Carolan PL. Cerebral abscess formation following ocular trauma: a hazard associated with common wooden toys. Pediatr Emerg Care 1993;9:285–288
39. Foy P, Sharr M. Cerebral abscesses in children after pencil-tip injuries. Lancet 1980;2:662–663
40. Seider N, Gilboa M, Lautman E, Miller B. Delayed presentation of rbito-cerebral abscess caused by a pencil-tip injury. Ophthal Plast Reconstr Surg 2006;22:316–317
41. Aarabi B, Taghipour M, Alibaii E, Kamgarpour A. Central nervous system infections after military missile head wounds. Neurosurgery 1998;42:500–509
42. Gonul E, Baysefer A, Kahraman S, et al. Causes of infections and management results in penetrating craniocerebral injuries. Neurosurg Rev 1997;20:177–181
43. Tunkel AR. Brain abscess. In: Mandell GL, Bennett JE, Dolin R, eds. Mandell, Douglas and Bennett's Principle of Infectious Diseases. Philadelphia: Elsevier Churchill Livingstone; 2005:1150–1163
44. Mathisen GE, Johnson JP. Brain abscess. Clin Infect Dis 1997;25:763–781
45. Kao PT, Tseng HK, Liu CP, Su SC, Lee CM. Brain abscess: clinical analysis of 53 cases. J Microbiol Immunol Infect 2003;36:129–136
46. Rath SA, Knoringer P. Late brain abscess years after severe cerebrocranial trauma with fronto-orbitobasal fracture. Childs Nerv Syst 1989;5:121–123
47. Dolan RW, Chowdhury K. Diagnosis and treatment of intracranial complications of paranasal sinus infections. J Oral Maxillofac Surg 1995;53:1080–1087
48. Haimes AB, Zimmerman RD, Morgello S, et al. MR imaging of brain abscesses. AJR Am J Roentgenol 1989;152:1073–1085
49. Boom WH, Tuazon CU. Successful treatment of multiple brain abscesses with antibiotics alone. Rev Infect Dis 1985;7:189–199
50. Barsoum AH, Lewis HC, Cannillo KL. Nonoperative treatment of multiple brain abscesses. Surg Neurol 1981;16:283–287
51. Carpenter JL. Brain stem abscesses: cure with medical therapy, case report, and review. Clin Infect Dis 1994;18:219–226
52. Sandermann J, Haase J, Bartholdy NJ, Udesen H. Nonsurgical treatment of a traumatic brain abscess in a child. Childs Nerv Syst 1986;2:49–51
53. Rosenblum ML, Hoff JT, Norman D, et al. Nonoperative treatment of brain abscesses in selected high-risk patients. J Neurosurg 1980;52:217–225
54. Mamelak AN, Mampalam TJ, Obana WG, Rosenblum ML. Improved management of multiple brain abscesses: a combined surgical and medical approach. Neurosurgery 1995;36:76–86
55. Tunkel AR. Bacterial Meningitis. Philadelphia: Lippincott Williams & Wilkins; 2001
56. Marion DW. Complications of head injury and their therapy. Neurosurg Clin N Am 1991;2:411–423
57. Kaufman BA, Tunkel AR, Pryor JC, Dacey RE. Meningitis in the neurosurgical patient. Infect Dis Clin North Am 1990;4:677–701
58. Helling TS, Evans LL, Fowler DL, et al. Infectious complications in patients with severe head injury. J Trauma 1988;28:1575–1577
59. Chandler JR. Traumatic cerebrospinal fluid leakage. Otolaryngol Clin North Am 1983;16:623–632
60. Baltas I, Tsoulfa S, Sakellariou P, Vogus V, Fylaktakis M, Kondodimou A. Posttraumatic meningitis: bacteriology, hydrocephalus and outcome. Neurosurgery 1994;35:422–427
61. MacGee EE, Cauthern JC, Brackett CE. Meningitis following CSF fistula. J Neurosurg 1970;33:312–316
62. Chen KT, Chen CT, Mardini S, Tsay PK, Chen YR. Frontal sinus fractures: a treatment algorithm and assessment of outcomes based on 78 clinical cases. Plast Reconstr Surg 2006;118:457–468
63. Appelbaum E. Meningitis following trauma to the head and face. JAMA 1960;173:1818–1822
64. Schlech WF III, Ward JI, Band JD, Hightower A, Fraser DW, Broome CV. Bacterial meningitis in the United States, 1978 through 1981. The National Bacterial Meningitis Surveillance Study. JAMA 1985;253:1749–1754
65. Villalobos T, Arango C, Kubilis P, Rathore M. Antibiotic prophylaxis after basilar skull fractures: a meta-analysis. Clin Infect Dis 1998;27:364–369
66. Tunkel AR, Scheld WM. Acute infectious complications of head trauma. In: Braakman R, ed. Handbook of Clinical Neurology: Head Injury. Amsterdam: Elsevier Science Publishing; 1990:317–326
67. Hyslop NE, Montgomery WW. Diagnosis and management of meningitis associated with cerebrospinal fluid leaks. In: Remington JS,

Swartz MN, eds. Current Clinical Topics in Infectious Diseases. Vol. 3. New York: McGraw-Hill; 1982:254–285
68. Ratilal B, Costa J, Sampaio C. Antibiotic prophylaxis for preventing meningitis in patients with basilar skull fractures. Cochrane Database Syst Rev 2006;1:CD004884
69. Eftekhar B, Ghodsi M, Nejat F, Ketabchi E, Esmaeeli B. Prophylactic administration of ceftriaxone for the prevention of meningitis after traumatic pneumocephalus: results of a clinical trial. J Neurosurg 2004;101:757–761
70. Eljamel MS. Antibiotic prophylaxis in unrepaired CSF fistulae. Br J Neurosurg 1993;7:501–505
71. Caldicott WJH, North JB, Simpson DA. Traumatic cerebrospinal fluid in fistulas in children. J Neurosurg 1973;38:1–9
72. Korinek AM, Baugnon T, Golmard JL, van Effenterre R, Coriat P, Puybasset L. Risk factors for adult nosocomial meningitis after craniotomy: role of antibiotic prophylaxis. Neurosurgery 2006;59:126–133
73. Laws ER Jr, Thapar K. Surgical management of pituitary adenomas. Baillieres Clin Endocrinol Metab 1995;9:391–405
74. van Aken MO, de Marie S, van der Lely AJ. Risk factors for meningitis after transsphenoidal surgery. Clin Infect Dis 1997;25:852–856
75. Roos KL, Tunkel AR, Scheld WM. Acute bacterial meningitis in children and adults. In: Scheld WM, Whitley RJ, Durack DT, eds. Infections of the central nervous system. 2nd ed. Philadelphia: Lippincott-Raven; 1997:335–401
76. Narotam PK, van Dellen JR, du Trevou MD, Gouws E. Operative sepsis in neurosurgery: a method of classifying surgical cases. Neurosurgery 1994;34:409–415
77. Haines SJ. Antibiotic prophylaxis in neurosurgery: the controlled trials. Neurosurg Clin N Am 1992;3:355–358
78. Forgacs P, Geyer CA, Friedberg SR. Characterization of chemical meningitis after neurological surgery. Clin Infect Dis 2001;32:179–185
79. Leib SL, Boscacci R, Gratzl O, Zimmerli W. Predictive value of cerebrospinal fluid (CSF) lactate level versus CSF/blood glucose ratio for the diagnosis of bacterial meningitis following neurosurgery. Clin Infect Dis 1999;29:69–74
80. Tunkel AR, Hartman BJ, Kaplan SL, et al. Practice guidelines for the management of bacterial meningitis. Clin Infect Dis 2004;39: 1267–1284
81. Briggs S, Elis-Pegler R, Raymond N, Thomas M, Wilkinson L. Gram-negative bacillary meningitis after cranial surgery or trauma in adults. Scand J Infect Dis 2004;36:165–173
82. Barker FG. Efficacy of prophylactic antibiotics for craniotomy: a meta-analysis. Neurosurgery 1994;35:484–492
83. Korinek AM, Golmard JL, Elcheick A, et al. Risk factors for neurosurgical site infections after craniotomy: a critical reappraisal of antibiotic prophylaxis on 4,578 patients. Br J Neurosurg 2005;19:155–162
84. van Aken MO, Feelders RA, de Marie S, et al. Cerebrospinal fluid leakage during transsphenoidal surgery: posteroperative external lumbar drainage reduces the risk of meningitis. Pituitary 2004;7:89–93
85. Kaufman BA. Infections of the cerebrospinal fluid shunts. In: Scheld WM, Whitley RJ, Durack DT, eds. Infections of the Central Nervous System. 2nd ed. Philadelphia: Lippincott-Raven; 1997:555–577
86. Tunkel AR, Kaufman BA. Cerebrospinal fluid shunt infections. In: Mandell GL, Bennett JE, Dolin R, eds. Mandell, Douglas and Bennett's Principle of Infectious Diseases. Philadelphia: Elsevier Churchill Livingston; 2005:1126–1131
87. Govender ST, Nathoo N, van Dellen JR. Evaluation of an antibiotic impregnated shunt system for the treatment of hydrocephalus. J Neurosurg 2003;99:831–839
88. Flibotte JJ, Lee KE, Koroshetz WJ, Rosand J, McDonald CT. Continuous antibiotic prophylaxis and cerebral spinal fluid infection in patients with intracranial pressure monitors. Neurocrit Care 2004;1:61–68
89. Kulkarni AV, Rabin D, Lamberti-Pasculli M. Cerebrospinal fluid shunt infection: a prospective study of risk factors. J Neurosurg 2001;94: 195–201
90. Mcgirt MJ, Zaas A, Fuchs HE, George TM, Kaye K, Sexton DJ. Risk factors for pediatric ventriculoperitoneal shunt infection and predictors of infectious pathogens. Clin Infect Dis 2003;36:858–862
91. Lozier AP, Sciacca RR, Romagnoli MF, Connolly ES Jr. Ventriculostomy-related infections: a critical review of the literature. Neurosurgery 2002;51:170–172
92. Schade RP, Schinkel J, Visser LG, Van Dijk JM, Voormolen JH, Kuijper EJ. Bacterial meningitis caused by the use of ventricular or lumbar cerebrospinal fluid catheters. J Neurosurg 2005;102:229–234
93. Lyke KE, Obasanjo OO, Williams MA, O'Brien M, Chotani R, Perl TM. Ventriculitis complicating use of intraventricular catheters in adult neurosurgical patients. Clin Infect Dis 2001;33:2028–2033
94. Aucoin PJ, Kotilainen JR, Gantz NM, et al. Intracranial pressure monitors, epidemiologic study of risk factors and infections. Am J Med 1986;80:369–376
95. Forward KR, Fewer HD, Stiver HG. Long-term analysis of cerebrospinal fluid shunt infections: a review of 35 infections in 32 patients. J Neurosurg 1983;59:389–394
96. Noetzel MJ, Baker RP. Shunt fluid examination: risks and benefits in the evaluation of shunt malfunction and infection. J Neurosurg 1984; 61:328–332
97. Schoenbaum SC, Gardner P, Shillito J. Infections of cerebrospinal fluid shunts: epidemiology, clinical manifestations and therapy. J Infect Dis 1975;131:543–552
98. Davis SE, Levy ML, McComb JG, Masri-Levine L. Does age or other factors influence the incidence of ventriculoperitoneal shunt infections? Pediatr Neurosurg 1999;30:253–257
99. Gelabert-Gonzalez M, Ginesta-Galan V, Sernamito-Garcia R, Allut AG, Bandin-Dieguez J, Rumbo RM. The Camino intracranial pressure device in clinical practice: assessment in 1000 cases. Acta Neurochir (Wien) 2006;148:435–441
100. Greene KA, Clark RJ, Zabramski JM. Ventricular CSF shunt infections associated with *Corynebacterium jeikeium*: report of three cases and review. Clin Infect Dis 1993;16:139–141
101. Knudsen JD, Nielsen CJ, Espersen F. Treatment of shunt-related cerebral ventriculitis due to *Corynebacterium jeikeium* with vancomycin administered intraventricularly: case report. APMIS 1994;102:317–320
102. James HE, Walsh JW, Wilson HD, Connor JD, Bean JR, Tibbs PA. Prospective randomized study of therapy in cerebrospinal fluid shunt infection. Neurosurgery 1980;7:459–463
103. James HE, Walsh JW, Wilson HD, Connor JD. The management of cerebrospinal fluid shunt infections: a clinical experience. Acta Neurochir (Wien) 1981;59:157–166
104. Sutherland GE, Palitang EG, Marr JJ, Luedke SL. Sterilization of Ommaya reservoir by instillation of vancomycin. Am J Med 1981;71:1068–1070
105. Brown EM, Edwards RJ, Pople IK. Conservative management of patients with cerebrospinal fluid shunt infections. Neurosurgery 2006; 58:657–665
106. McLaurin RL, Frame PT. Treatment of infections of cerebrospinal fluid shunts. Rev Infect Dis 1987;9:595–603
107. Chamberlain MC, Kormanik PA, Barba D. Complications associated with intraventricular chemotherapy in patients with leptomeningeal metastases. J Neurosurg 1997;87:694–699
108. Bayston R, Penny SR. Excessive production of mucoid substance in *Staphylococcus* SIIA: a possible factor in colonization of Holter shunts. Dev Med Child Neurol Suppl 1972;27:25–28
109. Younger JJ, Christensen GD, Bartley DL, Simmons JC, Barrett FF. Coagulase negative staphylococci isolated from cerebrospinal fluid shunts: importance of slime production, species identification, and shunt removal to clinical outcome. J Infect Dis 1987;156:548–554
110. Bell WO. Management of infected cerebrospinal fluid shunts in children. Contemp Neurosurg. 1992;14:1–6
111. Tunkel AR, Hartman BJ, Kaplan SL, et al. Practice guidelines for the management of bacterial meningitis. Clin Infect Dis 2004;39:1267–1284
112. Wong GK, Poon WS, Wai S, Yu LM, Lyon D, Lam JMK. Failure of regular external ventricular drain exchange to reduce cerebrospinal fluid infection: result of a randomised controlled trial. J Neurol Neurosurg Psychiatry 2002;73:759–761
113. Alleyne CH Jr, Hassan M, Zabramski JM. The efficacy and cost of prophylactic and periprocedural antibiotics in patients with external ventricular drains. Neurosurgery 2000;47:1124–1127

114. Poon WS, Ng S, Wai S. CSF antibiotic prophylaxis for neurosurgical patients with ventriculostomy: a randomized study. Acta Neurochir Suppl (Wien) 1998;71:146–148
115. Zabramski JM, Whiting D, Darouiche RO, et al. Efficacy of anti-microbial impregnated external ventricular drain catheters: a prospective, randomized, controlled trial. J Neurosurg 2003;98:725–730
116. Sloffer CA, Augspurger LA, Wagenbach A, Lanzino G. Antimicrobial-impregnated external ventricular catheters: does the very low infection rate observed in clinical trials apply to daily clinical practice? Neurosurgery 2005;56:1041–1044
117. Prabhu VC, Kaufman HH, Voelker JL, et al. Prophylactic antibiotics with intracranial pressure monitors and external ventricular drains: a review of the literature. Surg Neurol 1999;52:226–237
118. Haines SJ, Walters BC. Antibiotic prophylaxis for cerebrospinal fluid shunts: a metaanalysis. Neurosurgery 1994;34:87–92
119. Guidelines for the management of adults with hospital acquired, ventilator-associated and healthcare-associated pneumonia. Am J Respir Crit Care Med 2005;171:388–416
120. Kollef MH. Prevention of hospital-associated pneumonia and ventilator-associated pneumonia. Crit Care Med 2004;32:1396–1405
121. Craven DE, Palladino R, McQuillen DP. Healthcare-associated pneumonia in adults: management principles to improve outcomes. Infect Dis Clin North Am 2004;18(4):939–962
122. Chastre J, Wolff M, Fagon JY, et al. Comparison of 8 vs. 15 days of antibiotic therapy for ventilator-associated pneumonia in adults: a randomized trial. JAMA 2003;290:2588–2598
123. Celis R, Torres A, Gatell JM, Almela M, Rodriguez-Roisin R, Agusti-Vidal A. Nosocomial pneumonia-a multivariate analysis of risk and prognosis. Chest 1988;93:318–324
124. Niederman MS. The clinical diagnosis of ventilator-associated pneumonia. Respir Care 2005;50:788–796
125. Kollef MH, Morrow LE, Niederman MS. Clinical characteristics and treatment patterns among patients with ventilator-associated pneumonia. Chest 2006;129:1210–1218
126. Wisplinghoff H, Bischoff T, Tallent SM, Seifert H, Wenzel RP, Edmond MB. Nosocomial bloodstream infections in US hospitals: analysis of 24,179 cases from a prospective nationwide surveillance study. Clin Infect Dis 2004;39:309–317
127. Rosen AB, Fowler VG Jr, Corey GR, et al. Cost-effectiveness of transesophageal echocardiography to determine the duration of therapy for intravascular catheter-associated *Staphylococcus aureus* bacteremia. Ann Intern Med 1999;130:810–820
128. Mermel LA, Farr BM, Sherertz RJ, et al. Guidelines for the management of intravascular catheter-related infections. Clin Infect Dis 2001;32:1249–1272
129. Donahue SP, Greven CM, Zuravleff JJ, et al. Intraocular candidiasis in patients with candidemia: clinical implications derived from a prospective multicenter study. Ophthalmology 1994;101:1302–1309
130. Bryan CS, Reynolds KL. Hospital acquired bacteremic urinary tract infections: epidemiology and outcome. J Urol 1984;132:494–498
131. Wagenlehner FM, Naber KG. Hospital-acquired urinary tract infections. J Hosp Infect 2000;46:171–181
132. Tambyah PA, Maki DG. The relationship between pyuria and infection in patients with indwelling urinary catheters: a prospective study of 761 patients. Arch Intern Med 2000;160:673–677
133. Trautner BW, Darouiche RO. Role of biofilm in catheter-associated urinary tract infection. Am J Infect Control 2004;32:177–183
134. Bartlett JG. Antibiotic associated diarrhea. N Engl J Med 2002;346: 334–339
135. McDonald LC, Killgore GE, Thomson A, et al. An epidemic, toxin gene-variant strain of *Clostridium difficile*. N Engl J Med 2005;353:2433–2441
136. Teasley DG, Geding DN, Olson MM, et al. Prospective randomized trial of metronidazole versus vancomycin for *Clostridium difficile* associated diarrhea and colitis. Lancet 1983;2:1043–1046
137. Wenisch C, Parschalk B, Hasenhundl M, Hirschl AM, Graninger W. Comparison of vancomycin, teicoplanin, metronidazole and fusidic acid for the treatment of *Clostridium difficile* associated diarrhea. Clin Infect Dis 1996;22:813–818
138. Cunha BA. Fever in the critical care unit. Crit Care Clin 1998;14:1–14
139. Hirsch DR, Ingenito EP, Goldhaber SZ. Prevalence of deep venous thrombosis among patients in medical intensive care. JAMA 1995; 274:335–337
140. Stein PD, Afzal A, Henry JW, Villareal CG. Fever in acute pulmonary embolism. Chest 2000;117:39–42
141. Cooper MS, Stewart PM. Corticosteroid insufficiency in acutely ill patients. N Engl J Med 2003;348:727–734

20 Fluids/Electrolytes

Jim Hitt and Jack Jallo

Management of patients with traumatic injuries begins with the basics: airway, breathing, and circulation. After assessment of a patient's ability to protect his or her airway and insertion of an endotracheal tube, if necessary, fluid resuscitation is the next step in treating a patient who presents with compromised circulation.

Despite the fundamental role of fluid resuscitation in the "ABC's" of trauma assessment, controversies surround many basic aspects of fluid resuscitation (e.g., whether colloids are superior to crystalloids). Although standard treatment algorithms simplify management of patients with traumatic injuries, the specific nature of the injuries will dictate the course of treatment. Whereas the basic approach to patients with traumatic brain injury (TBI) overlaps with the management strategy of patients without brain injury, head-injured patients require modifications to the basic approach.

In either case, hypotension must be treated and oxygen delivery to the body's tissues must be restored. Head trauma presents an additional challenge because injury to the brain can create hemorrhage and edema, which can cause dangerous increases in intracranial pressures (ICPs). Fluid resuscitation strategies must optimize cerebral perfusion by increasing arterial pressure and decreasing ICP.

Resuscitation with normal saline is widely used for patients with and without brain injury. Colloid fluids have the advantage that they increase the osmolarity of the intravascular space and can expand intravascular volume more effectively than crystalloids. However, recent data suggest that although albumin is safe to use in patients without brain injury, it is associated with increased mortality in those with TBI. In addition, although hypertonic saline (HTS) is not routinely used in cases of general trauma, it has favorable effects on both intravascular volume and cerebral water content, which decrease ICP. Mannitol is another fluid administered to patients with TBI, although the osmotic diuretic effects of mannitol are not generally desirable when treating trauma patients. Mannitol's effects on both ICP and cerebral blood flow (CBF) make it beneficial to some patients with head trauma.

Although there are many options for resuscitation of patients with TBI, there is a lack of randomized, controlled trials that compare the efficacy of various resuscitation fluids. In addition, the diverse nature of traumatic injuries makes it difficult to control for all of the variables that could affect outcome, and very large comparative trials are needed to conclusively demonstrate the relative efficacy of fluid resuscitation strategies.

Goals of Fluid Resuscitation (see Table 20.1)

Patients with traumatic injuries can present with significant blood loss. Blood volume can be estimated based on body weight, being ~66 mL/kg for males and 60 mL/kg for females or 4.62 L and 4.2 L for a 70 kg male and female, respectively.[1] The cardiovascular system is sensitive to blood loss with 30 to 40% losses of blood volume causing severe hemodynamic compromise.

Classification of hemorrhagic shock is classically divided into four stages: compensated, mild, moderate, and severe. Compensated hemorrhagic shock (class I) typically occurs with less than 1,000 mL of blood loss and represents a state where hemodynamics are maintained by mild tachycardia (heart rate >100 bpm), vasoconstriction, and activation of the rennin-angiotensin-aldosterone system. Mild hemorrhagic (class II) shock typically occurs with 1,000 to 1,500 mL of blood loss and is characterized by increasing tachycardia (heart rate between 100 and 120 bpm) and oliguria (20 to 30 mL/h). Blood pressure is typically normal in the supine position, but orthostatic hypotension may be observed. Moderate hemorrhagic shock (class III) is observed with 1,500 to 2,000 mL of blood loss and manifests with increasing tachycardia (heart rate >120 bpm), oliguria (5 to 20 mL/h), moderate tachypnea, and a marked drop in blood pressure. Severe hemorrhagic shock (class IV) occurs with more than 2,000 mL of blood loss and presents with profound circulatory collapse (tachycardia, anuria, hypotension).

Whereas monitoring vital signs is simple and routine, this is not the most reliable means of assessing volume loss because changes in heart rate are not specific for

Table 20.1 Goals of Fluid Resuscitation

- Hemodynamic compromise is a late sign of hemorrhagic shock
- Invasive monitoring (arterial catheters, central venous pressure monitors, Swan-Ganz catheters) can help guide resuscitation efforts
- Cerebral perfusion pressure of 60 to 70 mm Hg is a general goal when managing a patient with severe traumatic brain injury

hemorrhage and hypotension occurs only after development of severe blood loss. Although restoring hemodynamic stability is a major goal of fluid resuscitation, the effects of resuscitation can be measured with invasive monitors that measure different aspects of hemodynamics. Central venous pressure is measured by a catheter in the superior vena cava and reflects the patient's volume status and indirectly represents the filling pressure in the right side of the heart (i.e., preload).

In addition to monitoring central venous pressure, pulmonary artery catheters allow for the measurement and calculation of more specific parameters of cardiac function during treatment and resuscitation of traumatically injured patients. When the balloon at the tip of a pulmonary artery catheter is inflated, there is theoretically a column of blood that extends from the catheter tip to the left ventricle at end diastole, and the pressure measured at the catheter tip equals the pressure in the left ventricle. It is then assumed that end diastolic left ventricular volume reflects left end diastolic pressure, which is the left ventricular preload. That assumption fails if the left ventricular compliance changes, and if compliance decreases, a given ventricular volume will result in a higher pressure and an overestimation of volume. It has been shown that hypovolemia results in decreased ventricular compliance, which would result in an overestimation of left end diastolic volume.[2]

Pulmonary artery catheters can measure other aspects of cardiac function. Cardiac output can either be measured by hemodilution or calculated with the Fick equation, and systemic vascular resistance can be calculated when the cardiac output is known. In addition, knowledge of the cardiac output allows for calculation of oxygen delivery. Pulmonary artery catheters also allow for sampling of mixed venous blood, which provides information about oxygen extraction.

The primary goal of fluid resuscitation is restoration or maintenance of adequate oxygen delivery to the body's tissues. In compensated hypovolemia, oxygen delivery decreases but tissue oxygen uptake remains constant due to increased oxygen extraction. Hypovolemic shock occurs when tissue oxygen uptake declines in the face of decreasing delivery, resulting in tissue hypoxia, increased anaerobic metabolism, and increased production of lactic acid. Whereas serum lactate levels can rise as a result of hypovolemic shock, an elevated serum lactate is not specific to shock.

Whereas the previous discussion applies to all patients with traumatic injuries, similar concerns are faced when considering a patient with TBI. The basic goals of resuscitation in TBI involve maintaining arterial pressure and reducing ICP. Adequate cerebral oxygenation relies on maintaining cerebral perfusion pressure (CPP), defined as the mean arterial pressure (MAP) minus the ICP. To recognize decreased CPP, the ICP must be monitored in patients with severe head trauma. This monitoring can be accomplished with either an intraparenchymal or an intraventricular device. Although intraparenchymal monitors are more easily placed, they do not offer a means of treating intracranial hypertension, whereas intraventricular catheters allow for both the measurement of pressure and drainage of cerebrospinal fluid (CSF) when ICPs rise.

Increasing CPP can be accomplished by either increasing MAP or decreasing ICP, and the focus of therapy will vary for each individual patient. Cerebral autoregulation functions to maintain CPP across a range of arterial pressures (typically from 60 to 120 mm Hg), through vasodilatation when arterial pressures are low and vasoconstriction when arterial pressures are high. Rosner and colleagues have postulated that elevated ICP causes decreased perfusion pressure, which triggers a vasodilatory cascade, worsening the intracranial hypertension.[3] They emphasized that increasing cerebral perfusion by increasing arterial pressure, rather than decreasing ICP, will break that cascade and ultimately reduce ICP. Others have suggested that increasing perfusion by decreasing ICP provides better treatment by minimizing the transcapillary pressure and decreasing cerebral edema.

Many studies have examined the optimal CPP in TBI. A perfusion pressure of 60 to 70 mm Hg typically provides adequate global cerebral perfusion in patients with TBI.[4] Although maintaining cerebral hemodynamics is important, the ultimate goal of resuscitation is to maintain adequate cerebral tissue oxygen delivery and uptake. A retrospective review of patients (n = 25) with severe TBI examined the effects of conventional treatments aimed at optimizing ICP and CPP on cerebral tissue oxygenation.[5] Study patients were monitored with an intraparenchymal monitor that measured ICP, brain temperature, and brain tissue oxygenation. Patients were resuscitated with crystalloid or colloid fluids and managed according to the Advanced Trauma Life Support and Severe Traumatic Brain Injury guidelines. The authors reported that one-third of patients with a CPP >60 mm Hg had evidence of severe cerebral hypoxia and that persistent cerebral hypoxia resulted in higher mortality. Although it is apparent that persistent cerebral hypoxia indicates a worse prognosis, it is not known if cerebral oxygenation measurement can guide resuscitation and treatment to improve mortality risk and neurological outcomes in severe TBI.

Fluid Resuscitation Treatments

Hypertonic Saline (see Table 20.2 and Fig. 20.1)

HTS has been used to treat intracranial hypertension. Although HTS is a crystalloid fluid, it can expand intravascular volume better than isotonic saline, and it has beneficial effects on cerebral water content and ICP

Table 20.2 Hypertonic Saline Treatment for Fluid Resuscitation

- Hypertonic saline increases intravascular volume and decreases both cerebral water content, cerebral bulk, and intracranial pressure. Due to the favorable effect of hypertonic saline on intravascular volume, it should be the fluid of choice in patients with intracranial hypertension and systemic hypotension.
- No standard concentration or dosing schedule of hypertonic saline has been established. Studies have investigated hypertonic saline concentrations ranging from 1.6 to 29.2%.
- Studies comparing hypertonic saline to crystalloid or mannitol have failed to show significant differences in terms of neurological outcome or mortality.
- Investigation of hypertonic saline administration in the prehospital setting by paramedics failed to show significant benefit over normal saline usage.

in patients with TBI. It is difficult to draw general conclusions about HTS because many of the published studies have used different concentrations and dosing schedules. Whereas many experiments have demonstrated that patients with shock and TBI can benefit from treatment with HTS because of beneficial effects on hemodynamics, ICP, and cerebral oxygenation, large-scale studies that compare HTS with other resuscitation fluids are lacking. Currently available studies used various HTS regimens and differing control fluids, and lack significant effects in long-term neurological outcome.

Intravascular infusion of HTS increases the osmolarity of blood plasma and subsequently increases the osmotic gradient between the brain and blood. This increased osmotic gradient draws water from the brain parenchyma into the blood and thereby decreases cerebral water volume and ICP. This increase in plasma osmolarity helps offset the increases in osmolarity in cerebral tissue following TBI that result from cell lysis and metabolic derangements in damaged cerebral tissue.[6,7]

The increased osmotic gradient created by HTS therapy also expands intravascular volume, which can be beneficial in patients with TBI who are hemodynamically unstable. Animal and human studies of shock (i.e., hemorrhagic,

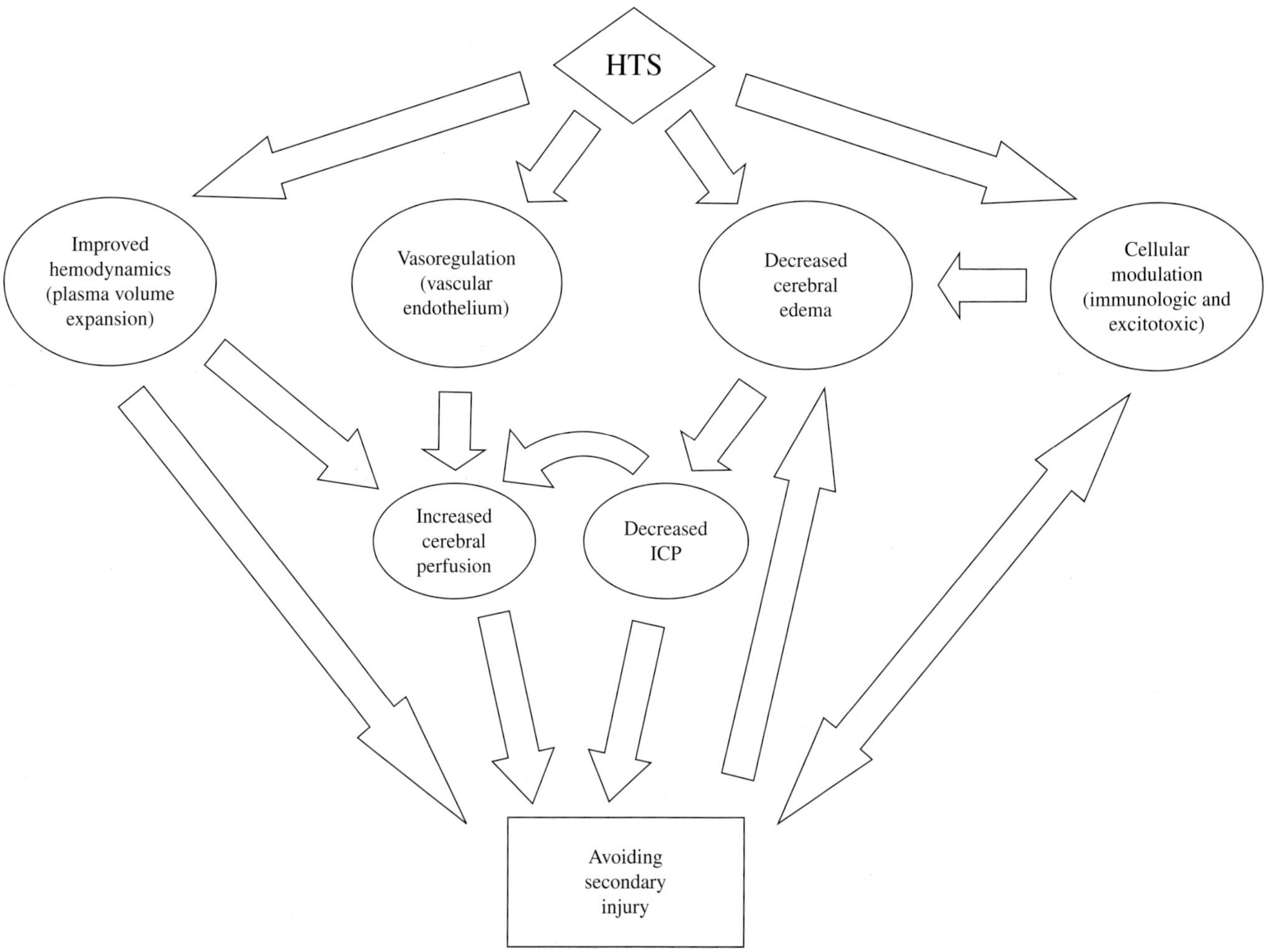

Fig. 20.1 Proposed mechanism of action for hypertonic saline. (From Doyle JA, Davis DP, Hoyt DB. The use of hypertonic saline in the treatment of traumatic brain injury. J Trauma 2001;50:367–383.) HTS, hypertonic saline; ICP, intracranial pressure.

septic, and cardiogenic) have demonstrated that treatment with HTS has beneficial effects on hemodynamics.[8–13] In addition to the benefits on intravascular volume expansion, HTS also improves hemodynamics by stimulating the release of adrenocorticotropic hormone (ACTH) and cortisol.[14–16] Ischemic injury also alters microcirculation by inducing erythrocyte swelling, and treatment with hypertonic and hyperosmolar solutions has been shown to reverse acidosis-induced erythrocyte swelling in vitro.[17] HTS may have other beneficial effects on microcirculation, including decreased leukocyte migration and adherence to the endothelium[18–21] (see **Fig. 20.2**).

Experiments of animal models of TBI and intracranial hemorrhage have demonstrated benefits of HTS therapy. Using a porcine model of epidural hemorrhage and hemorrhagic shock, Ducey and colleagues found that resuscitation with 6% NaCl was more effective than normal saline, hetastarch, or whole blood transfusion in restoring hemodynamics, reducing ICP, and normalizing CPP.[22] Prough and colleagues used a radiolabeled microsphere technique to demonstrate that 7.2% NaCl not only improved ICP and CPP but also improved regional blood flow in dogs with hemorrhagic shock and subdural hemorrhage.[23] Taylor and colleagues used a cryogenic model of TBI in the presence of hemorrhagic shock and compared the effects of lactated ringers (LR) and 7.5% NaCl on hemodynamics (cardiac output, MAP), ICP, and tissue oxygenation at the site of cryogenic brain injury.[24] The results demonstrated that LR and HTS had similar restorative effects on hemodynamics, but HTS had significant benefits in lowering ICP and increasing cerebral oxygenation in the damaged tissue.

Results of noncomparative studies of HTS are presented in **Table 20.3**. A case series of two patients demonstrated that a 20 to 50 mL bolus of 29.2% HTS resulted in an immediate and prolonged decline of ICP and an improvement in renal function.[25] Several prospective, observational studies have demonstrated that bolus injection of HTS (7.5 to 10%) resulted in a decrease in ICP of ~40% and an increase in CPP to values near 70 mm Hg.[26–28] Munar and colleagues treated 14 patients with TBI and intracranial hypertension (ICP >15 mm Hg) with a 1.5 mL/kg bolus of 7.2% HTS.[29] They reported that ICP declined ~70% from pretreatment values ($p < 0.0001$) and CPP and CI increased, whereas MAP remained stable. They also found the ateriovenous oxygen difference did not change with HTS treatment, suggesting that despite improved CPP, there was no significant change on CBF.[29]

In addition to studies that have shown the efficacy of HTS, some studies have compared HTS with other fluids. Gemma and colleagues compared the effects of 7.5% HTS and 20% mannitol on CSF pressure and cerebral bulk in patients undergoing elective intracranial procedures.[30]

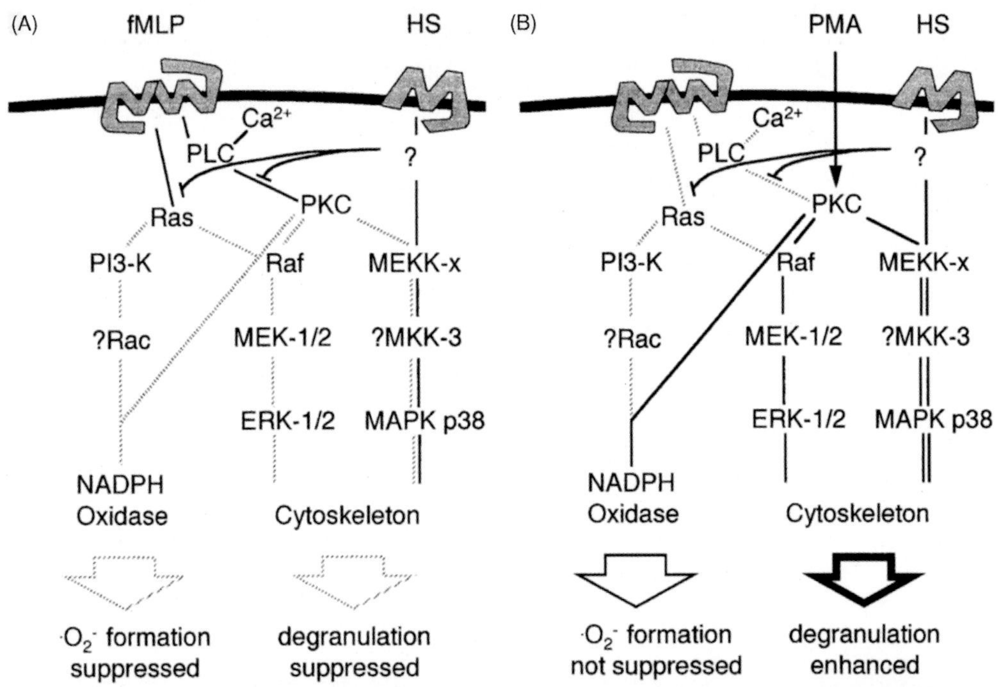

Fig. 20.2 Proposed mechanisms of modulation of neutrophil degranulation and superoxide production by HS. **(A)** Addition of HS before or at the time of stimulation with fMLP blocks superoxide formation and degranulation by uncoupling of several upstream signaling steps originating from the fMLP-receptor. **(B)** When these upstream signaling steps are circumvented by using PMA instead of fMLP or by adding HS after fMLP, HS does not affect superoxide formation but enhances degranulation by amplifying the p38 signaling pathway. (From Junger WG, Hoyt DB, Davis RE et al. Hypertonicity regulates the function of human neutrophils by modulating chemoattractant receptor signaling and activating mitogen-activated protein kinase p38. J Clin Invest 1998;101(12):2768–2779.)

Table 20.3 Noncomparative Studies of Hypertonic Saline for Treatment of Intracranial Hypertension in Humans

Citation	Study Design	Injury	Hypertonic Fluid Regimen	Dose	Outcomes
Worthley et al, 1988[25]	Case series ($n = 2$)	TBI	29.2% NaCl	20 mL and 50 mL bolus	Immediate decrease in ICP
Hartl et al, 1997[26]	Prospective observational ($n = 6$, 32 episodes)	Severe TBI (GCS 3 to 8)	7.5% NaCl and HES	≤250 mL bolus	Decreased ICP (44%) and increased CPP (38% to >70 mm Hg)
Schatzmann et al, 1998[28]	Prospective observational ($n = 6$, 42 episodes)	Severe TBI	10% NaCl	100 mL bolus	Decreased ICP (43% for an average of 93 minutes)
Horn et al, 1999[27]	Prospective observational ($n = 10$, 48 episodes)	TBI or SAH (with treatment-resistant ICH)	7.5% NaCl	2 mL/kg bolus	Decreased ICP (42%, 33 ± 9 to 19 ± 6 mm Hg; $p < 0.05$) and increased CPP (68 ± 11 to 79 ± 11 mm Hg; $p < 0.05$)
Munar et al, 2000[29]	Prospective observational ($n = 14$)	Moderate to severe TBI (GCS ≤13) and ICH (ICP >15 mm Hg)	7.2% NaCl	1.5 mL/kg bolus	Decreased ICP (70%; $p = 0.0001$), increased CPP and CI, and stable MAP and CBF (measured by arteriovenous O_2 difference)

Abbreviations: CBF, cerebral blood flow; CPP, cerebral perfusion pressure; GCS, Glasgow Coma Scale; HES, hydroxyethyl starch; ICH, intracranial hemorrhage; MAP, mean arterial pressure; SAH, subarrachnoid hemorrhage; TBI, traumatic brain injury.

The results showed that HTS and mannitol similarly reduced the CSF pressure and objective brain bulk during the neurosurgical procedure. Other results of studies that compare the results of HTS with isoosmolar volumes of crystalloid (normal saline [NS] or LR) or mannitol are presented in **Table 20.4**.

Shackford and colleagues compared 1.6% HTS with LR in a prospective, randomized trial of 34 patients with TBI (Glasgow Coma Scale [GCS] score ≤13) who required an ICP monitor.[31] Patients either received bolus injections of HTS or LR for hemodynamic instability or decreased urine output. Episodes of intracranial hypertension were

Table 20.4 Comparative Studies of Hypertonic Saline for Treatment of Intracranial Hypertension in Humans

Citation	Study Design	Injury	Hypertonic Fluid Regimen	Control Fluid	Dose	Outcomes
Shackford et al, 1998[31]	Prospective randomized ($n = 34$)	TBI (GCS ≤13 requiring ICP monitor)	1.6% NaCl	LR	Bolus HTS PRN	Similar ICP-lowering effect in two groups; HTS group had more severe injury (lower GCS and higher ICP at baseline)
Qureshi et al, 1999[32]	Retrospective review with case controls ($n = 82$)	Severe head injury (GCS ≤8)	2 or 3% NaCl with acetate	NS	Continuous infusion	Higher use of barbiturate coma (7 vs. 2; $p = 0.04$) and higher in-hospital mortality (OR, 3.1; 1.1 to 10.2 95% CI)
Vialet et al, 2003[33]	Prospective randomized ($n = 20$)	TBI associated with persistent coma	7.5% NaCl	20% mannitol	2 mL/kg bolus of either solution	Decreased number of and duration of ICH events for patients given HTS; similar mortality and neurological outcomes
Cooper et al, 2004[34]	Prospective randomized ($n = 229$)	Blunt TBI, coma (GCS <9), and hypotension	7.5% NaCl	LR	250 mL bolus of either fluid	Trends to lower ICP and higher CPP; no difference in mortality or neurological outcome

Abbreviations: CI, confidence interval; CPP, cerebral perfusion pressure; GCS, Glasgow Coma Scale; HTS, hypertonic saline; ICP, intracranial pressure; LR, lactated ringers; NS, normal saline; PRN, pro re nota: TBI, traumatic brain injury.

treated with head elevation, hyperventilation, CSF drainage, mannitol infusion, and barbiturate coma, if the intracranial hypertension was refractory to other interventions. Patients in the HTS group had significantly higher maximum ICP and presented with lower GCS at the beginning of the study, but, after treatment was initiated, there was no statistically significant difference in ICP between the groups on study days 2 through 5. Patients in the HTS arm required more interventions to control their ICP, but this may reflect the difference in the two groups at initial presentation. The results of this study showed similar treatment effects between patients treated with 1.6% HTS and LR, but because of the significant difference in baseline ICP and GCS, it is difficult to conclude that the two treatments are equally effective in lowering ICP.

Qureshi and colleagues conducted a retrospective review of the use of continuous infusion of 2 to 3% HTS in patients with severe TBI (GCS ≤8) and compared those cases with ones in which patients received continuous normal saline infusion.[32] Baseline characteristics (i.e., age and presenting GCS) were similar, but patients who received HTS were more likely to have penetrating head injury or an intracranial mass lesion. Although they found no difference between the groups in terms of the frequency of hyperventilation, CSF drainage, mannitol infusion, or vasopressor usage, they did report a significant increase in the use of pentobarbital coma in HTS-treated patients ($n = 7$ vs. $n = 2$, respectively; $p = 0.04$) and an increase in the incidence of in-hospital mortality (odds ratio of 3.1; 95% confidence interval [CI], 1.1 to 10.2).

Vialet and colleagues compared HTS to mannitol in a prospective, randomized trial of 20 patients with TBI and persistent coma, who required ICP monitoring.[33] Patients were randomly assigned to receive boluses (2 mL/kg) of either 7.5% HTS or 20% mannitol for treatment of refractory intracranial hypertension (i.e., with hyperventilation, CSF drainage, and hemodynamic support if necessary). Patients treated with HTS had fewer episodes of intracranial hypertension (6.8 ± 5.5 vs. 13.3 ± 14.2, respectively; $p = 0.02$) and a shorter total daily duration of intracranial hypertension (62 ± 81 vs. 95 ± 92 minutes, respectively; $p = 0.04$). Treatment failures were also less common in the patients treated with HTS (10% vs. 70%, respectively; $p = 0.01$).[33] Although the study was limited in scale, the results of this randomized, prospective trial support the use of HTS to treat episodes of intracranial hypertension. Although patients in the HTS arm experienced less intracranial hypertension, the study did not show any difference in mortality or neurological recovery in the two groups.

Cooper and colleagues conducted a prospective, randomized trial to compare the effects of HTS and LR in prehospital resuscitation of patients with blunt head injury, a GCS <9, and hypotension (systolic blood pressure <100 mm Hg).[34] Patients ($n = 229$) were randomized to receive a single 250 mL intravenous bolus of either 7.5% HTS or LR in addition to standard resuscitation fluids, and the primary end point was neurological function at 6 months as determined by the extended Glasgow Outcome Score (GOSe). Baseline patient characteristics were well balanced between the two groups in terms of demographics and injury severity. Not all patients enrolled in the study received ICP monitors (37 patients in the HTS group and 49 patients in the LR group), but there was a trend toward lower ICP in the HTS group as compared with the LR group (10 mm Hg [range 6 to 17 mm Hg] vs. 15 mm Hg [range 8.5 to 22]; $P = 0.08$). There was also a trend toward shorter duration of CPP <70 mm Hg (9.5 vs. 17 hours, respectively; $p = 0.6$), but no difference in duration of ICP >20 mm Hg (5.3 vs. 5.5 hours; $P = 0.40$).[34] Despite trends toward lower ICP and higher CPP in patients treated with HTS, there were no differences in neurological outcomes in terms of functional disability or GOSe, suggesting that administration of a 250 mL bolus of 7.5% HTS does not benefit outcomes at 6 months.

Mannitol (see Table 20.5)

Similar to HTS, mannitol administration increases serum osmolarity and causes cellular dehydration, but, in contrast to HTS, mannitol is an inert sugar alcohol that causes an osmotic diuresis. The osmotic gradient created by intravascular infusion of mannitol and subsequent reduction in cerebral water volume is a key mechanism that contributes to the decrease in ICP observed after administration.[35,36] In addition to osmotic reductions in cerebral water volume, mannitol infusion results in a decrease in blood viscosity (23%) at 10 minutes and a narrowing of pial arterioles.[37] The combination of decreased blood viscosity and decreased arteriole diameter results in a decrease in CBF and a reduction of ICP. The reduction of blood viscosity is most significant when erythrocytes are subjected to high shear rates (i.e., as they pass through

Table 20.5 Mannitol Treatment for Fluid Resuscitation

- Mannitol administration results in increased plasma osmolarity, decreased blood viscosity, reduced cerebral water content, and osmotic diuresis. Intravascular volume is increased immediately after mannitol administration, followed by diuresis and volume loss.
- Because of the diuretic effect, mannitol should be used in patients with intracranial hypertension and stable hemodynamics. Fluids lost through diuresis should be carefully replaced to avoid hypovolemia.
- Mannitol is not more effective than normal saline in the prehospital setting in terms of hemodynamic stability or mortality outcomes.

small arterioles and capillaries), and mannitol-coated red blood cells have decreased rigidity, which reverses when the mannitol is washed off the red blood cell membranes.[38]

Despite the evidence that supports the role of mannitol in reducing ICP and the widespread usage of mannitol to reduce ICP, there are relatively few studies that demonstrate the optimal dosing schedule for mannitol or demonstrate the relative efficacy of mannitol compared with other agents. Recent controversy has arisen surrounding results published on the beneficial effect of high-dose mannitol on death and severe disability at 6 months postinjury.[39] Cruz and colleagues presented results from three groups of patients with nonpenetrating TBI and acute subdural, intraparenchymal hemorrhage, or diffuse cerebral edema and impending death, that indicate high-dose mannitol therapy (~1.4 g/kg) significantly reduces death and disability.[40–42] Questions have been raised over the dramatic results, and, because the data were not able to be confirmed, they have been removed from the Cochrane review of mannitol trials.[39,43]

Table 20.6 lists comparative trials of mannitol therapy. The Cochrane review focuses on four randomized, controlled trials of mannitol[43]; three studies compare mannitol with other agents (pentobarbital, NS, and 7.5% HTS) and one compares with treatment approaches (one where treatment is guided by ICP and the other where it is based on neurological symptoms).[33,44–46] Schwartz and colleagues compared 20% mannitol with pentobarbital in patients with intracranial hypertension following TBI.[45] Patients were randomly selected to receive either pentobarbital or mannitol as initial therapy and were treated with the other agent if they exhibited refractory intracranial hypertension. In patients who did not need surgical evacuation of a hematoma, mortality was lower in those who were initially treated with mannitol than pentobarbital (41% vs. 77%, respectively), but this difference was not observed in those who underwent surgical evacuation of a hematoma (43% vs. 40%).[45] This difference in the nonsurgical group corresponds to a relative mortality risk of 0.85 (95% confidence interval of 0.52 to 1.38).[43]

Smith and colleagues compared ICP-directed mannitol therapy (i.e., treatment with 20% mannitol when ICP >20 mm Hg) with empirically based therapy (i.e., mannitol treatment when a neurological decline was evident).[46] They reported no difference in death or disability between the two groups,[46] with the relative mortality risk of ICP-directed treatment of 0.88 (95% confidence interval of 0.55 to 1.38).[43]

Sayre and colleagues compared prehospital administration of mannitol with normal saline in patients with multitrauma and TBI.[44] Patients were eligible if they were evaluated by paramedics within 6 hours of injury, had not received prior diuretic treatment, were not undergoing cardiopulmonary resuscitation (CPR), and were not pregnant. No significant difference in hemodynamics or mortality outcomes was observed between the two treatment groups.[43,44]

Vialet and colleagues compared isovolumic doses of 20% mannitol with 7.5% HTS as osmotic agents for the treatment of intracranial hypertension in patients with TBI and persistent coma.[33] Patients treated with mannitol had more episodes of intracranial hypertension (13.3 ± 14.2 vs.

Table 20.6 Clinical Trials of Mannitol Treatment for Fluid Resuscitation

Citation	Study Design	Injury	Mannitol Regimen	Dose	Control Therapy	Relative Risk of Death, Mannitol vs Control
Schwartz et al, 1984[45]	Prospective, randomized (*n* = 59)	Severe TBI (GCS <8)	20% mannitol	Escalating dose to keep ICp <20	Pentobarbital	0.85 (95% CI 0.52 to 1.38)
Smith et al, 1986[46]	Prospective, randomized (*n* = 77)	Severe TBI (GCS <8)	20% mannitol	Escalating dose to keep ICp <25	Nannitol therapy using neurological signs (GCS, ABG, neuro deficits)	0.83 (95% CI 0.47 to 1.46)
Sayre et al, 1996[44]	Prospective, randomized (*n* = 41)	Moderate to severe TBI (GCS <11)	Prehospital treatment 20% mannitol	5 mL/kg	NS	1.75 (95% CI 0.48 to 6.38)
Vialet et al, 2003[33]	Prospective, randomized (*n* = 20)	Severe TBI (GCS <8) and ICH	20% mannitol	2 mL/kg	7.5% HTS	1.25 (95% CI 0.47 to 3.33)
Battison et al, 2005	Prospective, randomized, crossover (*n* = 9)	Brain injury; TBI (*n* = 6) or SAH (*n* = 3)	20% mannitol	200 mL	7.5% HTS/6% dextran	N/A

Abbreviations: ABG, arterial blood gas; CI, confidence interval; GCS, Glascow Coma Scale; HTS, hypertonic saline; ICH, intracerebral hemorrhage; ICP, intracranial pressure; NS, normal saline; TBI, traumatic brain injury.

6.8 ± 5.5, respectively; $p = 0.02$), longer durations of intracranial hypertension (95 ± 92 vs. 62 ± 81 minutes, respectively; $p = 0.04$), and more treatment failures (70% vs. 10%, respectively; $p = 0.01$). Patients treated with mannitol also had a trend toward an increased risk of death (relative risk of 1.25 [95% confidence interval of 0.47 to 3.33]).[43]

Although there are abundant data and clinical experience that support the use of mannitol in the treatment of intracranial hypertension, questions remain about the optimal dosage, schedule, and relative efficacy of mannitol therapy. In the early phase of mannitol therapy intravascular volume is expanded, due to the favorable osmotic gradient; the eventual diuresis results in a contraction of the intravascular volume. Although the consequences of diuresis can be avoided by careful repletion of urinary losses, this effect can have unfavorable consequences in the setting of hypotension and should be avoided. The use of a volume expanding hyperosmolar agent (i.e., HTS) may be the preferred treatment for intracranial hypertension in a hemodynamically unstable patient.

Colloids (see Table 20.7)

In comparison with crystalloid fluids, colloids contain large, solute molecules that do not readily cross an intact capillary membrane, and, as a consequence, they help maintain the osmotic gradient that keeps water in the intravascular space. Crystalloid fluids are primarily composed of sodium chloride and evenly distribute between the intravascular and extravascular spaces. The intravascular volume is ~20% of the total body water, and, because crystalloids readily diffuse across capillary membranes, only ~20% of the volume of a crystalloid infusion remains in the vascular space.

In contrast, the solute molecules in colloid fluids do not diffuse through the endothelial barrier and, as a consequence, ~70% of the infused volume remains in the plasma in the few hours following the infusion. In addition to more effectively expanding the intravascular volume, colloid fluids have also been shown to more effectively increase cardiac output in hypovolumic patients.[47] Colloids increase cardiac output by both expanding intravascular volume, which increases cardiac preload, and by reducing the viscosity of blood, which decreases afterload.

Table 20.7 Colloids and Hydroxyethyl Starch Treatment for Fluid Resuscitation

- Results from the SAFE trial demonstrated a significant increase in mortality associated with albumin administration to patients with traumatic brain injury. This result was not seen in trauma patients without brain injury.
- Hydroxyethyl starches are colloids that expand intravascular volume and are slowly degraded by plasma amylase. The main drawback of HES fluids is the detrimental effect on coagulation, although newer HES fluids have less of a negative impact on coagulation
- Large-scale trials of HES fluids in patients with traumatic brain injury are needed to define safety parameters and optimal dosing.

Abbreviations: HES, hydroxyethyl starch; SAFE, Saline versus Albumin Fluid Evaluation study.

Animal studies have shown that combination therapy with hypertonic and hyperosmolar agents may have benefit in treating TBI and subarrachnoid hemorrhage (SAH). Elliott and colleagues compared the effects of 7.5% HTS, 7.5%HTS plus 4% albumin, and NS in rats in a controlled cortical impact model of TBI.[48] They compared the effects of immediate and delayed (6 hours) treatment with the three fluids (dose of 4 mL/kg) in terms of cortical injury volume and ipsilateral brain water content. Although immediate treatment with HTS showed a trend toward increased injury volume, delayed treatment with HTS resulted in significantly smaller injury volume as compared with immediate treatment. Immediate treatment with 4% albumin and 7.5% HTS resulted in a significant reduction in injury volume as compared with immediate treatment with HTS alone, and the delayed, combination treatment group showed the greatest reduction in injury volume, with a significant reduction as compared with control animals.[48]

Zausinger and colleagues reported results from a similar study of hypertonic/hyperosmolar therapy in a rat model of SAH.[21] They compared the effects of treatment with NS, 7.5% HTS, and 7.5% HTS plus 6% dextran-70 on ICP, CBF, histomorphological damage, and neurological recovery. Animals were treated with 4 mL/kg of each solution 30 minutes after injury. Although treatment with both HTS alone and HTS in combination with dextran significantly reduced the intracranial hypertension observed after induced SAH, the animals in the combination therapy group exhibited better neurological outcome and increased histomorphology of neurons. There was also a trend toward increased survival in the animals treated with hypertonic/hyperosmolar therapy.

Despite the theoretical advantages of colloid fluids, large-scale trials have failed to demonstrate improved outcomes in patients treated with colloid fluids. The Cochrane Injuries Group Albumin Reviewers conducted a metaanalysis of 24 studies that included 1,419 patients and calculated that patients who received albumin had a 6% increase in the absolute risk of death over those patients who received crystalloid fluids.[49] A subsequent larger metaanalysis conducted by Wilkes and Navickis contradicted those results showing no significant increase in mortality risk in patients treated with albumin.[50]

The Saline versus Albumin Fluid Evaluation (SAFE) study was a large, multicenter, randomized, double-blind trial conducted with the primary goal of comparing the

28 day mortality rate of patients treated with NS versus those treated with 4% albumin.[51] The SAFE study enrolled 6997 patients to either receive 4% albumin or 0.9% saline for fluid resuscitation, in addition to maintenance fluids, replacement fluids, enteral or parentral nutrition, and blood products. Although patients treated with albumin received significantly less total fluid volume and exhibited increased central venous pressure (CVP), the study group reported no overall difference in 28 day mortality, intensive care unit (ICU) stay length, or number of body organs in failure. However, subgroup analysis demonstrated that patients with TBI had a significant increase in mortality when treated with albumin compared with saline. In patients with TBI who were treated with albumin, 59 of 241 died as compared with 38 of 251 treated with saline, which corresponds to a relative risk of death of 1.62 (95% confidence interval, 1.12 to 2.34; $p = 0.009$).

The SAFE study investigators conducted a post hoc study of the subgroup of patients with TBI, examining baseline characteristics of the two groups and long-term outcomes at 24 months.[52] The baseline characteristics of the two groups were well balanced in terms of initial GCS, the proportion of patients with severe injury (GCS 3 to 8), severity of injury on computed tomography (CT) scan, and initial intracranial hypertension. Primary outcomes were reported for 214 patients treated with albumin and 206 patients treated with saline. Patients with severe injury who were treated with albumin had a significantly increased risk of death at 24 months (relative risk 1.88, 95% confidence interval, 1.31 to 2.70; $p < 0.001$), but no significant difference was seen in patients with an initial GCS of 9 to 12 (relative risk 0.74, 95% confidence interval, 0.31 to 1.79; $p = 0.50$). A majority of the deaths in both groups occurred within the initial 28 days of the study.

Hydroxyethyl Starch (see Table 20.8)

In contrast to albumin, hydroxyethyl starch (HES) is a synthetic colloid fluid comprising modified amylopectin starches, which are modified by hydroxyethyl bonds added to the glucose subunits at the C2, C3, or C6 carbon atoms. Hydroxyethylation limits the ability of serum amylase to break down the molecule, which prolongs the duration that the starch remains in the intravascular space. HES polymers are characterized by the amount of molar substitution (mole of hydroxyethyl per mole of glucose subunits), the C2:C6 hydroxyethylation ratio, the range of molecular weight, and mean molecular weight (see **Table 20.9**).

HES solutions are a polydisperse collection of molecular weights, and after intravenous administration, the smaller molecular weight molecules are rapidly excreted by the kidneys.[53] HES fluids can be grouped by their mean molecular weight (high, medium, and low, corresponding to ≥400 kd, 200 to 400 kd, and <200 kd, respectively). The larger molecules are progressively hydrolyzed by serum amylase, and the resulting smaller HES fragments are excreted. The degree and pattern of hydroxyethylation also determines the rate of hydrolysis. Highly substituted molecules (hetastarch; 0.62 to 0.75 molar substitution) are more slowly degraded than medium-substituted (pentastarch; 0.5) and the newest low-substituted (tetrastarch; 0.4 molecules).[53] Elimiation of tetrastarch is ~20 times faster than hetastarch and pentastarch.[54] In general, HES solutions with either high molecular weight or medium molecular weight with high molar substitution are more slowly degraded than those with low molecular weight or medium molecular weight with low molar substitution (see **Table 20.10**).

Maximum daily doses of HES solutions have been set to limit the adverse events, including impaired renal function, splanchnic perfusion, reticular endothelial cell function, inflammatory response, and coagulation.[53] Coagulopathy is of particular concern for patients with TBI. Slowly degradeable HES solutions have been shown to decrease the plasma concentrations of von Willebrand factor (vWF) and factor VIII up to 80% over healthy controls.[55,56] More rapidly degraded HES solutions have been shown to have less adverse impact on coagulation factors, demonstrating that tetrastarch can be administered in higher doses than hetastarch (50 to 70 mL/kg compared with 20 mL/kg, respectively).[53,56–58]

A retrospective review examined the use of pentastarch (10% HES 200/0.5; mean molecular weight 200 kd and 0.5 molar substitution) in patients with severe head injury.[59]

Table 20.8 Hydroxyethyl Starch Treatment for Fluid Resuscitation

- Synthetic colloid fluid comprising modified amylopectin starches
- HES solutions are a polydisperse collection of molecular weights.
- Smaller molecular weight molecules are rapidly excreted by the kidneys.[53]
- Larger molecules are hydrolyzed by serum amylase, resulting in smaller HES fragments that are excreted.
- Highly substituted molecules (hetastarch) are more slowly degraded than medium-substituted (pentastarch) and low-substituted (tetrastarch) molecules.[53]

Abbreviations: HES, hydroxyethyl starch.

Table 20.9 Types of Hydroxyethyl Starch Used for Fluid Resuscitation

Degree of Molecular Substitution	Hydroethyl Starch	Molar Substitution
Highly substituted molecules	Hetastarch	0.62–0.75
Medium-substituted molecules	Pentastarch	0.5
Low-substituted molecules	Tetrastarch	0.4

Table 20.10 Hydroethyl Starch Treatment Side Effects

- Adverse events include: impaired renal function, splanchnic perfusion, reticular endothelial cell function, inflammatory response, and coagulation.[53]
- Slowly degradable HES solutions have been shown to decrease the plasma concentrations of von Willebrand factor (vWF) and factor VIII up to 80% over healthy controls.[55,56]
- Rapidly degraded HES solutions have been shown to have less adverse impact on coagulation factors, demonstrating that tetrastarch can be administered in higher doses than hetastarch (50 to 70 mL/kg compared with 20 mL/kg, respectively).[53,56–58]

Abbreviations: HES, hydroxyethyl starch.

Patients ($n = 78$) were given 1,000 mL of HES daily in addition to crystalloid fluids, and the authors reported no adverse bleeding events associated with HES administration and an elevated activated partial thromboplastin time in only seven of 234 blood samples (2.65%). This study demonstrates the feasibility of using limited doses of pentastarch in the resuscitation of patients with severe head injury, but it is not possible to draw general conclusions about the safety and relative utility of HES versus other fluids from those data.

A randomized, controlled trial compared high-dose tetrastarch (70 mL/kg of 6% HES 130/0.4) with lower-dose pentastarch (33 mL kg of 6% HES 200/0.5) and albumin in patients with severe head injury.[58] The authors reported no difference in coagulation parameters (partial thromboplastin time, prothrombin time, fibrinogen levels, or platelet function analysis) or renal function between the two groups. Patients who received high-dose tetrastarch had fewer ICP peaks above 30 or 35 mm Hg compared with those who received pentastarch plus albumin, but there was no statistically significant difference in Glasgow Outcome Scale (GOS) score at 3 months and 6 months between the groups. Intercranial bleeding complications were noted in 5 of 16 patients in the tetrastarch group and 5 of 15 patients in the pentastarch group; however, these bleeding complications were not associated with measured coagulopathy, and the authors concluded that the events were related to underlying trauma and not due to the administration of HES.

Newer HES solutions are more rapidly degraded because of lower molecular weights and lower molar hydroxyethyl substitution. These HES molecules retain the volume-expanding properties of other colloids and may reduce the adverse events associated with HES fluid administration. Large-scale, comparative studies of HES fluids and other fluids used in the resuscitation of patients are lacking, and given the potential complications of inhibiting coagulation in patients with TBI, HES fluids should be used with caution until more complete safety data are available.

Effects of Administering Blood Products on Fluid Resuscitation (see Table 20.11)

Because blood products (i.e., whole blood, packed red blood cells, fresh frozen plasma, cryoprecipitate, platelets, etc.) contain many different proteins and cellular components, the administration of blood products has the same beneficial effects on intravascular volume as infusing other colloid solutions. Blood products are typically used to treat specific hematological abnormalities (i.e., anemia, thrombocytopenia, coagualopathy, etc.). Transfusion of blood products carries risks of infections and infusion reactions, and the decision to transfuse must be customized for each patient's specific situation.

Transfusing red blood cells to patients with TBI, either in the form of packed red blood cells or whole blood, carries certain risks and benefits. Raising the hematocrit increases the oxygen carrying capacity of the blood, but this benefit comes at the expense of higher viscosity. Although blood plasma has a viscosity 1.2-fold greater than water, whole blood with a hematocrit of 45% has a viscosity 2.4-fold greater than water.[60] The Hagen-Poiseuille equation ascertains that, for a newtonian fluid, the flow of the fluid is inversely proportional to its viscosity, and halving the viscosity of a fluid will double its flow. And although reducing the hematocrit will increase CBF, this comes at the cost of reducing oxygen delivery. It is generally believed that the optimal hematocrit that balances viscosity and oxygen carrying capacity lies in the range of 30 to 35%.[60]

Transfusion of blood products is sometimes essential for patients with traumatic injuries. The administration of red blood cells results in volume expansion similar to other colloid fluids and increases the oxygen carrying capacity, which is an essential intervention in the face of severe hemorrhagic shock. The commonly associated risks of blood transfusion include infectious complications from transfusions ranging from 1 in 2,000 for bacterial

Table 20.11 Effects of Administering Blood Products in TBI

- A hematocrit of 30% balances oxygen carrying capacity of blood with viscosity. This is the most commonly used transfusion threshold for patients with traumatic brain injury.
- Studies of the effects of blood transfusions in cardiac surgery patients have raised concerns about adverse effects of transfusions, including infection, ischemia, and mortality. More conservative transfusion thresholds are being advocated by some clinicians for this patient population.
- Although patients with traumatic injuries often present with significant blood loss and are in need of transfusion, the optimal transfusion threshold for hemodynamically stable patients with traumatic brain injury has not been determined.

infections to 1 in 1.4–2.4 million for HIV and immunologic reactions vary from 1 in 100 for febrile reactions to 1 in 600,000 for fatal reactions.[61] It is known that blood transfusions affect the immune response, although the mechanism and severity of immunomodulation are controversial. It has been reported that the use of leukocyte-reduced transfusions is associated with a 50% reduction in multiorgan failure in ICU patients and decreased postoperative infection and mortality in patients undergoing cardiac surgery.[61,62]

Recently, a large (n = 8500), prospective, randomized trial of liberal and conservative transfusion strategies in cardiac surgery demonstrated that blood transfusion was associated with a dose-dependent increase in postoperative infection risk, a sixfold increase in 30 day mortality, and an increased risk of ischemic events (myocardial and cerebral infarcts and renal injury).[63] The increased risk of ischemic events seems to contradict the general premise that administering red blood cells increases oxygen carrying capacity. It has been speculated that the increased risk of ischemia associated with blood transfusions is due to the fact that stored red blood cells are depleted of 2,3-diphosphoglycerate (2,3-DPG), which impairs their ability to release bound oxygen and decreases the ability of the red cell membrane to deform and pass through capillaries.[64]

Patients who present with TBI may have other injuries that result in significant blood loss, and in the face of hemorrhagic shock the benefits of blood transfusion far outweigh the risks; however, the transfusion threshold in hemodynamically stable patients whose hematocrit is less than 30% is less clear. The increased complication rate and mortality associated with blood transfusion in cardiac surgery suggests that blood transfusions should be approached with caution in patients with TBI, and further research will help define the optimal transfusion threshold in TBI.

Conclusion (see Table 20.12)

Treatment of patients with traumatic brain injury begins with an overall assessment of all traumatic injuries and addressing acute concerns over the patient's airway, breathing, and circulation. In situations with considerable acute blood loss, initial resuscitation with normal saline and blood products may be necessary, and all immediate life-threatening injuries should be addressed. After initial evaluation by physical exam and radiological studies, neurosurgical interventions should be evaluated.

Patients with severe head injury may benefit from the use of traditional invasive hemodynamic monitors (arterial, central venous, and pulmonary artery catheters), which can help gauge response to resuscitation. ICP monitors (intraparenchymal or intraventricular) can be used to identify episodes of intracranial hypertension and to calculate CPP. A CPP of 60 to 70 mm Hg is generally accepted as the minimal pressure goal when treating patients with head trauma. Although a low CPP indicates that CBF may be compromised, adequate cerebral oxygen uptake is the ultimate goal of TBI management. Brain tissue oxymetry allows for measurement of cerebral oxygenation with fine intraparenchymal probes, but this technique is of limited use in the routine management of head trauma.

Brain tissue oximetry provides information about the oxygenation of a limited area around the probe, which is dependent on local oxygen diffusion and presents risks of local damage and microbial infection. Although recent data illustrate that these monitors may provide prognostic information, more research needs to be done to determine their utility as tools that guide treatment strategies. These monitors do provide a valuable tool for monitoring treatment effects in clinical trials, and ultimately may be used in routine clinical practice.

The most commonly used fluids in resuscitation are HTS and mannitol. Both agents help decrease cerebral water volume and ICP through passive diffusion of water out of brain parenchyma. Mannitol also causes unique rheological effects that promote increased CBF and oxygen delivery. The main difference is that mannitol administration results in an osmotic diuresis, whereas HTS results in expansion of intravascular volume. This difference makes HTS the treatment of choice in patients who are hemodynamically unstable.

There is insufficient evidence from comparative studies to make firm conclusions about the relative utility of

Table 20.12 Overview of Fluid Resuscitation for TBI

- Cerebral perfusion pressure of 60 to 70 mm Hg as the minimal pressure goal when treating patients with head trauma
- Adequate cerebral oxygen uptake is the ultimate goal of traumatic brain injury management
- Mannitol and HTS causes unique rheological effects that promote increased cerebral blood flow and oxygen delivery, as well as osmotic diuresis
- Hypertonic saline results in expansion of intravascular volume
- Albumin administration is associated with an increased mortality in head trauma patients
- Paradoxical ischemia was found to be associated with transfusions; mortality increased in a dose-dependant manner with each unit of transfused blood, in cardiac surgery patients
- Hemoglobin of ~ 30% represents the theoretical optimal balance between oxygen carrying capacity and oxygen delivery for patients with traumatic brain injury, although the ideal threshold may be lower

one fluid over another, and many of the available studies compare different dosages and schedules of administration for each agent. Oftentimes, treatment with HTS or mannitol is initiated to treat intracranial hypertension, and although these agents can decrease ICP, the ultimate impacts of treatment on survival and long-term neurological recovery are unknown.

In addition, new hetastarch solutions (i.e., pentastarch and tetrastarch) may prove to be safe and effective volume expanders in head trauma. Use of these colloid fluids can help promote higher arterial pressures and better CBF. Because hetastarch solutions have been shown to cause coagulation disorders, they should be used with caution in patients with head trauma until they are proven safe by definitive clinical trials. The results from the SAFE study demonstrate that albumin should be used with caution in patients with head trauma due to increased mortality associated with albumin administration, although it is not known why this increased mortality is seen.

Similarly, blood transfusions have been shown to have significant risks in the population of patients undergoing cardiac surgery. Paradoxical ischemia was found to be associated with transfusions, and mortality increases with each unit of transfused blood in a dose-dependant manner. A hemoglobin of ~30% represents the theoretical optimal balance between oxygen carrying capacity and oxygen delivery for patients with TBI, but the ideal threshold for transfusion may indeed be lower. The risks of transfusion versus the potential benefits must be weighed for each patient, and further research efforts on the effects of blood transfusion in patients with TBI will help define the optimal transfusion threshold.

References

1. Marino PL, Sutin KM. The ICU Book. 3rd ed. Philadelphia: Lippincott Williams and Wilkins; 2006
2. Walley KR, Cooper DJ. Diastolic stiffness impairs left ventricular function during hypovolemic shock in pigs. Am J Physiol 1991;260(3 Pt 2): H702–H712
3. Rosner MJ, Rosner SD, Johnson AH. Cerebral perfusion pressure: management protocol and clinical results. J Neurosurg 1995;83(6): 949–962
4. Hlatky R, Robertson CS. Does raising cerebral perfusion pressure help head-injured patients? In: Andrews BT, Valadka AB, es. Neurotrauma: Evidence-Based Answers to Common Questions. New York: Thieme Medical Publishers; 2005, pp. 75–82
5. Stiefel MF, Udoetuk JD, Spiotta AM, et al. Conventional neurocritical care and cerebral oxygenation after traumatic brain injury. J Neurosurg 2006;105(4):568–575
6. Nonaka M, Yoshimine T, Kohmura E, Wakayama A, Yamashita T, Hayakawa T. Changes in brain organic osmolytes in experimental cerebral ischemia. J Neurol Sci 1998;157(1):25–30
7. Olson JE, Banks M, Dimlich RV, Evers J. Blood–brain barrier water permeability and brain osmolyte content during edema development. Acad Emerg Med 1997;4(7):662–673
8. Hjelmqvist H, Ullman J, Gunnarsson U, Hamberger B, Rundgren M. Increased resistance to haemorrhage induced by intracerebroventricular infusion of hypertonic NaCl in conscious sheep. Acta Physiol Scand 1992;145(2):177–186
9. Holcroft JW, Vassar MJ, Perry CA, Gannaway WL, Kramer GC. Use of a 7.5% NaCl/6% Dextran 70 solution in the resuscitation of injured patients in the emergency room. Prog Clin Biol Res 1989;299:331–338
10. Kien ND, Reitan JA, White DA, Wu CH, Eisele JH. Cardiac contractility and blood flow distribution following resuscitation with 7.5% hypertonic saline in anesthetized dogs. Circ Shock 1991;35(2):109–116
11. Ogata H, Luo XX. Effects of hypertonic saline solution (20%) on cardiodynamics during hemorrhagic shock. Circ Shock 1993;41(2):113–118
12. Ramires JA, Serrano Junior CV, Cesar LA, Velasco IT, Rocha e Silva Junior M, Pileggi F. Acute hemodynamic effects of hypertonic (7.5%) saline infusion in patients with cardiogenic shock due to right ventricular infarction. Circ Shock 1992;37(3):220–225
13. Walsh JC, Zhuang J, Shackford SR. A comparison of hypertonic to isotonic fluid in the resuscitation of brain injury and hemorrhagic shock. J Surg Res 1991;50(3):284–292
14. Bertone JJ, Shoemaker KE. Effect of hypertonic and isotonic saline solutions on plasma constituents of conscious horses. Am J Vet Res 1992; 53(10):1844–1849
15. Cudd TA, Purinton S, Patel NC, Wood CE. Cardiovascular, adrenocorticotropin, and cortisol responses to hypertonic saline in euvolemic sheep are altered by prostaglandin synthase inhibition. Shock 1998; 10(1):32–36
16. Tollofsrud S, Tonnessen T, Skraastad O, Noddeland H. Hypertonic saline and dextran in normovolaemic and hypovolaemic healthy volunteers increases interstitial and intravascular fluid volumes. Acta Anaesthesiol Scand 1998;42(2):145–153
17. Kempski O, Behmanesh S. Endothelial cell swelling and brain perfusion. J Trauma 1997;42(5, Suppl):S38–S40
18. Bauer M, Marzi I, Ziegenfuss T, Seeck G, Buhren V, Larsen R. Comparative effects of crystalloid and small volume hypertonic hyperoncotic fluid resuscitation on hepatic microcirculation after hemorrhagic shock. Circ Shock 1993;40(3):187–193
19. Hartl R, Medary MB, Ruge M, Arfors KE, Ghahremani F, Ghajar J. Hypertonic/hyperoncotic saline attenuates microcirculatory disturbances after traumatic brain injury. J Trauma 1997;42(5, Suppl):S41–S47
20. Spera PA, Arfors KE, Vasthare US, Tuma RF, Young WF. Effect of hypertonic saline on leukocyte activity after spinal cord injury. Spine 1998; 23(22):2444–2448
21. Zausinger S, Thal SC, Kreimeier U, Messmer K, Schmid-Elsaesser R. Hypertonic fluid resuscitation from subarachnoid hemorrhage in rats. Neurosurgery 2004;55(3):679–686
22. Ducey JP, Mozingo DW, Lamiell JM, Okerburg C, Gueller GE. A comparison of the cerebral and cardiovascular effects of complete resuscitation with isotonic and hypertonic saline, hetastarch, and whole blood following hemorrhage. J Trauma 1989;29(11):1510–1518
23. Prough DS, Whitley JM, Taylor CL, Deal DD, Dewitt DS. Regional cerebral blood flow following resuscitation from hemorrhagic shock with hypertonic saline: influence of a subdural mass. Anesthesiology 1991;75(2):319–327
24. Taylor G, Myers S, Kurth CD, et al. Hypertonic saline improves brain resuscitation in a pediatric model of head injury and hemorrhagic shock. J Pediatr Surg 1996;31(1):65–70
25. Worthley LI, Cooper DJ, Jones N. Treatment of resistant intracranial hypertension with hypertonic saline: report of two cases. J Neurosurg 1988;68(3):478–481
26. Hartl R, Ghajar J, Hochleuthner H, Mauritz W. Hypertonic/hyperoncotic saline reliably reduces ICP in severely head-injured patients with intracranial hypertension. Acta Neurochir Suppl (Wien) 1997;70:126–129
27. Horn P, Munch E, Vajkoczy P, et al. Hypertonic saline solution for control of elevated intracranial pressure in patients with exhausted response to mannitol and barbiturates. Neurol Res 1999;21(8):758–764

28. Schatzmann C, Heissler HE, Konig K, et al. Treatment of elevated intracranial pressure by infusions of 10% saline in severely head injured patients. Acta Neurochir Suppl (Wien) 1998;71:31–33
29. Munar F, Ferrer AM, de Nadal M, et al. Cerebral hemodynamic effects of 7.2% hypertonic saline in patients with head injury and raised intracranial pressure. J Neurotrauma 2000;17(1):41–51
30. Gemma M, Cozzi S, Tommasino C, et al. 7.5% hypertonic saline versus 20% mannitol during elective neurosurgical supratentorial procedures. J Neurosurg Anesthesiol 1997;9(4):329–334
31. Shackford SR, Bourguignon PR, Wald SL, Rogers FB, Osler TM, Clark DE. Hypertonic saline resuscitation of patients with head injury: a prospective, randomized clinical trial. J Trauma 1998;44(1):50–58
32. Qureshi AI, Suarez JI, Castro A, Bhardwaj A. Use of hypertonic saline/acetate infusion in treatment of cerebral edema in patients with head trauma: experience at a single center. J Trauma 1999;47(4): 659–665
33. Vialet R, Albanese J, Thomachot L, et al. Isovolume hypertonic solutes (sodium chloride or mannitol) in the treatment of refractory posttraumatic intracranial hypertension: 2 mL/kg 7.5% saline is more effective than 2 mL/kg 20% mannitol. Crit Care Med 2003;31(6):1683–1687
34. Cooper DJ, Myles PS, McDermott FT, et al. Prehospital hypertonic saline resuscitation of patients with hypotension and severe traumatic brain injury: a randomized controlled trial. JAMA 2004;291(11):1350–1357
35. Marshall LF, Smith RW, Rauscher LA, Shapiro HM. Mannitol dose requirements in brain-injured patients. J Neurosurg 1978;48(2):169–172
36. Wise BL, Chater N. The value of hypertonic mannitol solution in decreasing brain mass and lowering cerebro-spinal-fluid pressure. J Neurosurg 1962;19:1038–1043
37. Muizelaar JP, Wei EP, Kontos HA, Becker DP. Mannitol causes compensatory cerebral vasoconstriction and vasodilation in response to blood viscosity changes. J Neurosurg 1983;59(5):822–828
38. Burke AM, Quest DO, Chien S, Cerri C. The effects of mannitol on blood viscosity. J Neurosurg 1981;55(4):550–553
39. Roberts I, Smith R, Evans S. Doubts over head injury studies. BMJ 2007;334(7590):392–394
40. Cruz J, Minoja G, Okuchi K. Improving clinical outcomes from acute subdural hematomas with the emergency preoperative administration of high doses of mannitol: a randomized trial. Neurosurgery 2001; 49(4):864–871
41. Cruz J, Minoja G, Okuchi K. Major clinical and physiological benefits of early high doses of mannitol for intraparenchymal temporal lobe hemorrhages with abnormal pupillary widening: a randomized trial. Neurosurgery 2002;51(3):628–637
42. Cruz J, Minoja G, Okuchi K, Facco E. Successful use of the new high-dose mannitol treatment in patients with Glasgow Coma Scale scores of 3 and bilateral abnormal pupillary widening: a randomized trial. J Neurosurg 2004;100(3):376–383
43. Wakai A, Roberts I, Schierhout G. Mannitol for acute traumatic brain injury. Cochrane Database Syst Rev 2007;(1):CD001049
44. Sayre MR, Daily SW, Stern SA, Storer DL, van Loveren HR, Hurst JM. Out-of-hospital administration of mannitol to head-injured patients does not change systolic blood pressure. Acad Emerg Med 1996;3(9): 840–848
45. Schwartz ML, Tator CH, Rowed DW, Reid SR, Meguro K, Andrews DF. The University of Toronto head injury treatment study: a prospective, randomized comparison of pentobarbital and mannitol. Can J Neurol Sci 1984;11(4):434–440
46. Smith HP, Kelly DL Jr, McWhorter JM, et al. Comparison of mannitol regimens in patients with severe head injury undergoing intracranial monitoring. J Neurosurg 1986;65(6):820–824
47. Shoemaker WC. Relation of oxygen transport patterns to the pathophysiology and therapy of shock states. Intensive Care Med 1987; 13(4):230–243
48. Elliott MB, Jallo JJ, Gaughan JP, Tuma RF. Effects of crystalloid-colloid solutions on traumatic brain injury. J Neurotrauma 2007;24(1):195–202
49. Cochrane Injuries Group. Human albumin administration in critically ill patients: systematic review of randomised controlled trials. Cochrane Injuries Group Albumin Reviewers. BMJ 1998;317(7153): 235–240
50. Wilkes MM, Navickis RJ. Patient survival after human albumin administration: a meta-analysis of randomized, controlled trials. Ann Intern Med 2001;135(3):149–164
51. Finfer S, Bellomo R, Boyce N, French J, Myburgh J, Norton R. A comparison of albumin and saline for fluid resuscitation in the intensive care unit. N Engl J Med 2004;350(22):2247–2256
52. Myburgh J, Cooper J, Finfer S, et al. Saline or albumin for fluid resuscitation in patients with traumatic brain injury. N Engl J Med 2007; 357(9):874–884
53. Kozek-Langenecker SA. Effects of hydroxyethyl starch solutions on hemostasis. Anesthesiology 2005;103(3):654–660
54. Jungheinrich C, Sauermann W, Bepperling F, Vogt NH. Volume efficacy and reduced influence on measures of coagulation using hydroxyethyl starch 130/0.4 (6%) with an optimised in vivo molecular weight in orthopaedic surgery: a randomised, double-blind study. Drugs R D 2004;5(1):1–9
55. de Jonge E, Levi M, Buller HR, Berends F, Kesecioglu J. Decreased circulating levels of von Willebrand factor after intravenous administration of a rapidly degradable hydroxyethyl starch (HES 200/0.5/6) in healthy human subjects. Intensive Care Med 2001;27(11):1825–1829
56. Jamnicki M, Bombeli T, Seifert B, et al. Low- and medium-molecular-weight hydroxyethyl starches: comparison of their effect on blood coagulation. Anesthesiology 2000;93(5):1231–1237
57. Kasper SM, Meinert P, Kampe S, et al. Large-dose hydroxyethyl starch 130/0.4 does not increase blood loss and transfusion requirements in coronary artery bypass surgery compared with hydroxyethyl starch 200/0.5 at recommended doses. Anesthesiology 2003;99(1):42–47
58. Neff TA, Doelberg M, Jungheinrich C, Sauerland A, Spahn DR, Stocker R. Repetitive large-dose infusion of the novel hydroxyethyl starch 130/0.4 in patients with severe head injury. Anesth Analg 2003;96(5): 1453–1459, table
59. Huang SJ, Chen YS, Hong WC, et al. Clinical experience of hydroxyethyl starch (10% HES 200/0.5) in cerebral perfusion pressure protocol for severe head injury. Surg Neurol 2006;66(Suppl 2):S26–S31
60. Deutsch H, Ullman JS. What is the optimal hematocrit and hemoglobin for head-injured patients? In: Valadka AB, Andrews BT, eds. Neurotrauma: Evidence-Based Answers to Common Questions. New York: Thieme; 2005:88–90
61. Ferraris VA, Ferraris SP, Saha SP, et al. Perioperative blood transfusion and blood conservation in cardiac surgery: the Society of Thoracic Surgeons and the Society of Cardiovascular Anesthesiologists clinical practice guideline. Ann Thorac Surg 2007;83(5, Suppl):S27–S86
62. Bilgin YM, van de Watering LM, Eijsman L, Versteegh MI, van Oers MH, Brand A. Is increased mortality associated with post-operative infections after leukocytes containing red blood cell transfusions in cardiac surgery? An extended analysis. Transfus Med 2007;17(4): 304–311
63. Murphy GJ, Reeves BC, Rogers CA, Rizvi SI, Culliford L, Angelini GD. Increased mortality, postoperative morbidity, and cost after red blood cell transfusion in patients having cardiac surgery. Circulation 2007; 116(22):2544–2552
64. Rawn JD. Blood transfusion in cardiac surgery: a silent epidemic revisited. Circulation 2007;116(22):2523–2524
65. Battison C, Andrews PJ, Graham C, Petty T. Randomized controlled trial on the effects of 20% mannitol solution and 7.5% saline-6% dextran solution on increased intracranial pressure after brain surgery. J Neurosurg 1977;46:227–232

V Outcome

21 Rehabilitation

Shane D. McNamee, Treven C. Pickett, Sharon M. Benedict, and David X. Cifu

Traumatic brain injury (TBI) produces a complex constellation of medical consequences including physical, emotional, and cognitive deficits. Because of the multidimensional impact of TBI, a similarly dynamic rehabilitation process is necessary to recover or compensate for lost functional abilities. Immediately postinjury, the most pressing concern is medical stabilization. Later in the recovery process other challenges often emerge requiring active and holistic intervention. Rehabilitation is a method of treatment that uses innovative medical care to help individuals overcome the effects of a brain injury. Rehabilitation aims to restore maximum independence within the framework of individual limitations. Although TBI has only recently become a focus of clinical care and rehabilitation research,[1] it is clear that treatment of brain injury varies according to the severity and type of injury, and rehabilitation treatment plans often change to meet patients' biopsychosocial needs.

Rehabilitation may span months to years from initial time of injury. The process of rehabilitation begins in critical care units and extends to outpatient physician and therapy clinics. In the natural course of recovery, patients with TBI are expected to face several challenges in neurobehavioral, interpersonal/relational, occupational, and community readjustment areas. Early intervention, close interdisciplinary communication, and a holistic understanding of cognitive and functional deficits for a particular patient are integral components in this goal-driven process.[2]

Phases of TBI Rehabilitation Treatment

Typically, only TBI patients classified as complicated-mild, moderate, or severe are hospitalized for initial medical stabilization. When acute medical or surgical care is no longer required, a definitive recommendation for a rehabilitation program should be made. The nature of the disposition depends on factors including medical acuity and functional need. Disposition is often based on the level of cognitive functioning. Cognitive recovery is most commonly measured by the Rancho Los Amigos Scale (RLAS) (**Table 21.1**).[3] Options for rehabilitation settings range from intensive inpatient programs to community-based settings. An uninterrupted, seamless transfer between treatment settings is the key to successful patient management.

Table 21.1 Rancho Los Amigos Levels of Cognitive Functioning Scale

Description	Level
No response	1
Patient is completely unresponsive to any environmental stimuli	
Generalized response	2
Patient reacts inconsistently and nonpurposefully to stimuli. Responses are limited in nature and often the same regardless of the stimuli presented. Pain evokes global response. Sleep/wake cycles exist.	
Localized response	3
Patient responds specifically but inconsistently to stimulus. Responses are directly related to the type of stimuli presented. Head may turn toward a sound or eyes will focus on an object when presented. The individual may follow simple commands and may respond better to some people (i.e., family and friends) than to others.	
Confused: agitated	4
Patient is confused, excited, and often cannot be directed. Will communicate though is often disoriented and confused; attention span is short; patient may cooperate with treatment irregularly	
Confused: inappropriate	5
Patient appears alert. Responds to simple commands consistently. Agitation may still be present. Inappropriate verbalizations and high distractibility are common. Memory is severely impaired, but the individual may do ADLs with supervision.	
Confused: appropriate	6
Patient expresses goal-oriented behavior that needs direction. Simple commands are followed consistently, though memory still impaired. Awareness of self, family, and basic needs is increased.	

(Continued on page 386)

Table 21.1 *(Continued)*

Description	Level
Automatic: appropriate	7
Patient is appropriate within hospital and home settings. Daily routine automatic and robot-like. No longer confused but lacks insight. In an unstructured atmosphere frequently demonstrates poor judgment and problem solving. Typically needs a sheltered home and work environment.	
Purposeful: appropriate	8
Patient is alert and oriented, able to recall and integrate past and recent events. Independent in the home and community. Carryover for new learning is present, and the need for supervision is absent once activities have been learned. Social, emotional, and cognitive abilities may still be decreased.	

Note: The Rancho Los Amigos Levels of Cognitive Functioning (RLA) were designed to measure and track an individual's progress early in the recovery period. They have been used as a means to develop level-specific treatment interventions and strategies designed to facilitate movement from one level to another. An RLA level is determined based on behavioral observations.

Abbreviation: ADLs, activities of daily living.

Intensive Care Units

An interdisciplinary team constituted of rehabilitation specialists should be involved in patient care as soon as clinically indicated. Initial assessments by physiatry (preferably a brain injury specialist), physical therapy (PT), occupational therapy (OT), and speech and language pathology (SLP) specialists are indicated. Ideally, detailed neurological and medical examinations should be performed by a physiatrist as soon as medical stability is achieved. Physiatrists then become increasingly involved in the general medical management of the patient in the intensive care unit (ICU) by conducting serial evaluations to inform disposition planning. Physiatrists pay particular attention to seizure prophylaxis, deep venous thrombosis (DVT) prevention, pain management, bowel and bladder functioning, management of pathologic tone, nutritional status, behavioral issues and sleep cycles. Initial PT and OT assessments include recommendations about positioning in the service of preventing contractures, pressure sores, and peripheral nerve compression injuries. PT and OT therapies involve bedside range of motion (ROM) exercises to maximize functional range in all major joints and to ensure proper positioning. Specific activity training such as toileting and ambulation may be delayed until later in the rehabilitation process. The SLP assessment provides information about baseline cognition, communication abilities, and swallowing safety. Importantly, all of the aforementioned activities are generally well tolerated after moderate to severe TBI and have little impact on management of airway patency and intracranial pressure (ICP).

Neurological Stepdown Units

The initial rehabilitation plan implemented in the ICU should be continued and expanded in the neurological stepdown unit. Sedating medications that are often necessary in the ICU treatment setting are weaned in favor of optimizing arousal and cognitive functioning. It is advisable that comprehensive assessment of cognitive and behavioral capabilities be conducted once sedating agents have been removed. Several commonly used medications may impede cognitive recovery (**Table 21.2**). A broader array of rehabilitation therapies are introduced in this setting, as strict bed rest is no longer necessary or beneficial. At this level of care; transfers' abilities, gait safety, strength, balance, activities of daily living (ADLs), and assistive devices are assessed.

Acute Inpatient Rehabilitation

The last 3 decades have witnessed the emergence of acute inpatient rehabilitation programs that have become the mainstay of care following moderate to severe TBI. These comprehensive, interdisciplinary programs define functional deficits, assess cognitive strengths and weaknesses, and develop individually tailored treatment plans to maximize functional independence in the least restrictive atmosphere. This programmatic approach leads to greater community functioning and self-awareness in the moderate to severely injured.[4–8] Greater intensity of therapy services, particularly cognitive rehabilitation, has been shown to improve outcomes.[9]

The principle aim of acute inpatient rehabilitation is to restore maximal functional independence. Prior to admission, it is necessary to determine the patient's ability to

Table 21.2 Common Medications That Impair Cognition Function

• Narcotics	• Beta-blockers
• Antiepileptic agents	• H2 blockers
• Benzodiazepines	• Paralytics
• Barbiturates	• Metoclopramide
• Antispasticity agents	• Alpha antagonists

Table 21.3 Inpatient Rehabilitation Admissions Criteria

- Acute brain injury related disability and subsequent functional decline
- Support system that allows discharge to the community
- Ability to tolerate 3+ hours of therapy per day
- Medical stability

tolerate and benefit from the intensity of a daily therapy regimen (**Table 21.3**). The intensity of therapy services must be balanced against the need for the least restrictive treatment environment. The pace and extent of recovery from brain injury can vary considerably, even between patients with similar injuries. Another important consideration is the resilience of the patient's support system. Presence of interested and committed family may determine whether a patient is admitted for rehabilitation. Strong psychosocial support expedites progress toward rehabilitation goals and is helpful in reinforcing discharge recommendations for residual cognitive and behavioral deficits.

Acute inpatient rehabilitation programs support cognitive recovery while maximizing safety. These facilities are preferably separate, and locked, as a way to ensure environmental control. Therapy services include, on average, 3 hours of structured therapy per day, 24-hour specialized nursing care, and daily physiatric services, within the framework of an interdisciplinary model. Physiatrists lead interdisciplinary teams in this setting which typically consist of specialists from rehabilitation nursing (CRRN), physical therapy, occupational therapy, speech-language pathology, psychology/ neuropsychology, social work/case management, and recreation therapy (**Table 21.4**). Other consultative services may be needed for targeted problems such as orthopedics, neurosurgery, wound care, and neuroophthalmology. Interdisciplinary team (IDT) meetings should occur on a regular basis. These meetings provide a forum to apprise staff of medical status, allow for revisions in rehabilitation goals, address psychosocial issues, and plan for discharge.

Subacute Rehabilitation Units

Not all individuals suffering a moderate to severe TBI are appropriate for acute rehabilitation programs. In particular, two patient subpopulations require other types of specialty care. Those who have yet to return to consciousness cannot actively participate in rehabilitation. However, they benefit from other specialty programs. Recommendations for the minimally conscious patient are discussed below. Second, those too frail to tolerate at least 3 hours of therapy per day, elderly patients with numerous comorbid medical problems, severely debilitated patients, minimally conscious patients, or those with medical restrictions

Table 21.4 Members of a Traumatic Brain Injury Rehabilitation Team

Integrated approach focused on improving cognitive, behavioral, and physical deficits with the goal of enhancing function and independence

Case manager/social worker

- Facilitates effective coordination of patient care and appropriate utilization of community resources
- Coordinates discharge planning and follow-up
- Treatment includes crisis intervention, family counseling, and patient/family support groups

Neuropsychologist

- Expert in diagnosis of cognitive impairments
- Detailed neuropsychological assessment provides global assessment of intellectual functioning
- Guides treatment of cognitive deficits and their functional impact
- Educates patient and family members about brain injury and coping skills

Occupational therapist

- Functional experts
- Range of motion, splinting, and strengthening of upper extremities
- Enhances self-management skills: ADLs (e.g., feeding, dressing, grooming) and IADLs (shopping, driving, school and work activities)
- Application of equipment (e.g., memory aids, utensils)

Physiatrist

- Physician rehabilitation specialist provides medical evaluations and establishes plan of care
- Treats physical, cognitive, and behavioral sequelae of TBI
- Provides leadership for rehabilitation therapies
- Coordinates treatment to maximize the level of function

(Continued on page 388)

Table 21.4 *(Continued)*

Physical therapist
• Assess and treat for functional mobility, balance disorders, strengthen, physical problems, and pain
• Advances mobility, increase strength, decrease joint stiffness, improve balance, and manage pain and discomfort
• Evaluates equipment needs for ambulation
Psychologist
• Addresses emotional and behavioral sequelae of patient and family
• Establish behavioral management program
Recreation therapist
• Focuses on resuming community life through participation in play and leisure activities
• Treat in everyday settings through community outings
Speech and language pathologist
• Detailed assessment and treatment of cognitive and communication deficits
• Gain optimal communication skills
• Appraise aspiration risk and teach safe swallowing techniques to advance diet
Certified registered rehabilitation nurses (CRRN)
• Participate in the development and implementation of the therapeutic plan
• Skin and positioning management
• Family education and support
Vocational rehabilitation counselor
• Details premorbid work skills and assesses skills for job placement
• Provides assistance in returning to work through collaboration with employer, patient, and case manager

Abbreviations: ADLs, activities of daily living; IADLs, instrumental activities of daily living; TBI, traumatic brain injury.

(i.e., numerous fractures with weight-bearing restrictions) may be more appropriate for subacute rehabilitation units. Such programs provide supportive nursing and therapy albeit at a reduced intensity relative to acute inpatient rehabilitation units. Physical and occupational therapy services are typically available; speech and intensive cognitive therapies are less commonly available. The goal for subacute rehabilitation programs is to build functional capability for eventual discharge to a community setting.

Postacute Management of TBI

Management Based on Severity of TBI

TBI is a heterogeneous construct with ranges of severity that have been outlined by the American Academy of Physical Medicine and Rehabilitation (AAPM&R). *Mild TBI* (mTBI) is defined as loss of consciousness (LOC) <30 minutes with normal computed tomography (CT) and/or magnetic resonance imaging (MRI) findings, posttraumatic amnesia (PTA) <24 hours, and Glasgow Coma Scale score (GCS) of 13 to 15. Complicated mTBI is defined as neuroimaging findings without measurable residual deficit. *Moderate TBI* is LOC <6 hours, GCS score of 9 to 12, and PTA <7 days. *Severe TBI* is LOC >6 hours, GCS score of <9, PTA >7 days.[10]

Mild TBI

An estimated 80% of individuals sustaining a TBI are classified as mTBI.[11] Most mTBI patients make a rapid recovery, suffer few postinjury complications, and, for these reasons, often bypass acute medical attention or hospitalization. Nevertheless, up to a third of mTBI patients develop chronic symptoms, and delayed symptom onset is not uncommon.[11–13]

Postconcussive Syndrome

Postconcussive syndrome (PCS) refers to an array of physical, emotional, and cognitive symptoms that can occur following mTBI. **Table 21.5** compares symptom frequency in PCS versus the general population.[14,15] Patients with PCS may complain of headaches, postural balance problems

Table 21.5 Frequency of Postconcussive Syndrome (PCS) Symptoms following mTBI and in the General Population

Symptoms	mTBI PCS Symptom Frequency (% of Patients)	Frequency in the General Population (% of People)	PCS Increase after MHI (% Increase over Baseline)
Poor concentration	71	14	57
Irritability	66	16	50
Tired a lot more	64	13	51
Depression	63	20	43
Memory problems	59	20	39
Headaches	59	13	46
Anxiety	58	24	34
Trouble thinking	57	6	51
Dizziness	52	7	35
Visual changes	45	8	37
Sensitivity to light	40	14	26

Abbreviations: MHI, mild head injury; mTBI, mild traumatic brain injury.

insomnia, memory problems, fatigue, irritability or depressed mood, or interpersonal conflict. PCS is challenging to diagnose using a detailed physical examination or neuroimaging alone. It is often the case, unfortunately, that misattributions of underlying psychopathology are made to PCS patients. In other instances PCS patients may be regarded as motivated solely by secondary gain.

Given the broad negative impact exerted by PCS in major life areas, it is vital that PCS symptoms be delineated and aggressively treated as early as possible postinjury. Treatment for PCS symptoms often includes recommendations for improved rest, education about the transient nature of symptoms, and headache management. A stance emphasizing "validation" of PCS symptoms, paired with setting reasonable expectations for recovery, is recommended.[16] Pharmacological interventions are indicated for headaches and sleep problems that are unresponsive to behavioral management strategies. Headaches generally respond to nonsteroidal antiinflammatory drugs (NSAIDs), Midrin (Carnrick Laboratories, Cedar Knolls, NJ), and tryptans. Refractory headache pain can be treated with botulinum toxin injections into the frontalis and temporalis muscles.[17] Sleep disturbance following concussions is particularly unappreciated as an event following mTBI.[18] These sleep problems can worsen other problems that frequently occur in mild head injuries such as inattention, poor concentration, depression, relationship difficulties, and decreased problem-solving abilities. Trazodone is the first-line agent for sleep disturbances; zolpidem is also effective. Selective serotonin reuptake inhibitors (SSRIs) may improve depression, anxiety, and irritability following mTBI.[19] Neurostimulants such as methylphenidate can improve fatigue, slowed processing, and attention deficits.

Moderate TBI

Moderate TBI patients will typically continue to experience cognitive, behavioral, and functional challenges in the months and years postinjury. These patients have generally been hospitalized as a consequence of their injuries, and most will require intensive inpatient acute rehabilitation services followed by a structured residential (or intensive outpatient) rehabilitation program. Typically, physical injuries heal, though cognitive and neurobehavioral problems linger and result in disability. Prominent cognitive sequelae following moderate TBI include those in attention and concentration, new learning and memory, and executive control.[20] Vocational reentry is often possible with moderate TBI patients with appropriate accommodations (adaptive equipment/devices, distraction-free environment), structured or modified schedule (for fatigue management), and available supervisory support. Gradual resumption of vocational activities, with a premium placed upon ensuring success experiences, is often recommended to help restore feelings of self-worth and efficacy. Clinicians should reinforce the idea of return to work as early as is clinically indicated as a way of promoting appropriate expectations for recovery, and concretizing long-term incentives. It is helpful for rehabilitation professionals to establish working relationships with vocational rehabilitation specialists to optimize odds for successful return to work.

Severe TBI

Severe TBI results in profound, long-term cognitive and neurobehavioral deficits. Compensatory strategies are necessary to manage environmental complexities that may have been routine preinjury. Cognitive deficits in attention/concentration, processing speed, new learning and memory, and executive functioning (problem solving, organization, self-monitoring, self-awareness) indicate the need for ongoing professional and often caregiver assistance. Neurobehavioral problems might include impulsivity, disinhibition, and reduced frustration tolerance, hypersensitivity to sound/light, apathy, poor initiation, and social inappropriateness. Mood symptoms could manifest as depression, anxiety, irritability, lability, and poorly modulated emotional expression. Severe TBI patients are generally only capable of working in highly structured employment situations requiring simple, repetitive, and routine tasks. Special supervision is necessary to monitor work completion and accuracy and to manage persisting neurobehavioral problems that might affect the quality of coworker relationships and employment longevity. Severe TBI patients are unlikely to return to independent living. Appropriate placement of these patients is often in supervised residential settings such as adult group homes. In the event that family assumes fulltime care for these patients, associated caregiver stress and burden should be monitored and interventions made as indicated. Pharmacological and behavioral interventions to improve patients' quality of life can also reduce caregiver burden. Common residual sequelae of severe TBI including spasticity, pain, contractures, and dysphagia also require vigilant management.

Minimally Conscious Patient with TBI

Patients at RLAS 3 and below have not yet achieved a return of consciousness that would indicate placement in an acute intensive inpatient rehabilitation program. To progress, at a minimum, a patient must be able to follow simple commands. Programs have been developed to provide supportive services to accelerate return to consciousness. These programs typically employ environmental control of stimuli as a way of bringing about increased cortical arousal. Sedating medications and other barriers to consciousness are removed along with pharmacologic stimulation. Numerous titles are given to this approach, including "coma stimulation" and "cortical stimulation." To date, the literature provides little support for acceleration to return to consciousness using this approach.[21]

Management of Functional Implications of TBI

Motor Disturbances and Recovery

Motor disturbances are common in TBI patients and present treatment challenges. The nature of the motor problems depends in part on injury locus. It is frequently the case that TBI patients also have motor problems unrelated to neurological damage (i.e., peripheral orthopedic fractures). Neurologically mediated motor impairment may result in reduced strength, coordination, dexterity, and/or speed. Formal gait or movement analysis may uncover specific impairments that help guide therapies. Prognosis for recovery of gross motor and complex coordination abilities (such as ambulation) is favorable. Katz found that 85% of severe TBI patients eventually ambulate independently, and most (95%) within the first 2 to 3 months postinjury.[22] Return of upper extremity motor function occurs under similar, although slightly prolonged, time frames.

Postural imbalance and motor problems due to vestibular dysfunction may also complicate gross motor functioning. These problems result from a variety of central and peripheral lesions. Benign positional vertigo must be investigated in all patients presenting with dizziness. Comprehensive assessment of motor functioning should be undertaken by a physiatrist with input from physical and occupational therapists.

Problems with muscular weakness respond well to progressive resistance exercises and active assisted ROM. Ataxia and tremors can be addressed therapeutically using arm weights and weighted walkers to decrease the amplitude of movement. Beta-blocking and dopaminergic agonist medications offer modest benefit.

Slowed motor responses have clear functional and vocational implications. These problems appear to be due to central processing delays and not necessarily to secondary effects of a motor deficit.[23] No consensus exists as to the most effective treatment approach for slowed motor responses. Neurostimulants (e.g., methylphenidate 0.3 mg/kg twice daily) that improve cognitive processing speed may provide some benefit.[24,25]

Sensory Deficits

Sensory deficits after TBI depend on lesion locus such that disturbances may occur with basic sensation (i.e., visual acuity), perceptual processing of stimuli (i.e., visual spatial perception), olfactory/taste, or auditory processing. Damage to the thalamic system can result in refractory central pain syndromes.[26] Self-report of sensory problems are affected by communication and underlying cognitive deficits. Neuropsychological evaluation may assist in delineating the nature of sensory-perceptual impairments. Heterogeneity of sensory deficits precludes standardized approaches to rehabilitation. Involvement of specialists in vision, hearing, and rehabilitation of varied sensory problems is warranted for many TBI patients.

Management of Medical Complications of TBI

Pain

TBI often exists in the context of multisystem trauma, fractures, nerve injuries, and other musculoskeletal injuries. Pain incidence 1 year after TBI is between 52 and 72.6% and may actually increase over time.[27–30] Given the complexity of these injuries, it is not unusual to have multiple pain generators.[31] Assessment and treatment of pain after TBI pose great challenges.[32] Poorly controlled pain can cause distraction and cognitive impairment and can serve as a barrier to functional recovery. Conversely, opiate and neuropathic medications often cause sedation.[33] In addition, as cognition and communication are often impaired after TBI, clinicians may have to rely on other signs or symptoms (e.g., agitation, deformity, swelling, hypertension, tachycardia) to assess the presence of pain.

Interestingly, a negative relationship between injury severity and pain reporting frequency has been reported by numerous sources.[27,29,34,35] Namely, those with mild injuries report higher rates of pain. Prevalence rates of the type of pain have not been detailed in the literature. As expected, the most common locations of pain are in the head and neck.[29,36,37] Though the differential diagnosis in chronic posttraumatic headaches is long, migraines, tension, and cervicogenic subtypes are the most common types.[38]

Detailed, serial pain assessments should be conducted, and frequent adjustments to the pain treatment regimen may be needed. If possible, pain should be classified into one of two broad entities, musculoskeletal or neuropathic. Physical modalities including heat, ultrasound, transcutaneous nerve stimulation, and cryotherapy should be tried initially. Scheduled administration of acetaminophen or ibuprofen can be effective for musculoskeletal pain with limited cognitive side-effects. Targeted narcotic regimens are generally well tolerated by patients, although the side effect profile is limiting. Antiepileptic medications and tricyclic antidepressants have been shown to be efficacious in the treatment of neuropathic pain. These medications should be initiated at night, as they can actually promote normalization of sleep cycles.

Use of nonpharmacological pain management strategies in TBI patients can also be challenging. Traditional cognitive and behavioral pain management tools, which presume an ability to comprehend, assess, rate, and track the chronic pain experience will be difficult to master for individuals who have problems with organization, memory, and planning. A basic, but effective, behavioral pain management strategy for TBI patients is the use of redirection or distraction, in conjunction with scheduled dosing of medication. Presenting tasks or activities (i.e., worksheets, puzzles, movies) and reinforcing adherence to therapy schedules serves to focus the patient on the external environment and reduce perseveration on pain. More complex tasks such as keeping a pain diary, pacing activity levels, and employing cognitive strategies to reframe the pain experience may be more effective when simplified to accommodate specific cognitive deficits. Even in the cognitively impaired, simple adaptive responses to pain (i.e., diaphragmatic breathing, basic visual imagery, tension reduction) can be learned with repetition, reinforcement, and patience. Although no strict clinical guidelines exist for the treatment of pain after TBI, regimens should be individualized and tailored to allow patients to continue to make functional gains. Ideally, design and implementation of a comprehensive pain management program for brain-injured individuals require close collaboration between a trained behavioral specialist (i.e., pain or rehabilitation psychologist) and the physiatrist.

Deep Venous Thrombosis Prophylaxis and Treatment

The incidence of DVT following TBI is between 16 to 54%.[39] Numerous factors associated with TBI, including immobility, extremity fractures, and neurological surgery, place individuals at high risk for the development of DVT. The morbidity of pulmonary embolism (PE) and postphlebitic syndrome is significant. PE places great stress upon the cardiopulmonary system, which can weaken an already frail individual. Postphlebitic syndrome is a chronic condition associated with pain, varicosities, edema, recurrent DVT, and skin integrity issues.

The symptom complex of swelling, pain, and provocative measures do not consistently present in DVT. Suspicion for occult DVT necessitates further workup. Venography represents the gold standard for DVT diagnosis, although it is seldom used due to the inherent risks associated with an invasive procedure. Doppler ultrasonography is a noninvasive, highly available, and sensitive diagnostic test. D-dimer testing demonstrates good correlation with ultrasonography, although its poor specificity limits it use.[40–43]

Given the high risk of DVT after TBI, prophylactic treatment is standard. The decision to delay chemical prophylaxis in the case of impending surgery or intracranial bleed must be weighed against the risk of developing a DVT. Recent studies in both TBI and neurosurgical populations support the safety of heparin products for chemical prophylaxis.[44–50] Unfractionated heparin sodium is typically given at 5000 units subcutaneously every 12 hours for all nonambulatory individuals. Patients with a history of DVT or long bone or pelvic fractures should be considered for more aggressive prophylaxis with low-molecular-weight heparin.[51,52] There is no evidence that TED hose or aspirin reduce the risk of developing DVT. Graded compression stockings are of low utility.[51] Early ambulation should be encouraged, and chemical prophylaxis should be continued until ambulation is initiated.

Treatment of DVT and PE requires anticoagulation for at least 3 and 6 months, respectively.[52] This holds true whether clots occur in the upper or lower limbs. There is no consensus on treatment of DVT proximal to the popliteal fossa. Bed rest is recommended until 24 hours after treatment has been initiated. Low-molecular-weight heparin is recommended once diagnosis has been made due to its rapid achievement of full anticoagulation. Over time, warfarin is introduced, with a target international normalized ratio (INR) between 2 and 3. Anticoagulation in individuals with high fall risk (i.e., elderly, cognitively impaired) should be closely monitored. Greenfield filters are restricted for those who have suffered a PE despite full anticoagulation or when anticoagulation is contraindicated.[52]

Spasticity

Spasticity, a type of hypertonicity, is defined as velocity-dependent increase in tone.[53] The term *spasticity* is often used to describe all types of hypertonicity, including rigidity and dystonia. Upper motor neuron syndrome is characterized by weakness, increase in muscle tone, and loss of dexterity.[54] Injury anywhere along the upper motor neuron (UMN) track leads to varying degrees of symptoms. Muscle hypertonicity is commonly seen after TBI and is due to the loss of supraspinal inhibition to the muscle stretch reflex.[55–57] The unique presentations of spasticity and its functional impact warrants individualized treatment plans and serial clinical monitoring. Common patterns seen after TBI include adduction of the shoulder, wrist flexion, hip adduction, knee extension, and ankle plantar flexion.[58] Specific goals of spasticity treatment include improvement in gait, efficiency of transfers, positioning, motor and pain control, hygiene, and prevention of contractures.

Initially, the clinician must distinguish spasticity from other causes of resistance to passive motion, including joint derangement, fractures, heterotopic ossification, and contractures. Spasticity can have positive, but more frequently negative, impact on patient function. It leads to fibrosis and contractures, which represent a great barrier to both function and therapy participation.[59] In particular, muscles that cross two joints carry the highest risk for contracture.[60,61] On the other hand, increased extensor tone in the lower extremities can be used beneficially in stand–pivot transfers and standing when volitional strength is inadequate.

The degree of spasticity can serve as a useful clinical marker. A sudden increase in spasticity may be the only sign of a change in the underlying homeostasis in severely injured patients. A detailed search for triggers should include infection (commonly urinary tract), ulcers, occult fractures, and metabolic disturbances.

Treatment of spasticity should be multimodal and include both therapeutic interventions and medications. A detailed assessment of the locations (focal versus global), severity, and functional impact cannot be overly stressed. Daily bedside ROM exercises to all major joints and proper positioning form the therapeutic foundation of treatment. Prolonged stretch employed through orthotics or serial casting can improve underlying tone as well as soft tissue elements. Improvements are seen in strength and balance in ambulatory individuals.[62]

All medications are limited by shared adverse effect, particularly some degree of sedation. Dantrolene sodium is typically recommended as a first-line agent. It acts on the peripheral muscle and theoretically has less cognitive-sedating effect. Tizanidine and diazepam are effective in controlling both upper and lower extremity tone,[63] although are rarely used due to their sedation. Oral baclofen mainly relieves lower extremity tone and likewise is limited by somnolence.[64] TBI patients generally tolerate low doses of oral baclofen. However, when TBI leads to severe, global spasticity, the patient typically often cannot tolerate the effective dose. Intrathecal delivery offers much lower systemic dose and higher concentration delivered to the site of action. Over time, these systems have been proven safe, effective, and well tolerated.[65–69] To assure success, patient selection and education are of utmost importance as frequent adjustments are necessary. Intrathecal baclofen has also shown the added benefit of positively impacting the symptoms of autonomic dysfunction.[68,70,71]

Injection techniques, such as intramuscular phenol and botulinum toxin are effective in the treatment of focal spasticity. Botulinum toxin seems particularly effective in the upper limbs.[72,73] Improvements in tone are typically transient and, if effective, treatment will need to be repeated. Orthopedic and neurosurgical management are occasionally indicated after TBI. Procedures include dorsal rhizotomy to decrease sensory stimuli and tendon or soft tissue releases in cases of severe, functionally limiting contracture. Any invasive approach should be complemented with ongoing therapies to maximize functional improvements.

Seizure Prophylaxis and Treatment

Moderate to severe TBI often leads to the development of posttraumatic seizures (PTSs). The literature suggests that effective prophylaxis against early seizures has no impact on late seizures.[74–78] Temkin demonstrated the effectiveness of decreasing the amount of early seizures with 7 days of phenytoin prophylaxis.[79] This practice is endorsed by both the American Association of Neurological Surgeons and the American Academy of Physical Medicine and Rehabilitation. Early glucocorticoid administration has no impact on late seizures and has actually been associated with increased early seizure activity.[77]

Seizures after TBI are generally categorized as immediate (<24 hours), early (24 hours to 7 days), and late (>7 days). Seizures may be triggered by direct brain trauma, hemorrhagic irritation, metabolic disturbances, and hypoxia. The incidence of late seizures affect from 14 to 53% of moderate to severe TBI survivors.[80] Most patients (75 to 80%) who develop posttraumatic epilepsy experience their first seizure within 2 years postinjury.[81]

Risk factors for developing posttraumatic epilepsy have been identified, including biparietal contusion, dural penetration, multiple intracranial surgeries, subdural hematoma with evacuation, focal temporal or frontal lesions, presence of apolipoprotein E (APOE), and midline shift >5 mm.[80,82,83]

Development of both early and late seizures warrants at least 12 months of antiepileptic treatment. Immediate seizures are not considered a risk factor and require only the 7-day universal prophylaxis. The literature supports the use of both carbamazepine and valproate in treatment of PTS.[84] These and other traditional treatments (i.e., phenytoin, phenobarbital) must be used with caution as they may have a negative effect on cognitive recovery.[85] Newer agents (e.g., lamotrigine), though less sedating, have yet to be established as an effective treatment for PTS.

Heterotopic Ossification

Abnormal bone formation in soft tissues or periarticular regions following TBI occurs in 11 to 77% of cases.[86–88] True neurogenic heterotopic ossification (HO), however, occurs in periarticular regions, whereas myositis ossificans is found in areas of direct trauma. Although the underlying pathophysiology of HO is unknown, prevailing theories propose a neuroendocrine alteration. Risk factors include central nervous system (CNS) damage, prolonged coma (>2 months), spasticity, and fractures. The symptoms of HO include pain, decreased ROM, warmth, palpable mass, and tenderness. The hips are overwhelmingly most affected followed by the shoulders, knees, and elbows. Complications include decreased ROM that often impairs gait, pain, and nerve compression. Not surprisingly, HO has been linked to poorer functional outcomes.[89,90]

Plain x-rays are useful in the diagnosis of HO once the lesion has calcified. Early readings are typically negative. With high clinical suspicion, a triple-phase bone scan is warranted and serves as a more reliable diagnostic test in the early phases. Serum alkaline phosphate may be used to monitor maturity of lesions but has limited utility in diagnosis.

There is no evidence supporting prophylaxis with either bisphosphonates or high-dose irradiation (as used in hip arthroplasty) in the treatment of HO after TBI.[1] Treatment of HO should be daily ROM exercises at a minimum. Progression may be halted with the use of etidronate and ibuprofen. Case reports suggest treatment efficacy with high-dose radiation[91] and continuous passive motion machines.[92] Surgical excision should be reserved for mature, functionally detrimental lesions. More research is needed to fully evaluate the benefits of these novel treatment modalities.

Bladder Management

The cerebral control center of micturition exists in the frontal lobe. Damage to this area leads to an uninhibited bladder and is common after TBI. Bladder emptying is due to detrusor hyperreflexia and is characterized by frequent and uncontrolled voids. Given the widespread use of internal catheters in the acute management phase, a urinary tract infection must be initially ruled out. If negative for UTI, retention can be evaluated with postvoid residuals. Timed voids during waking hours along with fluid management form the basis of a successful bladder retraining program. Anticholinergic medications decrease detrusor hyperreflexia, but are limited by side-effect profile (i.e., sedation, memory impairment, and orthostatic hypotension).

Neuroendocrine Dysfunction

TBI can result in abnormalities across the endocrine system. A 62% incidence of pituitary injury has been reported in an autopsy study.[93] From 36 to 69% of TBI survivors have abnormalities in at least one hormone level.[94,95]

Abnormal serum sodium is a common electrolyte abnormality, which necessitates serial measurement in the acute stage. Hyponatremia is typically due to a syndrome of inappropriate antidiuretic hormone secretion (SIADH) or cerebral salt wasting (CSW), although iatrogenic causes must be considered. Hyponatremia and SIADH must be distinguished, as SIADH requires fluid restriction and CSW calls for salt replacement. Hypernatremia due to diabetes insipidus (DI) responds well to fluid management in the acute stage. Late-onset DI typically requires the addition of synthetic ADH. Careful fluid and electrolyte management is usually effective in the acute stages.

Amenorrhea usually resolves within the first year. Pregnancy testing is strongly recommended in any patient of childbearing age. Galactorrhea and gynecomastia occur from elevations of prolactin and can be seen after TBI. Sexual dysfunction in men is also common, although psychoemotional factors should be considered.

With the exception of sodium monitoring, no guidelines exist for the screening of neuroendocrine dysfunction. Patients with confounding symptoms should be screened to determine 9 am cortisol, thyroid axis, follicle-stimulating hormone (FSH), luteinizing hormone (LH), testosterone (in men), and estrogen (in women) levels. An experienced neuroendocrinologist should be consulted for management.

Nutrition

Given the hypermetabolic state following TBI, it is imperative to provide early, adequate nutrition. This caloric expenditure in acute rehabilitation has been estimated at

40 to 69% above premorbid baseline.[96] Fewer complications are noted when appropriate nutrition is supplied during the first 24 hours postinjury.[97] Common complications including gastroparesis, gastric ulcers, cognitive impairment, and nausea compound nutritional deficit. Poor nutrition is associated with numerous morbidities (i.e., poor wound healing, pneumonia, increased cardiovascular workload) and is linked to poor rehabilitative outcomes.[98,99] Nutritional state should be monitored starting with serial weight assessments. Supplementing with serum protein product evaluations and/or 24-hour urea nitrogen levels can provide useful windows into the nitrogen balance. In general, 2 to 2.5 g protein/kg per day and 25 to 35 nonprotein kcal/kg per day are recommended.[97]

Swallowing

Dysphagia can affect 25 to 60% of TBI patients; frank aspiration is seen in up to 42% of the population.[100] Aspiration pneumonia represents a serious complication, with mortality in up to 10% of cases. Bedside swallow evaluations have poor sensitivity, missing up to 40% of "silent" aspirations.[98,99] Standard of care is therefore either dynamic radiologic testing (barium swallow) or fiberoptic endoscopic evaluation.[101] Once aspiration risk is determined, both liquid and solid consistencies typically need altering. Unfortunately, nasogastric feeding provides little protection against aspiration (up to 50% occurrence following TBI).[102] After 3 weeks of non-oral feeding, a percutaneous gastric or jejunal tube is recommended. Involvement of a speech-language pathologist (SLP) is helpful, as these professionals help to clarify the diagnostic picture and provide recommendations for diet modification and compensatory strategies to minimize aspiration risk.

Management of Behavioral and Emotional Dysfunction in TBI

Acute Management

Behavioral problems such as agitation, hypoarousal, and depression are common in the early stages following brain injury.[103–105] Though expected, these behaviors can be difficult to manage and present a significant barrier to functional recovery (**Table 21.6**). *Behavioral management* refers to a planned and coordinated process to increase the frequency of patients' adaptive behaviors.[106] This often involves the strategic use of rewards and punishments. Typically devised by the staff psychologist, behavioral management plans can be implemented by interdisciplinary team members and other individuals involved in the patient's care.

Agitation

Agitation has been defined as a special subtype of delirium specific to TBI, and includes PTA and behaviors such as disinhibition, emotional lability, aggression, and akathisia.[107] Agitation is among the most commonly reported behavioral problem in the acute care setting. Behaviors such as psychomotor restlessness, yelling or cursing, angry outbursts, striking out, and inappropriate sexual gestures (i.e., public masturbation) can be distressing to family members and clinicians who are unfamiliar with TBI sequelae. The emergence of such behaviors often signals neurologic recovery. Nevertheless, it is imperative to rule out other etiologies because several iatrogenic and physiologic

Table 21.6 Common Problems Observed by Medical Professionals during the Acute Stages Postinjury, and the Symptoms and Associated Problems Characterizing these Problems

Agitation
• Combativeness and verbal or physical aggression
• Irritability
• Confusion and disorientation
• Motor restlessness
• Limited self-awareness and insight
• Impulsivity
• Drooling or spitting
• Difficulties with verbal expression
• Sleep problems
Hypoarousal
• Problems awakening or remaining awake
• Decreased alertness
• Sleep problems
• Attention and concentration problems
Depression
• Depressed or labile mood
• Flat affect
• Crying spells
• Expressions suggesting feelings of hopelessness, pessimism, or worthlessness
• Anhedonia
• Psychomotor retardation
• Sleep problems
• Poor appetite or weight loss
• Hypoarousal
• Limited energy, persistence, or motivation

Source: Cifu DX, Kreutzer JS, Slater D, Taylor L. Issues in brain injury rehabilitation. In: Braddom R, ed. Physical Medicine and Rehabilitation, 3rd ed. Philadelphia: Saunders; 2006:1133–1174

causes are possible. These include hydrocephalus, intracranial bleeding, seizure, pulmonary embolism, electrolyte disturbance, infection, medications, undertreated pain, and disturbed sleep.[105]

The Agitated Behavior Scale (ABS)[108] and the Overt Agitation Severity Scale (OAS)[109] are two measures constructed to assess agitation. The ABS is a 40-point agitation rating scale that has the advantages of rapid administration (<5 minutes), internal consistency, and adequate interrater reliability. ABS scores can be utilized to inform clinical interventions, and serial measurements (e.g., 3 times per day) can provide valuable feedback about the effectiveness of these interventions. An ABS score >28, for example, falls in the "moderate" range and warrants medication intervention.

Nonpharmacologic approaches are recommended to manage agitation when the behaviors are not severe or dangerous. Physical restraints are the most restrictive mode of intervention and are generally discouraged save for those instances when agitation leads to self-harm or harm of others. In situations where physical restraints are necessary, it is strongly recommended that providers first refer to state laws and facility guidelines. Environmental manipulations that address sleep/wake cycles, noise levels, pain, and reorientation to reduce confusion, may have a behavioral calming effect. Redirection and time-out can be used by staff to divert agitated patients' attention from sources of irritation. Some authors also have suggested channeling nonpurposeful physical activity to safer and more adaptive behaviors.[106]

Pharmacologic approaches should be utilized when environmental and/or behavioral management strategies fail. Whereas numerous studies support the use of β-blockers for post-TBI agitation, less robust evidence exists for the use of tricyclic antidepressants, atypical antipsychotics, stimulants, narcotics, and anticonvulsants.[1] Suggested practice to pharmacologically manage post-TBI agitation is to be conservative with initial starting dose, and to slowly titrate upward. Monitoring response to treatment is possible using standardized scales such as the ABS or OAS. Polypharmacy is discouraged given the importance of promoting cognitive recovery as early as possible in acute rehabilitation.

Hypoarousal

Hypoarousal is especially problematic during hospitalization because the patient's ability to remain awake and alert during treatment is compromised. Motor restlessness, involuntary yawning, drowsiness, and waning attention over a therapy session may all suggest inadequate arousal. Consequently, patients with hypoarousal may only be able to tolerate short periods of active therapy and may opt out of therapeutic activities that require cognitive exertion.[106]

Frequent breaks, early discrimination of fatigue, and promoting sleep hygiene are all effective nonpharmacologic environmental strategies to improve arousal. Therapists should consider scheduling sessions during times of peak alertness. Within sessions, content should alternate between challenging and less intense tasks. Staff should be vigilant to patient arousal levels within treatment sessions and, importantly, reduce task demands in advance of fatigue onset. Pharmacologic interventions such as the use of psychostimulants (e.g., methylphenidate and amantadine sulfate) may complement environmental and behavioral strategies.[110]

Depression

Estimates of the frequency of depressive disorders ranges from 6 to 77% in the literature.[111–113] Patients with premorbid personal or family history of depression may be at greater risk to develop depressive symptoms subsequent to TBI. However, the majority of depressive episodes arise in patients with no such vulnerabilities. Depressive symptoms may be associated with lesion locus. Some researchers have found a correlation between depression and left anterior and subcortical injury at the 1-month time point.[114] Depressive symptoms can significantly contribute to disability subsequent to a TBI. In mTBI, depressive symptoms may either present as a component of postconcussive symptoms or as a discrete major depressive episode.

Findings suggest that rehabilitation outcomes are adversely affected by depression,[115] and for this reason evaluation and treatment of depression are vital in the acute rehabilitation stage. Depression interferes with patients' ability to participate in and benefit from rehabilitation.[106] Symptoms of depressed mood include sadness, irritability, hopelessness, tearfulness, anhedonia, suicidal ideation, and sleep/appetite disturbances. The assessment of post-TBI depression often requires an appreciation for the natural course of emotional recovery after a TBI, and determining whether there is presence of mood disorder beyond that which would be expected secondary to TBI. This presents a formidable clinical diagnostic challenge. TBI patients may have cognitive problems such as aphasia that interfere with the accuracy of symptom reporting. Also, the injury or the hospitalization process may bring about "depressive" symptoms such as low energy, fatigue, reduced motivation, or anhedonia. Taken together, TBI patients may endorse symptoms that may or may not reflect the presence of a true mood disorder. Many depression screening questionnaires have been developed such as the Beck Depression Inventory,[116] Hamilton Depression Inventory,[117] and Zung Depression Inventory.[118] Referral to neuropsychology is indicated when there are uncertainties regarding differential diagnosis or treatment approach.

Effective treatment strategies for depressive symptoms are multimodal. Normalization of post-TBI problems, shaping positive expectations regarding recovery, focusing on improvements, and psychotherapy are all useful intervention strategies. A positive, upbeat, environmental setting is important during hospitalization because this setting is incompatible with depressed mood. Staff behavior also plays an important role in managing patients' depression and should be forward thinking, encouraging, and improvement-focused. Use of humor and normalization of reactions to disability are helpful interventions. TBI patients should be encouraged to maintain a positive outlook about the treatment benefits and, importantly, to focus on accomplishments relative to *recent* status and not engage in comparisons to premorbid functioning. Group, individual, and family therapy are often recommended during inpatient hospitalization. Group therapy provides an avenue for peer-to-peer normalization of problems and social support and can facilitate return of self-awareness. Psychotherapy is utilized for emotional support of TBI patients and family members. Educational interventions empower patients and families in the short-term and may provide a buffer against negative emotional experiences in the long-term because they will have knowledge about their deficits (and compensatory strategies) in advance. Antidepressant medication may also serve as a useful adjunct to individual or group psychotherapy, but careful consideration of side effects is encouraged, and side-effect profiles should be reviewed regularly with the patient and family. Finally, TBI patients may experience depressive symptoms once confronted with cognitive or neurobehavioral deficits in the community setting (i.e., after hospital discharge). This can result in new onset or exacerbation of already existing depressive symptoms; for this reason patient and family education should focus on identifying warning signs for depression, coping strategies, and education about when/how to pursue treatment if needed.[106]

Postacute Management

Behavioral and emotional problems may be long-lasting and take a tremendous toll on family members, caregivers, and friends. Even subtle personality changes can erode relationships and familial structure. Premorbid psychiatric problems increase the risk for TBI. Impulse control difficulties, substance abuse, and family problems are unlikely to improve in the postacute period following TBI.[119–123] Emotional problems may surface more readily due to the increased adjustment-related stress inherent in the hospitalization and rehabilitation process. In addition, damage to the frontal lobe (or neural connections to the frontal lobe) can result in neurobehavioral problems. Difficulty tolerating frustration, irritability, aggression, and destructive behavior are common in individuals with frontal lobe injuries. These symptoms are common after motor vehicle accidents involving rapid acceleration–deceleration. Sometimes, emotional symptoms are the direct result of neurological damage rather than psychological reactions secondary to having a brain injury, despite similar clinical appearance.[124]

Not surprisingly, behavioral and emotional dysfunction in the postacute period often contributes to life-long disability. These problems often endure long after physical injuries have healed. A large percentage of individuals with mTBI change or lose their jobs within 6 months of the injury[125]; many are at risk for not understanding why they now are having problems in their life.[126] Finally, treatment providers should be aware that, for individuals with mTBI, emotional symptoms might go unreported until the symptoms have produced a significant negative impact on the person's life.

Postacute Management of Cognitive Problems after Moderate to Severe TBI

Cognitive problems in attention and concentration, new learning and memory, executive control, reasoning, judgment, and self-awareness are common cognitive sequelae following moderate to severe TBI.[127] In moderate–severe TBI, these problems impede functional recovery and resumption of a productive lifestyle. Use of compensatory strategies is necessary. It is noteworthy that cognitive problems are not necessarily reflective of deficits in *intelligence*, per se, because TBI patients' scores on standardized tests of intelligence begin to approximate population mean scores after sufficient time and recovery.

TBI tends to affect more fluid than crystallized intellectual abilities. However, cognitive problems may also be evident in areas of orientation, processing speed, language, visuo-perceptual skills, and motor dexterity and/or speed. Language problems may include those in verbal fluency, word finding, confrontational naming, and/or misnaming (paraphasic errors). Other communication-relevant skills may be impacted such as appreciation for subtle social and interpersonal nuances, often referred to as "pragmatics." Nonverbal aspects of communication such as voice volume, rate, tone, gestures, and body posture, and interpersonal/relational style may be sequelae that are not captured by scores on standardized neuropsychological measures but nonetheless impede resumption of adaptive social-relational functioning. **Table 21.7** presents common neurocognitive impairments after TBI.

Rehabilitation services for cognitive deficits are "directed to achieve functional changes by (1) reinforcing, strengthening, or reestablishing previously learned patterns of behavior, or (2) establishing new patterns of cognitive activity or compensatory mechanisms for impaired neurological systems."[128] Attention and concentration problems are responsive to some cognitive rehabilitation strategies. For instance, "attention process training" demonstrates improvements in attention, memory, and other neuropsychological measures. Interventions to teach time pressure management strategies facilitate compensation for slowed information processing and handling multiple information sources.[129–131] New learning and memory problems are common and occur after medial inferior temporal lobe damage. Persons with TBI may experience difficulty encoding new material, retaining it, and retrieving it after a delay. Provision of categorical, multiple choice, or even phonemic cues may be necessary to retrieve information that was previously encoded. Some evidence supports the use of compensatory strategies for mild memory impairment after TBI.[132–134] Memory notebooks are one strategy employed by rehabilitation therapists for an efficacious compensatory strategy, which lead to fewer everyday memory problems.[134]

Table 21.7 Common Neurocognitive Impairments Observed by Rehabilitation Professionals following Traumatic Brain Injury and Intervention Techniques

Attention and concentration problems

- Reduce distractions in the environment (e.g., wear ear plugs, sit facing wall, clear desk before beginning work)
- Avoid interruptions (e.g., use "Do Not Disturb" sign)
- Use self-coaching (or talking self through a task) to stay on track
- Schedule regular breaks throughout the day to reduce fatigue
- Alternate between cognitively challenging and less demanding tasks
- Set goals to sustain attention for longer periods of time, using timers to signify when time has elapsed
- Be sure you have the patient's full attention before beginning to present information (e.g., say the patient's name, make eye contact with the patient, and redirect the patient back to the task if attention wanes)
- Avoid multitasking when possible; if not possible, record information about stopping point before changing tasks
- Consider medication alternatives (e.g., psychostimulants)

Learning and memory deficits

- Use assistive devices such as memory books, calendars, "to do" lists, cameras, alarms, and tape recorders
- Establish routine and maintain structure
- Present information in many forms (e.g., auditory, visual, kinetic) and demonstrate tasks
- Request information
- Have patients tape record and replay information to listen to information several times
- Use pillboxes and alarms to aid in recall of medication
- Teach patients mnemonic strategies, imagery techniques, and rhymes to facilitate recall of important information
- Break tasks down into small steps and introduce new steps as earlier steps are accomplished

Planning and problem-solving deficits

- Ask patients how they plan to approach task prior to beginning, and help them evaluate potential for success with their plan
- Encourage patients to stop and think before acting
- Each patients to use structured problem-solving techniques (i.e., define the problem, brainstorm alternatives, evaluate options, select best option, assess success of solution)
- Encourage patients to develop and maintain mentor relationship with a trusted family member or friend who can provide constructive feedback

Language problems

- Use short, simple sentences and enunciate clearly when presenting information to the patient
- Provide instructions in multiple formats (e.g., oral and written)
- Teach the patient to repeat and paraphrase information to ensure they heard the information correctly
- Encourage the patient to ask others to repeat information and to speak slowly and clearly

(Continued on page 398)

Table 21.7 *(Continued)*

- Be patient and allow patients time to find words and complete sentences
- Provide contextual and phonemic cues
- Encourage patients to use gestures, drawings, and descriptions while speaking
- Support efforts to speak and be alert for social withdrawal
- Educate family members and caregivers about the nature of deficits and techniques to ensure successful communication

Academic impairments

- Teach patients to use a calculator for all but the most basic mathematical operations and check work carefully
- Rely on family for financial management
- Encourage patients to take notes and highlight or underline key words while they are reading
- Teach the PQRST method for reading comprehension (preview, question, read, study, test)
- To aid in spelling difficulties, encourage the use of electronic spelling aid, word processing spell checker, or speller's dictionary
- Encourage patients to make flashcards to review words frequently missed, play *Scrabble*, and work crossword and other puzzles
- Focus on quality versus quantity, and allow ample time for task completion

Source: Cifu DX, Kreutzer JS, Slater D, Taylor L. Issues in brain injury rehabilitation. In Braddom R, ed. Physical Medicine and Rehabilitation, 3rd ed. Philadelphia: Saunders; 2006:1133–1174

Deficits in executive control are often associated with damage to the frontal lobe, or neural circuits in association with the frontal lobe. Executive functioning represents a broad cognitive domain that includes abilities of abstraction, reasoning, problem solving and hypothesis testing, foresight and planning, organization, flexibility, initiation, behavioral inhibition, persistence, and self-awareness. Individuals with executive problems may lack spontaneity. They may also be impulsive, unable to shift flexibly between tasks, or perseverate. Impaired self-awareness is common and may result in the individual asserting unrealistic goals and seeing no purpose for the use of compensatory strategies. TBI patients with executive functioning deficits may not evidence problems in familiar or highly structured tasks. Rehabilitation teams may involve TBI patients in novel and complex real-world situations as part of treatment to assess for the presence of executive functioning problems (and intervene accordingly). Despite the prevalence of executive functioning deficits after TBI, few controlled studies have been performed in this area.

The Role of Mental Health Professionals

Referral to psychology services is appropriate when a more detailed diagnostic interview, cognitive and/or emotional testing, and/or psychotherapy are warranted. Consider a referral to psychiatric services to assess the appropriateness of medication management of emotional or behavioral problems. If uncertain as to whether the etiology of emotional/behavioral problems are neurologic versus psychogenic, referral to a neurologist or neuropsychologist may be indicated. A clinical neuropsychologist is a professional within the field of psychology with special expertise in the applied science of brain–behavior relationships, and who "uses this knowledge in the assessment, diagnosis, treatment, and/or rehabilitation of patients across the lifespan with neurological, medical, neurodevelopmental and psychiatric conditions, as well as other cognitive and learning disorders."[135] Comprehensive neuropsychological evaluations include measures of general intelligence, attention, and concentration, learning and memory, language, visuospatial abilities, executive functions, and emotional/personality functioning. Results of neuropsychological evaluations assist in differential diagnosis and inform rehabilitation approach for the TBI patient, family, and rehabilitation team.

Family Adjustment and Treatment

TBI affects not only the individual but the family as a whole.[136–140] Research has demonstrated that unrelenting stress on the family from caregiving demands, the uncertain course of recovery, and losses in social, emotional, financial, and functional domains places family caregivers at high risk for experiencing psychological distress.[141–147] Nevertheless, these effects are not inevitable.[148–151] In many cases following TBI, however, the psychological well-being of the family system is threatened and core values and resources are challenged.[148–151]

Table 21.8 Key Components of Family Intervention Programs

Psychoeducation

- Provide information about the cognitive, emotional, and behavioral effects of traumatic brain injury on the patient and family

Bibliotherapy

- Enhance understanding of medical information

Skills training

- Teach stress and time management, constructive problem-solving, and effective communication

Resource identification

- Provide information about community support groups, day rehab and residential programs; empower family to self-advocate

Emotional support

- Validate concerns, build resilience

Wellness

- Promote healthy lifestyle practices and encourage physical and emotional self-care

The process of family adjustment after TBI can be conceptualized as fluid stages or reaction patterns.[152–155] Stage theories suggest that a family's readiness to seek treatment may not occur for several months following the injury, when energy and optimism begin to wane. Families are often initially treated in outpatient settings, which interestingly have been associated with improved coping relative to residential treatment settings.[156] Research has demonstrated that holistic approaches that include several key components offer the support necessary for families to manage the difficult and persistent role of caregiving (**Table 21.8**).[105–157] Assisting the family to identify and build a repertoire of healthy coping skills to manage caregiver stress is crucial to restoring a sense of control and family balance. Likewise, encouraging the family to advocate for themselves and to identify community-based resources (while validating their need to do so) empowers the family system as a whole.[140,158]

Family adjustment to living with a relative with TBI is a lengthy cycle of adaptation, which often demands the reorganization and redistribution of family roles.[138,155] The resultant changes in family functioning, variously perceived by some as unwelcome, disruptive, or overwhelming, can have a significant impact on an individual's recovery and long-term functional outcomes.[105,159] Professional counseling is not always available to families beyond the acute-care phase of TBI treatment,[160] although it has been shown that professional support promotes effective coping and stress reduction.[138] If psychological assistance is available in the early stages of treatment, families are often unable or reluctant to adequately articulate their needs, process complex feelings, or engage in coping-based strategies.[155] Concrete written information (e.g., an information booklet), a social work liaison program, long-term follow-up, and peer support provide promising approaches to enhanced coping for families of TBI patients.[161–166]

Boss[158,167] has proposed a psychodynamic treatment paradigm based on the theory of *ambiguous loss*, or loss without resolution, that has relevance for families coping with brain injury. Two types of ambiguous loss are proposed: (1) physical absence with psychological presence, or (2) psychological absence with physical presence (as is the case for TBI). Psychological interventions for ambiguous loss focus on family and community-based interventions in which the fundamental goal is to build resiliency and competence. Cognitively based strategies are used to identify situational ambiguity (for example, the TBI patient who "is here but not here") as the primary source of stress. Normalizing the reaction to ambiguous loss mobilizes the family toward accepting a new but more realistic future.

References

1. Gordon WA, Zafonte R, Cicerone K, et al. Traumatic brain injury rehabilitation: state of the science. Am J Phys Med Rehabil 2006;85:343–382
2. Semlyen JK, Summers S, Barnes M. Traumatic brain injury: efficacy of multidisciplinary rehabilitation. Arch Phys Med Rehabil 1998;79(6): 678–683
3. Hagen C, Malkmus D, Durham P, Bowman K. (1979). Levels of cognitive functioning. In Rehabilitation of the head injured adult: Comprehensive physical management. Downey, CA: Professional Staff Association of Rancho Los Amigos Hospital
4. Goranson TE, Craves RE, Allison D, et al. Community integration following multidisciplinary rehabilitation for traumatic brain injury. Brain Inj 2003;17:759–774
5. Klonoff PS, Lamb DC, Henderson SW, et al. Outcome assessment after milieu-oriented rehabilitation: New considerations. Arch Phys Med Rehabil 1998;79:684–690
6. Salazar AM, Warden DL, Schwab K, et al. Cognitive rehabilitation for traumatic brain injury: a randomized trial. Defense and Veterans Head Injury Program (DVHIP) Study Group. JAMA 2000;283:3075–3081
7. Malec JF. Impact of comprehensive day treatment on societal participation for persons with acquired brain injury. Arch Phys Med Rehabil 2001;82:885–895
8. Seale GS, Caroselli JS, High WM Jr, et al. Use of community integration questionnaire (CIQ) to characterize changes in functioning for individuals with traumatic brain injury who participated in a post-acute rehabilitation programme. Brain Inj 2002;16:955–967
9. Cifu DX, Kreutzer JS, Kolakowsky-Hayner MA, et al. The relationship between therapy intensity and rehabilitative outcomes after traumatic brain injury: a multicenter analysis. Arch Phys Med Rehabil 2003;84:1441–1448
10. Veterans Administration Health Initiative. Traumatic Brain Injury. Washington, DC: Office of Veterans Affairs; 2003:9
11. Alexander MP. Mild traumatic brain injury: pathophysiology, natural history, and clinical management. Neurology 1995;45: 1253–1260
12. Binder LM. A review of mild head trauma, II: Clinical implications. J Clin Exp Neuropsychol 1997;19:432–457

13. Vanderploeg RD, Curtiss G, Luis CA. Resolving Controversies in Mild TBI: Neuropsychological, Psychosocial, and Psychiatric Outcomes. Paper presented at: Symposium at the Annual Convention of the American Psychological Association; August 2001; San Francisco, CA, August 12–28, 2001
14. Mittenberg W, DiGiulio DV, Perrin S, Bass AE. Symptoms following mild head injury: expectation as aetiology. J Neurol Neurosurg Psychiatry 1992;55:200–204
15. Veterans Administration Health Initiative. Traumatic Brain Injury. Washington, DC: Office of Veterans Affairs; 2003:24
16. Salazar A, Warden D. Traumatic brain injury. Sci Am 1999;11:1–8
17. Mauskop A. The use of botulinum toxin in the treatment of headaches. Curr Pain Headache Rep 2002;6(4):320–323
18. Kelly J. The diagnosis and management of concussion. Paper presented at: Pacific Coast Brain Injury Conference; October 2002; Vancouver, Canada, October 3–5, 2002
19. Fann JR, Uomoto JM, Katon WJ. Cognitive improvement with treatment of depression following mild traumatic brain injury. Psychosomatics 2001;42:48–54
20. Veterans Administration Health Initiative. Traumatic Brain Injury. Washington, DC: Office of Veterans Affairs; 2003:13
21. Lombardi F, Taricco M, De Tanti A, Telaro E, Liberati A. Sensory stimulation for brain injured individuals in coma or vegetative state. Cochrane Database Syst Rev 2002;(2):CD001427
22. Katz DI, White DK, Alexander MP, et al. Recovery of ambulation after traumatic brain injury. Arch Phys Med Rehabil 2004;85(6): 865–869
23. van Zommeren AH, Brower WH, Deelman BG. Attention deficits: the riddles of selectivity, speed, and alertness. In: Brooks N, ed. Closed Head Injury: Psychological, Social, and Family Consequences. Oxford: Oxford University Press; 1984:74–107
24. Whyte J, Hart T, Vaccaro M, et al. Effects of methylphenidate on attention deficits after traumatic brain injury: a multidimensional, randomized, controlled trial. Am J Phys Med Rehabil 2004;83(6): 401–420
25. Whyte J, Hart T, Schuster K, et al. Effects of methylphenidate on attentional function after traumatic brain injury: a randomized, placebo-controlled trial. Am J Phys Med Rehabil 1997;76:440–450
26. Canavero S, Bonicalzi V. The neurochemistry of central pain: evidence from clinical studies, hypothesis and therapeutic implications. Pain 1998;74:109–114
27. Lahz S, Bryant RA. Incidence of chronic pain following traumatic brain injury. Arch Phys Med Rehabil 1996;77(9):889–891
28. Hoffman JM, Pagulayan KF, Zawaideh N, Bell KR. Pain after traumatic brain injury: predictors and correlates. Poster presented at: American Congress of Rehabilitation Medicine; 2005; Chicago, IL September 28–October 1, 2005
29. Uomoto JM, Esselman PC. Traumatic brain injury and chronic pain: differential types and rates by head injury severity. Arch Phys Med Rehabil 1993;74(1):61–64
30. Olver JH, Ponsford JL, Curran CA. Outcome following traumatic brain injury: a comparison between 2 and 5 years after injury. Brain Inj 1996;10(11):841–848
31. Ivanhoe CB, Hartman ET. Clinical caveats on medical assessment and treatment of pain after TBI. J Head Trauma Rehabil 2004;19(1):29–39
32. Sherman KB, Goldberg M. Traumatic brain injury and pain. Phys Med Rehabil Clin N Am 2006;17(2):473–490
33. Killen SA, Huntoon E. Drugs for pain management. Phys Med Rehabil Clin N Am 1997;8:695–705
34. Beetar JT, Guilmette TJ, Sparadeo FR. Sleep and pain complaints in symptomatic traumatic brain injury and neurologic populations. Arch Phys Med Rehabil 1996;77(12):1298–1302
35. Couch JR, Bearss C. Chronic daily headache in the posttrauma syndrome: relation to extent of head injury. Headache 2001;41(6): 559–564
36. Yamaguchi M. Incidence of headache and severity of head injury. Headache 1992;32(9):427–431
37. Kasch H, Stengaard-Pedersen K, Arendt-Nielsen L, Staehelin Jensen T. Headache, neck pain, and neck mobility after acute whiplash injury: a prospective study. Spine 2001;26(11):1246–1251
38. Radanov BP, Di Stefano G, Augustiny KF. Symptomatic approach to posttraumatic headache and its possible implications for treatment. Eur Spine J 2001;10(5):403–407
39. Brain Trauma Foundation–American Association of Neurological Surgeons–Joint Section on Neurotrauma and Critical Care. Early indicators of prognosis in severe traumatic brain injury. J Neurotrauma 2000;17:449–554
40. Meythaler JM, DeVivo MJ, Hayne JB. Cost-effectiveness of routine screening for proximal deep venous thrombosis in acquired brain injury patients admitted to rehabilitation. Arch Phys Med Rehabil 1996;77(1):1–5
41. Yablon SA, Rock WA. Deep vein thrombosis: prevalence and risk factors in rehabilitation admission with brain injury. Neurology 2004;63:485–491
42. Akman MN, Centin N. Value of the D-dimer test in diagnosing deep vein thrombosis in rehabilitation inpatients. Arch Phys Med Rehabil 2004;85:1091–1094
43. Meythaler JM. Fisher. Screening for venous thromboembolism in traumatic brain injury: limitations of the D-dimer assay. Arch Phys Med Rehabil 2003;84:285–290
44. Agnelli G, Piovella F. Enoxaparin plus compression stockings compared with compression stockings alone in the prevention of venous thromboembolism after elective neurosurgery. N Engl J Med 1998; 339:80–85
45. Raabe A, Gerlach R. The risk haemorrhage associated with early postoperative heparin administration after intracranial surgery. Acta Neurochir (Wien) 2001;143:1–7
46. Wen DY, Hall WA. Complications of subcutaneous low-dose heparin therapy in neurosurgical patients. Surg Neurol 1998;50:521–525
47. Macdonald RL, Amidei C. Randomized, pilot study of intermittent pneumatic compression devices plus dalteparin versus intermittent pneumatic compression devices plus heparin for prevention of venous thromboembolism in patients undergoing craniotomy. Surg Neurol 2003;59:363–372
48. Iorio A, Agnelli G. Low molecular weight and unfractionated heparin for prevention of venous thromboembolism in neurosurgery: a meta-analysis. Arch Intern Med 2000;160:2327–2332
49. Kim J, Gearhart MM. Preliminary report on the safety of heparin for deep venous thrombosis prophylaxis after severe head injury. J Trauma 2002;53:38–42
50. Norwood SH, McAuley CE. Prospective evaluation of the safety of enoxaparin prophylaxis for venous thromboembolism in patients with intracranial hemorrhagic injuries. Arch Surg 2002;137: 696–701
51. Geerts WH, Heit JA, Clagett GP, et al. Prevention of venous thromboembolism. Chest 2001;119(Suppl):132S–175S
52. Hyers TM, Agnelli G, Hull RD, et al. Antithrombotic therapy for venous thromboembolic disease. Chest 2001;119(Suppl 1):176S–193S
53. Lance JW. Symposium synopsis. Spasticity. In: Disordered Motor Control. Chicago: Yearbook Medical; 1980:485–494
54. Lance JW. Pyramidal and extrapyramidal disorders. In: Electromyography in CNS Disorders: Central EMG. Boston: Butterworth; 1984:1–19
55. Burke D. Spasticity as an adaption to pyramidal tract injury. Adv Neurol 1988;47:401–423
56. Katz RT. Spastic hypertonia: mechanisms and measurement. Arch Phys Med Rehabil 1989;70:144–155
57. Pierrot DE, Maziers L. Spinal mechanisms underlying spasticity. In: Clinical Neurophysiology in Spasticity. Amsterdam: Elsevier; 1985:63–73
58. Mayer NH, Esquenazi A, Childers MK. Common patterns of clinical motor dysfunction. Muscle Nerve Suppl 1997;6:S21–S35
59. Yarkony GM, Sahgal V. Contractures: a major complication of craniocerebral trauma. Clin Orthop Relat Res 1987;219:93–96
60. Gage JR. Gait Analysis in Cerebral Palsy. London: Mackeith Press; 1991:101–117

61. Harburn KL, Potter PJ. Spasticity and contractures. In: State of the Art Medical Reviews: Physical Medicine and Rehabilitation. Vol. 8. Philadelphia: Hanley & Belfus, Inc.; 1993:441–541
62. Wilson DJ, Swaboda JL. Partial weight-bearing gait retraining for persons following traumatic brain injury: preliminary report and proposed assessment scale. Brain Inj 2002;16:259–268
63. Meythaler JM, Guin-Renfroe S, Johnson A, et al. Prospective assessment of tizanidine for spasticity due to acquired brain injury. Arch Phys Med Rehabil 2001;82:1155–1163
64. Meythaler JM, Clayton W, Davis LK, et al. Orally delivered baclofen to control spastic hypertonia in acquired brain injury. J Head Trauma Rehabil 2004;19:101–108
65. Meythaler JM, Cuin-Renfroe S, Grabb P, et al. Long-term continuously infused intrathecal baclofen for spastic-dystonic hypertonia in traumatic brain injury: 1-year experience. Arch Phys Med Rehabil 1999; 80:13–19
66. Meythaler JM, Guin-Renfroe S, Hadley MN. Continuously infused intratheca! baclofen for spastic/dystonic hemiplegia: a preliminary report. Am J Phys Med Rehabil 1999;78:247–254
67. Rawicki B. Treatment of cerebral origin spasticity with continuous intrathecal baclofen delivered via an implantable pump: long-term follow-up review of 18 patients. J Neurosurg 1999;91:733–736
68. Francois B, Vacher P, Roustan J, et al. Intrathecal baclofen after traumatic brain injury: early treatment using a new technique to prevent spasticity. J Trauma 2001;50:158–161
69. Dario A, Di Stefano MG, Grossi A, et al. Long-term intrathecal baclofen infusion in supraspinal spasticity of adulthood. Acta Neurol Scand 2002;105:83–87
70. Becker R, Benes L, Sure U, et al. Intrathecal baclofen alleviates autonomic dysfunction in severe brain injury. J Clin Neurosci 2000;7: 316–319
71. Cuny E, Richer E, Castel JP. Dysautonomia syndrome in the acute recovery phase after traumatic brain injury: relief with intrathecal baclofen therapy. Brain Inj 2001;15:917–925
72. Pavesi G, Brianti B, Medici D, et al. Botulinum toxin type A in the treatment of upper limb spasticity among patients with traumatic brain injury. J Neurol Neurosurg Psychiatry 1998;64(3):419–420
73. Francisco GE, Boake C, Vaughn A. Botulinum toxin in upper limb spasticity after acquired brain injury: a randomized trial comparing dilution techniques. Am J Phys Med Rehabil 2002;81:355–363
74. The Brain Trauma Foundation. The American Association of Neurological Surgeons. The Joint Section on Neurotrauma and Critical Care. Computed tomography scan features. J Neurotrauma 2000;17: 597–627
75. Schierhout G, Roberts I. Anti-epileptic drugs for preventing seizures following acute traumatic brain injury. Cochrane Database Syst Rev 2001;4:CD000173
76. Temkin NR, Dikmen SS. Valproate therapy for prevention of posttraumatic seizures: a randomized trial. J Neurosurg 1999;91:593–600
77. Watson NF, Barber JK. Does glucocorticoid administration prevent late seizures after head injury? Epilepsia 2004;45:690–694
78. Temkin NR. Antiepileptogenesis and seizure prevention trial with antiepileptic drugs: meta-analysis of controlled trials. Epilepsia 2001;42:515–524
79. Temkin NR, Dikmen SS, Wilensky AJ, et al. A randomized double-blind study of phenytoin for the prevention of post-traumatic seizures. N Engl J Med 1990;323:497–502
80. Englander J, Bushnik T, Duong T, et al. Analyzing risk factors for late posttraumatic seizures: a prospective, multicenter investigation. Arch Phys Med Rehabil 2003;84:365–373
81. Yablon S, Dostrow V. Post traumatic seizures and epilepsy. In: McDeavitt J, ed. State of the Art Reviews in Physical Medicine and Rehabilitation: Traumatic Brain Injury. Philadelphia, Hanley and Belfus, Inc; 2001:301–318
82. Angeleri F, Majkowski J, Cacchiò G, et al. Posttraumatic epilepsy risk factory: one year study after head injury. Epilepsia 1999;40: 1222–1230
83. Diaz-Arrastia R, Gong Y. Increased risk of late posttraumatic seizures associated with inheritance of APOE episilon 4 allele. Arch Neurol 2003;60:818–822
84. Yablon SA. Posttraumatic seizures. Arch Phys Med Rehabil 1993; 74(9):983–1001
85. Dodrill CB, Troupin AS. Neuropsychological effects of carbamazepine and phenytoin: a reanalysis. Neurology 1991;41:141–143
86. Burnett DM, Watanabe TK, Greenwald BD. Congenital and acquired brain injury, II: Brain injury rehabilitation: medical management. Arch Phys Med Rehabil 2003;84(Suppl 1):S8–S11
87. Flin C, Curalucci H, Duvocelle A, et al. Heterotopic ossification and brain injury. Ann Readapt Med Phys 2002;45(9):517–520
88. Garland DE, Blum CE, Waters RL. Periarticular heterotopic ossification in head-injured adults: incidence and location. J Bone Joint Surg Am 1980;62:1143–1146
89. Johns JS, Cifu DX, Keyser-Marcus L, et al. Impact of clinically significant heterotopic ossification on functional outcome after traumatic brain injury. J Head Trauma Rehabil 1999;14(3):269–276
90. Ebinger T, Roesch M. Influence of etiology in heterotopic bone formation of the hip. J Trauma 2000;48:1058–1062
91. Jang SH, Shin SW. Radiation therapy of heterotopic ossification in a patient with traumatic brain injury. Yonsei Med J 2000;41: 536–539
92. Linan E, O'Dell MW, Pierce JM. Continuous passive motion in the management of heterotopic ossification in a brain injured patient. Am J Phys Med Rehabil 2001;80:614–617
93. Kornblum RN, Fisher R. Pituitary lesions in craniocerebral injuries. Arch Pathol 1969;88:242–248
94. Kelly DF, Gonzalo I, Cohan P, et al. Hypopituitarism following traumatic brain injury and subarachnoid hemorrhage: a preliminary report. J Neurosurg 2000;93(5):743–752
95. Lieberman SA, Oberoi AL, Gilkison CR, Masel BE, Urban RJ. Prevalence of neuroendocrine dysfunction in patients recovering from traumatic brain injury. J Clin Endocrinol Metab 2001;86(6):2752–2756
96. Cuthbertson DP. Alterations in metabolism following injury: part 1. Injury 1980;11:175–189
97. Taylor SJ, Fettes SB, Jewkes C, et al. Prospective, randomized, controlled trial to determine the effect of early enhanced enteral nutrition on clinical outcome in mechanically ventilated patients suffering head injury. Crit Care Med 1999;27:2525–2529
98. Leder SB. Fiberoptic endoscopic evaluation of swallowing in patients with acute traumatic brain injury. J Head Trauma Rehabil 1999; 14(5):448–453
99. Wilson MS, Gibson CJ, Hamm RJ. Haloperidol, but not olanzapine, impairs cognitive performance after traumatic brain injury in rats. Am J Phys Med Rehabil 2003;82(11):871–879
100. Young B, Ott L, Twyman D, et al. The effect of nutritional support on outcome from severe head injury. J Neurosurg 1987;67:76–80
101. Groher ME, Picon-Nieto L. Evaluation of communication and swallowing disorders. In: Rosenthal M, Griffith ER, Kreutzer JS, et al, eds. Rehabilitation of the Adult and Child with Traumatic Brain Injury. 3rd ed. Philadelphia: FA Davis; 1999:183–198
102. Saxe JM, Ledgerwood AM, Lucas CF, et al. Lower esophageal sphincter dysfunction precludes safe gastric feeding after head injury. J Trauma 1994;37:581–584
103. Morton MV, Wehman P. Psychosocial and emotional sequelae of individuals with traumatic brain injury: a literature review and recommendations. Brain Inj 1995;9(1):81–92
104. Sohlberg M, Mateer C. Cognitive rehabilitation: an integrative neuropsychological approach. New York: Guilford Press; 2001
105. Cifu DX, Kreutzer JS, Slater D, Taylor L. Issues in brain injury rehabilitation. In: Braddom R, ed. Physical Medicine and Rehabilitation. 3rd ed. Philadelphia: Saunders; 2006:1133–1174
106. Matthies BK, Kreutzer JS, West DD. The Behavior Management Handbook: A Practical Approach to Patients with Neurological Disorders. Richmond: National Resource Center for Traumatic Brain Injury; 2004

107. Sandel ME, Mysiw MJ. The agitated brain injured patient, I: definitions, Differential diagnosis, and assessment. Arch Phys Med Rehabil 1996;77:617–623
108. Corrigan JD. Development of a scale for assessment of agitation following traumatic brain injury. J Clin Exp Neuropsychol 1989;11: 261–277
109. Yudofsky SC, Silver JM, Jackson W, et al. The overt aggression scale for the objective rating of verbal and physical aggression. Am J Psychiatry 1986;143:35–39
110. McEligott JM, Greenwald BD, Watanabe TK. Congenital and acquired brain injury, IV: New frontiers: neuroprotective agents, cognitive enhancing agents, new technology, and complementary medicine. Arch Phys Med Rehabil 2003; 84(3, suppl 1)S18–S22
111. Levin HS, Grossman RG. Behavioral sequelae of closed head injury: a quantitative study. Arch Neurol 1978;35:720–727
112. Rutherford WH. Sequelae of concussion caused by minor head injuries. Lancet 1977;1:1–4
113. Varney NR, Martzke JS, Roberts RJ. Major depression in patients with closed head injury. Neuropsychology 1987;1:7–9
114. Silver J, McAllister T, Yudofsky S, eds.Textbook of Traumatic Brain Injury. Arlington, VA: American Psychiatry Publishing; 2005
115. Jorge RE, Robinson RG, Moser D, et al. Major depression following traumatic brain injury. Arch Gen Psychiatry 2004;61:42–50
116. Beck AT, Steer RA, Brown GK. Manual for the Beck Depression Inventory. 2nd ed. San Antonio, TX: The Psychological Corporation; 1996
117. Hamilton M. Development of a rating scale for primary depressive illness. Br J Soc Clin Psychol 1967;6(4):278–296
118. Zung WWK. A self-rating depression scale. Arch Gen Psychiatry 1965;12:63–70
119. Bennett TL, Raymond MJ. Emotional consequences and psychotherapy for individuals with mild brain injury. Appl Neuropsychol 1997;4:55–61
120. Hanks RA, Tempkin N, Machamer J, Dikmen SS. Emotional and behavioral adjustment after traumatic brain injury. Arch Phys Med Rehabil 1999;80:991–997
121. Kersel DA, Marsh NV, Havill JH, Sleigh JW. Psychosocial functioning during the year following severe traumatic brain injury. Brain Inj 2001;15:683–696
122. McCauley SR, Boake C, Levin HS, Contant CF, Song JX. Postconcussional disorder following mild to moderate traumatic brain injury: anxiety, depression, and social support as risk factors and comorbidities. J Clin Exp Neuropsychol 2001;23:792–808
123. Sarapata M, Herrman D, Johnson T, Aycock R. The role of head injury in cognitive functioning, emotional adjustment, and criminal behavior. Brain Inj 1998;12:821–842
124. Judd T. Assessment and intervention for major symptoms of brain damage. Workshop presented in Managua, Nicaragua. Cited from secondary source (Sohlberg & Mateer, 1989).
125. Gasquoine PG. Postconcussion symptoms. Neuropsychol Rev 1997;7: 77–85
126. Prigatano GP. Commentary: beyond statistics and research design. J Head Trauma Rehabil 1999;14:308–311
127. Cicerone KD, Dahlberg C, Kalmar K, et al. Evidence-based cognitive rehabilitation: recommendations for clinical practice. Arch Phys Med Rehabil 2000;81:1596–1615
128. Harley JP, Allen C, Braciszewski TL, et al. Guidelines for cognitive rehabilitation. NeuroRehabilitation 1992;2:62–67
129. Sohlberg MM, Mateer CA. Effectiveness of an attentional training program. J Clin Exp Neuropsychol 1987;9:117–130
130. Sohlberg MM, McLaughlin KA, Pavese A, Heidrich A, Posner MI. Evaluation of attention process therapy training in persons with acquired brain injury. J Clin Exp Neuropsychol 2000;22:656–676
131. Fasotti L, Kovacs F, Eling PA, Brouwer WH. Time pressure management as a compensatory strategy training after closed head injury. Neuropsychol Rehabil 2000;10:47–65
132. Berg I, Konning-Haanstra M, Deelman B. Long-term effects of memory rehabilitation: a controlled study. Neuropsychol Rehabil 1991; 1:97–111
133. Kaschel R, Della Sala S, Cantagallo E, et al. Imagery mnemonics for the rehabilitation of memory: a randomized group controlled trail. Neuropsychol Rehabil 2002;12:127–153
134. Schmitter-Edgecombe M, Fahy J, Whelan J, Long C. Memory remediation after severe closed head injury: notebook training versus supportive therapy. J Consult Clin Psychol 1995;63:484–489
135. National Academy of Neuropsychology. Definition of a clinical neuropsychologist—NAN web site. Available at: www.nanonline.org. Accessed August 15, 2006
136. Duff D. Family impact and influence following severe traumatic brain injury. Axone 2006;27(2):9–23
137. Marks JP, Daggett LM. A critical pathway for meeting the needs of families of patients with severe traumatic brain injury. J Neurosci Nurs 2006;38(2):84–89
138. Verhaeghe S, Defloor T, Grypdonck M. Stress and coping among families of patients with traumatic brain injury: a review of the literature. J Clin Nurs 2005;14:1004–1012
139. Livingston MG, Brooks DN. The burden on families of the brain injured: a review. J Head Trauma Rehabil 1988;3:6–15
140. Lezak MD. Brain damage is a family affair. J Clin Exp Neuropsychol 1988;10(1):111–123
141. Kolalowsky-Hayner SA, Kishore R. Caregiver functioning after traumatic injury. NeuroRehabilitation 1999;13:27–33
142. Gillen R, Tennen H, Affleck G, et al. Distress, depressive symptoms, and depressive disorder among caregivers of patients with brain injury. J Head Trauma Rehabil 1998;13:31–43
143. Boyle GJ, Haines S. Severe brain injury: some effects on family caregivers. Psychol Rep 2002;90:415–425
144. Marsh NV, Kersel DA, Haveill JA, et al. Caregiver burden during the year following severe traumatic brain injury. J Clin Exp Neuropsychol 2002;24:434–447
145. Chronister J, Chan F. A stress model of caregiving for individuals with traumatic brain injury. Rehabil Psychol 2006;51(3):190–201
146. Machamer J, Temkin N, Dikmen S. Significant other burden and factors related to it in traumatic brain injury. J Clin Exp Neuropsychol 2002;24:420–433
147. Carnes SL, Quinn WH. Family adaptation to brain injury: coping and psychological distress. Fam Syst Health 2005;23(2):186–203
148. Perlesz A, Kinsella G, Crowe S. Impact of traumatic brain injury on the family: a critical review. Rehabil Psychol 1999;44(1):6–35
149. Knight RG, Devereux R, Godfrey HP. Caring for a family member with traumatic brain injury. Brain Inj 1998;12:467–481
150. Adams N. Positive outcomes in families following traumatic brain injury (TBI). Aust N Z J Fam Ther 1996;17(2):75–84
151. Camplair PS, Kreutzer JS, Doherty KR. Family outcome following traumatic brain injury: a critical review of the literature. In: Kreutzer JS, Wehman P, eds. Community Integration Following Traumatic Brain Injury. New York: Paul H. Brookes; 1990:207–222
152. Curtiss G, Klemz S, Vanderploeg RD. Acute impact of stress traumatic brain injury on family structure and coping responses. J Head Trauma Rehabil 2000;15:1113–1122
153. Degeneffe CE. Family caregiving and traumatic brain injury. Health Soc Work 2001;26:257–268
154. Rape RN, Busch JP, Slavin LA. Toward a conceptualization of the family's adaptation to a member's head injury: a critique of the developmental stage models. Rehabil Psychol 1992;37:3–22
155. Lezak M. Psychological implication of traumatic brain damage for the patient's family. Rehabil Psychol 1986;31(4):241–250
156. Mintz MC, VanHorn KR, Levine MJ. Developmental models of social cognition in assessing the role of family stress in relatives' predictions following TBI. Brain Inj 1995;9:173–186
157. Kreutzer JS, Kolakowsky-Hayner S, Demm S, et al. A structured approach to family intervention after brain injury. J Head Trauma Rehabil 2002;17(4):349–367
158. Boss P. Loss, trauma, and resilience: therapeutic work with ambiguous loss. New York: Norton; 2006
159. Bishop DS, Miller IW. Traumatic brain injury: empirical family assessment techniques. J Head Trauma Rehabil 1988;3(4):16–30

160. Kolakowsky-Hayner SA, Miner KD, Kreutzer JS. Long-term life quality and family needs after traumatic brain injury. J Head Trauma Rehabil 2001;16(4):374–385
161. Morris KC. Psychological distress in careers of head injured individuals: the provision of written information. Brain Inj 2001;15: 247–255
162. Albert SM, Im A, Brenner L, Smith M, Waxman R. Effect of a social work liaison program on family caregivers to people with brain injury. J Head Trauma Rehabil 2002;17:175–189
163. Armstrong K, Kerns KA. The assessment of parent needs following paediatric traumatic brain injury. Pediatr Rehabil 2002;5: 149–160
164. Hibbard MR, Cantor J, Charatz H, et al. Peer support in the community: initial findings of a mentoring program for individuals with traumatic brain injury and their families. J Head Trauma Rehabil 2002;17:112–131
165. Ergh TC, Hanks RA, Rapport LJ, Coleman RD. Social support moderates caregiver life satisfaction following traumatic brain injury. J Clin Exp Neuropsychol 2003;25:1090–1101
166. Hawley CA, Ward AB, Magnay AR, Long J. Parental stress and burden following traumatic brain injury amongst children and adolescents. Brain Inj 2003;17:1–23
167. Boss P. Ambiguous Loss: Learning to Live with Unresolved Grief. Cambridge, MA: Harvard University Press; 1999

22 Prognosis

Rosalyn Nguyen, Ross D. Zafonte, and Heechin Chae

The prognosis after a traumatic brain injury (TBI) is critical for patients, families, and health care providers. An accurate prognosis has to be considered by the metric it is measured against such as survival, functional outcome, or return to employment. Although the data available still renders prognosis a science only in the more extreme scenarios, new information from clinical trial datasets is contributing to an increasing base of knowledge. In this chapter, we will review several critical factors that affect prognosis.

Age

Older age has been associated with worse outcome and increased mortality in TBI patients.[1–4] Several studies assessed several prognostic factors and concluded that age was the strongest predictor of functional outcome.[5,6] In most studies, outcome was measured by the Glasgow Outcome Scale (GOS). Cremer et al found a linear association between age and functional outcome.[5] Older patients required more inpatient rehabilitation and had a lower mean discharge functional independence measure (FIM) score than their younger counterparts. At 6 months, there was less of a difference in FIM scores, but younger patients still fared better.[7]

Willemse-van Son et al[8] summarized findings from 35 studies examining 14 cohorts regarding prognostic factors on outcome after TBI. They concluded that older age was associated with continued disability at least 1 year post-TBI. Disability was defined as outcome measures related to activity limitations. However, they also looked at nonproductivity, which included inability to return to school or work. In this category, results were equivocal for older patients.[8]

In regard to identifying threshold ages, there has been inconclusive data. Some studies have cited 65 years as a threshold age,[9] whereas others have suggested the age of 50,[10] or 30.[4] Of note, the mean age in the latter study was lower than the others. Woertgen et al cited a mean age of 42.7 for patients with unfavorable outcome as opposed to a mean age of 28.9 for patients with favorable outcome.[11]

In an analysis of 5,600 adult patients with closed TBI, 74% of patients older than age 55 had poor outcome at 6 months compared with 39% of younger patients. However, this relationship was continuous and there was actually no clear threshold age. The investigators concluded that, for every 10 years of age, the odds of a negative outcome increased by 40 to 50%.[2]

Livingston et al published findings from the Western Trauma Association multicenter prospective study in 2005, which showed that patients above the age of 60 with GOS scores of ≤ 4 at discharge had less improvement and lower FIM scores at 1 year. The elder subset also had less severe injuries as reflected by higher Glasgow Coma Scale (GCS) scores on admission. Furthermore, this age-dependent trend was seen even in the group of patients ages 45 to 59 with isolated TBI. They also had less improvement in their GOS and FIM scores at 1 year post-TBI compared with the younger patients.[9]

Additionally, younger patients were more likely to achieve independent ambulation.[12] Age was also predictive of recovery of postural and equilibrium reactions in TBI patients.[13] However, there was no association of age with recovery of arm function in patients with upper extremity paresis after TBI.[14]

Upon review of pediatric studies, the results are variable. In one assessment of the long-term functional outcome of children with severe TBI (GCS scores of 8 or less) who were followed for 5 to 7 years postinjury, age was not associated with long-term outcome.[15] In another pediatric study of severe TBI patients requiring mechanical ventilation (age 1 month to 14 years), younger children had worse outcome and higher mortality. Poor outcome was defined as partially or fully dependent functional status. Median follow-up duration was 2 years. In this cohort, median GCS and Pediatric Risk of Mortality (PRISM) scores were 6 and 13, respectively.[16] Another study of children age 1 month to 15 years (mean age of 7) showed that 2 years of age or younger was a predictive of poor outcome (**Table 22.1**).[17]

Secondary Insults

Secondary insults that have been associated with poor outcome after TBI include hypotension (systolic blood pressure [SBP] $<$90 mm Hg), hypoxia (pO_2 $<$60 mm Hg), and hypothermia ($<$35°C). These secondary insults generally result in higher disability at discharge and longer hospital

Table 22.1 Age-Related Outcome in Traumatic Brain Injury

- Older age is associated with a worse outcome and increased mortality
- Age likely has a continuous relationship to outcome
- Very young children are also at increased risk for poor outcome

lengths of stay.[18] Occurrence of hypotension, hypoxia, and hypothermia are not uncommon. Prevalence can be between 10 to 40%. The odds of poor outcome are almost doubled for each factor. Moreover, combinations of secondary insults can result in worse outcome than an individual insult. The presence of these factors on admission or prior to admission was associated with poorer outcome. Patients with sustained hypotension or hypoxia were often found to have more severe features on computed tomography (CT; with shift, swelling, Marshall class III or IV). Among the secondary insults mentioned above, hypotension was the strongest prognostic factor.[6,18,19]

A retrospective review assessed the outcome of 11 secondary brain injury factors (SBIFs) in the first 24 hours post-TBI and found that hypotension, hypocapnia, and acidosis had the highest occurrence. Increased mortality was seen in patients with hypotension, hypothermia, and hyperglycemia.[20]

Hypotension

Hypotension was associated with poor outcome, longer hospital stays, and higher rates of discharge to a rehabilitation facility versus to home. In a review of eight randomized, controlled trials and a population-based series with over 6600 patients, a U-shaped relationship was found between blood pressure and functional outcome, but a clear threshold value was not evident. Nonetheless, SBPs of 120 to 150 mm Hg and mean arterial pressures (MAPs) of 85 to 110 mm Hg were associated with good outcome (best outcome was seen with SBP = 135 mm Hg and MAP = 90 mm Hg). Values above and below those were associated with poorer outcome, although when adjusted for other factors, the relationship was not significant.[20,21]

Low blood pressure was often associated with blood loss, anemia, and thrombocytopenia. Cerebral perfusion was likely decreased in these cases, as a drop in systemic blood pressure is typically seen later on. Higher blood pressure was often seen in association with poorer motor responses, mass lesions, and probable increased intracranial pressure (ICP). As such, these events reflected more severe clinical situations, which may account for the worse outcomes.[21]

White et al[22] also found that SBP ≥135 mm Hg was associated with lower mortality rates. Assuming that autoregulation was intact, the odds of survival increased by 5% for every 1 mm Hg increase in systolic blood pressure up to 135 mm Hg.[22]

In pediatric studies, poor outcome was seen in patients with early hypotension, which was described as an SBP less than the fifth percentile for age measured in the field or in the emergency room. Poor outcome was defined as GOS score <4, death, or discharge to a skilled nursing facility. Early hypotension was also associated with higher pediatric intensive care unit (PICU) and hospital length of stay (LOS). It had better predictive potential than delayed hypotension or blood pressure <90 mm Hg.[23] Another study found that age-appropriate SBP <75th percentile had a fourfold higher risk of unfavorable outcome (GOS <4) compared with patients in the >75th percentile group. Patients with age-appropriate SBP <75th percentile were more likely to have poor outcome even if SBP was >90 mm Hg.[24] One study found that hypotension was only weakly associated with outcome after 1 year.[5]

Hypothermia

Hypothermia has been controversial in the literature as some studies proposed that it provided cerebral protection. The National Acute Brain Injury Study on Hypothermia[25] found that hypothermia was associated with negative outcomes in patients >45 years of age but was beneficial in patients younger than 45 years of age with hypothermia on admission. However, they found many variables that confounded the data and led to increased intercenter variance. In contrast, Jeremitsky et al[20] found that there was a higher mortality for patients age <45 with hypothermia. In a multicenter trial in 2001 utilizing hypothermia treatment to induce body temperatures of 33°C within 8 hours after injury, hypothermia was found to be ineffective in improving outcomes.[26] In pediatric populations, there are no data to support the use of hypothermia in TBI patients.[27]

Studies of hyperthermia were inconclusive. One study suggested that it was not associated with mortality or longer hospital stay.[20] Another proposed that early hyperthermia correlated with lower GCS score at discharge and longer ICU LOS. Authors hypothesized that the hyperthermia seen was associated with TBI severity, rather than infectious etiology or body organ dysfunction.[28]

Hyperglycemia

Hyperglycemia was associated with increased mortality and prolonged hospital stay, although it was not an independent predictor of outcome in a study by Jeremitsky et al in 2003.[20] The IMPACT database from six phase III randomized, controlled trials and an observational study showed that glucose was a strong prognostic factor in predicting outcome. Hyperglycemia was associated with poor outcome. As circulation may already be affected in TBI, hyperglycemia can further injure the microvasculature.[6,29]

Hypoxia

Hypoxia was associated with longer ICU and hospital stays. Prehospital hypoxia was associated with higher mortality.[18,20] Hypocapnic patients with low GCS scores of 4 to 5 had worse outcome. When occurring between 15 to 24 hours, it was associated with longer ICU and hospital LOS.[20] Acidosis correlated with longer ICU and hospital LOS and patients were more likely to be discharged to a rehabilitation facility rather than to home.[20] Furthermore, it was associated with poorer functional outcome.[29]

Coagulopathy and Anemia

Increased prothrombin time (PT) was a strong independent predictor of outcome.[6,29] A meta-analysis published in 2008 reviewing 34 studies found a 32% prevalence of coagulopathy after TBI. Coagulopathy was associated with poorer outcome.[30] It is postulated that coagulopathy may worsen contusions.[29] Delayed injury with findings of new lesions on CT correlated with prolonged PT and partial thromboplastin time (PTT). However, in one study, increased international normalized ratio (INR) was not related to outcome.[20] Anemia was a strong prognostic factor associated with poorer outcome. Low hemoglobin and high glucose were the strongest predictors of outcome in the IMPACT database from 2007. If cerebral perfusion is already compromised, anemia can compound the effect and lead to further ischemia.[6,29] The need for emergent transfusion within the first 6 hours was also predictive of poorer outcome.[17] Thrombocytopenia on admission was associated with poorer functional outcome.[6,29]

Catecholamine Levels

Increased norepinephrine levels on admission have been associated with worse outcome at 1 week in TBI patients with GCS of 3 or 4. Highest levels were found in patients that had early brain death (within the first week postinjury).[31–33]

Sodium Levels

Sodium levels had a U-shaped relationship to outcome. Both high and low values were associated with poorer outcome. Hyponatremia may potentially worsen cerebral edema and hence can affect outcome.[29] In the IMPACT study from 2007, the patients with laboratory abnormalities that had the worst outcome at 6 months were the ones with hyperglycemia, coagulopathy, hyponatremia, and anemia, which were likely reflective of the severity of their injury (**Table 22.2**).[29]

Clinical Test Scores

The GCS score has been known to be a strong prognostic indicator in outcome studies of TBI patients.[3,5,6,15,16,22,34–38]

Table 22.2 Secondary Insults in Traumatic Brain Injury

- Hypotension (systolic blood pressure < 90 mm HG) and hypoxia ($pO_2 < 60$ mm Hg) are associated with poor outcome
- Hyperglycemia is associated with increased mortality and prolonged hospital stay
- High and low sodium levels are associated with poorer outcome

From results of the IMPACT database, which comprised 8,700 patients, there was a strong association between motor score and outcome as measured by the GOS score. GCS motor score was just behind age as the strongest prognostic factor. Secondarily, the eye and verbal components were also related to outcome, although their strength of association was less robust.

Best motor score at 6 hours after injury or on day 1, rather than on admission, has been cited as a suitable timeframe to use in prognostic models, although other authors suggest a longer poststabilization duration after injury to attain a moreappropriate score.[5,22,38] A large-scale study found a significant change in motor GCS score and pupil reactivity in the time interval between prehospital assessment and poststabilization after injury. Initial GCS scores may be influenced by factors such as sedation, intubation, increased ICP, decreased initial cerebral perfusion, periorbital swelling, vascular instability, hypoxia, and hypotension after injury. For prognostic purposes, it was proposed that using poststabilization scores would be more appropriate.[38]

Research looking at prehospital GCS scores compared with admission GCS scores in 12,000 TBI patients found that the two scores were highly correlated and were predictive of outcome. In terms of mortality and need for neurosurgical intervention, a change in GCS from prehospital to admission scores had predictive potential. In this study, Trauma Score and Injury Severity Score (TRISS) calculations to predict survival also showed prognostic promise.[39]

Among children, Massagli et al[15] assessed GCS scores in the field, and at 6, 24, and 72 hours postinjury. They found that early outcome (GOS scores at hospital discharge) correlated with GCS scores in the field and at 6, 24, and 72 hours postinjury. However, late outcome (GOS scores at 5 to 7 years after discharge) correlated with GCS scores at 24 and 72 hours, but not the earlier scores.[15] In a study by Michaud et al, GCS motor response at 72 hours was most predictive of disability severity. Flaccid, withdrawing, extensor or flexor posturing were associated with higher disability.[40]

GCS score of 3 to 5, motor score of 1 to 3, absent verbal response, absent pupillary reaction, or absent oculocephalic reflex were independently predictive of poor functional outcome as measured by GOS score.[41] Other research postulated a GCS threshold value of 5 or 6 for predicting poor outcome in children after TBI.[17,37] Relative risk of poor outcome with a GCS score of 5 or less was twice that of patients with GCS scores >5 (95% CI = 1.27 to 3.25).[16] Patients with initial GCS of 3 to 7 had significantly lower mean admission and discharge motor and cognitive FIM scores compared with patients with GCS of 13 to 15.[34] However, despite lower GCS scores, many patients with GCS ≤5 can still survive and be functional.[16] GCS scores have been correlated with functional and occupational (return to work) outcome.[35] Initial GCS score was also associated with severity of injury found on initial neuroimaging, which, in turn, correlated with functional outcome.[42]

In pediatric studies, the Pediatric Risk of Mortality (PRISM) score, which is an index of illness severity, has been shown to be a strong prognostic indicator.[16,36] Poor outcome is seen with higher PRISM scores. Nearly 80% of patients with PRISM scores ≥2 had poor outcome. The relative risk of unfavorable outcome with PRISM score ≥20 was 4 times higher (95% CI = 1.92 to 9.22). The relative risk of poor outcome was 10 times greater with a GCS score of ≤5 and PRISM score of ≥20 compared with GCS of ≤5, but PRISM score of <20 (95% CI = 1.4 to 69.3). Thakker et al concluded that PRISM scores in combination with GCS scores can enhance prognostication in pediatric patients with GCS scores ≤5.[16]

Abbreviated injury score (AIS) assesses severity of injury in seven body regions; head AIS uses neuroradiologic or operative findings in its assessment. The injury assessment score (ISS) reflects an assessment of the three most severely injured body regions. These anatomic measures have proven useful in prognostic models.[43] Analyses of prognostic significance comparing the head AIS upon admission, the ISS, and the GCS showed that ISS was the best predictor of functional outcome after TBI as measured by the extended GOS at 12 months postinjury. GCS score followed. ISS or AIS in combination with GCS resulted in modest improvement in prognostication.[43]

Head AIS and ISS scores were also associated with both early and long-term outcome at 5 to 7 years after discharge. Head AIS of 1 to 3 and ISS of <25 were predictive of good recovery compared with head AIS scores of 4 to 6 and ISS of ≥25. Higher ISS scores were also associated with higher mortality rates.[15,17] Michaud et al found that ISS and pupillary reaction were significantly predictive of survival.[40]

In contrast to the previous results that showed a strong relationship between GCS and outcome, Willemse-van Son et al[8] summarized findings from 35 published studies examining 14 cohorts and found that lower GCS scores were not consistently related to outcome. However, 20 different outcome measures were used including "disability, psychosocial distress, social integration, quality of life and independence," rather than a standard functional outcome measure.[8]

Table 22.3 Clinical Scores in Patients with Traumatic Brain Injury

- Glasgow Coma Score motor is a strong predictor of outcome
- Head AIS and ISS scores are associated with both early- and long-term outcome
- ISS scores and papillary response are strongly predictive of survival

FIM motor scores have also been found to be predictive of discharge FIM scores. Furthermore, baseline FIM scores at the beginning of rehabilitation can also be an independent predictor of 1-year outcome (**Table 22.3**).[3,34]

Radiologic Findings

Computed Tomography Findings

CT findings have been shown to be important factors in TBI prognosis.[5] The Marshall CT Classification has been used in many studies to correlate with functional outcome.[6,44]

Data from the large-scale IMPACT study from 2007 found that the Marshall CT Classification and individual CT characteristics were strong prognostic factors in predicting outcome, which was measured by the Glasgow Outcome Scale. Patients with diffuse injuries in class III or IV had worse outcomes. Among patients with mass lesions, the outcome was better for epidural hematomas compared with acute subdural hematomas.[6,44] Conversely, in a pediatric cohort followed for 5 to 7 years, the presence of subdural or intracerebral hemorrhage was not predictive of outcome.[15]

More data has been published in recent years showing that traumatic subarachnoid hemorrhage is a significant independent predictor.[6,41,44] Intraventricular hemorrhage has also been associated with poorer outcome.[44,45] Partial or full obliteration of the basal cisterns and midline shift were strong predictors of outcome as well.[6,44] Evidence of contusions only has a modest effect on prognosis.[6]

In pediatric studies, initial CT showing diffuse axonal injury, diffuse brain edema, complex lesions, or massive focal lesions were associated with poor outcome,[17] although other studies suggested that cerebral edema was unrelated to outcome[15] and an early CT scan or a single CT scan may not have significant prognostic implication in children with severe diffuse brain injury.[41]

Investigators from the International and North American tirilazad trials postulated a prediction model that took into account the Marshall CT classification, but they placed more emphasis on individual CT features. They refined the predictive value by incorporating intraventricular hemorrhage, traumatic subarachnoid hemorrhage, and further differentiating mass lesions (epidural versus intradural) and basal cisterns (absent or compressed cisterns). The resultant prediction trees and CT score charts have associated percentages or calculated probabilities for prognostic risk and mortality.[45]

In a pediatric study, neuroimaging results were categorized into two groups. The first included diffuse injury II, evacuated mass less or no visible CT pathology. The second included diffuse injury III and IV or nonevacuated mass lesion. Worse initial neuroimaging correlated with poorer outcome (GOS 1 to 2). Initial GCS was also found to be related to the initial neuroimaging category.[42]

Bigler et al[46] assessed ventricle-to-brain ratio (VBR) from MRI scans performed 25 or more days after injury as an index of cerebral atrophy. Comparing these later findings to the day-of-injury (DOI) CT, the presence of abnormalities on the DOI CT was associated with an increased VBR. There was no significant difference in VBR among the CT classifications (II-VII). Negative DOI CT scans correlated with minimal or insignificant change in VBR. Day of injury CT abnormalities were predictive of development of cerebral atrophy, which was associated with poorer outcome as assessed by discharge Disability Rating Scale (DRS) and FIM scores. In this study, CT classification did not result in significant differences in DRS and FIM outcome. However, patients with brainstem injury had higher DRS and lower FIM scores at discharge.[46]

Looking at LOS in acute and rehabilitation facilities, CT evidence of intracranial bleed with skull fracture correlated with longer total LOS.

Magnetic Resonance Imaging Findings

Traumatic microbleeds (TMBs) seen on T2-weighted gradient echo magnetic resonance imaging (MRI) have been postulated to be markers of diffuse axonal injury. Detection of TMBs was found to be better with MRI at 3 T (Tesla) compared with 1.5 T, which may be considered if the clinical suspicion of DAI is high, but MRI was unremarkable. There was also a negative correlation between the number of TMBs and the time interval between TBI and MRI. Median interval period after TBI was 61 months in this group (**Table 22.4**).[47]

Table 22.4 Radiologic Findings in Traumatic Brain Injury

- Marshall Computed Tomography Classification is strongly predictive of outcome
- Partial or full obliteration of basal cisterns and midline shift were strong predictors of outcome
- Subarachnoid hemorrhage is a significant independent predictor of outcome

Structural and Clinical Correlations

Brain stem involvement was also associated with poorer long-term outcome. Presence of brain stem injury also correlated with poorer "professional ability." Coordination problems, visual impairment, psychosis, and spasticity appeared to occur more frequently in these patients.[48]

Recovery of arm function after upper extremity paresis in TBI patients was found to be prolonged in patients with diffuse injury compared with patients with more focal injury. However, diffuse injuries were associated with continued recovery after 3 months. Therefore, it was concluded that even after 2 months, it was possible to have further recovery in persons with diffuse brain injury.[14]

MRI findings in children revealed that most lesions were in the corpus callosum and frontal lobes. Generally, neuropsychological evaluations at 1 year post-TBI did not correlate with total lesion volume, number of injured lobes, or extent of cerebral atrophy. However, certain areas did have some association with anatomic locations. Dyscalculia was found to be associated with cerebellar lesions, total lesion volume, and number of lobes affected. Cerebellar injury was associated with poorer visual recognition memory and poorer results on verbal and nonverbal tests. Worse cognitive results were found in children with the deepest lesions.[49]

Duration of Coma

Length of coma appeared to have some impact on both early functional outcome at time of discharge and long-term level of disability (GOS scores at 5 to 7 years post-TBI). It was shown to be a strong prognostic factor in predicting both functional and occupational long-term outcome.[35]

Patients with good functional outcome had a median length of coma of one day, whereas persons with moderate disability had a median length of 6 days in a coma. Lastly, patients with severe disability had a median of 62 days in a coma.[15] Moreover, duration of coma was also predictive of recovery of postural and equilibrium reactions, as well as recovery of arm function in TBI patients with upper extremity paresis.[13]

In contrast, some studies in the literature found that longer loss of consciousness was unrelated to eventual outcome.[8,14]

Posttraumatic Amnesia

Longer posttraumatic amnesia was associated with lower productivity in terms of vocational or educational pursuits post-TBI. It was also related to lower functional outcome, as measured by the GOS score.[8,35] Furthermore, there was a relationship between length of posttraumatic amnesia and independent ambulation.[12]

Intracranial Pressure/Cerebral Perfusion Pressure

Several studies found a significant association between ICP values and outcome.[10,50,51] Information from the Traumatic Coma Data Bank and the American Brain Injury Consortium database provided evidence that managing cerebral perfusion pressure (CPP) was associated with better outcome.[52]

Furthermore, ICP values and their response or lack of response to treatment were found to be associated with outcome.[50] Signorini et al found that ICP values in the first 72 hours after TBI were predictive of 1 year survival and resulted in poorer outcomes.[10]

In pediatric patients, initial CPP between 40 to 70 mm Hg has been found to be associated with better prognosis compared with higher or lower CPP values. In this cohort, over 60% of patients with initial CPP <40 mm Hg had poor outcome. In terms of ICP, 80% of the patients with initial ICPs of <20 mm Hg had good prognosis.[51] The current recommendation for pediatric patients is maintaining CPP of >40 mm Hg in children with severe TBI.[27]

However, there are also numerous studies in the literature that did not find a relationship between initial ICP, CPP, peak ICP, or duration of elevated ICP and outcome.[15–17,20]

Pupillary Reactivity

Pupil reactivity has been shown to be predictive of survival.[40] Recent results from over 8,700 patients from the IMPACT database revealed that the presence of at least one nonreactive pupil significantly correlated with poorer outcome.[53]

Some authors consider poststabilization pupil response to be superior to prehospitalization response in determining eventual functional outcome.[5,53] When finding sluggishly reactive or dilated pupils on initial exam, the etiology may be compromised perfusion of the brain stem after TBI and may not always be uncal herniation or direct third cranial nerve injury. After stabilization, pupil reactivity may change.[53]

Nonetheless, pupil reactivity in the field also appears to correlate with long-term outcome, as measured by GOS scores at 5 to 7 years after discharge (**Table 22.5**).[15]

Table 22.5 Clinical and Structural Abnormalities in Traumatic Brain Injury

- Length of coma appears to have an impact on early functional outcome
- Time to follow commands is also a strong predictor of outcome
- Longer posttraumatic amnesia is associated with lower productivity
- Elevated intracranial pressure is associated with worse global outcome

Markers of Injury

Admission serum levels of calcium-binding protein B (S-100B), glial fibrillary acidic protein (GFAP), and neuron specific enolase (NSE) were found to be elevated in TBI patients. Elevated levels were significantly predictive of poor functional outcomes or mortality.[54,55] Relationships were found between these markers and the injury severity score and CT findings. However, there was no correlation with GCS score.[54]

In pediatric cohorts, initial and peak NSE levels and initial myelin basic protein (MBP) levels were stronger predictors of outcome in children 4 years of age or younger. The correlation was weaker in older children.[55]

Biomarkers

Among the markers of neural injury, S-100B has received a notable amount of attention in the TBI literature. It is an astroglial cell protein that has been found to be elevated after TBI. In one prospective study, serum levels of S-100B were increased 18 times normal values in TBI patients.[54] Several studies have provided evidence for its strong association with functional outcome.[11,36]

Serum levels of S-100B measured within 1 to 6 hours of TBI has been found to have significant prognostic value in estimating functional outcome. Woertgen et al[11] compared the positive and negative predictive values of admission S-100B levels with the GCS score and Marshall CT Classification and found that S-100B level had superior predictive value over the other two prognostic factors. In a cohort of patients with initial GCS scores of <9, patients with poorer outcome (GOS 1 to 3) at 11 months had higher S-100B levels compared with patients with better outcome (GOS 4 to 5).[11]

Pertinent values cited in the literature that correlate with poorer outcomes range between 1.13 to 3.6. Vos et al found that levels >1.13 μg/L were associated with highest mortality rates.[54] Woertgen et al[11] cited a mean of 5.55 μg/L in their poor outcome group (GOS 1 to 3). The good outcome group (GOS 4 to 5) had a mean level of 0.96 μg/L.[11]

Spinella et al[36] also reported that levels ≥2 μg/L corresponded with poor outcome as measured by the Pediatric Cerebral Performance Category (PCPC) score in a pediatric cohort. Median level was 3.6 in the poor outcome group and ranged from 1.4 to 20 μg/L). Patients with good outcome had median levels of 0.85 μg/L and ranged between 0.008 and 4.8 μg/L. As a comparison, children without traumatic brain injury had a mean S-100B level of 0.3 μg/L. There was also an inverse relationship between S-100B levels and age in this pediatric population.[36]

Vos et al found that GFAP was increased over 4 times normal values in their group of TBI patients and a level >1.5 μg/L was associated with highest mortality rates.[54] Nylen et al[56] found a median 10-fold increase in serum GFAP levels in their group. The levels peaked during the initial days after TBI. Patients with poor outcome, as defined by GOS score 1 to 3, vegetative state or death, had higher peak GFAP levels in the range of 0.38 to 49.58 μg/L and median level of 2.72 μg/L. Patients with good outcome, defined as GOS score of 4 to 5 or moderate disability, had peak GFAP levels in the range of 0.14 to 6.98 μg/L with a median level of 0.85 μg/L. When comparing isolated TBI to patients with multitrauma, there was no major difference in the peak GFAP values.[56] Subsequently, in 2007, Nylen et al published findings that GFAP levels were independent predictors of outcome in aneurysmal subarachnoid hemorrhage. Furthermore, patients with focal lesions on imaging, secondary ischemic events, or rebleeds had higher maximum GFAP levels than those without these findings.[57] NSE levels have been evaluated in those with TBI. Patients with approximately double normal values and a level >21.7 μg/L were associated with higher mortality.[54]

Apolipoprotein E

In a Chinese cohort, investigators speculated that the apolipoprotein E (APOE-) 491AA promoter in epsilon 4 carriers was associated with poor clinical outcome in the first week after TBI as measured by decline in GCS score or worsening of CT findings.[58] Prior work has suggested APOE allele is likely to impact outcome among those with more severe injuries. Data regarding less severe injuries is mixed; however, one recent study suggests even a risk for concussion exists with this polymorphism.

Nature of Injury

Mechanism/Cause of Injury

Results collected from eight randomized, controlled trials from the IMPACT database showed that cause of injury was not an independent predictor of long-term outcome after TBI after adjusting for age. Falls generally had worse outcomes than motor vehicle accidents, sports injuries, or physical assault, but they tended to occur in elderly patients and moreover, were often found in conjunction with mass lesions.[59] Massagli et al also found that mechanism of injury was not associated with long-term outcome.[15]

Multitrauma

Injuries to the extremities in multitrauma patients were associated with poorer long-term outcome and higher disability, although these studies were not specific to the traumatic brain injury population.[60,61] Interestingly, Cowen et al noted that TBI patients with extremity fractures after motor vehicle accidents were found to have higher cognitive FIM scores at discharge.[34] In a pediatric study, chest injury was associated with poor outcome.[37] However, in other studies, chest or abdomen trauma was not predictive of long-term functional outcome.[15]

Medical Issues/Complications

Hospital Medical Complications in Multitrauma Patients

Results of over 1,000 trauma patients from the Trauma Recovery Project revealed that patients with major hospital complications had poorer outcome as measured by the Quality of Well-Being (QWB) Scale at 1 year postinjury. Ten percent of their patients had medical complications during the hospitalization. Poorer outcome was seen after pulmonary complications (e.g., pneumonia [PNA], pulmonary embolism [PE], adult respiratory stress syndrome [ARDS], etc.), gastrointestinal complications (e.g., gastrointestinal hemorrhage, small bowel obstruction [SBO], bowel injury, etc.), infections (septicemia, wound infection, etc.), and musculoskeletal issues (compartment syndrome, nonunion, etc.). Worse long-term outcome was most closely associated with pulmonary complications and infections. Although the population studied was comprised of multitrauma patients, awareness of such outcomes can be pertinent to our TBI patients—many of them also suffered multitrauma.[62]

Acute Lung Injury

Holland et al[66] followed a cohort of patients with isolated head injury prospectively over 4 years. About 30% of the group with severe TBI developed acute lung injury. It was speculated that acute lung injury may be a result of neurogenic pulmonary edema that occurred after activation of the sympathoadrenal axis.[63] Alternatively, it may be associated with the systemic inflammatory response,[64] or is a consequence of the hypertension induced to maintain a stable CPP in the setting of elevated ICP.[65,66]

Patients with acute lung injury had poorer outcome and higher mortality. Injury severity scores were also higher in these patients.[66]

Intubation

In patients that were initially intubated, the duration and reason behind intubation were not associated with outcome.[16]

Preinjury Status

Preinjury Unemployment

Willemse-van Son et al[8] compiled results from 35 studies reviewing TBI prognostic factors. Preinjury unemployment was found to be associated with continued disability (activity limitations) and nonproductivity (not returning to work or training) at least 1 year post-TBI.[8]

Substance Abuse

Willemse-van Son et al also found that substance abuse was associated with continued disability (activity limitations) and nonproductivity (not returning to work or training) at least 1 year post-TBI.[8] In particular, alcohol use was associated with poorer outcome.[58]

Cardiac Considerations

Cardiac Uncoupling and Beta-Blockers

The hyperadrenergic state and autonomic dysfunction associated with TBI can also manifest as decreased heart rate variability (HRV).[67,68] Higher severity of injury appears to have a greater degree of impact on autonomic control of heart rate. This reduced variability, particularly in the first 24 hours, and state of cardiac uncoupling has been associated with increased mortality and autonomic nervous system failure.[33,68,69]

Beta blockade in severe TBI patients appears to increase survival. Riordan et al[68] proposed stratifying mortality risk based on the amount of time that patients had cardiac uncoupling over 24 hours, which they defined as 5-minute heart rate standard deviation between 0.3 bpm and 0.6 bpm. They discovered that β blockade had the best effect on patients that were in a cardiac uncoupled state for >5% of the 24 hours. Hence, HRV and cardiac uncoupling may be useful in determining which patients could benefit most from β–blocker therapy.[68]

Rapenne et al[33] compared HRV during the awakening period in patients with good recovery and in patients with poor recovery (or worsened state as determined by GCS scores). Poorer outcome was associated with lower HRV and parasympathetic tone in the awakening period. However, when they compared HRV in sedated patients with early brain death to HRV in survivors, they found that preserved HRV on day one and higher parasympathetic tone was associated with early brain death.[33]

Serum Troponin and Beta-Blockers

Increased troponin (TnI) levels have been associated with lower GCS scores, higher ISS scores, and higher mortality in TBI patients. It has been found to be an independent predictor of poor outcome even after adjusting for injury severity. Beta-blocker treatment was associated with improved survival in patients with elevated TnI.[70]

Demographics

Race

Evidence for the relationship between race and outcome in TBI patients is inconclusive. Some resources established that race was not related to outcome.[15] However, data from the large-scale IMPACT database found that black patients had poorer outcome.[4]

Education

Lower educational level prior to TBI did not correlate with nonproductivity post-TBI in some studies.[8] However, others found that higher educational levels above 12 years had a weak correlation with better outcome.[4]

Gender

Gender was not found to be related to functional outcome in several studies.[4,8,15] In contrast, data from the Trauma Recovery Project using the QWB Scale showed that female trauma patients had significantly lower QWB scores. However, this was not specific to TBI patients (**Table 22.6**).[61] This issue remains controversial.

Table 22.6 Markers in Traumatic Brain Injury

- Elevated S-100B may be related to outcome but questions remain regarding its elevation in general polytrauma
- Neuron-specific enolase elevations appear associated with higher mortality
- Apolipoprotein E4 (APOE4) genotype is associated with worse outcome among those with severe injuries

Hospital Stays/Admission or Discharge Status

Acute-Care Length of Stay

Longer lengths of stay at the acute hospital have been associated with lower admission motor and cognitive FIM scores in some studies,[34] whereas others found no association with outcome.[8,16]

A large, prospective epidemiologic study comprised of trauma patients showed that lengths of stay 7 days or more at the acute hospital or 4 or more days in the ICU were associated with worse 12- and 18-month functional outcome as measured by the QWB Scale, which includes assessments of mobility and physical and social activity. However, this study was focused on trauma patients and was not specific to TBI patients.[61]

Discharge Site and Discharge Status

Site of discharge was a prognostic factor related to GOS scores at time of discharge and at 5 to 7 years after discharge. Discharge to home after acute care was predictive of good outcome.[15] Higher disability at discharge from rehabilitation, as indicated by the DRS, was associated with continued disability one year after TBI.[8]

Functional Status at Admission or Discharge

Functional status on admission to the rehabilitation facility was associated with eventual functional outcome as measured by DRS, level of care, FIM and functional assessment measure (FAM) scores.[71] Greater disability on admission to the rehabilitation facility was a prognostic indicator associated with future nonproductivity, which included work or school status post-TBI. Higher disability at discharge from rehabilitation was also found to be predictive of continued disability at 1 year post-TBI.[8]

Impairment level, as measured by the level of paresis on the Brunnstrom Stages of recovery (BS), ranging from 1, severe, to 6 in patients with upper extremity paresis was also predictive of recovery and time to recover.[14]

Length of Time between Injury and Rehabilitation Admission/Earlier Transfer to Rehabilitation

Length of time between TBI occurrence and admission to rehab was also related to functional outcome.[71] Earlier admission to rehab was associated with better outcome.[34]

Length of Stay in Rehabilitation

With longer lengths of stay in the rehabilitation hospital, there was less change in functional status during the latter part of the hospitalization. FIM and FAM scores did not change significantly after a 12-month rehabilitation program stay.

Postacute Community Reentry Program

High et al reported positive outcome results from a postacute community reentry program with an average duration of 4 months, which focused on adjustment issues, transition to community reintegration, and compensatory mechanisms for deficits. Improvement in productivity, functional ability, and independence was seen even in patients 12-months postinjury, although patients that started earlier (i.e., 6 months postinjury experienced continued improvement in independence after discharge from the program. This presents another facet of rehabilitation that can affect eventual functional outcome.[71]

Duration of Time Postinjury

In a pediatric study, 37% of the patients were functionally independent in the immediate aftermath postinjury, but after 2 years, 65% of patients were functionally independent. This highlights the plasticity of recovery in pediatric TBI patients and proposes that a tincture of time can better predict outcome. Many studies in the literature measure outcome after 6 to 12 months. However, follow-up over a longer period may uncover even further functional recovery and better outcomes.[16]

Severe Injury

Patients in a Vegetative State or Minimally Conscious

Prognosis for Survival

Most of the studies to date have examined patients with TBI of varying degrees of severity and have attempted to predict who will survive beyond the acute period.[72–74] As expected, severity of injury, other multiple comorbidities, and older age contribute to higher mortality.

Studies of long-term survival in the vegetative state are even more scarce because they require longitudinal follow-up for months or years. The following findings are seen in the existing literature: (a) overall life expectancy is shortened in the vegetative state population; (b) younger patients survive longer; and (c) patients in a vegetative state for longer intervals have greater chances for survival.[75–77]

Prognosis for Return of Consciousness

There is no definite temporal cut-off beyond which consciousness cannot return. However, the probability of regaining consciousness drops in a continuous fashion with increasing time after the injury.[78,79]

1. Children have a better chance of regaining consciousness than adults.
2. Anoxic or vascular events in addition to traumatic cause of injury leads to worse prognosis for return of consciousness.
3. Most of recovery of consciousness occurs during the first year postinjury. Recoveries after 1 year deal with severe disability for the rest of their lives.
4. Bilateral absence of cortical responses in somatosensory evoked potential (SSEPs) done within 7 days of injury has poor prognosis.

Prognosis for a Certain Level of Functioning

The literature is not clear about answering this question. Multiple factors affect the outcome. Unilateral brain injury, intact brain stem, how soon the improvement started to occur after the injury, the rate of functional change, and demonstration of insight by the person all play important roles in better outcomes. It is important to note that there is a significant amount of outcome variability; therefore, all decisions should be based on an individual basis.

Patients with Penetrating Injuries

Studies show that there is a high mortality rate associated with penetrating injury.[11,80,81] GCS and the bullet trajectory are associated with outcome. Lower GCS score (3 to 8) and CT findings of bilateral injury or transventricular injury were associated with poor outcome.[81]

Once a person survives the penetrating injury, the chance of good recovery is high. A significantly less number of people remain in a vegetative state or minimally conscious state compared with the population with closed head injury.

Conclusion

A myriad of variables interact to impact on the prognosis of the person with TBI. No clear formula exists to predict detailed functional outcome. Investigators have attempted to predict survival with good to moderate success. The ability to employ future technologies will enhance prognostic ability by making person-specific factors available. Thus, magnetic resonance spectroscopy, diffusion tensor imaging, and novel biomarkers will contribute to clinical and resource planning (**Tables 22.7** and **22.8**).

Table 22.7 Prognostic Factors Associated with Poorer Outcome

Prognostic Factor	Demographics Study
Older age	Gray and Burnham, 2000[1]; Hukkelhoven et al, 2003[2]; Poon et al, 2005[3]; Cremer et al, 2006[5]; Mushkudiani et al, 2007[4]; Willemse-van Son et al, 2007[8]
Black race	Mushkudiani et al, 2007[4]
Laboratories, Vital Signs, Clinical Measures	
Hypotension (systolic blood pressure < 90 mm Hg)	Jeremitsky et al, 2003[20]; Vavilala et al, 2003[24]; Coates et al, 2005[23]; Chi et al, 2006[18]; Ducrocq et al, 2006[17]; McHugh et al, 2007[19]; Butcher et al, 2007[21]; Murray et al, 2007[6]
Hypoxia (pO_2 < 60 mm Hg)	Jeremitsky et al, 2003[20]; Chi et al, 2006[18]
Hyperglycemia	Murray et al, 2007[6]; Van Beek et al, 2007[29]
Hypocapnia	Jeremitsky et al, 2003[20]
Increased prothrombin time	Murray et al, 2007[6]; Van Beek et al, 2007[29]; Harhangi et al, 2008[30]
Anemia	Murray et al, 2007[6]; Van Beek et al, 2007[29]
Thrombocytopenia on admission	Murray et al, 2007[6]; Van Beek et al, 2007[29]
Hyponatremia or Hypernatremia	Van Beek et al, 2007[29]
Increased norepinephrine on admission	Hamill et al, 1987[31]; Woolf et al, 1987[32]; Rapenne et al, 2001[33]
Increased S-100B levels	Woertgen et al, 1999[11]; Spinella et al, 2003[36]; Vos et al, 2004[54]
Increased serum glial fibrillary acidic protein (GFAP) levels	Vos et al, 2004[54]; Nylen et al, 2006[56]

(Continued on page 414)

Table 22.7 *(Continued)*

	Demographics
Increased neuron specific enolase (NSE) levels	Vos et al, 2004[54]
Higher intracranial pressures (ICP) values	Prat and Calatayud-Maldonado, 1998[50]; Signorini et al, 1999[10]; Catala-Temprano et al, 2007[51]
Initial cerebral perfusion pressure (CPP) lower or higher than 40–70 mm Hg in pediatric patients	Catala-Temprano et al, 2007[51]
Increased troponin (TnI) levels	Salim, Hadjizacharia et al. 2008[70]
Scores—Measures of Injury Severity	
Worse GCS scores	Cowen et al, 1995[34]; Massagli et al, 1996[15]; Thakker et al,1997[16]; Asikainen et al, 1998[33]; White et al, 2001[22]; Spinella et al, 2003[36]; Poon et al, 2005[3]; Chung et al, 2006[37]; Cremer et al, 2006[5]; Marmarou et al, 2007[53]; Murray et al, 2007[6]
Higher Pediatric Risk of Mortality (PRISM) score	Thakker et al, 1997[16]; Spinella et al, 2003[36]
Higher injury severity score (ISS)	Massagli et al, 1996[15]; Ducrocq et al, 2006[17]; Foreman et al, 2007[43]
Higher head abbreviated injury score (AIS)	Massagli et al, 1996[15]; Ducrocq et al, 2006[17]; Foreman et al, 2007[43]
Worse FIM scores at the beginning of rehabilitation	Cowen et al, 1995[34]; Poon et al, 2005[3]
Neuroimaging	
Worse Marshall CT Classification	Claret Teruel et al, 2007[42]; Maas et al, 2007[44]; Murray et al, 2007[6]
Presence of traumatic subarachnoid hemorrhage	Pillai et al., 2001[41]; Maas et al, 2007[44]; Murray et al, 2007[6]
Presence of intraventricular hemorrhage	Maas et al., 2005[45]; Maas et al. 2007[44]
Partial or full obliteration of the basal cisterns and midline shift	Maas et al. 2007[44]; Murray et al, 2007[6]
Presence of day of injury CT abnormalities	Bigler et al, 2006[46]
Brain stem injury	Wedekind and Lippert-Gruner, 2005[48]; Bigler et al, 2006[46]
Presence of deep lesions/ cerebellar damage (worse cognitive outcome in children)	Braga et al, 2007[49]
Other TBI Factors	
Longer duration of coma	Macpherson et al, 1992[13]; Massagli et al,1996[15]; Asikainen et al, 1998[33]
Longer posttraumatic amnesia	Asikainen et al, 1998[33]; Katz et al, 2004[12]; Willemse-van Son et al, 2007[8]
Non- or poorly reactive pupils	Massagli et al, 1996[15]; Marmarou et al, 2007[53]
Acute lung injury	Holland et al, 2003[66]
Lower heart rate variability and cardiac uncoupling	Rapenne et al, 2001[33]; Morris et al, 2006[69]; Riordan et al, 2007[68]
Higher disability at admission or discharge from rehabilitation	Willemse-van Son et al, 2007[8]
Later admission to rehabilitation	Cowen et al, 1995[34]; Gray and Burnham, 2000[1]

Abbreviations: CT, computed tomography; FIM, functional independence measure; GCS, Glasgow Coma Scale; TBI, traumatic brain injury.

Table 22.8 Multiple Variables' Impact on Outcome

Study	Prognostic Factor	Outcome Measure	Correlated with Poorer Outcome	Number of Subjects/Patients
Murray et al, 2007[6]	Age, GCS, pupil response, CT characteristics, blood pressure, laboratories, vital signs	6-Month GOS	Older age Worse GCS motor score Poor pupil response Worse Marshall CT classification Evidence of traumatic SAH on CT Hypotension Hypoxia Glucose Prothrombin time	8509 (for age, GCS), range 840–8,508 for other variables)
Mushkudiani et al, 2007[4]	Age, race, gender, education	6-Month GOS	Older age Black race Weak association: lower education	Age (8,719), gender (8,720), race (5,320), education (2,201)
Marmarou et al, 2007[53]	GCS, pupil reactivity	6-month GOS	Lower motor score on GCS, also eye and verbal components of GCS One or both unreactive pupils	8,721
Willemse-van Son et al, 2007[8]	Over 100 prognostic factors examined	20 outcome measures – divided into disability and nonproductivity	Older age Preinjury unemployment Preinjury substance abuse More disability at rehabilitation discharge or admission Longer posttraumatic amnesia	Review of 14 cohorts, 35 articles (range 21–2,771)
Ducrocq et al, 2006[17]	Many variables	Discharge and 6-month GOS	Initial hypotension GCS score ≤ 5 ISS score ≥ 28 Need for emergency transfusion on arrival Diffuse axonal injuries Complex lesion or Massive focal lesion on early CT scan Age ≤2	585 (pediatrics)
Katz et al, 2004[12]	Functional measures, injury severity measures, age	Recovery of independent ambulation and time to recover	Older age More severely injured, based on longer duration of posttraumatic amnesia, Poorer admission gait scores	116
Cremer et al, 2006[5]	Age, GCS, pupil response, CT findings, blood pressure	Extended GOS after ≥ 12 months	Older age Poorer GCS score (motor response on day one) Poor pupil reactivity Worse CT findings [Low blood pressure was only a weak predictor]	304 patient that remained comatose for > 24 hours after TBI
Massagli et al, 1996[15]	Many variables	GOS at discharge and at 5–7 years post-TBI	Discharge GOS: Poorer head AIS, ISS score, GCS score in the field and at 6, 24, 72 hours, longer length of coma, and initial discharge site (not to home). Long-term GOS: poorer head AIS score, ISS score, pupil responses in the field, GCS scores at 24 and 72 hours, longer length of coma, site of discharge (not to home), and early GOS scores	75 (pediatrics)

(Continued on page 416)

Table 22.8 (*Continued*)

Study	Prognostic Factor	Outcome Measure	Correlated with Poorer Outcome	Number of Subjects/Patients
White et al, 2001[22]	Pediatric Trauma Score, GCS score, many variables	Survival, PICU LOS, day at which GCS score was ≥14	Lower 6-hour GCS score (Mannitol use was associated with prolonged LOS. Survival was associated with maximum systolic blood pressure ≥135 mm Hg)	136 (pediatrics)
Chung et al, 2006[37]	GCS and other variables	GOS	GCS score ≤5 Also presence of subarachnoid hemorrhage with brain swelling and edema, subdural, intracerebral hemorrhage, and basal ganglion lesions, chest trauma	309
Poon et al, 2005[3]	Many variables	1 year GOS	Older age Poorer GCS score or baseline FIM at the beginning of rehabilitation	68
Holland et al, 2003[66]	Acute lung injury	3 and 12 month GOS	Development of acute lung injury	137
Braga et al, 2007[49]	MRI findings	Neuropsychological sequelae >1 year postinjury	Left frontal lesions (resulted in lower semantic verbal fluency), right occipital lesions (lower visual recognition task scores), cerebellar lesions (dyscalculia, lower cognitive performances and lower visual recognition memory)	23
Signorini et al, 1999[10]	Many clinical variables	Survival at 1 year (prognostic model)	Early intracranial hypertension	110
Neuroimaging				
Study	**Prognostic Factor**	**Outcome Measure**	**Correlated with Poorer Outcome**	**Number of Subjects/Patients**
Maas et al, 2007[44]	Marshall CT classifications and individual CT characteristics	6-month GOS	Diffuse injuries in CT class III or IV (Acute subdural hematoma Partial obliteration of basal cisterns Traumatic subarachnoid hemorrhage, or Midline shift	8,721: CT classification (5,209), basal cistern (3861), midline shift (4,698), tSAH (7,407), intracranial lesions (7,613)
Claret Teruel et al, 2007[42]	Marshall CT classifications	12-month GOS	Poorer initial neuroimaging patterns	156 (pediatrics)
Bigler et al, 2006[46]	Day of injury CT, Marshall CT classification, MRI 25 or more days postinjury	Disability Rating Scale (DRS), FIM measure	Increased ventricle-to-brain ratio at 25 or more days postinjury (also associated with day of injury CT abnormalities) Also: brainstem injury	240
Maas et al, 2005[45]	Marshall CT classification, individual CT predictors	6-month mortality	Midline shift > 5 mm Basal cisterns compressed/absent (CT class IV) Intraventricular blood Traumatic subarachnoid hemorrhage	2,269
Hou et al, 2007[82]	(ADC values—diffusion-weighted MRI	6–12-month GOS	Higher mean deep gray and white matter ADC values	72
Secondary Insults, Laboratories				
Study	**Prognostic Factor**	**Outcome Measure**	**Correlated with Poorer Outcome**	**Number of Subjects/Patients**
Butcher et al, 2007[21]	Admission blood pressure	6-month GOS	Hypotension or Hypertension (U-shaped relationship found with better outcome in patients with	6,801 (systolic blood pressure data), 6,647 (mean arterial blood pressure data)

Table 22.8 *(Continued)*

Study	Prognostic Factor	Outcome Measure	Correlated with Poorer Outcome	Number of Subjects/Patients
			SBP 120–150 mm Hg or MAP 85–110 mm Hg)	
Van Beek et al, 2007[29]	Glucose, sodium, pH, hemoglobin, platelet count, prothrombin time	6-month GOS	High glucose Low hemoglobin High prothrombin time Low platelets Low pH Low and high sodium	Glucose (4,834), sodium (5,270), pH (3,398), hemoglobin (3,875), platelet count (1,629), prothrombin time (840)
McHugh et al, 2007[19]	Hypoxia, hypotension, hypothermia	6-month GOS	Hypoxia Hypotension Hypothermia	Hypoxia (5,661), hypotension (6,629), hypothermia (4,195)
Jeremitsky et al, 2003[20]	Acidosis, coagulopathy, hypotension, hypoxia, hypocapnia, hypercapnia, hypothermia, hyperthermia, hyperglycemia, intracranial hypertension, seizure.	ICU and hospital LOS, mortality, discharge to rehabilitation rather than home	Hypotension (Hypothermia in patients age < 45 years Hypoxia (Hypocapnia, in hours 15–24) Acidosis	81
Coates et al, 2005[23]	Secondary insults— hypotension	Discharge GOS, disposition (death or discharge to a skilled nursing facility), PICU and hospital LOS	Early hypotension (systolic blood pressure < 5th percentile for age)	93 (pediatrics)
Vavilala et al, 2003[24]	Secondary insults—hypotension	Discharge GOS	Age-appropriate systolic blood pressure percentile < 75th percentile, even when systolic blood pressure was ≥ 90 mm Hg	172 (pediatrics)
Chi et al, 2006[18]	Secondary insults—hypoxia, hypotension	Mortality and DRS score at discharge	Hypoxia (affected mortality and DRS score) Hypotension (affected DRS score).	150
Natale et al, 2000	Secondary insults—hyperthermia	GCS score at PICU discharge, PICU LOS	Early hyperthermia	117
Salim et al, 2008[70]	Serum troponin	Mortality	Elevated serum troponin (TnI)	420
Nylen et al, 2006[56]	Serum GFAP	1-year GOS	Higher maximal s-GFAP levels in the acute phase	59
Spinella et al, 2003[36]	Serum S-100B, GCS, PRISM	PCPC score at discharge and at 6 months	Higher S-100B levels Poorer GCS and PRISM scores	163 (pediatrics)
Vos et al, 2004[54]	Serum GFAP, S-100B, NSE levels	6-month GOS	Higher GFAP, S-100B, NSE levels	85
Woertgen et al, 1999[11]	Serum S-100B and other variables	11-month GOS	Higher serum S-100B levels within 1–6 hours of severe head injury. Also: older age, lower GCS, poorer Marshall CT classification.	44
Berger et al, 2007	Serum S-100B, MBP, NSE	GOS or GOS-Extended Pediatric at varying time points from discharge to 12 months postinjury	Higher levels of S-100B, MBP, NSE (peak concentrations correlated more strongly)	152 (pediatrics)
Nylen et al, 2007[57]	Serum GFAP	Extended GOS at 1 year	Higher maximum GFAP levels	116

(Continued on page 418)

Table 22.8 (*Continued*)

Study	Prognostic Factor	Outcome Measure	Correlated with Poorer Outcome	Number of Subjects/Patients
Coma, Posttraumatic Amnesia				
Sherer et al, 2008	Posttraumatic confusion	Employability at rehabilitation discharge and productivity status at 1 year postinjury	More severely confused Longer time to follow commands Presence of psychotic-type symptoms	168
Asikainen et al, 1998[33]	GCS, LOC, PTA	GOS at the end of 5–20-year follow-up (mean 12 years), postinjury occupational outcome	Poorer GCS score on admission (functional outcome) Longer length of coma and duration of posttraumatic amnesia (work outcome and functional outcome).	508
Demographics, Scores				
Livingston et al, 2007[9]	Age	Discharge and 1-year GOS, discharge disposition, modified FIM score	Older age	241
Mosenthal et al, 2004[7]	Age	Discharge disposition, discharge and 6-month GOS and FIM score	Older age (but outcome was still relatively good)	235
Thakker et al, 1997[16]	Vital signs from day 1, PRISM score, GCS, other variables	Functional status based on locomotion, self-care, communication.	Younger age Lower GCS score Higher PRISM score on admission Higher PRISM adjusted heart rate Lower PRISM adjusted systolic blood pressure	105 (pediatrics)
Davis et al, 2006[39]	GCS scores	Mortality, need for neurosurgical care	Poorer field GCS and arrival GCS scores (change in field to arrival GCS also predicted outcome)	12,882
Foreman et al, 2007[43]	GCS, head AIS, ISS scores	Extended GOS at 12 months	Combination of poorer AIS or ISS and GCS scores. ISS > GCS > head AIS	270

Abbreviations: ADC, apparent diffusion coefficient; AIS, abbreviated injury score; CT, computed tomography; DRS, Disability Rating Scale; FIM, functional independence measure; GCS, Glasgow Coma Scale; GFAP, glial fibrillary acidic protein; GOS, Glasgow Outcome Scale; ISS, injury severity score; LOC, loss of consciousness; LOS, length of stay; MBP, myelin basic protein; MRI, magnetic resonance imaging; NSE, neuron specific enolase; PCPC, Pediatric Cerebral Performance Category; PICU, pediatric intensive care unit; PRISM, Pediatric Risk of Mortality; PTA, posttraumatic amnesia; SAH, subarachnoid hemorrhage; SBP, systolic blood pressure; TBI, traumatic brain injury; tSAH, traumatic subarachnoid hemorrhage.

References

1. Gray DS, Burnham RS. Preliminary outcome analysis of a long-term rehabilitation program for severe acquired brain injury. Arch Phys Med Rehabil 2000;81(11):1447–1456
2. Hukkelhoven CW, Steyerberg EW, Rampen AJ, et al. Patient age and outcome following severe traumatic brain injury: an analysis of 5600 patients. J Neurosurg 2003;99(4):666–673
3. Poon WS, Zhu XL, Ng SC, et al. Predicting one year clinical outcome in traumatic brain injury (TBI) at the beginning of rehabilitation. Acta Neurochir Suppl (Wien) 2005;93:207–208
4. Mushkudiani NA, Engel DC, Steyerberg EW, et al. Prognostic value of demographic characteristics in traumatic brain injury: results from the IMPACT study. J Neurotrauma 2007;24(2):259–269
5. Cremer OL, Moons KG, van Dijk GW, et al. Prognosis following severe head injury: development and validation of a model for prediction of death, disability, and functional recovery. J Trauma 2006;61(6): 1484–1491
6. Murray GD, Butcher I, McHugh GS, et al. Multivariable prognostic analysis in traumatic brain injury: results from the IMPACT study. J Neurotrauma 2007;24(2):329–337
7. Mosenthal AC, Livingston DH, Lavery RF, et al. The effect of age on functional outcome in mild traumatic brain injury: 6-month report of a prospective multicenter trial. J Trauma 2004;56(5):1042–1048
8. Willemse-van Son AH, Ribbers GM, et al. Prognostic factors of long-term functioning and productivity after traumatic brain injury: a systematic

review of prospective cohort studies. Clin Rehabil 2007;21(11): 1024–1037
9. Livingston DH, Lavery RF, Verhagen AP, et al. Recovery at one year following isolated traumatic brain injury: a Western Trauma Association prospective multicenter trial. J Trauma 2005;59(6):1298–1304
10. Signorini DF, Andrews PJ, Jones PA, et al. Predicting survival using simple clinical variables: a case study in traumatic brain injury. J Neurol Neurosurg Psychiatry 1999;66(1):20–25
11. Woertgen C, Rothoerl RD, Metz C, et al. Comparison of clinical, radiologic, and serum marker as prognostic factors after severe head injury. J Trauma 1999;47(6):1126–1130
12. Katz DI, White DK, Alexander MP, et al. Recovery of ambulation after traumatic brain injury. Arch Phys Med Rehabil 2004;85(6): 865–869
13. Macpherson V, Sullivan SJ, Lambert J. Prediction of motor status 3 and 6 months post severe traumatic brain injury: a preliminary study. Brain Inj 1992;6(6):489–498
14. Katz DI, Alexander MP, Klein RB. Recovery of arm function in patients with paresis after traumatic brain injury. Arch Phys Med Rehabil 1998;79(5):488–493
15. Massagli TL, Michaud LJ, Rivara FP. Association between injury indices and outcome after severe traumatic brain injury in children. Arch Phys Med Rehabil 1996;77(2):125–132
16. Thakker JC, Splaingard M, Zhu J, Babel K, Bresnahan J, Havens PL. Survival and functional outcome of children requiring endotracheal intubation during therapy for severe traumatic brain injury. Crit Care Med 1997;25(8):1396–1401
17. Ducrocq SC, Meyer PG, Orliaguet GA, et al. Epidemiology and early predictive factors of mortality and outcome in children with traumatic severe brain injury: experience of a French pediatric trauma center. Pediatr Crit Care Med 2006;7(5):461–467
18. Chi JH, Knudson MM, Vassar MJ, et al. Prehospital hypoxia affects outcome in patients with traumatic brain injury: a prospective multicenter study. J Trauma 2006;61(5):1134–1141
19. McHugh GS, Engel DC, Butcher I, et al. Prognostic value of secondary insults in traumatic brain injury: results from the IMPACT study. J Neurotrauma 2007;24(2):287–293
20. Jeremitsky E, Omert L, Dunham CM, Protetch J, Rodriguez A. Harbingers of poor outcome the day after severe brain injury: hypothermia, hypoxia, and hypoperfusion. J Trauma 2003;54(2):312–319
21. Butcher I, Maas AI, Lu J, et al. Prognostic value of admission blood pressure in traumatic brain injury: results from the IMPACT study. J Neurotrauma 2007;24(2):294–302
22. White JR, Farukhi Z, Bull C, et al. Predictors of outcome in severely head-injured children. Crit Care Med 2001;29(3):534–540
23. Coates BM, Vavilala MS, Mack CD, et al. Influence of definition and location of hypotension on outcome following severe pediatric traumatic brain injury. Crit Care Med 2005;33(11):2645–2650
24. Vavilala MS, Bowen A, Lam AM, et al. Blood pressure and outcome after severe pediatric traumatic brain injury. J Trauma 2003;55(6):1039–1044
25. Clifton GL, Choi SC, Miller ER, et al. Intercenter variance in clinical trials of head trauma: experience of the National Acute Brain Injury Study: hypothermia. J Neurosurg 2001;95(5):751–755
26. Clifton GL, Miller ER, Choi SC, et al. Lack of effect of induction of hypothermia after acute brain injury. N Engl J Med 2001;344(8):556–563
27. Knudson MM, McGrath J. Improving outcomes in pediatric trauma care: essential characteristics of the trauma center. J Trauma 2007; 63(6, Suppl)S140–S142
28. Natale JE, Joseph JG, Helfaer MA, Shaffner DH. Early hyperthermia after traumatic brain injury in children: risk factors, influence on length of stay, and effect on short-term neurologic status. Crit Care Med 2000;28(7):2608–2615
29. Van Beek JG, Mushkudiani NA, Steyerberg EW, et al. Prognostic value of admission laboratory parameters in traumatic brain injury: results from the IMPACT study. J Neurotrauma 2007;24(2):315–328
30. Harhangi BS, Kompanje EJ, Leebeek FW, Maas AI. Coagulation disorders after traumatic brain injury. Acta Neurochir (Wien) 2008;150(2): 165–175
31. Hamill RW, Woolf PD, McDonald JV, Lee LA, Kelly M. Catecholamines predict outcome in traumatic brain injury. Ann Neurol 1987;21(5): 438–443
32. Woolf PD, Hamill RW, Lee LA, Cox C, McDonald JV. The predictive value of catecholamines in assessing outcome in traumatic brain injury. J Neurosurg 1987;66(6):875–882
33. Rapenne T, Moreau D, Lenfant F, et al. Could heart rate variability predict outcome in patients with severe head injury? A pilot study. J Neurosurg Anesthesiol 2001;13(3):260–268
34. Cowen TD, Meythaler JM, DeVivo MJ, Ivie CS III, Lebow J, Novack TA. Influence of early variables in traumatic brain injury on functional independence measure scores and rehabilitation length of stay and charges. Arch Phys Med Rehabil 1995;76(9):797–803
35. Asikainen I, Kaste M, Sarna S. Predicting late outcome for patients with traumatic brain injury referred to a rehabilitation programme: a study of 508 Finnish patients 5 years or more after injury. Brain Inj 1998;12(2):95–107
36. Spinella PC, Dominguez T, Drott HR, et al. S-100beta protein-serum levels in healthy children and its association with outcome in pediatric traumatic brain injury. Crit Care Med 2003;31(3):939–945
37. Chung CY, Chen CL, Cheng PT, See LC, Tang SF, Wong AM. Critical score of Glasgow Coma Scale for pediatric traumatic brain injury. Pediatr Neurol 2006;34(5):379–387
38. Marmarou A, Lu J, Butcher I, et al. IMPACT database of traumatic brain injury: design and description. J Neurotrauma 2007;24(2):239–250
39. Davis DP, Serrano JA, Vilke GM, et al. The predictive value of field versus arrival Glasgow Coma Scale score and TRISS calculations in moderate-to-severe traumatic brain injury. J Trauma 2006;60(5): 985–990
40. Michaud LJ, Rivara FP, Grady MS, Reay DT. Predictors of survival and severity of disability after severe brain injury in children. Neurosurgery 1992;31(2):254–264
41. Pillai S, Praharaj SS, Mohanty A, Kolluri VR. Prognostic factors in children with severe diffuse brain injuries: a study of 74 patients. Pediatr Neurosurg 2001;34(2):98–103
42. Claret Teruel G, Palomeque Rico A, Cambra Lasaosa FJ, Català Temprano A, Noguera Julian A, Costa Clarà JM. Severe head injury among children: computed tomography evaluation as a prognostic factor. J Pediatr Surg 2007;42(11):1903–1906
43. Foreman BP, Caesar RR, Parks J, et al. Usefulness of the abbreviated injury score and the injury severity score in comparison to the Glasgow Coma Scale in predicting outcome after traumatic brain injury. J Trauma 2007;62(4):946–950
44. Maas AI, Steyerberg EW, Butcher I, et al. Prognostic value of computerized tomography scan characteristics in traumatic brain injury: results from the IMPACT study. J Neurotrauma 2007;24(2):303–314
45. Maas AI, Hukkelhoven CW, Marshall LF, Steyerberg EW. Prediction of outcome in traumatic brain injury with computed tomographic characteristics: a comparison between the computed tomographic classification and combinations of computed tomographic predictors. Neurosurgery 2005;57(6):1173–1182
46. Bigler ED, Ryser DK, Gandhi P, Kimball J, Wilde EA. Day-of-injury computerized tomography, rehabilitation status, and development of cerebral atrophy in persons with traumatic brain injury. Am J Phys Med Rehabil 2006;85(10):793–806
47. Scheid R, Ott DV, Roth H, Schroeter ML, von Cramon DY. Comparative magnetic resonance imaging at 1.5 and 3 Tesla for the evaluation of traumatic microbleeds. J Neurotrauma 2007;24(12):1811–1816
48. Wedekind C, Lippert-Gruner M. Long-term outcome in severe traumatic brain injury is significantly influenced by brainstem involvement. Brain Inj 2005;19(9):681–684
49. Braga LW, Souza LN, Najjar YJ, Dellatolas G. Magnetic resonance imaging (MRI) findings and neuropsychological sequelae in children after severe traumatic brain injury: the role of cerebellar lesion. J Child Neurol 2007;22(9):1084–1089
50. Prat R, Calatayud-Maldonado V. Prognostic factors in postraumatic severe diffuse brain injury. Acta Neurochir (Wien) 1998;140(12): 1257–1260, discussion 1261

51. Catala-Temprano A, Claret Teruel G, Cambra Lasaosa FJ, et al Intracranial pressure and cerebral perfusion pressure as risk factors in children with traumatic brain injuries. J Neurosurg 2007;106(6, Suppl):463–466
52. Marmarou A, Saad A, Aygok G, Rigsbee M. Contribution of raised ICP and hypotension to CPP reduction in severe brain injury: correlation to outcome. Acta Neurochir Suppl (Wien) 2005;95:277–280
53. Marmarou A, Lu J, Butcher I, et al. Prognostic value of the Glasgow Coma Scale and pupil reactivity in traumatic brain injury assessed prehospital and on enrollment: an IMPACT analysis. J Neurotrauma 2007; 24(2):270–280
54. Vos PE, Lamers KJ, Hendriks JC, et al. Glial and neuronal proteins in serum predict outcome after severe traumatic brain injury. Neurology 2004;62(8):1303–1310
55. Berger RP, Beers SR, Richichi R, Wiesman D, Adelson PD. Serum biomarker concentrations and outcome after pediatric traumatic brain injury. J Neurotrauma 2007;24(12):1793–1801
56. Nylen K, Ost M, Csajbok LZ, et al. Increased serum-GFAP in patients with severe traumatic brain injury is related to outcome. J Neurol Sci 2006;240(1–2):85–91
57. Nylen K, Csajbok LZ, Ost M, et al. Serum glial fibrillary acidic protein is related to focal brain injury and outcome after aneurysmal subarachnoid hemorrhage. Stroke 2007;38(5):1489–1494
58. Jiang Y, Sun X, Gui L, et al. Correlation between APOE-491AA promoter in epsilon4 carriers and clinical deterioration in early stage of traumatic brain injury. J Neurotrauma 2007;24(12):1802–1810
59. Butcher I, McHugh GS, Lu J, et al. Prognostic value of cause of injury in traumatic brain injury: results from the IMPACT study. J Neurotrauma 2007;24(2):281–286
60. Seekamp A, Regel G, Tscherne H. Rehabilitation and reintegration of multiply injured patients: an outcome study with special reference to multiple lower limb fractures. Injury 1996;27(2):133–138
61. Holbrook TL, Anderson JP, Sieber WJ, Browner D, Hoyt DB. Outcome after major trauma: 12-month and 18-month follow-up results from the Trauma Recovery Project. J Trauma 1999;46(5):765–771
62. Holbrook TL, Hoyt DB, Anderson JP. The impact of major in-hospital complications on functional outcome and quality of life after trauma. J Trauma 2001;50(1):91–95
63. Mascia L, Andrews PJ. Acute lung injury in head trauma patients. Intensive Care Med 1998;24(10):1115–1116
64. Eberhard LW, Morabito DJ, Matthay MA, et al. Initial severity of metabolic acidosis predicts the development of acute lung injury in severely traumatized patients. Crit Care Med 2000;28(1):125–131
65. Contant CF, Valadka AB, Gopinath SP, Hannay HJ, Robertson CS. Adult respiratory distress syndrome: a complication of induced hypertension after severe head injury. J Neurosurg 2001;95(4):560–568
66. Holland MC, Mackersie RC, Morabito D, et al. The development of acute lung injury is associated with worse neurologic outcome in patients with severe traumatic brain injury. J Trauma 2003;55(1):106–111
67. Goldstein B, Toweill D, Lai S, Sonnenthal K, Kimberly B. Uncoupling of the autonomic and cardiovascular systems in acute brain injury. Am J Physiol 1998;275(4 Pt 2):R1287–R1292
68. Riordan WP Jr, Cotton BA, Norris PR, Waitman LR, Jenkins JM, Morris JA Jr. Beta-blocker exposure in patients with severe traumatic brain injury (TBI) and cardiac uncoupling. J Trauma 2007;63(3):503–510
69. Morris JA Jr, Norris PR, Ozdas A, et al. Reduced heart rate variability: an indicator of cardiac uncoupling and diminished physiologic reserve in 1,425 trauma patients. J Trauma 2006;60(6):1165–1173
70. Salim A, Hadjizacharia P, Brown C, et al. Significance of troponin elevation after severe traumatic brain injury. J Trauma 2008;64(1):46–52
71. High WM Jr, Roebuck-Spencer T, Sander AM, Struchen MA, Sherer M. Early versus later admission to postacute rehabilitation: impact on functional outcome after traumatic brain injury. Arch Phys Med Rehabil 2006;87(3):334–342
72. Vapahlati M, Troupp H. Prognosis for patients with severe head injuries. BMJ 1971;3:404–407
73. Jennett B, Snock J, Bond MR, Brooks N. Disability after severe head injury: observations on the use of the Glasgow Outcome Scale. J Neurol Neurosurg Psychiatry 1981;44:285–293
74. Born JD, Albert A, Hans P, Bonnal J. Relative prognostic value of best motor response and brain stem reflexes in patients with severe head injury. Neurosurgery 1985;16:595–600
75. Shavelle RM, Strauss D, Whyte J, Day SM, Yu YL. Longterm causes of death after traumatic brain injury. Am J Phys Med Rehabil 2001;80: 510–516
76. Higashi K, Hatano M, Abiko S, et al. Five-year follow up study of patients with persistent vegetative state. J Neurol Neurosurg Psychiatry 1981;44:552–554
77. Strauss DJ, Shavell RM, Ashwal SA. Life expectancy and median survival time in the permanent vegetative state. Pediatr Neurol 1999;21:626–631
78. Whyte J, Katz D, DiPasquale MC, et al. Predictors of outcome and effect of psychoactive medications in prolonged posttraumatic disorders of consciousness: a multicenter study. Arch Phys Med Rehabil 2005; 86(3):453–462
79. Zafonte RD, Wood D, Harrison-Felix C, et al. Severe penetrating head injury: a study of outcomes. Arch Phys Med Rehabil 2001;82:306–310
80. Kim KA, Wang M, McNatt S, et al. Vector analysis correlating bullet trajectory to outcome after civilian through and through gunshot wound to the head: using imaging cues to predict fatal outcome. Neurosurgery 2005;57(4):737–747
81. Williams AJ, Ling G, Tortella F. Severity level and injury track determine outcome following a penetrating ballistic like brain injury in the rat. Neurosci Lett 2006;408:183–188
82. Hou DJ, Tong KA, Ashwal S, et al. Diffusion weighted magnetic resonance imaging improves outcome prediction in adult traumatic brain injury, J Neurotrauma 2007;24:1558–1569

VI Socioeconomics

23 Ethics: Life and Death Choices

Paul J. Ford and Abhishek Deshpande

Difficult life and death choices regularly occur in neurotrauma treatment. The choices surrounding whether, how quickly, and by what method to treat always have strong ethical dimensions. These ethical dimensions play important roles at the time of treatment, in structuring the policy and environment before the treatment, and in revising policies based on experiences. The time-sensitive nature and uncertainty in neurotrauma treatments create exceptions to some medical ethics guidelines we use in more elective situations. Further, the centrality of the brain in personality and cognition adds important textures to our ethical considerations. For this chapter, we briefly review a basic ethical framework in which to discuss the variety of standard and special issues faced in treating patients with traumatic brain injury (TBI). In exploring these issues we hope to provide tools for careful consideration of challenging circumstances in patient care. Neurotrauma research ethics will be discussed in detail in the second volume of this set. In this chapter, we will simply mention some of the research challenges. The framework for clinical ethics and neurotrauma discussed below are intended to help guide clinicians in their practice as well as to alert them of the need for occasional ethical assistance from an ethics committee or a clinical ethicist.

Clinical Ethics: The Basics

Clinical ethics becomes an issue when a necessary value loss occurs based on the treatment decision. These are dilemmas where, to some degree, one important value must be sacrificed to preserve another important value. The most troubling cases are those where reasonable people could choose to weigh values differently such that more than one course of action may be ethically permissible. However, viable solutions always must fall into an ethically permissible range for them to be acceptable. Often, this range includes those actions that are also legally permissible. There are scenarios with absolute wrong answers and absolute right answers: these situations do not need careful analysis. Because we (doctors, nurses, patients, and families) interact with one another in a community, there must be ways of discussing and justifying to one another our controversial or troubling actions. All situations are neither totally relative nor totally absolute; however, we do need ways of communicating why some course of action is ethically permissible or ethically preferable over other courses of action.

Take the scenario of a patient arriving at your emergency room (ER) with a large iron rod piercing through his frontal lobes. He is awake and communicating. The patient says to the ER physician that he does not want to have the rod removed because he knows of a historical character, Phineus Gage, who had this type of injury.[1] Since Phineus Gage's life "turned out rotten" because of his frontal lobe damage, your patient believes his life also will be rotten if he survives. As a matter of quality of life, he does not wish to have the rod removed. Further, your patient proclaims to be a Jehovah's Witness who will not accept any blood products. Finally, he threatens that if anyone attempts to prepare him for the removal of the metal bar, he will do physical harm to that person. Now, there are many values at stake in this short hypothetical description. You value allowing patients to make their own decisions. You value respecting a patient's core beliefs. You value saving this patient's life. You value reducing this patient's suffering. You value your own safety. Finally, you value providing a standard of care for this patient, which would be to remove the metal bar and transfuse him if necessary. In **Table 23.1**, we have outlined this set of values that are at play for both the physician and the patient in this type of situation.

In an ideal scenario, we would be able to preserve all values at stake. However, given the current limitations and facts of the case, something must be lost to maximize the outcome. Possible solutions include ignoring

Table 23.1 Values in the Phineus Gage Patient

Value	Patient	Physician
Life saving		X
Quality of life (short-term suffering)		X
Quality of life (no executive impairment)	X	
No blood (religious)	X	
Professional standards		X
Personal safety		X
Patient autonomy (consent)	X	X

Table 23.2 Loss and Preservation of Values in Treatment Options

Value	Follow Patient	Ignore Patient	Best Interest/No Transfusion
Life saving	–	+	+
Quality of life (short–term suffering)	+	–	+
Quality of life (no executive impairment)	+	–	–
No blood (religious)	+	–	+
Professional standards	–	+	+
Personal safety	+	–	–
Patient autonomy (consent)	+	–	+/–

the patient by acting in his "best" interest by removing the rod and transfusing if necessary. Or, another solution would be to follow the patient's articulation of wishes very literally by not providing any treatment. As always, there may be several intermediate positions one could take between these polar extremes that would provide a better solution. For instance, one could respect the patient's wish not to have blood products, but believe he currently does not have decision-making capacity with respect to the removal of the metal rod. On this last balance, a surgeon could believe it justifiable to remove the rod, but not give blood products. We have given a brief summary of these three options with some of the values gained and lost in **Table 23.2**. As we can see from the last entry in **Table 23.2**, some values may be partially lost and preserved at the same time. One could argue that the patient has a longstanding overriding religious belief about not accepting blood products that is well considered and should be respected, while still arguing that the patient's belief about the removal of the metal rod is transitory and impaired by his injury. In this way, you would respect his autonomous choice about blood products, but not about the rod removal because other values override this weaker belief. This is a very tricky ground to navigate because it can quickly lead to an undesirable overemphasis on physician paternalism in decision making.

There is no absolute way to calculate the best action. However, there needs to be at least an explicit justification why one would preserve one set of values at the expense of another. In this vein, **Table 23.2** is provided as a guide to the type of explicit choices that must be made in challenging clinical situations. It is not intended to be a simple arithmetic calculation where each value is assigned a positive or negative point depending on the column, with the most positive choice being the most ethically permissible. That type of enumeration does not work in this scenario because each of our values has a significantly different weight. For instance, the saving of someone's life generally has greater importance than putting one's safety at a very small risk because of a vague threat. Although no one expects physicians to sit down and write out a table of values at the time of assessing a trauma case, when a particularly ethically complex case arises there is an expectation that a moment of consideration will be given as to the best path. This could be thought of as yet another step in reducing errors, although this is an error of a different kind than those usually discussed as medical errors. By taking a breath and considering what value is being given up and gained globally by any of several paths, we can facilitate good decision making and as a corollary provide clear documentation. In challenging cases that are not particularly time sensitive, it might be helpful to seek the advice of a colleague or someone who is trained in ethics. Almost every hospital has a clinical ethics consultation service available either for advice at the time of a case or to retrospectively review a case to assist in improving processes. These consultation services are usually provided through a hospital ethics committee.

If a more structured way of discussing problems is desired, we could use a classical method of four ethical principles. This is a tool for enumerating important aspects of ethically troubling cases that is commonly taught in all medical schools in the United States. The four principles as proposed by Tom Beauchamp and James Childress are beneficence, nonmaleficence (do no harm), justice, and respect for autonomy (**Table 23.3**).[2] These categories

Table 23.3 Ethical Principles and Guidelines for Protection of Human Subjects in a Research Study

One method for weighing difficult challenges is to evaluate the challenges in these four categories:

- Beneficence (benefit patient)
- Nonmaleficence (do no harm)
- Justice
- Respect for autonomy

Find the solution that best balances these categories given patient values and medical standards were adapted from a foundational research ethics document entitled the Belmont Report.[3] Simply, when faced with an ethical dilemma this system requires an analysis of how each of the four principles could be applied to the case. Although traditionally we think of ethical dilemmas occurring when these four principles come into conflict with one another, they can also contain conflicts within the categories. For instance, a respect for autonomy of the patient may conflict with a respect for autonomy of the physician to make a moral judgment. Alternatively, a respect for autonomy of the Phineus Gage–like patient may ignore a short-term goal in favor of preserving a long-term goal. This system can be a very useful shorthand tool for quickly articulating ethical challenges. However, it is only one among many ways of approaching the value conflicts.

Independent of the way in which values are enumerated, articulated, and balanced, informed consent has become a central element of contemporary medical ethics. Informed consent has its foundation in the belief that respecting autonomy means that the patient is in the best position to balance risks for any particular therapeutic choice (benefit and harm). Further, it finds a foundation in a belief that informed consent propagates a good therapeutic relationship through trust and transparency (justice). The traditional criteria for informed consent require that a patient be given all relevant information, understand the given information, appreciate the ramifications of the decision, and decide voluntarily on a course of treatment (**Table 23.4**). The relevant information involves what a "reasonable person" would want to know about the risks and benefits. How to measure or judge whether a patient really understands the information and can appreciate the consequences is very difficult. Even patients who are globally competent may not have the appropriate capacity to give informed consent for a particularly complex medical decision. Informed consent presents special challenges in neurotrauma given that many injuries induce alterations in cognition. Although there are many tools that have recently been developed to address whether a patient has the capacity to give consent, they are often time consuming and untested for neurotrauma patients.[4] In general, it is the professional judgment of the attending physician as to whether a patient has the capacity to consent to any particular treatment.

Table 23.4 Conditions for Informed Consent

Good informed consent entails
• All relevant information provided
• Patient understands information
• Patient appreciates ramifications
• Patient voluntarily agrees
Collaborative process that includes expert advice from physician

Informed consent is not a document or a single conversation. Rather, it is a process in which continuous patient participation should be elicited. Because a patient's capacity to consent may fluctuate during the entire treatment process, periodic reevaluation of the treatment course and patient's participation may be necessary. When it is not reasonably possible to attain informed consent from a patient, then an advance directive is consulted, a surrogate decision maker is relied upon, or a physician decides on treatment options. Because it is common in neurotrauma for a patient to lack decision-making capacity, we will further discuss this topic later in this chapter. Under special circumstances, informed consent may be overridden. Usually, this is referred to as a therapeutic privilege being exerted by the clinician in the rare circumstances that a course of action is obligatory because of fiduciary duty. There is considerable debate concerning whether iatrogenic complications compose a special class of such cases.[5]

Before proceeding to the particular challenges of ethics in neurotrauma treatment, we must briefly discuss futility, withdrawing treatment, and withholding treatment. The most important part of any futility discussion concerns the ends to which something is futile. For instance, a cranial decompression may be futile to the end of preserving life or futile to the end of preserving a certain level of quality of life. In one case you could argue that the intervention is physiologically futile because the increased intracranial pressure has already caused a herniation and the relief of this pressure will have no medical benefit. In the second invocation of futility there may be a medical effect, but that effect will be futile toward reaching an intended goal. This second use of *futile* is the most controversial one because it explicitly makes a value judgment about which kinds of lives are worth living. In general, we leave judgment about goals to the patient. The medical community plays a role in giving judgments about whether the proposed therapies have a reasonable chance of attaining those goals. These judgments, whether at the bedside, in a courtroom, or during a media interview, should be given on the basis of best scientific/medical knowledge and not be based upon ideology or politics.[6] If a physician finds that a patient's goals are incompatible with the physician's conscience, then the physician has an obligation to transfer the patient to another physician, rather than unreasonably obstructing the treatment. In these cases there is a fine line between holding true to a personal/professional standard and abandoning a patient. Physicians remain moral agents who must preserve the integrity of their fundamental values, while respecting patient values that significantly vary from their own. Again, when a violation of either physician or patient values must occur, then consultation with an ethics service to be of particular use in the guiding process. Futility cases are instances in which ethics committees can be of particular assistance.

There has been considerable discussion of whether withholding and withdrawing life-sustaining treatments are morally equivalent actions. Philosophically it is a relatively settled answer in that there is no moral distinction between not starting a therapy or later taking it away as long as the condition of the patient is similar at both times.[7,8] However, viscerally and psychologically these actions feel very different to the physician actually withdrawing or withholding a therapy. For instance, to allow intraventricular pressures to rise and not to do a ventriculostomy appears very different than undoing a ventriculostomy after successfully controlling intracranial pressures. In general, there is a greater hesitancy about actively taking away a therapy than in not initially introducing it. In both cases, the action, by either commission or omission, will result in the patient's death despite the availability of possible effective therapy. This is not to say that it is always morally right to either withhold or withdraw therapy. Simply, if you are willing to do one in a given circumstance, then you should be willing to do the other in similar circumstances.

In neurotrauma, there actually may be a stronger obligation to initiate therapy to preserve the choices of the patient than withholding the therapy and closing off those possibilities. In those cases where significant uncertainty about the range of outcomes exists, a more conservative approach is to act in a way to preserve function and life. However, in attaining consent to initiate a therapy there needs to be transparency regarding whether the medical team will be willing to withdraw a treatment once it is started. Some patients and families may opt not to start a therapy so that they will not later be embroiled in a battle with medical staff or other family members regarding withdrawing that treatment. The Terri Schiavo case in Florida, which ended in 2005, provides an important insight into the challenges in certain types of withholding and withdrawing of therapy.[5] In the Schiavo case, the family members were at great odds about the removal of a feeding tube in a permanent vegetative state (PVS) patient. Although Ms. Schiavo's ischemic brain injury was not due to trauma, the case provides an important warning about the challenges that can arise in difficult brain injury cases where initial therapeutic choices have long-term implications.

Curing or Palliating: Broad Issues in Neurotrauma

Now that we have discussed clinical ethics issues in general, let us turn our attention to selected topics of particular relevance to neurotrauma. Specifically, we will discuss quality of life, triaging, proxy decision making, advanced directives, and do not resuscitate (DNR) orders. Although many of these issues arise most prominently in the acute phases of injury, they have significant implications for later treatment.

The decisions made at the time of initial treatment narrow the ethically permissible actions later in the course of care. As discussed previously, withdrawing and withholding are thought to be morally equivalent when patients' conditions are similar. However, this becomes a trickier concept when an intervention is successful and a patient regains some function but not enough for a good-quality outcome. For example, a patient with severe intracerebral hemorrhage may have a devastating cognitive prognosis and may need to be placed on a ventilator. During the time the patient needs a ventilator, one could argue that ventilator removal would be equivalent to not having implemented the therapy in the first place. However, at the point that the patient begins to breathe on his own, a "window of opportunity" may have been lost for the avoidance of living a certain type of life. Simply, we are relatively comfortable with allowing a disease process to take a natural course toward death. We are not comfortable with anything that will actively shorten a patient's life in ways unrelated to the disease course, i.e., euthanasia. At times this distinction can be unclear, but it remains an important political and ethical boundary. To not provide ventilation for a patient who is unable to breathe because of neurotrauma is very different ethically than later giving that patient a lethal dose of medication. Although the results may be similar, the process is deemed to be ethically problematic. The particular values given up through actively shortening life are too great to sustain good medical practice. A major value at stake in this discussion is the trust needed by the medical profession to maximize the goods that can be done. To maintain public and patient trust, physicians need to avoid any suggestion that they are willing to cross the boundary between killing a patient and letting a patient die. The many ethical arguments within the question of euthanasia cannot be addressed in the space provided in this chapter. Simply, a therapy can be withdrawn ethically when the prognosis is grim and unacceptable to the patient, but the process of dying cannot be actively helped along through the administration of therapies unrelated to the disease process.

A second interesting question arises in the justice of limited resources. Any physician can directly care for one patient at a time. When faced with multiple patients all vying for the same operating room and surgeon, how does one go about prioritizing who ought to be treated first? Although this might seem like an easy task, a great deal hinges on what one considers to be fair and just. There are significant disaster scenarios where triaging becomes very

Table 23.5 Ideas of Justice and Implication to Triage

Justice	Implication to Triage
Most in need	The sickest person treated first independent of diminishing possibility of success
Most likely to benefit	Treat those with most time-sensitive treatments
Most likely to benefit system	Person with most influence, money, or skills is treated first
Minimize suffering	Treat those experiencing the greatest pain
Everyone has equal chance	Treat patients in the order they arrive or by lottery (avoidance of judgment)

real. Consider the various understandings of justice outlined in **Table 23.5**. Depending on which ideal of justice one applies, one may first treat the sickest, the most likely to survive, or the wealthiest. Our idea of fairness is more than a theoretical construct. It has significant utility in making triage judgment in all cases. That we should act consistently is a general ethical tenet that applies equally to triage as to other medical care. Our ideas of fairness should be reflected in our general practice and procedures that we develop in anticipation of disaster situations. Part of this philosophy becomes clear in societal choices regarding funding levels for neurotrauma. If society truly values the lives of the relatively young population most affected by neurotrauma, then resources should be put in place to avoid the general need for significant triage of cases. This final issue is an ethical issue of policy and politics that may not be in the control of the individual surgeon. However, the politics may create circumstances in which the surgeon is forced to make difficult decisions about which patient to treat. The surgeon has a moral obligation to advocate change of the system so as to avoid the situation and to initiate processes for deciding between cases in a suboptimal system.

As previously discussed, ideal medical decision making involves a patient making his or her own decisions regarding health care values in treatments. Often with neurological injuries, patients are unable to make complex health care decisions themselves. Health care providers must call upon surrogate decision makers to give consent or permission to proceed with a particular health care treatment. Any person taking on a surrogate role, whether as a health care proxy, family member, or physician, is expected to set aside personal preferences and to articulate choices the patient would have made. There are at least three standards for surrogate decision making: substituted judgment, best interest, and reasonable treatment.[9] These are summarized in **Table 23.6**. The generally preferred method, substituted judgment, requires the surrogate to communicate how the patient would choose in such a situation, even if it is contrary to the surrogate's wishes or benefit. In this standard, the surrogate brings to bear all past knowledge about the patient to make a health care choice. This knowledge should include any previous conversations with the patient explicitly about health care choices. If the surrogate knows nothing about the patient's explicit health care preferences, then the surrogate is expected to use a best interest standard. In this standard, the surrogate uses all that is known about what the patient found important in life to predict how the patient would make these particular decisions. In this model, the surrogate attempts to preserve those values that most significantly structure the patient's life. Finally, if there is little known about a patient's values and goals, then a reasonable treatment standard would be used. In this the surrogate attempts to decide what a reasonable person would expect to have done. Often, this last standard results in a conservative approach that favors preservation of function and life. There are times when the reasonable treatment standard will result in decisions toward palliation in cases of extreme suffering or a devastating prognosis. In general, a surrogate should not be asked what he or she wants, but rather what the patient would have wanted. When decisions are to be made for a patient who is decisionally incapacitated, we must be

Table 23.6 Proxy Decision-Making Models

Model	Strengths	Weaknesses	When to Apply
Substituted judgment	Most direct expression of patient	Prior wishes about a therapy may not be relevant to current context	Patient wishes known
Best interest	Respect for the unique individual	Difficult to apply to individual therapeutic choices	Patient values known
Reasonable treatment	Often based on standard practices	Does not account well for individual desires and goals	Little known of patient's values and wishes

clear concerning which model is to be used. Finally, the surrogate should only be given choices that will actually be undertaken. If a therapy is deemed inappropriate for the patient, then it should not be offered as a real option.

Advance Directives and Do Not Resuscitate Orders

In trauma treatment, the issue of advance directives documents and DNR orders can be particularly challenging and have significant influence on whether a patient lives or dies. Advance directives are a way in which patients document their health care wishes prior to becoming decisionally incapacitated. These directives are premised on valuing patient participation in decision making and the importance of autonomous choice. Two types of documents, the living will and the health care proxy, are available for patients to complete in case they become decisionally incapacitated. The living will usually take effect when a patient can no longer make health care decisions for him- or herself and is in a terminal condition or a permanent vegetative state. These documents specify what kind of treatment a patient in such a condition will accept and what kind he or she will not. Generally, patients in the hope of avoiding futile artificial life support measures complete these documents.

The health care proxy document, sometimes called a durable power for health care, names a surrogate decision maker for when a patient is decisionally incapacitated. It is expected that the health care proxy has been informed by the patient of his or her values and wishes concerning treatment options. The named proxy is expected to use the substituted judgment model as outlined above. Considerable debate continues concerning the usefulness and ethical appropriateness of advance directives.[10,11] In particular, it is difficult to prospectively anticipate the decisions that will be needed in any particular trauma scenario. Although these documents may work well for a progressive disease like cancer or amyotrophic lateral sclerosis, trauma cases are so varied and have such great uncertainty that it would be impractical to attempt specification of treatment wishes that would apply to all possible instances. These documents can be useful in guiding discussions with families and health care providers in most circumstances. They give a window into patient values.

It needs to be emphasized that advance directives are not DNR orders (**Table 23.7**) Advance directives are expressions of patient wishes. DNR is a physician order. When a patient is admitted with an advance directive, it is up to the treating team to decide which specific therapies are appropriate for treatment in the context of the advance directive (if the patient lacks decision-making capacity). A DNR order is a written physician order which specifies that under particular circumstances resuscitative measures should not be undertaken. The DNR should be treated with the same respect as any other physician order on the patient's medical chart. This distinction is fundamentally important in treating patients in an ethical manner.

Further, a DNR order does not necessarily mean that a patient has decided on comfort or palliative care only. Some patients opt for aggressive treatment while still having a DNR order to cover scenarios where they actually have cardiac and/or pulmonary arrest. This point is particularly important for trauma. Just because a patient has a DNR order written prior to the trauma does not mean that aggressive surgery should be withheld. The DNR simply means that the medical team, if time permits, should discover why the DNR order was written and how any further interventions might fit with a patient's overall health care plan. When there is any question about the relevance of the order to the particular situation, the safest path is to

Table 23.7 Distinctions between Advance Directives and Do Not Resuscitate Orders

- Advanced directives *are not* physician orders, but express the patient's wishes about resuscitative measures.
- Living wills occasionally will specify a patient's desire for aggressive resuscitation to always be attempted.
- DNR orders are physician orders reflecting patient values and standards of medical treatment related to whether (and which) resuscitative measures should be undertaken in the case of cardiac arrest.
- Patients cannot demand physicians attempt resuscitation if it is judged to be outside proper medical practice.
- A DNR order does not necessarily exclude the possibility of aggressive treatment because it only applies to resuscitation. Separate orders cover all other treatments.

	Lack Decision Making	Terminal/PVS	Physician Order
Living will	X	X	
Health care proxy	X	?	
Do not resuscitate		?	X

Abbreviations: DNR, do not resuscitate; PVS, permanent vegetative state.

treat first and gain clarity as soon as possible. Once there is reasonable clarity that a DNR order continues to be consistent with the situation, then all unwanted therapy should be withheld and withdrawn. Again, this becomes difficult when an iatrogenic event occurs.[12]

Given that trauma comes unexpectedly and may have interventions that are needed in a transitory manner, it often calls into question the relevance of advance directives and preexisting DNR orders in general. As an ethical principle we must not assume too much when faced with these documents. Unreflectively following documents may create instances of self-fulfilling prophecies. Many ventilator-dependent patients become terminal with the withdrawal of a ventilator who otherwise could have recovered if they had remained on a ventilator for a longer time. One must be very careful in a judgment about what constitutes a terminal condition. It is an open question as to whether a terminal patient is one who will die in the near term despite aggressive therapy or one who will die in the near term if aggressive therapy is not chosen. Therefore, withdrawal of therapies such as ventilators must be done with a great deal of attention to justice and ethics.[13]

Special Ethical Issues in Neurotrauma

Several instances in neurotrauma have special ethical issues and concerns that are worth mentioning briefly. Below we will raise the three primary issues of pregnancy, pediatrics, and neurological criteria for death. Each topic increases the ethical complexity of cases.

Pregnant Patients

A pregnant patient with a brain injury is in a unique clinical situation because there are more vested interests than her own body. As the fetus develops toward viability, the obligations of a mother-to-be increase and the ethical pull of fathers becomes more relevant. A patient could reasonably choose to risk her own function and health for the health of her unborn child. The ethics get even trickier if a pregnant patient does not have decision-making capacity and needs surgery for functional preservation that at the same time will put her unborn child at risk. Often the next of kin decision maker for such a patient is a husband or the father to be. The husband may have conflicting interests depending on the circumstances. Although some cultures will always act in favor of preserving the life and function of the pregnant woman over the unborn child, it is not unreasonable that decisions may be made to maximize the health of the unborn child. This does not only apply to the potential for curative surgery, it also may apply to choices about withdrawing life support. At the extreme is the case of Susan Torres who in 2005, despite severe brain damage due to an advanced tumor, was kept alive in a coma long enough to gestate her 6-month fetus to viability. Ms. Torres's husband consented to have advance life-support continued while the mother was in a coma progressing toward neurological criteria for death, for the sole purpose of birthing the baby. After the birth, the ventilator was disconnected. One could argue that the mother was being used as a means only. Whenever decisions are being made regarding a pregnant patient, extra care needs to be taken regarding which interests and values are being preserved and the potential conflicts that arise.

Pediatric Patients

Pediatric patients pose special ethical challenges because of physiological differences as well as challenges in obtaining consent. Younger children's brains behave differently than adults. For instance, greater plasticity is seen in younger children in their recovery from neurological injury. This makes prognosis particularly uncertain and complicated. Further, children have not yet had the opportunity to develop their own preferences and robust values. Hence, the decision-making model of substituted judgment cannot be applied in such cases. We rely on the parents to give permission for treatment and on physicians to protect children from undue burdens placed by parents. For instance, a 10-year-old would be given lifesaving blood products even if his family were Jehovah's Witness and were against the procedure. Although there may be a loss of valued trust, a lack of respect for the value of family autonomy and religious beliefs, this is justified because we value preserving children's future ability to make their own decisions based on their own values. On the opposite end of the spectrum, children may need protection from overly aggressive treatment that moves toward futility. Also, any time that the child's injuries could reasonably be due to abuse, physicians more strongly play the role of protector of the patient. Finally, the adolescent female trauma surgery case may become particularly sensitive if the patient tests positive for pregnancy. Again, in treating pediatric cases we need to prospectively be aware of the various ethical challenges posed by this segment of the population.

Neurological Criteria for Brain Death and Declaring Brain Death

A patient with severe brain injury may progress to death while being on advanced life support. Neurological criteria for death, formally referred to as brain death, can be

Table 23.8 Criteria for Brain Death

- Neurological criteria for death include
  - Coma or complete unresponsiveness
  - Absence of cerebral and brain stem function
  - Absence of spontaneous breathing
- Declaration of death by neurological criteria is important in scenarios of appropriate allocation of health care resources, organ donation, and societal concerns
- Organ donation potentially complicates the declaration of death because of the implied conflict of interest between the patient's family and the potential recipient of the organ

Source: Wijdicks EM. The diagnosis of brain death. N Engl J Med. 2001; 344:1215–1221

used to pronounce a patient dead even when the body continues to be oxygenated by ventilators and other artificial means. The neurological criteria for death are the complete and irreversible cessation of all brain activity, including a lack of spontaneous respiration owing to irreversible brain damage. The three essential findings for death by neurological criteria are coma, absence of brain stem reflexes, and absence of spontaneous breathing (**Table 23.8**). The judgment of irreversibility of cessation of all brain function is difficult because we must rely on inductive assumptions based on past experiences that certain injuries will not spontaneously heal. As dead patients continue to be perfused by artificial means, they remain warm and lifelike. There may be great confusion and misunderstandings from families about these patients actually being dead. This confusion is shared by many physicians, including neurointensivists.[14]

Several ethical issues arise surrounding this methodology of declaring death related to organ transplantation and religious/cultural clashes. Several cultures and religions do not accept neurological criteria as validly indicating death. These traditions generally rely on a cardiopulmonary cessation as the standard for indicating death. Examples of these views can be found in Japanese and Indian cultures as well as in Orthodox Judaism.

The declaration of death by neurological criteria becomes important for at least two resource issues. First, continuing to perfuse a dead body is a poor use of health care resources and a poor use of medical expertise. However, given that we spend excessive amounts of resources on less serious and sacred matters, this value should not be the only argument for insisting on applying neurological criteria for death. The more compelling issue is that candidates to donate lifesaving organs are generally those who are pronounced dead using these neurological criteria. We have a particularly important use and need of body parts to help those with failing organs. The status is somewhat unclear regarding who controls the body parts of a dead person. Some societies, such as those in Belgium presume that dead people's organs should be distributed to others who are sick. The law of the land presumes consent for the use of these organs. Other societies believe that citizens can irrevocably agree to donate organs in advance. The state of Pennsylvania aggressively harvests organs, independent of family member wishes, from those who advance-sign donor cards. Most commonly, decisions concerning whether to donate organs or not are left to families of the deceased patients. The actual conversation regarding the donation of organs should be left to those trained in approaching this topic.

One reluctance of patients toward donating organs stems from a fear of premature declaration of death so that organ harvesting can occur. This classic conflict of interest scenario should be avoided. Although the treating physician of a patient may have the closest relationship with the family, the treating physician generally should not initiate a discussion of organ donation. The decisions about patient care, which includes declaring the patient dead, need to be undertaken by a medical team primarily interested in the patient's well-being. Similarly, the discontinuation of therapies that might lead to a patient progressing to fill the neurological criteria for death should be made on the basis of patient care. There is a very tricky overlap here when the patient has expressed a strong desire to be an organ donor and treatment options may be different depending on whether preserving organs or life are in the balance.

Conclusion

In this chapter, we have discussed the important need to consider carefully what types of values may be lost and those gained in challenging situations. That a therapy can be physiologically successful does not necessarily mean that it will be successful in achieving the patient's articulated goals. The surgeon must respect the autonomy of patients, but he or she also has an obligation to act in the patient's best interest. Brain trauma poses many interesting and difficult situations where treatment decisions must be made with a limited knowledge about the likely outcomes and the values of the patient. It is our obligation to prospectively consider which of them are the most important values to preserve and how to respect the value judgments of others. These initial treatment choices become increasingly complex when combined with research, innovation, and long-term care.

References

1. Harlow JM. Recovery from the passage of an iron bar through the head. Boston Medical and Surgical Journal. 1848;39:389–392
2. Beauchamp TL, Childress JF. Principles of biomedical ethics. 5th ed. New York: Oxford University Press; 2001
3. The Belmont Report. Ethical Principles and Guidelines for the Protection of Human Subjects or Research. Report of the National Commission for the Protection of Human Subjects of Biomedical and Behavioral Research. Washington, DC: U.S. Department of Health, Education and Welfare; 1979
4. Dunn LB, Nowrangi MA, Palmer BW, Jeste DV, Saks ER. Assessing decisional capacity for clinical research or treatment: a review of instruments. Am J Psychiatry 2006;163:1323–1334
5. Casarett D, Ross LF. Overriding a patient's refusal of treatment after an iatrogenic complication. N Engl J Med 1997;336(26):1908–1910
6. Cranford R. Facts, lies, and videotapes: the permanent vegetative state and the sad case of Terri Schiavo. J Law Med Ethics 2005;33(2): 363–371
7. Rachels J. Active and passive euthanasia. N Engl J Med 1975;292:78–80
8. Thomson JJ. Killing, letting die, and the trolley problem. Monist 1976;59:204–217
9. Devettere RJ. Deciding for others. In: Practical Decision Making in Health Care Ethics. 2nd ed. Washington, DC: Georgetown University Press; 2000:127–161
10. Fagerlin A, Schneider CE. Enough. The failure of the living will. Hastings Cent Rep 2004;34(2):30–42
11. Tulsky JA. Beyond advance directives: importance of communication skills at the end of life. JAMA 2005;294(3):359–365
12. Christensen JA, Orlowski JP. Iatrogenic cardiopulmonary arrests in DNR patients. J Clin Ethics 2000;11(1):14–20
13. Toms SA. Outcome predictors in the early withdrawal of life support: issues of justice and allocation for the severely brain injured. J Clin Ethics 1993;4:206–211
14. Boissy AR, Provencio JJ, Smith CA, Diringer MN. Neurointensivists' opinions about death by neurological criteria and organ donation. Neurocrit Care 2005;3:115–121

24 Medicolegal Issues

Frederick Levy and Nisha C. Wagle

Unfortunately, like all physicians in today's litigious climate, neurosurgeons must be aware of some complex legal rules that have developed over recent years. The most important is the comprehensive, yet confusing federal law known as the Emergency Medical Treatment and Labor Act (EMTALA). However, even if they are in full compliance with EMTALA, neurosurgeons may still be faced with traditional state malpractice suits.

EMTALA is a broad and sweeping law that has evolved to encompass many aspects of a physician's practice. However, the issue that is of greatest concern to most neurosurgeons is how EMTALA applies to the following controversial issue:

What *exactly* are the on-call obligations of the neurosurgeon responding to the emergency department (ED) consult call?

When patients with traumatic brain injury (TBI) present to a local ED or are transferred from that ED to a tertiary hospital, EMTALA governs the duties of the neurosurgeon's on-call response to the ED. Unfortunately, most neurosurgeons have limited knowledge of EMTALA, which makes the controversy even more difficult to resolve. The case that follows is illustrative of this major problem facing neurosurgeons today.

The Case

In 1985, Eugene "Red" Barnes came out of an abandoned "crack house" with a stab wound to his head and collapsed in front of bystanders. When he arrived at the local hospital, the emergency physician examined him and called the on-call neurosurgeon, but the neurosurgeon refused to consult on the patient. The emergency physician called another neurosurgeon who was not on call; he also refused to care for the patient at the receiving hospital unless the emergency physician performed burr holes in the patient in the ED. A third hospital finally agreed to accept the patient, but care was ultimately delayed. Even with surgery, the patient died 3 days later.[1]

The History and Definition of the Emergency Medical Treatment and Labor Act

The History

In 1986, Congress enacted EMTALA to ensure public access to emergency services regardless of ability to pay. This was not Congress's first attempt to deal with this issue. Forty years prior to the enactment of EMTALA, Congress made its first attempt to deal with this problem. It did so by enacting the Hill–Burton Act (HBA), which was only partially successful. In return for federal loans and grant guarantees, HBA required hospitals to provide care free, or at reduced cost, to indigent patients.[2] Even with this act, unstable patients were still being transferred to other facilities based on a lack of insurance. Ultimately, HBA amounted to a set of guidelines and was not able to enforce the proscription of the "dumping" of uninsured patients.

The combination of press reports, the obvious ineffectiveness of HBA, and the increasing presence of the federal government in all things health care related, led to the ultimate enactment of EMTALA. Congressman Pete Stark of California, one of the leading proponents of EMTALA said, "(p)atient dumping is but a symptom of a much larger problem. Thirty-seven million Americans are without health insurance."[3] Because of the increasing number of reports that EDs were refusing to accept or treat patients who did not have insurance, Congress passed EMTALA.[4]

The tipping point occurred with two highly publicized reports detailing the extent of patient dumping in the Chicago area. In these reports, the authors first defined patient dumping as "the denial of, or limitation in, the provision of medical services to a patient for economic reasons and the referral of that patient elsewhere."[5,6,50] In one study, 87% of transfers by the sending hospital were due to a lack of insurance. These studies also reported that nearly a quarter of the patients that were transferred were unstable at the time of transfer. Additionally, these patients were twice as likely to die compared with those who were treated at the transferring hospital. This practice was not limited to the Chicago area, but extended to public hospitals in most large cities.[6]

EMTALA was finally passed in 1986 as part of the Consolidated Omnibus Budget Reconciliation Act of 1985 (COBRA). COBRA dealt entirely with Medicare issues and EMTALA was added almost as an afterthought. Although EMTALA was originally only four pages in length, it created a storm of controversy over the ensuing 2 decades. Even though the initial language covered the care of emergency medical conditions (EMCs), interpretations from the Center for Medicare Services (CMS) as well as various court decisions, EMTALA now applies to potentially all aspects of patient care in the *hospital* setting.

All physicians on the hospital staff, including neurosurgeons, need to be familiar with EMTALA's general requirements. The law and the subsequent final status regulations passed in 2003 include discussions of on-call physicians' responsibilities under EMTALA, penalties, and enforcement procedures. It also applies to any member of the hospital staff who admits or discharges patients from the hospital.[7]

The Definition

The Basic Principles of EMTALA

Before examining the details of EMTALA and the clarifying regulations, it is worthwhile exploring some of the basic principles that are critical in gaining a deeper understanding of this complex Act (**Table 24.1**). One of the key elements that must be satisfied to come into compliance with EMTALA is the notion of giving all patients that request an examination or treatment a screening examination to rule out an EMC.

If an EMC exists, the transferring hospital must stabilize the patient before transfer. This is not limited only to diagnostic testing, but may include subspecialty consultation. If the patient is unstable, then the benefits of transfer to the accepting hospital must exceed the risks of remaining at the sending facility. This must all be clearly documented in the medical record, including a discussion with the physician in charge of accepting patient transfers.

Another principle mandated by EMTALA is that any participating Medicare hospital that has specialized capabilities or facilities shall not refuse to accept an appropriate transfer if the hospital has the capacity to treat the individual. This section of EMTALA has come to be known as the "reverse dumping" part of the statute. It prevents the specialized accepting hospital from rejecting transfers based on their inability to pay for services.

This reverse dumping provision only applies to the accepting hospital. If the receiving facility feels that the transfer is inappropriate, they should accept the patient anyway and investigate the appropriateness of the transfer at a later date. The only exception to this principle of mandatory acceptance is if the hospital is full to capacity or if, for whatever reason, the on-call specialty physician is not available to care for the patient.

Table 24.1 Basic Principles of the Emergency Medical Treatment and Active Labor Act (EMTALA)

Medical screening examination (MSE)	Given to all those patients that request an MSE
	Purpose: Rule out emergency medical condition
	Includes ancillary services
	Cannot delay for inquiry into insurance status
	Continue until emergency excluded or stabilized
Emergency medical condition	Severe condition that without immediate medical attention places patient health in jeopardy
Appropriate transfer	Legal if patient cannot be stabilized
	Several criteria must be met:
	• Sending hospital has provided its best care
	• Benefits of transfer outweigh risks
	• Accepting hospital agrees to accept patient
	• Transfer with qualified personnel and equipment
Stable patients	Once patient stabilized EMTALA does not apply
	No obligation for transferring or receiving hospital

With respect to on-call specialists, physicians must realize that they are not just on call for their practice but on call for the hospital. Therefore, they are legally acting on behalf of the hospital. In exchange for hospital privileges, they must agree to take a certain amount of on-call responsibility, the details of which are confusing but somewhat clarified by the new regulations set forth in 2003.

Review of the basics of EMTALA is inadequate to fully appreciate the scope and reach of the law. On-call physicians, including neurosurgeons, should be aware of the details of EMTALA even though many of these details apply primarily to ED physicians.

The Details

Medical Screening Examination

The exact language that defines the medical screening examination (MSE) is clear. An MSE states that "if any individual comes to the ED requesting an exam, the hospital must provide a screening exam within the capabilities of the ED, including ancillary services to determine if an EMC exists."[8] This examination cannot be delayed to inquire about a patient's method of payment or insurance status. However, CMS has determined that it is acceptable to obtain demographic information prior to the MSE as long as this documentation does not delay the MSE.

This screening examination, when it describes ancillary services, is aimed particularly at the more advanced ED diagnostics like a computed tomography (CT) scan or a specialty consultation. The MSE continues until there is a determination that no emergency exists or until the patient has been stabilized. If an emergency condition exists that cannot be stabilized, this triggers the requirement of transfer to a facility that possesses a higher level of care.[9] Exactly what defines an EMC is addressed below.

Emergency Medical Condition

The law defines an EMC differently from the common understanding of that term. Under EMTALA, an EMC is defined as "a condition manifesting itself by acute symptoms of sufficient severity (including pain) that in the absence of immediate medical attention could reasonably be expected to result in placing the patient's health in serious jeopardy."[8] This differs from the commonly understood definition of the term. For example, a sprained ankle or an ear infection may both be characterized as an emergency because they present to the ED, but neither of these would fall under the legal definition as stated above.

Appropriate Transfer

In many cases, a legally appropriate transfer can occur even if the patient cannot be stabilized. However, several criteria must be met. Chief among them is that the sending hospital has treated the patient to the best of its capabilities. Additionally, the medical risks of the transfer are outweighed by the benefits. This risk/benefit notion must be clearly documented in the medical record. Under this scenario, the accepting hospital has agreed to accept the patient in transfer, and copies of the medical records are sent along with the patient. Finally, the transfer must be performed by qualified personnel and transportation equipment as required by the circumstances.[10]

Stable Patients

Once the patient has been stabilized or it has been determined that no EMC exists, EMTALA ceases to apply. Neither the transferring nor receiving hospital has any obligation whatsoever under EMTALA to transfer or accept stable patients. As a matter of fact, either hospital may transfer or accept stable patients for economic reasons, although any patient movement for this reason may be subject to a higher level of scrutiny.[11] In fact, when transferring a stable patient, the government only requires that "no material deterioration of the EMC that has been stabilized is likely, within a reasonable medical probability, to result from this transfer."[12]

It soon became evident that despite the best of intentions, EMTALA was leading to more and more confusion. Accordingly, Congress delegated the CMS, formerly known as the Health Care Financing Administration (HCFA), to define the exact role of subspecialists with regard to taking ED calls.

The 2003 Clarifying Regulations for EMTALA

The Rationale for the Final Clarifying Regulations

As noted earlier, EMTALA was crafted with the best of intentions. However, like many such measures, it soon caused more problems than it solved. Anecdotes describing arbitrary and illogical interpretations of EMTALA, as well as tales of draconian penalties imposed on hospitals and physicians who allegedly violated the law, created so much fear and insecurity that many physicians sought ways to avoid providing emergency care. One of those ways was to avoid taking night call for the hospital.[13]

As a result, there has been considerable friction between on-call physicians and the EDs. Many on-call specialists do not understand the ramifications of EMTALA and feel that they do not have to come in to see a patient at the "whim" of the emergency physician. EMTALA makes the hospital responsible for maintaining daily on-call lists through the hospital's medical bylaws. Generally, any hospital that offers routine surgeries must maintain this list.[9] It has become increasingly difficult, however, for EDs to find specialists who will agree to be on call for the ED. The resulting shortages have had dire and sometimes tragic consequences.[14]

As evidence of this, a California study revealed that neurosurgeons were the fifth least likely subspecialty (22%) to respond to on-call coverage call from the ED. The authors of the study theorized that this relatively poor response to on-call obligations was the insurance status of the patient. The authors concluded that the on-call situation in California had reached crisis proportions.[15]

In addition to the lack of insurance of indigent patients, an additional reason for the unwillingness of the subspecialties to respond to ED call was the lack of available subspecialists. According to the American Hospital Association, there are 5,810 registered hospitals in the United States and only 3,900 practicing neurosurgeons (**Fig. 24.1**). There is a tremendous gap between the number

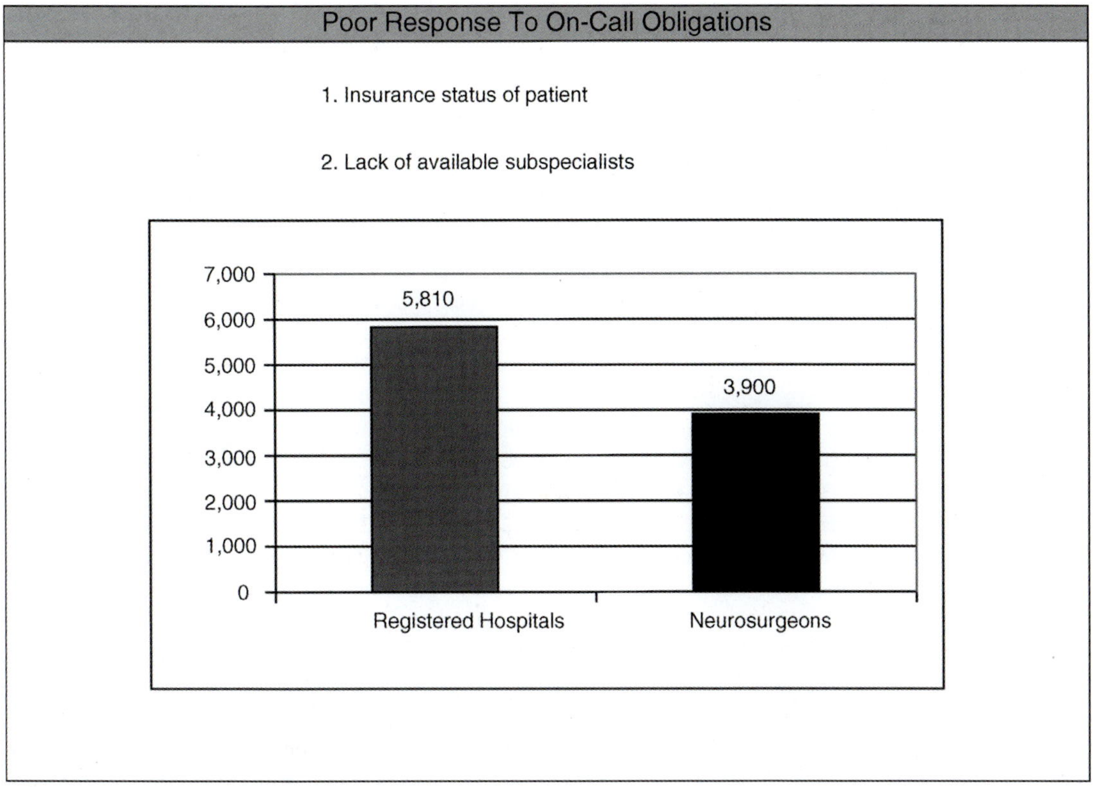

Fig. 24.1 Graph depicting factors responsible for poor response to on-call obligations.

of available neurosurgeons and those hospitals in need of neurosurgical services. This applies to some extent to the other specialties as well.[16] In a national survey conducted by the Office of the Inspector General (OIG) in 2002, neurosurgery ranked number one of all the subspecialty areas facing on-call shortages.[17]

CMS Interpretive Guidelines

After EMTALA was passed in 1986, the growing contentions and confusion among clinicians led to a series of interim regulations by the CMS. In November 2003, CMS promulgated a final set of regulations, which have seemingly relaxed the requirements of the on-call specialties, although several controversies still remain. This is the direct result of the inconsistencies of the federal law and its regulations, and most important, the interpretation of the rules by the CMS whose officers enforce the law.

Hospitals and medical professionals have repeatedly charged that EMTALA obligations are burdensome, complex, and unclear. To help promote its consistent application, in 2003 the CMS published "Clarifying policies related to the responsibilities of Medicare participating hospitals in treating individuals with an EMC" (**Table 24.2**).[18] The most

Table 24.2 Center for Medicare Services (CMS) Interpretive Guidelines: Responsibilities of Medicare Participating Hospitals

Relaxation of on-call requirements for on-call panels	Services only have to match the resources
	Flexibility of no longer requiring 24/7 call coverage
	• "Rule of Three" — if hospital has at least three physicians to take calls, required to provide 24/7 coverage
Local decision	Decide number of physicians needed to fulfill call duty
	Individual hospitals decide what best meets the needs of patients (factoring in resources)
Other circumstances	Beyond control of the physician that prevents prompt response
	• CMS recognizes this (no elaboration)
Simultaneous call and other duties	Acceptable to CMS as long as back-up plan in place
Violation	Any hospital with capacity to treat but refuses to do so
	Penalties: termination of provider agreement or civil monetary fines

relevant change for the neurosurgeon is that the on-call requirements for on-call panels have been relaxed.[19]

The key regulation dealt with the definition of what "best meets the needs of the hospital's patients." The CMS changed its interpretation of this definition to be less restrictive. Rather than mandating a certain number of on-call physicians at all times, this definition requires only that the services match the resources and allows for the flexibility of no longer requiring 24 hours a day, 7 days a week (24/7) call coverage. This was formerly known as "the rule of three"—if the hospital had at least three physicians able to take calls, then the hospital was required to provide 24/7 coverage.[20]

The CMS felt that proscriptive rules should not mandate such matters; rather, that the number of physicians needed to fulfill call duties should be a local decision at the discretion of the individual hospital through coordination of that hospital and its staff of physicians. The new regulation states that "each hospital has the discretion to maintain call lists in a manner that best meets the needs of the hospital's patients which include factoring the resources of the hospital."[21]

The CMS further acknowledged that there may be circumstances beyond a physician's control that may prevent the on-call person from responding promptly to the call. However, the CMS declined to elaborate on those conditions. With respect to simultaneous call and performance of other services while on call, the CMS accepts this practice, provided that the hospital has a back-up plan in place. Furthermore, all hospitals involved must be aware of the on-call situation as each hospital has its own independent EMTALA obligation.[22]

A participating hospital with specialized capabilities that has the capacity to treat those complex patients requiring specialized care but refuses to do so would still be in violation of EMTALA. They could therefore be liable for termination of the provider agreement or civil monetary penalties or both. However, with the new regulations, a closer look reveals that the hospitals' fear of citations and litigation may be overstated. As long as hospitals have proper procedures in place, the new regulations suggest that facilities are not likely to be in violation of EMTALA.[23]

Why On-Call Neurosurgeons Should Be Concerned about EMTALA

Current Level of Neurosurgeons' Awareness of EMTALA

It is hardly surprising that many physicians are either unaware or are incompletely aware that EMTALA even exists. In today's milieu of increasing legal liability, this seems difficult to believe but, in fact, there have been several studies to suggest that this is the case[24, 25]. These studies were retrospective chart reviews and questionnaire type studies and as such, possess the usual limitations inherent to these types of studies. Still, they correlate with what most physicians might believe about true knowledge and understanding of EMTALA. One such study was designed to determine what percentage of the medical staff at a university medical center had ever heard of EMTALA and if so, what was the extent of their knowledge.

The results of this study, as it relates to the knowledge of on-call physician responsibilities, were that only 29.3% had ever heard of EMTALA. There was a significant linear correlation between those that took at least monthly call and knowledge of the law, but even that subset of on-call specialists knew only half of what EMTALA encompassed. The result of this study suggests that hospitals need to better educate their physicians in an effort to reduce liability exposure to EMTALA violations.[24]

A later study confirmed these findings and further suggested that many on-call physicians did not know some of the subtleties of EMTALA's requirements. Additionally, physicians did not know the requirements regarding prompt consultation and the differences between on-campus and off-campus referrals. Although a very small percentage of respondents indicated that they could decline an ED consult while on call (1%), 8% indicated that they could send a resident to the ED and not see the patient themselves. In fact, one-third of the respondents thought that they could see the patient in an off-campus office instead of the ED. An even higher percentage felt that they could delay seeing an ED patient until completing their office hours—averaging delays of up to 4 hours. These findings reflect the state of knowledge at a teaching facility. It should be recognized that the level of knowledge would likely vary at nonteaching hospitals, where the role of attending physicians is different given the lack of in-house residents.[25]

With regard to sending residents to evaluate an ED consult, the wording of EMTALA specifies that the consult attending must see the patient in person. However, informal advice from the CMS suggests that the practice of sending residents to see the ED patient may be acceptable. Although the promulgated 2003 regulations do not address the resident issue, they do expressly state that sending a physician assistant to see the ED patient is acceptable (**Table 24.3**).

The Connection between EMTALA and On-Call Physicians

As previously stated, with the enactment of EMTALA, Congress decreed universal access to hospital services for all. In so doing, EMTALA also forced providers to assume

Table 24.3 Current Level of Neurosurgeons' Awareness about the Emergency Medical Treatment and Active Labor Act (EMTALA)

Either unaware or incompletely aware	In one study, 29.3% of on-call physicians had never heard of EMTALA
	Later study: • Confirmed that many do not know the subtleties of EMTALA requirements • Also unaware of requirements regarding prompt consultation and differences between on-campus and off-campus referrals
	• 1% said they could decline an ED consult while on call
	• 8% said they could send a resident to see the patient instead of themselves
	• 33.3% said they could see patient at off-campus office rather than ED
	• Even higher % said could delay seeing ED patient until office hours complete
EMTALA specifies that	Consult attending must see patient in person
	Sending resident may be acceptable
	Sending physician assistant is acceptable

Abbreviation: ED, emergency department.

fiscal responsibility for care of the poor under threat of civil liability or loss of participation in the Medicare system, largely considered a financial "death sentence" for hospitals and physicians.[26] Hospitals must now be responsible for the actions taken by all of their medical staff. It is their responsibility to ensure that all medical staff is willing to provide on-call services or accept patients in transfer on the hospital's behalf. In essence, EMTALA amounts to an enormous unfunded mandate, which, like numerous laws in the past and present, has many unintended consequences.[27]

At its core, EMTALA requires hospitals that participate in the Medicare program (which amounts to 98% of all hospitals in the United States) to provide a screening examination. It also requires hospitals to provide the necessary stabilizing treatment to persons presenting with emergency medical conditions. A hospital must also accept transfers from other facilities if it has the ability to care for such patients and if the sending hospital declares that it cannot care for them.

Because EMTALA itself does not provide for reimbursement, a physician who is required to provide a patient with emergency treatment will not receive payment for those services. Ironically, this is true even if a patient has insurance because, in a true emergency, there may not be time to obtain preauthorization from the insurance carrier. Waiting for preauthorization is permissible only if it does not delay treatment. If it does delay treatment, it could be inferred that the treatment was delayed for financial reasons, which would subject the hospital and physician to a potential EMTALA violation. Although the number of physicians who have ever been fined for EMTALA violations is quite small, the pervasive fear that "it could happen to me" has made many physicians very cautious about taking ED calls.[13] Yet less than 2% of neurosurgeons report they have been investigated for a violation.[13]

Even with the expansion of EMTALA to include on-call physicians, the Department of Health and Human Services (DHSS) conducted a nationwide survey in 2001 that identified neurosurgery, cardiovascular surgery, pediatrics, orthopedics, obstetrics, neurology, and plastic surgery (in that order) as the most problematic services to respond to ED on-call obligations (**Table 24.4**). Soaring premiums and fear of litigation were identified as the major factors in this survey.[18]

The Obligations of Neurosurgeons under EMTALA

Under EMTALA, a hospital that offers its services for an EMC agrees to maintain a list of on-call physicians who are on duty after the initial examination to provide necessary treatment to stabilize a patient with an EMC. CMS suggests response time to be on the order of 30 minutes although the regulations also permit a "reasonable response time should be addressed in the medical staff bylaws." This roster must be posted in the ED with dated lists with specifics on each of the on-call physicians.[29] This essentially amounts to pro bono health care that is unparalleled in any other profession.

The law specifically holds that the hospital is primarily responsible for coverage; the hospital can force on-call participation by clearly requiring subspecialty calls in the medical staff bylaws and hospital policies. Like other unfunded mandates, there are no specific provisions in the law to fund on-call services. Lack of funding has seriously damaged the infrastructure of specialty backup to the ED. In addition, the lack of payment, lifestyle of nighttime availability, local scarcity, medicolegal risks, and excessive professional demands all play a role in the reluctance to take calls.[30]

What Happens When an EMTALA Violation Occurs

Process

The chance of a neurosurgeon or other specialist unwittingly violating EMTALA is low; nevertheless, the punishment is severe (**Table 24.5**). Typically, the process begins

Table 24.4 The Connection between EMTALA and On Call

EMTALA enacted	Universal access to care for all
	Fiscal responsibility for care of the poor placed on provider
	• Under threat of civil liability or loss of participation in Medicare system—financial "death sentence" for hospitals and physicians
Hospital responsibilities (all Medicare participating institutions = 98% of all U.S. hospitals)	Responsible for actions taken by entire medical staff
	Must provide screening examination
	Necessary stabilizing treatment to those with EMC
	Must accept transfers if it has the ability to care and if sending hospital states it cannot
Payment and care	EMTALA does not provide for reimbursement
	Physician required to provide emergency treatment and will not be compensated for those services
	• Even true if patient has insurance, as there are times physician cannot delay care to obtain preauthorization from carrier
	• Acquiring preauthorization only permissible if it does not delay treatment
	• Delaying treatment for financial reasons places hospital and doctor in violation of EMTALA
	• 2% of neurosurgeons report they have been investigated for violation
ED on-call comparison to other medical fields	Department of Health and Human Services nationwide survey, 2001
	In order of the most problematic to least problematic services to respond to ED on-call obligations:
	1. Neurosurgery
	2. Cardiovascular surgery
	3. Pediatrics
	4. Orthopedics
	5. Obstetrics
	6. Neurology
	7. Plastic surgery
	Reason: Soaring premiums and fear of litigation

Abbreviations: ED, emergency department; EMC, emergency medical condition; EMTALA, the Emergency Medical Treatment and Active Labor Act.

with an inside "whistleblower" or "snitch rule" whereby an anonymous complaint is filed with the OIG at the CMS.[31] The OIG dispatches an investigation to the hospital in question and a federal investigation ensues. Every involved party is interviewed, including emergency physicians, on-call physicians, and the medical staff of the hospital. These investigations are usually unannounced.[32] One of the goals of the investigator is to determine if the hospital has policies and procedures to address the EMTALA provisions. As this investigation relates to on-call physicians, the first verification is whether or not the hospital maintains a call list. Specifically, it investigates the group practice names and the specific individual on the date under investigation. If a violation has occurred, stiff penalties are handed down to the hospital and the violating physician. Moreover, the hospital can sue the violating physician for placing the hospital in jeopardy.

Fines

If a facility is issued a citation, a fine may be administered. A hospital that negligently violates the statute may be subject to a civil monetary penalty of up to $50,000 per violation. If the hospital has fewer than 100 beds, the maximum penalty is $25,000. In the larger facilities, physicians may be subject to a civil monetary penalty of up to $50,000 and there may be malpractice liability.[33]

For instance, the OIG successfully fined an Oklahoma hospital $25,000 for an EMTALA violation. In this case, an administrative law judge determined that the hospital did not articulate a clear transfer acceptance policy, which assured compliance with EMTALA, nor did it educate its staff and on-call physicians as to their responsibilities.[34]

Table 24.5 EMTALA Violation: Investigation Process

Process	"Whistleblower" or "snitch" rule
	• Anonymous complaint filed with OIG at CMS
	OIG starts hospital investigation and federal investigation ensues
	• Almost always unannounced
	Every party involved is interviewed
	Determine if hospital has EMTALA policies
	• Verify if hospital maintains a call list
	• Investigates group practice names and specific person on-call the date under investigation
	If violation occurred, penalties against hospital and physician
	Hospital can sue the physician
Fines	Hospital: monetary penalty up to $50,000/violation
	• If fewer than 100 beds, maximum penalty is $25,000
	Physician: monetary penalty up to $50,000
	• Potential malpractice liability as well

Abbreviations: CMS, Center for Medical Services; ED, emergency department; EMC, emergency medical condition; EMTALA, the Emergency Medical Treatment and Active Labor Act; OIG, Office of General Counsel.

Neurosurgeons' Response to EMTALA

The result of EMTALA's unfunded mandate can be summarized as follows: There has been an increasing work burden on those neurosurgeons who continue to take ED call. They have appropriately questioned what they receive in return for the increased demands. The unfortunate answer has been that they receive less money and more risk of liability. The increase in liability exposure comes from higher insurance premiums associated with taking ED call and the potential catastrophic exposure in the case of a lawsuit against them.

As a result, neurosurgeons have responded with two different strategies: contracting with hospitals for on-call stipends or avoiding ED calls altogether. Larger hospital centers have had to develop economic and social mechanisms of coping with the increased burden. Incentives in the form of hospital stipends for taking neurosurgical call have been one such approach. However, this does not address the medicolegal concerns or other issues that come from this increased workload.

Contracting for On-Call Stipends

The benefits to hospitals and neurosurgeons are obvious. With respect to hospitals, neurosurgeons improve the individual institution's ability to meet their EMTALA obligations. Stipends help alleviate the double burden of providing mandatory uncompensated care even as reliably compensated elective practice is negatively impacted. Without these types of contractual stipends, there may come a day when administrators are forced to pay "in-house hospital neurosurgeons" to cover the ED because staff neurosurgeons will be forced to leave. The lack of contractual stipends have been greatest in the larger, academic centers where surveys suggest that they are half as likely as private practice neurosurgeons to receive stipends.[35]

Neurosurgeons as "Spinal Surgeons"

Another neurosurgical response that has produced considerable controversy is that some neurosurgeons have declared themselves "spinal surgeons." This strategy is to avoid ED calls in an effort to focus on elective cases and decrease exposure to malpractice suits. In 2002, the American Association of Neurological Surgeons (AANS) wrote a letter to the CMS to advance this concept. The AANS noted that neurosurgeons in many cases have been forced to eliminate emergent procedures because of the increasing liability exposure and rising premiums.[36]

Additionally, neurosurgeons feel that in calling themselves spine surgeons, taking emergency calls would technically be performing procedures "outside the scope of their practice." Therefore, they have requested that the CMS further clarify the rules by declaring several "safe harbor" regulations. Chief among them is for the CMS to recognize that spinal surgeons should only be on call for emergencies that are within the scope of their practice.

The difficulty with this position, however, has been that most neurosurgeons are generally credentialed to perform all types of procedures (**Table 24.6**). Hospitals responded to this position by countering that credentialing is a conferred privilege and as such, surgeons are working as agents of the hospital. Many hospitals have threatened the neurosurgeons with potential EMTALA violations and have essentially forced the neurosurgeons to rethink, or in some cases abandon this position altogether.

Orthopedists have made a similar argument. What if the hospital performs complex spine surgeries, but the particular orthopedist on call states that he does not do these procedures and requests that the patient be transferred elsewhere? This would likely be considered an EMTALA violation, especially if CMS investigates and finds evidence that these complex procedures are done at this hospital and this particular patient was refused such care. Hospitals are ultimately responsible for the violation and are unwilling to accept liability in allowing this practice to occur.[15]

In a later AANS bulletin, although neurosurgeons have maintained that decreasing their scope of practice

Table 24.6 Neurosurgeons' Response to EMTALA

Result of EMTALA's unfunded mandate	Increasing work burden on neurosurgeons who take ED calls
	Receive less money and more risk of liability
	Higher insurance premiums associated with ED calls
	Potential catastrophic exposure in the case of a lawsuit
Neurosurgical response	Contracting for on-call stipends • Incentives in form of hospital stipend for taking neurosurgical calls
	• Helps alleviate burden of providing uncompensated care
	• May help avoid paying the day when forced to pay in house hospital neurosurgeons to cover ED because of neurosurgical staff shortage
	Neurosurgeons identifying themselves as "spinal surgeons"
	• To avoid ED calls to focus on elective cases and minimize exposure to malpractice suits
	• ED calls would technically be performing procedures "outside the scope of their practice"
	• Requested CMS make "safe harbor" regulations—"spinal surgeons" only on call for emergencies within their scope of practice
	• Difficult because neurosurgeons are credentialed to perform all types of procedures

Abbreviations: ED, emergency department; EMC, emergency medical condition; EMTALA, the Emergency Medical Treatment and Active Labor Act.

decreases their risks and concomitant premium rates, this "cherry picking" technique is fraught with potential risk of violating the CMS position. Specifically, physicians who practice in a narrow subspecialty should still be competent in their larger specialty. Under any scenario, neurosurgeons possess more skill and expertise than emergency physicians do when it comes to dealing with neurosurgical emergencies. For example, a spinal surgeon may still be expected to have more expertise than an ED physician does when it comes to treating a subdural hematoma.[13] It is unclear whether this practice of neurosurgeons labeling themselves as spine surgeons is wise. The risk of an EMTALA violation may be lessened if the neurosurgical community did not continue this practice until this issue is clearly resolved by the CMS.

EMTALA Case Law

Which physician should accept the transfer is another area of controversy. Whereas it ostensibly makes sense that the on-call specialist be the one to accept the patient, the specialist should probably make this decision in conjunction with the emergency attending physician working that shift. It is easy to understand how an on-call subspecialist would have little idea about critical acceptance factors, like bed availability throughout the specialized areas of the hospital. Additionally, the on-call physician is unlikely to be familiar with the nuances of EMTALA and may make decisions based on erroneous information. Citations usually result from on-call physicians' improper rejections of appropriate transfers. A hospital is legally liable for the actions of this physician, *even* if the hospital was totally unaware of the rejection. According to court decisions, any EMTALA violation by a physician is a violation by the hospital.[38]

A specialty consultant must be wary of refusing patients in transfer. In *Inspector General v St. Anthony Hospital*, the on-call thoracic surgeon refused to accept an appropriate transfer of a trauma victim from a nearby hospital. The judge agreed with the OIG and fined the hospital $35,000 holding that the physician was the hospital's agent and therefore subjected the hospital to an EMTALA violation for reverse dumping. The court went on to hold that the main defense for an *appropriate* refusal is that the accepting facility does not have the capacity to safely accommodate the patient.[34]

This trend appears to be expanding to holding every on-call physician liable as well. In *Millard v Corrado*, a Missouri appellate court found a thoracic surgeon liable for abandonment. The rationale in this case was that the physician's on-call status constituted a physician–patient relationship. Therefore, the surgeon was responsible for the care of the patient.[39]

In 1991, another court held that an on-call physician had entered into a contract with his hospital to take call for obstetrical emergencies. As such, he was obligated to consult on a patient to be transferred and his failure to adequately do so was a violation of federal law.[38]

As indicated by other court cases, the transferring hospital may be subject to liability as well. In *Huckaby et al v East Alabama Medical Center et al*, a brain-injured patient was ultimately transferred to a tertiary facility despite the fact that the on-call accepting neurosurgeon had the reputation for refusing to accept patients. The transfer was eventually arranged even though the patient was not stable and died shortly after arrival to the facility. The accepting hospital was held liable for this refusal. The transferring hospital and physician were also held liable for failing to adequately stabilize the patient prior to transfer.[40]

Even though many courts have ruled in favor of the plaintiff, one court held in favor of the defendant. In 1999,

Table 24.7 The Emergency Medical Treatment and Active Labor Act (EMTALA) Case Law

Ruling in favor of plaintiff	Inspector General v St. Anthony Hospital	On-call thoracic surgeon refused *appropriate* transfer of trauma patient
		Hospital fined $35,000
		• Physician was the hospital's agent
		• Subject to EMTALA violation of "reverse dumping"
		Appropriate refusal only when facility does not have capacity to safely accommodate patient
	Millard v Colorado	Thoracic surgeon found liable for abandonment
		• On-call status constituted patient–physician relationship
		• Therefore, he was responsible for care of patient
	Huckaby v E. Alabama Medical Center	Brain-injured patient transferred to tertiary hospital knowing that the accepting neurosurgeon had reputation for refusing to accept transfers
		• Transfer made with unstable patient and patient died
		Accepting hospital: held liable for refusal
		Transferring hospital and physician: held liable for failing to stabilize patient prior to transfer
Ruling in favor of defendant	Cherukuri v Shalala	Held that a surgeon's transfer of two seriously injured patients from small local facility to teaching hospital equipped for brain surgery did not violate EMTALA

the United States Court of Federal Appeals for the Sixth Circuit held that a surgeon's transfer of two seriously injured patients from a small local hospital to a teaching hospital equipped to perform brain surgery did not violate EMTALA (**Table 24.7**).[41]

According to most of the case law involving other specialties, it is likely that the on-call neurosurgeon would have an obligation to treat an unstable or transferred patient. This is particularly true when the patient has been transferred for the *sole* purpose of receiving neurosurgical care. However, even if neurosurgeons manage to escape federal liability exposure, they will still be subject to state malpractice law.

The Difference between EMTALA Case Law and State Malpractice Case Law

EMTALA Malpractice Law

EMTALA was not meant to be a federal malpractice law. Despite the complexities of the MSE, courts have generally found that the MSE does not guarantee an accurate diagnosis, but merely establishes a uniform standard of evaluation and care, thereby keeping EMTALA from becoming a federal malpractice law.[42,51–53] However, if a doctor is *negligent* in the treatment, that negligence is not actionable under EMTALA but must be brought under a traditional medical malpractice suit.

Claims for medical malpractice arise under state law and vary from state to state. EMTALA does not take the place or limit any malpractice claim under state law. Instead, it offers another way for a plaintiff to make a claim for damages and a way to get his claims removed to a federal court. Inevitably, plaintiff attorneys will allege a violation of EMTALA as part of their medical malpractice claim. However, a medical malpractice claim is almost always based on the defendant physician's violation of the standard of care.[43]

State Malpractice Case Law

Background

Even if a hospital or provider is cleared of any EMTALA violation, they may still be subject to a potential state malpractice suit. In effect, this means that the case will be retrospectively scrutinized and expert testimony allowed. Normal objective standards will be applied to make a factual determination of a breach in the standard of care. This burden is often more rigorous than the evaluation of an EMTALA violation. EMTALA does not require the physician to make the correct diagnosis. It simply requires *equal* treatment for all patients regardless of their ability to pay for the service rendered.[44]

Negligence Elements That Comprise a State Malpractice Lawsuit

Negligence does not only require an accurate diagnosis, but a timely one. There are more and more malpractice suits in which the physician has made the correct diagnosis but been found liable for failing to implement treatment in a timely manner.

As a threshold element, the plaintiff must first prove that there was a duty to treat the patient. This duty is almost implied by virtue of the contract formed when the physician agrees to care for the patient. From a practical standpoint, the most important element to be proven is that the physician breached that duty by caring for the patient in substandard fashion. This breach of care is always one of omission or commission. The breach is almost always proven with expert testimony—the so-called battle of the experts. The third element of negligence is that of proximate cause. This means that the breach in the standard must have been the proximate cause of any alleged injury. Without demonstrating that the substandard care led to a tangible injury, the claim of negligence will fail.[45]

Current State Case Law Involving On-Call Issues

Fortunately for subspecialists in general, and neurosurgeons in particular, no state case law is directly on point. A search was conducted via PUBMED and LEXIS search engines but at present, litigation of the on-call issue seems to be only at the federal level. A likely explanation for this is that even though EMTALA has been the law of the land for 2 decades, the final 2003 regulations that attempted to clarify this issue are relatively recent. However, there may be state claims that remain unreported because an appeal has not had the chance to reach a final decision. This should be cold comfort for neurosurgeons who can expect that before too long, plaintiff attorneys will seek to add a state malpractice cause of action that attempts to litigate this issue in state courts.

State Malpractice Data Involving Neurosurgeons

National surveys have shown that over 50% of all neurosurgeons in the United States face a malpractice claim every year. Neurosurgery is one of three most frequently sued specialties and faces the highest average premiums in the country.[46] In comparison, one-third of orthopedists, obstetricians, and trauma surgeons get sued in a given year.[47]

Professional liability premiums mirror these malpractice data. The AANS reports that professional liability carriers have raised their rates for neurosurgeons that perform emergency procedures. The past 2 years have seen a 24% increase in premiums for neurosurgeons practicing in New York.[13] Conversely, some carriers are offering "discounted" rates for those neurosurgeons who limit their practice to less risky procedures. In Texas, for example, some insurers lowered their rates for neurosurgeons that did not perform craniotomies.

For the moment, this may be a regional trend that has localized to the states experiencing a malpractice crisis. This is likely to spread to other states if the current trend in "lottery" verdicts suits continues throughout the country.[49] The staggering reality of what drives these figures begins with the fact that the average jury award is 3.5 million dollars, with a large percentage of this going toward "pain and suffering." The mean annual malpractice premiums for neurosurgeons in 2002 increased from $35,000 to $71,000. As a result, 33% of neurosurgeons have switched carriers, and 19% report that they have moved to other states with more stable premiums.[49]

Neurosurgery is an inherently high-risk specialty given the nature of the surgical procedures that are performed. This even applies to many elective cases and with even more force to emergency cases. The impression among many neurosurgeons is that they are more frequently sued than any other subspecialty. Unfortunately, although this may not have always been the case, the latest data corroborate that neurosurgery is now one of the most common specialties facing malpractice suits today (**Table 24.8**).

Conclusion

The difficulty with the issue of ED on call for the neurosurgeon has been an ongoing controversy that has been well documented. The thrust of the problem seems to be the tension created by EMTALA and the neurosurgical obligations that arise from this federal law. At its core, EMTALA is an unfunded mandate that forces neurosurgeons to take ED call for high-risk emergency cases.

Naturally, this has resulted in significant pushback from the neurosurgical community. One partial solution to this problem has been to create on-call contractual stipends between the neurosurgeons and the hospital administration. Interestingly, other neurosurgeons have tried to avoid ED calls entirely by labeling themselves as elective spine surgeons.

As if EMTALA was not concerning enough, state malpractice laws have had an adverse impact on this problem as well. Physicians can still be sued in state court even if they are in full compliance with EMTALA. Malpractice suits are on the rise, in part owing to huge

Table 24.8 EMTALA Case Law versus State Malpractice Case Law

EMTALA "malpractice" law	MSE does not guarantee accurate diagnosis
	Merely establishes uniform standard of evaluation and care
	Negligence is not actionable under EMTALA
	• Must be brought under a traditional malpractice suit
	EMTALA does not take the place or limit malpractice claim under state law
	• Rather, it is another way for plaintiff to make a claim for damages and get his claims removed to federal court
Four elements required to establish the claim of negligence	1. Duty to treat
	2. Breach of duty by violating standard of care
	3. Standard of care violation caused the injury
	4. Tangible injury also known as damage
	No state case laws involving "on-call" issue
State malpractice data involving neurosurgeons	Is 1 of 3 most frequently sued specialties • 50% of U.S. neurosurgeons face a malpractice claim every year
	• Compared with 33.3% of orthopedists, obstetricians, and trauma surgeons
	Faces the highest average premiums in the country
	• 24% increase in premiums in last few years in New York state
	• Some carriers offering "discounted" rates to those willing to limit practice to less risky procedures
	Average jury award is 3.5 million dollars
	• Large % of this going toward "pain and suffering"
	In 2002, mean annual malpractice premium for neurosurgeon increased from $35,000 to $71,000
	• As result, 33% of neurosurgeons have switched carriers
	• 19% have moved to other states with more stable premiums
State law malpractice	Even if the hospital or provider is cleared under EMTALA, they are not exempt from state malpractice suit.

Abbreviation: ED, emergency department; EMTALA, the Emergency Medical Treatment and Active Labor Act.
Source: American Association of Neurological Surgeons and Congress of Neurological Surgeons, 2004 survey. Federal medical liability reform. Alliance of Specialty Medicine, July 2005

awards, which in turn increases malpractice premium rates. As a result, neurosurgeons have been either cutting back from fulltime hospital status, decreasing or limiting their practice, moving to different states with more favorable state laws, or in some instances, retiring from clinical practice.

At the moment, a permanent solution seems out of reach. Neurosurgeons, federal and state governments, insurance companies, and hospital executive staffs must find a way to work together. Ultimately, any solution will have to be acceptable to all parties while fulfilling the current government mandate.

References*

1. American College of Surgeons (ACS). Advocacy and health policy. ACS Cross Country (ACS Monthly State Affairs Newsletter); 2004. Available at: http://www.facs.org/ahp/feb04crosscountry.html. Accessed September 30, 2006
2. Pub. L. No. 79–725, 42 U.S.C. §§ 291 *et seq*
3. Kusske JA. Neurosurgical practice in the current regulatory environment. Neurosurg Focus 2002;12(4):e11
4. Teshome G, Closson F. Emergency Medical Treatment and Labor Act: the basics and other medicolegal concerns. Pediatr Clin North Am 2006;53:139–155
5. Gionis TA, Camargo CA, Zito AS. The intentional tort of patient dumping: a new state cause of action to address the shortcomings of the Federal Emergency Medical Treatment and Active Labor Act (EMTALA). Am Univ L Rev 2002;52:173–308
6. Schiff RL, Ansell DA, Schlosser JE, et al. Transfers to a public hospital: a prospective study of 467 patients. N Engl J Med 1986;314:552–557
7. Bitterman RA. Transferring and accepting patients under EMTALA. In: Bitterman RA, ed. Providing Emergency Care under Federal Law: EMTALA: With New Supplement. Dallas: American College of Emergency Physicians 2000;7:103–123

8. 42 U.S.C. § 1395dd (1986) (an examination and treatment for emergency medical conditions and women in labor)
9. Zibulewsky J. The Emergency Medical Treatment and Active Labor Act (EMTALA): what it is and what it means for physicians. Proc (Bayl Univ Med Cent) 2001;14:339–346
10. Department of Health and Human Services, Center for Medicare Services. Medicare Program: clarifying policies related to the responsibilities of Medicare-participating hospitals in treating individuals with emergency medical conditions. 68 Fed. Reg. 174 (Sept. 9, 2003) codified as 42 C.F.R. §§ 413, 482, 489
11. *Green v. Touro Infirmary*, 992 F.2d 537 (5th Cir.1993)
12. Center for Medicare Services. Interpretive Guidelines–Responsibilities of Medicare Participating Hospitals in Emergency Cases. State Operations Manual, V-25. Washington, DC: Department of Health and Human Services, Center for Medicare Services
13. Valadka AB. The ER, who is answering call? AANS Bulletin 2004;13:6–12
14. Harrington TR. Future of emergency care in the US health system. Ann Emerg Med 2006;48(2):117
15. Rudkin SE, Oman J, Langdorf MI, et al. The state of ED on-call coverage in California. Am J Emerg Med 2004;22:575–581
16. Heros, RC, Papadapoulos, SM. AANS letter to Scully TA, Administrator, Department of Health and Human Services, Center for Medicare Services; www.neurosurgeon.org. May 30, 2002
17. Office of the Inspector General (OIG). EMTALA: survey of hospital emergency department. Washington, DC: Department of Health and Human Services; 2001
18. 68 Fed. Reg. 53222 (2003)
19. Teshome G, Closson FT. EMTALA: the basics and other medicolegal concerns. Pediatr Clin North Am 2006;53:139–155
20. 42 C.F.R. § 489.24(j)
21. 42 C.F.R. § 489.24(e)
22. 42 C.F.R. § 489.24(d)
23. McHugh EM. The new EMTALA regulations and on-call physician shortage: in defense of the regulations. J Health Law 2004;37(1):61–84

A number of references in this chapter use legal citations for statutes, regulations, and court cases. The styles of legal citation are explained in The Bluebook: A Uniform System of Citation *(published and distributed by The Harvard Law Review Association, Cambridge, MA). The 18th edition, published in 2005, was used as a reference. A court case is referenced as follows: 385 F.3d 113 (6th Cir. 2006), where the initial number and letter combination is the reporter volume number and reporter abbreviation, the second three-digit number is the first page of the case, the third citation is the deciding court, and the fourth is the year of publication. Reporters refer to bound publications that print only cases.*
Citation by an individual provision of the United States Code is illustrated in the following example: 42 U.S.C. § 1395y(e) where 42 is the volume number, followed by the code abbreviation and then the specific section and subsections cited. Citation of a particular provision in the Code of Federal Regulations is as follows: 42 C.F.R. § 1008.5, where 42 is the C.F.R. number, C.F.R. is the abbreviation of the set of regulations followed by the section symbol and specific section cited. Citations of the Federal Register *are as follows: 66 Fed. Reg. 856–965, where 66 is the volume number followed by the abbreviation and the page numbers of interest.*

24. Zibulewsky J. Medical staff knowledge of EMTALA at a large, tertiary care hospital. Am J Emerg Med 2003;21(1):8–13
25. Cone DC, Alexander V, Myint W. EMTALA knowledge among on-call specialists at an academic medical center. J Emerg Med 2006;30(4):444–446
26. Bitterman RA. A critical analysis of the federal COBRA hospital “antidumping law”: ramifications for hospitals, physicians, and the effects on access to healthcare. Univ Detroit Mercy Law Rev 1992;70:125–190
27. Bitterman RA. Transferring and accepting patients under EMTALA. In: Bitterman RA, ed. Providing emergency care under federal law: EMTALA: with new supplement. Dallas: American College of Emergency Physicians; 2000;7:1–6
29. Johnson LA, Taylor TB, Lev R. The emergency department on-call crisis: finding remedies for a serious public health problem. Ann Emerg Med 2001;37(5):495–499
30. Taylor TB, Bitterman RA, Ghezzi K, et al. On-call duties and responsibilities. Emerg Physicians Monthly. 2000;7:4
31. Fosmire, MS. Frequently Asked Questions about the Emergency Medical Treatment and Active Labor Act (EMTALA). Available at: http://www.emtala.com/faq.htm. Accessed September 30, 2006
32. 42 C.F.R. §§ 489.24(m),(q), and (r)
33. Linzer JF. EMTALA: a clearer road to the future? Clin Pediatr Emerg Med 2003;4:249–255
34. *St. Anthony Hosp. v U.S. Dept. of HHS*, 309 F.3d 680 (10th Cir. 2002); *appealed from Inspector General v St. Anthony Hosp.*, DAB No. C-98–460, Depart. of HHS, Depart. Appeals Board, Civil Remedies Division (Oct. 5, 1999)
35. Harrington TR. Neurosurgical manpower needs: achieving a balance. Surg Neurol 1997;47:316–320
36. AANS and College of Neurological Surgeons, EMTALA Technical Advisory Group. Comments, aans.org. March 20, 2005
38. *Burditt v U.S. Dept. of HHS*, 934 F.2d 1362 (5th Cir. 1991)
39. *Millard v Corrado*, No. ED 75420 RD (Mo. App. 1999)
40. *Huckaby et al v East Alabama Medical Center et al*, 830 F. Supp. 1399 (U.S. Dist. 1993)
41. *Cherukuri v Shalala*, 175 F.3d 446 (6th Cir. 1999)
42. *Collins v DePaul Hos.*, 963 F.2d 303 (10th Cir. 1992)
43. Hudson T. Attorneys fear patient transfer claims in malpractice cases. Hospitals 1991;65(7):44–48
44. *Richardson v Rohrbaugh*, 857 S.W.3d 415 (Mo. App. 1993)
45. Comodeca JA, Maggio MM, Truax PJ, Bilz JM. Tort reform article: killing the golden goose by evaluating medical care through the retroscope: tort reform from the defense perspective. Dayton L Rev 2004;31:206–207
46. Anderson RE. Effective legal reform and the malpractice insurance crisis. Yale J Health Policy Law Ethics 2005;1:343–355
47. New York State Neurological Society. Statement to the Press. Paper presented at: New York State Neurological Society Medical Tort Reform Symposium; New York, NY September 20, 2004:1–3
49. Neurosurgeons to Preserve Health Care Access. Available at: http://www.neuros2preservecare.org. Accessed September 30, 2006
50. Ansell DA, Schiff RL. Patient dumping: status, implications and policy recommendations. JAMA 1987;257:1500–1502
51. *Barber v Hosp. Corp. of Am.*, 977 F.2d 872 (4th Cir. 1992)
52. *Brooks v Md Gen. Hosp.*, 996 F.2d 708 (4th Cir. 1993)
53. *Williams v Birkness*, 34 F.3d 695 (8th Cir. 1994)

25 Cost of Traumatic Brain Injury and Return on Helmet Investment in the United States

Ted R. Miller, Eduard Zaloshnja, and Delia Hendrie

Setting priorities for injury prevention and control and allocating scarce resources between alternative uses involve difficult choices. Programs targeting different injury causes and programs in related areas compete for funding. The associated funding choices are challenging. Resource allocation decisions must account for the complex interplay of social, economic, and political factors. At the same time, policy makers and program managers face the challenge of having to allocate resources to areas that provide the best value for the money. Simply choosing programs that work or even those that work best is no longer acceptable. Economic evaluation can contribute information on the costs and benefits of alternative interventions to these decisions and summarize this information in cost-outcome measures.[1]

In addition to their use in benefit-cost analysis, injury costs represent the code that makes injury burden estimates understandable. Cost offers a major advantage over incidence by reducing disparate outcomes—for example, deaths, skull fractures, broken jaws, anoxias, and dog-bitten faces—to a single compact metric. Compactness eases comprehension. That makes cost data valuable for problem size and risk assessment, broad priority-setting, health and safety advocacy, regulatory analysis, and performance comparison. Cost data describe how injuries affect society and drive analyses of the potential to reduce injuries cost effectively.

Increasingly, this basic health services research tool is a focal point for debate and decision making. Cost is a powerful persuader. The Press and politicians understand a savings of $1 billion in medical and work loss costs far better than a statistically significant 1% reduction in injury deaths and hospital admissions.

In this chapter, we analyze the total cost of traumatic brain injury (TBI) in the United States in 2000. We describe cost concepts and categories, and how we estimated different cost components. We present the comprehensive cost of TBI by cost category, severity, nature of injury, level of treatment, age and gender, and cause. A framework for conducting economic evaluation with injury cost data is provided, as well as an overview of the types of economic evaluation that are possible. To illustrate how to apply the methods we describe, we include a benefit-cost analysis of bicycle helmets. Finally, we discuss the limitations of our estimates and offer some concluding remarks.

Analyzing Costs

Cost Concepts

Costs can be incidence- or prevalence-based (**Table 25.1**). *Incidence-based costs* sum the lifetime costs that are expected to result from injuries that occur during a single year. For example, the incidence-based cost of TBI in 2000 estimates present and future medical spending associated with all TBIs that occurred in 2000. Incidence-based costs are computed by multiplying the number of injury victims times lifetime cost per victim. They measure the savings that prevention can yield. This chapter presents incidence-based costs stated in 2006 dollars.

Prevalence-based costs measure all injury-related expenses during 1 year, regardless of when the injury occurred. For example, the prevalence-based cost of TBI in 2000 measures the total health care spending on head injuries during 2000, including spending on victims injured many years earlier. Prevalence-based costs are computed by summing all costs incurred during the year. They are used to project health care spending and evaluate cost controls.

Investments earn interest. In incidence-based costing, therefore, future costs must be discounted to present value. This procedure shows the amount that would be invested today to pay future costs as they arise. The U.S.

Table 25.1 Cost Concepts

Incidence-based costs	• Sum lifetime costs expected to result from injuries during a single year (future costs must be discounted to present value) • Computed by: number of injury victims * lifetime cost per victim • They measure the savings that prevention can yield
Prevalence-based costs	• Measure all injury-related expenses during one year, regardless of when injury occurred • Computed by: summing all costs incurred during the year • Used to project health care spending and evaluate cost controls

Panel on Cost-Effectiveness in Health and Medicine[2] recommends that all cost savings analyses include an estimate at a 3% discount rate to accommodate cross-study comparisons. Real rates of return on investment and discount rates that individuals apply when making health decisions suggest this discount rate is a conservative upper bound in the United States[3–5] and elsewhere.[6] Governments around the world, however, often require use of higher discount rates of 5 to 7% in regulatory analysis. Implicitly, they use the discounting process to lessen the influence of optimistic benefit estimates.

Cost Categories

TBI burden falls into three categories: medical costs, work loss costs, and quality of life costs (**Table 25.2**).

Medical costs include emergency transport, medical, hospital, rehabilitation, mental health, pharmaceutical, ancillary, and related treatment costs, as well as funeral/coroner expenses for fatalities and administrative costs of processing medical payments to providers.

Work loss costs value productivity losses. They include victims' lost wages and the replacement cost of lost household work, as well as fringe benefits and the administrative costs of processing compensation for lost earnings through litigation, insurance, or public welfare programs like food stamps and disability income. In addition to victim work losses from death or permanent disability and from short-term disability, this category includes work losses by family and friends who voluntarily care for the injured.

Quality of life costs include the value of pain, suffering, and quality of life loss to victims and their families. This factor can be included in dollars or in unmonetized form. Monetizing is controversial because it assumes that the monetary value per quality-adjusted life year (QALY, defined in the next section) is constant across the lifespan and that proportionate values for different health states are independent of income (e.g., that people of all income levels value the mobility loss from needing a walker at half the loss from needing a wheelchair). It also requires using a value of fatal risk reduction from one of several meta-analyses on the amount people routinely pay or are willing to pay in the expectation of saving one statistical life, but the meta-analyses disagree about this value.

Some aspects of injury burden are readily measured in monetary terms. These include medical costs and work losses. Together, they are called economic costs or human capital costs. Costs that include the value of pain and lost quality of life are called comprehensive costs or willingness-to-pay costs. In this chapter, we report the comprehensive costs of TBI.

Table 25.2 The Three Cost Categories for Traumatic Brain Injury

Medical costs	Includes emergency transport, medical, hospital, rehabilitation, mental health, pharmaceutical, ancillary, related treatment costs, funeral/coroner expenses, and administrative costs
Work loss costs (value of productivity losses)	• Victims lost wages and work losses due to death or disability • Replacement cost of lost household work • Fringe benefits • Administrative costs of processing compensation for lost earnings through litigation, insurance, or public welfare programs • Work losses by family and friends who voluntarily care for injured
Quality of life costs	• Value of pain, suffering, and quality-adjusted life year (QALY) losses to victims and families • Monetizing these costs is controversial
Some aspects of injury burden are tangible and thus, readily measured in monetary terms: medical costs, work losses = economic costs or human capital costs	
Some are intangible and difficult to monetize, including those that value pain and lost quality of life = comprehensive costs or willingness-to-pay costs	

Computing Costs

Medical Costs

Medical cost estimates are computed best *bottom-up* (**Table 25.3**), by multiplying estimated medical spending per case or visit by diagnosis times corresponding

Table 25.3 Methods Used to Factor Costs

Medical costs	Bottom-up	• Multiply estimated medical spending per case (or visit) times corresponding estimated cases (or visits)
	Top-down	• Obtain prevalence-based national medical spending • Apportion it according to hospital days by diagnosis group • Used when comparing spending on injury and illness
	Factoring	• Calculate local costs by adjusting a national cost per case to local prices, multiplied by a local case count • Often used to make state or provincial cost estimates • Inexpensive

Table 25.4 Bottom-Up Estimation of U.S. Medical Costs for Traumatic Brain Injury

Nonhospitalized injury	• Used MEPS to quantify medical costs in the first 18 months postinjury
Hospitalized injury: inpatient costs	• Inpatient facility costs: HCUP-National Inpatient Sample charge data times facility-specific cost-to-charge ratios from Agency for Healthcare Research and Quality • Nonfacility costs during inpatient admission: Medstat's Marketscan database
Hospitalized injury: postdischarge treatment in first 18 months after injury	• Multiplied total inpatient costs times the MEPS ratio of all costs during first 18 months postinjury to inpatient costs for that kind of injury
All nonfatal injury: medical costs beyond 18 months	• Used multipliers from longitudinal 1979–88 Detailed Claims Information data on workers compensation claims
Fatalities	• Computed medical costs for five separate places of death: ◦ Death on scene/at home ◦ Death on arrival to hospital ◦ Death at ED ◦ Death at hospital after inpatient admission ◦ Death at nursing home

Abbreviations: ED, emergency department; HCUP, Healthcare Cost and Utilization Project; MEPS, Medical Expenditure Panel Survey.

estimated case or visit counts (**Table 25.4**). Two coarser approaches are possible.

Top-down. One can obtain total national medical spending, then apportion it according to hospital days by diagnosis group. This prevalence-based approach often is taken when comparing spending on injury and illness.[7,8]

Factoring. One can adjust a national cost per case to local prices (and preferably local length of hospital stay), then multiply times a local case count to get local costs. We often use this method to make state or provincial cost estimates. It is inexpensive, yet yields reasonably credible numbers.

We used the bottom-up approach in estimating incidence-based TBI medical costs. Our methods closely follow those employed by Finkelstein et al.[9] We used Medical Expenditure Panel Survey (MEPS) data to quantify medical costs for nonhospitalized injuries. For hospitalized injuries, because of the small sample size of admitted injuries in MEPS, we primarily relied on other data sources. We used Healthcare Cost and Utilization Project Nationwide Inpatient Sample (HCUP-NIS) data and cost-to-charge ratios from the Agency for Healthcare Research and Quality to compute inpatient facility costs. We then used Medstat's Marketscan (MEDSTAT Group, Inc., Ann Arbor, MI) data to quantify nonfacility costs incurred during an inpatient admission.

Most injuries that require a hospitalization will also require additional treatment after discharge. To estimate short- to medium-term medical costs for injuries requiring an inpatient admission, we multiplied total inpatient costs derived from the HCUP-NIS/Marketscan data by the ratio of all costs during the first 18 months of injury, on average, to the total inpatient costs for that kind of injury. We derived these ratios from 1996 to 1999 MEPS data.

We used an identical strategy to Rice et al[10] for estimating long-term medical costs (18+ months). We used multipliers derived from longitudinal 1979–1988 Detailed Claims Information (DCI) data on 463,174 Worker's Compensation claims. The DCI file was unique and nothing similar has subsequently become available[11]. This method implicitly assumes that while treatment costs vary over time, the ratio of 18-month costs to total lifetime costs has remained constant between the time the DCI data were reported and 2000.

For fatalities, we computed medical costs separately for five places of death identified in the 2000 National Vital Statistics System (NVSS) data[12]: death-on-scene/at home, death-on-arrival to the hospital, death at the ED, death at the hospital after inpatient admission, and death at a nursing home. Depending on place of death, the medical costs incurred might include coroner/medical examiner (C/ME), medical transport, ED, inpatient hospital, or nursing home. Generally, the cost calculations paralleled those for nonfatal injury.

Work Loss Costs

Work or productivity loss has two components: short-term losses during acute injury recovery and lifetime losses due to death or permanent work-related disability (**Table 25.5**). We quantify temporary or short-term work loss for nonfatal injuries using the approach presented by Finkelstein et al,[9] where the probability of an injury that resulted in lost workdays was combined with the mean workdays lost (conditional on having missed at least 1 day) per injury estimated. We computed work loss durations for injuries separately for admitted and nonadmitted cases for each age category, sex, and mechanism.

To apply a monetary value to temporary work loss, we multiplied estimated work loss days by the average daily wage and fringe benefit costs stratified by age group and sex from the Current Population Survey[13]. Following numerous other studies,[14–16] we relied on survey data that showed household work is lost on 90% of days that wage work is lost to injury. Using this ratio and the value of household work,[17] we also imputed a value for household work lost.

Table 25.5 Estimation of National Work Loss Costs from Traumatic Brain Injury

Short-term losses	• Multiplied estimated work loss days by the average daily wage and fringe benefit costs • Also imputed value for household work loss	
Permanent or long-term disability losses	• Considered permanent total disability and permanent partial disability separately (a sum total of both)	
	Permanent total disability	Multiplied present value of age- and sex-specific lifetime earnings and household production times probability of permanent disability for each injury type
	Permanent partial disability	Multiplied present value of lifetime earnings times probability of permanent partial disability times an additional factor that identified % of disability that resulted from that type of injury

To compute productivity loss due to permanent or long-term disability, we considered permanent total disability and permanent partial disability separately. For death and other permanent total disability, we multiplied the present value of age- and sex-specific lifetime earnings and household production[14] by the probability of permanent disability for each type of injury. For permanent partial disability, we multiplied the earnings estimate by the probability of permanent partial disability and an additional factor that identified the percentage of disability that resulted from that type of injury. We then summed the results to compute the net productivity loss associated with permanent disability, including total and partial disability. The probabilities of permanent and partial disability and the percentage disabled (by body part and nature of injury) were computed from DCI data by Lawrence et al.[11] Application of these estimates to our analysis assumes that these probabilities are the same for injuries that do and do not occur on-the-job and that they have not changed significantly over time.

Quality of Life Costs

Our method of estimating quality of life costs followed closely those employed by Miller et al.[18] It based quality of life loss on physicians' estimates of the functional capacity lost over time by injury diagnosis and a systematic review of the survey literature on the loss in value of life that results from different functional losses. These losses were determined based on meta-analyses[19–21] that examine what people pay for small changes in fatality risk and surveys on what they state they are willing to pay. Following Zaloshnja et al,[16] we monetize QALYs using the value of $4.17 million per life saved (in 2006 dollars) from Miller[19] that is incorporated into regulatory analyses throughout the U.S. Department of Transportation. For compactness, we provide monetized QALY estimates here. To obtain unmonetized QALYs, divide the monetized estimates by $140,366 (**Table 25.6**).

Table 25.6 Estimation of Quality of Life Loss Costs from Traumatic Brain Injury in the U.S.

- Based quality of life loss on physicians' estimates of the functional capacity lost over time by injury diagnosis and a systematic review of literature on loss of life from different functional losses
- Costs were placed on these losses based on what people pay for small changes in fatality risk and what they say they are willing to pay
- Monetize quality-adjusted life years (QALYs) using value of $4.17 million/life saved

The Comprehensive Cost of TBI

More than 1.3 million Americans suffered TBIs in 2000. Their injuries cost more than $206 billion (in 2006 dollars). Of the victims, 40,000 died and the QALYs lost by other victims amounted to another 20,000 lifetimes lost. Approximately $135 billion of TBI cost was for fatal injuries, $54 billion for nonfatal TBIs that required hospitalization, and the remaining $17 billion for nonhospitalized TBIs (**Table 25.7**). TBI costs were dominated by quality of life losses (over $129.5 billion) and work losses (over $63 billion). Medical costs exceeded $13 billion.

TBI costs represented 15% of total U.S. injury costs in 2000. TBI caused 1% of total U.S. medical spending (computed from Bureau of the Census,[22] **Table 25.7**).

The Barell Injury Diagnosis Matrix[23–24] maps the International Classification of Diseases 9th Revision Clinical Modification (ICD-9-CM) codes into 36 body parts and 12 natures of injury. It defines three types of head injury: it is a type 1 injury if there is recorded evidence of an intracranial injury with moderate or prolonged loss of consciousness (LOC) or injuries to the optic nerve pathways; type 2 applies to injuries with no recorded evidence of intracranial damage, but with LOC of less than 1 hour, LOC of unknown duration, or unspecified level of consciousness; and type 3 refers to patients with no evidence of intracranial injury and no LOC. Correcting a mapping

Table 25.7 U.S. Comprehensive Costs of Traumatic Brain Injury by Level of Treatment (M 2006$) in 2000

Level of Treatment	Incidence	Medical Cost (Millions)	Work Loss Cost (Millions)	Quality of Life Loss (Millions)	Total Cost (Millions)	% of Total
Fatal	40,148	490	47,588	86,789	134,868	65.4
Hospitalized	155,587	10,770	12,423	30,701	53,894	26.1
Nonhospitalized	1,147,485	2,203	3,207	12,052	17,462	8.5
Total	1,343,220	13,463	63,218	129,542	206,224	100.0
% of Total	6.5	30.7	62.8	100.0		

error in Finkelstein et al,[9] we include unspecified head injuries (ICD-9-CM code 959.01) in type 3 (rather than in the Barell "other head injury" category).

TBI type 1 was responsible for 86% of the total cost of TBI (**Table 25.8**). This high injury burden is explained by its high incidence and high cost per case ($174,357 as opposed to the average cost of $153,529 per case). Internal organ and open wound TBIs were responsible for $59.6 billion and $52.7 billion, respectively (**Table 25.9**).

Table 25.10 presents TBI total costs by severity of injury. Severity is measured by the Abbreviated Injury Scale (AIS) score, a scale that bases its threat-to-life estimates primarily on the nature and degree of damage to different body regions. It ranges from 1, a minor injury with a high likelihood of survival, to 6, an injury that is virtually unsurvivable. Among nonfatal TBIs, AIS 4 injuries had the highest injury burden (~27.4 billion). They were more common than AIS 5 injuries (which are more costly) and more costly than AIS score 1 to 3 injuries (which are more common).

Falls represented the main cause of TBI (**Table 25.11**). However, road incidents had the highest injury burden, followed by firearms (comprehensive cost: approximately $79.8 billion and $60.2, respectively). The same pattern was true for men but not for women. In terms of the burden of injury, falls followed road incidents among women but followed road incidents and firearms among men.

The 25 to 44 age group had the highest incidence of TBIs and the highest injury burden, followed by the 15 to 24 age group (**Table 25.12**). The same pattern held for women. Among men, the 5 to 14 age group had the highest incidence, but not the highest injury burden. Women suffered slightly more TBIs than men did, but their total cost was 3 times lower.

Table 25.8 U.S. Comprehensive Costs of Traumatic Brain Injury (TBI) by TBI Type (M 2006$) in 2000

		Costs			
TBI Type	Incidence	Medical	Work Loss	Quality of Life	Total
TBI 1	1,022,480	11,952	58,524	107,801	178,277
TBI 2	315,258	1,369	4,225	21,501	27,095
TBI 3	5,483	142	470	240	852
Total	1,343,220	13,463	63,128	129,542	206,224

Table 25.9 U.S. Comprehensive Costs of Traumatic Brain Injury by Nature of Injury (M 2006$) in 2000

Nature of		Costs			
Injury	Incidence	Medical	Work Loss	Quality of Life	Total
Fracture	55,923	3,595	5,706	23,214	32,515
Internal organ	444,738	7,756	15,638	36,251	59,646
Open wound	14,560	60	19,318	33,337	52,714
Crushing	213	1	326	582	908
Nerve	493	1	122	16	139
Unspecified	827,295	2,051	22,109	36,141	60,301
Total	1,343,220	13,463	63,218	129,542	206,224

Table 25.10 U.S. Comprehensive Costs of Traumatic Brain Injury by Threat-to-Life Severity (M 2006$) in 2000

Severity	Incidence	Costs			
		Medical	Work Loss	Quality of Life	Total
AIS-1	284,584	708	1,051	206	1,965
AIS-2	334,656	1,335	3,363	17,712	22,409
AIS-3	45,909	902	2,375	7,790	11,068
AIS-4	95,261	6,450	5,817	15,112	27,379
AIS-5	7,316	2,424	1,790	1,649	5,863
AIS-6	40,148	490	47,588	86,789	134,868
Unknown	535,346	1,155	1,234	282	2,671
Total	1,343,220	13,463	63,218	129,542	206,224

Abbreviations: AIS, abbreviated injury scale.

Framework for Conducting an Economic Evaluation with Injury Cost Data

This section and the next explain how costs can be used to evaluate preventive measures. An economic evaluation has several interrelated components. The study question must be specified, costs must be calculated, the effectiveness of the alternatives must be determined, and finally cost-outcome measures must be computed. Within each component, several steps can be identified (**Table 25.13**). A summary of the steps is presented here and illustrated in the Bicycle Helmets and Head Injury: A Benefit-Cost Analysis section with an analysis of the potential of the return on investment in child and adult bicycle helmets. Our method (drawn from Miller and Levy,[25]) loosely follows widely cited guidelines for conducting economic evaluation.[2]

Define the Intervention

The first step in conducting an economic evaluation is to define the intervention to be evaluated. This includes deciding on the objectives of the evaluation, alternatives to be compared, the target population, the setting of the intervention, the time horizon over which the costs and outcomes will be calculated, and the type of economic evaluation.

Determine the Perspective(s) of the Analysis

An important practical dimension in any economic evaluation is to determine the perspective of the study (e.g., a societal perspective can be adopted for the analysis.)

Adjust for Differential Timing

Many interventions have costs and benefits extending over several years. Inflation results in money prices changing over time even though the amount of resources used (or saved) and their opportunity cost remain the same. An economic evaluation must measure all costs and benefits in a common base year. In addition, costs of an intervention incurred in the future, or benefits received in the future, are argued to be of lesser value because (1) money can earn interest when invested, and (2) the future is uncertain. The way of incorporating this phenomenon into a study is to reduce or discount future cost and benefit streams to reflect their present value. This discounting procedure has the effect of giving less weight to future events. We used a 3% discount rate.

Estimate the Costs of Alternative Options

The costs of interventions must be estimated. Absent a "status quo" alternative, costs common to all interventions being compared need not be considered as they will not affect the choice of intervention.

Select the Relevant Outcome Measure(s)

The outcome measure selected depends on the type of economic evaluation, the intervention being evaluated, and the availability of effectiveness data. Outcome measures often used in public health are number of injuries or illnesses prevented or QALY or injury cost savings per dollar spent on prevention.

Estimate the Effectiveness of the Alternative Options

Data on the effectiveness of an intervention can be obtained from epidemiological studies, existing research, or expert professional opinion. The latter should only be used in situations where epidemiological studies are unethical, unfeasible, or too costly, and where there has been little or no research conducted.

Table 25.11 U.S. Comprehensive Costs of Traumatic Brain Injury by Gender and Cause (M 2006$) in 2000

Cause	Incidence	Comprehensive Cost
All		
MV occupants/other road users	322,829	79,795
Falls	397,877	31,220
Struck by/against	336,977	12,639
Cut/pierce	7,223	555
Fire/burn	947	67
Machinery/tools	929	682
Firearm/gunshot	17,441	60,180
Other/unknown	258,998	21,086
Total	1,343,220	206,224
Males		
MV occupants/other road users	147,542	57,571
Falls	199,333	20,550
Struck by/against	191,998	9,233
Cut/pierce	1,758	431
Fire/burn	908	43
Machinery/tools	887	643
Firearm/gunshot	14,834	51,629
Other/unknown	102,582	14,726
Total	659,843	154,827
Females		
MV occupants/other road users	175,286	22,224
Falls	198,544	10,670
Struck by/against	144,979	3,405
Cut/pierce	5,464	123
Fire/burn	39	24
Machinery/tools	42	39
Firearm/gunshot	2,607	8,551
Other/unknown	156,416	6,361
Total	683,377	51,397

Abbreviations: MV, motor vehicle.

Table 25.12 U.S. Comprehensive Costs of Traumatic Brain Injury by Gender and Age (M 2006$) in 2000

Age Group	Incidence	Comprehensive Cost
All		
00–04	159,087	11,066
05–14	296,169	17,484
15–24	231,607	52,939
25–44	314,877	72,614
45–64	161,166	35,360
65–74	40,206	7,333
75+	140,109	9,427
Total	1,343,220	206,224
Males		
00–04	73,460	6,202
05–14	186,879	12,451
15–24	115,195	42,022
25–44	143,899	57,297
45–64	86,001	26,643
65–74	19,826	4,824
75+	34,583	4,757
Total	659,843	154,827
Females		
00–04	85,627	4,865
05–14	109,290	5,034
15–24	116,411	10,917
25–44	170,978	14,686
45–64	75,165	8,717
65–74	20,380	2,509
75+	105,526	4,669
Total	683,377	51,397

Calculate the Outcomes of the Alternative Options

The outcomes of an intervention include the health gains and cost savings from the reduction in the number of injuries.

Compute the Cost-Outcome Measure

The ultimate aim of an economic evaluation is to bring together and interpret the results on the costs and outcomes of interventions to determine which option provides the best value for the money. In calculating cost-outcome measures, an incremental approach is generally adopted in which the additional costs that one alternative imposes over another is compared with the additional benefits provided.

Describe Any Unquantified Costs and Benefits

Interventions may produce costs and benefits that are not included in the economic evaluation, such as those (1) occurring outside the time frame of the analysis, (2) affecting other than the target population, or (3) resulting from more widespread adoption of an intervention. These costs and benefits should be identified in the economic evaluation, even if they cannot be quantified.

Table 25.13 Economic Evaluation Using Injury Cost Data

Define the intervention	• Objectives of evaluation • Alternatives to be compared • Target population • Setting of the intervention • Time horizon • Type of economic evaluation
Determine perspective of the analysis	• Most commonly societal • External, individual, health care system, and government also may be relevant
Adjust for differential timing	• Adjust for inflation—costs and benefits must be measured in a common base year • Discount future costs to reflect their present value (3% discount rate)
Estimate the costs of alternative options	• Include overhead costs and the value of volunteer time
Select relevant outcome measures	• Type of economic evaluation • Type of intervention • Availability of effectiveness data
Estimate effectiveness of alternative options	• Intervention effectiveness obtained from epidemiological studies, existing research, or expert opinion
Calculate outcomes of alternative options	• Include health gain, cost savings
Compute cost-outcome measures	• Take incremental approach—additional costs of an alternative compared with additional benefits provided
Describe any unquantified costs and benefits	• Outside time frame of study • Affect other target population • Resulting from more widespread adoption of an intervention

Table 25.14 Types of Economic Evaluation Analysis

Cost-effectiveness analysis	• Most straightforward • Takes into account differences in outcomes in clarifying choices (one-dimensional) • Comparisons made between different injury prevention programs in terms of cost per unit of outcome • Those with lowest cost per unit of outcome are most efficient
Cost-utility analysis	• More advanced • Special form of cost-effectiveness analysis • Costs per unit of utility (person's well-being) are calculated • Most common unit of health-related utility is quality-adjusted life years (QALYs), which incorporate quality of life and years of life into one measure. • QALYs measure physical, emotional, mental health, and social aspects relevant and important to an individual's well-being.
Cost-benefit analysis	• Divides total benefits by intervention costs, yielding a return on investment of the intervention • Supports direct comparison across diverse interventions with different objectives • Advantage: clearly indicates whether an intervention is worthwhile implementing • Disadvantage: requires putting a dollar value on a QALY, which is difficult and which some find distasteful
Net-benefit analysis	• A companion to a cost-benefit analysis • Net benefit = benefits – costs • Some interventions where benefits > costs may not be worthwhile as (1) investments that offer a larger return may be available, and (2) uncertainty means that return will vary up or down from the average.

Types of Economic Evaluation Analyses

An overview of the different types of economic evaluation analyses is presented in **Table 25.14**.

Cost-Effectiveness Analysis

Cost-effectiveness analysis is the most straightforward type of economic evaluation to take account of differences in outcomes. In cost-effectiveness analysis, outcomes are measured in naturally occurring units, which can be generic units (e.g., fatalities prevented) that can be compared across all injury causes or more specific units (e.g., falls prevented) that can only be used to compare interventions with the same objective. In cost-effectiveness analysis, comparisons are made between different injury prevention programs in terms of their cost per unit of outcome, such as cost per fatality prevented or cost per fall prevented. Interventions with the lowest cost per unit of outcome are the most efficient. Separating those interventions that represent value for money from those that do not requires some judgment, as no threshold or cut-off values exist. Approaches that can be used to derive these cut-off values include comparing the cost per unit of outcome with other programs, "rules of thumb," and inferences from past decisions.[26]

Cost-Utility Analysis

Cost-utility analysis is more advanced than cost-effectiveness analysis. Information from cost-effectiveness analyses is useful in clarifying choices between different programs on the basis of an outcome measure that is one dimensional. However, a limitation of cost-effectiveness analysis is if comparisons need to be made between interventions for different injury causes where the unit of outcome varies across the alternative options. In addition, if outcomes are measured using a generic unit such as life years saved then cost-effectiveness analysis does not account for differences in quality of life resulting from the intervention. This makes it inappropriate for comparing programs that are primarily life saving with those for which the major objective is an improvement in quality of life.

Cost-utility analysis was developed as a special form of cost-effectiveness analysis, in which the costs per unit of utility (units that relate to a person's well-being) are calculated.[2] The most commonly used unit of health-related utility is quality-adjusted life years (QALYs). QALYs incorporate some components of quality of life as well as quantity (or length) of life into a single measure. The number of life years (quantity of life) gained because of an intervention is combined with some judgment on the quality of those life years to calculate the number of QALYs gained. Quality of life is a multidimensional concept measuring the physical, emotional, mental health, and social aspects that are relevant and important to a person's well-being. Conventionally, quality is measured on a scale from 0 to 1 where 0 is equivalent to death and 1 is equivalent to good health. An alternative measure popularized by the World Health Organization[27] is a disability-adjusted life year or DALY. It equals one minus a QALY. Results are presented in terms of cost per QALY gained from the alternative options, and the option with the lowest cost per QALY gained is the most efficient. Because outcomes are being measured in commensurate units of utility in cost-utility analysis, comparisons can be made across diverse interventions for different injury causes. Again, no threshold or cut-off values exist below which the cost per QALY represents value for money and a similar assessment must be made as for cost-effectiveness analysis, based on comparisons with other programs, rules of thumb, or inferences from past decisions. As a general guide, around the world, interventions that cost more than $40,000 to $60,000 per QALY saved generally would not be implemented.

Cost-Benefit Analysis

Cost-benefit analysis divides total benefits by intervention costs, yielding the return on investment in the intervention. In this analysis, all benefits are either monetized or omitted from the calculation. Cost-benefit analysis supports direct comparison across diverse interventions with different objectives. Also, as with cost-utility analysis, multiple benefits can be captured in cost-benefit analysis if the interventions under consideration produce multidimensional outcomes. An advantage of cost-benefit analysis over cost-effectiveness analysis and cost-utility analysis is that it clearly indicates whether an intervention is worthwhile implementing.

Net Benefit Analysis

Net benefit analysis generally is a companion to a cost-benefit analysis. The net benefit equals the benefits minus the costs. Any intervention where the benefits are greater than the costs is worthwhile (i.e., net benefits greater than 0 or benefit-cost ratio greater than 1). When comparing two alternatives, depending on budget constraints, the intervention with the greatest net benefit or the one with the highest cost-benefit ratio may be the preferred option.

Bicycle Helmets and Head Injury: A Cost-Benefit Analysis

In this section, we present an example of a cost-benefit analysis of an intervention to encourage the use of bicycle helmets by both children (under 15 years old) and adults (**Table 25.15**). The example updates the estimate for child bicycle helmets in Miller and Levy[22] and adds an adult estimate. We follow the steps suggested in the preceding section.

Define the Intervention

The intervention is a bicycle helmet purchase for every pedalcyclist in the United States, which equates to analyzing the average return on investment in a helmet. We examine the benefits over a 5-year period, over which we assume a helmet would be used.

What Is the Perspective?

A societal perspective is adopted to reflect the fact that the program is motivated in the public interest. This perspective includes cost savings from avoiding lost work and pain and suffering. We also present breakdowns from an insurer's perspective.

How Are Future Values Adjusted?

A 3% discount rate was used to discount future injury cost savings. Cost savings were adjusted for inflation using

Table 25.15 Bicycle Helmets and Head Injury: An Example of a Cost-Benefit Analysis

<table>
<tr><td>Intervention defined</td><td colspan="3">• Bicycle helmet purchase for every cyclist in the U.S. (analyzing average return on investment in a helmet over a 5-year period)</td></tr>
<tr><td>Perspective</td><td colspan="3">• Societal perspective—everyone's costs and benefits count
• Perspective includes cost savings from avoiding lost work and pain and suffering</td></tr>
<tr><td>Future values adjusted</td><td colspan="3">• 3% discount rate used to discount future injury cost savings</td></tr>
<tr><td>Cost of helmets</td><td colspan="3">• Analysis uses $18 (adult) and $11.50 (child) helmets
• In U.S., 36.2% of the estimated 85.3 million bicycle riders were children under 15 years
• With a 5-year average helmet life, # of helmets purchased would be $^1/_5$ of this rider count
• Annual helmet spending:
◦ $71 million for children <15 years
◦ $190 million for ages ≥15 years</td></tr>
<tr><td>Bicycle-related head injury toll</td><td colspan="3">Year 2000 study of bicycle crashes:
• 426 fatal head injuries
• 43,049 nonfatal TBIs
• 132,606 nonfatal other head injuries</td></tr>
<tr><td>Cost of bicycle head injuries</td><td colspan="3">Lifetime comprehensive costs:
1. Child:
• $0.575 billion for fatal head injuries
• $1.4 billion for nonfatal TBIs
• $0.65 billion for nonfatal scalp injuries
2. Adult:
• $1.1 billion for fatal head injuries
• $1.6 billion for nonfatal TBIs
• $0.476 billion for nonfatal scalp injuries</td></tr>
<tr><td>Effectiveness of helmets</td><td colspan="3">• Prevent 49–56% of fatal head injuries
• Prevent 68–80% of nonfatal TBIs
• Prevent 65% of other head injuries</td></tr>
<tr><td>Prevention of cyclist death and injury via helmet use</td><td colspan="3">• Estimated 180 TBI deaths in children in 2000 if no helmets used
• Estimated 86 TBI deaths in children in 2000 if every child wore a helmet
• If universal helmet use by child cyclists had been instituted in 2000, the estimated effects would have been:
◦ Prevented 94 deaths
◦ Prevented 46,400 nonfatal TBIs
◦ Prevented 106,600 other nonfatal head injuries</td></tr>
<tr><td>Cost savings and cost-benefit ratio of universal helmet use</td><td colspan="3"></td></tr>
<tr><td></td><td>Children</td><td>Cost savings</td><td>• Injury cost saving = $3.3 bill
• Medical cost saving = $.3 bill
• Work loss saving = $1.2 bill
• QALY saving = $1.8 bill</td></tr>
<tr><td></td><td></td><td>Cost-benefit ratio (= 47)</td><td>$11.50 spent on a helmet:
• Saves $53 in medical spending
• Prevents $194 of work loss
• Preserves QALYs valued at $292</td></tr>
</table>

Table 25.15 *(Continued)*

	Adult	Cost savings	• Injury cost saving = $2.8 bill • Medical cost saving = $.4 bill • Work loss saving = $0.8 bill • QALY saving = $1.6 bill
		Benefit-cost ratio (= 15)	$18 spent on a helmet: • Saves $32 in medical spending • Prevents $79 of work loss • Preserves QALYs valued at $150
Uncosted outcomes	• Parents spend less time and expense caring for injured children • Lawyers file fewer lawsuits seeking compensation for cyclists • Ride bike less often because helmet is uncomfortable: ◦ Increase in obesity ◦ Decrease in bicycle-related injuries		
Changes in insurance payments	• Save approximately $53 per child helmet • Save approximately $32 per adult helmet • Auto insurers process less claims		

Abbreviations: TBIs, traumatic brain injuries; QALY, quality-adjusted life year.

medical spending, wage, and consumer price indices calculated from the 2007 Economic Report of the President[28].

What Would the Helmets Cost?

Prices for bicycle helmets that meet U.S. Consumer Product Safety Commission (Bethesda, MD) standards came from a search of the Web sites of the two largest retail companies that currently sell helmets in the United States. Prices ranged from $14.47 to $19.99 plus sales tax (4 to 7% in many states) for adult helmets and ranged as low as $9.75 for child helmets. Some helmets cost much more. The analysis uses an $18 price (with sensitivity analysis at $15 and $40) for adults and $11.50 (with sensitivity analysis at $10 and $25) for children.

In the United States, an estimated 85.3 million people rode bicycles in 1998, of which 36.2% were under 15 years old.[24] The number of helmets purchased per year would be one-fifth of this rider count (assuming a 5-year life span for helmets). Annual helmet-related spending would be $71 million for children under 15 years old (85.3 million/5 * 36.2% * $11.5) and $190 million for older cyclists (85.3 million/5 * (1 – 36.2%) * $18).

How Large Is the Bicycle-Related Head Injury Toll?

In 2000, bicycle crashes caused 426 fatal head injuries, 43,049 nonfatal TBIs, and 132,606 other nonfatal head injuries.[30] These statistics come from a time period with 69% helmet use among children under 15 years old and 38% use among adults.[29]

What Do Bicycle-Related Head Injuries Cost?

Lifetime comprehensive costs (in 2006 dollars) totaled $575 million for child fatal head injuries, over $1.4 billion for child nonfatal TBIs, and $650 million for child nonfatal scalp injuries (**Table 25.16**). For adults, the respective totals were $1.1 billion, $1.6 billion, and $476 million (**Table 25.17**). These costs are from Miller et al,[30] which closely follows the costing methods employed here and in Finkelstein et al.[9]

Lifetime medical spending due to bicycle-related head injuries approached $239 million annually for children under 15 years old. The other losses were much larger—$973 million in future work loss and approximately $1.4 billion in lost quality of life. For adults, the respective totals were $342 million, $983 million, and $1.8 billion.

How Effective Are Helmets?

If universally used, helmets prevent 49 to 56% of bicycle-related head injury deaths, 68 to 80% of nonfatal TBIs, and 65% of other head injuries.[31–33] We used midpoint estimates for helmet effectiveness (i.e., we assumed that helmets prevent 53.5% of bicycle-related head injury deaths, 74% of nonfatal TBIs, and 65% of other head injuries). Given that only 69% of children and 38% of adults

Table 25.16 U.S. Costs of Traumatic Brain Injury (TBI) and Other Head Injuries in Child Cyclists (M 2006$) in 2000

		Incidence	Medical	Work Loss	Quality of Life	Total
TBI	Fatal	115	3	191	381	575
	Nonfatal	30,673	134	349	886	1,369
Other head	Fatal	0	0	0	0	0
	Nonfatal	90,467	102	432	125	660
Total		121,255	239	973	1,392	2,604
If no cyclist used their helmet						
TBI	Fatal	180	5	300	597	902
	Nonfatal	62,675	273	714	1,810	2,797
Other head	Fatal	0	0	0	0	0
	Nonfatal	164,038	185	784	227	1,197
Total		226,893	463	1,798	2,634	4,896
If every cyclist used their helmet						
TBI	Fatal	86	2	143	284	429
	Nonfatal	16,295	71	186	471	727
Other head	Fatal	0	0	0	0	0
	Nonfatal	57,413	65	274	79	419
Total		73,794	138	603	834	1,575
Savings		153,099	325	1,195	1,801	3,321

Table 25.17 U.S. Costs of Traumatic Brain Injury (TBI) and Other Head Injuries in Adult Cyclists (M 2006$) in 2000

		Incidence	Medical	Work Loss	Quality of Life	Total
TBI	Fatal	277	7	365	618	990
	Nonfatal	12,376	251	397	915	1,562
Other head	Fatal	34	0	45	75	120
	Nonfatal	42,139	84	176	216	476
Total		54,826	342	983	1,824	3,149
If no cyclist used their helmet						
TBI	Fatal	346	8	456	772	1,237
	Nonfatal	17,218	349	552	1,273	2,174
Other head	Fatal	42	0	56	94	151
	Nonfatal	55,961	112	234	287	632
Total		73,568	470	1,298	2,426	4,193
If every cyclist used their helmet						
TBI	Fatal	164	4	217	367	588
	Nonfatal	4,477	91	144	331	565
Other head	Fatal	20	0	27	45	72
	Nonfatal	19,587	39	82	100	221
Total		24,248	134	469	843	1,445
Savings		49,320	336	829	1,583	2,748

who own bicycles regularly used helmets, it was assumed that only 69% of the effectiveness was achieved in children and 38% in adults.

How Many Cyclist Deaths and Injuries Can Helmet Use Prevent?

If no child cyclist used a helmet in 2000, 180 TBI deaths would have occurred in this population (**Table 25.16**). This estimate was derived using the equation 115/(1 – 0.537 * 0.69) with 115 actual fatal injuries, 53.7% helmet effectiveness, and 69% helmeted. Using a parallel calculation for nonfatal injuries, we estimated that a total of 226,893 child head injuries would have occurred if no helmets were used by child cyclists.

If every child cyclist wore a helmet in 2000, only 86 TBI deaths would have occurred in this population. This estimate was derived by multiplying the number of injuries at 0% helmet use times 1 minus percentage effectiveness in reducing head injury deaths [180 * (1 – 0.537)]. Similarly, only 73,794 child head injuries would have occurred if no child cyclists rode helmeted. Thus, universal helmet use by child cyclists (as opposed to no use at all) would have prevented 94 deaths, 46,379 nonfatal TBIs, and 106,625 other nonfatal head injuries in 2000. **Table 25.17** presents parallel estimates for adults.

What Cost Savings and Cost : Benefit Ratio Would Helmet Use Yield?

Universal helmet use by child cyclists (as opposed to no use at all) would have resulted in over $3.3 billion in injury cost savings. Helmet use by children would have saved medical costs, work loss, and quality of life valued at $0.3 billion, $1.2 billion, and $1.8 billion, respectively. The benefit:cost ratio of buying and using child bicycle helmets is 47. On average, an $11.50 child bicycle helmet saves $53 in medical spending, prevents $194 of work loss, and preserves quality of life valued at $292.

Universal helmet use by adult cyclists (as opposed to no use at all) would have resulted in over $2.8 billion in injury cost savings, including $0.4 billion in medical spending, $829 million in work loss, and $1.6 billion in quality of life. The cost : benefit ratio of buying and using adult bicycle helmets is 15. The average $18 adult bicycle helmet saves $32 in medical spending, saves $79 in work loss, and preserves quality of life valued at $150.

What Uncosted Outcomes Will Result?

- Parents will spend less time and expense caring for injured children.
- Lawyers will file fewer lawsuits seeking compensation for bicyclist injuries.
- Some people will find helmets uncomfortable or inconvenient, which may cause them to ride their bicycles less often, possibly increasing obesity or preventing other bicycle-related injuries.

How Will Insurance Payments Change?

Health insurers, public and private, will save almost all of the medical payments, saving an estimated $53 per child helmet and $32 per adult helmet. Auto insurers also will process less claims. Twenty-five percent of injured bicyclists were in motor vehicle crashes.[28] Miller et al[34] find auto insurers compensate 36% of the work losses in highway crashes and 18% of the medical costs. That implies auto insurers will save an estimated $19.50 per child helmet and $8.50 per adult helmet.

How Sensitive Are the Results?

The cost : benefit ratios here are for low-cost helmets. Bulk purchase program prices would be lower. At a $10 price, the cost : benefit ratio would be 54. Conversely, families buying fancier $25 child bicycle helmets can expect a return of $21.50 for each dollar spent. If adults buy $40 high-end helmets, the return would be $6.50 for each dollar spent and if they buy $15 helmets, the return would be $17.50.

Our estimate of the cost : benefit ratio assumes an average 5-year life span for helmets. If an 8-year life span is assumed for adult helmets instead, the benefit : cost ratio would rise from 15 to 23. We used midpoint estimates for helmet effectiveness. If high-point estimates were used instead, the cost : benefit ratio would be 53 for child helmets and 16 for adult helmets. If low-point estimates were used, the cost : benefit ratio would be 42 for child helmets and 13 for adult helmets.

How Do the Savings Compare with Savings from Other Helmets?

Cost : benefit ratios are available for two types of more costly helmets.[30] All-terrain vehicle (ATV) helmets cost an average of $120, have an estimated cost : benefit ratio of 4. Motorcycle helmets typically cost at least $200. They have a cost : benefit ratio of 19 if worn voluntarily. When a law mandates their use, discomfort and inconvenience costs reduce the cost : benefit for new users to 3.

Limitations of the Analysis

No single data source for calculating TBI costs exists. Consequently, we were forced to combine information from myriad data sources, each with limitations. Some sources were old, others were based on non-nationally representative samples, and all were subject to reporting and measurement error. These limitations not only increase

Table 25.18 Study Limitations

Factors making cost estimates conservative	Treatment by mental health and alternative medicine providers may be omitted
	Hard to track TBI follow-up care
	Sequelae of minor TBI often are missed

Abbreviations: TBI, traumatic brain injury.

the lack of precision around the estimates, but may result in additional bias (**Table 25.18**).

Several factors make our cost estimates conservative. First, injury treatment by mental health professionals and alternative medicine providers may be omitted. Second, it is hard to fully track TBI follow-up care. A good life care plan might identify many unmet needs omitted from the costs. Third, sequelae of minor TBI often are missed in our datasets. Moreover, physician ratings of prognosis deal with typical outcomes, not the occasional bad-outcome case.

The helmet benefit-cost analysis deals with averages. Benefits for individual riders will vary widely with exposure (miles or hours bicycled), skill, risk-taking behavior, and where the bicycle is ridden (e.g., along busy roads, on paved bicycle paths, on unpaved trails). Still, the cost: benefit ratios are so high that even occasional riders who are not daredevils are likely to benefit from helmet use.

Conclusion

Economic analysis provides a compact way to measure the burden that TBI imposes on individuals and society. It also supports comparison of the return on competing investments in preventive measures.

TBI is a large problem costing U.S. society more than $206 billion a year, almost twice the cost of impaired driving. The comprehensive cost of TBI represented 15% of the total cost of injury in the United States in 2000. Moreover, TBI caused 1% of total U.S. medical spending. Leading causes of TBI in terms of costs were motor vehicle crashes, falls, and for men, firearms.

As the bicycle helmet benefit-cost analysis illustrates, prevention can be much cheaper than the consequences of not preventing. Preventive measures can specifically target TBI as helmets do. Alternatively, they can target broader objectives like reducing falls or road crashes that frequently cause TBI or better protecting vehicle occupants in crashes.

More research on TBI consequences is needed, especially on less-than-catastrophic TBIs. The disability associated with such injuries result in high costs to society.

References

1. Hendrie D, Miller TR. Economic evaluation of injury prevention and control programs. In: McClure R, Stevenson M, McEvoy S, eds. The Scientific Basis of Injury Prevention and Control. Sydney, Australia: IP Communications; 2004:372–390
2. Gold MR, Siegel JE, Russell LB, Weinstein MC, eds. Cost-effectiveness in Health and Medicine. New York, NY: Oxford University Press; 1996
3. *Jones and Laughlin Steel Corp. v Pfeifer*, 462 U.S. 523, 103 (SCt 1983)
4. U.S. Office of Management and Budget. Guidelines and discount rates for benefit-cost analysis of federal programs. Washington, DC: Office of Management and Budget; 1994. Circular A-94
5. Viscusi WK. Discounting health effects for medical decisions. In: Sloan FA, ed. Valuing Health Care: Costs, Benefits, and Effectiveness of Pharmaceuticals and Medical Technology. New York: Cambridge University Press; 1995
6. Murray CJL, Lopez AD. Global Comparative Assessments in the Health Sector: Disease Burden, Expenditures and Intervention Packages. Geneva: World Health Organization; 1994
7. Rice DP, Hodgson TA, Kopstein AN. The economics of illness: a replication and update. Health Care Financ Rev 1985;7:61–80
8. Moore R, Mao Y, Zhang J, Clarke K. Economic Burden of Illness in Canada, 1993. Ottawa, Ontario, Canada: Canadian Public Health Association; 1997
9. Finkelstein EA, Corso PC, Miller TR, Fiebelkorn IA, Zaloshnja E, Lawrence BA. Incidence and Economic Burden of Injuries in the United States, 2000. New York: Oxford University Press; 2006
10. Rice DP, MacKenzie EJ, Jones AS, et al. Cost of Injury in the United States: A report to Congress. San Francisco, CA: Institute for Health & Aging, University of California, and Injury Prevention Center, The Johns Hopkins University; 1989
11. 1979-1988 Detailed Claims Information. National Council on Compensation Insurance
12. 2000 Current Population Survey. U.S. National Center for Health Statistics
13. 2000 Current Population Survey. U.S. Bureau of Labor Statistics
14. Lawrence BA, Miller TR, Jensen AF, Fisher DA, Zamula WW. Estimating the costs of non-fatal consumer product injuries in the United States. Inj Control Saf Promot 2000;72:97–113
15. Miller TR, Romano EO, Spicer RS. The cost of childhood unintentional injuries and the value of prevention. Future Child 2000;10(1):137–163
16. Zaloshnja E, Miller TR, Romano EO, Spicer RS. Crash costs by body part injured, fracture involvement, and threat to life severity, United States, 2000. Accid Anal Prev 2004;36(3):415–427
17. Haddix AC, Teutsch SM, Corso PS. Prevention Effectiveness: A Guide to Decision Analysis and Economic Evaluation. 2nd ed. New York: Oxford University Press; 2003
18. Miller TR, Pindus NM, Douglass JB, Rossman SB. Databook on Nonfatal Injury: Incidence, Costs, and Consequences. Washington, DC: Urban Institute Press; 1995
19. Miller TR. The plausible range for the value of life: red herrings among the mackerels. Journal of Forensic Economics. 1990;3(3):17–39
20. Miller TR. Variations between countries in values of statistical life. Journal of Transport Economics and Policy. 2000;34(2):169–188
21. Viscusi WK, Aldy JE. The value of statistical life: a critical review of market estimates throughout the world. J Risk Uncertain 2003;27(1):5–76
22. U.S. Census Bureau. Statistical abstract of the United States. Washington, DC: U.S. Department of Commerce. Available at: http://www.census.gov/prod/2003pubs/02statab/health.pdf. Accessed
23. Barell V, Aharonson-Daniel L, Fingerhut LA, et al. An introduction to the Barell body region by nature of injury diagnosis matrix. Inj Prev 2002;8(2):91–96
24. Clark DE, Ahmad S. Estimating injury severity using the Barell matrix. Inj Prev 2006;12:111–116

25. Miller TR, Levy DT. Cost-outcome analysis in injury prevention and control: a primer on methods. Inj Prev 1997;3(4):288–293
26. Weinstein M. From cost-effectiveness ratios to resource allocation: Where to draw the line? In: Sloan FA, ed. Valuing Health Care: Costs, Benefits, and Effectiveness of Pharmaceuticals and Other Medical Technologies. Cambridge: Cambridge University Press; 1996:77–97
27. Murray CJ, Lopez AD. 1994. Global comparative assessments in the health sector: Disease Burden, Expenditures an Intervention Packages. Geneva, Switzerland: World Health Organization.
28. Bush GW. 2007. Economic Report of the President transmitted to Congress February 2007, Washington DC. U.S. Government Printing Office
29. Rodgers GB. Bicycle and bicycle helmet use patterns in the United States in 1998. J Safety Res 2000;31:149–153
30. Miller TR, Zaloshnja E, Lawrence BA, Crandall J, Ivarsson J, Finkelstein AE. Pedestrian and pedalcyclist injury costs in the United States by age and injury severity. 48th Proceedings of the Association for the Advancement of Automotive Medicine. Barrington, IL: Association for the Advancement of Automotive Medicine; 2004:265–284
31. Thompson DC, Thompson RS, Rivara FP. Effectiveness of bicycle safety helmets in preventing head injuries. JAMA 1996;276(24):1968–1973
32. Thompson DC, Nunn ME, Thompson RS, Rivara FP. Effectiveness of bicycle safety helmets in preventing serious facial injury. JAMA 1996; 276(24):1974–1975
33. Sacks JJ, Holmgren P, Smith S, Scain DM. Bicycle-associated head injuries and deaths in the United States from 1984 through 1988. JAMA 1991;266:3016–3018
34. Miller TR, Viner JG, Rossman SB, et al. The Costs of Highway Crashes. Washington, DC: Urban Institute; 1991
35. Miller TR, Finkelstein AE, Zaloshjna E, Hendrie D. The cost of child and adolescent injuries and the savings from prevention. In: Liller K, ed. Injury Prevention for Children and Adolescents: Research, Practice, and Advocacy. Washington, DC: American Public Health Association; 2005:15–64

Index

Note: Page numbers followed by *f* and *t* indicate figures and tables, respectively.

D

E

F

G

I

Q

R

S

X

Z